Nonmelanocytic Tumors of the Skin

AFIP Atlas of Tumor Pathology

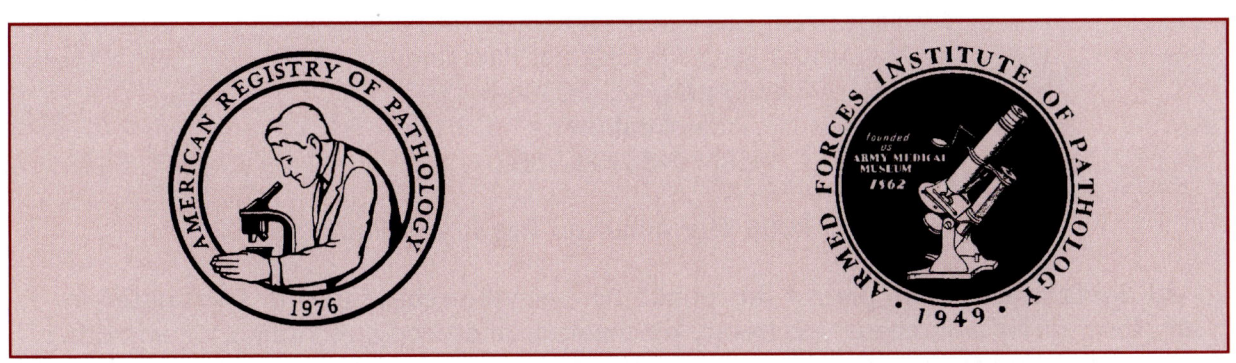

ARP PRESS

Silver Spring, Maryland

Editorial Director: Kelley S. Hahn
Production Editor: Dian S. Thomas
Editorial/Scanning Assistant: Mirlinda Q. Caton
Copy Editor: Audrey Kahn
Scanning Technician: Kenneth Stringfellow

Available from the American Registry of Pathology
Armed Forces Institute of Pathology
Washington, DC 20306-6000
www.afip.org
ISBN 1-881041-98-0

Copyright © 2006 The American Registry of Pathology

All rights reserved. No part of this publication may be reproduced or transmitted in any form or by any means: electronic, mechanical, photocopy, recording, or any other information storage and retrieval system without the written permission of the publisher.

AFIP ATLAS OF TUMOR PATHOLOGY

Fourth Series
Fascicle 4

NONMELANOCYTIC TUMORS OF THE SKIN

by

JAMES W. PATTERSON, MD, FACP
Professor of Pathology and Dermatology
Director of Dermatopathology
Department of Pathology
University of Virginia Health System
Charlottesville, Virginia

MARK R. WICK, MD, FASCP
Professor of Pathology and Dermatology
Director of Pathology Residency Training Program
Department of Pathology
University of Virginia Health System
Charlottesville, Virginia

Published by the
American Registry of Pathology
Washington, DC
in collaboration with the
Armed Forces Institute of Pathology
Washington, DC
2006

AFIP ATLAS OF TUMOR PATHOLOGY

EDITOR
Steven G. Silverberg, MD
Department of Pathology
University of Maryland School of Medicine
Baltimore, Maryland

ASSOCIATE EDITOR
Leslie H. Sobin, MD
Armed Forces Institute of Pathology
Washington, DC

EDITORIAL ADVISORY BOARD

Jorge Albores-Saavedra, MD	Louisiana State University Health Sciences Center Shreveport, Louisiana
Ronald A. DeLellis, MD	Lifespan Academic Medical Center Providence, Rhode Island
William J. Frable, MD	Medical College of Virginia/Virginia Commonwealth University Richmond, Virginia
William A. Gardner, Jr, MD	American Registry of Pathology Washington, DC
Kim R. Geisinger, MD	Wake Forest University School of Medicine Winston-Salem, North Carolina
Donald West King, MD	National Library of Medicine Bethesda, Maryland
Leonard B. Kahn, MD	Long Island Jewish Medical Center New Hyde Park, New York
James Linder, MD	Cytyc Corporation Marlborough, Massachusetts
Virginia A. LiVolsi, MD	University of Pennsylvania Medical Center Philadelphia, Pennsylvania
Elizabeth Montgomery, MD	Johns Hopkins University School of Medicine Baltimore, Maryland
Juan Rosai, MD	Instituto Nazionale Tumori Milano, Italy
Mark H. Stoler, MD	University of Virginia Health Sciences Center Charlottesville, Virginia
William D. Travis, MD	Memorial Sloan-Kettering Cancer Center New York, New York
Noel Weidner, MD	University of California San Diego Medical Center San Diego, California
Mark R. Wick, MD	University of Virginia Medical Center Charlottesville, Virginia

Manuscript Reviewed by:
Clay J. Cockerell, MD
William J. Frable, MD
Bruce R. Smoller, MD

EDITORS' NOTE

The Atlas of Tumor Pathology has a long and distinguished history. It was first conceived at a Cancer Research Meeting held in St. Louis in September 1947 as an attempt to standardize the nomenclature of neoplastic diseases. The first series was sponsored by the National Academy of Sciences-National Research Council. The organization of this Sisyphean effort was entrusted to the Subcommittee on Oncology of the Committee on Pathology, and Dr. Arthur Purdy Stout was the first editor-in-chief. Many of the illustrations were provided by the Medical Illustration Service of the Armed Forces Institute of Pathology (AFIP), the type was set by the Government Printing Office, and the final printing was done at the Armed Forces Institute of Pathology (hence the colloquial appellation "AFIP Fascicles"). The American Registry of Pathology (ARP) purchased the Fascicles from the Government Printing Office and sold them virtually at cost. Over a period of 20 years, approximately 15,000 copies each of nearly 40 Fascicles were produced. The worldwide impact of these publications over the years has largely surpassed the original goal. They quickly became among the most influential publications on tumor pathology, primarily because of their overall high quality but also because their low cost made them easily accessible the world over to pathologists and other students of oncology.

Upon completion of the first series, the National Academy of Sciences-National Research Council handed further pursuit of the project over to the newly created Universities Associated for Research and Education in Pathology (UAREP). A second series was started, generously supported by grants from the AFIP, the National Cancer Institute, and the American Cancer Society. Dr. Harlan I. Firminger became the editor-in-chief and was succeeded by Dr. William H. Hartmann. The second series' Fascicles were produced as bound volumes instead of loose leaflets. They featured a more comprehensive coverage of the subjects, to the extent that the Fascicles could no longer be regarded as "atlases" but rather as monographs describing and illustrating in detail the tumors and tumor-like conditions of the various organs and systems.

Once the second series was completed, with a success that matched that of the first, ARP, UAREP, and AFIP decided to embark on a third series. Dr. Juan Rosai was appointed as editor-in-chief, and Dr. Leslie H. Sobin became associate editor. A distinguished Editorial Advisory Board was also convened, and these outstanding pathologists and educators played a major role in the success of this series, the first publication of which appeared in 1991 and the last (number 32) in 2003.

The same organizational framework will apply to the current fourth series, but with UAREP no longer in existence, ARP will play the major role. New features will include a hardbound cover, illustrations almost exclusively in color, and an accompanying electronic version of each Fascicle. There will also be increased emphasis (wherever appropriate) on the cytopathologic (intraoperative, exfoliative, and/or fine needle aspiration) and molecular features that are important in diagnosis and prognosis. What will not change from the three previous series, however, is the goal of providing the practicing pathologist with thorough, concise, and up-to-date information on the nomenclature and classification; epidemiologic, clinical, and pathogenetic features; and, most importantly, guidance in the diagnosis of the tumors and tumor-like lesions of all major organ systems and body sites.

As in the third series, a continuous attempt will be made to correlate, whenever possible, the nomenclature used in the Fascicles with that proposed by the World Health Organization's Classification of Tumors, as well as to ensure a consistency of style throughout. Close cooperation between the various authors and their respective liaisons from the Editorial Board will continue to be emphasized in order to minimize unnecessary repetition and discrepancies in the text and illustrations.

Particular thanks are due to the members of the Editorial Advisory Board, the reviewers (at least two for each Fascicle), the editorial and production staff, and—first and foremost—the individual Fascicle authors for their ongoing efforts to ensure that this series is a worthy successor to the previous three.

Steven G. Silverberg, MD

Leslie H. Sobin, MD

PREFACE

The purpose of this volume is to provide a complete survey of the nonmelanocytic tumors of the skin in as concise a manner as possible. We hope that the information provided will be of practical help in day-to-day diagnosis. At the same time, both the text and the extensive list of references should provide the interested reader the foundation for further study or perhaps inspire further investigations in the field.

It is no secret that a number of the conditions discussed in this book are covered in other Fascicles in the series. We have tried to emphasize those aspects of disease that are pertinent to the skin, while placing them in the broader context of general medicine.

A fact of life in the book writing business is that as time passes between completion of a manuscript and actual publication, new medical studies continue unabated. In an attempt to compensate for this, we have included key references that have appeared since our manuscript was first submitted. We hope that these additions will be of further interest to our readers and extend the useful life of this book.

James W. Patterson, MD, FACP
Mark R. Wick, MD, FASCP

ACKNOWLEDGMENTS

Having completed a work of this type, it is customary to reflect upon one's own educational background and to acknowledge the role that teachers have played in making it all possible. As much as we are indebted to these individuals, we also wish to pay tribute to the various schools of surgical pathology and dermatopathology that they have so ably represented. Dr. Francis H. McMullan trained at Johns Hopkins University during the era in which Drs. Lloyd W. Ketron, Maurice Sullivan, and Francis A. Ellis were major forces. Dr. Saul Kay served under Dr. Arthur Purdy Stout at Columbia University, whereas Dr. William J. Frable received a portion of his training at Memorial Sloan-Kettering Cancer Center. Dr. Edward Abell studied under Edward Wilson Jones at London's St. John's Hospital for Diseases of the Skin. We have benefitted directly from the teaching of Drs. Elson B. Helwig and James H. Graham of the Armed Forces Institute of Pathology. Other mentors include Drs. Richard K. Winkelmann, John P. Goellner, and W.P. Daniel Su—who were all trained at the Mayo Clinic under the influence of one of the "founders" of dermatopathology, Dr. Hamilton Montgomery—as well as two renowned acolytes of Dr. Lauren V. Ackerman at Washington University, namely, Dr. Juan Rosai and Dr. Louis P. Dehner.

We also wish to make special note of the numerous investigators whose works are cited in this volume. Many are close colleagues and friends. All of them have made and continue to make contributions that keep dermatopathology a living, vibrant subspecialty. In particular, the many professional accomplishments of Dr. A. Bernard Ackerman, Dr. Christopher D. Fletcher, and Dr. Philip E. LeBoit are gratefully recognized.

We would also like to acknowledge those who have played a more direct role in the production of this volume. We wish to particularly thank Dr. Philip H. Cooper, not only for his important contributions to dermatopathology, but also for his help and support over the years and for his collection of teaching slides, which was most helpful in the preparation of this work. We are likewise grateful to all of our colleagues in the Division of Surgical Pathology at the University of Virginia for their encouragement and advice. Special recognition goes to Drs. Mark H. Stoler and Stacey E. Mills. Drs. Jon H. Meyerle, CPT, MC, USAR and Eric C. Parlette, LT, MC, USNR kindly provided examples of superficial acral fibromyxoma and blastic NK-cell lymphoma, respectively, for inclusion as photomicrographs. Finally, we are thankful for the love and support of our families and friends, the impact of which cannot be overstated.

James W. Patterson, MD, FACP
Mark R. Wick, MD, FASCP

CONTENTS

1. **Epidermal Tumors** 1
   - **Epithelial Cysts** 1
     - Epidermal Cyst and Milium 1
     - Human Papillomavirus-Associated Cyst (Verrucous Cyst) 2
     - Proliferating Epidermal Cyst 2
     - Pigmented Follicular Cyst 3
     - Cutaneous Keratocyst 3
     - Epithelial Cysts in Gardner's Syndrome 3
     - Trichilemmal Cyst (Pilar Cyst, Isthmus-Catagen Cyst) 4
     - Proliferating Trichilemmal Cyst (Proliferating Trichilemmal Tumor, Pilar Tumor, Proliferating Pilar Tumor) 5
     - Steatocystoma 6
     - Dermoid Cyst 7
     - Eruptive Vellus Hair Cyst 8
     - Cutaneous Cysts and Related Structures that May Be Ciliated 8
     - Other Cutaneous Cysts 11
   - **Benign Epidermal Tumors** 14
     - Epidermal Nevus 14
     - Acantholytic Acanthoma 17
     - Epidermolytic Acanthoma 17
     - Warty Dyskeratoma 18
     - Seborrheic Keratosis and its Variants 19
     - Large Cell Acanthoma 24
     - Clear Cell Acanthoma 25
     - Clear Cell Papulosis 26
     - Pseudoepitheliomatous Hyperplasia 26
   - **Premalignant and Malignant Epidermal Tumors** 27
     - Actinic Keratosis 27
     - Porokeratosis 31
     - Bowen's Disease (Squamous Cell Carcinoma In Situ) 32
     - Erythroplasia of Queyrat 35
     - Bowenoid Papulosis 36
     - Squamous Cell Carcinoma 37
     - Verrucous Carcinoma 40
     - Keratoacanthoma 42
     - Adenosquamous Carcinoma 44

	Sarcomatoid Carcinoma (Carcinosarcoma, Metaplastic Carcinoma)	45
	Lymphoepithelioma-Like Carcinoma	46
	Basal Cell Carcinoma	46
2.	Neoplastic and Pseudoneoplastic Lesions of the Hair Follicles	71
	Benign Follicular Neoplasms with Nongerminative Cellular Differentiation	71
	Tumor of the Follicular Infundibulum	71
	Pilar Sheath Acanthoma	72
	Winer's Pore	72
	Trichoadenoma	73
	Trichilemmoma	73
	Benign Proliferating Pilar Tumor	75
	Benign Follicular Neoplasms with Germinative-Type Differentiation	76
	Trichofolliculoma	77
	Trichoepithelioma	78
	Desmoplastic Trichoepithelioma	81
	Pilomatricoma	82
	Trichogerminoma	85
	Mixed Epithelial and Mesenchymal Follicular Proliferations	86
	Basaloid Follicular Hamartoma	86
	Trichoblastoma	87
	Neoplasms Showing Differentiation Towards Follicle-Related Mesenchyme	89
	Trichodiscoma	89
	Perifollicular Fibroma	89
	Fibrofolliculoma	90
	Follicular Myxoma	91
	Pilar Leiomyoma	91
	Malignant Pilar Neoplasms	92
	Trichilemmal Carcinoma	92
	Malignant Proliferating Pilar Tumor	95
	Pilomatrix Carcinoma	97
	Adnexal Carcinomas with Mixed Differentiation	98
	Pilar Leiomyosarcoma	98
	Pseudoneoplastic Proliferations of Hair Follicles and Follicle-Related Mesenchyme	99
	Hair Follicle Nevus	99
	Linear Basal Cell Nevus	100
	Steatocystoma Multiplex and Simplex	101
	Eruptive Vellus Hair Cyst	101
	Neurofollicular and Pilar Neurocristic Hamartomas	102

3. Tumors and Tumor-Like Conditions with Predominantly Sebaceous Differentiation .. 117
   - Pseudoneoplastic Sebaceous Proliferations.. 117
     - Sebaceous Hyperplasia.. 117
     - Nevus Sebaceus 117
   - Benign Sebaceous Neoplasms 119
     - Sebaceous Adenoma 119
     - Superficial Epithelioma with Sebaceous Differentiation 122
     - Sebaceoma 123
   - Borderline Sebaceous Neoplasms 124
     - Basal Cell Carcinoma with Sebaceous Differentiation 124
   - Malignant Sebaceous Neoplasms 126
     - Sebaceous Carcinoma 126

4. Neoplasms and Pseudoneoplastic Proliferations of the Sweat Glands, and Primary
   Neuroendocrine (Merkel Cell) Carcinoma 137
   - Benign Eccrine Sweat Gland Neoplasms... 137
     - Eccrine Cylindroma.. 137
     - Eccrine Spiradenoma... 138
     - Syringoma 139
     - Eccrine Poroma 139
     - Eccrine Syringofibroadenoma 141
     - Papillary Eccrine Adenoma (Tubulopapillary Eccrine Hidradenoma) 143
     - Eccrine Acrospiroma (Solid and Cystic Hidradenoma, Nodular Eccrine
       Hidradenoma 143
   - Benign Apocrine Sweat Gland Neoplasms 146
     - Syringocystadenoma Papilliferum 147
     - Hidradenoma Papilliferum 148
     - Tubular Apocrine Adenoma 149
   - Sweat Gland Tumors with Mixed Differentiation... 149
     - Benign Mixed Tumors of the Skin (Chondroid Syringoma) 149
     - Other Mixed Lineage Adnexal Tumors... 151
   - Malignant Sweat Gland Tumors 152
     - Eccrine Carcinomas.. 152
     - Eccrine Carcinomas that Are Histologically Definable as Primary Tumors 152
     - Eccrine Carcinomas that Histologically Simulate Metastatic Tumors 164
     - Apocrine Carcinomas 168
     - Apocrine Carcinomas that Are Histologically Definable as Primary Tumors 169
     - Apocrine Carcinomas that May Histologically Simulate Metastases 172
   - Adnexal Carcinomas of Uncertain or Mixed Lineage, with Sweat Glandular
     Elements 175

Lymphoepithelioma-Like Carcinoma 175
Adnexal Carcinoma with Mixed Differentiation 177
Primary Neuroendocrine (Merkel Cell) Carcinoma 177
Pseudoneoplastic Lesions of Sweat Glands. 184
Eccrine and Apocrine Nevi 184
Syringometaplasia 184
Eccrine and Apocrine Hidrocystomas 185

5. Metastatic Neoplasms 201
Visceral Carcinomas that Involve the Skin 201
Clinical Features 201
Pathologic Findings 203
Specific Visceral Sources of Cutaneous Metastasis 204
Immunohistochemistry in the Determination of Primary Site 209
Primary Nonadnexal Epithelial Skin Tumors that May Resemble Metastatic Lesions. 209
Other Metastatic Neoplasms 209

6. Fibrous Tissue Tumors 215
Benign Fibrous Tissue Tumors 215
Fibroepithelial Polyps 215
Connective Tissue Nevus 216
Fibrous Hamartoma of Infancy 217
Dermatofibroma 218
Dermatomyofibroma 223
Angiofibroma and Related Lesions 223
Plexiform Fibrohistiocytic Tumor 226
Superficial Acral Fibromyxoma 227
Pleomorphic Fibroma 227
Sclerotic Fibroma 228
Collagenous Fibroma (Desmoplastic Fibroblastoma) 229
Postoperative Spindle Cell Nodule 230
Inflammatory Pseudotumor 230
Keloid 231
Elastofibroma Dorsi 233
Giant Cell Tumor of Tendon Sheath 234
Peripheral Giant Cell Granuloma (Giant Cell Epulis) 235
Fibroma of Tendon Sheath 236
Fibromatosis 237
Recurrent Infantile Digital Fibroma 238
Myofibroma 238

      Juvenile Hyaline Fibromatosis 240

      Nodular Fasciitis 241

   Fibrous Tissue Tumors of Intermediate Malignancy 243

      Solitary Fibrous Tumor 243

      Dermatofibrosarcoma Protuberans 244

      Bednar's Tumor (Pigmented Dermatofibrosarcoma Protuberans) 247

      Giant Cell Fibroblastoma 248

      Aggressive Angiomyxoma, Superficial Angiomyxoma, and
            Angiomyofibroblastoma 249

      Low-Grade Fibromyxoid Sarcoma 252

      Atypical Fibroxanthoma 253

   Malignant Fibrous Tissue Tumors 255

      Malignant Fibrous Histiocytoma 255

      Epithelioid Sarcoma 256

      Synovial Sarcoma 258

      Fibrosarcoma 258

7. Vascular Tumors and Pseudotumors 277

   Vascular Nevus 277

   Benign Vascular Neoplasms 277

      Lymphangioma 278

      Cavernous and Capillary Hemangiomas 279

      Lobular Capillary Hemangioma (Pyogenic Granuloma) and Related Lesions 281

      Kimura's Disease 283

      Epithelioid (Histiocytoid) Hemangioma 283

      Acral Arteriovenous Tumor/(Arterio-)Venous Hemangioma 285

      Hobnail/Targetoid/"Atypical" Hemangioma 287

      Other Cutaneous Hemangioma Variants 289

      Angiokeratoma 291

   Borderline Vascular Tumors 292

      Papillary Endovascular (Intralymphatic?) Angioendothelioma 292

      Epithelioid Hemangioendothelioma 294

      Spindle Cell Hemangioendothelioma (Hemangioma) 296

      Kaposiform Hemangioendothelioma 297

      Retiform Hemangioendothelioma 298

      Other Hemangioendotheliomas 299

   Malignant Vascular Neoplasms 299

      Kaposi's Sarcoma 300

      Angiosarcoma 304

Tumefactive Non-Neoplastic Vascular Proliferations 309
    Lesions that Simulate Kaposi's Sarcoma 309
    Potential Simulators of Angiosarcoma 313
    Other Reactive Vascular Proliferations 314

8. Tumors and Tumor-Like Conditions Showing Neural, Nerve Sheath, and Adipocytic Differentiation 329
    Neural Lesions 329
        Neuroma and Ganglioneuroma 329
        Neurofibroma 330
        Neurilemmoma 333
        Neurothekeoma 335
        Benign Granular Cell Tumor 337
        Peripheral Neuroepithelioma/Primitive Neuroectodermal Tumor 339
        Nonepithelioid Malignant Peripheral Nerve Sheath Tumor 341
        Epithelioid Malignant Peripheral Nerve Sheath Tumor 344
        Malignant Granular Cell Tumor 345
    Pseudotumors of the Skin Related to the Nervous System 345
        Rudimentary Meningocele (Primary Cutaneous Meningioma, Meningotheliomatous Hamartoma) 345
        Cutaneous Glial Heterotopia (Nasal Glioma) 347
    Tumors with Adipocytic Differentiation 348
        Lipoma Variants 348
        Lipoblastoma 353
        Hibernoma 353
    Adipocytic Pseudotumors 353
        Nevus Lipomatosus 353
        Tumefactive Localized Lipedema 355

9. Tumors of Muscle, Cartilage, and Bone 365
    Smooth Muscle Tumors 365
        Smooth Muscle Hamartoma 365
        Leiomyoma 366
        Cutaneous Angiomyolipoma (Angiolipoleiomyoma) 369
        Leiomyosarcoma 370
    Striated Muscle Tumors and Rhabdoid Tumor 372
        Rhabdomyomatous Mesenchymal Hamartoma 372
        Rhabdomyosarcoma 373
        (Extrarenal) Malignant Rhabdoid Tumor 374
    Cartilaginous Tumors and Parachordoma 375
        Extraskeletal Chondroma 375

	Subungual Osteochondroma and Exostosis	376
	Parachordoma	376
	Chondrosarcoma	377
Calcifying and Ossifying Tumors		377
	Ossifying Fibromyxoid Tumor	377
	Fibro-osseous Pseudotumor of the Digits	378
	Calcifying Aponeurotic Fibroma	379
	Osteosarcoma	380
10. Histiocytic Proliferations		389
Non-Langerhans Cell Histiocytic Infiltrates		389
	(Juvenile) Xanthogranuloma	389
	Benign Cephalic Histiocytosis	392
	Progressive Nodular Histiocytosis	393
	Generalized Eruptive Histiocytoma	394
	Xanthoma Disseminatum	395
	Reticulohistiocytosis	396
	Familial Histiocytic Dermatoarthritis	399
	Rosai-Dorfman Disease (Sinus Histiocytosis with Massive Lymphadenopathy)	399
Malignant Histiocytosis		401
Langerhans Cell Histiocytosis and Indeterminate Cell Histiocytosis		402
	Langerhans Cell Histiocytosis	402
	Congenital Self-Healing Reticulohistiocytosis	404
	Indeterminate Cell Histiocytosis	404
11. Plasmacellular Infiltrative Disorders		415
Multiple Myeloma		415
Extraosseous Plasmacytoma		416
Macroglobulinemia of Waldenström		417
Castleman's Disease		419
12. Cutaneous Mastocytosis		425
Systemic Mastocytosis		425
Cutaneous Mastocytosis (Urticaria Pigmentosa)		426
13. Lymphoid Infiltrates, Lymphoma, and Hematopoietic Proliferations		431
Lymphoid Infiltrates and Lymphomas		431
Lymphocytoma Cutis (Reactive Lymphoid Infiltrate, Cutaneous Lymphoid Hyperplasia, Pseudolymphoma, Lymphadenosis Benigna Cutis)		432
B-Cell Neoplasms		435
Cutaneous Marginal Zone B-Cell Lymphoma (Mucosa-Associated Lymphoid Tissue [MALT] Lymphoma)		435

      Follicular Lymphoma 438
      Diffuse Large B-Cell Lymphoma 440
      Intravascular Large B-Cell Lymphoma 442
      Lymphomatoid Granulomatosis 444
      Other B-Cell Lymphomas Involving the Skin 445
   T-Cell and NK-Cell Neoplasms 447
      Precursor T-Cell Lymphoblastic Lymphoma 447
      Adult T-Cell Leukemia/Lymphoma 448
      Extranodal NK/T-Cell Lymphoma, Nasal Type 451
      Subcutaneous Panniculitis-Like T-Cell Lymphoma 453
      Mycosis Fungoides 456
      Pagetoid Reticulosis 464
      Granulomatous Slack Skin 465
      Sézary's Syndrome 466
      Primary and Secondary Cutaneous Anaplastic Large Cell Lymphoma 469
      Peripheral T-Cell Lymphoma, Not Further Specified (Including Lennert's
         Lymphoma) 472
      Angioimmunoblastic T-Cell Lymphoma 475
      Lymphomatoid Papulosis 477
      Other T-Cell and NK-Cell Lymphomas Involving the Skin 480
   Cutaneous Involvement in Hodgkin's Disease 480
   Leukemia Cutis 483
   Extramedullary Hematopoiesis 486
Index 513

1 EPIDERMAL TUMORS

Tumors and cysts of epidermal origin or differentiation are among the most common lesions that arise in skin. In fact, just five of them, namely, seborrheic keratosis, epidermal cyst, actinic keratosis, basal cell carcinoma, and squamous cell carcinoma, comprise a large percentage of lesions seen in any dermatopathology practice. This situation is likely to continue, particularly considering our aging, ultraviolet-exposed population. There is also a wide variety of malformations, cysts, and some less common or rare tumors, both benign and malignant, of which the pathologist needs to be aware. Even among the five common entities mentioned above, there are histopathologic variants that can create considerable diagnostic confusion. In this chapter we review the salient clinical and histopathologic features of epidermal tumors.

EPITHELIAL CYSTS

Epidermal Cyst and Milium

Clinical Features. The *epidermal cyst* is a smooth, dome-shaped, freely movable, somewhat fluctuant subcutaneous swelling, sometimes attached to the skin by a central pore. These lesions are common on the face, neck, and trunk but can occur in virtually any anatomic location. The cyst may rupture, either spontaneously or due to trauma, with resultant inflammation and tenderness. Epidermal cysts are sometimes associated with other anomalies, such as nevus comedonicus or the Favre-Racouchot syndrome. They are also a cutaneous manifestation of Gardner's syndrome. It is likely that some epidermal cysts constitute a developmental anomaly of the follicular infundibulum, although in other instances traumatic implantation is probably also a cause (producing the "epidermal inclusion cyst").

A *milium* is a smaller version of an epidermal cyst, measuring from 1 to 4 mm in diameter. It may derive from the outer root sheath of vellus follicles. Milia are frequently multiple and tend to develop in areas of trauma, e.g., following abrasive injuries. They are particularly common in the infraorbital region. They also accompany several bullous disorders, notably porphyria cutanea tarda and dominant dystrophic epidermolysis bullosa.

Pathologic Findings. Epidermal cysts are lined by a stratified squamous epithelium that resembles epidermis or follicular infundibulum. Therefore, a granular cell layer is found adjacent to the keratin-containing cyst lumen (fig. 1-1). The cyst wall may be thinned or acanthotic, with a smooth-contoured base or with irregular budding. The keratin contents are usually loosely woven, typically more so than the overlying epidermis. Rupture is accompanied by neutrophilic or granulomatous inflammation, or both (fig. 1-2), and scar is found adjacent to older inflamed lesions. The cyst epithelium may respond to such events with marked acanthosis, but in other instances the cyst wall is obliterated or replaced by granuloma. The presence of flakes of keratin surrounded by granuloma or within multinucleated giant cells

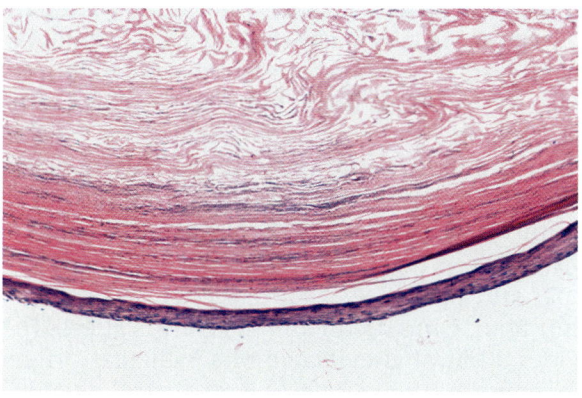

Figure 1-1

EPIDERMAL CYST

The thinned epithelial lining possesses a granular cell layer.

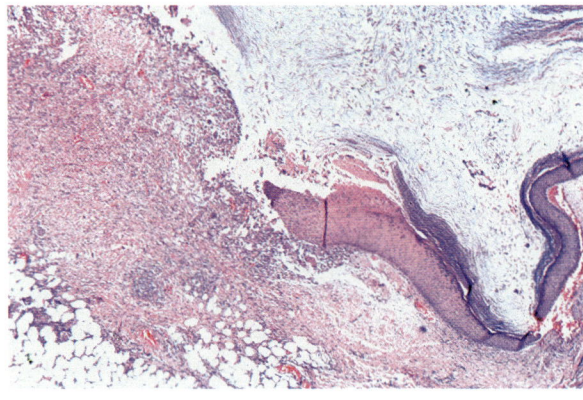

Figure 1-2

EPIDERMAL CYST

Rupture of the cyst wall as well as acute and granulomatous inflammation are seen.

provides a clue to the diagnosis of a ruptured cyst. Milia manifest as smaller, thin-walled epidermal cysts that are located in the superficial dermis.

There have been rare reports of Bowen's disease, basal cell carcinoma, or squamous cell carcinoma arising in epidermal cysts. Squamous cell carcinomas that have been partly biopsied or treated occasionally form cyst-like configurations without apparent connection to the overlying epidermis.

Differential Diagnosis. Although epidermal cysts and milia are among the most readily diagnosable lesions in dermatopathology, occasional problems can arise. Superficial shave biopsies showing changes of epidermal cyst may miss deeper foci that would point to a different diagnosis such as warty dyskeratoma, branchial cleft cyst, or syringocystadenoma papilliferum. Pilar cysts (trichilemmal cysts) are usually easily recognized by their distinctly palisaded basilar layer, swollen periluminal keratinocytes with sparse or absent keratohyaline granules, and homogeneous eosinophilic keratin. Occasional hybrid cysts have areas resembling both epidermal and pilar cysts. The presence of both infundibular and trichilemmal keratinization provides additional evidence of a follicular origin for these epithelial cysts. Markedly inflamed lesions may be difficult to distinguish from foreign body or infectious granulomas. In such instances, careful search for cyst wall fragments or keratin flakes can be decisive.

Milia-like formations may be observed in the periphery of keratoacanthomas, and a partial biopsy of the edge of such a lesion can create confusion. A clinical history of a rapidly advancing keratotic lesion may then raise suspicion of keratoacanthoma and prompt more complete sampling of the tumor.

Human Papillomavirus-Associated Cyst (Verrucous Cyst)

In recent years, a type of epidermal cyst has been described with microscopic features consistent with human papillomavirus (HPV) infection. These cysts most commonly arise in the plantar areas of the foot (20), although similar lesions have been reported on the scalp, face, back, and extremities (66,85). Clinically, the lesions resemble conventional cysts, or suggest dermatofibroma or basal cell carcinoma (85). Microscopically, the cysts are of the infundibular type, and feature varying degrees of papillomatosis, hypergranulosis, parakeratosis, and squamous eddy formation. Koilocytic changes with large keratohyaline granules are noted (21,66,85). The presence of HPV has been documented by immunohistochemistry (21), hybridization studies (20,38), and by polymerase chain reaction (PCR) methods that detect HPV DNA sequences (45). To date, both HPV types 57 and 60 have been found in these cysts (39,45). There is, at present, uncertainty about whether these lesions result from traumatic implantation of verrucae or from secondary infection of preexisting epidermal cysts.

Proliferating Epidermal Cyst

Although the proliferating trichilemmal cyst is a well-established entity (see below), a similar proliferative cystic lesion characterized by infundibular keratinization, with formation of a granular cell layer and laminated keratin, is not as widely recognized (62,64). The *proliferating epidermal cyst* has now been well documented by Sau et al. (75,76). In contrast to proliferating trichilemmal cysts, these lesions show a male predominance, and most occur in locations other than the scalp. They usually have a cyst-like clinical appearance.

Microscopically, several patterns have been described: papillomatous and acanthotic epithelium with squamous eddy formation and

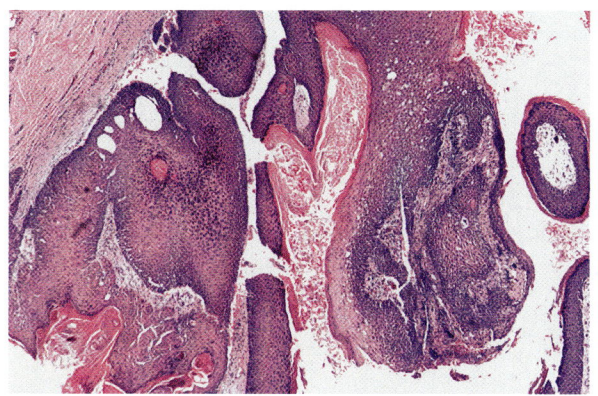

Figure 1-3

PROLIFERATING EPIDERMAL CYST

This example has acanthotic and focally papillomatous changes.

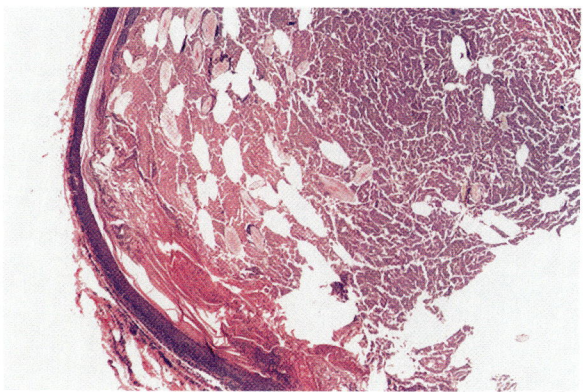

Figure 1-4

PIGMENTED FOLLICULAR CYST

Several pigmented hair shaft fragments are present in spaces (arrows) within the cyst lumen.

connection to the surface through a narrow opening; inverted follicular keratosis-like changes; a multiloculated cystic pattern lined by basaloid epithelium, with peripheral palisading of nuclei; pseudoepitheliomatous hyperplasia of the cyst lining; anastomosing bands reminiscent of proliferating trichilemmal cysts; conglomerations of numerous microcysts; and verrucous projections of lining epithelium into the cyst lumen reminiscent of HPV-induced cysts (fig. 1-3) (76). In most of these lesions, at least focal portions of the cyst wall resemble a typical epidermal cyst. An example of a proliferating tumor that showed both trichilemmal and infundibular keratinization has been described (62). Seven of the 33 tumors reported by Sau et al. (76) showed carcinomatous histopathologic features, and lesions with these changes were particularly prone to local aggressiveness (recurrence), although metastases were not reported.

Pigmented Follicular Cyst

This unusual cyst was first described by Mehregan and colleagues in 1982 (52). It usually presents as a solitary lesion in the head and neck region of adult men (73). A patient with multiple lesions has been reported; the lesions were present on the chest and abdomen (72).

Clinically, these cysts have a distinctly blue appearance, suggestive of blue nevus. Microscopically, they are typically cysts of infundibular type; the cyst lining maintains a rete ridge pattern. Within the lumen of the cyst are multiple pigmented hair shafts (fig. 1-4), and hair follicles or sebaceous lobules may attach to the cyst wall (52,72). Some of these lesions appear to be hybrid cysts, showing both infundibular and trichilemmal keratinization (72).

Cutaneous Keratocyst

Barr et al. (6) discovered that two of four cutaneous cysts removed from patients with the basal cell nevus syndrome had features resembling those of the odontogenic keratocysts that characteristically occur in that syndrome. Subsequently, a similar lesion was reported by Baselga et al. (7). Microscopically, the epithelia of these cysts have festooned configurations, are lined by two to five squamous cell layers, and keratinize without the formation of a granular cell layer. One of the cysts of Barr et al. also showed a small follicular bud and contained lanugo hairs, features reminiscent of steatocystoma, although sebaceous glands were absent. Additional reports will be necessary to determine if cutaneous cysts with these features are characteristic of the nevoid basal cell carcinoma syndrome.

Epithelial Cysts in Gardner's Syndrome

Gardner's syndrome is a dominantly inherited disorder consisting of premalignant colonic polyps, fibromas and desmoid tumors, osteomatosis, and cutaneous cysts. The cysts largely have the microscopic characteristics of epidermal cysts, but pilomatrixoma-like changes have been described in a number of them (17,50,57,70).

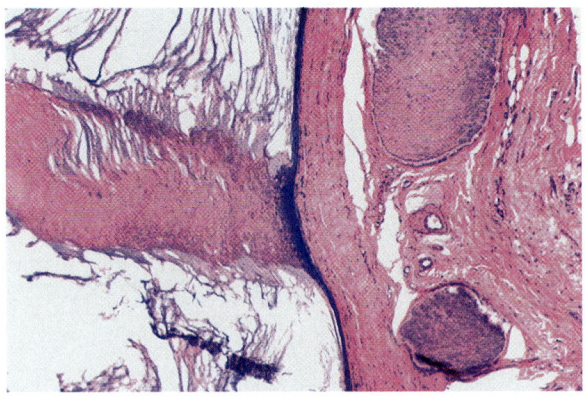 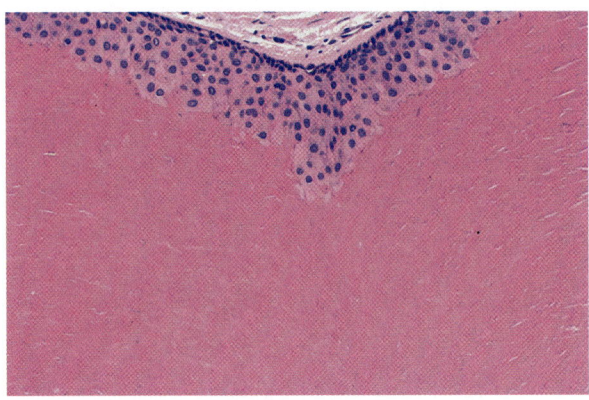

Figure 1-5

EPITHELIAL CYST IN GARDNER'S SYNDROME

A column of shadow cells projects into the cyst lumen. At its base are basaloid cells reminiscent of hair matrix. Aggregates of shadow cells are also present within the pericystic connective tissue.

Figure 1-6

TRICHILEMMAL CYST

Swollen, pale epithelial cells; absence of a granular cell layer; and homogeneous eosinophilic keratin are within the cyst lumen.

There are aggregates of shadow cells that are arranged as columns projecting into cyst lumens, lying free within the lumens, or present within pericystic connective tissue and associated with granuloma formation (17). When arranged as columns, the shadow cells appear to arise from basaloid, hair matrix-like cells within the cyst lining (fig. 1-5) (17). Narisawa and Kohda (57) have also reported trichilemmal keratinization, sebaceous glands attached to the cyst wall, and epithelial islands that are cytokeratin (CK) 19 positive and contain CK20-positive Merkel cells. The latter changes are consistent with the "bulge area" of follicular epithelia, and suggest that these cysts could arise from stem cells within the bulge.

Trichilemmal Cyst (Pilar Cyst, Isthmus-Catagen Cyst)

Clinical Features. The *trichilemmal*, or *pilar, cyst* commonly arises on the scalp, although it may also develop on the face, trunk, or extremities. Multiple cysts are not uncommon, particularly on the scalp, and the development of these cysts may be inherited as an autosomal dominant trait. Chromosomal mosaicism has been detected in a case of epidermal nevi associated with trichilemmal cysts (36).

The microscopic appearance of trichilemmal cysts suggests that they originate from the midportion, or isthmus, of the hair follicle, the zone located between the follicular entry of the sebaceous duct and the insertion of the arrector pili muscle. Ultrastructural studies indicate a close resemblance between these cysts and the trichilemmal sac surrounding catagen follicles (43), hence the alternative name, isthmuscatagen cyst. These cysts are distinguishable from most epidermal cysts because of the relative ease of their surgical enucleation.

Pathologic Findings. Histologically, there is keratinization of the wall of a trichilemmal cyst without the formation of a granular cell layer (although a few keratohyaline granules are occasionally identified). Instead, cells progress from a distinctly palisaded basilar layer to a swollen, pale cell layer adjacent to a cyst lumen that contains homogeneous, eosinophilic keratin material (fig. 1-6). As pointed out, this configuration closely resembles that of the follicular isthmus. Hybrid cysts have mixed features of trichilemmal and epidermal (infundibular) cysts (12). Foci of calcification occur within the cyst lumen in about 25 percent of cases. Occasionally, rupture of the cyst wall is observed, associated with a granulomatous response to the cyst contents. Cystic rupture may be followed by repair of the defect: by marsupialization to the epidermis, with partial or complete resolution of the cyst, or by proliferation of the cyst wall. The latter change may account for the *proliferating trichilemmal cyst (proliferating trichilemmal tumor)* (51).

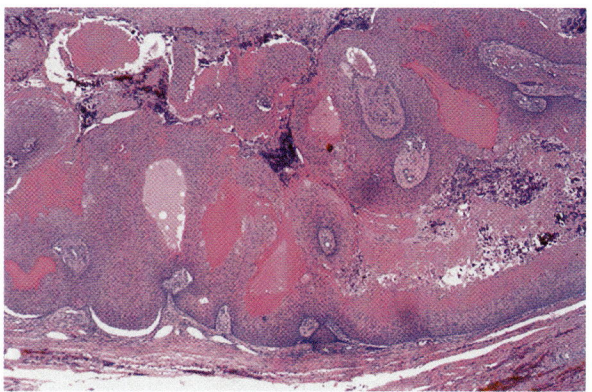

Figure 1-7

PROLIFERATING TRICHILEMMAL CYST

The epithelium is lobulated and there are foci of trichilemmal keratinization.

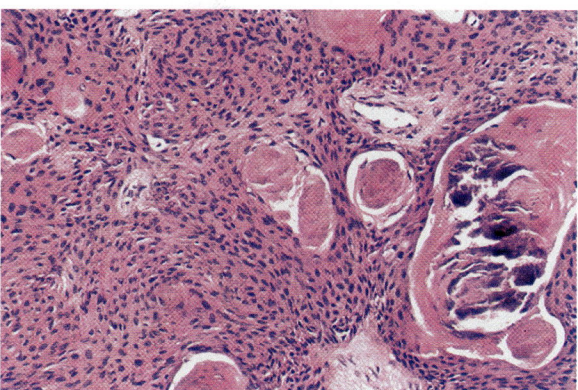

Figure 1-8

PROLIFERATING TRICHILEMMAL CYST

This high-power view shows foci of trichilemmal keratinization, one with calcium deposition, and lobules of relatively bland-appearing epithelium.

Proliferating Trichilemmal Cyst (Proliferating Trichilemmal Tumor, Pilar Tumor, Proliferating Pilar Tumor)

Clinical Features. The *proliferating trichilemmal cyst* is usually a solitary tumor that most often occurs on the scalp, particularly in middle-aged or elderly women. These lesions may occur in multiples (8,32,98); arise in locations such as the trunk (76), arm (98), or hand (46); and are occasionally encountered in young persons (98). They occur in men in about 30 percent of cases (76).

Proliferating trichilemmal cysts present as subcutaneous nodules or lobulated masses that may ulcerate or "marsupialize." As the name implies, it is widely believed that these lesions result from repeated episodes of rupture and re-epithelialization of trichilemmal (pilar) cysts (13,51). Massive cutaneous horns of the scalp have been reported to arise from proliferating trichilemmal tumors (53).

Pathologic Findings. Microscopically, there are lobules of squamous epithelium of varying sizes, some of which demonstrate peripheral palisading and are surrounded by basement membrane material. Sometimes, these changes arise in the wall of a trichilemmal cyst (13). The formation of amorphous eosinophilic keratin without the interposition of a granular cell layer in islands of squamous epithelium is the characteristic feature of trichilemmal keratinization (figs. 1-7, 1-8). Occasionally, keratinization of the infundibular type can also be identified, resulting in the configuration of a "hybrid" proliferating cyst (62). Other findings include apocrine or sebaceous (primary epithelial germ) differentiation (71), squamous eddy formation, calcification, and foci of clear cell change that demonstrate differentiation towards outer root sheath epithelium. Nuclear pleomorphism, a mitotic rate of up to one per high-power field, and small foci of stromal infiltration may be seen. Such findings occur in lesions that otherwise show benign biologic behavior. Since recurrences have been reported, complete excision is indicated for these lesions.

The malignant proliferating trichilemmal (pilar) tumor (giant hair matrix tumor, trichochlamydocarcinoma) shows considerable clinical overlap with the proliferating trichilemmal cyst, although it is most common in older women and averages 4 cm or more in diameter. Histologically, this tumor also resembles the proliferating trichilemmal cyst, or may even arise from a proliferating trichilemmal cyst. There are several characteristic features, however, that set malignant proliferating trichilemmal tumor apart: squamoid or basaloid cells showing little tendency toward pilar differentiation, conspicuous nuclear atypia, high mitotic activity (4 to 5 per high-power field), dyskeratotic cells, foci of necrosis, and stromal invasion (97). One metastasizing tumor showed areas of transition from proliferating trichilemmal cyst to spindle

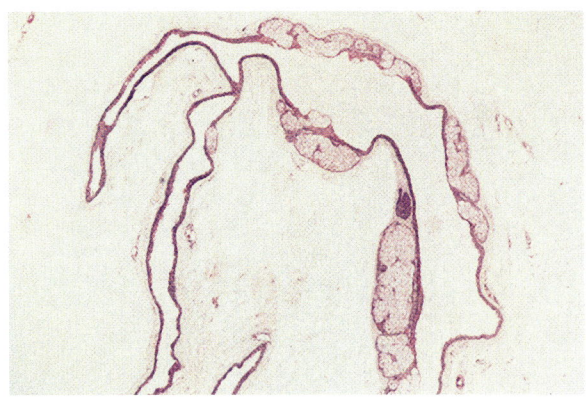

Figure 1-9

STEATOCYSTOMA

The thin-walled cyst has undulating contours. Small, flattened sebaceous lobules are present along the outer portion of the cyst wall.

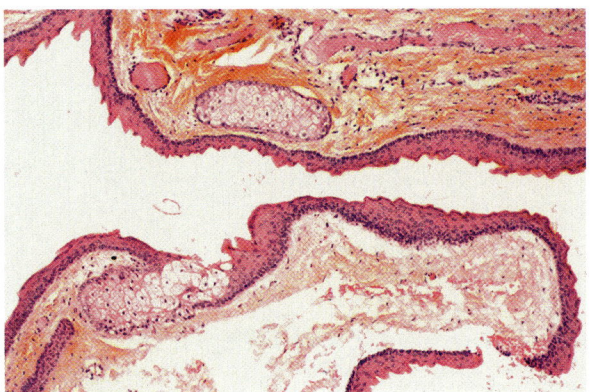

Figure 1-10

STEATOCYSTOMA

A sebaceous lobule is present in the cyst wall. There is a cuticular layer lining the luminal surface of the cyst.

cell carcinoma (56). Recognition of these tumors is important since they are capable of regional lymph node metastasis or visceral spread, and therefore wide local excision and close clinical follow-up are indicated.

Recent studies have demonstrated p53 positivity in a proliferating trichilemmal cyst as well as in a malignant proliferating trichilemmal tumor (96). Nondiploid DNA has been detected by flow cytometry in two of four proliferating trichilemmal cysts, and these results appeared to correlate with higher mitotic counts and increased staining with the Ki-67 monoclonal antibody (83). Takata and colleagues (89) used PCR-based microsatellite loss of heterozygosity (LOH) analysis to demonstrate complete loss of the wild type p53 in a trichilemmal carcinoma arising from a proliferating trichilemmal cyst. These analyses may eventually permit early identification of those histologically borderline proliferating trichilemmal tumors that are capable of greater biologic aggressiveness.

Differential Diagnosis. Proliferating trichilemmal tumor can be mistaken for squamous cell carcinoma, and in the past some of these cases may have accounted for reports of "squamous cell carcinomas arising in pilar cysts." Foci of trichilemmal keratinization, an adjacent pilar cyst, and limited cytologic atypia or mitotic activity are all features that tend to support a diagnosis of proliferating trichilemmal tumor.

Steatocystoma

Clinical Features. Steatocystoma consists of one or more cystic papules or nodules that measure between 1 and 3 cm in diameter. The multiple form, *steatocystoma multiplex,* can be inherited as an autosomal dominant trait. The lesions arise most often on the trunk, scalp, face, and arms; tend to manifest during adolescence or early adult life; and occur equally in both sexes. They are generally flesh colored, and when incised, discharge an oily fluid. An association with pachyonychia congenita has repeatedly been described (27,34,42), and recently, missense mutations in keratin 17 have been linked to both pachyonychia congenita type 2 and steatocystoma multiplex (18,84).

Pathologic Findings. The steatocystoma often has folded or undulating contours (fig. 1-8). It is lined by several layers of epithelial cells; a distinct, eosinophilic, cuticular layer lines the luminal surface. There are small, flattened sebaceous lobules along the outer layer of the cyst wall (figs. 1-9, 1-10). Pale-staining flocculent material is present within the cyst lumen, and occasionally, small hair shafts. These features in aggregate suggest differentiation towards sebaceous ductal epithelium (44).

Differential Diagnosis. Steatocystomas, as a rule, are easily distinguished microscopically from epidermal (infundibular) or trichilemmal cysts. Steatocystoma does resemble a dermoid cyst

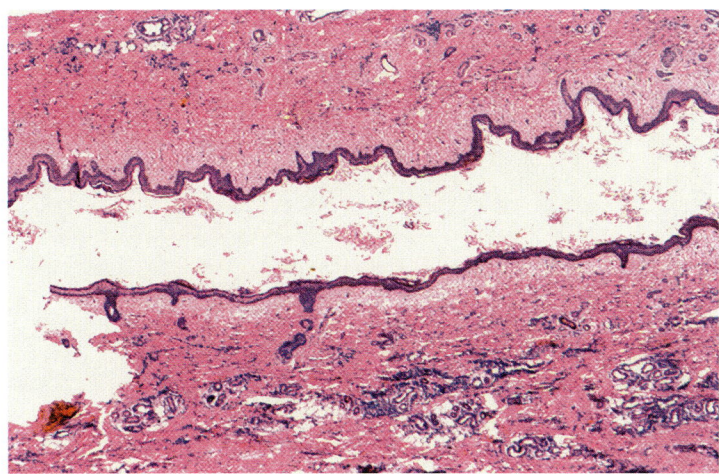
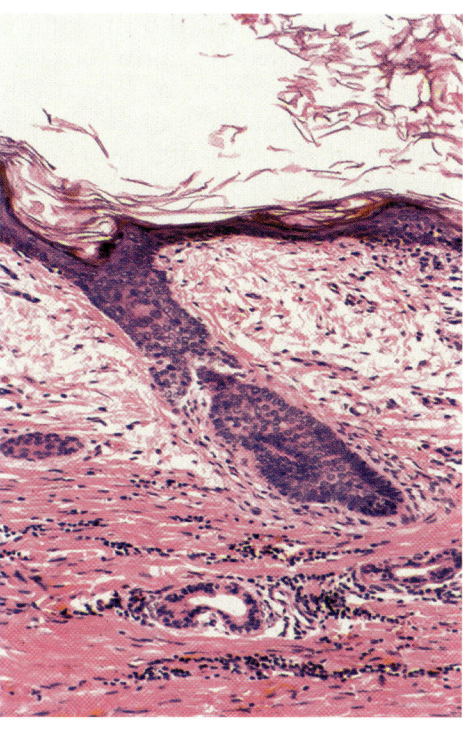

Figure 1-11

DERMOID CYST

Above: This cyst is lined by stratified squamous epithelium and contains keratin debris.

Right: A hair follicle enters the cyst wall. Sweat glands can be identified in the vicinity.

(see below). Dermoid cysts, however, are larger, tend to occur along embryonic lines of closure, have thicker walls, lack the thick cuticular luminal border, and contain prominent pilosebaceous and sometimes other adnexal elements. Eruptive vellus hair cysts (see below) resemble steatocystoma clinically, but clearly have a structural relationship to the vellus follicle. Coexistence of vellus hair cysts and steatocystomas (41,54), and even hybrids of the two (1,35), have been described. The notion of a relationship between the two cysts is not conceptually difficult, given the primary epithelial germ derivation of both hair follicle and sebaceous duct. This is further supported by the reported patterns of keratin expression for these cysts (keratin 17 for eruptive vellus hair cysts, keratins 10 and 17 for steatocystoma) (91).

Dermoid Cyst

Clinical Features. *Dermoid cysts* are subcutaneous cysts of ectodermal origin that arise along embryonic lines of closure. They are believed to be congenital lesions, but they may not become apparent until the second or third decades of life, due to episodes of rapid growth, inflammation, or trauma. They are most common in the head and neck area, particularly the supraorbital region, brow, upper eyelid, glabella, and scalp. They constitute the most common cause of periorbital mass lesions in infants and children (40). Dermoid cysts are more common in males than females. Sequestration of cutaneous epithelium during embryonic life is widely believed to explain the origin of these cysts; this may occur by several mechanisms, depending in part upon the location of the cyst (5,11).

Dermoid cysts present as subcutaneous swellings, with either an intact overlying epidermis or a depression connecting to a draining sinus tract. A collar of tufted hairs may surround scalp lesions. Cysts may be immobile due to attachment to periosteum, and those that rest on the dura or extend intracranially may fluctuate when a child cries. Infection, including bacterial meningitis, may be a complication, depending upon the location of the cyst and its associated sinus tracts.

Pathologic Findings. On gross examination, the dermoid cyst is a firm, tan, cystic mass with protruding hair shafts; it contains a yellow, oily material. Microscopic features include a cyst lined by stratified squamous epithelium, into which are inserted a number of small hair follicles (fig. 1-11). The cyst lumen contains keratin debris and hair shaft fragments. Sebaceous glands are associated with the follicles and are usually not flattened against the cyst wall, as is the case in steatocystoma. Sweat glands, both eccrine and apocrine, can be identified in the vicinity of the cyst (fig. 1-11), and smooth muscle is present in up to one third of cases. This constellation of findings usually allows distinction from steatocystoma.

Differential Diagnosis. In addition to steatocystoma, the dermoid cyst should be distinguished from the recently described folliculosebaceous cystic hamartoma. The latter is more superficially located in the dermis, is less cystic, has more prominent sebaceous glands, and is not associated with hair follicles or other adnexal structures (44). Cystic teratoma is sometimes casually called a "dermoid," but this lesion is rare in skin (55,94), or in the head and neck region in general, and has tissues derived from all three germ layers. Dermoid cysts also differ from the corneal and epibulbar "dermoids" that are associated with a variety of syndromes; these lesions consist mainly of dense, hyalinized connective tissue that may contain pilosebaceous units.

Eruptive Vellus Hair Cyst

Clinical Features. *Eruptive vellus hair cysts,* first reported by Esterly et al. in 1977 (22), are characterized by an eruption of yellow to brown papules over the chest and proximal extremities of children and young adults. Lesions may be localized to the face, and a solitary lesion was associated with a melanocytic nevus and a conventional epidermal cyst (95). Spontaneous clearing after several years has been reported. The condition may be inherited as an autosomal dominant disorder (87).

Pathologic Findings. The epithelial-lined cyst contains keratin and sections of vellus hairs (fig. 1-12). In addition to these vellus hairs, evidence of a follicular origin includes invagination of the cyst wall by follicle-like elements or the presence of portions of a telogen follicle or arrectores pilorum muscle, which may extend beneath the cyst. The cysts may communicate with the skin surface, discharging their contents and causing granulomatous inflammation; the latter changes may explain the crusting that is associated with some lesions (10). The microscopic findings suggest a developmental

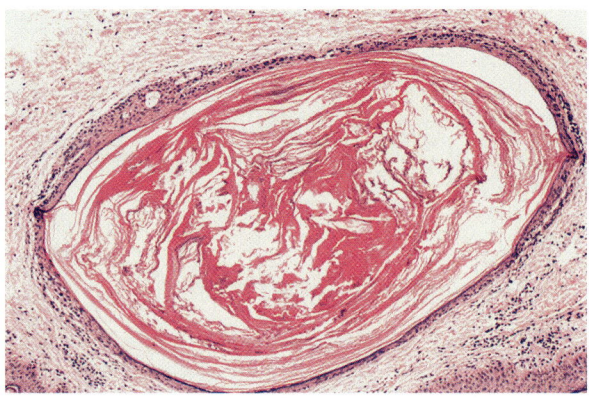

Figure 1-12
ERUPTIVE VELLUS HAIR CYST
This epithelial-lined cyst contains keratin material and sections of vellus hairs. There is an adjacent cord of epithelium containing a few sebaceous cells.

anomaly involving vellus follicles, with occlusion and cystic dilatation (14,22).

Differential Diagnosis. The microscopic features of eruptive vellus hair cysts are characteristic. The clinical resemblance to and occasional histopathologic association with steatocystoma multiplex has already been discussed.

Cutaneous Cysts and Related Structures that May Be Ciliated

There is a group of cysts or related structures that uncommonly occur in the skin and may feature ciliated epithelium. These include structures of possible müllerian or urogenital sinus origin (endometriosis, endosalpingiosis, mucinous and ciliated vulvar cyst, and cutaneous ciliated cyst), bronchogenic cyst, thyroglossal duct cyst, branchial cleft cyst, and thymic cyst. Median raphe cysts of the penis have also been reported to contain cilia on rare occasion. Despite their differing modes of origin, these cysts are discussed here collectively because of their common microscopic feature of ciliated epithelium (see separate discussion of the median raphe cyst below).

Cilia have a characteristic cross-sectional appearance on ultrastructural examination: two central fibrils surrounded by nine double fibrils. This 9+2 arrangement is constant in cilia throughout the plant and animal kingdoms (15,24). Cilia, however, are not normal constituents of

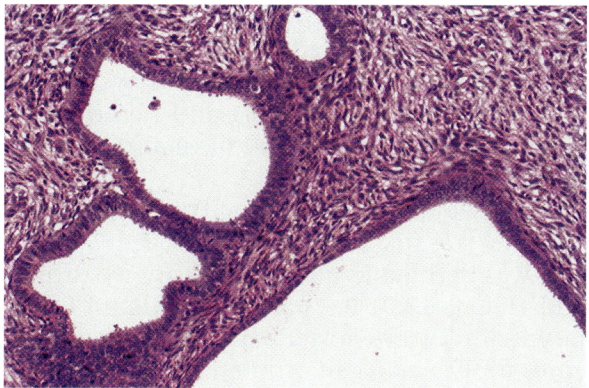 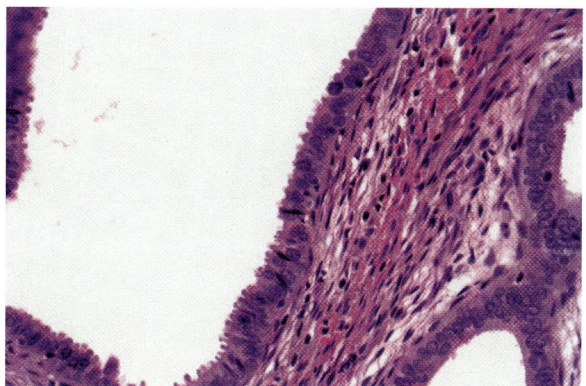

Figure 1-13

CUTANEOUS ENDOMETRIOSIS

Left: Endometrial glands and stroma in a cutaneous lesion.
Right: Cilia can sometimes be identified in the glandular epithelium.

cutaneous epithelia, and their presence in the skin is distinctly unusual.

There are several possible explanations for finding ciliated epithelia. Sequestration and migration during embryogenesis have been invoked as explanations for the cutaneous ciliated cyst, which often arises in the lower extremities, and for the cutaneous bronchogenic cyst. Cutaneous ciliated cysts are believed by some to be of müllerian origin, as are the fallopian tubes, uterus, and upper third of the vagina. Their appearance in the lower extremities may be explained by the common coelomic wall origin of limb buds and müllerian ducts during embryogenesis, with later migration of these müllerian elements within the developing limb (29), although other explanations have also been proposed. In the case of bronchogenic cysts, bronchial epithelium is known to derive from the ventral portion of the primitive foregut, and sequestrations from the foregut may migrate into the developing skin or be pinched off by the subsequent fusing of sternal bars.

Failure of regression of embryonic structures could play a role in the formation of some ciliated cysts. Dysontogenesis, or defective embryonic development, is theoretically possible. Embryonic sweat ducts and glands feature cilia at 16 weeks' gestation (30), and, therefore, arrested sweat gland development could theoretically result in persistence of ciliated epithelia.

Prosoplasia, or abnormal development resulting in a "higher" state of organization, has been suggested as an explanation for vaginal adenosis, the appearance of ciliated glandular epithelium in the vagina or vulva (68,81). Transplantation of tissue could occur following surgical procedures, via either direct inoculation or lymphatic or hematogenous metastasis. This mechanism has been proposed for cutaneous endometriosis.

Finally, metaplasia of pluripotential cells to form ciliated epithelia is a theoretical explanation that has been proposed for the development of endometriosis (86) and ciliated odontogenic keratocysts (65). However, hard evidence for the role of metaplasia in producing ciliated cysts in skin is lacking.

Endometriosis. First described in the latter part of the 19th century, endometriosis occasionally arises in skin. Locations include the umbilicus, lower abdomen, inguinal region, labia, or perineum. The lesions are often present within surgical scars (especially cesarean section or laparotomy scars). They are typically papules to small nodules (approximately 5 mm in diameter) and brownish in color, although they may appear blue-black due to cyclical bleeding.

Microscopically, there are combinations of glands and stroma, the former showing the characteristic features of uterine endometrium expected during the proliferative, secretory, or menstruation phases of the menstrual cycle. Cilia may sometimes be identified (fig. 1-13). One study has shown a poor correlation between the histologic features of these lesions and the actual stage of the menstrual cycle (90).

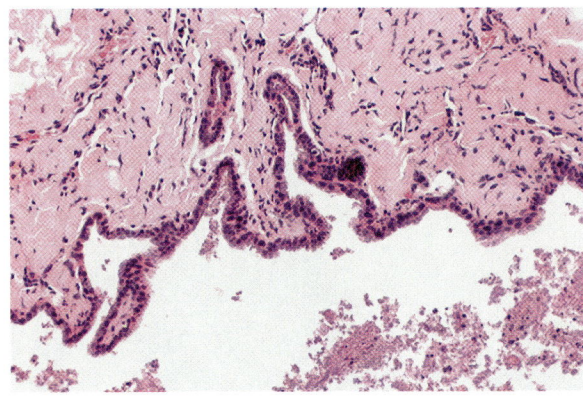

Figure 1-14

MUCINOUS AND CILIATED VULVAR CYST

This cyst features low columnar epithelium.

Decidualized changes can sometimes be encountered, particularly in lesions detected during pregnancy, and such lesions may be confused with malignancy by the unwary pathologist. Similar problems can arise when fine-needle aspiration biopsies are performed (4).

Endosalpingiosis. This rare condition is characterized by the development of brown papules (resembling nonhemorrhagic lesions of cutaneous endometriosis) in a periumbilical distribution following salpingectomy. Microscopically, there is a cyst lined by columnar epithelial cells, some of which are ciliated. Papillary projections are present within the lumen. These features resemble fallopian tube as well as the cutaneous ciliated cyst (see below) (19).

Mucinous and Ciliated Vulvar Cyst. Mucinous and ciliated cysts occur in the vulvar region. Their origin has been the subject of debate. Robboy et al. (68) found small mucinous glands in 53 percent of vulvas examined at autopsy, and, in addition, encountered 11 cysts in clinical practice that featured varying combinations of mucinous and ciliated epithelium. They suggested that glands lined by mucinous or ciliated epithelium are normal vulvar constituents, and that cysts develop due to inflammation and obstruction of their outlets (68). They and others (58) favor an origin from entoderm of the urogenital sinus, although a müllerian origin or metaplasia of apocrine glands have also been considered (37).

The cysts are lined by cuboidal to tall columnar or pseudostratified columnar epithelium with variable amounts of mucin and/or cilia (fig. 1-14). Squamous metaplasia and neutrophilic infiltration of the cyst wall have also been reported (37,58,68).

Cutaneous Ciliated Cyst. This type of ciliated cyst was first reported by Hess in 1890 (33), and was defined as a distinct entity by Farmer and Helwig (23). It usually presents as a solitary lesion on the lower extremities, and most commonly occurs in women. Similar lesions have been reported on the sole of the foot, buttock, scapular area, and scalp, and there has been one reported case in a male (93). The cysts may extend to several centimeters in diameter, are unilocular or multilocular, and on incision contain clear or serous fluid.

Microscopically, the cyst is lined by cuboidal or columnar ciliated epithelium, arranged in folds or papillary projections (fig. 1-15). Mucinous cells are usually not observed but have been reported (88). The lining resembles that of fallopian tube. Immunohistochemical staining is positive for epithelial membrane antigen, CAM5.2, and AE1/AE3, and negative for carcinoembryonic antigen, similar to the results seen in normal fallopian tube; positive staining for estrogen or progesterone receptors has been reported (80).

Bronchogenic Cyst. Bronchogenic cysts occur in both males and females, and are usually first recognized early in life. They typically occur as solitary dermal or subcutaneous nodules over the suprasternal notch or manubrium sterni, but other locations have been reported, including the scapular area, shoulder (26), chin (2), and back (92). The cysts have a firm wall and contain clear fluid. Bronchogenic cysts are lined by cuboidal to columnar ciliated epithelium that may be pseudostratified (fig. 1-16, left) and form folds or papillary projections into the lumen. Goblet cells are usually present (fig. 1-16, right), and the stroma may include smooth muscle, mucous glands, or cartilage. A mixed inflammatory infiltrate is sometimes present (63).

Thyroglossal Duct Cyst, Branchial Cleft Cyst, and Thymic Cyst. These cysts normally do not fall within the purview of the dermatologist or dermatopathologist, but they occasionally have cutaneous manifestations and

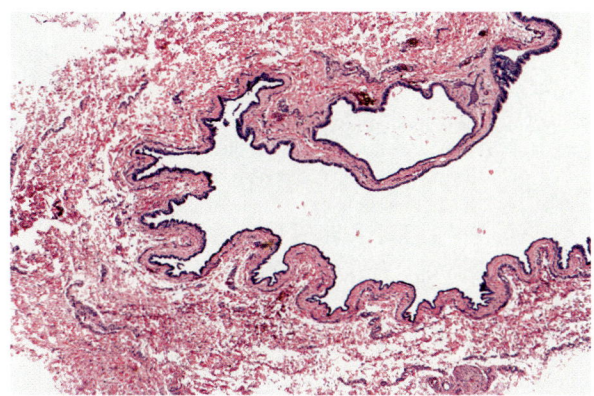 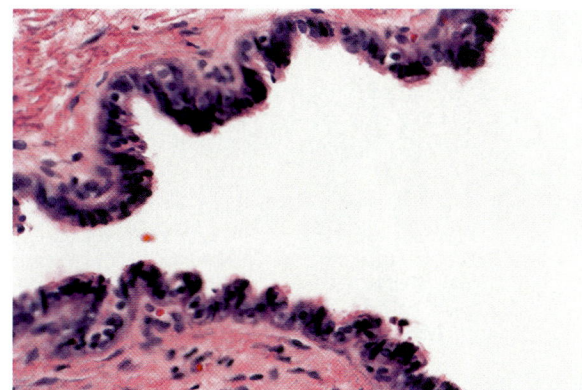

Figure 1-15

CUTANEOUS CILIATED CYST

Left: The epithelium is folded and has papillary projections.
Right: At high power, cilia can be identified.

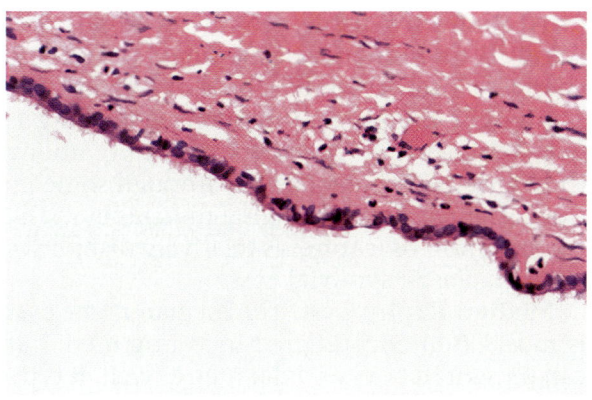 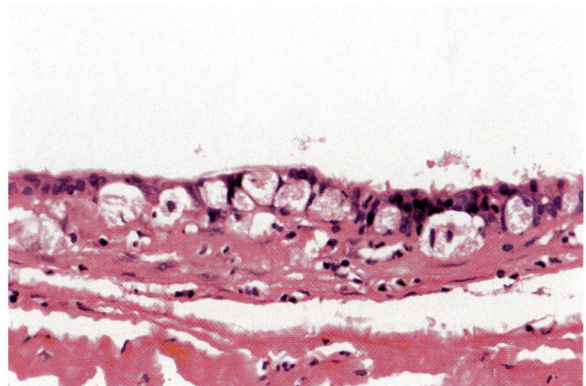

Figure 1-16

BRONCHOGENIC CYST

Left: Ciliated epithelium is evident.
Right: Goblet cells are often in the lining epithelium.

each may contain cilia. The thyroglossal duct cyst arises from embryonic remnants of the duct that remain after the descent of the developing thyroid gland. The cyst is usually located near the hyoid bone, and is brought to the attention of the patient and physician due to infection or formation of a cutaneous fistula. These cysts may be associated with thyroid follicles and lack smooth muscle or cartilage in their walls (fig. 1-17) (78). Branchial cleft cysts typically occur on the lateral neck, are lined by stratified squamous and/or columnar epithelium, and have walls containing lymphoid tissue (fig. 1-18) (60). Thymic cysts are believed to arise from embryonic remnants of the thymopharyngeal duct and may be present in the neck. Microscopically, they resemble the bronchogenic cyst but lack goblet cells; thymic tissue is present and cholesterol granulomas are in the surrounding stroma (74).

Other Cutaneous Cysts

Metaplastic Synovial Cyst. This recently described cutaneous lesion arises most often in areas subjected to surgical or other types of trauma, although one reported case was associated with a basal cell carcinoma and no history

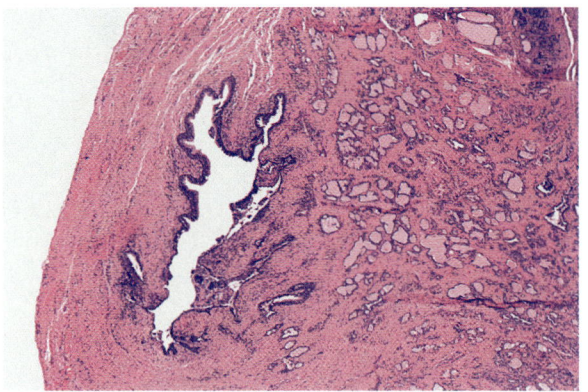 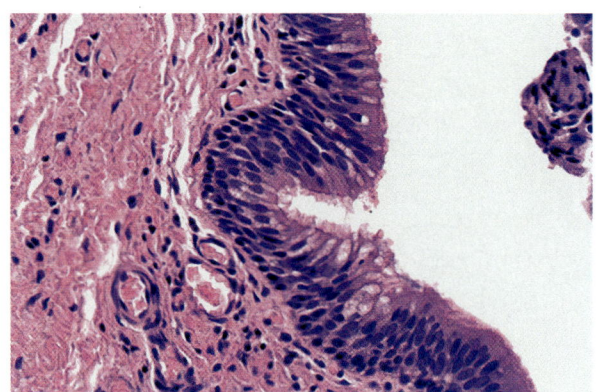

Figure 1-17

THYROGLOSSAL DUCT CYST

Left: Portion of a cyst associated with thyroid tissue.
Right: The epithelium of the cyst is ciliated.

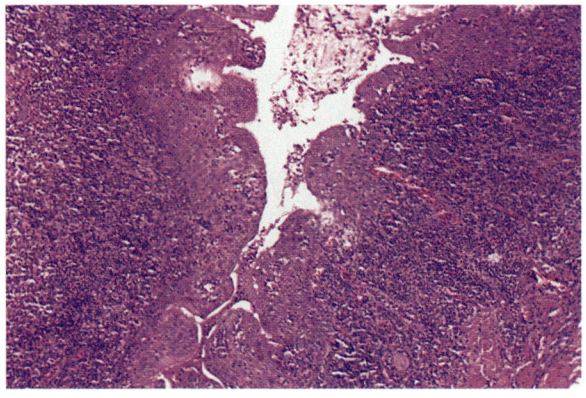

Figure 1-18

BRANCHIAL CLEFT CYST

Focally stratified epithelium and lymphoid tissue are seen.

of trauma (9). Other associations include chronic inflammatory states such as rheumatoid arthritis (82) or heritable disorders of connective tissue such as Ehlers-Danlos syndrome (59). Similar lesions have been identified in soft tissue, usually related to prior surgery or experimental induction (28).

Microscopically, the changes characteristic of metaplastic synovial cyst are identified at varying levels of the dermis and may extend to the cutaneous surface. These consist of cystic structures with villous protrusions within lumens, lined by a thin fibrinous exudate and a connective tissue core consisting of loosely organized connective tissue, prominent vessels, and spindled to epithelioid cells (fig. 1-19). These changes closely resemble those of hyperplastic synovium. Immunohistochemical staining is generally negative except for vimentin among the lining and stromal cells. Although some lesions slightly resemble digital mucous cyst, the constellation of features is relatively distinctive for metaplastic synovial cyst.

Median Raphe Cyst. The median raphe cyst is most often encountered in young men, but can present in boys or older men as well. It typically occurs along the ventral portion of the penis, particularly in the region of the glans, but can arise anywhere along the median raphe, including the perianal region (77). The lesions are usually solitary, but multiple lesions occur (79). The presenting complaint is usually that of a mass or distortion of penile contour.

Histologically, these cysts are lined by pseudostratified columnar epithelium that variably contains mucous cells (fig. 1-20) (3,16). Cilia have also been reported (69). Thus, the cysts have a urothelial lining, a conclusion supported by positive staining for cytokeratins (13, 67). Serotonin-containing cells have also been reported in these cysts (25). Theories of their origin have included failure of closure of the median raphe or derivation from the periurethral glands of Littre. Sequestration of ectopic urethral mucosa during embryonic development seems a reasonable explanation (16).

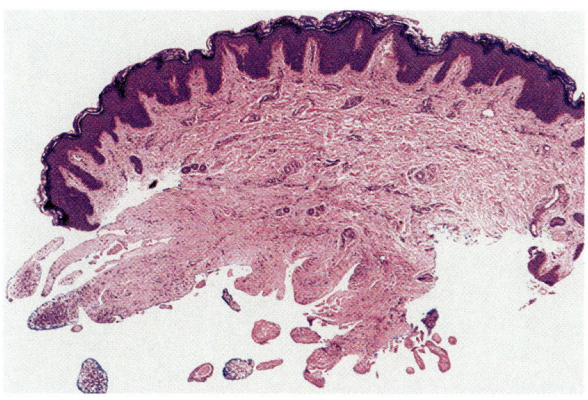 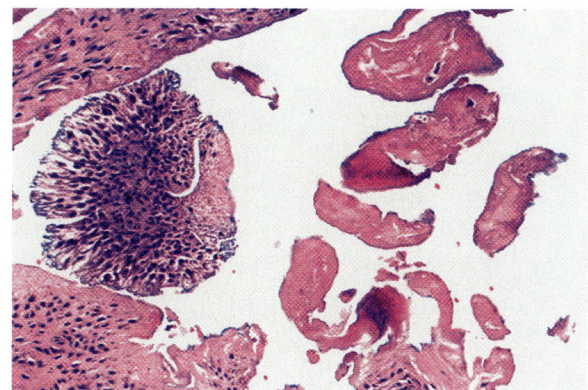

Figure 1-19

METAPLASTIC SYNOVIAL CYST

Left: There is an ill-defined cystic structure in the subcutis.
Right: Within the lumen are several villous structures. One of these contains numerous spindled to epithelioid cells.

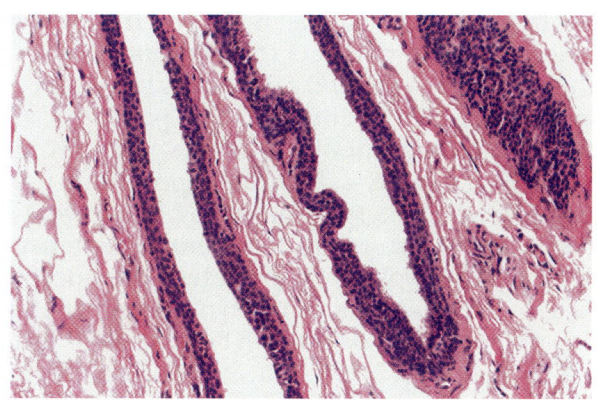 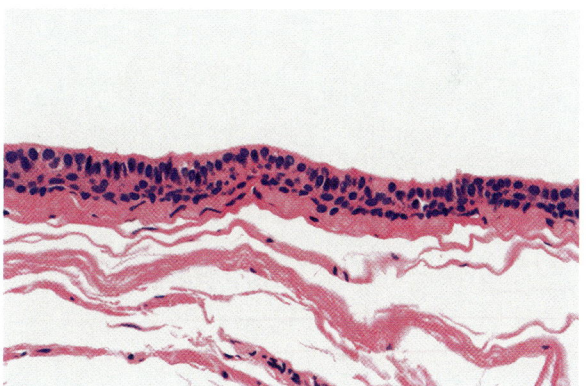

Figure 1-20

MEDIAN RAPHE CYST

Left: Low-power view of a cyst.
Right: The cyst is lined by pseudostratified columnar epithelium. Rare cilia can be identified.

Omphalomesenteric Duct Polyp. During early embryonic development, the omphalomesenteric duct communicates between the midgut and the yolk sac. It typically disappears during the seventh week of development, but persistence results in polyp, sinus, or cyst formation. This may present as a red umbilical polyp that is usually noted soon after birth or in early childhood. A central depression indicates an underlying sinus or cyst. Pyogenic granuloma is sometimes suspected clinically, although bleeding and exudation are not typical features (49).

Histologically, the polyp contains branching epithelium that may have the appearance of gastric or small or large intestinal mucosa, sometimes with connections to the epidermal surface (fig. 1-21). Aberrant pancreatic tissue has been reported in one case (47). Other findings include smooth muscle, lymphoid nodules (99), and varying degrees of erosion, acanthosis, inflammation, and vascular proliferation (31). Definitive removal of these lesions should be preceded by studies to rule out associated anomalies, such as enteric fistulae and Meckel's diverticulum (48,49). There has also been a rare report of an umbilical polyp associated with urachal rather than omphalomesenteric remnants (61).

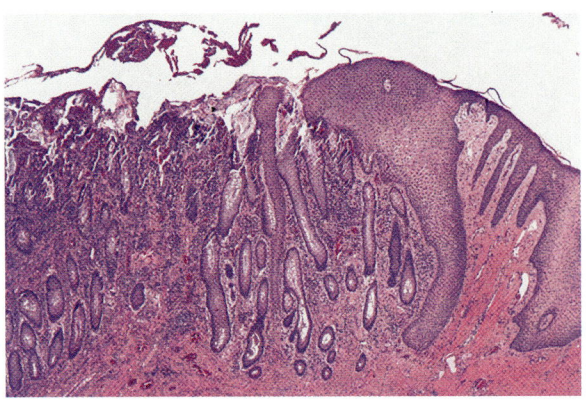
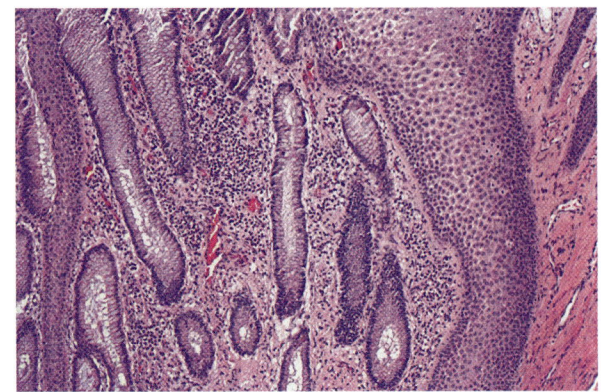

Figure 1-21

OMPHALOMESENTERIC DUCT POLYP

Left: This polyp extends to the epidermal surface.
Right: The polyp is composed of intestinal epithelium.

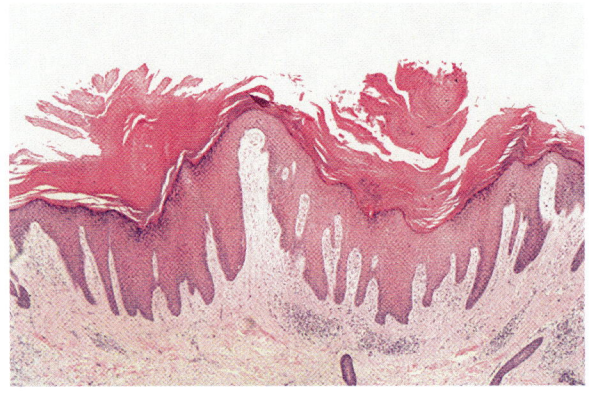

Figure 1-22

EPIDERMAL NEVUS

This lesion displays hyperkeratosis, regular papillomatosis, and acanthosis.

BENIGN EPIDERMAL TUMORS

Epidermal Nevus

Clinical Features. *Epidermal nevi* generally present as verrucous papules that are either present at birth or develop during early childhood, although adult onset has been documented. Papules may be solitary or arranged in clusters that often assume a linear configuration. Extensive linear lesions are said to follow Blaschko's lines. Several names have been applied to clinical variants, including *nevus unius lateris* for unilateral lesions and *ichthyosis hystrix* for bilateral systematized lesions. An epidermal nevus syndrome has been proposed, linking extensive epidermal nevi with abnormalities of the central nervous and cardiovascular systems, eyes, and skeleton. Some of these patients also have other cutaneous findings, including nevocellular nevi, café au lait spots, and hemangiomas. This syndrome may be congenital or show autosomal dominant inheritance (142,143). Happle (118) disputes the concept of a single "epidermal nevus syndrome," as several different birth defects can be associated with epidermal nevi.

Other variants of epidermal nevi include *nevoid hyperkeratosis of the nipple*, *nevus comedonicus*, and *inflammatory linear verrucous epidermal nevus* (ILVEN). In nevoid hyperkeratosis of the nipple, verrucous change resembling epidermal nevus involves one or both areolae (111,133). Nevus comedonicus consists of linear arrangements of comedones, sometimes with small cysts, abscesses, or fistulae that tend to form on the trunk. An association with other stigmata of the epidermal nevus syndrome has been reported. Lesions of ILVEN commonly occur on the lower extremities of females but can be seen in other locations and in males. These lesions are typically inflamed and pruritic, and clinically resemble psoriasis.

Pathologic Findings. The most typical features of epidermal nevi are hyperkeratosis, acanthosis, and papillomatosis (figs. 1-22, 1-23). The papillomatosis may be irregular (fig. 1-24), and flattening of the surfaces of the papillary

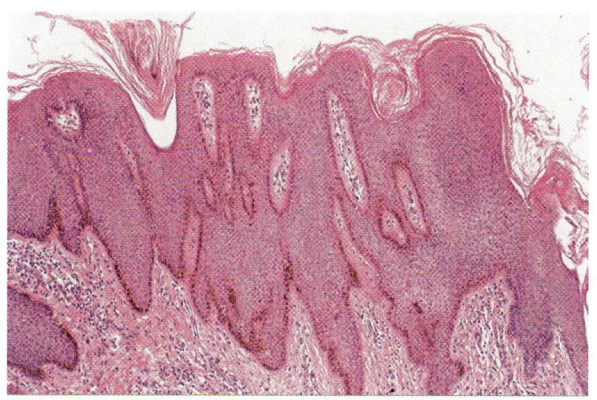

Figure 1-23

EPIDERMAL NEVUS

Papillomatosis and pronounced acanthosis are the major findings.

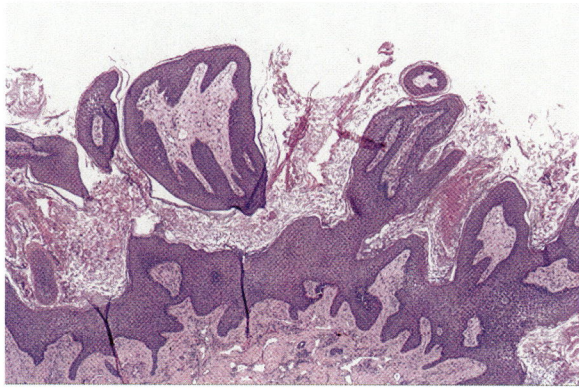

Figure 1-24

EPIDERMAL NEVUS

This epidermal nevus displays marked irregular papillomatosis.

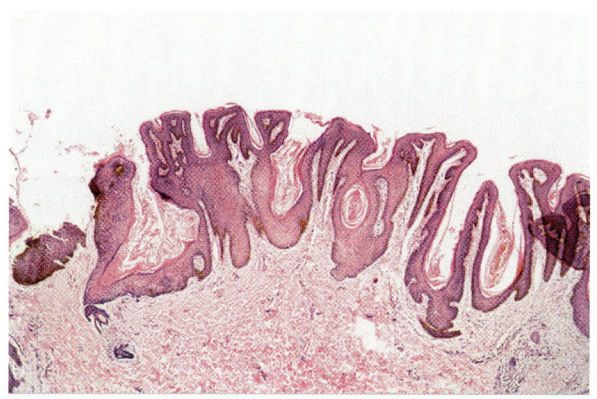
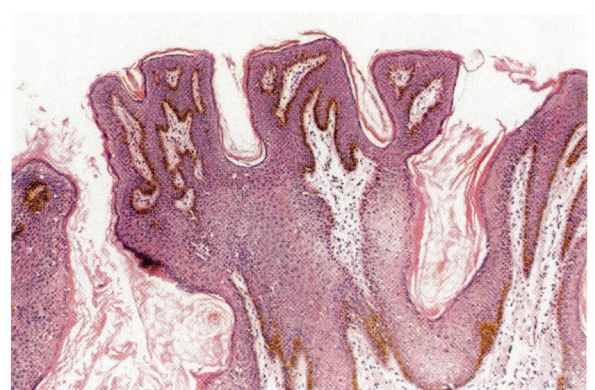

Figure 1-25

EPIDERMAL NEVUS

Low-power (left) and high-power (right) views show flattening of the papillary projections (the "mesa" sign).

projections (the "mesa" sign) is sometimes encountered (fig. 1-25). Regular, "church-spired" papillomatosis, such as encountered in acrokeratosis verruciformis of Hopf or stucco keratosis, is sometimes observed. Changes of epidermolytic hyperkeratosis are sometimes present, especially in the clinical variant known as ichthyosis hystrix. Less commonly, there are changes of acantholytic dyskeratosis resembling Darier's disease. These include suprabasilar acantholysis and formation of dyskeratotic keratinocytes (113,144). Such lesions have sometimes been designated *acantholytic, dyskeratotic epidermal nevus*. In a study by Submoke (145), 62 percent of epidermal nevi had the typical hyperkeratosis-papillomatosis-acanthosis configuration, while 16 percent showed changes of epidermolytic hyperkeratosis.

Nevoid hyperkeratosis of the nipple shows varying degrees of hyperkeratosis, acanthosis, and papillomatosis (fig. 1-26). In nevus comedonicus, there are dilated follicles filled with keratin in the manner of comedones, sometimes with milia or proliferations of the lining epithelium (fig. 1-27). Changes of epidermolytic hyperkeratosis have also been reported in these

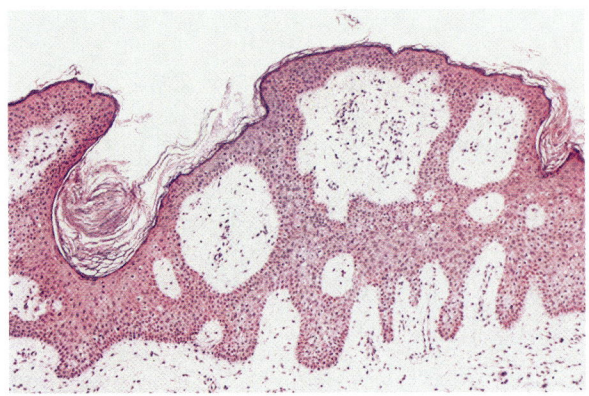

Figure 1-26

NEVOID HYPERKERATOSIS OF THE NIPPLE

There are focal hyperkeratosis, papillomatosis, and irregular acanthosis.

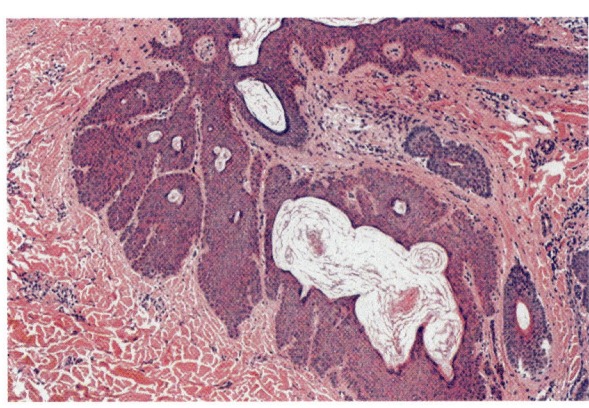

Figure 1-27

NEVUS COMEDONICUS

This comedo-like structure shows proliferations of its wall, resembling a dilated pore of Winer.

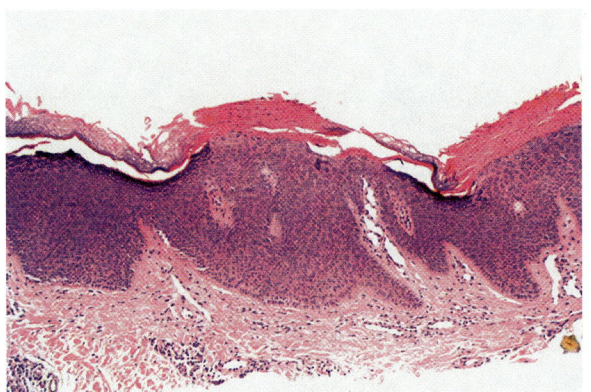
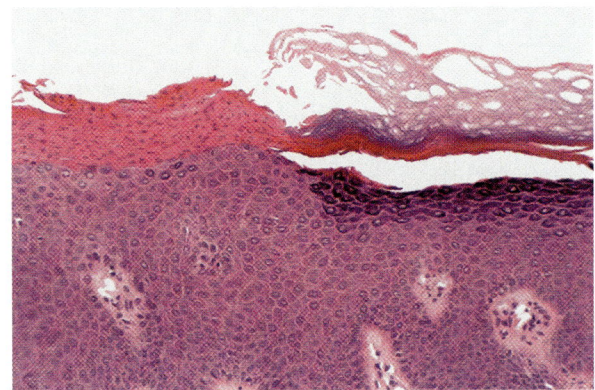

Figure 1-28

INFLAMMATORY LINEAR VERRUCOUS EPIDERMAL NEVUS

Left: Psoriasiform acanthosis with alternating orthokeratosis and parakeratosis. Hypergranulosis is present in the epidermal invaginations, while parakeratosis surmounts papillary projections of epidermis.

Right: High-power view shows abrupt transition between orthokeratosis and parakeratosis.

lesions (114). Lesions of ILVEN show psoriasiform acanthosis with an underlying perivascular lymphohistiocytic infiltrate. Spongiosis may be present. A characteristic feature of these lesions is the presence of alternating orthokeratosis and parakeratosis. Parakeratosis is associated with papillary projections of epidermis and absence of a granular layer, while orthokeratosis is found in adjacent epidermal invaginations, accompanied by hypergranulosis (fig. 1-28). With immunohistochemical staining, there is increased involucrin expression in orthokeratotic areas and negative expression in parakeratotic areas (121).

Differential Diagnosis. The differential diagnosis of conventional epidermal nevi includes verrucae, seborrheic keratoses, and other papillomatous lesions such as acanthosis nigricans and confluent and reticulated papillomatosis of Gougerot and Carteaud. Old verrucae may lack the typical viropathic changes or the "in-bowing" of epithelial margins seen in well-developed viral lesions, while at the same time the papillomatosis can closely mimic that of epidermal nevi. Changes of epidermolytic hyperkeratosis can also superficially mimic the viropathic changes of human papillomavirus infection. In such cases, the absence of characteristic koilocytic cells with "raisinoid" nuclei, and possible extension of vacuolated changes deep within the epidermis favor epidermal nevus.

The close-set basaloid cells and pseudohorn cysts of seborrheic keratosis are usually characteristic, but hyperkeratotic varieties with marked papillomatosis and lacking horn cysts can resemble epidermal nevi. Some regard seborrheic keratosis as a kind of "tardive" epidermal nevus. Nevertheless, a diagnosis of seborrheic keratosis should not be made in children, and only with caution in young adults; most lesions in these age groups probably represent either epidermal nevi or verrucae.

Acanthosis nigricans and confluent and reticulated papillomatosis have lesser degrees of hyperkeratosis and papillomatosis than ordinarily encountered in epidermal nevi, and clinical data should help to exclude these diagnoses in most instances. Nevoid hyperkeratosis of the nipple can mimic one of the distribution patterns of acanthosis nigricans; greater degrees of epidermal change and lack of involvement in other locations tend to exclude acanthosis nigricans in such cases.

ILVEN can resemble psoriasis microscopically as well as clinically. The presence of alternating orthokeratosis and parakeratosis, however, is not typical of psoriasis, and the pattern of involucrin expression differs as well, since in psoriasis most suprabasilar keratinocytes are involucrin positive (105).

Acantholytic Acanthoma

Acantholytic acanthoma is an uncommon lesion that presents as a papule or small nodule. It is often a solitary lesion, but multiple lesions have been reported in the genital region. It is not surprising that the diagnosis is rarely made clinically, as it has no distinctive clinical features.

Microscopically, acantholytic changes can mimic those of pemphigus vulgaris, pemphigus vegetans, pemphigus foliaceus, or Hailey-Hailey disease (familial benign chronic pemphigus) (fig. 1-29). Changes of acantholytic dyskeratosis, as seen in Darier's disease, were not emphasized in original reports but definitely occur and may even be common (fig. 1-30). Thus, this lesion can show a spectrum of changes analogous to those of transient acantholytic

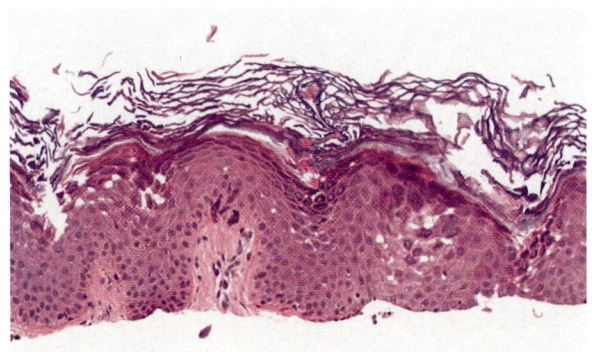

Figure 1-29

ACANTHOLYTIC ACANTHOMA

This lesion shows foci that are somewhat spongiotic, but with a degree of dyskeratosis.

dermatosis (Grover's disease). The clinical presentation of one or a few lesions usually allows an accurate diagnosis. Direct immunofluorescence may be helpful in the rare instance when there are multiple lesions that microscopically resemble pemphigus: a negative immunofluorescent study would be expected for acantholytic acanthoma (106,109,110).

Epidermolytic Acanthoma

Epidermolytic acanthoma is usually a solitary lesion that is less than 1 cm in diameter. There may be a few lesions or, rarely, disseminated, small, flat, brown papules located over the trunk.

The microscopic changes seen in epidermolytic acanthoma are characteristic of a dominantly inherited form of ichthyosis that is also known as *epidermolytic hyperkeratosis* (formerly, bullous congenital ichthyosiform erythroderma). These changes include hyperkeratosis and vacuolization of cells of the granular and suprabasilar layers of the epidermis with formation of large, irregularly shaped keratohyaline granules (fig. 1-31). Such changes may be observed in epidermal nevi (see above), forms of hyperkeratosis of palms and soles, or skin biopsy specimens as an incidental finding.

The clinical presentation of the lesion rules out other disorders that show changes of epidermolytic hyperkeratosis. Microscopically, verrucae have similar features; however, unlike verrucae, epidermolytic acanthoma typically lacks parakeratosis and may show vacuolization that extends close to the basilar layer (131,141).

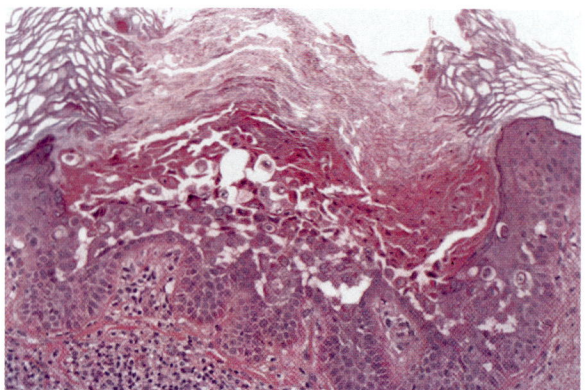 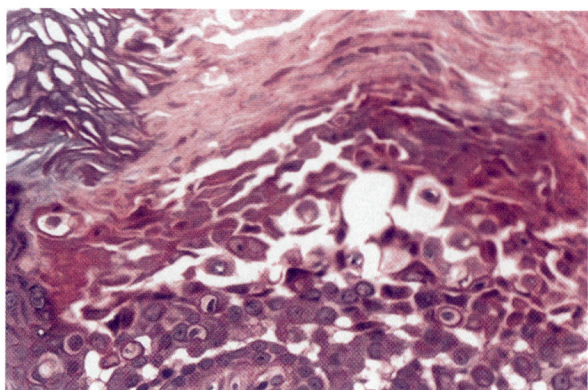

Figure 1-30

ACANTHOLYTIC ACANTHOMA

Left: There is marked acantholysis, such as may be seen in Hailey-Hailey disease, however, dyskeratosis is readily apparent.

Right: High-power view shows corps ronds (cells with pyknotic nuclei, perinuclear halos, and deeply eosinophilic cytoplasm) and grains (large variants of parakeratotic cells). These dyskeratotic elements are characteristic of Darier's disease and related disorders.

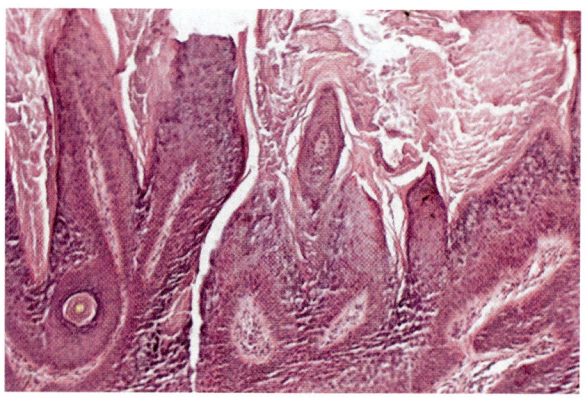 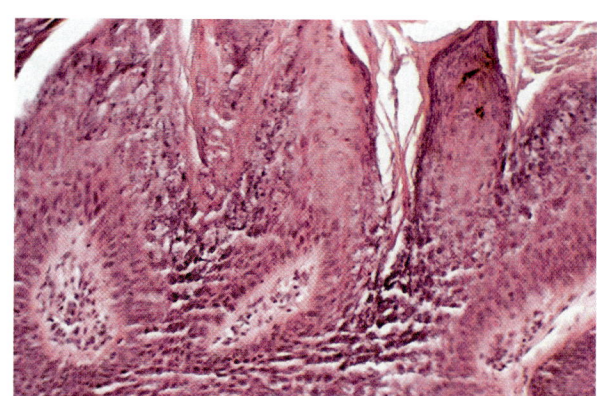

Figure 1-31

EPIDERMOLYTIC ACANTHOMA

Left: Marked hyperkeratosis and papillomatosis are seen. Vacuolated keratinocytes and irregularly shaped keratohyaline granules occupy much of the viable epidermis.

Right: Detail of vacuolated cells and irregular keratohyaline.

Warty Dyskeratoma

Clinical Features. *Warty dyskeratoma* is a crusted papule or small nodule with a central keratotic plug. This lesion commonly occurs on the face, neck, and scalp, or in the axilla (107). Oral mucosal lesions have been frequently described in the literature (101,132,148), and a subungual lesion has been reported (104). Although warty dyskeratoma is most often solitary, multiple lesions can occur (103,117).

Pathologic Findings. There is a cup-shaped invagination of epidermis, filled with keratin. The epithelial lining shows suprabasilar acantholysis with villus formation, and dyskeratotic cells along its surface (fig. 1-32) (146,147). The two best-known forms of dyskeratosis are the *corps rond* and *grain*. Corps rond cells feature a pyknotic nucleus surrounded either by a clear halo or by dense eosinophilic material. Grain cells resemble plump parakeratotic nuclei. Both cell types are typical of lesions characterized by

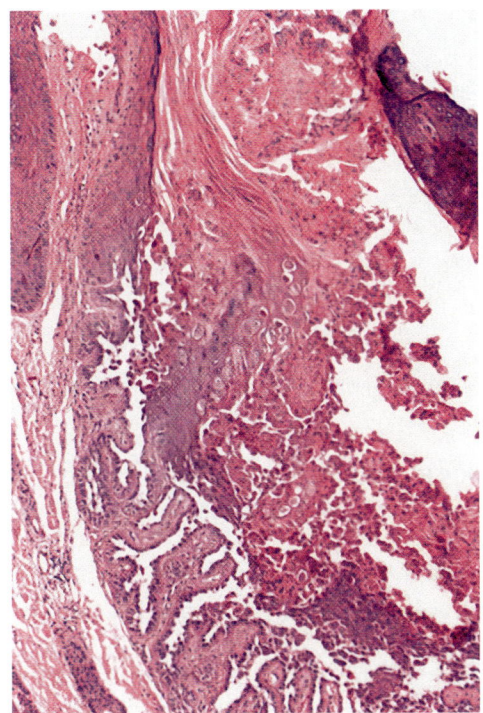
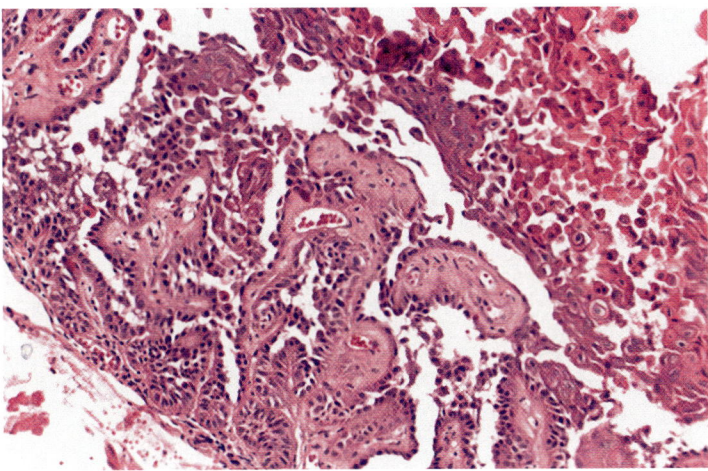

Figure 1-32

WARTY DYSKERATOMA

Left: An invagination of epidermis is filled with keratin. The lining epithelium demonstrates acantholysis.

Above: Detail of acantholytic lining epithelium shows the formation of villi and dyskeratosis.

acantholytic dyskeratosis, including warty dyskeratoma (fig. 1-33); the prototype genodermatosis, Darier's disease (keratosis follicularis); Grover's disease (transient acantholytic dermatosis); certain epidermal nevi (acantholytic, dyskeratotic epidermal nevi); and some acantholytic acanthomas. Focal acantholytic dyskeratosis can also be encountered as an incidental finding in biopsy specimens obtained for unrelated reasons.

Differential Diagnosis. The characteristic cystic invagination of the epidermis, combined with acantholytic and dyskeratotic changes, gives the warty dyskeratoma a diagnostic appearance. Shallow lesions may resemble, or in fact be examples of, dyskeratotic acantholytic acanthomas, while a cystic invagination of proliferative epidermis without acantholytic or dyskeratotic changes may actually represent a dilated pore or pilar sheath acanthoma.

Seborrheic Keratosis and its Variants

Clinical Features. *Seborrheic keratoses* are extremely common lesions among adults. They are benign lesions that are often removed, even by nonsurgical means, for cosmetic reasons. They may clinically mimic both premalignant and malignant lesions. In addition, they some-

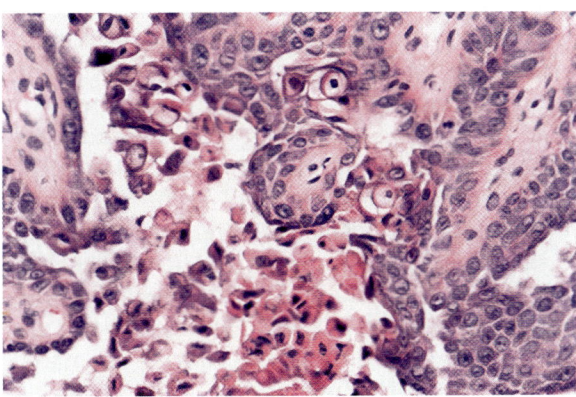

Figure 1-33

WARTY DYSKERATOMA

This high-power view shows corps rond and grain formation.

times show histologic features that raise concerns about malignancy, and occasionally malignant cutaneous tumors (e.g., squamous cell carcinoma, malignant melanoma) actually do arise in association with seborrheic keratosis. These facts underscore the importance of a familiarity with the microscopic appearance of seborrheic keratosis and its variants.

Seborrheic keratosis is a rough-surfaced papule, nodule, or plaque that occurs especially on

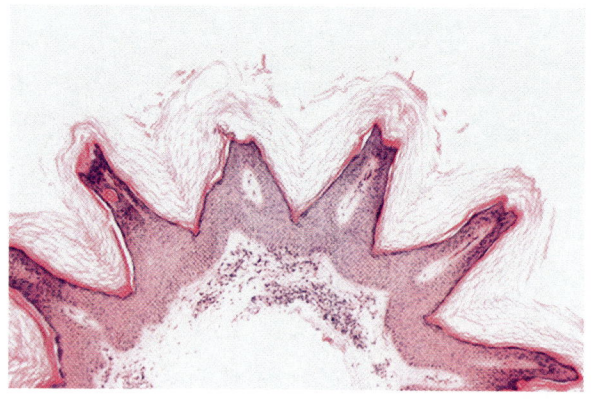

Figure 1-34

SEBORRHEIC KERATOSIS, HYPERKERATOTIC TYPE

There is pronounced "church-spired" papillomatosis. This feature is seen in stucco keratosis.

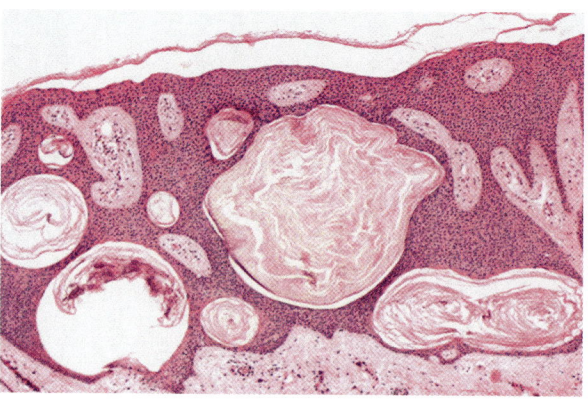

Figure 1-35

SEBORRHEIC KERATOSIS, ACANTHOTIC TYPE

There are close-set basaloid cells and pseudohorn cysts.

the trunk but can involve virtually any cutaneous surface except palms and soles. These lesions typically begin to develop during the fourth or fifth decades, and may become quite numerous. Although they usually do not exceed 3 cm in diameter, they can occasionally form annular plaques that are considerably larger. Seborrheic keratoses arise de novo or from preexisting lentigines. Increased numbers of keratoses may develop, even in an eruptive fashion, in association with weight gain or exfoliative erythroderma. The sign of Leser-Trélat is the rapid appearance of pruritic seborrheic keratoses in association with internal malignancy, most often adenocarcinomas of the gastrointestinal tract; this sign is also often associated with acanthosis nigricans (140).

Several clinical variants of seborrheic keratosis have been described. Tag-like seborrheic keratoses that are heavily pigmented are commonly found in the malar regions of African-American individuals, and are termed *dermatosis papulosa nigra*. Multiple, small, slightly elevated, flesh-colored papules termed *stucco keratoses* are frequently observed over the distal extremities. Other variants are defined mainly by their unique histopathologic features; these include *irritated seborrheic keratosis, inverted follicular keratosis, nested ("clonal") seborrheic keratosis,* and *melanoacanthoma.*

Pathologic Findings. Seborrheic keratosis is characterized by varying combinations of hyperkeratosis, acanthosis, and papillomatosis. The involved epidermis is often sharply demarcated at its base, forming a straight line that is continuous with the adjacent, uninvolved epidermis; this is a reflection of the exophytic nature of most of these lesions. Characteristically, seborrheic keratosis is composed of close-set basaloid cells and pseudohorn cysts. The latter are cystic invaginations of the epithelium that are filled with surface keratin, which in a given microscopic section may be cut in cross-section, thereby appearing as "cysts" within the involved epidermis.

Seborrheic keratosis is often divided into three major types: hyperkeratotic, acanthotic, and reticulated. *Hyperkeratotic seborrheic keratosis* has pronounced papillomatosis, which may be digitate or "church-spired" in type, the latter showing regular, pointed epidermal projections (fig. 1-34). *Acanthotic* lesions are mainly typified by marked epidermal thickening (fig. 1-35). *Reticulated* lesions show downgrowth of interconnecting narrow epidermal tracts (fig. 1-36). The latter type often arises in association with solar lentigines. As might be expected, mixtures of these three configurations occur.

The lesions of *dermatosis papulosa nigra* combine features of seborrheic keratosis and fibroepithelial polyp, with basilar hypermelanosis (fig. 1-37). *Stucco keratosis* features regular, church-spired papillomatosis, thereby qualifying as a hyperkeratotic seborrheic keratosis variant (fig. 1-34). Seborrheic keratoses are often inflamed or irritated. Hemorrhagic scale-crust

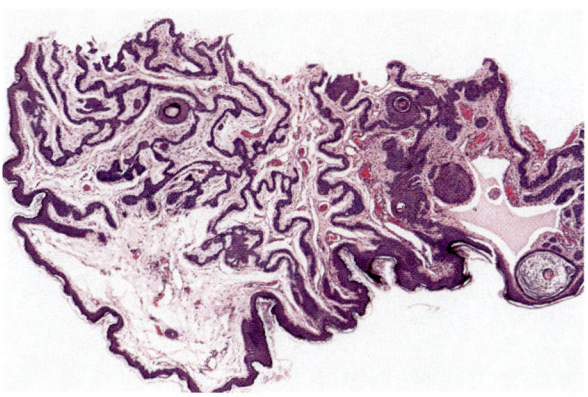 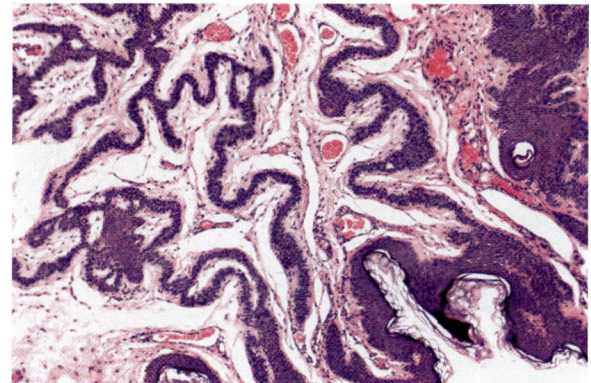

Figure 1-36

SEBORRHEIC KERATOSIS, RETICULATED TYPE

This type shows narrow, interconnecting epithelial cords that at times can be quite elaborate.
Left: Low-power view.
Right: Detail of interconnecting epithelial cords.

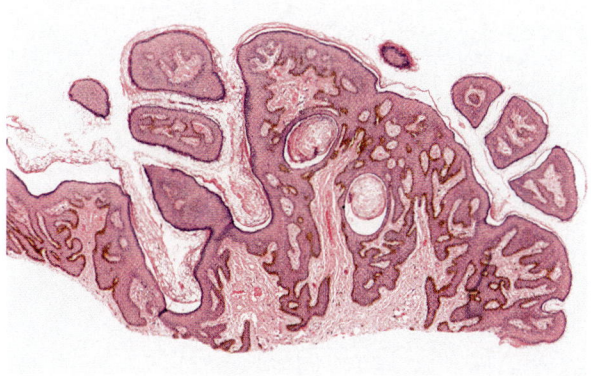 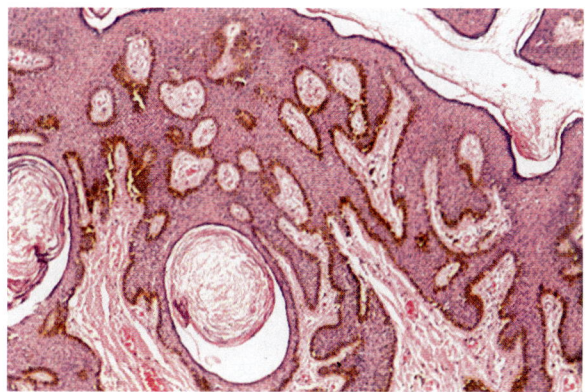

Figure 1-37

DERMATOSIS PAPULOSA NIGRA

Left: There is a papillomatous, focally polypoid configuration.
Right: High-power detail includes reticulated features, basilar hypermelanosis, and pseudohorn cysts.

formation, surface neutrophilic accumulation (sometimes producing spongiform pustulation), erosion or ulceration, and dermal inflammation with exocytosis are often encountered (fig. 1-38). Other lesions have minimal inflammation but show marked spongiosis, sometimes sufficient to result in mild acantholysis and "squamous eddies," whorls of flattened keratinocytes with a superficial resemblance to the "horn pearls" of squamous cell carcinoma (fig. 1-39). Lesions with the latter changes are known as *irritated seborrheic keratoses*. A distinction has been made between "inflamed" and "irritated" seborrheic keratoses, since lesions with spongiosis and squamous eddies can be produced by experimental irritation in the absence of inflammation. *Inverted follicular keratosis* also features spongiosis and squamous eddy formation, with a distinctly endophytic growth pattern arrayed about a central keratin-filled invagination. This endophytic configuration is a reasonably unique feature of these lesions, although some authors consider it simply a variant of the irritated seborrheic keratosis (128). *Nested ("clonal") seborrheic keratosis* contains discrete clusters of keratinocytes, reminiscent of the Borst-Jadassohn phenomenon

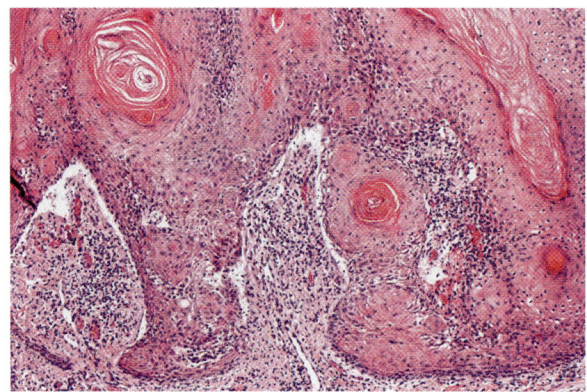 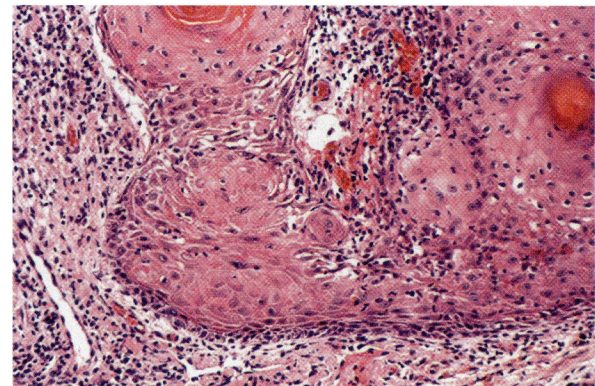

Figure 1-38

IRRITATED, INFLAMED SEBORRHEIC KERATOSIS

Left: Squamous eddy formation and spongiosis are associated with the inflammation that permeates the epidermis.
Right: Squamous eddies and nuclear disorganization can raise concerns about squamous cell carcinoma.

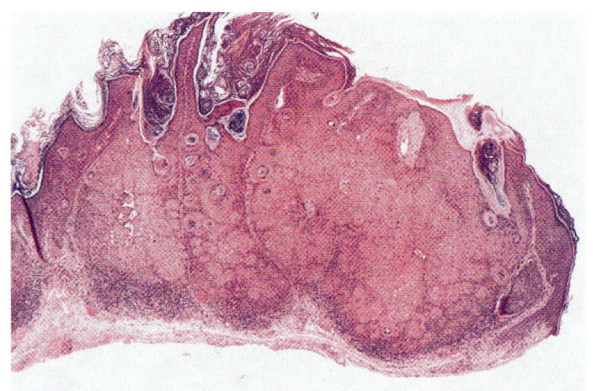 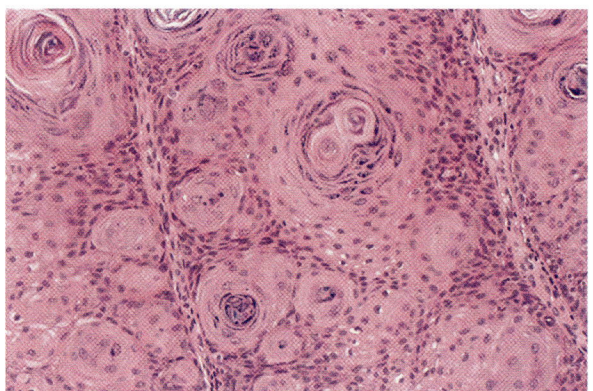

Figure 1-39

IRRITATED SEBORRHEIC KERATOSIS

Left: The lobulated growth features whorls of keratinocytes. There is a degree of band-like lymphocytic inflammation beneath the epidermis, but permeation of the epidermis by inflammatory cells is not observed.
Right: Squamous eddies are prominent.

(fig. 1-40). Some authors prefer the modifier "nested" to "clonal," since there is no evidence that the keratinocyte nests represent true clones of cells as genetically defined. *Melanoacanthomas* are seborrheic keratoses that contain numerous dendritic melanocytes, accentuated by their melanin content (fig. 1-41). Melanosomes fill the cytoplasm and the dendritic processes of melanocytes, but there is little, if any, transfer of pigment to surrounding keratinocytes (the "constipated melanocyte"), a feature nicely demonstrated with the Fontana-Masson stain (139).

Since a similar process occurs in a variety of other clinical settings, e.g., as a mucous membrane lesion, in clear cell acanthomas (see below), or as a manifestation of the hypopigmentation in sarcoidosis, it may be best to regard melanoacanthoma as a phenomenon rather than a specific clinicopathologic entity.

Differential Diagnosis. The majority of seborrheic keratoses are readily diagnosable, but there are differential diagnostic considerations, some of which are relatively trivial but a few of which are diagnostically important.

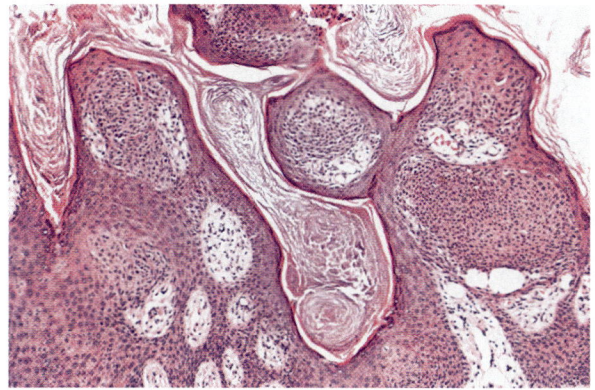
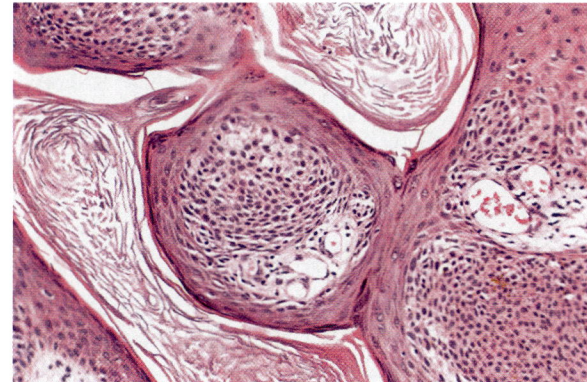

Figure 1-40

NESTED ("CLONAL") SEBORRHEIC KERATOSIS

Discrete nests of cells are present within the acanthotic papillomatous epidermis.
Left: Low-power view.
Right: High-power view of one of the cellular nests.

The lesions of acrokeratosis verruciformis of Hopf, a dominantly inherited lesion characterized by verrucous papules on distal extremities, typically show the church-spired papillomatosis that is virtually indistinguishable from the hyperkeratotic forms of seborrheic keratosis, especially stucco keratosis. The clinical history is important here, since lesions of acrokeratosis verruciformis begin at birth, during childhood, or at puberty, while seborrheic keratoses have a much later time of onset.

Flegel's disease (hyperkeratosis lenticularis perstans) consists of flat, hyperkeratotic papules that commonly arise on the lower legs and feet (116). Autosomal dominant transmission has been reported. Microscopically, these may closely resemble hyperkeratotic seborrheic keratoses. Lesions showing compact orthokeratosis, flattening of the underlying epidermis, and acanthosis or papillomatosis at their margins are reasonably characteristic of Flegel's disease. There may also be a dense lichenoid infiltrate in the upper dermis. In addition, a family history may be of some diagnostic help.

Inverted follicular keratosis resembles trichilemmoma architecturally, another lobulated, endophytic epithelial tumor that may be arranged about a central follicular structure. However, the latter tumor features clear cells (due to the presence of glycogen), a distinctly palisaded basilar layer, and a surrounding cuticular basement membrane. Although a distinction be-

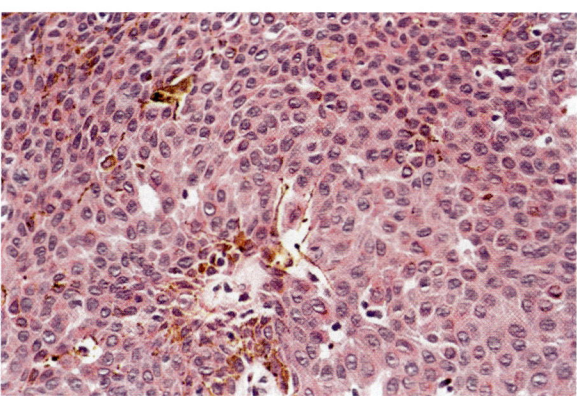

Figure 1-41

MELANOACANTHOMA

There is dense pigment within the melanocytic dendrites that does not transfer to the surrounding keratinocytes.

tween these two lesions per se is not crucial, recognition of trichilemmoma may be important because of its occurrence in the cancer-associated syndrome, Cowden's disease.

Many of the seborrheic keratosis variants resemble verrucae, particularly since the latter do not always possess easily recognizable viral inclusions or other viropathic changes. As an example of this dilemma, studies of "seborrheic keratoses" of the genital region have revealed the presence of HPV in these lesions (152). On the other hand, similar investigations of inverted follicular keratoses have generally been negative. In the absence of supporting data, it is probably best to acknowledge the possibility of verruca when faced with borderline lesions. Seborrheic keratosis-like lesions in children are more likely to be either verrucae or epidermal nevi (see section on epidermal nevus above).

Dermatopathologists frequently encounter hyperkeratotic lesions that are more squamoid than basaloid, that lack pseudohorn cysts, and that may have varying degrees of irregular papillomatosis, acanthosis, or scale-crust formation. These less than diagnostic lesions are often diagnosed as seborrheic keratoses, verrucae, or simply as "acanthomas." This would seem to be a reasonable approach in the absence of clinical data to the contrary. Of greater concern are those seborrheic keratoses that mimic premalignant or malignant epidermal tumors. Acanthotic seborrheic keratosis composed of close-set basaloid cells can resemble the occasional lesion of Bowen's disease that features minimal pleomorphism of keratinocytes. In such instances, careful evaluation of lesional keratinocytes is crucial: subtle loss of maturation, variability of nuclear size, formation of multinucleate cells, and frequent mitotic figures at all levels of the epidermis point to Bowen's disease as the correct diagnosis.

Nested seborrheic keratosis resembles other lesions typified by the formation of intraepidermal nests, or the Borst-Jadassohn phenomenon, especially benign or malignant hidroacanthoma or Bowen's disease with a nested configuration. Hidroacanthomas are basically intraepidermal poromas. The nests are composed of close-set cells with small nuclei that contain glycogen, which is not the case in seborrheic keratosis. Special staining variably demonstrates the sweat gland differentiation of these tumors. Significant pleomorphism and atypia among nested cells may indicate malignant hidroacanthoma, and Bowen's disease with nesting often shows foci of more typical, non-nested Bowen's disease in other portions of the lesion.

Another concern is differentiating irritated seborrheic keratosis from hypertrophic actinic keratosis or squamous cell carcinoma. Occasionally, a lesion with scale-crusting, squamous eddy formation, and spongiosis will also show degrees of keratinocyte atypia, mostly manifested by nuclear hyperchromasia, variation in nuclear size, and scattered mitotic figures. In such instances, distinction from squamous cell carcinoma can be problematic. In our experience, this situation most often arises in elderly individuals. These lesions require particularly close attention to architectural and cytologic details. Irritated seborrheic keratosis shows limited pleomorphism, absence of atypical mitoses, and lack of significant atypia among the lower epidermal layers and basilar keratinocytes. On the other hand, significant nuclear enlargement, atypical mitoses, acantholytic changes not associated with obvious spongiosis, and basilar keratinocyte atypia favor squamous cell carcinoma. Most often, the diagnosis can be established with confidence using these guidelines, but undoubtedly there will be occasional lesions that defy accurate identification. This often occurs in the case of shaved lesions, where the entire base cannot be evaluated. In these instances, it is probably best to identify the lesion as an irritated seborrheic keratosis with atypical features, and recommend complete removal. As further support for this conservative approach, malignancies including basal cell carcinomas, Bowen's disease, and well-differentiated squamous cell carcinomas, have been reported to arise within, or adjacent to, seborrheic keratoses (108,130,151).

Large Cell Acanthoma

Large cell acanthoma is a relatively common lesion of middle-aged to older adults. The lesions are flat to barely elevated, hyperpigmented patches with sharply demarcated borders, measuring less than 1 cm in diameter (138). One or several (135) lesions may be present, typically arising on the head and neck, trunk, and extremities.

Microscopically, large cell acanthomas show basket-woven hyperkeratosis and a prominent granular cell layer. Lesions may be papillomatous and have plump rete ridges, or may be relatively flat both at the surface and along the dermal-epidermal interface (138). A key feature is the nuclear and cytoplasmic enlargement of involved keratinocytes, which are sharply demarcated from normal adnexa (follicular infundibula and acrosyringia) and adjacent epidermis (fig. 1-42). Slightly increased basilar pigmentation may be seen.

There is some controversy regarding the histogenesis of these lesions. They are regarded by

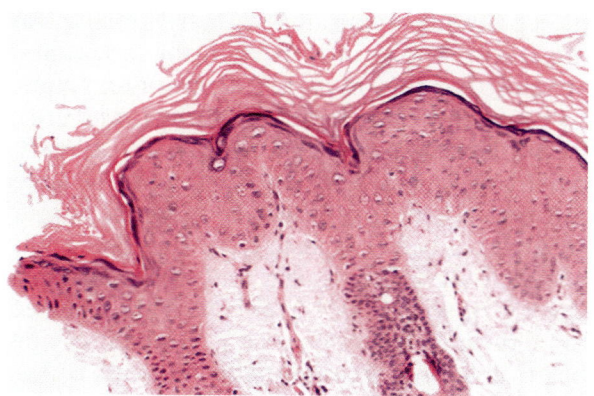

Figure 1-42

LARGE CELL ACANTHOMA

The basket-woven hyperkeratosis and keratinocytes with enlarged nuclei and increased cytoplasm are sharply demarcated from adjacent, underlying follicular epithelium.

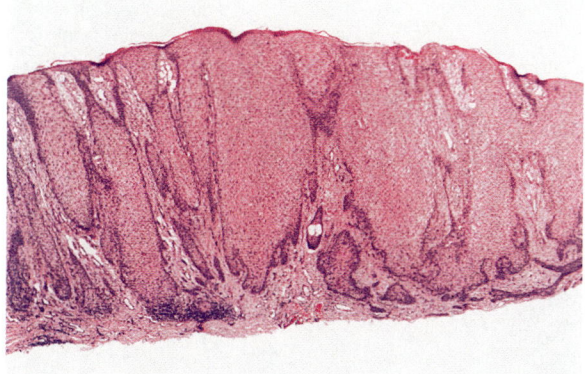

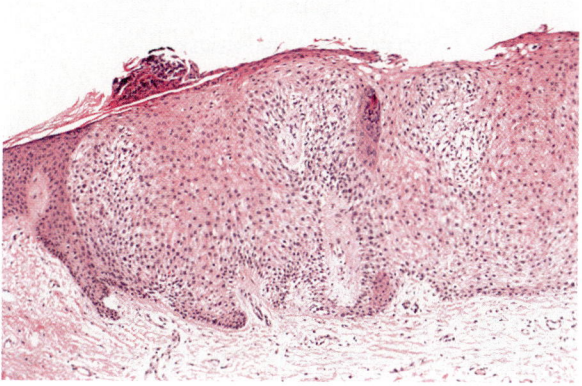

Figure 1-43

CLEAR CELL ACANTHOMA

Top: Acanthotic pale-staining epithelium with an overlying thin layer of parakeratosis.

Bottom: The lesional epithelium is sharply demarcated from adjacent uninvolved acrosyringium and normal epidermis.

some as variants of solar lentigines (136), while others believe they reflect a degree of keratinocyte atypia analogous to actinic (solar) keratosis (137). Image analysis cytometry by Argenyi et al. (102) has shown significant aneuploidy in large cell acanthoma lesions, but a lack of evidence of significant proliferation by immunohistochemistry and a mean DNA index between that of actinic keratosis and Bowen's disease. The authors concluded that the results do not resolve the classification controversy regarding large cell acanthoma.

Clear Cell Acanthoma

Clinical Features. *Clear cell acanthoma*, or *pale cell acanthoma* (an alternative and probably preferable designation), was first described by Degos (112). It manifests as a circumscribed red nodule with a peripheral scale, measuring about 1 cm in diameter. It usually arises in adults over the age of 40 years, presenting as a slowly growing, asymptomatic lesion on the leg. Other sites of involvement include the abdomen and scrotum. Clear cell acanthoma is often solitary, but multiple lesions can occur (120,149). The red, exudative surface with a collarette of scale clinically resembles pyogenic granuloma (lobular capillary hemangioma) (115).

Pathologic Findings. The acanthotic epithelium is composed of cells with pale-staining cytoplasm. Prominently pigmented melanocytic dendrites may be present, a finding indicative of the "melanoacanthoma" phenomenon (126). The configuration of the involved epidermis may be acanthotic, exophytic, or psoriasiform (fig. 1-43, top) (129). The involved epithelium is particularly sharply demarcated from adjacent normal epidermis and from adnexal epithelium, a feature of great diagnostic importance (fig. 1-43, bottom). At the surface there may be parakeratosis or erosion, and collections of neutrophils may be observed (122). The dermis features vasodilatation and a lymphocytic infiltrate of variable intensity. The keratinocytes of clear cell acanthoma contain glycogen, and show an absence or decrease of respiratory enzymes such as phosphorylase, cytochrome oxidase, and succinic dehydrogenase (150). More

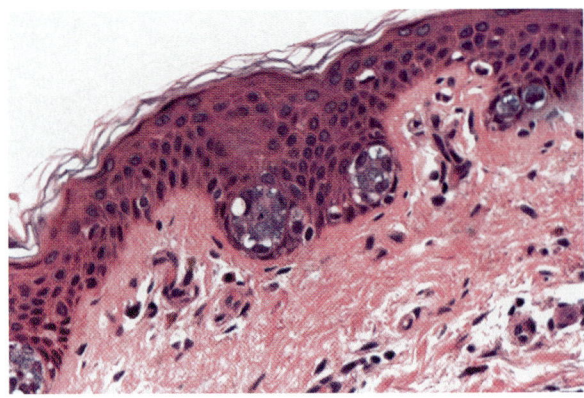

Figure 1-44
CLEAR CELL PAPULOSIS
Clear cells containing mucin are present within the basilar layer of the epidermis.

recent studies showing positive involucrin (119) and negative carcinoembryonic antigen (134) staining argue against a sweat gland origin for this tumor, while lectin binding sites are similar to those of normal epidermis (100).

Differential Diagnosis. The microscopic features of clear cell acanthoma are unique. Lesions can closely resemble psoriasis, but the sharp demarcation from the adjacent epidermis and sparing of the adnexa are not features of psoriasis. Seborrheic keratoses lack pale-appearing keratinocytes, possess pseudohorn cysts, and are often hyperkeratotic and hypergranulotic; furthermore, they do not show the sharp demarcation that is the hallmark of clear cell acanthoma. Eccrine poroma can have similar clinical features, including a location on the distal extremities, and microscopically, sharp demarcation of tumor from adjacent epidermis. However, in contrast to clear cell acanthoma, these lesions are typically composed of small, close-set, cuboidal cells.

Clear Cell Papulosis

Only a few cases of this unusual lesion have been reported, having been described among children in Taiwan (123,125,127). Whitish papules develop along the milk lines, over the abdomen and pubis; lesions of the lumbar area and buttocks have also been reported.

Microscopically, the lesions are comprised of pagetoid clear cells within the basilar layer of the epidermis, associated with hypomelanosis (fig. 1-44). The clear cells stain for mucin and are positive for AE1/AE3, carcinoembryonic antigen, epithelial membrane antigen, and gross cystic disease fluid protein-15 (124,125), thereby having the characteristics of the cells of Paget's disease and of Toker clear cells of the nipple (124). It has been suggested that these cells may be precursors of mammary and extramammary Paget's disease (127). Melanocytes are reported to be normal, although a lack of melanosomes has been noted in superficial portions of the epidermis (127).

Pseudoepitheliomatous Hyperplasia

Clinical Features. Proliferation of the epidermis, with extension deep into the dermis, can be sufficiently pronounced in *pseudoepitheliomatous hyperplasia* to raise concerns about a well-differentiated squamous cell carcinoma. Such extensive epidermal proliferation can be a manifestation of halogen ingestion (halogenoderma, including bromoderma and iododerma) or associated with infectious diseases. The prototypical infection showing pseudoepitheliomatous hyperplasia is North American blastomycosis, but virtually identical changes can occur in other deep fungal infections (South American blastomycosis, cryptococcosis, coccidioidomycosis, chromomycosis, sporotrichosis) as well as infections due to bacteria (blastomycosis-like pyoderma, atypical mycobacterial infection) or achloric alga (protothecosis). Other lesions that show pseudoepitheliomatous hyperplasia include hidradenitis suppurativa, skin adjacent to chronic ulcers, prurigo nodularis, and tumors such as Spitz's nevus, basal cell carcinoma, and granular cell tumors. Marked acanthosis and pseudoepitheliomatous hyperplasia can also accompany true squamous cell carcinomas; such changes are often observed in lesions from acral sites, such as the dorsa of the hands or lower legs.

Pathologic Findings. There is marked proliferation of the epidermis, the base of which may have irregular, jagged contours (figs. 1-45, 1-46). Horn pearls are sometimes present, and mitotic figures may be numerous. Infiltration of involved epidermis by neutrophils, eosinophils, or both, sometimes with intraepidermal microabscess formation, is a feature of

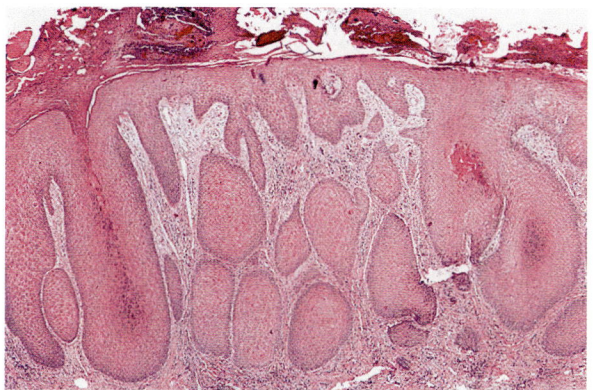

Figure 1-45

PSEUDOEPITHELIOMATOUS HYPERPLASIA ASSOCIATED WITH PRURIGO NODULARIS

This condition is associated with persistent rubbing and scratching of the skin.

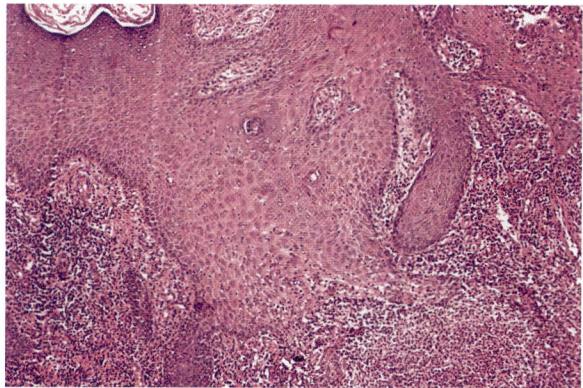

Figure 1-46

PSEUDOEPITHELIOMATOUS HYPERPLASIA ACCOMPANYING NORTH AMERICAN BLASTOMYCOSIS

Considerable acute and granulomatous inflammation accompanies this lesion.

pseudoepitheliomatous hyperplasia, and is especially common among those cases caused by infectious agents or drugs. Accompanying granulomatous inflammation also favors infection, as this finding is characteristic of North American blastomycosis and related infectious diseases.

Differential Diagnosis. The presence of unexplained pseudoepitheliomatous hyperplasia should prompt a search for associated tumors, such as granular cell tumor. True squamous cell carcinomas accompanied by pseudoepitheliomatous change can easily be missed, especially in a superficial shave biopsy. Careful search may reveal narrow cords of atypical keratinocytes, sometimes arising at the angle of intersection of the proliferative epidermis and acanthotic follicular epithelium. Verrucous carcinoma can be particularly difficult to distinguish from pseudoepitheliomatous hyperplasia, but the former is suspected when the lesion is exophytic as well as endophytic, contains deeply extending crypts filled with neutrophils and keratinous debris, and shows bulbous "pushing" deep margins.

PREMALIGNANT AND MALIGNANT EPIDERMAL TUMORS

Actinic Keratosis

Clinical Features. *Actinic keratosis* (*solar keratosis*) is a common lesion that occurs in any chronically sun-exposed site, including the head and neck, forearms, and dorsa of the hands. Lesions from the lower legs have also been identified with increasing frequency. Lesions are often multiple, presenting as flat to elevated keratotic areas that may be flesh-colored, pigmented, or erythematous. They are relatively discrete, but may have ill-defined borders and can coalesce to form large patches, particularly in severely sun-damaged individuals. A spreading, pigmented type ranges from 1 to 2 cm in diameter. Cutaneous horn formation is common.

These keratoses most frequently occur in fair complected individuals who have had considerable outdoor exposure. Many of these patients also present with prominent elastotic changes, telangiectases, and solar lentigines. Although clearly a condition of middle-aged to older adults, similar keratoses occur in young individuals who suffer from the recessively inherited "experiment of nature," xeroderma pigmentosum. In a related condition, keratoses arise in patients receiving PUVA (psoralen-ultraviolet A) therapy, typically for psoriasis; these are termed *PUVA keratoses*. Similar lesions occur in individuals who have been exposed to inorganic, pentavalent arsenic in the form of contaminated well water or as constituents of old therapies such as Fowler's solution or "asiatic pills." Arsenical keratosis can develop 6 years or more following exposure, and not only in sun-exposed sites but also in locations such as the palms and soles, trunk, and proximal extremities.

Although the term actinic, or solar, keratosis may imply something less than a malignant process, it has been recognized for some time that these lesions represent intraepidermal malignancies. Drawing an analogy to similar lesions of the uterine cervix, some authors have suggested renaming these lesions "solar keratotic intraepidermal squamous cell carcinoma" (169). Recent basic studies have shed some light on the relationship of actinic keratosis to squamous cell carcinomas. Actinic keratosis tends to show aberrant expression of p53 protein (244), is positive for proliferating cell nuclear antigen (PCNA) (206), and has intermediate levels of Ki-67 expressed as growth fraction (GF) when compared to seborrheic keratosis (low GF) and squamous cell carcinoma (high GF) (210). These features show that actinic keratosis represents a stage of neoplastic transformation. On the other hand, actinic keratosis is differentiated from squamous cell carcinoma by negative or weak staining for the oncoprotein c-erb-2 (155), positive cyclin E expression (161), and more frequent loss of heterozygosity (200). The latter studies suggest that, despite a close morphologic association, distinct changes in gene expression occur with progression to invasive squamous cell carcinoma.

Estimates of the rate of progression of actinic keratosis to invasive squamous cell carcinoma range from 0.1 to 10.0 percent. Differences in study design probably account for much of the variability in these figures, but a realistic estimate of lifetime risk is 6 to 10 percent (185,238). Clinical experience and available statistics suggest that the risk of metastasis of invasive squamous cell carcinoma arising from actinically damaged skin is low, ranging from 0.5 to 3.0 percent (207,216). Nevertheless, such metastases are well documented (182), and in one study of metastatic cutaneous squamous cell carcinomas, changes of actinic keratosis were present in the original lesion in 44 percent of cases (174).

Pathologic Findings. Actinic keratosis shows basilar keratinocyte atypia, which first manifests as "crowding" of basal keratinocytes and variability in nuclear size. The adnexal epithelium is initially spared, as are the more superficial portions of the epidermis. The apparent normal maturation of the surface epidermis in many actinic keratoses is explained by the contribution

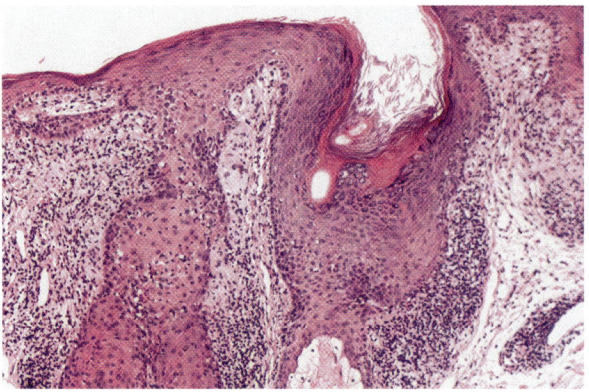

Figure 1-47

ACTINIC KERATOSIS

This lesion shows basilar keratinocyte atypia, with early extension along superficial portions of the follicular units. The surface epidermis appears to be uninvolved at this point.

to the epidermis of normal keratinocytes from adjacent, uninvolved adnexal structures, and this epithelium forms an "umbrella" over the atypical basilar keratinocytes (213). Atypical basilar keratinocytes, however, may proliferate along the basilar layer of adnexal epithelium (fig. 1-47). With progression, more and more of the epidermis and adnexal epithelium take on an atypical appearance, with marked nuclear pleomorphism, formation of multinucleated cells, and mitotic figures, some of which are atypical in configuration. Full thickness epithelial atypia can develop, resulting in an appearance called *bowenoid actinic keratosis* (fig. 1-48) (see Differential Diagnosis and section on Bowen's disease below). Basilar pigmentation can be increased (164,195), sometimes with exaggerated "budding" of the rete ridges in the manner of lentigo, changes associated with the *spreading, pigmented actinic keratosis*. The involved epidermis may be atrophic, or markedly thickened and hypertrophic. *Hypertrophic actinic keratosis* may simply represent an acanthotic version of conventional actinic keratosis, with prominent budding of atypical basilar epithelium, or may feature broad acanthosis comprised of cells with distinctly eosinophilic cytoplasm (fig. 1-49).

The parakeratosis overlying such lesions is often interrupted by columns of blue-staining keratin arising from the relatively spared intraepidermal portions of sweat ducts; this change is particularly common in hypertrophic lesions on

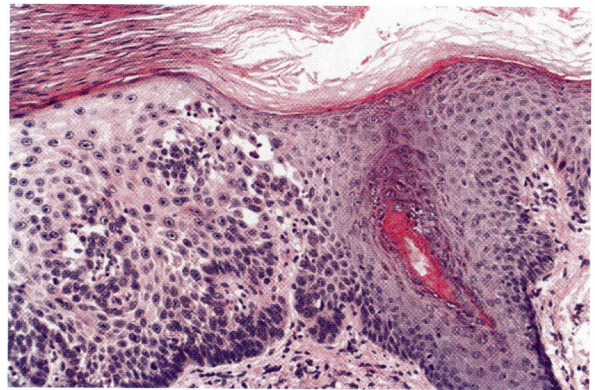

Figure 1-48

BOWENOID ACTINIC KERATOSIS

On the left is full-thickness epithelial atypia. The follicle to the right is still largely uninvolved.

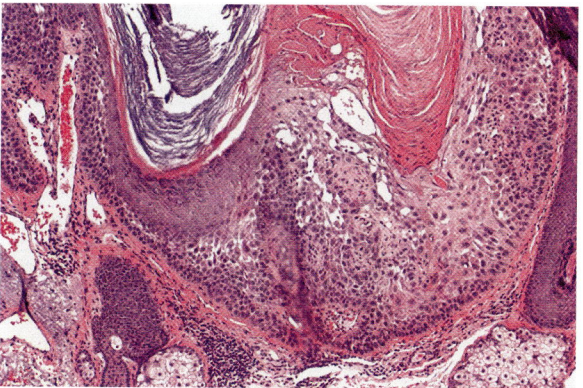

Figure 1-49

HYPERTROPHIC ACTINIC KERATOSIS

The epidermis is thickened by a proliferation of atypical keratinocytes with overlying hyperkeratosis.

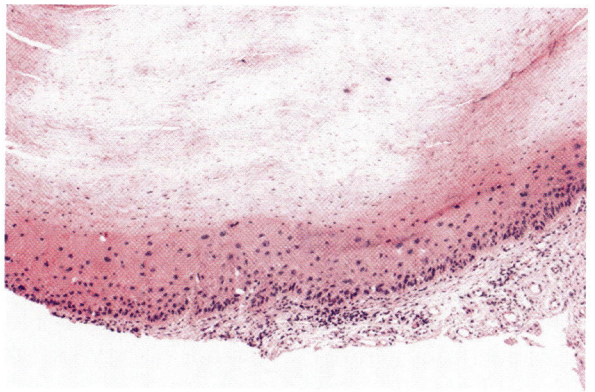

Figure 1-50

ACTINIC KERATOSIS WITH CUTANEOUS HORN FORMATION

Cytologic atypia may be subtle. Clues to the diagnosis include pronounced cytoplasmic eosinophilia and nuclear crowding among keratinocytes.

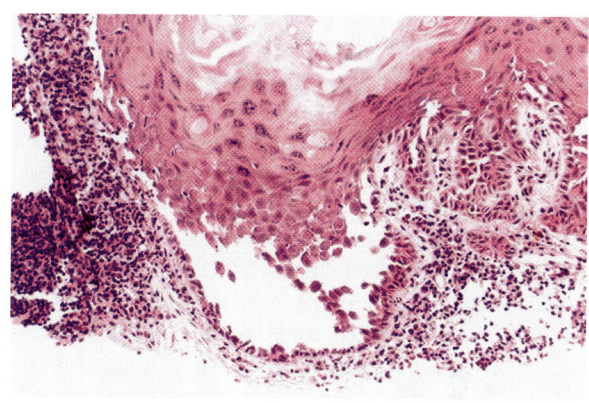

Figure 1-51

ACANTHOLYTIC ACTINIC KERATOSIS

There is dyshesion among the atypical lesional keratinocytes.

the dorsa of the hands. In areas subjected to trauma or irritation, such as forearms, dorsa of hands, and lower legs, bland hyperkeratosis, acanthosis, or pseudoepitheliomatous hyperplasia may predominate; then, careful inspection of the angles formed by follicular units and adjacent epidermis may show small foci of atypical basilar budding, allowing a diagnosis of actinic keratosis with secondary changes. Actinic keratosis with cutaneous horn formation often displays surprisingly bland epithelium. Pronounced cytoplasmic eosinophilia and nuclear crowding are clues to the correct diagnosis (fig. 1-50).

Suprabasilar acantholysis is common in actinic keratosis (fig. 1-51), and at times mimics other, nonpremalignant acantholytic disorders (168). These lesions can give rise to acantholytic (pseudoglandular) squamous cell carcinomas (see below).

Actinic keratosis, and lesions of actinic cheilitis, have been reported to have epidermolytic changes of the superficial epidermis (154,252). Varying degrees of inflammation are associated with actinic keratosis, with a predominance of lymphocytes and, at times, a plasmacytic component. Actinic keratosis with vacuolar degeneration of the basilar layer and band-like infiltrates that

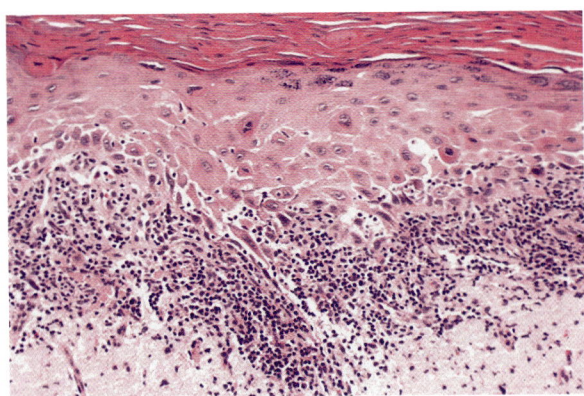

Figure 1-52
LICHENOID ACTINIC KERATOSIS
The changes of actinic keratosis are combined with vacuolar degeneration of the basilar layer and a band-like infiltrate.

may obscure the dermal-epidermal interface is termed *lichenoid actinic keratosis* (fig. 1-52) (248). Such changes are not confined to hypertrophic actinic keratoses, as has been implied in the past.

Arsenical keratosis shows varying degrees of hyperkeratosis, papillomatosis, and acanthosis. Cytologic atypia among keratinocytes may be virtually absent, but there may also be degrees of atypia comparable to those in actinic keratosis or Bowen's disease (266). The configuration of PUVA keratosis is similar, consisting of hyperkeratosis with focal parakeratosis, papillomatosis, and acanthosis. Atypia among keratinocytes is present in only about half of cases and tends to be mild, consisting of nuclear hyperchromasia and variability of nuclear size (253).

Dermal invasion indicates transition to squamous cell carcinoma, and may require examination of multiple levels for confirmation. It should be realized, however, that small groups of keratinocytes confined to the papillary dermis may simply represent cross-sections of budding basilar epithelium, as can be demonstrated with leveling, and such lesions may best be labeled actinic keratosis. Evolution to invasive squamous cell carcinoma often occurs without the development of full-thickness epithelial atypia (i.e., formation of a bowenoid actinic keratosis).

Differential Diagnosis. At times, actinic keratosis must be distinguished from a variety of other conditions. These include acantholytic dermatoses such as Darier's disease and related disorders, benign lichenoid keratosis and, rarely, other interface dermatoses such as lupus erythematosus, irritated seborrheic keratosis (basosquamous acanthoma), solar lentigo (including large cell acanthoma) and lentigo maligna, superficial basal cell carcinoma, and porokeratosis.

A key to the recognition of actinic keratosis is the identification of keratinocyte atypia that most often involves the lower portions of the epidermis and occurs in a background of solar elastosis. This feature aids in distinguishing actinic keratosis from other acantholytic dermatoses that show either no keratinocyte atypia (e.g., some examples of Grover's disease [transient acantholytic dermatosis] or nondyskeratotic forms of acantholytic acanthoma) or atypia concentrated in superficial rather than deep portions of the epidermis. The latter feature is associated with corps rond and grain formation, as would be the case, for example, in lesions of Darier's disease or warty dyskeratoma.

Benign lichenoid keratosis can closely mimic actinic keratosis: the mild basilar keratinocyte atypia of the former sometimes makes differentiation from lichenoid actinic keratosis difficult. The basilar atypia in benign lichenoid keratosis is usually confined to areas of most intense inflammation. Evidence of origin in a lentigo or seborrheic keratosis may be observed. Lichenoid actinic keratosis usually shows unequivocal basilar atypia, often extending beyond foci of band-like inflammation, and suprabasilar acantholysis may be present.

Forms of lupus erythematosus (LE) have been included in the differential diagnosis of actinic keratosis, particularly the atrophic variety. We have not generally found this to be a difficult diagnostic problem, due to the lack of keratinocyte atypia in most examples of LE and the presence of other features not generally found in actinic keratosis: orthokeratosis with follicular plugging, distinctive thickening of the basement membrane zone, dermal mucin deposition, and periadnexal inflammation. The difficulties in distinguishing hypertrophic actinic keratosis from some irritated seborrheic keratoses (basosquamous acanthomas), especially those that occur in elderly individuals (see differential diagnosis of seborrheic keratosis above), have been discussed. Careful attention to cytologic detail is important, particularly with regard to basilar keratinocyte atypia, the presence of which favors hypertrophic actinic keratosis. Occasional cases defy accurate categorization, and management appropriate for actinic keratosis or superficial squamous cell carcinoma may be warranted.

Large cell acanthoma is a controversial lesion that some consider to be a variant of actinic keratosis. Lesions with sharply demarcated borders, enlarged keratinocyte nuclei and increased cytoplasm, flattening of the rete ridge pattern, and basket-woven hyperkeratosis and hypergranulosis are probably best classified as large cell acanthomas.

Traditional solar lentigo and even lentigo maligna may be associated with degrees of keratinocyte atypia and, similarly, actinic keratosis may be accompanied by lentiginous changes and junctional melanocytic hyperplasia. In such circumstances, a judgment must be made regarding which abnormal cell type predominates. This can sometimes be aided by immunohistochemical staining for cytokeratins, S-100 protein, Melan-A, or tyrosinase. The proliferation of atypical melanocytes along the outer root sheaths of hair follicles favors lentigo maligna. Clinical data is helpful, although a spreading pigmented actinic keratosis may easily be confused with lentigo maligna.

Exaggerated or broad-based basilar budding of actinic keratosis can occasionally be difficult to distinguish from superficial basal cell carcinoma. Islands of the latter tend to show exaggerated peripheral palisading of nuclei or cleft-like spaces separating the cells from the underlying dermis, but these changes are not always obvious. Immunohistochemical staining for BerEP4 (249) or for the gene product of bcl-2 (214) have been reported to be helpful in this regard; both markers are positive in superficial basal cell carcinomas and negative in actinic keratosis.

Differentiating actinic keratosis from forms of porokeratosis can be a challenge, as the cornoid lamella, the parakeratotic column that is the diagnostic hallmark for porokeratosis (see below), can occur in actinic keratosis, and degrees of keratinocyte atypia are observed in porokeratosis. Keratinocyte atypia in porokeratosis, however, is concentrated at the base of cornoid lamellae (representing an abnormal clone of keratinocytes), while the atypia in actinic keratosis tends to be more radially extensive.

Porokeratosis

Clinical Features. *Porokeratosis* is traditionally described as a genodermatosis with autosomal dominant inheritance, but it clearly occurs sporadically as well. There are several clinical types, including the plaque type (*porokeratosis of Mibelli*), disseminated (*disseminated superficial actinic porokeratosis* [DSAP]), *linear porokeratosis, porokeratosis palmaris, plantaris et disseminata,* and *punctate porokeratosis* confined to the palms and soles. There is considerable clinical overlap among some of these conditions, particularly the plaque and disseminated types, and sometimes the classifications are arbitrary. Lesions tend to be keratotic, with atrophic centers and raised, keratotic or "thread-like" borders; the latter represents the cornoid lamella, the clinical and histopathologic hallmark of these lesions. They occur in virtually any location, although central face and genital involvement are rare. The development of squamous cell carcinomas in these lesions has been reported on numerous occasions, particularly in lesions of the disseminated and Mibelli types. This is consistent with the notion that a clone of abnormal keratinocytes is responsible for the production of the cornoid lamella. Disease associations are uncommon, but development of lesions has followed hemodialysis and renal transplantation (198) as well as various forms of ultraviolet or radiation exposure.

Pathologic Findings. Biopsies should incorporate the edges of the lesions, where the diagnostic features are found. There are one or more keratin-filled epidermal invaginations featuring parakeratotic columns, the cornoid lamella. The underlying epidermis features an absent granular layer and irregularly distributed and focally vacuolated keratinocytes with pyknotic nuclei.

The cornoid lamella is prominent in the plaque type of porokeratosis, but may be small and inconspicuous in DSAP, seen only as a slight focal condensation of horny material and a few parakeratotic nuclei (fig. 1-53). The parakeratotic column migrates peripherally, and often enters the epidermis at an angle that points away from the center of the lesion (233). If initial sectioning occurs tangentially, the cornoid

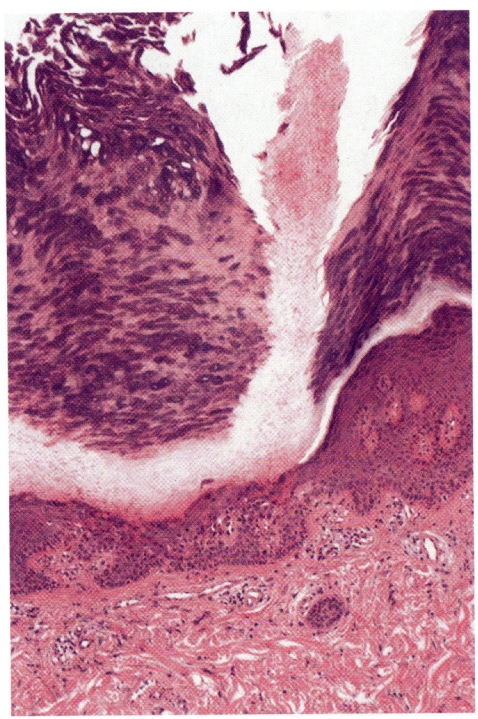

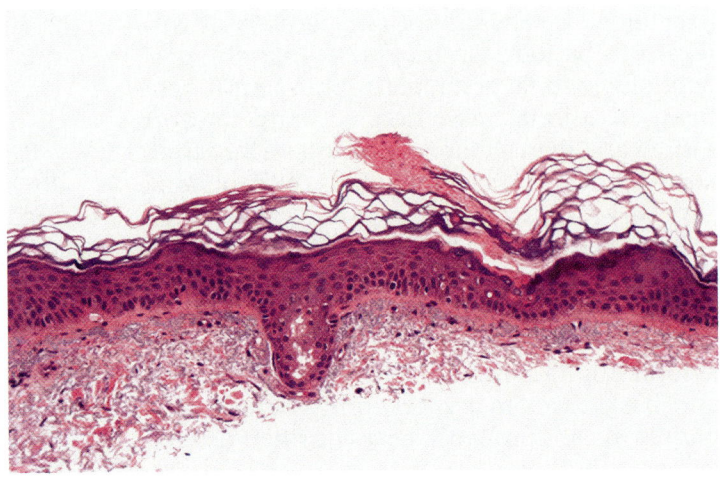

Figure 1-53

POROKERATOSIS

Left: A prominent cornoid lamella is seen in the plaque type porokeratosis (Mibelli).

Above: A somewhat more subtle cornoid lamella is seen in disseminated superficial actinic porokeratosis. The underlying keratinocytes in both lesions are vacuolated and have pyknotic nuclei.

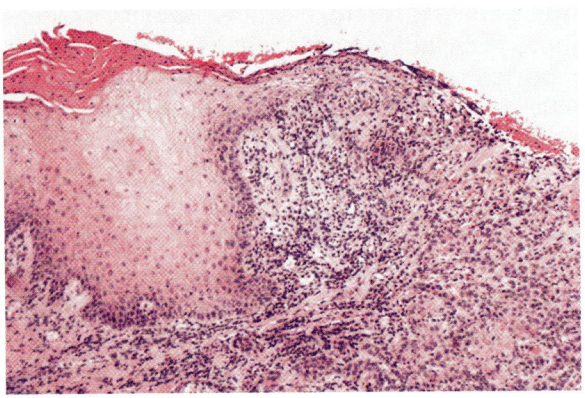

Figure 1-54

SQUAMOUS CELL CARCINOMA IN POROKERATOSIS

An ulcerated, well-differentiated squamous cell carcinoma has developed in a lesion of porokeratosis.

lamella may be cut en face, and instead of a parakeratotic column there may be a linear stretch of parakeratosis along the surface of the lesion. In such a case, further sectioning deeper into the specimen will generally show the typical epidermal invagination and columnar arrangement of the cornoid lamella. Squamous cell carcinomas may arise from the altered epidermis at the base of cornoid lamellae (fig. 1-54).

The epidermis in the midportion of the lesion is often thinned but may be normal in appearance or acanthotic. A loosely organized lymphocytic infiltrate is often present in the underlying dermis, and at times there may be a distinctly band-like infiltrate that partly obscures the dermal-epidermal interface, giving the lesion a lichenoid appearance. The latter changes have been observed in the Mibelli, disseminated, and linear types.

Differential Diagnosis. The cornoid lamella is characteristic of porokeratosis, but similar structures can be observed in actinic keratosis and verrucae (254). In such instances, finding significant basilar keratinocyte atypia not confined to the parakeratotic column (in actinic keratosis) or the presence of viral inclusions (in verrucae) is diagnostically important. The porokeratotic eccrine ostial and dermal duct nevus can closely mimic porokeratosis, especially the linear type, but the parakeratotic columns in the former are associated with dilated eccrine ducts (153).

Bowen's Disease
(Squamous Cell Carcinoma In Situ)

Clinical Features. *Bowen's disease* is the eponym commonly applied to *squamous cell carcinoma in situ* when it involves the skin. It typically

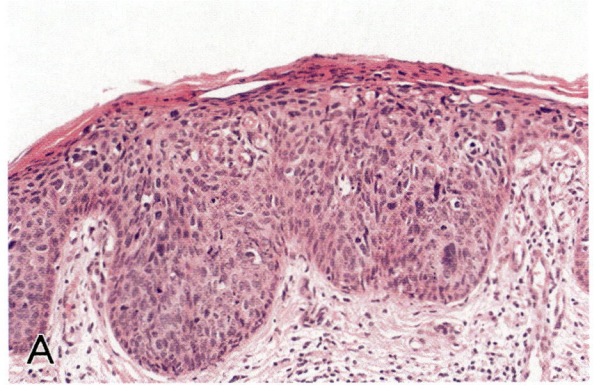
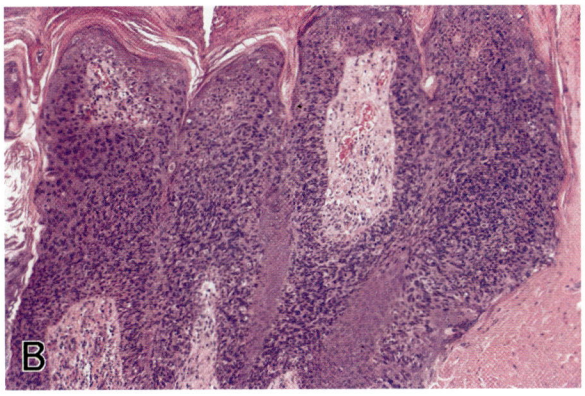
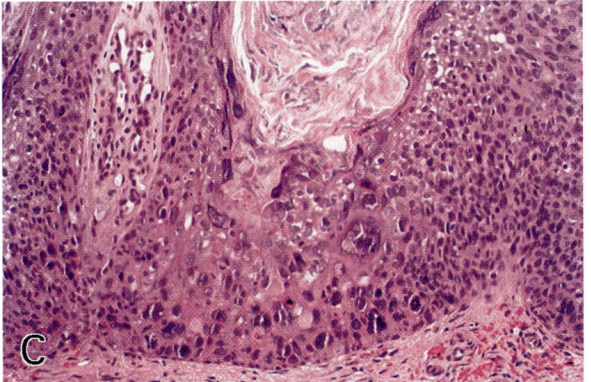

Figure 1-55

BOWEN'S DISEASE

A: A lesion with moderate acanthosis.
B: A more acanthotic example.
C: Full-thickness atypia with loss of normal epidermal maturation.

presents as a sharply marginated, erythematous, scaly or verrucous plaque with varying amounts of pigment, and can occur anywhere on the cutaneous surface, in both sun-exposed and sun-protected sites. Ultraviolet exposure plays a role in the former, but other factors may also be responsible, particularly exposure to inorganic arsenic and certain HPV types. The latter include HPV types 16 and 18 (also responsible for lesions of bowenoid papulosis, see below) and HPV 5, implicated in the lesions that occur in the genetically determined disorder, epidermodysplasia verruciformis. About 3 to 5 percent of lesions become invasive squamous cell carcinomas. Once invasive, there is a risk of metastasis, although figures on the degree of risk vary from 13 to 37 percent. An association with internal malignancy had been supported by some authors, but the prevailing opinion is that there is not an increased association with internal malignancy. There may be some increase in risk when lesions occur in nonsun-exposed sites or are associated with inorganic arsenic exposure.

Pathologic Findings. The lesions of Bowen's disease are variably hyperkeratotic and parakeratotic. There is often acanthosis that may be quite pronounced, although the epidermis, at times, is virtually normal in thickness. There is full-thickness loss of maturation of keratinocytes, with cells showing large, hyperchromatic nuclei. Multinucleated epithelial cells and mitotic figures are identified throughout the epidermis, producing what has been termed a "windblown" appearance (fig. 1-55). Individual cell keratinization and apoptosis are frequently observed. Scattered vacuolated cells may be present, giving these lesions a pagetoid configuration (fig. 1-56). Occasionally, sharply demarcated nests of atypical cells are identified within the epidermis, an example of the Borst-Jadassohn phenomenon (fig. 1-57). Skip areas may occur, characterized by short, uninvolved stretches of epidermis within the confines of the lesion. Areas of atypia confined to basilar layers, resembling actinic keratosis, may be present and merge with foci of full-thickness atypia. Lesions with these features usually occur in sun-exposed sites

Nonmelanocytic Tumors of the Skin

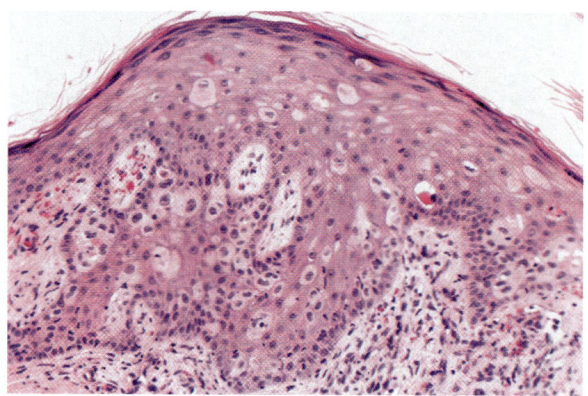

Figure 1-56
PAGETOID BOWEN'S DISEASE
Widely scattered atypical cells are in all layers of the epidermis.

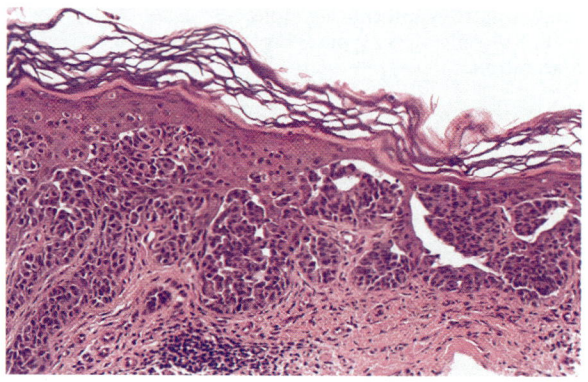

Figure 1-57
NESTED BOWEN'S DISEASE
This is an example of the Borst-Jadassohn phenomenon. Some of these cases may have been labeled "intraepidermal epithelioma" in the past.

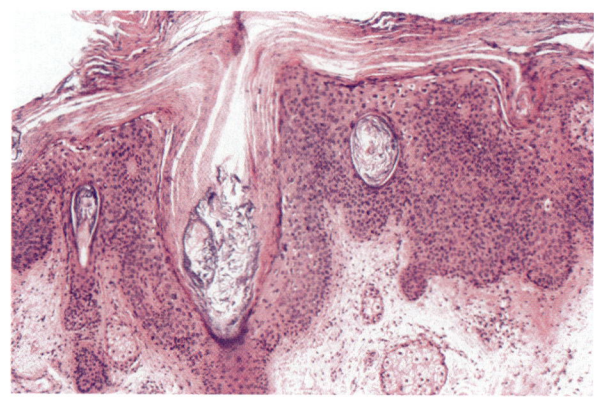

Figure 1-58
BOWEN'S DISEASE
Follicular involvement is evident.

and are sometimes termed *bowenoid actinic keratosis*. It is not clear whether the biologic behavior of these lesions (in terms of likelihood of invasion or metastasis) differs from that of Bowen's disease elsewhere. There is frequent involvement of follicular epithelium, extending to the level of the sebaceous duct (fig. 1-58). Sweat duct involvement is less common but has been reported. This adnexal involvement raises important therapeutic issues, since superficially destructive methods may miss deep foci of tumor within adnexa.

Invasive carcinoma arising from Bowen's disease often has a distinctive appearance. It consists of basaloid tumor islands, each of which shows the same type of pleomorphism and lack of organization observed in the in situ portions of the lesion (fig. 1-59). These tumor islands superficially resemblance basal cell carcinoma but lack the distinct peripheral palisading and generally do not display the clefting artifact that separates tumor from stroma in basal cell carcinoma. In addition, invasive tumors arising from Bowen's disease may have the appearance of adnexal carcinomas, and lesions showing sebaceous (176,193) or sweat gland (197,237) differentiation have been reported.

Differential Diagnosis. Lesions of Bowen's disease sometimes resemble seborrheic keratosis. Both lesions can have a plaque-like configuration and horn cysts. Some cases of Bowen's disease have closely crowded basaloid cells with limited pleomorphism (fig. 1-60), while the irritated seborrheic keratosis (basosquamous acanthoma), with its squamous eddies and loss of cohesion of keratinocytes, can give the impression of atypia (see differential diagnosis of seborrheic keratosis above). Lesions with overlapping features of Bowen's disease and seborrheic keratosis do occur, particularly in elderly patients, and cases of Bowen's disease deriving from seborrheic keratoses have been reported (162,209,217,265).

Bowen's disease with invasive carcinoma can show adnexal differentiation, raising the possibility of sebaceous or, less commonly, sweat gland carcinoma. The finding of typical bowenoid changes in the overlying epidermis would obviously be helpful in identifying the true source of

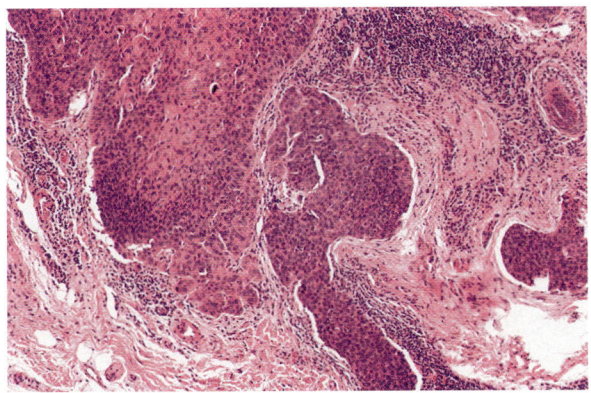

Figure 1-59

BOWEN'S DISEASE WITH INVASIVE SQUAMOUS CELL CARCINOMA

Invasive tumor islands display the same degree of pleomorphism and disorganization.

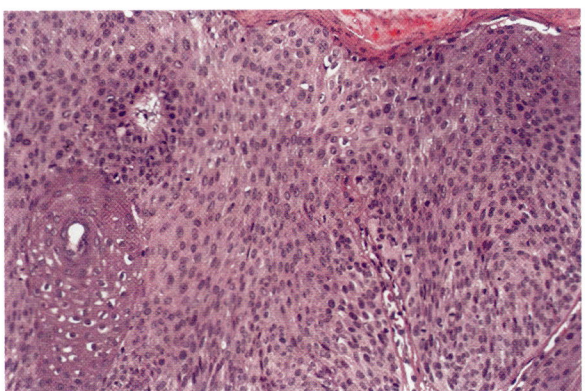

Figure 1-60

BOWEN'S DISEASE

This lesion shows minimal pleomorphism.

the tumor. It is still an open question, however, as to whether bowenoid squamous cell carcinoma with adnexal differentiation behaves any differently from primary sebaceous or sweat gland carcinoma.

Bowen's disease with pagetoid features can resemble other tumors that have similar changes, including pagetoid melanoma and pagetoid reticulosis (or cutaneous T-cell lymphoma with marked epidermotropism) as well as mammary and extramammary Paget's disease. The recognition of substantial pleomorphism and dyskeratosis among keratinocytes is the key to recognizing Bowen's disease. Positive staining of vacuolated cells for mucin (mucicarmine, Alcian blue, colloidal iron, aldehyde fuchsin) supports a diagnosis of Paget's or extramammary Paget's disease. Differential immunohistochemical staining can be of great help in difficult cases, since Paget's cells are carcinoembryonic antigen and low molecular weight cytokeratin positive; melanoma cells are S-100 protein, HMB45, and tyrosinase positive; and pagetoid reticulosis/T-cell lymphoma cells are positive for lymphocyte markers. Bowen's disease cells tend to stain for higher molecular weight cytokeratins, although overlap with Paget's disease does exist, and examples of pagetoid Bowen's disease cells staining for cytokeratin 7 (usually considered a marker for Paget's disease) have been reported (263).

The presence of discrete nests of cells within the epidermis raises the issue of a controversial entity called intraepidermal epithelioma. It appears that most authors now consider this to be a pattern of epidermal change that can occur in a variety of conditions, rather than a distinct clinicopathologic entity. In addition to Bowen's disease, intraepidermal nesting can be observed in "clonal" seborrheic keratosis, the variant of intraepidermal poroma known as hidroacanthoma simplex, some melanocytic nevi, basal cell carcinoma, Merkel cell carcinoma, epidermotropic metastasis, and malignant hidroacanthoma, an intraepidermal porocarcinoma. The latter lesion may have sufficient cytologic atypia to be confused with Bowen's disease with intraepidermal nesting, but it can be distinguished immunohistochemically from Bowen's disease because of its reactivity for S-100 protein and carcinoembryonic antigen.

Erythroplasia of Queyrat

Clinical Features. *Erythroplasia of Queyrat* is squamous cell carcinoma in situ that develops on the glans penis, corona, inner prepuce, or urethral meatus in uncircumcised or late circumcised men. Typically, these lesions present as red, velvety plaques. Similar lesions have been reported in the vulva and oral or ocular mucosa. In one study, invasion occurred in as many as 30 percent of cases, with metastases in 20 percent of invasive cases (186). These figures are probably somewhat elevated since the study was performed at a referral center for

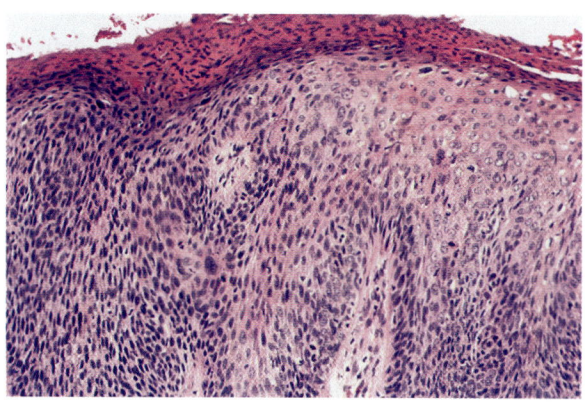

Figure 1-61

ERYTHROPLASIA OF QUEYRAT

The configuration of the lesion is virtually identical to that of Bowen's disease.

pathology. Recent studies indicate a relationship with oncogenic HPV types, including type 16 (215). Co-infection with oncogenic HPV types and HPV type 8 (associated with the precancerous condition epidermodysplasia verruciformis) has been reported (261).

Pathologic Findings. Erythroplasia of Queyrat is almost microscopically identical to Bowen's disease, with perhaps fewer dyskeratotic or multinucleated cells (186) and, due to its mucosal location, without significant appendageal involvement (fig. 1-61). Inflammation may be pronounced, often with a high percentage of plasma cells.

Differential Diagnosis. Erythroplasia clinically resemblances a benign condition known as Zoon's plasmacellular balanitis. These conditions can be easily distinguished on biopsy, although there has been a case of Zoon's balanitis that eventually showed features of erythroplasia of Queyrat (172).

Bowenoid Papulosis

Clinical Features. For a number of years, it has been recognized that solitary or multiple, pigmented, flat-topped papules to small plaques arise in the anogenital region, with clinical features reminiscent of nevi, seborrheic keratosis, or flat verrucae but with atypical histopathologic changes reminiscent of squamous cell carcinoma in situ. Clinical experience indicated that these lesions would often respond to conservative therapies and would even spontaneously regress (175). The term *bowenoid papulosis* was applied to such lesions (256,257). Unfortunately, the microscopic findings often prompted aggressive and sometimes mutilating surgery. Since then, numerous articles have been published concerning bowenoid papulosis and its relationship to Bowen's disease and invasive squamous cell carcinoma.

Although predominantly a lesion of the anogenital region, identical lesions occur in other locations, including the face (158). Young people are predominantly involved, with a marked decline in incidence over the age of 40 years. Early suspicions that the lesion was related to HPV infection have been confirmed, and an association with oncogenic HPV types, especially 16 and 18, has been repeatedly demonstrated (191). These same HPV types have been linked to Bowen's disease and cervical cancer (163,191,224).

Since the initial descriptions of bowenoid papulosis, cases transitioning to frank squamous cell carcinoma in situ and invasive squamous cell carcinoma occasionally have been reported (190,230). There has been a trend towards incorporating bowenoid papulosis into the concept of vulvar intraepithelial neoplasia (VIN) and its male equivalent, penile intraepithelial neoplasia (PIN). Nevertheless, recent studies have indicated some differences between bowenoid papulosis and Bowen's disease, including significant nuclear morphometric differences among keratinocyte nuclei (225) and a much lower incidence of invasive carcinoma in bowenoid papulosis (173). The lessons from all of these studies are that bowenoid papulosis: 1) can be associated with invasive cancer, and therefore requires careful management and diligent followup; 2) is a diagnosis that requires clinicopathologic correlation; 3) should be diagnosed with caution in individuals over the age of 40 years; and 4) normally responds to conservative therapies, and overly aggressive surgery should generally be avoided.

Pathologic Findings. The lesions of bowenoid papulosis show full-thickness epithelial atypia, but this manifests as widely scattered atypical keratinocytes on a background of orderly epithelial maturation. Scattered dyskeratotic cells and numerous same-stage mitotic figures are observed (fig. 1-62). Large keratohyaline granules and plump, rounded, pyknotic

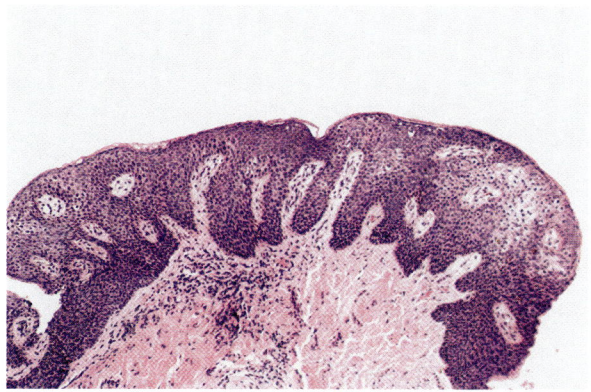 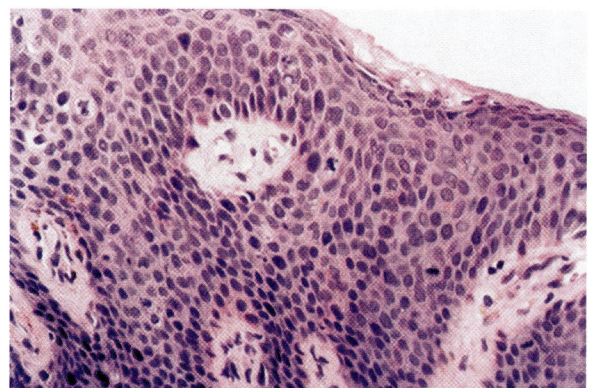

Figure 1-62

BOWENOID PAPULOSIS

Left: Low-power view of a papular lesion. Note the acanthosis and focal band-like dermal infiltrate.
Right: High-power view shows scattered dyskeratotic cells and mitotic figures.

parakeratotic nuclei are suggestive of the lesion's HPV origins.

Differential Diagnosis. In contrast to typical Bowen's disease, follicular infundibula are usually spared, while intraepidermal portions of eccrine sweat ducts tend to be involved (227). Band-like lymphoplasmacytic infiltrates are often present. Some of these findings are also observed following podophyllin therapy for genital warts, but epithelial changes resulting from this form of therapy are markedly diminished 72 hours after application (255).

Squamous Cell Carcinoma

Clinical Features. *Squamous cell carcinoma* is a common cutaneous malignancy, second only to basal cell carcinoma in frequency, that often presents as an elevated, indurated lesion with varying degrees of ulceration and crusting. These tumors sometimes resemble basal cell carcinoma. Squamous cell carcinoma can arise from any cutaneous site, but is most common in actinically damaged skin. It also frequently occurs in mucocutaneous sites, where predisposing factors include ultraviolet light (the lips) or HPV infection (the genitalia). Squamous cell carcinomas also arise in burn scars, stasis ulcers, sinus tracts, or occasionally, in conditions characterized by chronic inflammation or scarring, such as lupus erythematosus, lichen planus (particularly in the oral mucosa), or dystrophic forms of epidermolysis bullosa. Although usually a disease of adults, rare cases occur at an early age, in patients with conditions such as the recessively inherited xeroderma pigmentosum. Squamous cell carcinoma occurs with increased frequency in immunocompromised individuals (e.g., in renal transplant patients), and in this setting it may display greater biologic aggressiveness. Cutaneous metastasis from squamous cell carcinomas arising in other tissues also occurs; the oral mucous membrane is a common source of these metastatic cancers.

The frequency of metastasis of cutaneous squamous cell carcinoma varies, depending in part upon the mode of origin. As indicated in the section on actinic keratosis above, the metastatic rate for squamous cell carcinoma arising from actinically damaged skin is low, ranging from 0.5 percent to 3.0 percent. There is evidence for greater biologic aggressiveness among acantholytic (pseudoglandular) squamous cell carcinomas, which typically arise in actinically damaged skin. The incidence is also higher for lesions arising from the lip, or from burn scars, areas of radiation injury, or sinus tracts.

Pathologic Findings. The tumors consist of varying sized masses of epithelial cells with nuclear pleomorphism, individual cell keratinization, and atypical mitotic figures (fig. 1-63). Horn pearls are present, characterized by small aggregates of keratinocytes in concentric arrangements with varying degrees of keratinization at their centers (fig. 1-64). Loss of cohesion of keratinocytes can create a pseudoglandular appearance: tumor islands

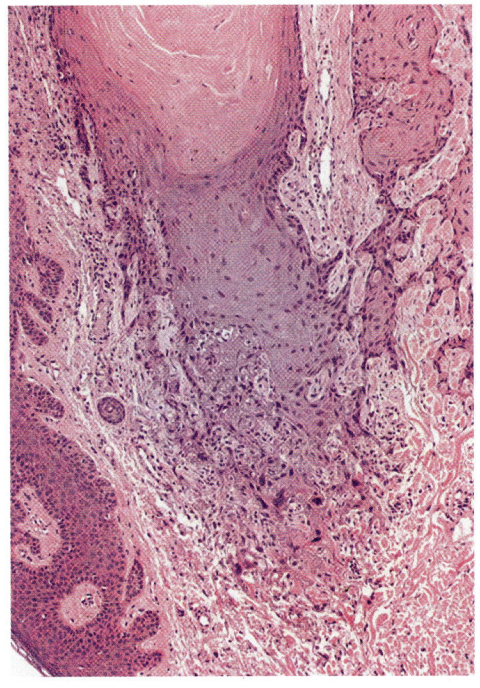
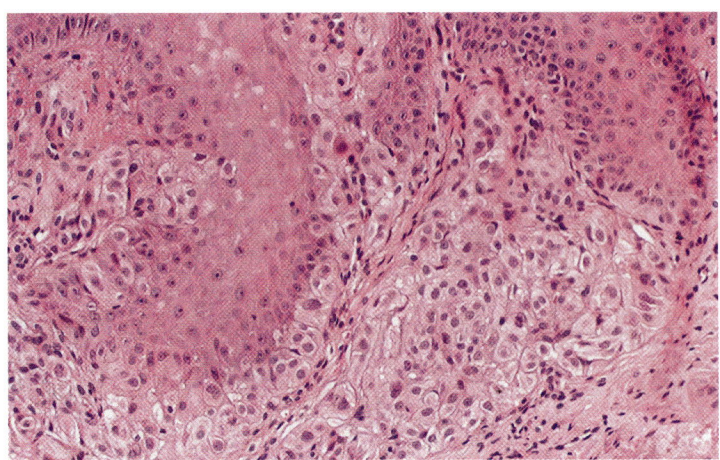

Figure 1-63

SQUAMOUS CELL CARCINOMA

This is a superficially invasive tumor.
Left: Infiltrative islands of atypical keratinocytes.
Above: Cells near the base of the tumor are moderately to poorly differentiated.

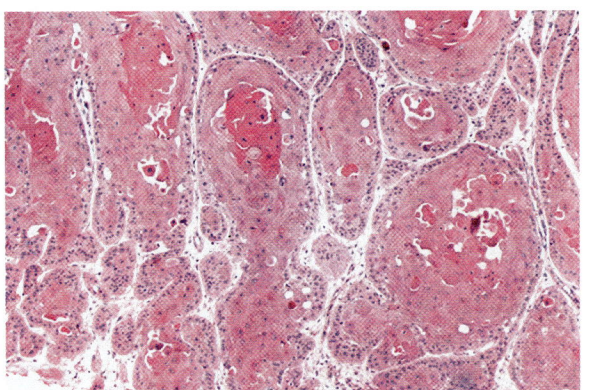

Figure 1-64

SQUAMOUS CELL CARCINOMA

Horn pearls are numerous.

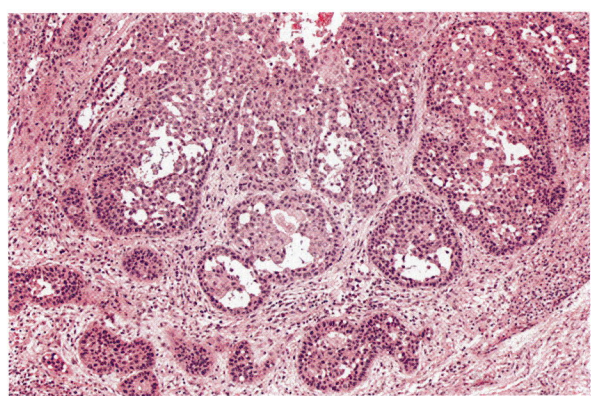

Figure 1-65

SQUAMOUS CELL CARCINOMA, PSEUDOGLANDULAR TYPE

Acantholytic cells create the false impression of gland formation.

with cohesive outer layers and false "lumens" created by central acantholytic cells (fig. 1-65). These *acantholytic, adenoid,* or *pseudoglandular squamous cell carcinomas* often derive from acantholytic actinic keratoses.

A variant of this type of squamous cell carcinoma can closely mimic angiosarcoma, and has been termed *pseudovascular adenoid squamous cell carcinoma*. Recognizing the true nature of this tumor requires identification of foci of epidermal origin or an immunohistochemical profile that includes cytokeratin and epithelial membrane antigen positivity in the face of negative factor VIII and (usually) CD34 staining. Nevertheless, these appear to be biologically aggressive tumors, and deaths have been reported (218). Invasive carcinomas arising from Bowen's disease often maintain the distinctive histopathologic attributes of this lesion, although carcinomas with evidence of adnexal differentiation also occur.

Epidermal Tumors

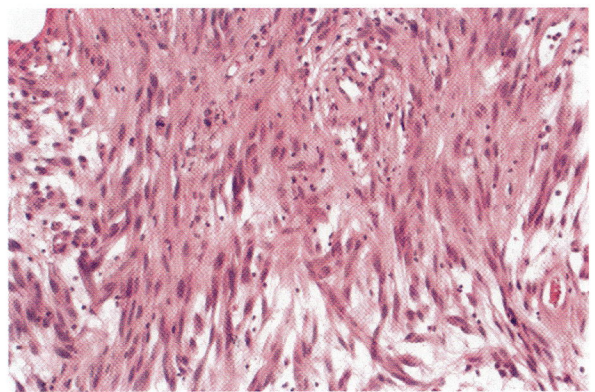

Figure 1-66

SQUAMOUS CELL CARCINOMA, SPINDLE CELL TYPE

Atypical spindled cells intermingle with connective tissue. The borders of such lesions are often indistinct.

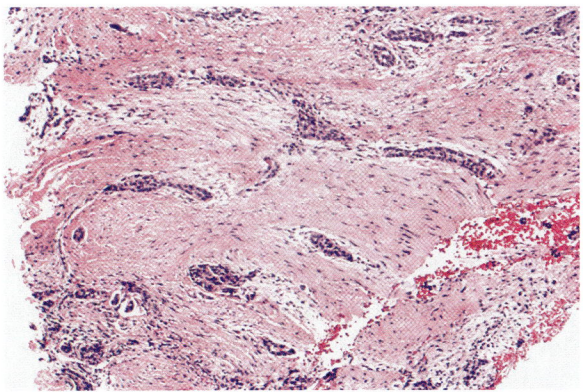

Figure 1-67

SQUAMOUS CELL CARCINOMA, DESMOPLASTIC TYPE

Cords of atypical squamous cells are present within a desmoplastic matrix.

Spindle cell squamous cell carcinoma most often arises in sun-damaged skin. The spindled cells have large, vesicular nuclei and indistinct cell borders created, in part, by intermingling with dense connective tissue (fig. 1-66). Pleomorphism, atypical giant cell formation, and frequent mitoses are observed, creating a close resemblance to atypical fibroxanthoma. There may be evidence of origination from the overlying epidermis or foci of squamous differentiation. Surprisingly, these apparently poorly differentiated tumors tend to have a favorable prognosis, although metastases have been reported, and may be more common in those tumors arising from radiation exposure.

The cells of *desmoplastic squamous cell carcinoma* have a trabecular growth pattern, with cords of atypical cells proliferating in a desmoplastic matrix (fig. 1-67). One study suggested a much higher incidence of local recurrence and metastasis among these tumors compared to a group of squamous cell carcinomas lacking desmoplasia (165).

A rare variant of squamous cell carcinoma is comprised of numerous individual tumor cells with a *signet ring* appearance, thereby resembling the cells of adenocarcinoma (170,212). The cytoplasm of these cells contains glycogen, and the cells express a variety of keratins (fig. 1-68). The cytoplasmic vacuoles may result from markedly dilated endoplasmic reticulum (212).

Various grading systems for squamous cell carcinomas have been devised, with the Broders

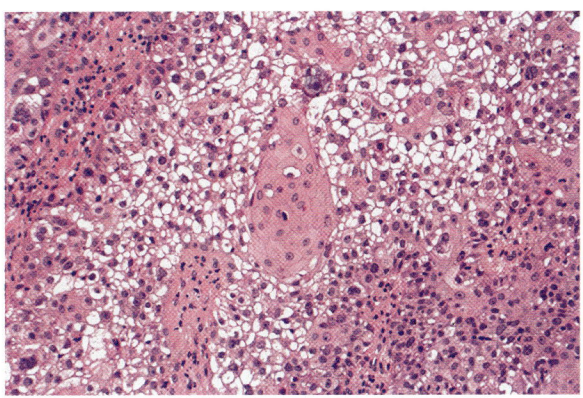

Figure 1-68

SQUAMOUS CELL CARCINOMA WITH CLEAR CELL FEATURES

Cytoplasmic vacuoles impart a signet ring appearance to some of the cells.

system being the oldest and best known. In practice, many pathologists use a three-tiered system of well differentiated, moderately differentiated, and poorly differentiated, based upon the proportion of differentiated cells and the configuration of invasive portions of the tumor. In squamous cell carcinoma of the lip (and, by extrapolation, squamous cell carcinoma arising in the skin), important histologic findings associated with metastasis include perineural invasion, lesions greater than 6 mm in thickness, dispersed pattern, and high cytologic grade (181). Other important factors determining prognosis include location (statistically greater likelihood for recurrence and metastasis in lesions arising at mucocutaneous junctions) and immunosuppression.

Differential Diagnosis. Several problems arise in the diagnosis of squamous cell carcinoma, even when faced with an obvious keratinocyte neoplasm. One is determining the point at which an actinic keratosis has progressed to a superficially invasive squamous cell carcinoma. The key to diagnosis is the recognition that invasive tumor is truly present, and that clusters of atypical keratinocytes do not simply represent cross-sectional profiles of prominent budding rete ridges. This distinction is at times somewhat arbitrary and probably makes little difference in terms of management, but determining invasion may be impossible when superficially shaved specimens are submitted for review. In such cases, a diagnosis of "at least actinic keratosis" is appropriate. Another issue is the handling of large, bulky, keratinocyte neoplasms that are completely connected to the epithelial surface. Such lesions are probably best designated squamous cell carcinoma even if unequivical invasive tumor islands are not detectable.

Acantholytic, adenoid, or pseudoglandular squamous cell carcinomas can be distinguished from true adenocarcinomas by the focal changes of more typical squamous cell carcinoma, by the absence of epithelial mucin, and by a typical immunohistochemical profile for squamous cell carcinoma. The latter also facilitates distinction from angiosarcoma (see above).

The close clinical and histopathologic resemblance of spindle cell squamous cell carcinoma to atypical fibroxanthoma can be problematic, and in fact, prior to the advent of immunohistochemistry some experts believed they were the same. As noted above, demonstration of connections to the surface epidermis or foci of more typical squamous differentiation can aid in distinction, and positive cytokeratin staining of tumor cells may be decisive.

The absence of intracellular mucin aids in differentiating the rare signet ring cell squamous cell carcinoma from similar-appearing adenocarcinomas. Another potential source of diagnostic confusion is the rare signet ring cell carcinoma of the eyelids. The latter is thought to be a tumor of sweat gland origin, presents in middle-aged or elderly men as diffuse induration of the lids, and is biologically aggressive, with a high rate of regional or distant metastases (194,264). Tumor cells proliferate within a sclerotic stroma, but may be positive for estrogen and progesterone receptors and for milk fat globule protein (264).

Occasionally, squamous cell carcinoma can be confused with basal cell carcinoma. This problem can arise in several situations: 1) Bowen's disease with invasive carcinoma (see discussion of Bowen's disease above); 2) pseudoepitheliomatous hyperplasia overlying a basal cell carcinoma; 3) true collision lesions with both basal and squamous cell carcinomas; and 4) tumors with mixed features of basal and squamous cell carcinomas, sometimes termed *basosquamous carcinoma* or *metatypical basal cell carcinoma* (177). Differentiation of the latter from a moderately to poorly differentiated squamous cell carcinoma may be largely academic; the more important consideration is the recognition that these tumors are biologically aggressive, with a high rate of recurrence and metastasis.

Differentiating squamous cell carcinoma from pseudoepitheliomatous hyperplasia, keratoacanthoma, and irritated seborrheic keratosis (basosquamous acanthoma) is discussed in the sections concerning these lesions.

Verrucous Carcinoma

Clinical Features. *Verrucous carcinoma* is a particularly well-differentiated variant of squamous cell carcinoma that is characterized by an exophytic, warty appearance; slow but relentless growth; and rare metastasis (211,241). First described as a lesion of the oral cavity by L.V. Ackerman in 1948 (199a), it also occurs with frequency in the anogenital region or on the plantar surface of the foot. Lesions in the latter location are also termed *epithelioma cuniculatum* (cuniculus is a Latin word meaning "rabbit burrow," a reference to the deep crypts that are frequently present in these lesions). Occasionally, these lesions occur in other cutaneous locations or in association with chronic ulcers and sinuses.

Invasion and destruction of deep structures do occur, explaining the necessity for complete removal of these tumors despite the rarity of metastasis. Although the early literature reported anaplastic transformation of verrucous carcinoma of the oral cavity following X irradiation (228), this does not always occur, and there are reports

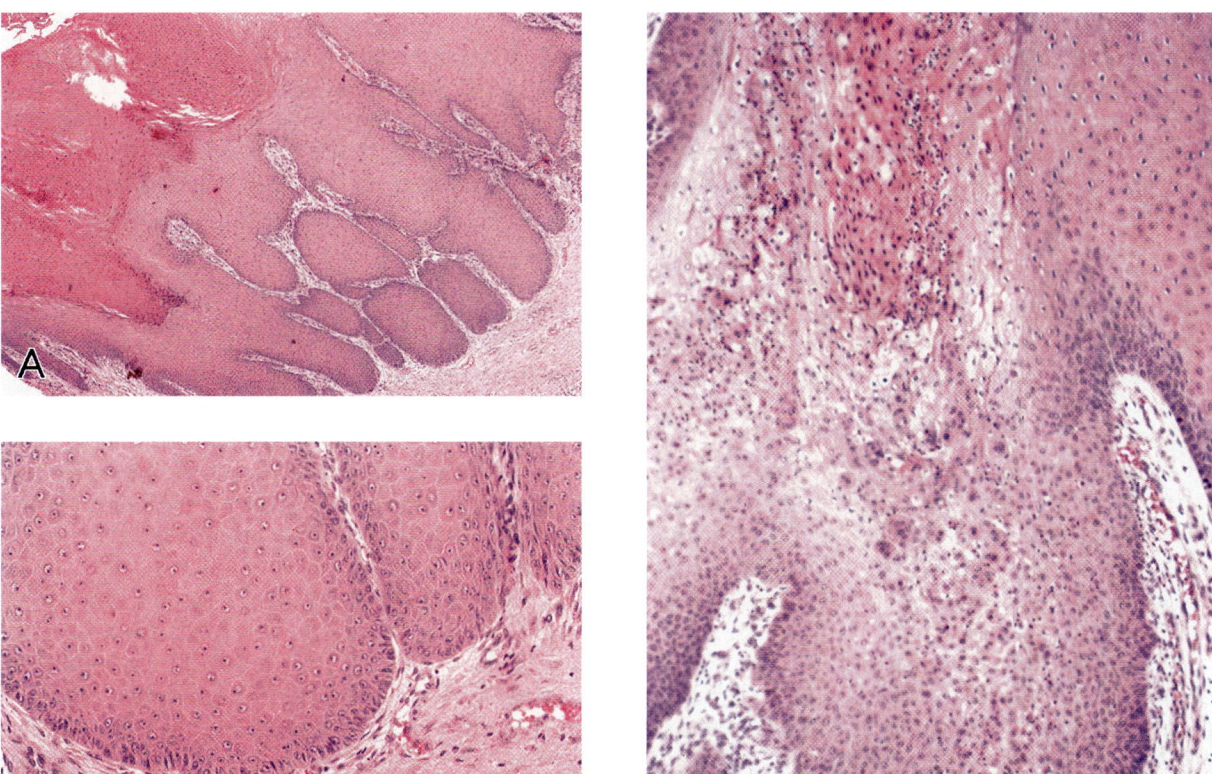

Figure 1-69
VERRUCOUS CARCINOMA
A: Low-power view shows both exophytic and endophytic components.
B: This is a well-differentiated tumor with rounded, "pushing" contours.
C: There are keratin-filled crypts that contain neutrophils.

in the literature regarding the benefits of radiotherapy as a treatment for verrucous carcinoma (223,242). De novo anaplastic transformation of these lesions has been reported (267).

Proposed causes of verrucous carcinoma have included various forms of trauma, but most work has focused on the relationship to infection by HPV. Initially, this relationship was suggested by a clinical resemblance to or association with verrucae (262), but this has been further supported by the detection of a variety of HPV types in these tumors, particularly types 6/11 and 16/18 (171, 239,243) but also types 1 (222) and 2 (221).

Pathologic Findings. Verrucous carcinomas show hyperkeratosis, parakeratosis, and marked acanthosis, and have both exophytic and endophytic components (fig. 1-69A). Proliferations of epithelium typically have blunt contours that appear to "push" and compress the underlying connective tissues rather than to infiltrate between them (fig. 1-69B). Keratin-filled crypts that contain neutrophils are frequently present (fig. 1-69C). Although some of the granular cells give the impression of vacuolization, unequivocal viropathic changes are not observed. The underlying dermis features varying degrees of vasodilation and acute and chronic inflammation. The development of substantial cytologic atypia and invasive features suggests transformation to a biologically more aggressive squamous cell carcinoma. Expression of proliferating cell nuclear antigen and overexpression of p53 oncoprotein have been reported in verrucous carcinoma, both with distribution patterns concentrated in the basilar layers at the periphery of the tumor (204,219,220).

Differential Diagnosis. The chief problem in the differential diagnosis is created by biopsy specimens that are too shallow and fail to include the entire base of the lesion. Such cases may be difficult or impossible to distinguish from verrucae, keratoacanthoma, or forms of pseudoepitheliomatous hyperplasia. The clinical history is important for a full evaluation, in that lesions in characteristic locations that are of long duration or that may have been previously treated as verrucae are particularly good candidates for verrucous carcinoma.

Keratoacanthoma

Clinical Features. *Keratoacanthoma* has been a controversial entity for years, mainly because of its relationship to squamous cell carcinoma. The recognition by Rook and Whimster (235a), Musso (217a), and others of a self-healing "epithelioma" with characteristic clinical and histopathologic features was certainly an important contribution. This has been tempered by the considerable clinical and histopathologic overlap with squamous cell carcinoma, by the occasional aggressive behavior of these lesions, including metastases, and by a general failure of investigators to detect reliable ultrastructural, immunohistochemical, or genetic differences between keratoacanthoma and squamous cell carcinoma. The cause of keratoacanthoma is unknown, but there is both histopathologic and experimental (184,229) evidence that it may arise from cells of the follicular infundibulum. A relationship with HPV infection has been supported by some studies (183,189,229,240) but not by others (205).

Keratoacanthomas are found most often in middle-aged to elderly adults, and frequently develop on sun-exposed skin. They consist of dome-shaped nodules that range from 1 to 3 cm in diameter and have central keratin craters. Keratoacanthomas typically arise rapidly (within 6 to 8 weeks), remain stationary for a time, and then involute over a period ranging from 6 months to 1 year. Involuted lesions typically leave behind a ragged, somewhat crateriform scar. They are most often solitary, but several lesions may develop, and occasionally multiple lesions arise in surgical scars or around graft sites. Special locations for these lesions include the subungual region and the orbit. In contrast to keratoacanthomas in other locations, subungual tumors are not prone to spontaneously regress, and they may actually be more destructive than traditional squamous cell carcinomas occurring in the same location (245). In addition, rapid and extensive involvement of orbital tissues has been documented (156,234). Keratoacanthomas also display greater biologic aggressiveness in immunosuppressed individuals.

There are several other types of keratoacanthoma: *multiple self-healing epitheliomas of Ferguson-Smith,* which may begin in childhood and may be inherited; *eruptive keratoacanthoma of Grzybowski,* in which there may be hundreds of small lesions and mucous membrane involvement; and *keratoacanthoma centrifugum marginatum,* a lesion that spreads by peripheral extension, producing a giant annular lesion with central atrophy.

Pathologic Findings. Since recognition of the overall configuration of a keratoacanthoma is the key to accurate diagnosis, adequate sampling of a lesion is essential. Whenever possible, removal of the entire lesion (by traditional elliptical excision or "saucerization") is preferred, and sections through the midportion of the lesion should be obtained. In large lesions, an adequate incisional biopsy through the midportion of the lesion and including its base is acceptable.

A fully developed keratoacanthoma shows a central keratin crater with underlying islands of squamous epithelium that extend into the dermis; there is a buttress-like arrangement of adjacent, otherwise normal-appearing epidermis at either side of the crater (fig. 1-70). Cells comprising the epithelial proliferations feature generous amounts of glassy-appearing cytoplasm and bland-appearing nuclei, producing low nuclear to cytoplasmic ratios (fig. 1-70). Some nuclear pleomorphism and mitotic activity may be identified at the base of the lesion, particularly in evolving lesions. Perineural infiltration can be observed in these tumors, a finding that does not necessarily indicate an adverse prognosis (202). Intraepidermal neutrophilic microabscesses are common (fig. 1-71), and the underlying dermal infiltrate may include fairly numerous eosinophils. Involuting lesions may feature numerous apoptotic keratinocytes, a shallow crater, thinning of the underlying epithelium, and dermal scar with varying degrees of inflammation (fig. 1-72).

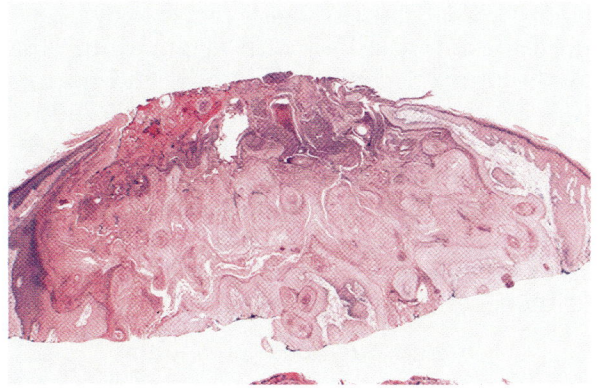 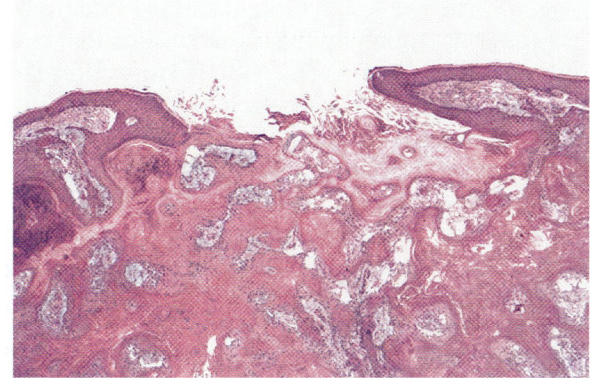

Figure 1-70

KERATOACANTHOMA

Left: Low-power view shows a keratin-filled crater with islands of squamous epithelium extending into the underlying dermis.

Right: There is a buttress-like arrangement of adjacent epidermis at either side of the crater.

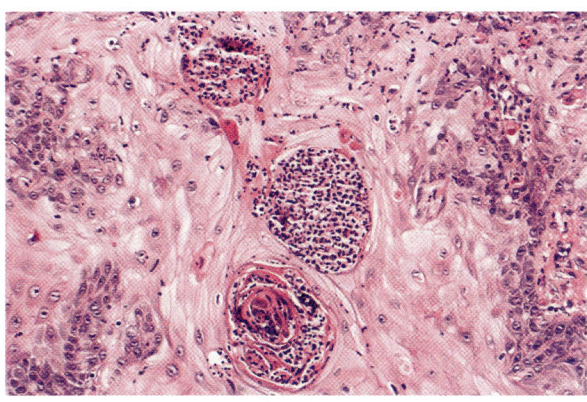 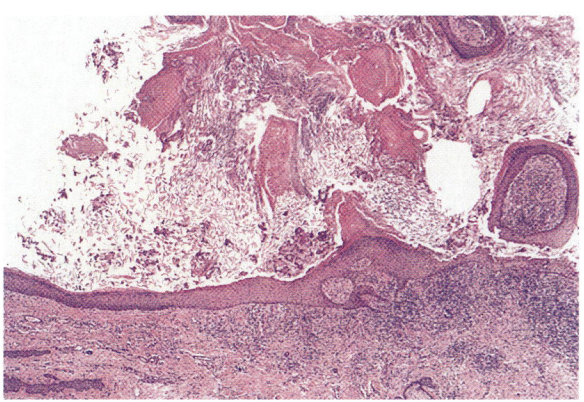

Figure 1-71	Figure 1-72
KERATOACANTHOMA	**INVOLUTING KERATOACANTHOMA**
Glassy-appearing cytoplasm with a low nuclear to cytoplasmic ratio and intraepidermal neutrophilic microabscesses.	A shallow crater, thinned epithelium, dermal scar, and lymphocytic inflammation are seen.

There are slight variations in the microscopic appearance of the special forms of keratoacanthoma. Subungual tumors may show extensive apoptosis and a sparsity of neutrophils and eosinophils in the accompanying infiltrate (245). We have observed numerous well-formed horn cysts in a case of rapidly progressing keratoacanthoma of the eyelid. Tangential sections of the border of keratoacanthoma centrifugum marginatum may show broad acanthosis and a less than ideal demonstration of the central keratin crater, while the keratin craters may be inconspicuous in lesions of eruptive keratoacanthoma of Grzybowski.

Differential Diagnosis. Partial or improperly oriented biopsies of keratoacanthoma may make distinction from verrucae, verrucous carcinoma, or forms of pseudoepitheliomatous hyperplasia extremely difficult. The most significant problem is the differentiation of keratoacanthoma from squamous cell carcinoma. Although the features of keratoacanthoma are characteristic, there may be substantial overlap with squamous cell carcinoma, even in terms of the degree of cytologic atypia. Metastasis of lesions originally diagnosed as keratoacanthoma has been reported (188). Features that favor squamous cell carcinoma include: atypia (including changes of actinic keratosis or squamous cell carcinoma in situ) in the epidermis immediately adjacent to the lesion; severe degrees of cytologic atypia, including cells with high nuclear to cytoplasmic ratios, marked nuclear pleomorphism, and atypical mitotic figures; and foci of acantholysis, including pseudoglandular changes. Squamous metaplasia of the underlying eccrine sweat glands is indicative of a lesion of longer duration and therefore tends to favor squamous cell carcinoma over keratoacanthoma. The composition of the dermal infiltrate is generally not helpful, as neutrophils and eosinophils, complete with intraepithelial microabscess formation, can be seen in both.

Since none of these findings is absolute, extensive investigations have been performed over the years in an attempt to identify some marker that might reliably distinguish keratoacanthoma from squamous cell carcinoma. Studies have focused on c-erbB-2/neu/HER-2 (155), cyclin E (161), proliferating cell nuclear antigen, p53 oncoprotein (167), and Ki-67 (206). Investigators have evaluated DNA content and proliferative index via flow cytometry (232), oncostatin M expression (250), and beta-2-microglobulin expression (187). For the most part, none of these studies allows clear separation of the two lesions. Somewhat more promising results have been obtained with peanut agglutinin binding (uniformly positive cytoplasmic membrane staining in keratoacanthomas, not generally seen in well-differentiated squamous cell carcinomas without prior neuraminidase digestion) (196), and with loss of heterozygosity analysis (258).

There is no known absolutely reliable means of distinguishing keratoacanthoma from squamous cell carcinoma. The current trend is to regard keratoacanthoma as a variant form of squamous cell carcinoma, one that is capable of self-healing, and to advocate complete if conservative removal of all such lesions (159,188,208). While we generally agree with this viewpoint, we still make a diagnosis of keratoacanthoma provided that certain conditions are met. There should be a clear-cut clinical description (preferably from a dermatologist) of a rapidly evolving crateriform lesion, with keratoacanthoma as the primary clinical diagnosis, and no history of immunosuppression. Adequate biopsy material should be submitted, allowing complete visualization of the lesion. Finally, the microscopic findings should be absolutely classic for keratoacanthoma. Otherwise, a diagnosis of squamous cell carcinoma with features of keratoacanthoma is preferred.

Adenosquamous Carcinoma

Clinical Features. In recent years there have been several publications describing a primary carcinoma of the skin with features of squamous cell carcinoma but also with areas of true glandular differentiation. It is clear that this tumor differs from the acantholytic, or pseudoglandular, squamous cell carcinoma that commonly arises in actinically damaged skin and that sometimes bears the confusing designation "adenoid squamous cell carcinoma."

Adenosquamous carcinoma is prone to occur in the central facial region of middle-aged to elderly adults (157,259). Tumors on the scalp and hand have also been identified. They present as indurated, slightly elevated keratotic plaques, but these features are not distinctive, and the correct diagnosis depends upon histopathologic findings. The evidence suggests that this is an aggressive neoplasm, with a propensity to local recurrence or regional nodal metastasis, but there is potential for a favorable outcome among small, dermally located tumors (180).

Pathologic Findings. Microscopic changes include a multifocal epidermal origin, deep infiltrative growth with accompanying desmoplasia, and perineural infiltration. Superficial portions of the tumor have an appearance most consistent with squamous cell carcinoma, but in deeper portions there is evidence of glandular differentiation, with formation of lumens lined by vacuolated, mucin-containing cells (fig. 1-73). The mucin has staining characteristics of epithelial mucin (sialomucin), and is typically Alcian blue positive, hyaluronidase resistant, and sialidase sensitive. These glandular areas are also positive for low molecular weight cytokeratin (CAM5.2) and carcinoembryonic antigen. Cytologic atypia may be pronounced and mitotic figures plentiful; however, cases have been

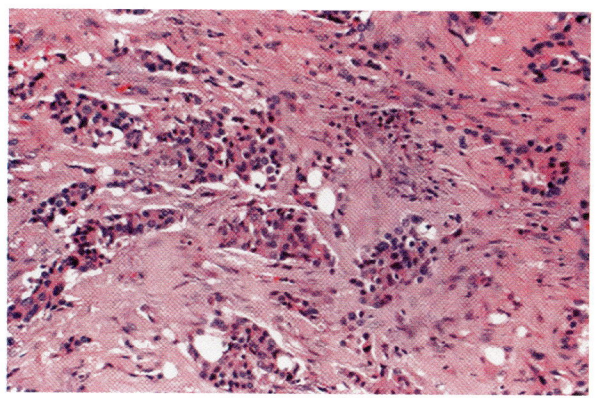

Figure 1-73

ADENOSQUAMOUS CARCINOMA

There are infiltrative tumor islands with glandular differentiation.

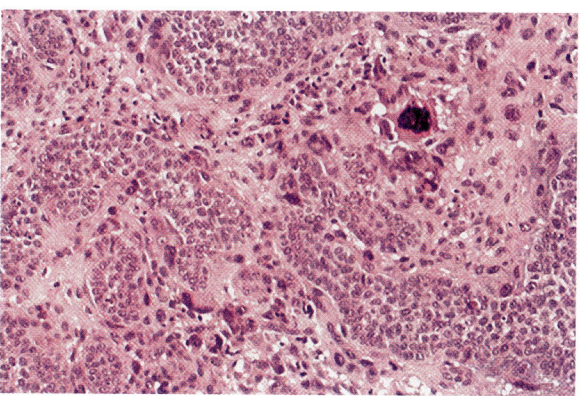

Figure 1-74

CARCINOSARCOMA OF THE SKIN

This tumor had a basal cell carcinoma-like epithelial component and stromal changes of an undifferentiated spindle cell sarcoma.

reported in which the cytologic atypia was mild to moderate (179,180) or in which only superficial dermal invasion was noted (180). It is unclear whether this lesion represents divergent differentiation within a squamous cell carcinoma or a variant of sweat gland carcinoma (157).

Differential Diagnosis. Adenosquamous carcinoma must be distinguished from acantholytic, or pseudoglandular, squamous cell carcinomas, in which gland-like formations result from central acantholysis or necrosis of tumor cells. Some cases with the microscopic characteristics of adenosquamous carcinoma have been termed mucoepidermoid carcinoma (179). Banks and Cooper (157), however, feel that the latter term should be reserved for tumors of salivary gland origin, and that most lesions reported as primary mucoepidermoid carcinoma of the skin are actually malignant acrospiromas with mucin production. Adenosquamous carcinoma also has features in common with microcystic adnexal carcinoma, in that both are prone to develop in the central facial region, and both show superficial keratotic features and a deeply infiltrative growth pattern. Microcystic adnexal carcinoma, however, does not produce mucin and has lesser degrees of cytologic atypia and mitotic activity (157).

Sarcomatoid Carcinoma (Carcinosarcoma, Metaplastic Carcinoma)

Clinical Features. *Sarcomatoid carcinoma (carcinosarcoma)* is a tumor composed of malignant epithelial and mesenchymal elements. It has been reported in a variety of organs, including the skin, but primary carcinosarcoma arising in skin is particularly rare. Skin lesions most often arisen in the head and neck region or on the trunk; at least one case occurred on the upper arm (160,166,192,226,231,236,251). The tumors lack diagnostic characteristics, and have been described as red, rapidly growing, or ulcerated. Recurrences and metastases have been reported (166), but it remains to be seen whether or not this statistic will bear out over the long term. Theories regarding the origin of these lesions include: 1) "collision" of two separate tumors; 2) epithelial induction of sarcomatous change in the surrounding stroma; 3) induction of malignant transformation of epithelium by sarcomatous tissue; and 4) metaplastic differentiation of epithelial tumor cells into sarcomatous elements (226).

Pathologic Findings. The epithelial component of primary cutaneous carcinosarcoma has included basal cell carcinoma, squamous cell carcinoma, and sweat gland carcinoma. Sarcomatous components have shown osteoblastic, chondroid, or skeletal or smooth muscle differentiation, although occasionally only the changes of undifferentiated spindle cell sarcoma are present (fig. 1-74) (192). Intermingling of epithelial and mesenchymal elements is often observed. Currently, a diagnosis of carcinosarcoma often depends upon the finding of

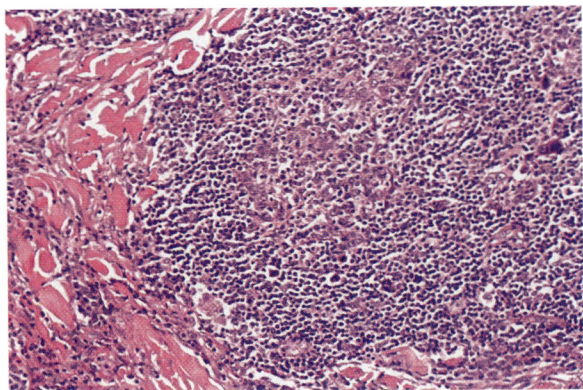

Figure 1-75
LYMPHOEPITHELIOMA-LIKE CARCINOMA OF THE SKIN
Atypical polygonal cells are permeated by lymphocytes.

heterologous elements (e.g., osteoblastic or chondroid differentiation), although there is no logical reason why the diagnosis cannot be applied to tumors with areas of spindle cell sarcoma that lack these heterologous elements.

Differential Diagnosis. The differential diagnosis for carcinosarcoma is limited. True "collision" of separate epithelial and mesenchymal tumors is a rare event. Metastasis of carcinosarcoma from an internal site is possible, but could be excluded by demonstrating epidermal connections to the malignant epithelial component (226).

Lymphoepithelioma-Like Carcinoma

Clinical Features. In recent years, there have been reports of a primary cutaneous tumor with microscopic similarities to undifferentiated carcinoma (lymphoepithelial carcinoma) of the nasopharynx and other organs. This tumor, designated *lymphoepithelioma-like carcinoma of the skin,* usually arises in sun-exposed skin of the face in middle-aged or older adults. The lesions are solitary nodules that may be pearly or flesh colored. Patients often have a good prognosis following complete excision, although recurrences and metastases have been reported (246,247). Unlike nasopharyngeal lymphoepithelioma, these cutaneous tumors are invariably negative for Epstein-Barr virus genomic sequences (178,201,203,235,260).

Pathologic Findings. Lymphoepithelioma-like carcinoma of the skin is composed of islands of polygonal cells, which are infiltrated and "cuffed" by lymphocytes (fig. 1-75). The polygonal cells possess large vesicular nuclei, prominent nucleoli, and mitotic figures, some of which are atypical. These tumor islands lack connections to the surface epidermis. Foci of keratinization or duct formation are also observed. The cells are typically positive for cytokeratin cocktail and epithelial membrane antigen, and they may express "hard keratins" (demonstrated by positive staining with AE14) or show focal positivity for carcinoembryonic antigen, S-100 protein, and leu-M1. The lymphocytic infiltrates contain admixtures of B and T cells (235). The findings suggest that these are poorly differentiated adnexal carcinomas with the capability of follicular or sweat gland differentiation (199,235,246,260).

Differential Diagnosis. The microscopic differential diagnosis includes lymphoma and Merkel cell carcinoma. Identification of the atypical epithelial component argues against rules out lymphoma, as does the bland appearance of the lymphocytes and their lack of phenotypic evidence for clonality. Merkel cell carcinoma is composed of small cells with evenly dispersed chromatin, and lacks the intense admixture of lymphocytes seen in lymphoepithelioma-like carcinoma. The dot-like paranuclear cytokeratin staining among cells of Merkel cell carcinoma is also distinctive. Cutaneous metastasis from a nasopharyngeal carcinoma would also be a diagnostic consideration, but negativity for Epstein-Barr virus genomic sequences or evidence of cutaneous adnexal differentiation would favor a primary cutaneous lesion.

Basal Cell Carcinoma

Clinical Features. Basal cell carcinoma (BCC) is, by far, the most common cutaneous malignancy, representing about 70 percent of malignant lesions involving the skin (279). The tumor was recognized at least as early as 1897, when it was described in Hyde and Montgomery's text on cutaneous diseases (301) as "superficial epithelioma," "rodent ulcer," or (histopathologically) "tubular epithelioma." Krompecher (310), however, is generally given credit for designating these tumors "basal cell" (*Der Basalzellenkrebs*) due to their resemblance to epidermal basal keratinocytes. These early works demonstrated an accurate understanding of both the biologic behavior and treatment of these tumors. From that time to the present, much has been written about the origins and growth characteristics of BCC and its various microscopic configurations. It is now known that BCC exhibits a spectrum of biologic behavior, ranging from local persistence and destructiveness to less common, but well-documented, metastasis, and at least some indication of its behavior can be discerned from the histopathologic features of a particular tumor (288,298).

BCC is most commonly seen in sun-exposed skin, especially (but not invariably) in individuals with fair complexions. Middle-aged to older adults are particularly affected, but young adults can also develop the tumor. BCCs occasionally arise in children, but are then most often associated with a syndrome or nevus (see below). The development of BCC mainly in sun-exposed skin implies a failure of keratinocytic stem cells to repair solar damage to DNA (294,296, 353,366), however, numerous reports have documented the occurrence of BCC in sun-protected or unusual cutaneous sites. These locations include the abdomen, back, buttocks, perineum and genitalia, proximal extremities, plantar surfaces, and interdigital areas (272,308, 322,325,329,335,342). In patients who have received organ transplants, BCC usually occurs in sites other than the head and neck; it also appears at a younger age and is associated with a higher frequency of superficial growth (307).

The development of BCC in nonsun-exposed locations suggests that factors other than solar damage play a role in its development. Some patients with BCC in unusual locations have received prior radiotherapy to the tumor site for unrelated conditions. Recent studies have also implicated several strains of HPV as possible agents for producing BCC (350). In any event, karyotypic analyses have shown aberrations in chromosome 9 in tumor cells in the majority of cases (290,338). Abnormalities of the *p53* gene also may play a role in producing a subset of BCC (299,311,316,330). Recently, attention has been directed toward the sonic hedgehog signaling pathway, which is involved in embryonic patterning. Dysregulation of this pathway is believed to be important for tumor growth, and has been detected not only in BCC but also in related conditions such as basal cell nevus syndrome, nevus sebaceus, and familial basaloid follicular hamartoma (287,306,347, 361). Among types of BCC there is some variability in the expression of the two transmembrane proteins that are components of the sonic hedgehog signaling pathway, ptc (patched) and smo (smoothened). In one study, enhanced expression of ptc and smo was found in nodular BCC, but these proteins were undetectable in superficial BCC (361). There is evidence that the cellular localization of beta-catenin may correlate with the current classification of histologic types of BCC (see below); in addition, this molecule may also affect the invasiveness of the tumors (346), perhaps in part due to its role in cell-cell adhesion. BCC can also develop in areas of skin subjected to chronic inflammation, infection, or trauma such as with hidradenitis suppurativa, stasis dermatitis and venous ulcers, smallpox vaccinations, amputation stumps, lupus vulgaris, cutaneous gummas, and onchocerciasis (268,273).

There are several clinical subtypes of BCC, demonstrating the considerable variability in appearance of which these tumors are capable. The classic noduloulcerative lesion has a pearly, telangiectatic appearance, often with a central ulcer. Papulonodular lesions may lack ulceration and show minimal, if any, telangiectatic change. Superficial BCC presents as an erythematous scaly patch. Pigmentation sometimes occurs in BCC, especially in nodular and superficial types; these lesions can clinically mimic malignant melanoma. Fibroepithelioma of Pinkus most often takes the form of an erythematous nodule that occasionally can be pedunculated. Sclerotic or morpheaform BCC manifests as an indurated plaque. Unusual variants include the "horrifying" BCC, which is a particularly large, mutilating tumor with nodulocystic or infiltrating microscopic features (298,354), and "keratopurpuric" BCC, a lesion with a central scale and peritumoral blush that on biopsy shows parakeratosis and peritumoral granulation tissue (312).

Uncommonly, perineural infiltration by BCC produces clinical neuropathies (327). Regression, usually partial, occurs in about 5 percent of cases (283). In practice, this is most commonly observed when reexcision follows a partial biopsy of the tumor, and is accompanied histopathologically by inflammation and apoptosis.

BCC is encountered congenitally in the form of *linear basal cell nevus*. This is a unilateral, zosteriform eruption of papulonodular BCC with comedones and cutaneous atrophy (274). Syndromes featuring BCC as an essential element include basal cell nevus syndrome, Bazex's syndrome, and xeroderma pigmentosum. The basal cell nevus syndrome, or Gorlin's syndrome, is dominantly inherited and consists of multiple cutaneous BCCs. They arise in childhood and are associated with keratocysts of the jawbones; similar cysts also arise in the skin. Bifid ribs, neurologic abnormalities, palmar-plantar pits, and characteristically unusual facies are also part of Gorlin's syndrome (269,354). Bazex's syndrome combines BCCs with hypotrichosis, follicular atrophoderma, and hypohidrosis (336). Xeroderma pigmentosum is associated with premature actinic damage resulting from abnormalities in DNA repair.

Efforts have been made to identify those clinicopathologic features that correlate with frequent recurrence and persistent growth, in order to allow complete removal at an early stage. Lang and Maize (313) and Jacobs et al. (305) found that initial excision specimens showing infiltrative or micronodular patterns tended to pursue an aggressive subsequent clinical course. BCCs that lack peripheral nuclear palisading also have shown a greater tendency to recur (313). This is true also of basosquamous carcinomas, which are tumors that have a propensity to metastasize (275,286). Perineural invasion in BCC appears to correlate with tumor aggressiveness (340).

According to Vico et al. (362), there are three major determinants of adverse prognosis in BCC: maximum size of greater than 1 cm, more than two recurrences, and growth of tumor beneath the subcutis. Immunocompromised individuals are also at greater risk for tumor-related morbidity (365). About 0.1% of nonsquamoid BCCs metastasize, most often to regional lymph nodes, lung, and bone (289,352, 363). About 230 cases of metastasizing BCC have been reported (343). Metastasis appears to be more likely among large, neglected tumors, especially in immunocompromised or malnourished individuals (363).

Pathologic Findings. BCC displays a considerable diversity of microscopic appearances. Histologic variants include nodulocystic, superficial, adenoid, morpheaform, infiltrative, keratotic, and pigmented forms as well as some uncommon variants. The specific histologic types of BCC are described below, but in clinical practice, various combinations of these types are often encountered.

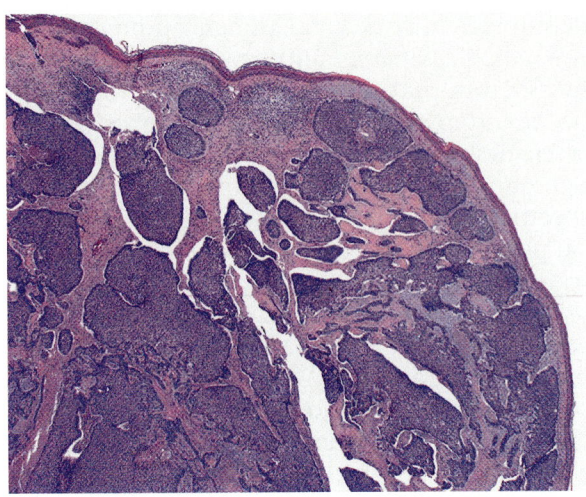

Figure 1-76

NODULOCYSTIC BASAL CELL CARCINOMA

Branching lobules of small hyperchromatic cells and peripheral palisading of nuclei are observed.

Nodulocystic BCC is the most common histologic type (approximately 70 percent of cases). It is composed of rounded or bluntly branched lobules of small hyperchromatic cells that are connected to the overlying epidermis by narrow cords or broad trabeculae. The cellular clusters vary in size and shape, but are characterized by peripheral nuclear palisading (fig. 1-76). The tumor cells are uniform in size and polygonal in shape, with generally oval nuclei and inconspicuous nucleoli. Occasionally, spindled or giant dysplastic (anaplastic) nuclear forms may be observed, although they appear to have no prognostic significance (331). Cytoplasm is scanty and amphophilic, and mitotic activity is variable. The stroma in this form of BCC is fibromyxoid, and characteristically retracts from tumor cell clusters in formalin-fixed specimens. Solar elastosis is almost invariably seen in the surrounding dermis.

Zamecnik et al. (373) described the occasional formation of collagenous crystalloids in the matrix of BCC. Necrosis within tumor nodules

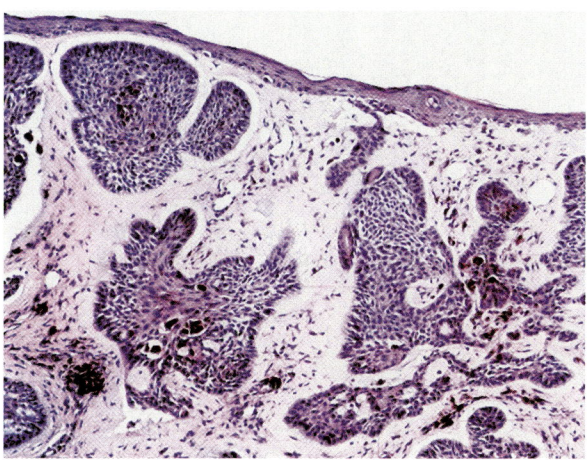 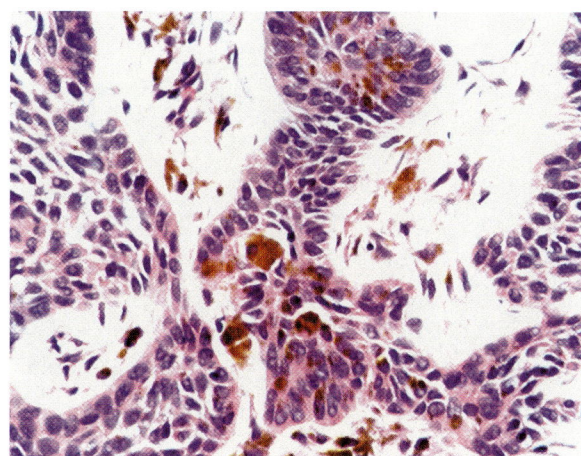

Figure 1-77

PIGMENTED NODULOCYSTIC BASAL CELL CARCINOMA

Left: Low-power view.
Right: High-power view. Melanocytes are admixed with nonpigmented tumor cells, and melanophages are present in the stroma.

may produce a cystic quality that can be appreciated both clinically and microscopically. Confluent necrotic areas in adjacent cellular lobules may produce broad areas of anucleate debris. The overlying epidermis may ulcerate, producing the classic clinical image of a "rodent ulcer." Another feature of some BCCs with a nodulocystic or superficial growth pattern is the presence of abundant intratumoral melanocytes (fig. 1-77) (319,334). These may reflect "divergent differentiation" in BCC. The melanocytes are usually evenly admixed with nonpigmented tumor cells, but have dendritic individual profiles. Pigment-containing melanophages are found in the stroma, and probably account for most of the color noted clinically in these lesions, since the melanocytes themselves contain only a scant amount of finely granular melanin (334).

Superficial BCC differs from nodulocystic BCC by the downward, bud-like growth of tumor lobules from the basal epidermis (fig. 1-78). Although seeming to be multifocal, serial sectioning indicates that the tumor islands are interconnected, suggesting a unicentric origin for this variant of BCC (314,318). Tumor islands seldom extend more deeply than the papillary dermis, but they have the same cellular composition as nodulocystic lesions. The surrounding stroma often has a scar-like appearance,

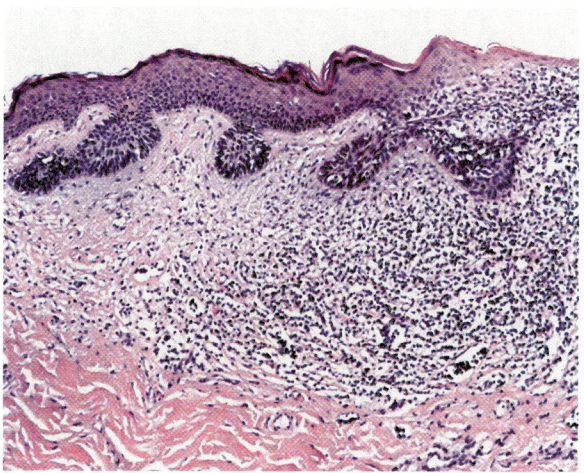

Figure 1-78

SUPERFICIAL BASAL CELL CARCINOMA

Bud-like tumor lobules extend from the basilar epidermis.

which is a useful clue to the diagnosis when tumor islands are not identified in initial sections. Overlying ulceration is infrequent, but epidermal atrophy is common. Although acantholysis is generally uncommon in BCC, the superficial subtype is most likely to demonstrate that finding (321).

The fibroepithelioma of Pinkus combines the features of intracanalicular fibroadenoma of the

Nonmelanocytic Tumors of the Skin

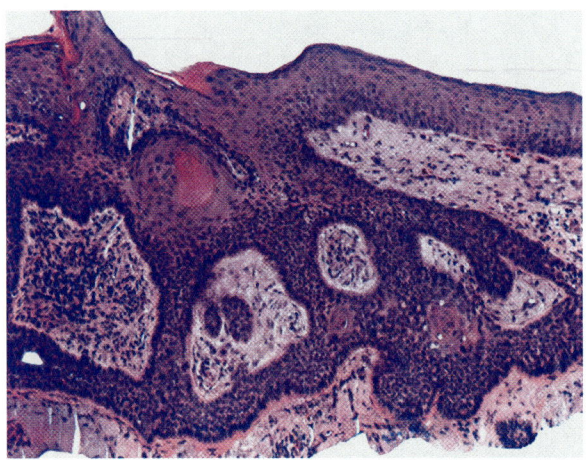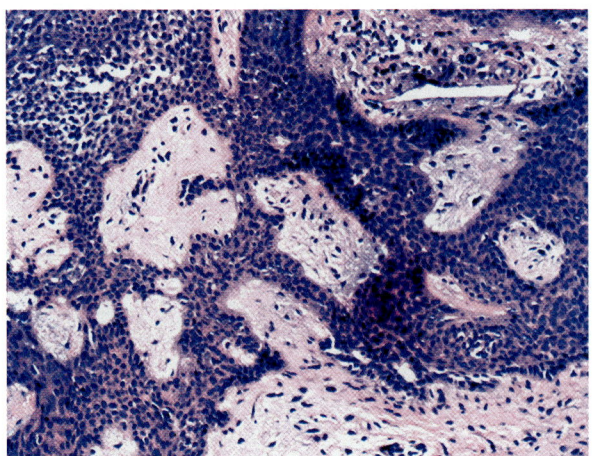

Figure 1-79

FIBROEPITHELIOMA OF PINKUS

Left: Branching strands of keratinocytes extend from the epidermis and are embedded in a fibromyxoid matrix.
Right: Buds of palisaded basaloid cells protrude from some of the branching cellular cords.

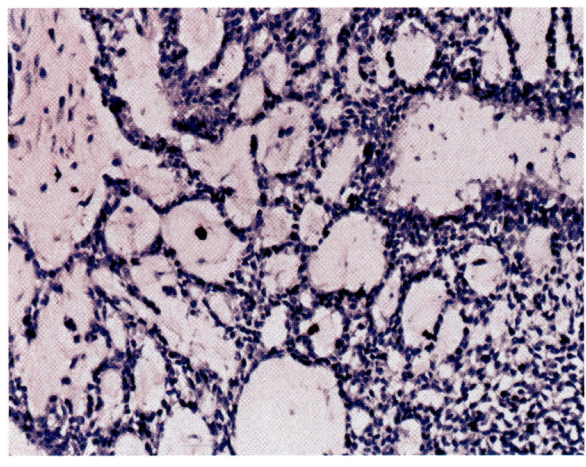

Figure 1-80

ADENOID BASAL CELL CARCINOMA

The reticulated arrangement of tumor cells forms spaces containing amorphous, granular or colloid-like material.

breast, seborrheic keratosis, and superficial BCC. Elongated branching strands of keratinocytes in reticulated arrays are connected to the epidermal surface and surrounded by a fibromyxoid matrix. Buds of palisaded basaloid cells sometimes protrude from these branching cords of cells (fig. 1-79).

Roughly 20 percent of BCCs have a reticulated and gland-like growth pattern within tumor cell clusters, a configuration termed *adenoid BCC* (fig. 1-80). The spaces formed in these lesions may contain amorphous, granular or colloid-like material; alternatively, they may consist only of fibromyxoid stroma. Connections between the dermal tumor mass and the overlying epidermis are invariably present in adenoid BCC, but they are more focal than in other variants, and step sections may be required in order to demonstrate them. The most helpful features in distinguishing this form of BCC from true glandular tumors of the skin are the retention of peripheral nuclear palisading and the presence of stromal retraction. Basaloid tumors with eccrine differentiation have been labeled "eccrine epitheliomas," but some of these may actually represent adenoid cystic carcinoma of sweat glands (102). Occasional BCCs also have focal apocrine features (345), and it is possible that BCC containing mucicarmine-positive signet ring cells also reflect apocrine differentiation (fig. 1-81).

Adnexal differentiation is also observed in keratotic (pilar) and basosebaceous BCCs. *Keratotic (pilar) BCCs* feature keratinous horn cysts and clusters of parakeratotic cells with eosinophilic cytoplasm (fig. 1-82). A small percentage contain papillary mesenchymal bodies, fibroblastic aggregations that mimic the structures responsible for hair induction. Those bodies are found in most trichoepitheliomas, and their presence in occasional keratotic BCCs provides

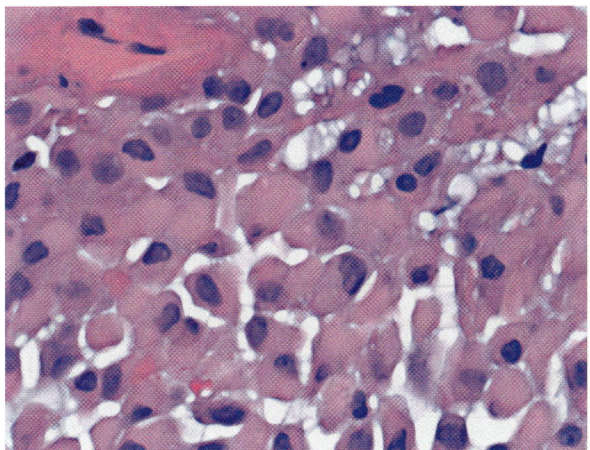
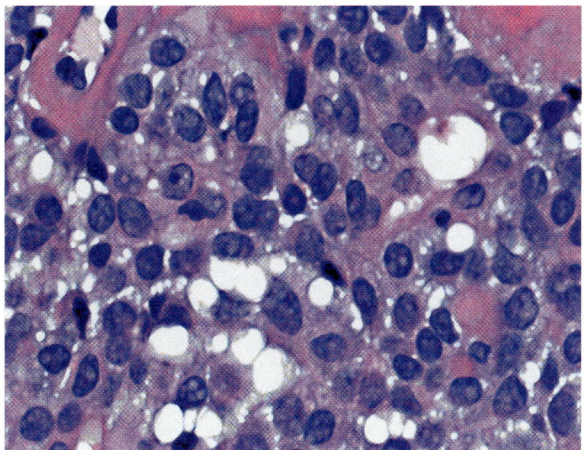

Figure 1-81
BASAL CELL CARCINOMA WITH SIGNET RING CELLS
Two examples of basal cell carcinoma with signet ring change. This may reflect apocrine differentiation.

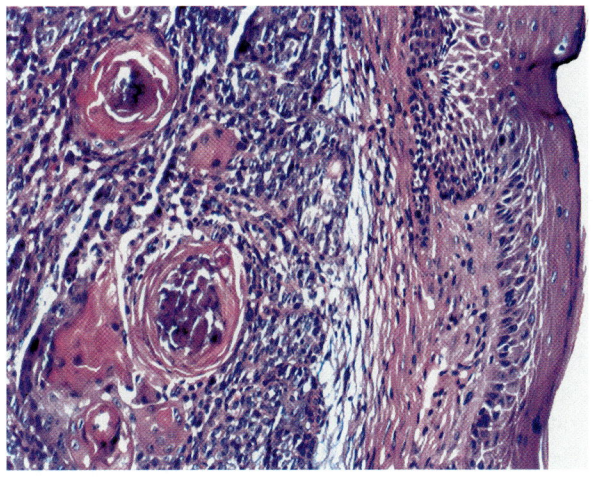

Figure 1-82
KERATOTIC (PILAR) BASAL CELL CARCINOMA
There are horn cysts and clusters of parakeratotic cells with eosinophilic cytoplasm.

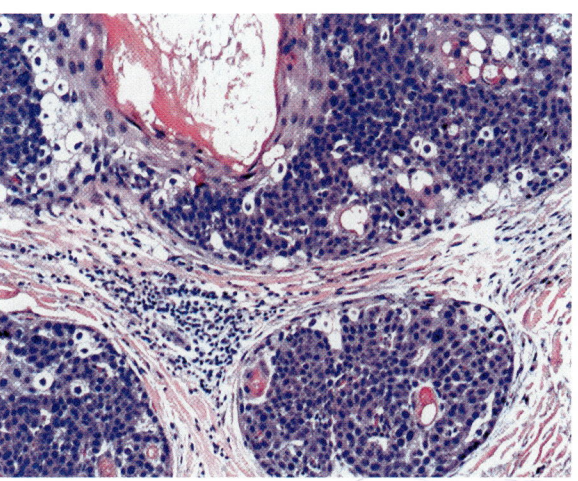

Figure 1-83
BASOSEBACEOUS BASAL CELL CARCINOMA
Mature sebaceous cells are readily identified. In this example, sebaceous cells are located near the periphery of tumor islands rather than in their central portion.

some evidence of follicular differentiation (276). The presence of citrulline, a component of pilar keratin, in these lesions lends further support to this interpretation (300).

Basosebaceous BCCs contain mature sebaceous cells within basal cell nests, without transitional forms (fig. 1-83). The basaloid elements of basosebaceous BCC are larger than those of ordinary BCC, and stromal retraction and peripheral nuclear palisading are not as pronounced. The sebocytes tend to be concentrated in the central portion of the tumor cell aggregate. These neoplasms have been called "sebaceous epitheliomas" in the past, but that term is inaccurate and confusing.

Morpheaform BCC accounts for approximately 15 percent of all BCCs. This variant derives its name from the dense, collagenized, hypocellular matrix that resembles the skin changes seen in morphea (364). Within the stroma are

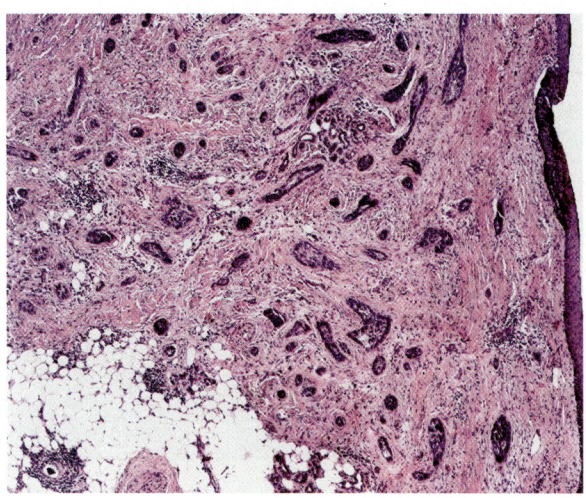

Figure 1-84

MORPHEAFORM BASAL CELL CARCINOMA

Narrow cords of tumor cells are present within a dense stroma.

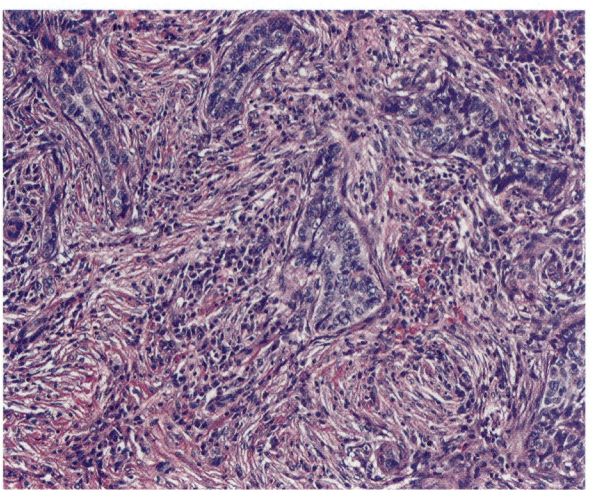

Figure 1-85

INFILTRATIVE BASAL CELL CARCINOMA

Tumor cells with jagged contours are observed within a cellular stroma.

narrow cords of tumor cells that are often slightly branched; however, linear, single cell profiles also are frequently observed (fig. 1-84). As a result, peripheral nuclear palisading is not readily apparent and stromal retraction is usually inconspicuous. Step sections may be required to demonstrate a connection between the tumor and the epidermis, since it is usually focal. Morpheaform BCC is characterized by its deep invasion of the dermis and occasional extension into the subcutis. The overlying skin surface may be atrophic, ulcerated, or relatively normal in appearance.

Infiltrative BCCs are hybrids of the nodulocystic and morpheaform varieties, combining expansile nodules with branched, sharply angulated, and linear cell groupings (351). Jacobs et al. (305) described the irregular and acutely tapered contours of the tumor cells in this lesion as "spiky." Deep dermal invasion is typical, and epidermal ulceration is common. The stroma is more cellular than that associated with nodulocystic or morpheaform tumors (fig. 1-85). Infiltrative BCC may be the best *in vivo* example of the interdependency between the tumor cells and stroma in this epithelial neoplasm. Its fibroblast-rich stroma is unlike that seen in other BCC variants and is intimately attached to basaloid cell aggregates. As a result, retraction artifact is not particularly notable in these lesions.

There is controversy in the literature regarding which tumors should best be classified as basosquamous BCC. Some authors include cases that show a gradual transition between basaloid elements and cell nests with more abundant eosinophilic cytoplasm, larger nuclei, and concentric arrangements ("pearls"), while others restrict the term to lesions with admixed components of both BCC and squamous cell carcinoma (275,286,349). We favor the latter definition, since the distinction between the former and either keratotic or metatypical BCC is otherwise unclear. In order to avoid confusion with areas of simple squamous metaplasia in BCC, the squamous cell carcinoma element of basosquamous carcinoma should demonstrate nuclear anaplasia, dyskeratosis, nucleolar prominence, and mitotic activity (fig. 1-86). The BCC component may exhibit a nodulocystic, adenoid, superficial, or infiltrative growth patterns. This variant of BCC comprises less than 0.5 percent of all cases.

Metatypical BCC also has been defined in various ways by several authors (275,286,289). In our opinion, this term encompasses a variant of BCC that lacks peripheral palisading within cellular lobules, and has larger nuclei, more abundant eosinophilic cytoplasm, and a somewhat spindled cell growth pattern with focally prominent intercellular bridges. Cell nests are

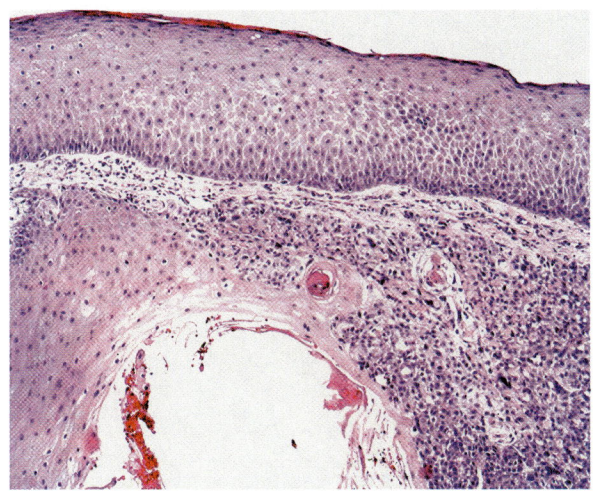

Figure 1-86

BASOSQUAMOUS BASAL CELL CARCINOMA

The squamous cell carcinoma element shows significant nuclear anaplasia and dyskeratosis.

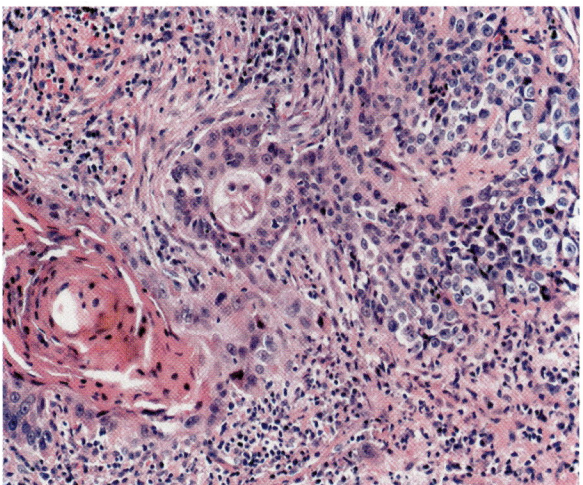

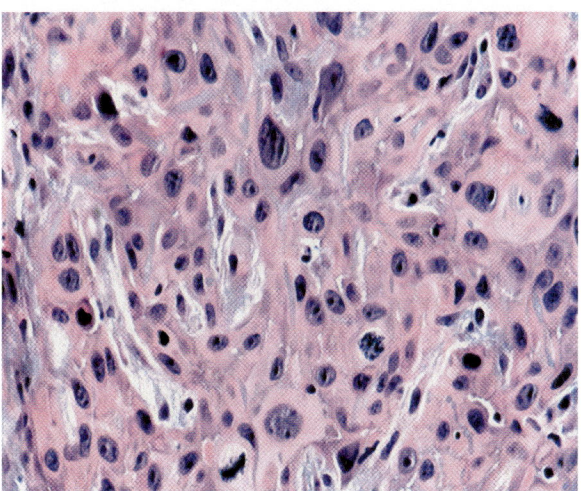

Figure 1-87

METATYPICAL BASAL CELL CARCINOMA

Top: There is a lack of peripheral palisading. The cells have pale cytoplasm and relatively enlarged nuclei.

Bottom: High-power view of another lesion shows cytologic details.

often more elongated than those in nodulocystic BCC, and the stroma is variably fibroblastic (fig. 1-87). It has been suggested that metatypical BCC is cytologically intermediate between nodulocystic BCC and squamous cell carcinoma (286). Perineural and lymphatic permeation are more frequent in metatypical BCC than in other variants.

Unusual forms of BCC include a *clear cell type* (fig. 1-88) (270,332,355) and *BCC with granular cells* (271,291,328). Both are associated with the fibromyxoid stroma characteristic of other types of BCC. *Adamantinoid BCC* is composed of stellate rather than polygonal cells, enclosing amorphous, amphophilic intercellular material. These tumors resemble adamantinoma and ameloblastoma (315). "Dedifferentiated," or *carcinosarcomatous BCC* combines BCC with malignant mesenchymal tissues (see discussion of carcinosarcoma earlier in this chapter) (285,304,337). This form of clonal evolution probably does not affect the biologic behavior of BCC adversely, in contrast to what intuition might suggest.

BCC can arise in association with other lesions, including nevus sebaceus, congenital nevus, linear epidermal nevus, onchocercoma, and seborrheic keratosis. BCC-like changes in dermatofibroma most likely represent basaloid hyperplasia, perhaps a manifestation of "stromal induction." Several apparent examples of true BCC arising in association with dermatofibroma have been reported, however (295).

Conventional special stains are infrequently used in diagnosing BCC, but mucin stains can help identify both epithelial and stromal mucins, e.g., in adenoid tumors. Keratin-derived amyloid is identified with appropriate stains in those tumors that show a high level of apoptosis (297,317,333). Immunohistochemically, BCCs are cytokeratin positive, particularly for types 5, 14, and 17, a profile similar to that of normal basal keratinocytes and follicular epithelium (320, 360). Trichogenic tumors and squamous

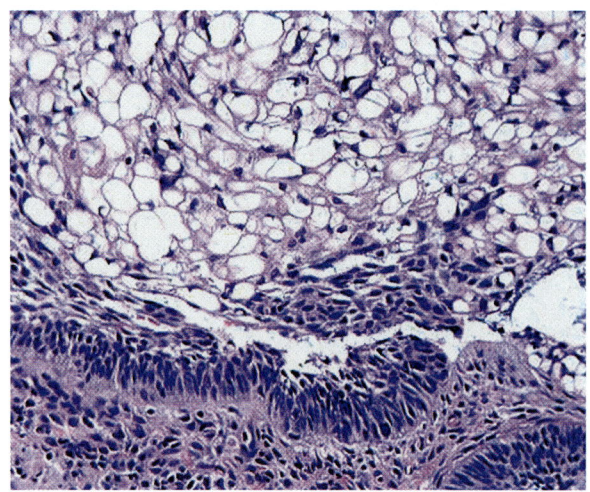

Figure 1-88

CLEAR CELL BASAL CELL CARCINOMA

The clear cells lack the multivacuolated appearance of the sebaceous cells seen in basosebaceous basal cell carcinoma.

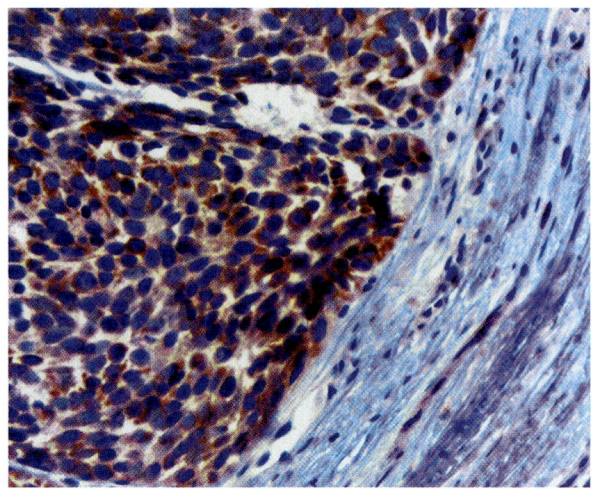

Figure 1-89

BASAL CELL CARCINOMA

Diffuse positivity for bcl-2 protein is seen.

cell carcinomas usually express a broader range of keratins. One might anticipate that these profiles could distinguish trichoepithelioma or small cell squamous cell carcinoma from BCC, but unfortunately that expectation has not been consistently realized. Other adnexal tumors of the skin also have a keratin profile similar to that of BCC (323,372).

Diffuse positivity has been demonstrated for the apoptosis inhibitor bcl-2 protein (326,330); this is a paradoxical result, given the obvious apoptosis seen in these tumors (fig. 1-89). The expression of bcl-2 varies among different types of BCC, however, being strong in superficial and nodular tumors, weak in infiltrative subtypes, and variable or intermediate in *micronodular* lesions (339). BerEP4, an antibody that recognizes a cell membrane glycoprotein, is uniformly positive in BCC (fig. 1-90) (358). On the other hand, CD44, a participant in intercellular adhesion, is absent in BCC but present in cutaneous squamous cell carcinomas (371). Some BCCs are positive for the neuroendocrine markers CD56, chromogranin, and synaptophysin. In one study, neuroendocrine differentiation was confirmed by reverse transcriptase polymerase chain reaction (RT-PCR) for chromogranin-A (281). Smooth muscle (alpha-isoform) actin expression is seen in some BCCs, particularly the micro-

nodular and morpheaform types; actin is involved in cellular motility and may be a marker of aggressive biologic potential in these tumors (280). Positive results are also observed in BCC with stains for transferrin receptor proteins (292), beta-2 microglobulin, proliferating cell nuclear antigen (293), and Ki-67; at present, these have limited practical diagnostic importance.

Variable reactivity has been obtained for p63 protein. In one study that used antibody 4A4 raised against six p63 isoforms, all BCCs were immunopositive (341). However, in another evaluation of chronic ulcerative stomatitis protein (CUSP), the most abundant cutaneous isoform of p63, CUSP was frequently undetectable in BCC using immunofluorescence detection. That was true even though CUSP-mRNA and its translated protein were found in the study cases using Northern and Western blot analyses (287).

Matrix metalloproteinases (MMP) have been implicated in cancer growth and metastasis. One of these, stromelysin-3, is expressed in the dermal fibroblasts surrounding some BCCs, with a particularly high frequency in morpheaform and deeply invasive tumors (282). Another, MMP-19, is expressed in proliferative epidermal cells but is downregulated in invasive tumor cell islands of BCC (302).

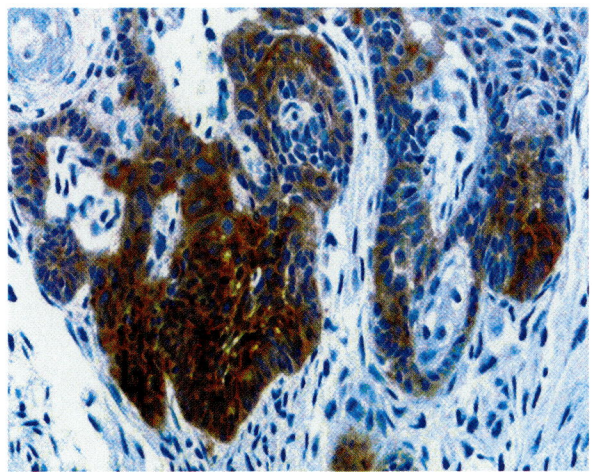

Figure 1-90
BASAL CELL CARCINOMA
Staining is positive for BerEP4.

Electron microscopy shows a heterogeneous population of tumor cells that vary considerably in their content of intracytoplasmic organelles (303). Ishibashi et al. (303) suggested that amorphous granular material within the rough endoplasmic reticulum of BCC cells may correlate with the presence of extracellular mucopolysaccharide around these tumors. Filaments with the characteristics of amyloid have been identified in the stroma of BCCs (297). In accord with the occasional ability to demonstrate neuroendocrine differentiation by immunohistochemistry, ultrastructural examination has shown neurosecretory granules in the cytoplasm of some BCC cells (284).

Differential Diagnosis. The differential diagnosis of BCC includes cutaneous adnexal tumors with follicular, sebaceous, or sweat glandular differentiation, as well as certain types of squamous cell carcinoma. Trichoepitheliomas (including classic and variant forms), which are composed of cellular lobules of similar size, usually exhibit a more organoid growth pattern than that of BCC. Broad connections to the epidermis are uncommon in dermal hair sheath tumors, including trichoepithelioma, but they are regularly present in cases of BCC. The fibrous matrix of trichoepithelioma has a different appearance from the fibromyxoid stroma of BCC, and stromal retraction is not a prominent feature. It has been reported that immunostains for bcl-2 protein and CD34 (human hematopoietic progenitor cell antigen) are capable of distinguishing between BCC and trichoepithelioma, because bcl-2 is preferentially expressed diffusely in the tumor cells of BCC, and CD34 is localized to the stroma immediately adjacent to the cellular lobules of trichoepithelioma (309,326). Our laboratory, however, has been unable to confirm those findings, and we have observed substantial overlap in the immunophenotypes of these two lesions (357). There are certainly times when a clear-cut distinction between BCC and trichoepithelioma is difficult or impossible to discern. This is particularly the case among isolated lesions in older adults in the absence of a known predisposing clinical syndrome, such as with the epithelioma adenoides cysticum complex. When the differential diagnosis revolves around BCC and trichoepithelioma, we favor rendering a "default" interpretation of BCC. That approach assures the patient of receiving optimal therapy for the more aggressive of the two lesions.

One particular subtype of trichoepithelioma, desmoplastic trichoepithelioma, usually can be distinguished from morpheaform BCC in excisional biopsies because of the striking differences in overall tumor image. Desmoplastic trichoepithelioma shows a plate-like, circumscribed configuration in the dermis that usually includes overlying epidermal hyperplasia, horn cysts, and blunt-ended narrow strands of basaloid cells with an absence of irregularly expansile cell nests. Desmoplastic trichoepithelioma also occurs in a younger patient population than is typical for morpheaform BCC (278), and unlike the latter lesion, it is epithelial membrane antigen positive. In one recent study, stromelysin-3 was found in the stromal cells surrounding islands of morpheaform BCC in 68 percent of cases, but was absent in all examples of desmoplastic trichoepithelioma (359).

Basaloid follicular hamartoma is another follicular proliferation that has some histopathologic similarities to trichoepithelioma, organoid BCC, and fibroepitheliomatous BCC (Pinkus tumor). It may be seen as an autosomal dominant disorder, manifesting as multiple 1 to 2 mm, smooth papular lesions on the face, or as a unifocal sporadic lesion (277). The cells of basaloid follicular hamartoma are somewhat larger than those of conventional trichoepithelioma or comparable BCC variants. They have a more distinctly squamoid appearance and assume a more prominent anastomosing growth pattern, with interspersed horn cysts. Pigmented variants of this lesion also occur. Immunohistochemical staining for proliferating cell nuclear antigen and Ki-67 is more limited in these tumors than is the case in BCC (306). Nevertheless, in small biopsies, or when there is incomplete clinical information, a distinction from BCC may be difficult or impossible. In such cases, diagnostic preference should again be given to BCC, although we commonly mention the possibility of basaloid follicular hamartoma in an accompanying note.

Basaloid sebaceous carcinoma must be distinguished from the basosebaceous type of BCC. This distinction is largely based on assessment of the differentiated sebocytes in each lesion. BCC with sebaceous features contains easily found clusters of well-developed sebaceous cells that are typically, but not invariably, located towards the center of tumor cell islands. In contrast, basaloid sebaceous carcinoma shows very few, if any, mature sebocytes, and these have a random distribution throughout the tumor mass. Unfortunately, both tumors have the capacity for nuclear palisading (370). Pagetoid involvement of the epidermis favors an interpretation of sebaceous carcinoma, but this change is not invariably present. The diagnosis may be aided by lipid stains done on frozen sections or immunostains for epithelial membrane antigen: sebaceous carcinomas show diffuse positivity with both methods (344,367), whereas basosebaceous BCCs are reactive only in areas of obvious sebaceous differentiation. Ultrastructural studies reveal the widespread presence of intracytoplasmic lipid droplets only in sebaceous carcinoma (370).

Basaloid variants of sweat gland carcinoma usually lack the epidermal connections that are evident in adenoid BCC. Still, the distinction between these entities can be extremely challenging; for example, several reported examples of "eccrine" BCC actually appear to represent true adenoid cystic carcinoma. Sweat gland carcinomas do not manifest the fibromyxoid stroma or matrical retraction artifact of BCC. The finding of even a few melaninized cells or rudimentary foci of pilar keratinization in an adenoid basal cell tumor argues strongly against the diagnosis of a sudoriferous carcinoma. Immunostains for carcinoembryonic antigen and epithelial membrane antigen are also helpful, because they are consistently positive in sweat gland carcinoma and negative in BCC (367,369). Mino et al. (324) have recently found significantly less c-kit (CD117) expression in BCC than in adenoid cystic carcinoma (324), and our experience has confirmed the value of that marker in separating the two lesions diagnostically. On ultrastructural examination, glandular (microvillous) differentiation is seen in sweat gland tumors but not in BCC.

Small cell (basaloid) squamous cell carcinoma (SCSCC) shows a lesser degree of nuclear palisading than BCC, and typically lacks a fibromyxoid stroma. Tumor cell nuclei in SCSCC are vesicular with prominent nucleoli, as opposed to the generally compact, anucleolated forms of BCC (368). The distinction between basaloid squamous cell carcinoma and BCC is particularly important in the perianal skin, where true BCC must be differentiated from "cloacogenic" carcinoma. The latter tumor is highly aggressive as compared to BCC. When confronting this diagnostic dilemma, immunostaining for BerEP4 can be helpful because of the strong, diffuse expression of this antigen in BCC and consistently negative results in squamous cell carcinomas (358).

Clear cell BCC can mimic a variety of other tumors, including balloon cell melanoma, trichilemmal carcinoma, sebaceous carcinoma, and clear cell eccrine tumors (356). The fibromyxoid stroma of BCC is usually distinctive. In addition, the lack of intracytoplasmic compartmentalization in clear cell BCC differs from the multivacuolated appearance of the tumor cells in sebaceous carcinoma. Granular cell BCC can be distinguished from true granular cell tumor not only by its typical fibromyxoid stroma but also by its cytokeratin positivity. A variant of BCC with central nuclear palisading may resemble schwannoma; however, peripheral palisading of tumor cell nuclei and stromal retraction are usually also present, and in contrast to true schwannoma, the tumor cells are cytokeratin positive and S-100 protein negative (348).

REFERENCES

Epithelial Cysts

1. Ahn SK, Chung J, Lee WS, Lee SH, Choi EH. Hybrid cysts showing alternate combination of eruptive vellus hair cyst, steatocystoma multiplex, and epidermoid cyst, and an association among the three conditions. Am J Dermatopathol 1996;18:645–9.
2. Ambiavagar PC, Rosen Y. Cutaneous ciliated cyst of the chin. Probable bronchogenic cyst. Arch Dermatol 1979;115:895–6.
3. Asarch RG, Golitz LE, Sausker WF, Kreye GM. Median raphe cysts of the penis. Arch Dermatol 1979;115:1084–6.
4. Ashfaq R, Molberg KH, Vuitch F. Cutaneous endometriosis as a diagnostic pitfall of fine needle aspiration biopsy. A report of three cases. Acta Cytol 1994;38:577–81.
5. Barkovich AJ, Vandermarck P, Edwards MS, Cogen PH. Congenital nasal masses: CT and MR imaging features in 16 cases. AJNR Am J Neuroradiol 1991;12:105–16.
6. Barr RJ, Headley JL, Jensen JL, Howell JB. Cutaneous keratocysts of nevoid basal cell carcinoma syndrome. J Am Acad Dermatol 1986;14:572–6.
7. Baselga E, Dzwierzynski WW, Neuburg M, Troy JL, Esterly NB. Cutaneous keratocyst in naevoid basal cell carcinoma syndrome. Br J Dermatol 1996;135:810–2.
8. Bengoechea-Beeby MP, Velasco-Oses A, Casado-Perez C. Multiple proliferating trichilemmal tumors and cysts involving the scalp: report of a case. J Oral Maxillofac Surg 1994;52:985–6.
9. Bhawan J, Dayal Y, Gonzalez-Serva A, Eisen R. Cutaneous metaplastic synovial cyst. J Cutan Pathol 1990;17:22–6.
10. Bovenmyer DA. Eruptive vellus hair cysts. Arch Dermatol 1979;115:338–9.
11. Bradley PJ. The complex nasal dermoid. Head Neck Surg 1983;5:469–73.
12. Brownstein MH. Hybrid cyst: a combined epidermoid and trichilemmal cyst. J Am Acad Dermatol 1983;9:872–5.
13. Brownstein MH, Arluk DJ. Proliferating trichilemmal cyst: a simulant of squamous cell carcinoma. Cancer 1981;48:1207–14.
14. Burns DA, Calnan CD. Eruptive vellus hair cysts. Clin Exp Dermatol 1981;6:209–13.
15. Clark JV. Ciliated epithelium in a cyst of the lower limb. J Pathol 1969;98:289–90.
16. Cole LA, Helwig EB. Mucoid cysts of the penile skin. J Urol 1976;115:397–400.
17. Cooper PH, Fechner RE. Pilomatricoma-like changes in the epidermal cysts of Gardner's syndrome. J Am Acad Dermatol 1983;8:639–44.
18. Covello SP, Smith FJ, Sillevis Smitt JH, et al. Keratin 17 mutations cause either steatocystoma multiplex or pachyonychia congenita type 2. Br J Dermatol 1998;139:475–80.
19. Dore N, Landry M, Cadotte M, Schurch W. Cutaneous endosalpingiosis. Arch Dermatol 1980;116:909–12.
20. Egawa K, Honda Y, Inaba Y, Ono T, De Villiers EM. Detection of human papillomaviruses and eccrine ducts in palmoplantar epidermoid cysts. Br J Dermatol 1995;132:533–42.
21. Elston DM, Parker LU, Tuthill RJ. Epidermoid cyst of the scalp containing human papillomavirus. J Cutan Pathol 1993;20:184–6.
22. Esterly NB, Fretzin DF, Pinkus H. Eruptive vellus hair cysts. Arch Dermatol 1977;113:500–3.
23. Farmer ER, Helwig EB. Cutaneous ciliated cysts. Arch Dermatol 1978;114:70–3.
24. Fawcett DW, Porter KR. A study of the fine structure of ciliated epithelia. J Morphol 1954;94:221–81.
25. Fetissof F, Lorette G, Dubois MP, Philippe A, Tharanne MJ, Jobard P. Endocrine cells in median raphe cysts of the penis. Pathol Res Pract 1985;180:644–6.
26. Fraga S, Helwig EB, Rosen SH. Bronchogenic cysts in the skin and subcutaneous tissue. Am J Clin Pathol 1971;56:230–8.
27. Giustini S, Amorosi B, Canci C, et al. Pachyonychia congenita with steatocystoma multiplex. A report of two cases and a discussion of the classification. Eur J Dermatol 1998;8:158–60.
28. Gonzalez JG, Ghiselli RW, Santa Cruz DJ. Synovial metaplasia of the skin. Am J Surg Pathol 1987;11:343–50.
29. Gruenwald P. Origin of endometriosis from the mesenchyme of the coelomic walls. Am J Obstet Gynecol 1942;44:470–4.
30. Hashimoto K, Gross BG, Lever WF. The ultrastructure of human embryo skin. II. The formation of intradermal portion of the eccrine sweat duct and of the secretory segment during the first half of embryonic life. J Invest Dermatol 1966;46:513–29.
31. Hejazi N. Umbilical polyp: a report of two cases. Dermatologica 1975;150:111–5.
32. Hendricks DL, Liang MD, Borochovitz D, Miller T. A case of multiple pilar tumors and pilar cysts involving the scalp and back. Plast Reconstr Surg 1991;87:763–7.

33. Hess K. Ueber eine subcutane flimmercyste. Beitr Pathol 1890;8:98.
34. Hohl D. Steatocystoma multiplex and oligosymptomatic pachyonychia congenita of the Jackson-Sertoli type. Dermatology 1997;195:86–8.
35. Hurlimann AF, Panizzon RG, Burg G. Eruptive vellus hair cyst and steatocystoma multiplex: hybrid cysts. Dermatology 1996;192:64–6.
36. Iglesias Zamora ME, Vazquez-Doval FJ. Epidermal naevi associated with trichilemmal cysts and chromosomal mosaicism. Br J Dermatol 1997;137:821–4.
37. Kang IK, Kim YJ, Choi KC. Ciliated cyst of the vulva. J Am Acad Dermatol 1995;32:514–5.
38. Kashima M, Adachi M, Honda M, Niimura M, Nakabayashi Y. A case of peculiar plantar warts. Human papillomavirus type 60 infection. Arch Dermatol 1994;130:1418–20.
39. Kawase M, Honda M, Niimura M. Detection of human papillomavirus type 60 in plantar cysts and verruca plantaris by the in situ hybridization method using digoxigenin labeled probes. J Dermatol 1994;21:709–15.
40. Kersten RC. The eyelid crease approach to superficial lateral dermoid cysts. J Pediatr Ophthalmol Strabismus 1988;25:48–51.
41. Kiene P, Hauschild A, Christophers E. Eruptive vellus hair cysts and steatocystoma multiplex. Variants of one entity? Br J Dermatol 1996;134:365–7.
42. Kim JU, Nogita T, Terajima S, Kawashima M. Pachyonychia congenita associated with steatocystoma multiplex. J Dermatol 1998;25:479–81.
43. Kimura S. Trichilemmal cysts. Ultrastructural similarities to the trichilemmal sac. Dermatologica 1978;157:164–70.
44. Kimura T, Miyazawa H, Aoyagi T, Ackerman AB. Folliculosebaceous cystic hamartoma. A distinctive malformation of the skin. Am J Dermatopathol 1991;13:213–20.
45. Kitasato H, Egawa K, Honda Y, Ono T, Mizushima Y, Kawai S. A putative human papillomavirus type 57 new subtype isolated from plantar epidermoid cysts without intracytoplasmic inclusion bodies. J Gen Virol 1998;79(Pt 8):1977–81.
46. Komuro Y, Takedai T, Tagawa K. Proliferating trichilemmal tumor on the dorsum of the hand. Ann Plast Surg 1995;34:657–9.
47. Kondoh S, Taniki T, Umemoto A, et al. [A case of umbilical polyp with aberrant pancreas and small intestinal mucosa—analysis of cases of umbilical polyp reported in Japan.] Nippon Geka Gakkai Zasshi 1994;95:786–9. (Japanese.)
48. Kutin ND, Allen JE, Jewett TC. The umbilical polyp. J Pediatr Surg 1979;14:741–4.
49. Larralde de Luna M, Cicioni V, Herrera A, Casas JG, Magnin PH. Umbilical polyps. Pediatr Dermatol 1987;4:341–3.
50. Leppard BJ, Bussey HJ. Gardner's syndrome with epidermoid cysts showing features of pilomatrixomas. Clin Exp Dermatol 1976;1:75–82.
51. Leppard BJ, Sanderson KV. The natural history of trichilemmal cysts. Br J Dermatol 1976;94:379–90.
52. Mehregan AH, Medenica M. Pigmented follicular cysts. J Cutan Pathol 1982;9:423–7.
53. Michal M, Bisceglia M, Di Mattia A, et al. Gigantic cutaneous horns of the scalp: lesions with a gross similarity to the horns of animals: a report of four cases. Am J Surg Pathol 2002;26:789–94.
54. Moon SE, Lee YS, Youn JI. Eruptive vellus hair cyst and steatocystoma multiplex in a patient with pachyonychia congenita. J Am Acad Dermatol 1994;30(Pt 1):275–6.
55. Moreno A, Muns R. A cystic teratoma in skin. Am J Dermatopathol 1985;7:383–6.
56. Mori O, Hachisuka H, Sasai Y. Proliferating trichilemmal cyst with spindle cell carcinoma. Am J Dermatopathol 1990;12:479–84.
57. Narisawa Y, Kohda H. Cutaneous cysts of Gardner's syndrome are similar to follicular stem cells. J Cutan Pathol 1995;22:115–21.
58. Newland JR, Fusaro RM. Mucinous cysts of the vulva. Nebr Med J 1991;76:307–10.
59. Nieto S, Buezo GF, Jones-Caballero M, Fraga J. Cutaneous metaplastic synovial cyst in an Ehlers-Danlos patient. Am J Dermatopathol 1997;19: 407–10.
60. Ninomiya T, Hosaka M, Higashiyama H, Kurenuma S, Mori M. Branchial cleft cysts. Histologic and immunohistochemical aspects. Acta Histochem 1989;85:143–53.
61. Oguzkurt P, Kotiloglu E, Tanyel FC, Hicsonmez A. Umbilical polyp originating from urachal remnants. Turk J Pediatr 1996;38:371–4.
62. Patterson JW. Infundibular and trichilemmal keratinization of a pilar tumor. Cutis 1985;36:330–2.
63. Patterson JW, Pittman DL, Rich JD. Presternal ciliated cyst. Arch Dermatol 1984;120:240–2.
64. Perwein E, Maciejewski W. [Proliferating epidermal cysts.] Hautarzt 1986;37:102–6. (German.)
65. Piecuch JF, Eisenberg E, Segal D, Carlson R. Respiratory epithelium as an integral part of an odontogenic keratocyst: report of case. J Oral Surg 1980;38:445–7.
66. Reis MD, Tellechea O, Baptista AP. Verrucous cyst. Eur J Dermatol 1998;8:186–8.
67. Richard-Lallemand MA, Choux R, Szekeres G, Bacquie N, Chamlian A, Bonerandi JJ. [Immunohistochemical characterization of a median raphe cyst of the penis.] Ann Pathol 1994;14:174–6. (French.)

68. Robboy SJ, Ross JS, Prat J, Keh PC, Welch WR. Urogenital sinus origin of mucinous and ciliated cysts of the vulva. Obstet Gynecol 1978;51:347–51.
69. Romani J, Barnadas MA, Miralles J, Curell R, de Moragas JM. Median raphe cyst of the penis with ciliated cells. J Cutan Pathol 1995;22:378–81.
70. Rutten A, Wenzel P, Goos M. [Gardner syndrome with pilomatrixoma-like hair follicle cysts.] Hautarzt 1990;41:326–8. (German.)
71. Sakamoto F, Ito M, Nakamura A, Sato Y. Proliferating trichilemmal cyst with apocrine-acrosyringeal and sebaceous differentiation. J Cutan Pathol 1991;18:137–41.
72. Salopek TG, Lee SK, Jimbow K. Multiple pigmented follicular cysts: a subtype of multiple pilosebaceous cysts. Br J Dermatol 1996;134:758–62.
73. Sandoval R, Urbina F. Pigmented follicular cyst. Br J Dermatol 1994;131:130–1.
74. Sanusi ID, Carrington PR, Adams DN. Cervical thymic cyst. Arch Dermatol 1982;118:122–4.
75. Sau P, Graham JH. The diagnosis is proliferating epidermoid cyst. Mil Med 1983;148:818, 20–2.
76. Sau P, Graham JH, Helwig EB. Proliferating epithelial cysts. Clinicopathological analysis of 96 cases. J Cutan Pathol 1995;22:394–406.
77. Scelwyn M. Median raphe cyst of the perineum presenting as a perianal polyp. Pathology 1996;28:201–2.
78. Shapira A, Porat M, Ophir D. [Thyroglossal duct cyst.] Harefuah 1989;116:138–9. (Hebrew.)
79. Shibagaki N, Ohtake N, Furue M. Spontaneous regression of congenital multiple median raphe cysts of the raphe scroti. Br J Dermatol 1996;134:376–8.
80. Sickel JZ. Cutaneous ciliated cyst of the scalp. A case report with immunohistochemical evidence for estrogen and progesterone receptors. Am J Dermatopathol 1994;16:76–9.
81. Siders D, Parrott MH, Abell MR. Gland cell prosoplasia (adenosis) of vagina. Am J Obstet Gynecol 1965;91:190–203.
82. Singh SR, Ma AS, Dixon A. Multiple cutaneous metaplastic synovial cysts. J Am Acad Dermatol 1999;41(pt 2):330–2.
83. Sleater J, Beers B, Stefan M, Kilpatrick T, Hendricks J. Proliferating trichilemmal cyst. Report of four cases, two with nondiploid DNA content and increased proliferation index. Am J Dermatopathol 1993;15:423–8.
84. Smith FJ, Corden LD, Rugg EL, et al. Missense mutations in keratin 17 cause either pachyonychia congenita type 2 or a phenotype resembling steatocystoma multiplex. J Invest Dermatol 1997;108:220–3.
85. Soyer HP, Schadendorf D, Cerroni L, Kerl H. Verrucous cysts: histopathologic characterization and molecular detection of human papillomavirus-specific DNA. J Cutan Pathol 1993;20:411–7.
86. Steck WD, Helwig EB. Cutaneous endometriosis. Clin Obstet Gynecol 1966;9:373–83.
87. Stiefler RE, Bergfeld WF. Eruptive vellus hair cysts—an inherited disorder. J Am Acad Dermatol 1980;3:425–9.
88. Tachibana T, Sakamoto F, Ito M, Ito K, Kaneko Y, Takenouchi T. Cutaneous ciliated cyst: a case report and histochemical, immunohistochemical, and ultrastructural study. J Cutan Pathol 1995;22:33–7.
89. Takata M, Rehman I, Rees JL. A trichilemmal carcinoma arising from a proliferating trichilemmal cyst: the loss of the wild-type p53 is a critical event in malignant transformation. Hum Pathol 1998;29:193–5.
90. Tidman MJ, MacDonald DM. Cutaneous endometriosis: a histopathologic study. J Am Acad Dermatol 1988;18(Pt 1):373–7.
91. Tomkova H, Fujimoto W, Arata J. Expression of keratins (K10 and K17) in steatocystoma multiplex, eruptive vellus hair cysts, and epidermoid and trichilemmal cysts. Am J Dermatopathol 1997;19:250–3.
92. Tresser NJ, Dahms B, Berner JJ. Cutaneous bronchogenic cyst of the back: a case report and review of the literature. Pediatr Pathol 1994;14:207–12.
93. Trotter SE, Rassl DM, Saad M, Sharif H, Ali M. Cutaneous ciliated cyst occurring in a male. Histopathology 1994;25:492–3.
94. Tsai TF, Chuan MT, Hsiao CH. A cystic teratoma of the skin. Histopathology 1996;29:384–6.
95. Tsuruta D, Nakagawa K, Taniguchi S, Kobayashi H, Hamada T, Ishii M. Combined cutaneous hamartoma encompassing benign melanocytic naevus, vellus hair cyst and epidermoid cyst. Clin Exp Dermatol 2000;25:38–40.
96. Urano Y, Oura H, Sakaki A, et al. Immunohistological analysis of P53 expression in human skin tumors. J Dermatol Sci 1992;4:69–75.
97. Wick MR, Swanson PE. Cutaneous adnexal tumors: a guide to pathologic diagnosis. Chicago: ASCP Press; 1991:117–8, 24–25.
98. Yamaguchi J, Irimajiri T, Ohara K. Proliferating trichilemmal cyst arising in the arm of a young woman. Dermatology 1994;189:90–2.
99. Zappi E, Berry RS. Cutaneous remnants of the omphalomesenteric duct. Arch Dermatol 1983;119:538–9.

Benign Epidermal Tumors
100. Akiyama M, Hayakawa K, Watanabe Y, Nishikawa T. Lectin-binding sites in clear cell acanthoma. J Cutan Pathol 1990;17:197–201.

101. Anneroth A, Isacsson G. Warty dyskeratoma. Acta Derm Venereol 1975;55:227–32.
102. Argenyi ZB, Huston BM, Argenyi EE, Maillet MW, Hurt MA. Large-cell acanthoma of the skin. A study by image analysis cytometry and immunohistochemistry. Am J Dermatopathol 1994;16:140–4.
103. Azuma Y, Matsukawa A. Warty dyskeratoma with multiple lesions. J Dermatol 1993;20:374–7.
104. Baran R, Perrin C. Focal subungual warty dyskeratoma. Dermatology 1997;195:278–80.
105. Bernard BA, Reano A, Darmon YM, Thivolet J. Precocious appearance of involucrin and epidermal transglutaminase during differentiation of psoriatic skin. Br J Dermatol 1986;114:279–83.
106. Brownstein MH. Acantholytic acanthoma. J Am Acad Dermatol 1988;19(Pt 1):783–6.
107. Calandra P, Lattanzi M. [Warty dyskeratoma. Analysis and case reports.] Minerva Med 1978; 69:1551–9. (Italian.)
108. Cascajo CD, Reichel M, Sanchez JL. Malignant neoplasms associated with seborrheic keratoses. An analysis of 54 cases. Am J Dermatopathol 1996;18:278–82.
109. Chorzelski TP, Kudejko J, Jablonska S. Is papular acantholytic dyskeratosis of the vulva a new entity? Am J Dermatopathol 1984;6:557–60.
110. Coppola G, Muscardin LM, Piazza P. Papular acantholytic dyskeratosis. Am J Dermatopathol 1986;8:364–5.
111. D'Souza M, Gharami R, Ratnakar C, Garg BR. Unilateral nevoid hyperkeratosis of the nipple and areola. Int J Dermatol 1996;35:602–3.
112. Degos R, Civatte J. Clear-cell acanthoma. Experience of 8 years. Br J Dermatol 1970;83: 248–54.
113. Demetree JW, Lang PG, St Clair JT. Unilateral, linear, zosteriform epidermal nevus with acantholytic dyskeratosis. Arch Dermatol 1979;115: 875–7.
114. Dudley K, Barr WG, Armin A, Massa MC. Nevus comedonicus in association with widespread, well-differentiated follicular tumors. J Am Acad Dermatol 1986;15(Pt 2):1123–7.
115. Fine RM, Chernosky ME. Clinical recognition of clear-cell acanthoma (Degos'). Arch Dermatol 1969;100:559–63.
116. Flegel H. Hyperkeratosis lenticularis perstans. Hautarzt 1958;9:362–4.
117. Griffiths TW, Hashimoto K, Sharata HH, Ellis CN. Multiple warty dyskeratomas of the scalp. Clin Exp Dermatol 1997;22:189–91.
118. Happle R. How many epidermal nevus syndromes exist? A clinicogenetic classification. J Am Acad Dermatol 1991;25:550–6.
119. Hashimoto T, Inamoto N, Nakamura K, Harada R. Involucrin expression in skin appendage tumours. Br J Dermatol 1987;117:325–32.
120. Innocenzi D, Barduagni F, Cerio R, Wolter M. Disseminated eruptive clear cell acanthoma— a case report with review of the literature. Clin Exp Dermatol 1994;19:249–53.
121. Ito M, Shimizu N, Fujiwara H, Maruyama T, Tezuka M. Histopathogenesis of inflammatory linear verrucose epidermal naevus: histochemistry, immunohistochemistry and ultrastructure. Arch Dermatol Res 1991;283:491–9.
122. Jones EW, Wells GC. Degos' acanthoma (acanthome a cellules claires). A clinical and histological report of nine cases. Arch Dermatol 1966;94:286–94.
123. Kim YC, Bang D, Cinn YW. Clear cell papulosis: case report and literature review. Pediatr Dermatol 1997;14:380–2.
124. Kuo TT, Chan HL, Hsueh S. Clear cell papulosis of the skin. A new entity with histogenetic implications for cutaneous Paget's disease. Am J Surg Pathol 1987;11:827–34.
125. Kuo TT, Huang CL, Chan HL, Yang LJ, Chen MJ. Clear cell papulosis: report of three cases of a newly recognized disease. J Am Acad Dermatol 1995;33(Pt 1):230–3.
126. Langer K, Wuketich S, Konrad K. Pigmented clear cell acanthoma. Am J Dermatopathol 1994;16:134–9.
127. Lee JY, Chao SC. Clear cell papulosis of the skin. Br J Dermatol 1998;138:678–83.
128. Lund HZ. The nosologic position of inverted follicular keratosis is still unsettled. Am J Dermatopathol 1983;5:443–5.
129. Lupton GP, Graham, JH. Clear cell acanthoma. J Cutan Pathol 1986;13:85.
130. Mikhail GR, Mehregan AH. Basal cell carcinoma in seborrheic keratosis. J Am Acad Dermatol 1982;6(Pt 1):500–6.
131. Miyamoto Y, Ueda K, Sato M, Yasuno H. Disseminated epidermolytic acanthoma. J Cutan Pathol 1979;6:272–9.
132. Neville BW, Coleman PJ, Richardson MS. Verruciform xanthoma associated with an intraoral warty dyskeratoma. Oral Surg Oral Med Oral Pathol Oral Radiol Endod 1996;81:3–4.
133. Okan G, Baykal C. Nevoid hyperkeratosis of the nipple and areola: treatment with topical retinoic acid. J Eur Acad Dermatol Venereol 1999;13:218–20.
134. Penneys NS, Nadji M, Ziegels-Weissman J. Clear cell acanthoma: not of sweat gland origin. Acta Derm Venereol 1981;61:569–70.
135. Rabinowitz AD. Multiple large cell acanthomas. J Am Acad Dermatol 1983;8:840–5.

136. Roewert HJ, Ackerman AB. Large-cell acanthoma is a solar lentigo. Am J Dermatopathol 1992;14:122–32.
137. Sanchez Yus E, de Diego V, Urrutia S. Large cell acanthoma. A cytologic variant of Bowen's disease? Am J Dermatopathol 1988;10:197–208.
138. Sanchez Yus E, del Rio E, Requena L. Large-cell acanthoma is a distinctive condition. Am J Dermatopathol 1992;14:140–7; discussion 148.
139. Schlappner OL, Rowden G, Philips TM, Rahim Z. Melanoacanthoma. Ultrastructural and immunological studies. J Cutan Pathol 1978;5:127–41.
140. Schwartz RA. Sign of Leser-Trelat. J Am Acad Dermatol 1996;35:88–95.
141. Shapiro L, Baraf CS. Isolated epidermolytic acanthoma. A solitary tumor showing granular degeneration. Arch Dermatol 1970;101:220–3.
142. Solomon LM. Hemangiomas in the epidermal nevus syndrome. Mod Probl Paediatr 1976;20:38–9.
143. Solomon LM, Fretzin DF, Dewald RL. The epidermal nevus syndrome. Arch Dermatol 1968;97:273–85.
144. Starink TM, Woerdeman MJ. Unilateral systematized keratosis follicularis. A variant of Darier's disease or an epidermal naevus (acantholytic dyskeratotic epidermal naevus)? Br J Dermatol 1981;105:207–14.
145. Submoke S, Piamphongsant T. Clinico-histopathological study of epidermal naevi. Australas J Dermatol 1983;24:130–6.
146. Szymanski FJ. Warty dyskeratoma, a benign cutaneous tumor resembling Darier's disease microscopically. Arch Dermatol 1957;75:567–72.
147. Tanay A, Mehregan AH. Warty dyskeratoma. Dermatologica 1969;138:155–64.
148. Tomich CE, Burkes EJ. Warty dyskeratoma (isolated dyskeratosis follicularis) of the oral mucosa. Oral Surg Oral Med Oral Pathol 1971;31:798–807.
149. Trau H, Fisher BK, Schewach-Millet M. Multiple clear cell acanthomas. Arch Dermatol 1980;116:433–4.
150. Wells GC, Wilson-Jones E. Degos' acanthoma (acanthome a cellules claires). A report of five cases with particular reference to the histochemistry. Br J Dermatol 1967;79:249–58.
151. Yap WM, Tan PH, Ong BH. Malignancy arising in seborrheic keratosis: a report of two cases. Ann Acad Med Singapore 1997;26:235–7.
152. Zhu WY, Leonardi C, Penneys NS. Detection of human papillomavirus DNA in seborrheic keratosis by polymerase chain reaction. J Dermatol Sci 1992;4:166–71.

Premalignant and Malignant Epidermal Tumors

153. Abell E, Read SI. Porokeratotic eccrine ostial and dermal duct naevus. Br J Dermatol 1980;103:435–41.
154. Ackerman AB, Reed RJ. Epidermolytic variant of solar keratosis. Arch Dermatol 1973;107:104–6.
155. Ahmed NU, Ueda M, Ichihashi M. Increased level of c-erbB-2/neu/HER-2 protein in cutaneous squamous cell carcinoma. Br J Dermatol 1997;136:908–12.
156. Alyahya GA, Heegaard S, Prause JU. Malignant changes in a giant orbital keratoacanthoma developing over 25 years. Acta Ophthalmol Scand 2000;78:223–5.
157. Banks ER, Cooper PH. Adenosquamous carcinoma of the skin: a report of 10 cases. J Cutan Pathol 1991;18:227–34.
158. Bart RS. Bowenoid papulosis of the chin. J Dermatol Surg Oncol 1984;10:821–3.
159. Beham A, Regauer S, Soyer HP, Beham-Schmid C. Keratoacanthoma: a clinically distinct variant of well differentiated squamous cell carcinoma. Adv Anat Pathol 1998;5:269–80.
160. Biernat W, Kordek R, Liberski PP, Wozniak L. Carcinosarcoma of the skin. Case report and literature review. Am J Dermatopathol 1996;18:614–9.
161. Bito T, Ueda M, Ito A, Ichihashi M. Less expression of cyclin E in cutaneous squamous cell carcinomas than in benign and premalignant keratinocytic lesions. J Cutan Pathol 1997;24:305–8.
162. Bloch PH. Transformation of seborrheic keratosis into Bowen's disease. J Cutan Pathol 1978;5:361–7.
163. Bohmer B, Hamm H, Jackisch C, Bonsmann G. [Cervix cancer in HPV16-associated Bowenoid papulosis]. Geburtshilfe Frauenheilkd 1992;52:438–41. (German.)
164. Braun-Falco O, Schmoeckel C, Geyer C. [Pigmented actinic keratoses.] Hautarzt 1986;37:676–8. (German.)
165. Breuninger H, Schaumburg-Lever G, Holzschuh J, Horny HP. Desmoplastic squamous cell carcinoma of skin and vermilion surface: a highly malignant subtype of skin cancer. Cancer 1997;79:915–9.
166. Brown TJ, Tschen JA. Primary carcinosarcoma of the skin: report of a case and review of the literature. Dermatol Surg 1999;25:498–500.
167. Cain CT, Niemann TH, Argenyi ZB. Keratoacanthoma versus squamous cell carcinoma. An immunohistochemical reappraisal of p53 protein and proliferating cell nuclear antigen expression in keratoacanthoma-like tumors. Am J Dermatopathol 1995;17:324–31.

168. Carapeto FJ, Garcia-Perez A. Acantholytic keratosis. Dermatologica 1974;148:233–9.
169. Cockerell CJ. Histopathology of incipient intraepidermal squamous cell carcinoma ("actinic keratosis"). J Am Acad Dermatol 2000;42 (Pt 2):11–7.
170. Cramer SF, Heggeness LM. Signet-ring squamous cell carcinoma. Am J Clin Pathol 1989; 91:488–91.
171. Cuesta KH, Palazzo JP, Mittal KR. Detection of human papillomavirus in verrucous carcinoma from HIV-seropositive patients. J Cutan Pathol 1998;25:165–70.
172. Davis-Daneshfar A, Trueb RM. Bowen's disease of the glans penis (erythroplasia of Queyrat) in plasma cell balanitis. Cutis 2000;65:395–8.
173. de Belilovsky C, Lessana-Leibowitch M. [Bowen's disease and bowenoid papulosis: comparative clinical, viral, and disease progression aspects.] Contracept Fertil Sex 1993;21:231–6. (French.)
174. Dinehart SM, Nelson-Adesokan P, Cockerell C, Russell S, Brown R. Metastatic cutaneous squamous cell carcinoma derived from actinic keratosis. Cancer 1997;79:920–3.
175. Eisen RF, Bhawan J, Cahn TH. Spontaneous regression of bowenoid papulosis of the penis. Cutis 1983;32:269–72.
176. Escalonilla P, Grilli R, Canamero M, et al. Sebaceous carcinoma of the vulva. Am J Dermatopathol 1999;21:468–72.
177. Farmer ER, Helwig EB. Metastatic basal cell carcinoma: a clinicopathologic study of seventeen cases. Cancer 1980;46:748–57.
178. Ferlicot S, Plantier F, Rethers L, Bui AD, Wechsler J. Lymphoepithelioma-like carcinoma of the skin: a report of 3 Epstein-Barr virus (EBV)-negative additional cases. Immunohistochemical study of the stroma reaction. J Cutan Pathol 2000;27:306–11.
179. Fernandez-Figueras MT, Fuente MJ, Bielsa I, Ferrandiz C. Low-grade mucoepidermoid carcinoma on the vermilion border of the lip. Am J Dermatopathol 1997;19:197–201.
180. Friedman KJ. Low-grade primary cutaneous adenosquamous (mucoepidermoid) carcinoma. Report of a case and review of the literature. Am J Dermatopathol 1989;11:43–50.
181. Frierson HF Jr, Cooper PH. Prognostic factors in squamous cell carcinoma of the lower lip. Hum Pathol 1986;17:346–54.
182. Fukamizu H, Inoue K, Matsumoto K, Okayama H, Moriguchi T. Metastatic squamous-cell carcinomas derived from solar keratosis. J Dermatol Surg Oncol 1985;11:518–22.
183. Gassenmaier A, Pfister H, Hornstein OP. Human papillomavirus 25-related DNA in solitary keratoacanthoma. Arch Dermatol Res 1986;279:73–6.
184. Ghadially FN. The role of the hair follicle in the origin and evolution of some cutaneous neoplasms of man and experimental animals. Cancer 1961;14:801–16.
185. Glogau RG. The risk of progression to invasive disease. J Am Acad Dermatol 2000;42(Pt 2):23–4.
186. Graham JH, Helwig EB. Erythroplasia of Queyrat. A clinicopathologic and histochemical study. Cancer 1973;32:1396–414.
187. Graham RM, MacFarlane AW, Curley RK, Nash JR. Beta 2 microglobulin expression in keratoacanthomas and squamous cell carcinoma. Br J Dermatol 1987;117:441–9.
188. Hodak E, Jones RE, Ackerman AB. Solitary keratoacanthoma is a squamous-cell carcinoma: three examples with metastases. Am J Dermatopathol 1993;15:332–42; discussion 343–52.
189. Hsi ED, Svoboda-Newman SM, Stern RA, Nickoloff BJ, Frank TS. Detection of human papillomavirus DNA in keratoacanthomas by polymerase chain reaction. Am J Dermatopathol 1997;19:10–5.
190. Hurwitz RM, Egan WT, Murphy SH, Pontius EE, Forster ML. Bowenoid papulosis and squamous cell carcinoma of the genitalia: suspected sexual transmission. Cutis 1987;39:193–6.
191. Ikenberg H, Gissmann L, Gross G, Grussendorf-Conen EI, zur Hausen H. Human papillomavirus type-16-related DNA in genital Bowen's disease and in bowenoid papulosis. Int J Cancer 1983;32:563–5.
192. Izaki S, Hirai A, Yoshizawa Y, et al. Carcinosarcoma of the skin: immunohistochemical and electron microscopic observations. J Cutan Pathol 1993;20:272–8.
193. Jacobs DM, Sandles LG, Leboit PE. Sebaceous carcinoma arising from Bowen's disease of the vulva. Arch Dermatol 1986;122:1191–3.
194. Jakobiec FA, Austin P, Iwamoto T, Trokel SL, Marquardt MD, Harrison W. Primary infiltrating signet ring carcinoma of the eyelids. Ophthalmology 1983;90:291–9.
195. James MP, Wells GC, Whimster IW. Spreading pigmented actinic keratoses. Br J Dermatol 1978;98:373–9.
196. Kannon G, Park HK. Utility of peanut agglutinin (PNA) in the diagnosis of squamous cell carcinoma and keratoacanthoma. Am J Dermatopathol 1990;12:31–6.
197. Kao GF. Carcinoma arising in Bowen's disease. Arch Dermatol 1986;122:1124–6.
198. Knoell KA, Patterson JW, Wilson BB. Sudden onset of disseminated porokeratosis of Mibelli in a renal transplant patient. J Am Acad Dermatol 1999;41(Pt 2):830–2.

199. Ko T, Muramatsu T, Shirai T. Lymphoepithelioma-like carcinoma of the skin. J Dermatol 1997;24:104–9.
199a. Kraus FT, Perezmesa C. Verrucous carcinoma. Clinical and pathologic study of 105 cases involving oral cavity, larynx and genitalia. Cancer 1966;19:26–38.
200. Kushida Y, Miki H, Ohmori M. Loss of heterozygosity in actinic keratosis, squamous cell carcinoma and sun-exposed normal-appearing skin in Japanese: difference between Japanese and Caucasians. Cancer Lett 1999;140(1-2):169–75.
201. Kutzner H, Schwenzer G, Embacher G, Kutzner U, Schroder J. [Lymphoepithelioma-like carcinoma of the skin.] Hautarzt 1991;42:575–9. (German.)
202. Lapins NA, Helwig EB. Perineural invasion by keratoacanthoma. Arch Dermatol 1980;116:791–3.
203. Lind AC, Breer WA, Wick MR. Lymphoepithelioma-like carcinoma of the skin with apparent origin in the epidermis—a pattern or an entity? A case report. Cancer 1999;85:884–90.
204. Lopez-Amado M, Garcia-Caballero T, Lozano-Ramirez A, Labella-Caballero T. Human papilloma-virus and p53 oncoprotein in verrucous carcinoma of the larynx. J Laryngol Otol 1996;110:742–7.
205. Lu S, Syrjanen SL, Havu VK, Syrjanen S. Known HPV types have no association with keratoacanthomas. Arch Dermatol Res 1996;288:129–32.
206. Lu S, Tiekso J, Hietanen S, Syrjanen K, Havu VK, Syrjanen S. Expression of cell-cycle proteins p53, p21 (WAF-1), PCNA and Ki-67 in benign, premalignant and malignant skin lesions with implicated HPV involvement. Acta Derm Venereol 1999;79:268–73.
207. Lund HZ. How often does squamous cell carcinoma of the skin metastasize? Arch Dermatol 1965;92:635–7.
208. Manstein CH, Frauenhoffer CJ, Besden JE. Keratoacanthoma: is it a real entity? Ann Plast Surg 1998;40:469–72.
209. Marschall SF, Ronan SG, Massa MC. Pigmented Bowen's disease arising from pigmented seborrheic keratoses. J Am Acad Dermatol 1990;23(Pt 1):440–4.
210. Matsuta M, Kimura S, Kosegawa G, Kon S. Immunohistochemical detection of Ki-67 in epithelial skin tumors in formalin-fixed paraffin-embedded tissue sections using a new monoclonal antibody (MIB-1). J Dermatol 1996;23:147–52.
211. McKee PH, Wilkinson JD, Corbett MF, Davey A, Sauven P, Black MM. Carcinoma cuniculatum: a cast metastasizing to skin and lymph nodes. Clin Exp Dermatol 1981;6:613–8.
212. McKinley E, Valles R, Bang R, Bocklage T. Signet-ring squamous cell carcinoma: a case report. J Cutan Pathol 1998;25:176–81.
213. Mehregan AH. Pinkus' guide to dermato-histopathology. Norwalk, Conn: Appleton-Century-Crofts: 1986.
214. Mills AE. Solar keratosis can be distinguished from superficial basal cell carcinoma by expression of bcl-2. Am J Dermatopathol 1997;19:443–5.
215. Mitsuishi T, Sata T, Iwasaki T, et al. The detection of human papillomavirus 16 DNA in erythroplasia of Queyrat invading the urethra. Br J Dermatol 1998;138:188–9.
216. Moller R, Reymann F, Hou-Jensen K. Metastases in dermatological patients with squamous cell carcinoma. Arch Dermatol 1979;115:703–5.
217. Monteagudo JC, Jorda E, Terencio C, Llombart-Bosch A. Squamous cell carcinoma in situ (Bowen's disease) arising in seborrheic keratosis: three lesions in two patients. J Cutan Pathol 1989;16:348–52.
217a. Musso L. Spontaneous resolution of molluscum sebaceum. Proc Roy Soc Med 1950;43:838–9.
218. Nappi O, Wick MR, Pettinato G, Ghiselli RW, Swanson PE. Pseudovascular adenoid squamous cell carcinoma of the skin. A neoplasm that may be mistaken for angiosarcoma. Am J Surg Pathol 1992;16:429–38.
219. Noel JC, Heenen M, Peny MO, et al. Proliferating cell nuclear antigen distribution in verrucous carcinoma of the skin. Br J Dermatol 1995;133:868–73.
220. Noel JC, Peny MO, De Dobbeleer G, et al. p53 protein overexpression in verrucous carcinoma of the skin. Dermatology 1996;192:12–5.
221. Noel JC, Peny MO, Detremmerie O, et al. Demonstration of human papillomavirus type 2 in a verrucous carcinoma of the foot. Dermatology 1993;187:58–61.
222. Noel JC, Peny MO, Goldschmidt D, Verhest A, Heenen M, De Dobbeleer G. Human papillomavirus type 1 DNA in verrucous carcinoma of the leg. J Am Acad Dermatol 1993;29:1036–8.
223. O'Sullivan B, Warde P, Keane T, Irish J, Cummings B, Payne D. Outcome following radiotherapy in verrucous carcinoma of the larynx. Int J Radiat Oncol Biol Phys 1995;32:611–7.
224. Obalek S, Jablonska S, Beaudenon S, Walczak L, Orth G. Bowenoid papulosis of the male and female genitalia: risk of cervical neoplasia. J Am Acad Dermatol 1986;14:433–44.
225. Olemans C, Pierard-Franchimont C, Delvenne P, Pierard GE. Comparative karyometry in Bowen's disease and bowenoid papulosis. Derivation of a nuclear atypia index. Anal Quant Cytol Histol 1994;16:284–6.

226. Patel NK, McKee PH, Smith NP, Fletcher CD. Primary metaplastic carcinoma (carcinosarcoma) of the skin. A clinicopathologic study of four cases and review of the literature. Am J Dermatopathol 1997;19:363–72.
227. Patterson JW, Kao GF, Graham JH, Helwig EB. Bowenoid papulosis. A clinicopathologic study with ultrastructural observations. Cancer 1986;57:823–36.
228. Perez CA, Kraus FT, Evans JC, Powers WE. Anaplastic transformation in verrucous carcinoma of the oral cavity after radiation therapy. Radiology 1966;86:108–15.
229. Pfister H, Gassenmaier A, Fuchs PG. Demonstration of human papillomavirus DNA in two keratoacanthomas. Arch Dermatol Res 1986;278:243–6.
230. Planner RS, Andersen HE, Hobbs JB, Williams RA, Fogarty LF, Hudson PJ. Multifocal invasive carcinoma of the vulva in a 25-year-old woman with bowenoid papulosis. Aust N Z J Obstet Gynaecol 1987;27:291–5.
231. Quay SC, Harrist TJ, Mihm MC Jr. Carcinosarcoma of the skin. Case report and review. J Cutan Pathol 1981;8:241–6.
232. Randall MB, Geisinger KR, Kute TE, Buss DH, Prichard RW. DNA content and proliferative index in cutaneous squamous cell carcinoma and keratoacanthoma. Am J Clin Pathol 1990;93:259–62.
233. Reed RJ, Leone P. Porokeratosis—a mutant clonal keratosis of the epidermis. I. Histogenesis. Arch Dermatol 1970;101:340–7.
234. Requena L, Romero E, Sanchez M, Ambrojo P, Sanchez Yus E. Aggressive keratoacanthoma of the eyelid: "malignant" keratoacanthoma or squamous cell carcinoma? J Dermatol Surg Oncol 1990;16:564–8.
235. Requena L, Sanchez Yus E, Jimenez E, Roo E. Lymphoepithelioma-like carcinoma of the skin: a light-microscopic and immunohistochemical study. J Cutan Pathol 1994;21:541–8.
235a. Rook A, Whimster I. Keratoacanthoma—a thirty year retrospect. Br J Dermatol 1979;100:41–7.
236. Saboorian MH, Kenny M, Ashfaq R, Albores-Saavedra J. Carcinosarcoma arising in eccrine spiradenoma of the breast. Report of a case and review of the literature. Arch Pathol Lab Med 1996;120:501–4.
237. Saida T, Okabe Y, Uhara H. Bowen's disease with invasive carcinoma showing sweat gland differentiation. J Cutan Pathol 1989;16:222–6.
238. Salasche SJ. Epidemiology of actinic keratose 238 and squamous cell carcinoma. J Am Acad Dermatol 2000;42(1 Pt 2):4–7.
239. Sasaoka R, Morimura T, Mihara M, Hagari Y, Aki T, Miyamoto T. Detection of human papillomavirus type 16 DNA in two cases of verrucous carcinoma of the foot. Br J Dermatol 1996;134:983–4.
240. Scheurlen W, Gissmann L, Gross G, zur Hausen H. Molecular cloning of two new HPV types (HPV 37 and HPV 38) from a keratoacanthoma and a malignant melanoma. Int J Cancer 1986;37:505–10.
241. Schrader M, Laberke HG, Jahnke K. [Lymphatic metastases of verrucous carcinoma (Ackerman tumor).] HNO 1987;35:27–30. (German.)
242. Schwade JG, Wara WM, Dedo HH, Phillips TL. Radiotherapy for verrucous carcinoma. Radiology 1976;120:677–9.
243. Shroyer KR, Greer RO, Fankhouser CA, McGuirt WF, Marshall R. Detection of human papillomavirus DNA in oral verrucous carcinoma by polymerase chain reaction. Mod Pathol 1993;6:669–72.
244. Sim CS, Slater S, McKee PH. Mutant p53 expression in solar keratosis: an immunohistochemical study. J Cutan Pathol 1992;19:302–8.
245. Stoll DM, Ackerman AB. Subungual keratoacanthoma. Am J Dermatopathol 1980;2:265–71.
246. Swanson SA, Cooper PH, Mills SE, Wick MR. Lymphoepithelioma-like carcinoma of the skin. Mod Pathol 1988;1:359–65.
247. Takayasu S, Yoshiyama M, Kurata S, Terashi H. Lymphoepithelioma-like carcinoma of the skin. J Dermatol 1996;23:472–5.
248. Tan CY, Marks R. Lichenoid solar keratosis—prevalence and immunologic findings. J Invest Dermatol 1982;79:365–7.
249. Tope WD, Nowfar-Rad M, Kist DA. Ber-EP4-positive phenotype differentiates actinic keratosis from superficial basal cell carcinoma. Dermatol Surg 2000;26:415–8.
250. Tran TA, Ross JS, Sheehan CE, Carlson JA. Comparison of oncostatin M expression in keratoacanthoma and squamous cell carcinoma. Mod Pathol 2000;13:427–32.
251. Tschen JA, Goldberg LH, McGavran MH. Carcinosarcoma of the skin. J Cutan Pathol 1988;15:31–5.
252. Vakilzadeh F, Happle R. Epidermolytic leukoplakia. J Cutan Pathol 1982;9:267–70.
253. van Praag MC, Bavinck JN, Bergman W, et al. PUVA keratosis. A clinical and histopathologic entity associated with an increased risk of nonmelanoma skin cancer. J Am Acad Dermatol 1993;28:412–7.
254. Wade TR, Ackerman AB. Cornoid lamellation. A histologic reaction pattern. Am J Dermatopathol 1980;2:5–15.
255. Wade TR, Ackerman AB. The effects of resin of podophyllin on condyloma acuminatum. Am J Dermatopathol 1984;6:109–22.

256. Wade TR, Kopf AW, Ackerman AB. Bowenoid papulosis of the penis. Cancer 1978;42:1890–903.
257. Wade TR, Kopf AW, Ackerman AB. Bowenoid papulosis of the genitalia. Arch Dermatol 1979;115:306–8.
258. Waring AJ, Takata M, Rehman I, Rees JL. Loss of heterozygosity analysis of keratoacanthoma reveals multiple differences from cutaneous squamous cell carcinoma. Br J Cancer 1996;73:649–53.
259. Weidner N, Foucar E. Adenosquamous carcinoma of the skin. An aggressive mucin- and gland-forming squamous carcinoma. Arch Dermatol 1985;121:775–9.
260. Wick MR, Swanson PE, LeBoit PE, Strickler JG, Cooper PH. Lymphoepithelioma-like carcinoma of the skin with adnexal differentiation. J Cutan Pathol 1991;18:93–102.
261. Wieland U, Jurk S, Weissenborn S, Krieg T, Pfister H, Ritzkowsky A. Erythroplasia of Queyrat: coinfection with cutaneous carcinogenic human papillomavirus type 8 and genital papillomaviruses in a carcinoma in situ. J Invest Dermatol 2000;115:396–401.
262. Wilkinson JD, McKee PH, Black MM, Whimster IW, Lovell D. A case of carcinoma cuniculatum with coexistant viral plantar wart. Clin Exp Dermatol 1981;6:619–23.
263. Williamson JD, Colome MI, Sahin A, Ayala AG, Medeiros LJ. Pagetoid Bowen disease: a report of 2 cases that express cytokeratin 7. Arch Pathol Lab Med 2000;124:427–30.
264. Wollensak G, Witschel H, Bohm N. Signet ring cell carcinoma of the eccrine sweat glands in the eyelid. Ophthalmology 1996;103:1788–93.
265. Yap WM, Tan PH, Ong BH. Malignancy arising in seborrheic keratosis: a report of two cases. Ann Acad Med Singapore 1997;26:235–7.
266. Yeh S. Skin cancer in chronic arsenicism. Hum Pathol 1973;4:469–85.
267. Youngberg GA, Thornthwaite JT, Inoshita T, Franzus D. Cytologically malignant squamous-cell carcinoma arising in a verrucous carcinoma of the penis. J Dermatol Surg Oncol 1983;9:474–9.

Basal Cell Carcinoma

268. Aram H, Barsky S. Pigmented basal cell epithelioma arising in the scar of an onchocerciasis nodule. Int J Dermatol 1984;23:658–60.
269. Bale AE, Gailani MR, Leffell DJ. Nevoid basal cell carcinoma syndrome. J Invest Dermatol 1994;103(Suppl):126S–30S.
270. Barr RJ, Alpern KS, Santa Cruz DJ, Fretzin DF. Clear cell basal cell carcinoma: an unusual degenerative variant. J Cutan Pathol 1993;20:308–16.
271. Barr RJ, Graham JH. Granular cell basal cell carcinoma. A distinct histopathologic entity. Arch Dermatol 1979;115:1064–7.
272. Bhagchandani L, Sanadi RE, Sattar S, Abbott RR. Basal cell carcinoma presenting as finger mass. A case report. Am J Clin Oncol 1995;18:176–9.
273. Black MM, Walkden VM. Basal cell carcinomatous changes on the lower leg: a possible association with chronic venous stasis. Histopathology 1983;7:219–27.
274. Bleiberg J, Brodkin RH. Linear unilateral basal cell nevus with comedones. Arch Dermatol 1969;100:187–90.
275. Borel DM. Cutaneous basosquamous carcinoma. Review of the literature and report of 35 cases. Arch Pathol 1973;95:293–7.
276. Brooke JD, Fitzpatrick JE, Golitz LE. Papillary mesenchymal bodies: a histologic finding useful in differentiating trichoepitheliomas from basal cell carcinomas. J Am Acad Dermatol 1989;21(Pt 1):523–8.
277. Brownstein MH. Basaloid follicular hamartoma: solitary and multiple types. J Am Acad Dermatol 1992;27(Pt 1):237–40.
278. Brownstein MH, Shapiro L. Desmoplastic trichoepithelioma. Cancer 1977;40:2979–86.
279. Casson P. Basal cell carcinoma. Clin Plast Surg 1980;7:301–11.
280. Christian MM, Moy RL, Wagner RF, Yen-Moore A. A correlation of alpha-smooth muscle actin and invasion in micronodular basal cell carcinoma. Dermatol Surg 2001;27:441–45.
281. Collina G, Macri L, Eusebi V. [Endocrine differentiation in basocellular carcinoma.] Pathologica 2001;93:208–12. (Italian.)
282. Cribier B, Noacco G, Peltre B, Grosshans E. Expression of stromelysin 3 in basal cell carcinomas. Eur J Dermatol 2001;11:530–3.
283. Curson C, Weedon D. Spontaneous regression in basal cell carcinomas. J Cutan Pathol 1979;6:432–7.
284. Dardi LE, Memoli VA, Gould VE. Neuroendocrine differentiation in basal cell carcinomas. J Cutan Pathol 1981;8:335–41.
285. Dawson EK. Carcino-sarcoma of the skin. J R Coll Surg Edinb 1972;17:243–6.
286. de Faria J. Basal cell carcinoma of the skin with areas of squamous cell carcinoma: a basosquamous cell carcinoma? J Clin Pathol 1985;38:1273–7.
287. Dellavalle RP, Walsh P, Marchbank A, et al. CUSP/p63 expression in basal cell carcinoma. Exp Dermatol 2002;11:203–8.
288. Dellon AL. Host-tumor relationships in basal cell and squamous cell cancer of the skin. Plast Reconstr Surg 1978;62:37–48.

289. Farmer ER, Helwig EB. Metastatic basal cell carcinoma: a clinicopathologic study of seventeen cases. Cancer 1980;46:748–57.
290. Gailani MR, Leffell DJ, Ziegler A, Gross EG, Brash DE, Bale AE. Relationship between sunlight exposure and a key genetic alteration in basal cell carcinoma. J Natl Cancer Inst 1996; 88:349–54.
291. Garcia Prats MD, Lopez Carreira M, Martinez-Gonzalez MA, Ballestin C, Gil R, De Prada I. Granular cell basal cell carcinoma. Light microscopy, immunohistochemical and ultrastructural study. Virchows Arch A Pathol Anat Histopathol 1993;422:173–7.
292. Gatter KC, Pulford KA, Vanstapel MJ, et al. An immunohistological study of benign and malignant skin tumours: epithelial aspects. Histopathology 1984;8:209–27.
293. Geary WA, Cooper PH. Proliferating cell nuclear antigen (PCNA) in common epidermal lesions. An immunohistochemical study of proliferating cell populations. J Cutan Pathol 1992;19: 458–68.
294. Gloster HM Jr, Brodland DG. The epidemiology of skin cancer. Dermatol Surg 1996;22:217–26.
295. Goette DK, Helwig EB. Basal cell carcinomas and basal cell carcinoma-like changes overlying dermatofibromas. Arch Dermatol 1975; 111:589–92.
296. Goldberg LH, Joseph AK, Tschen JA. Proliferative actinic keratosis. Int J Dermatol 1994;33: 341–5.
297. Hashimoto K, Brownstein MH. Localized amyloidosis in basal cell epitheliomas. Acta Derm Venereol 1973;53:331–9.
298. Hauben DJ, Zirkin H, Mahler D, Sacks M. The biologic behavior of basal cell carcinoma: Part I. Plast Reconstr Surg 1982;69:103–9.
299. Helander SD, Peters MS, Pittelkow MR. Expression of p53 protein in benign and malignant epidermal pathologic conditions. J Am Acad Dermatol 1993;29(Pt 1):741–8.
300. Holmes EJ, Bennington JL, Haber SL. Citrulline-containing basal cell carcinomas. Differentiation toward hari structures with induction of dermal hair papillae. Cancer 1968;22:663–70.
301. Hyde JN, Montgomry FH. Diseases of the skin, 4th ed. Philadelphia: Lea Brothers; 1897:669–88.
302. Impola U, Toriseva M, Suomela S, et al. Matrix metalloproteinase-19 is expressed by proliferating epithelium but disappears with neoplastic dedifferentiation. Int J Cancer 2003;103:709–16.
303. Ishibashi A, Kasuga T, Tsuchiya E. Electron microscopic study of basal cell carcinoma. J Invest Dermatol 1971;56:298–304.
304. Izaki S, Hirai A, Yoshizawa Y, et al. Carcinosarcoma of the skin: immunohistochemical and electron microscopic observations. J Cutan Pathol 1993;20:272–8.
305. Jacobs GH, Rippey JJ, Altini M. Prediction of aggressive behavior in basal cell carcinoma. Cancer 1982;49:533–7.
306. Jih DM, Shapiro M, James WD, et al. Familial basaloid follicular hamartoma: lesional characterization and review of the literature. Am J Dermatopathol 2003;25:130–7.
307. Kanitakis J, Alhaj-Ibrahim L, Euvrard S, Claudy A. Basal cell carcinomas developing in solid organ transplant recipients: clinicopathologic study of 176 cases. Arch Dermatol 2003;139: 1133–7.
308. Kim ED, Kroft S, Dalton DP. Basal cell carcinoma of the penis: case report and review of the literature. J Urol 1994;152(Pt 1):1557–9.
309. Kirchmann TT, Prieto VG, Smoller BR. CD34 staining pattern distinguishes basal cell carcinoma from trichoepithelioma. Arch Dermatol 1994;130:589–92.
310. Krompecher E. Der Basalzellenkrebs. Jena: Fischer; 1903.
311. Kubo Y, Urano Y, Yoshimoto K, et al. p53 gene mutations in human skin cancers and precancerous lesions: comparison with immunohistochemical analysis. J Invest Dermatol 1994;102: 440–4.
312. Kuflik EG. Basal-cell carcinoma: an unusual clinical and histologic variant. J Dermatol Surg Oncol 1980;6:730–2.
313. Lang PG Jr, Maize JC. Histologic evolution of recurrent basal cell carcinoma and treatment implications. J Am Acad Dermatol 1986;14(Pt 1):186–96.
314. Lang PG Jr, McKelvey AC, Nicholson JH. Three-dimensional reconstruction of the superficial multicentric basal cell carcinoma using serial sections and a computer. Am J Dermatopathol 1987;9:198–203.
315. Lerchin E, Rahbari H. Adamantinoid basal cell epithelioma. A histological variant. Arch Dermatol 1975;111:586–8.
316. Lo Re G, Canzonieri V, Veronesi A, et al. Extrapulmonary small cell carcinoma: a single-institution experience and review of the literature. Ann Oncol 1994;5:909–13.
317. Looi LM. Localized amyloidosis in basal cell carcinoma. A pathologic study. Cancer 1983; 52:1833–6.
318. Madsen A. Studies on basal-cell epithelioma of the skin.The architecture, manner of growth, and histogenesis of the tumours. Whole tumours examined in serial sections cut parallel to the skin surface. Acta Pathol Microbiol Scand 1965:177(Suppl):173–63.

319. Maloney ME, Jones DB, Sexton FM. Pigmented basal cell carcinoma: investigation of 70 cases. J Am Acad Dermatol 1992;27:74–8.
320. Markey AC, Lane EB, Macdonald DM, Leigh IM. Keratin expression in basal cell carcinomas. Br J Dermatol 1992;126:154–60.
321. Mehregan AH. Acantholysis in basal cell epithelioma. J Cutan Pathol 1979;6:280–3.
322. Mehregan AH. Aggressive basal cell epithelioma on sunlight-protected skin. Report of eight cases, one with pulmonary and bone metastases. Am J Dermatopathol 1983;5:221–9.
323. Miettinen M, Lehto VP, Virtanen I. Antibodies to intermediate filament proteins. The differential diagnosis of cutaneous tumors. Arch Dermatol 1985;121:736–41.
324. Mino M, Pilch BZ, Faquin WC. Expression of KIT (CD117) in neoplasms of the head and neck: an ancillary marker for adenoid cystic carcinoma. Mod Pathol 2003;16:1224–31.
325. Mizushima J, Ohara K. Basal cell carcinoma of the vulva with lymph node and skin metastasis—report of a case and review of 20 Japanese cases. J Dermatol 1995;22:36–42.
326. Morales-Ducret CR, van de Rijn M, LeBrun DP, Smoller BR. bcl-2 expression in primary malignancies of the skin. Arch Dermatol 1995;131:909–12.
327. Morris JG, Joffe R. Perineural spread of cutaneous basal and squamous cell carcinomas. The clinical appearance of spread into the trigeminal and facial nerves. Arch Neurol 1983;40:424–9.
328. Mrak RE, Baker GF. Granular cell basal cell carcinoma. J Cutan Pathol 1987;14:37–42.
329. Nahass GT, Blauvelt A, Leonardi CL, Penneys NS. Basal cell carcinoma of the scrotum. Report of three cases and review of the literature. J Am Acad Dermatol 1992;26:574–8.
330. Nakagawa K, Yamamura K, Maeda S, Ichihashi M. bcl-2 expression in epidermal keratinocytic diseases. Cancer 1994;74:1720–4.
331. Okun MR, Blumental G. Basal cell epithelioma with giant cells and nuclear atypicality. Arch Dermatol 1964;89:598–600.
332. Oliver GF, Winkelmann RK. Clear-cell, basal cell carcinoma: histopathological, histochemical, and electron microscopic findings. J Cutan Pathol 1988;15:404–8.
333. Olsen KE, Westermark P. Amyloid in basal cell carcinoma and seborrheic keratosis. Acta Derm Venereol 1994;74:273–5.
334. Ono T, Fallas VH, Higo J. Basal cell epithelioma with dermal melanocytes: a case report. J Dermatol 1986;13:63–6.
335. Perrone T, Twiggs LB, Adcock LL, Dehner LP. Vulvar basal cell carcinoma: an infrequently metastasizing neoplasm. Int J Gynecol Pathol 1987;6:152–65.
336. Plosila M, Kiistala R, Niemi KM. The Bazex syndrome: follicular atrophoderma with multiple basal cell carcinomas, hypotrichosis and hypohidrosis. Clin Exp Dermatol 1981;6:31–41.
337. Quay SC, Harrist TJ, Mihm MC Jr. Carcinosarcoma of the skin. Case report and review. J Cutan Pathol 1981;8:241–6.
338. Quinn AG, Healy E, Rehman I, Sikkink S, Rees JL. Microsatellite instability in human non-melanoma and melanoma skin cancer. J Invest Dermatol 1995;104:309–12.
339. Ramdial PK, Madaree A, Reddy R, Chetty R. bcl-2 protein expression in aggressive and non-aggressive basal cell carcinomas. J Cutan Pathol 2000;27:283–91.
340. Ratner D, Lowe L, Johnson TM, Fader DJ. Perineural spread of basal cell carcinomas treated with Mohs micrographic surgery. Cancer 2000;88:1605–13.
341. Reis-Filho JS, Torio B, Albergaria A, Schmitt FC. p63 expression in normal skin and usual cutaneous carcinomas. J Cutan Pathol 2002;29:517–23.
342. Robins P, Rabinovitz HS, Rigel D. Basal-cell carcinomas on covered or unusual sites of the body. J Dermatol Surg Oncol 1981;7:803–6.
343. Robinson JK, Dahiya M. Basal cell carcinoma with pulmonary and lymph node metastasis causing death. Arch Dermatol 2003;139:643–8.
344. Rulon DB, Helwig EB. Cutaneous sebaceous neoplasms. Cancer 1974;33:82–102.
345. Sakamoto F, Ito M, Sato S, Sato Y. Basal cell tumor with apocrine differentiation: apocrine epithelioma. J Am Acad Dermatol 1985;13(Pt 2):355–63.
346. Saldanha G, Fletcher A, Slater DN. Basal cell carcinoma: a dermatopathological and molecular biological update. Br J Dermatol 2003;148:195–202.
347. Saldanha G, Shaw JA, Fletcher A. Evidence that superficial basal cell carcinoma is monoclonal from analysis of the Ptch1 gene locus. Br J Dermatol 2002;147:931–5.
348. San Juan J, Monteagudo C, Navarro P, Terradez JJ. Basal cell carcinoma with prominent central palisading of epithelial cells mimicking schwannoma. J Cutan Pathol 1999;26:528–32.
349. Schuller DE, Berg JW, Sherman G, Krause CJ. Cutaneous basosquamous carcinoma of the head and neck: a comparative analysis. Otolaryngol Head Neck Surg 1979;87:420–7.

350. Shamanin V, zur Hausen H, Lavergne D, et al. Human papillomavirus infections in nonmelanoma skin cancers from renal transplant recipients and nonimmunosuppressed patients. J Natl Cancer Inst 1996;88:802–11.
351. Siegle RJ, MacMillan J, Pollack SV. Infiltrative basal cell carcinoma: a nonsclerosing subtype. J Dermatol Surg Oncol 1986;12:830–6.
352. Snow SN, Sahl W, Lo JS, et al. Metastatic basal cell carcinoma. Report of five cases. Cancer 1994;73:328–35.
353. Sober AJ, Burstein JM. Precursors to skin cancer. Cancer 1995;75(Suppl):645–50.
354. Southwick GJ, Schwartz RA. The basal cell nevus syndrome: disasters occurring among a series of 36 patients. Cancer 1979;44:2294–305.
355. Starink TM, Blomjous CE, Stoof TJ, Van Der Linden JC. Clear cell basal cell carcinoma. Histopathology 1990;17:401–5.
356. Suster S. Clear cell tumors of the skin. Semin Diagn Pathol 1996;13:40–59.
357. Swanson PE, Fitzpatrick MM, Ritter JH, Glusac EJ, Wick MR. Immunohistologic differential diagnosis of basal cell carcinoma, squamous cell carcinoma, and trichoepithelioma in small cutaneous biopsy specimens. J Cutan Pathol 1998;25:153–9.
358. Tellechea O, Reis JP, Domingues JC, Baptista AP. Monoclonal antibody Ber EP4 distinguishes basal-cell carcinoma from squamous-cell carcinoma of the skin. Am J Dermatopathol 1993;15:452–5.
359. Thewes M, Worret WI, Engst R, Ring J. Stromelysin-3: a potent marker for histopathologic differentiation between desmoplastic trichoepithelioma and morpheaike basal cell carcinoma. Am J Dermatopathol 1998;20:140–2.
360. Thomas P, Said JW, Nash G, Banks-Schlegel S. Profiles of keratin proteins in basal and squamous cell carcinomas of the skin. An immunohistochemical study. Lab Invest 1984;50:36–41.
361. Tojo M, Mori T, Kiyosawa H, et al. Expression of sonic hedgehog signal transducers, patched and smoothened, in human basal cell carcinoma. Pathol Int 1999;49:687–94.
362. Vico P, Fourez T, Nemec E, Andry G, Deraemaecker R. Aggressive basal cell carcinoma of head and neck areas. Eur J Surg Oncol 1995;21:490–7.
363. von Domarus H, Stevens PJ. Metastatic basal cell carcinoma. Report of five cases and review of 170 cases in the literature. J Am Acad Dermatol 1984;10:1043–60.
364. Wade TR, Ackerman AB. The many faces of basal-cell carcinoma. J Dermatol Surg Oncol 1978;4:23–8.
365. Wang CY, Brodland DG, Su WP. Skin cancers associated with acquired immunodeficiency syndrome. Mayo Clin Proc 1995;70:766–72.
366. Wei Q, Matanoski GM, Farmer ER, Hedayati MA, Grossman L. DNA repair capacity for ultraviolet light-induced damage is reduced in peripheral lymphocytes from patients with basal cell carcinoma. J Invest Dermatol 1995;104:933–6.
367. Wick MR, Kaye VN. The role of diagnostic immunohistochemistry in dermatology. Semin Dermatol 1987;5:136–47.
368. Wick MR, Scheithauer BW. Primary neuroendocrine carcinoma of the skin. In: Wick MR, ed. Pathology of unusual malignant cutaneous tumors. New York: Marcel Dekker; 1985:107–80.
369. Wick MR, Swanson PE. Primary adenoid cystic carcinoma of the skin. A clinical, histological, and immunocytochemical comparison with adenoid cystic carcinoma of salivary glands and adenoid basal cell carcinoma. Am J Dermatopathol 1986;8:2–13.
370. Wolfe JT 3rd, Wick MR, Campbell RJ. Sebaceous carcinomas of the oculocutaneous adnexa and extraocular skin. In: Wick MR, ed. Pathology of unusual malignant cutaneous tumors. New York: Marcel Dekker; 1985:77–106.
371. Yasaka N, Furue M, Tamaki K. CD44 expression in normal human skin and skin tumors. J Dermatol 1995;22:88–94.
372. Yoshikawa K, Katagata Y, Kondo S. Relative amounts of keratin 17 are higher than those of keratin 16 in hair-follicle-derived tumors in comparison with nonfollicular epithelial skin tumors. J Invest Dermatol 1995;104:396–400.
373. Zamecnik M, Skalova A, Michal M. Basal cell carcinoma with collagenous crystalloids. Arch Pathol Lab Med 1996;120:581–2.

SUPPLEMENTAL REFERENCES

Epidermal Cyst and Milium
Fujiwara M, Nakamura Y, Ozawa T, et al. Multilocular giant epidermal cyst. Br J Dermatol 2004;151:943–5.

Hattori H. Epidermal cyst containing numerous spherules of keratin. Br J Dermatol 2004;151:1286–7.

Sudhakar N, Stephenson GC. Swelling on the head—a forgotten lesson: a case report of an intradiploic epidermal cyst with an iatrogenic complication. Br J Oral Maxillofac Surg 2004;42:155–7.

Human Papillomavirus–Associated Cyst
Egawa K, Egawa N, Honda Y. Human papillomavirus-associated plantar epidermoid cyst related to epidermoid metaplasia of the eccrine duct epithelium: a combined histological, immunohistochemical, DNA-DNA in situ hybridization and three-dimensional reconstruction analysis. Br J Dermatol 2005;152:961–7.

Misago N, Narisawa Y. Verrucous trichilemmal cyst containing human papillomavirus. Clin Exp Dermatol 2005;30:38–9.

Cutaneous Keratocyst
Cassarino DS, Linden KG, Barr RJ. Cutaneous keratocyst arising independently of the nevoid basal cell carcinoma syndrome. Am J Dermatopathol 2005;27:177–8.

Trichilemmal Cyst
Eiberg H, Hansen L, Hansen C, Mohr J, Teglbjaerg PS, Kjaer KW. Mapping of hereditary trichilemmal cyst (TRICY1) to chromosome 3p24-p21.2 and exclusion of beta-CATENIN and MLH1. Am J Med Genet A 2005;133:44–7.

Steatocystoma
Mortazavi H, Taheri A, Mansoori P, Kani ZA. Localized forms of steatocystoma multiplex: case report and review of the literature. Dermatol Online J 2005;11:22.

Eruptive Vellus Hair Cyst
Mieno H, Fujimoto N, Tajima S. Eruptive vellus hair cyst in patients with chronic renal failure. Dermatology 2004;208:67–9.

Endometriosis
De Giorgi V, Massi D, Mannone F, Stante M, Carli P. Cutaneous endometriosis: non-invasive analysis by epiluminescence microscopy. Clin Exp Dermatol 2003;28:315–7.

Endosalpingiosis
Perera GK, Watson KM, Salisbury J, Du Vivier AW. Two cases of cutaneous umbilical endosalpingiosis. Br J Dermatol 2004;151:924–5.

Ciliated Cyst
Santos LD, Mendelsohn G. Perineal cutaneous ciliated cyst in a male. Pathology 2004;36:369–70.

Thymic Cyst
Chetty R, Reddi A. Rhabdomyomatous multilocular thymic cyst. Am J Clin Pathol 2003;119:816–21.

Metaplastic Synovial Cyst
Choonhakarn C, Tang S. Cutaneous metaplastic synovial cyst. J Dermatol 2003;30(6):480–4.

Lin YC, Tsai TF. Cutaneous metaplastic synovial cyst: unusual presentation with "a bag of worms." Dermatol Surg 2003;29:198–200.

Epidermal Nevus
Alpsoy E, Durusoy C, Ozbilim G, Karpuzoglu G, Yilmaz E. Nevus comedonicus syndrome: a case associated with multiple basal cell carcinomas and a rudimentary toe. Int J Dermatol 2005; 44:499–501.

Sugarman JL. Epidermal nevus syndromes. Semin Cutan Med Surg 2004;23:145–57.

Vissers WH, Muys L, Erp PE, de Jong EM, van de Kerkhof PC. Immunohistochemical differentiation between inflammatory linear verrucous epidermal nevus (ILVEN) and psoriasis. Eur J Dermatol 2004;14:216–20.

Seborrheic Keratosis
Bai H, Cviko A, Granter S, Yuan L, Betensky RA, Crum CP. Immunophenotypic and viral (human papillomavirus) correlates of vulvar seborrheic keratosis. Hum Pathol 2003;34:559–64.

Large Cell Acanthoma
Mehregan DR, Hamzavi F, Brown K. Large cell acanthoma. Int J Dermatol 2003;42:36–9.

Clear Cell Acanthoma
Bugatti L, Filosa G, Broganelli P, Tomasini C. Psoriasis-like dermoscopic pattern of clear cell acanthoma. J Eur Acad Dermatol Venereol 2003;17:452–5.

Clear Cell Papulosis
Kumarasinghe SP, Chin GY, Kumarasinghe MP. Clear cell papulosis of the skin: a case report from Singapore. Arch Pathol Lab Med 2004;128:e149–52.

Actinic Keratosis
Anwar J, Wrone DA, Kimyai-Asadi A, Alam M. The development of actinic keratosis into invasive squamous cell carcinoma: evidence and evolving classification schemes. Clin Dermatol 2004;22: 189–96.

Salama ME, Mahmood MN, Qureshi HS, Ma C, Zarbo RJ, Ormsby AH. p16INK4a expression in actinic keratosis and Bowen's disease. Br J Dermatol 2003;149:1006–12.

Satchell AC, Barnetson RS, Halliday GM. Increased Fas ligand expression by T cells and tumour cells in the progression of actinic keratosis to squamous cell carcinoma. Br J Dermatol 2004;151:42–9.

Stanimirovic A, Cupic H, Bosnjak B, Kruslin B, Belicza M. Expression of p53, bcl-2 and growth hormone receptor in actinic keratosis, hypertrophic type. Arch Dermatol Res 2003;295:102–8.

Porokeratosis

Arranz-Salas I, Sanz-Trelles A, Ojeda DB. p53 alterations in porokeratosis. J Cutan Pathol 2003;30:455–8.

Bowen's Disease

Bayer-Garner IB, Reed JA. Immunolabeling pattern of syndecan-1 expression may distinguish pagetoid Bowen's disease, extramammary Paget's disease, and pagetoid malignant melanoma in situ. J Cutan Pathol 2004;31(2):169–73.

Bowenoid Papulosis

Degener AM, Laino L, Pierangeli A, Accappaticcio G, Innocenzi D, Pala S. Human papillomavirus-32-positive extragenital Bowenoid papulosis (BP) in a HIV patient with typical genital BP localization. Sex Transm Dis 2004;31:619–22.

Hama N, Ohtsuka T, Yamazaki S. Elevated amount of human papillomavirus 31 DNA in a squamous cell carcinoma developed from bowenoid papulosis. Dermatology 2004;209:329–32.

Yu DS, Kim G, Song HJ, Oh CH. Morphometric assessment of nuclei in Bowen's disease and bowenoid papulosis. Skin Res Technol 2004;10:67–70.

Squamous Cell Carcinoma

Brown VL, Harwood CA, Crook T, Cronin JG, Kelsell DP, Proby CM. p16INK4a and p14ARF tumor suppressor genes are commonly inactivated in cutaneous squamous cell carcinoma. J Invest Dermatol 2004;122:1284–92.

Huang CC, Boyce SM. Surgical margins of excision for basal cell carcinoma and squamous cell carcinoma. Semin Cutan Med Surg 2004;23:167–73.

Khanna M, Fortier-Riberdy G, Dinehart SM, Smoller B. Histopathologic evaluation of cutaneous squamous cell carcinoma: results of a survey among dermatopathologists. J Am Acad Dermatol 2003;48:721–6.

Lyakhovitsky A, Barzilai A, Fogel M, Trau H, Huszar M. Expression of e-cadherin and beta-catenin in cutaneous squamous cell carcinoma and its precursors. Am J Dermatopathol 2004;26:372–8.

Satchell AC, Barnetson RS, Halliday GM. Increased Fas ligand expression by T cells and tumour cells in the progression of actinic keratosis to squamous cell carcinoma. Br J Dermatol 2004;151:42–9.

Stelow EB, Skeate R, Wahi MM, Langel D, Jessurun J. Invasive cutaneous verruco-cystic squamous cell carcinoma. A pattern commonly present in transplant recipients. Am J Clin Pathol 2003;119:807–10.

Wheeler DL, Li Y, Verma AK. Protein kinase C epsilon signals ultraviolet light-induced cutaneous damage and development of squamous cell carcinoma possibly through induction of specific cytokines in a paracrine mechanism. Photochem Photobiol 2005;81:9–18.

Verrucous Carcinoma

Ouban A, Dellis J, Salup R, Morgan M. Immunohistochemical expression of Mdm2 and p53 in penile verrucous carcinoma. Ann Clin Lab Sci 2003;33:101–6.

Wu M, Putti TC, Bhuiya TA. Comparative study in the expression of p53, EGFR, TGF-alpha, and cyclin D1 in verrucous carcinoma, verrucous hyperplasia, and squamous cell carcinoma of head and neck region. Appl Immunohistochem Mol Morphol 2002;10:351–6.

Keratoacanthoma

Biesterfeld S, Josef J. Differential diagnosis of keratoacanthoma and squamous cell carcinoma of the epidermis by MIB-1 immunohistometry. Anticancer Res 2002;22:3019–23.

Putti TC, Teh M, Lee YS. Biological behavior of keratoacanthoma and squamous cell carcinoma: telomerase activity and COX-2 as potential markers. Mod Pathol 2004;17:468–75.

Carcinosarcoma

Bigby SM, Charlton A, Miller MV, Zwi LJ, Oliver GF. Biphasic sarcomatoid basal cell carcinoma (carcinosarcoma): four cases with immunohistochemistry and review of the literature. J Cutan Pathol 2005;32(2):141–7.

Lymphoepithelioma-Like Carcinoma

Clarke LE, Ioffreda MD. Lymphoepithelioma-like carcinoma of the skin with spindle cell differentiation. J Cutan Pathol 2005;32(6):419–23.

Basal Cell Carcinoma

Alpsoy E, Durusoy C, Ozbilim G, Karpuzoglu G, Yilmaz E. Nevus comedonicus syndrome: a case associated with multiple basal cell carcinomas and a rudimentary toe. Int J Dermatol 2005;44:499–501.

Grimbaldeston MA, Green A, Darlington S, et al. Susceptibility to basal cell carcinoma is associated with high dermal mast cell prevalence in non-sun-exposed skin for an Australian populations. Photochem Photobiol 2003;78:633–9.

Hatta N, Hirano T, Kimura T, et al. Molecular diagnosis of basal cell carcinoma and other basaloid cell neoplasms of the skin by the quantification of Gli1 transcript levels. J Cutan Pathol 2005;32:131–6.

Huang CC, Boyce SM. Surgical margins of excision for basal cell carcinoma and squamous cell carcinoma. Semin Cutan Med Surg 2004;23:167–73.

Hutchin ME, Kariapper MS, Grachtchouk M, et al. Sustained Hedgehog signaling is required for basal cell carcinoma proliferation and survival: conditional skin tumorigenesis recapitulates the hair growth cycle. Genes Dev 2005;19:214–23.

Saladi RN, Singh F, Wei H, Lebwohl MG, Phelps RG. Use of Ber-EP4 protein in recurrent metastatic basal cell carcinoma: a case report and review of the literature. Int J Dermatol 2004;43:600–3.

Saldanha G, Ghura V, Potter L, Fletcher A. Nuclear beta-catenin in basal cell carcinoma correlates with increased proliferation. Br J Dermatol 2004;151:157–64.

Yada K, Kashima K, Daa T, Kitano S, Fujiwara S, Yokoyama S. Expression of CD10 in basal cell carcinoma. Am J Dermatopathol 2004;26:463–71.

2 NEOPLASTIC AND PSEUDONEOPLASTIC LESIONS OF THE HAIR FOLLICLES

Because the hair follicles are complicated at a microanatomic level, the nosologic scheme for pilar neoplasms is extensive. Hair follicle tumors can be divided into those that differentiate towards the outer hair sheath epithelium; those whose target is the germinative epithelium; and lesions with mixed epithelial-mesenchymal features or lineages resembling those of the follicle-related mesenchymal tissues. It must be admitted before discussing pilar neoplasms, that their classification is perhaps the most contentious area of cutaneous adnexal pathology at the present time. Several competing classification schemes for pilar tumors have been advocated in the past and new variations continue to appear, often with little more to recommend them than rather theoretical considerations. We have used a relatively orthodox approach in this section, because it seems to correlate well with morphologic observations.

BENIGN FOLLICULAR NEOPLASMS WITH NONGERMINATIVE CELLULAR DIFFERENTIATION

Tumor of the Follicular Infundibulum

Clinical Features. *Tumor of the follicular infundibulum* (TFI) is also known as *basal cell hamartoma with follicular differentiation* and *infundibuloma* (1,3,5–7). It is an uncommon lesion that shows a marked predilection for middle-aged or elderly women. TFI presents as a solitary papulonodular tumor measuring less than 1 cm in greatest dimension; multiplicity and an eruptive pattern are less common but have been reported. There may be a clinical association with nevus sebaceus, Schopf-Schulze-Passarge syndrome (keratoderma, apocrine hidrocystomas, nail and tooth abnormalities, and hypotrichosis), or Cowden's syndrome (1,8).

Pathologic Findings. TFI demonstrates a subepidermal plate of compact polyhedral cells that form a lattice-work pattern and connect with the surface epithelium multifocally (fig. 2-1). The lesion is sharply demarcated and has been described as "fenestrated." Peripheral cells in the lesion may show nuclear palisading and can be glycogenated, resembling the trichilemmal sheath (1,3,5–7). A prominent layer of eosinophilic basement membrane material is often seen surrounding the cords as well. Nuclei are bland, and mitotic activity and apoptosis are consistently absent (fig. 2-2). Hair is not formed in TFI, but "bystander" follicles may be entrapped in the tumor, and intralesional acrosyringia and sebaceous glands are seen in some examples (2,4). Cribier and Grosshans (1) have found a deposition of elastic tissue immediately beneath TFIs in the corium. An infundibular nature for this tumor is hypothetical, and based mainly on the relationship of TFI to the acrotrichium.

TFI is typically nonimmunoreactive with Ber-EP4, which is a monoclonal antibody that decorates the majority of basal cell carcinomas. Other special techniques have not as yet been applied to the specific recognition of this tumor.

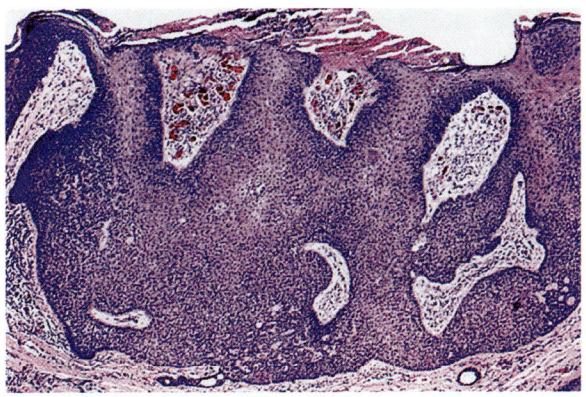

Figure 2-1

TUMOR OF THE FOLLICULAR INFUNDIBULUM

Fenestrated plates of keratinocytes are centered on a pilar unit.

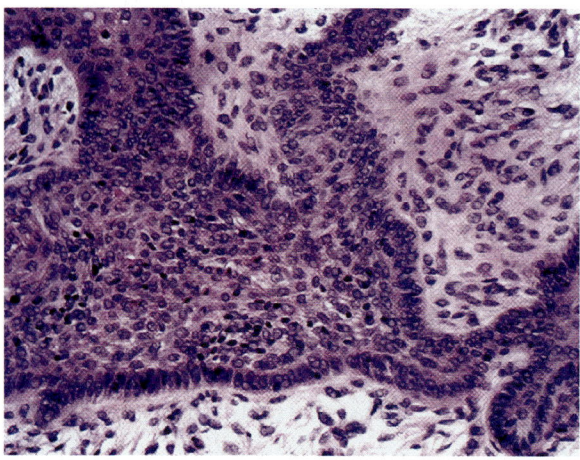

Figure 2-2

TUMOR OF THE FOLLICULAR INFUNDIBULUM

There is a bland cellular constituency, with no apoptosis. Basement membrane material surrounds the cellular lobules.

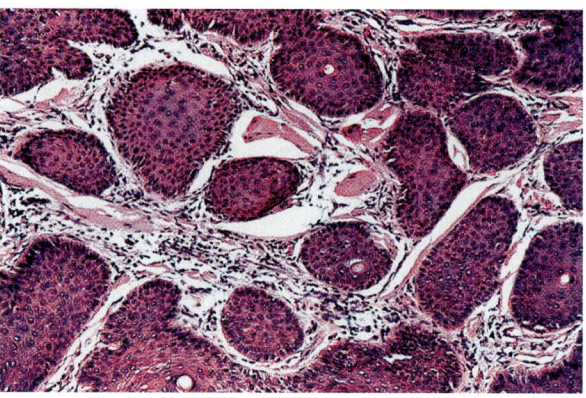

Figure 2-4

PILAR SHEATH ACANTHOMA

The tumor cells are bland, and are grouped into lobules of relatively equal size.

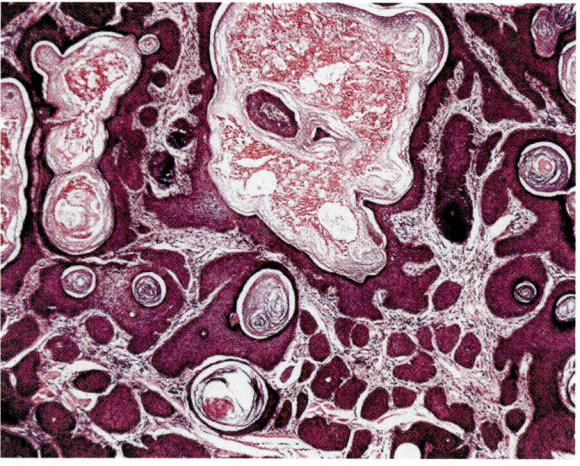

Figure 2-3

PILAR SHEATH ACANTHOMA

The centrally dilated pilar unit has proliferating lobules of polygonal cells budding away from it into the dermis.

Differential Diagnosis. Distinguishing TFI from superficial basal cell carcinoma may be challenging in selected cases. The former is highly differentiated, with regular formation of basement membrane and more voluminous cytoplasm.

Pilar Sheath Acanthoma

Clinical Features. Middle-aged or elderly patients usually develop *pilar sheath acanthoma* (PSA). The lesion is a single tan-pink papule or plaque, typically on the upper lip or the central face. A small, central keratotic plug is often apparent (9,11–14). PSA is curable by simple excision.

Pathologic Findings. Microscopically, a central infundibular microcyst harboring keratinous material and opening to the skin surface is observed. The cyst wall is keratinocytic and proliferative, with lobular buds extending radially into the corium (figs. 2-3, 2-4). Tumor cells are either polyhedral, with pale eosinophilic or clear cytoplasm, or basaloid. The cellular projections may enclose small horn cysts. Hair is not formed in PSA.

Because of the probable presence of infundibular and isthmic differentiation in PSA, Hurt (10) has suggested that it be called *lobular infundibuloisthmicoma*. The older of the two names has the benefit of greater familiarity and brevity.

There is no need for the use of adjuvant pathologic assessments in the diagnosis of PSA.

Differential Diagnosis. The only tenable entity in the differential diagnosis of PSA is Winer's pore. In reality, these two entities likely represent points in the same pathologic spectrum.

Winer's Pore

Winer's pore is a relatively common clinical entity, seen as a single nodular lesion on the head and neck in adults (16). The conceptual separation of Winer's pore and PSA, however, is a dubious one. The only differences between these proliferations are that Winer's pore has a larger cystic opening to the skin surface, commonly exhibits small sebaceous glands or vellus hairs in its base, and manifests a lesser degree of peripheral epithelial proliferation with the appearance of accentuated rete ridges. Lesions resembling Winer's pore have been reported together with other pilar proliferations in association with nevus comedonicus (15).

Trichoadenoma

Clinical Features. *Trichoadenoma (of Nikolowski)* is an infrequently encountered neoplasm that is represented clinically by a nondescript solitary nodule in the skin of the head, neck, or trunk (20–22,24). It generally measures less than 1 cm in greatest dimension. Occasional lesions said to resemble trichoadenoma have been reported in extracutaneous sites including the salivary glands and palate (19,23), but we consider that these are other metaplastic or hamartomatous proliferations.

Pathologic Findings. The histologic image features a proliferation of microcystic arrays of pilar-type keratinizing epithelium, separated from one another by fibroblastic stroma in the dermis, without any attachment to the epidermis. The keratin-filled cysts are composed of polyhedral cells that often contain keratohyaline granules and eosinophilic or clear cytoplasm. Nuclei are bland, without nucleoli or mitotic figures (fig. 2-5). There are no basaloid elements, and only a minor component of noncyst-forming epithelial cells, in the form of solid buds from the microcysts, is apparent.

Trichoadenoma lacks immunoreactivity for carcinoembryonic antigen (CEA), epithelial membrane antigen (EMA), chromogranin A, and CD15, distinguishing it from its differential diagnostic mimics.

Differential Diagnosis. The principal alternative choices to a diagnosis of trichoadenoma include desmoplastic trichoepithelioma and microcystic adnexal carcinoma (17,18). Desmoplastic trichoepithelioma is positive for EMA and chromogranin in approximately 85 percent of cases; roughly the same proportion of microcystic adnexal carcinomas are positive for CEA and CD15. Moreover, desmoplastic trichoepithelioma demonstrates the proliferation of much narrower cords of epithelial cells than those seen in trichoadenoma, and microcal-

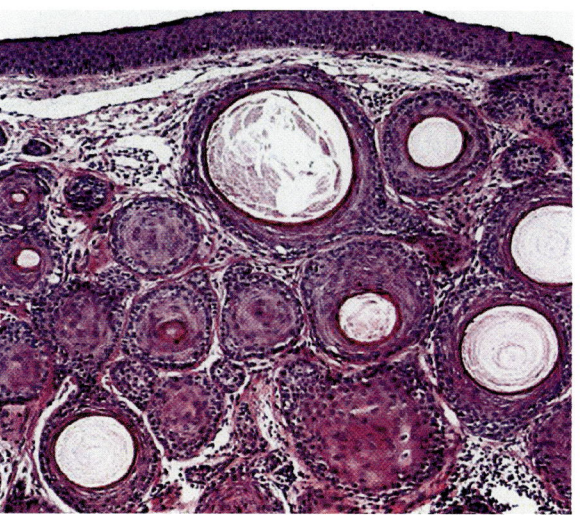

Figure 2-5

TRICHOADENOMA

A congerie of cytologically bland microcysts is seen in the dermis, each of which contains trichilemmal-type keratin.

cification is an expected feature of the former but not the latter of those lesions. Microcystic adnexal carcinoma shows deep infiltration of subjacent tissue, unlike the circumscribed growth of trichoadenoma (18).

Trichilemmoma

Clinical Features. *Trichilemmoma* is a tumor of the face or neck that shows a predilection to arise in adults (27,28,31,36). A potential association exists between multiple lesions and Cowden's syndrome (25,26). That condition includes the autosomally determined presence of multifocal hamartomatous intestinal polyps, an increased risk of breast carcinoma or other visceral malignancies, and additional proliferations of the skin such as sclerotic fibromas (collagenomas) and adnexal hamartomas or nevi (26).

Pathologic Findings. No matter whether trichilemmoma is solitary or syndromic, its morphologic characteristics are the same. It is typified by a lobular, follicle-centered proliferation of bland, amitotic, uniform polyhedral cells with clear glycogenated cytoplasm, surrounded by cuffs of basement membrane material (fig. 2-6) (26–29,31,36). Tumor cells commonly demonstrate peripheral nuclear palisading in the cellular lobules (fig. 2-7); the interfollicular

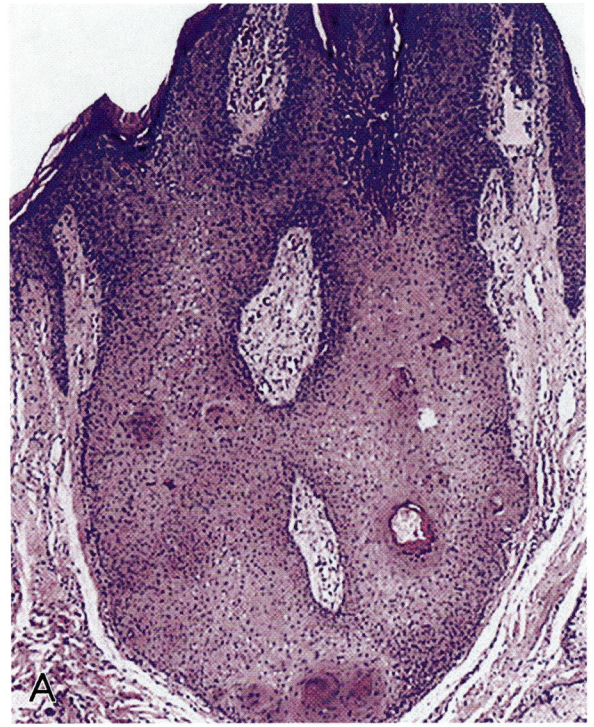
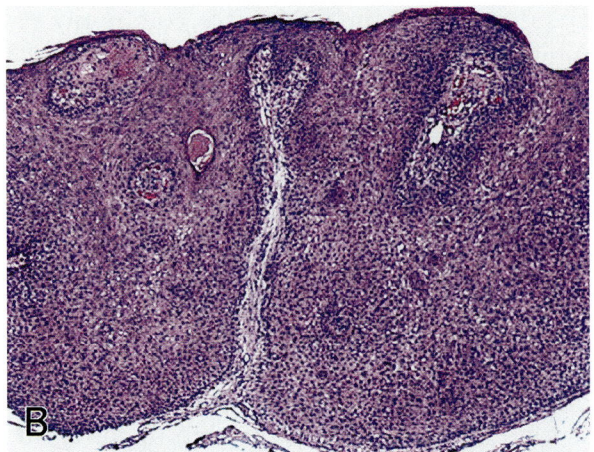
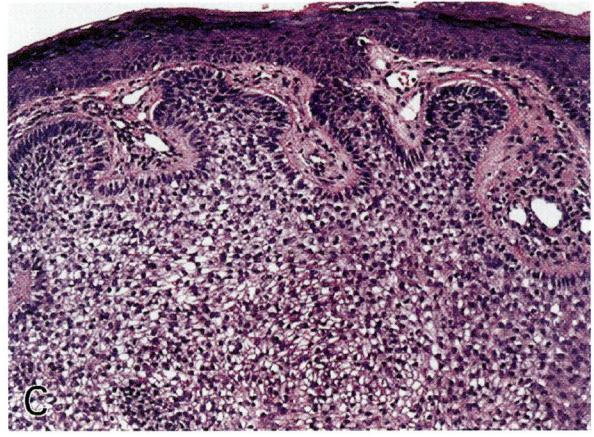

Figure 2-6

TRICHILEMMOMA

A,B: Bulbous lobular expansion of the pilar epithelium is seen.

C: The tumor is surrounded by a cuff of basement membrane material.

epidermis is unremarkable. Lobular profiles often coalesce, producing a nodular mass in the dermis. Squamous eddies are absent in this neoplasm, as is overt keratinization.

Hunt et al. (32) and others (29,35,38) have documented a type of trichilemmoma in which there is a pseudoinfiltrative junction between the tumor and the surrounding stroma, instead of a "pushing" interface (fig. 2-8). The tumor cells have a fusiform appearance and the dermis beneath such lesions shows a fibromyxoid response, explaining the proposed name of *desmoplastic tricholemmoma*. Some mitoses may be present in such tumors, and this feature, in conjunction with the growth pattern, may result in an erroneous diagnosis of basal cell or squamous cell carcinoma. To complicate matters further, Crowson and Magro (29) have reported four examples of basal cell carcinoma that were associated with desmoplastic tricholemmomas.

A helpful clue to the correct diagnosis of desmoplastic trichilemmoma is the peritumoral basement membrane in that tumor, which is retained in spite of the other disturbing histologic findings (32). It is potentially highlighted with the periodic acid–Schiff (PAS) stain or immunostains for collagen type IV or laminin. Despite the relative value of that finding, it is not definitive for excluding some basal cell carcinomas, as described by El-Shabrawi and LeBoit (30). Illueca et al. (33) documented CD34 reactivity in all trichilemmoma variants but not in other histologically similar neoplasms.

Differential Diagnosis. The differential diagnosis of trichilemmoma includes clear cell basal cell carcinoma, clear cell squamous cell carcinoma, and inverting follicular keratosis and follicular verruca, proliferations that are related to infection with the human papillomavirus (HPV). The first two entities can be

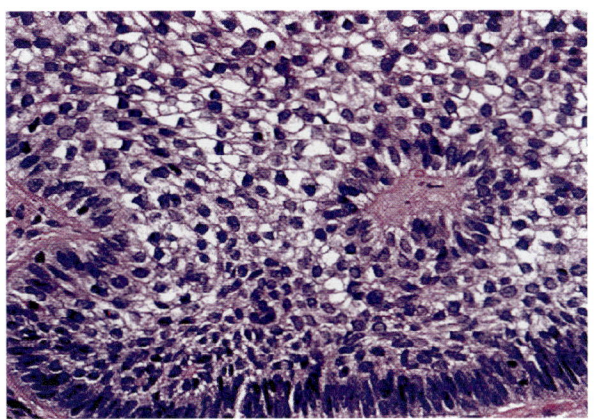

Figure 2-7
TRICHILEMMOMA
Nuclear palisading is seen.

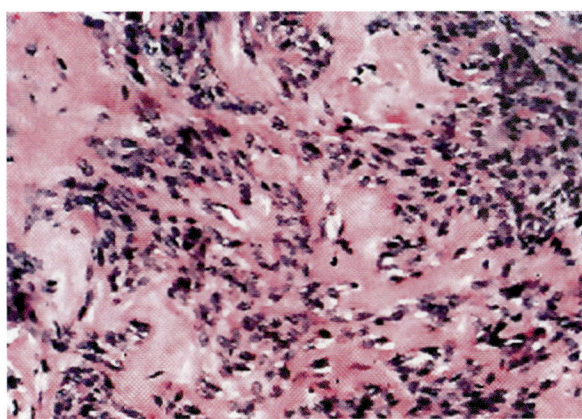

Figure 2-8
DESMOPLASTIC TRICHILEMMOMA
There is an ill-defined interface between fusiform tumor cells and fibroblastic stroma in the dermis. This image may result in the misinterpretation of such lesions as malignant.

separated effectively from trichilemmoma by their cytologic anaplasia; the latter two show formation of squamous eddies and lack evidence of HPV DNA in the lesional cells (34,37).

Benign Proliferating Pilar Tumor

Clinical Features. *Benign proliferating pilar tumor* (BPPT), also known as *proliferating trichilemmal tumor, proliferating trichilemmal cyst,* and *pilar tumor,* typically is encountered in middle-aged or elderly patients, with a strong predilection for women (39–42,47–50,53,56). It is usually situated in the scalp, but examples of this neoplasm have been documented in other body sites as well (39,53). Associated organoid nevi have been recognized in some instances (44,52). BPPT arises in the deep corium and evolves gradually over several years, often attaining a size of several centimeters (fig. 2-9). Erosion of the overlying skin surface may be seen. Simple excision is usually curative.

Pathologic Findings. BPPT exhibits sharp circumscription on scanning microscopic examination. That feature is important because the architecture of proliferating pilar tumors is the major determinant of their biologic behavior (56,57). Understandably, therefore, piecemeal removal or curettage should be avoided if BPPT is suspected. Cords of polygonal tumor cells with squamoid characteristics are observed in this tumor, and they typically interconnect (figs. 2-10, 2-11); rarely, divergent differentia-

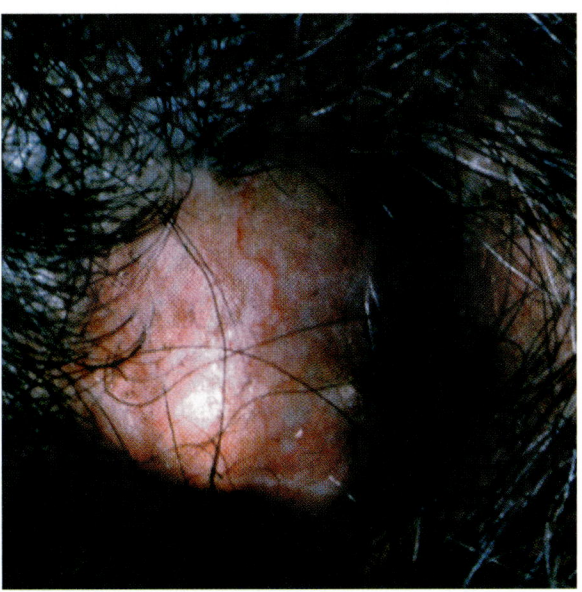

Figure 2-9
BENIGN PROLIFERATING PILAR TUMOR
A protuberant nodule in the scalp is seen.

tion, with ductal or sebaceous elements, may be seen (55). A central cystic area may be present in BPPT, filled with trichilemmal-type keratinous debris; this explains the common designation of this lesion as a clinical "cyst" (fig. 2-12). Clear cells are often apparent, and a cuff of basement membrane material may enclose the

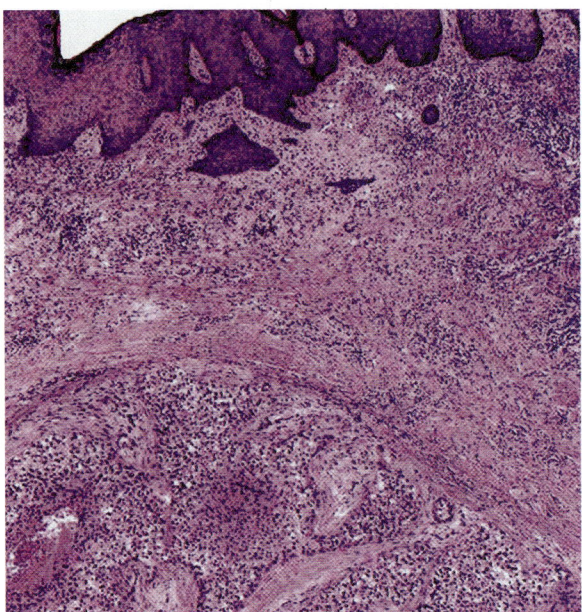

Figure 2-10

BENIGN PROLIFERATING PILAR TUMOR

There is a well-circumscribed, nodular dermal proliferation of mature keratinocytic cells.

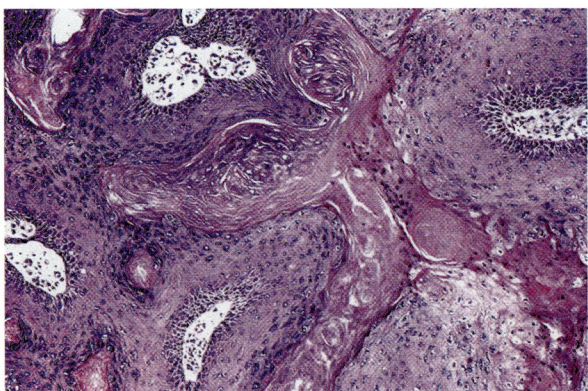

Figure 2-11

BENIGN PROLIFERATING PILAR TUMOR

Cords and lobules of interconnecting squamoid cells comprise this tumor.

peripheral aspects. These findings are common in other tumors of the hair sheath.

The cytologic features of BPPT are, however, potentially different from those of other benign follicular neoplasms, because they often include pleomorphic nuclei, vesicular nuclear chromatin, nucleolar prominence, and mitotic activity (fig. 2-13) (40,49). Because of such attributes, BPPTs have formerly been confused with squamous cell carcinomas; this is a particular problem in fine-needle aspiration biopsies (58). It must again be emphasized that the architectural configuration of a BPPT, rather than its cytomorphology, has the greatest prognostic significance. If the tumor is sharply demarcated, it will behave in a benign fashion; on the other hand, infiltrative growth into the surrounding tissue should cause concern for at least low-grade malignancy. Dystrophic calcifications are often evident in BPPTs, as are foci of trichilemmal-type keratinization. Rarely, infundibular keratinization is apparent as well (51).

In our judgment, special analyses of proliferating pilar tumors are not particularly contributory to diagnosis in individual cases. Some reports have applied quantitative DNA evaluations to the prognostication of these neoplasms, suggesting that DNA-diploid lesions are likely to be benign whereas DNA-aneuploid tumors are not (45,46,54,62). Others have implied that a lack of mutant p53 protein immunoreactivity is restricted to BPPTs (43,60,61). Our experience has shown these approaches to be less than reliable in regard to the differential diagnosis and the prediction of biologic behavior; Sleater et al. (59) concur in that opinion.

Differential Diagnosis. The differential diagnosis of BPPT principally concerns its separation from malignant proliferating pilar tumors and squamous cell carcinoma. The overall growth pattern of the latter two entities is invasive, unlike that of BPPT. That single point of disparity is sufficient to cull BPPT from its potential simulants. Clinical histories are also useful in this context, in that squamous cell carcinoma generally evolves more rapidly than does BPPT.

BENIGN FOLLICULAR NEOPLASMS WITH GERMINATIVE-TYPE DIFFERENTIATION

The germinative components of the follicle are the matrical cells, cortical cells, and cells of the inner hair sheath. Four neoplasms of the skin are felt to show similar cellular features: trichofolliculoma, trichoepithelioma, pilomatricoma, and trichogerminoma. Tumors resembling germinative follicular elements may reproduce the complete spectrum of hair formation as seen in embryonic and mature skin. A characteristic profile of maturation is apparent in a subset of

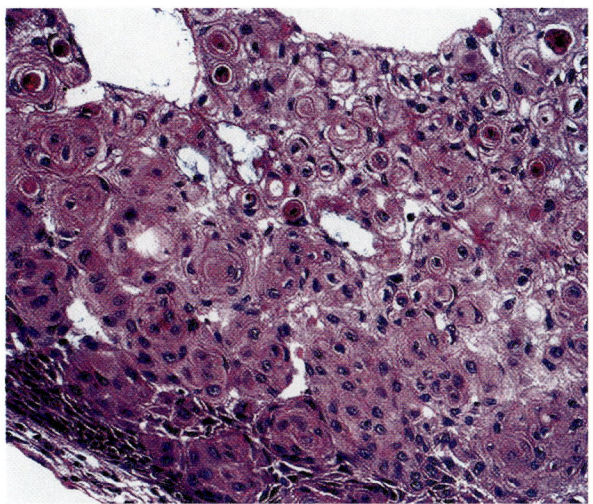 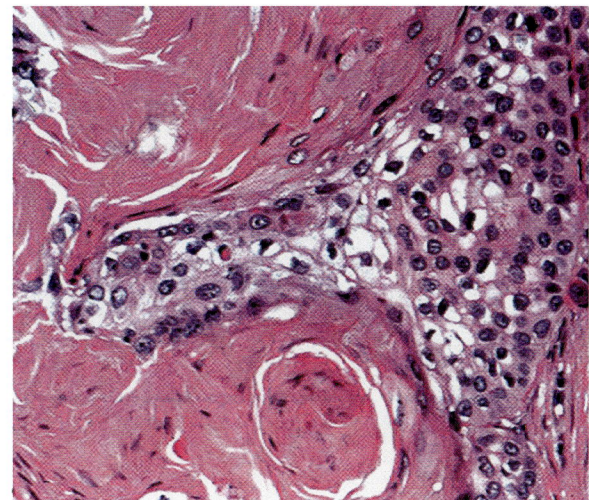

Figure 2-12

BENIGN PROLIFERATING PILAR TUMOR

The central aspect of many benign proliferating pilar tumors contains trichilemmal-type keratin, as seen here, and this feature is responsible for their being labeled as "cysts."

these lesions, in which immature matrical cells lose their organelles and simultaneously accumulate cytoplasmic keratin. Such elements are called "ghost" or "shadow" cells because they have ghost-like images and karyolytic nuclear profiles. Such cells are felt to signify the presence of matrical follicular differentiation (63) in neoplasms of the cutaneous appendages.

Trichofolliculoma

Clinical Features. *Trichofolliculoma* is a relatively uncommon lesion that is usually encountered in the head and neck. Examples in other skin sites have been reported, however; Peterdy et al. (67) described three cases of trichofolliculomas that were associated with vulvar intraepithelial neoplasia. This tumor typically arises in adults as a nonspecific, flesh-colored nodule, often with a central keratinous plug containing vellus hairs (64,65,70,71). Simple excision is adequate for cure.

Pathologic Findings. Trichofolliculoma is a proliferative keratinocytic lesion that is centered on a dilated primary follicle. The follicle is lined by infundibular or isthmic-type epithelium and opens to the skin surface (fig. 2-14). Secondary follicles bud from the "parent" in a centrifugal fashion, and these demonstrate germinative epithelial differentiation or form mature hairs

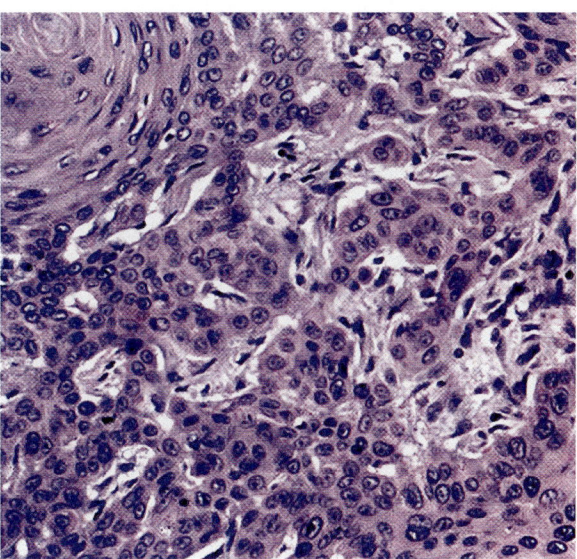

Figure 2-13

BENIGN PROLIFERATING PILAR TUMOR

Atypical cytologic features may be seen in the tumor cells of benign proliferating pilar tumor, as shown here. If a lesion such as this one is well-demarcated and circumscribed on low-power microscopy, it may be regarded as benign.

(fig. 2-15). The stroma in and around the lesion is densely collagenous and arranged in parallel layers. The tumor cells exhibit a spectrum of cytologic attributes, including isthmic,

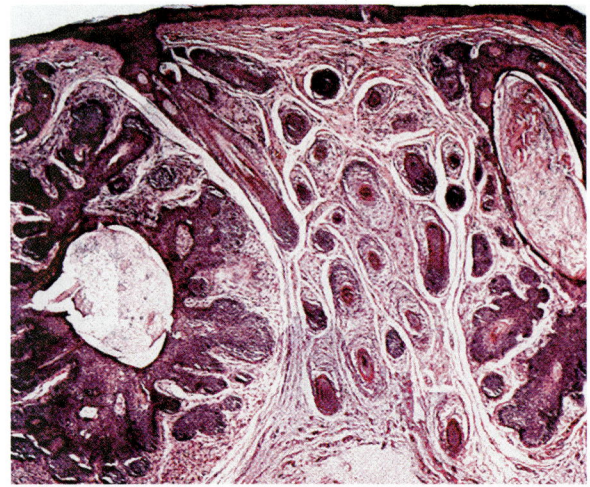

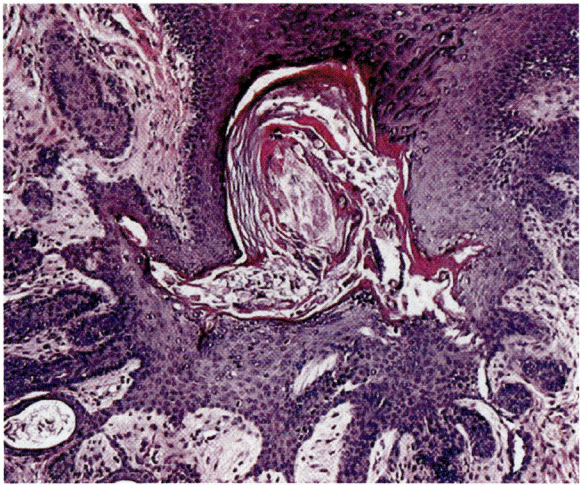

Figure 2-14

TRICHOFOLLICULOMA

Lobules of follicular epithelium extend outward from central pilar units.

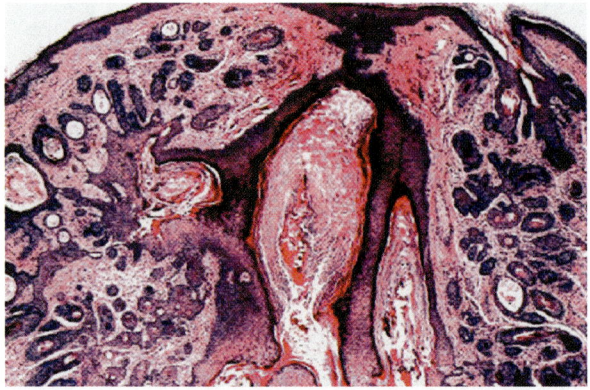

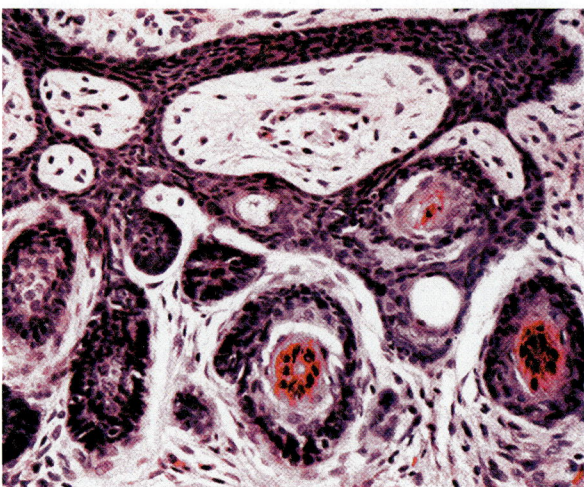

Figure 2-15

TRICHOFOLLICULOMA

The tumor cells may be germinative or form mature central hairs in each of the secondary follicles.

keratinizing elements; outer hair sheath features (clear cytoplasm and peripheral nuclear palisading); and a compact polyhedral or basaloid appearance. Some examples of trichofolliculoma show partial sebocytic differentiation in the secondary follicles, yielding the term *sebaceous trichofolliculoma* (66,68,69).

Differential Diagnosis. The differential diagnosis of trichofolliculoma principally centers on another pilar neoplasm, trichoepithelioma, and keratotic (pilar-type), or infundibulocystic, basal cell carcinoma (BCC) (72). Trichoepithelioma lacks dilated primary follicles and is composed almost solely of basaloid cells, in contrast to trichofolliculoma. The fibromyxoid stroma of BCC, and the apoptosis that is so common in these lesions, is not shared by trichofolliculoma.

Schulz and Hartschuh (69) have offered the opinion that a lesion known as *folliculosebaceous cystic hamartoma* (FCH) is in fact a trichofolliculoma with cystic changes. We endorse that construct, but we would add that mesenchymal proliferation in FCH is more marked than that of the usual trichofolliculoma, and the stroma of FCH may include neural, vascular, adipocytic, and fibrous components.

Trichoepithelioma

Clinical Features. Classic *trichoepithelioma* is a single, slowly growing, flesh-colored nodule

Neoplastic and Pseudoneoplastic Lesions of the Hair Follicles

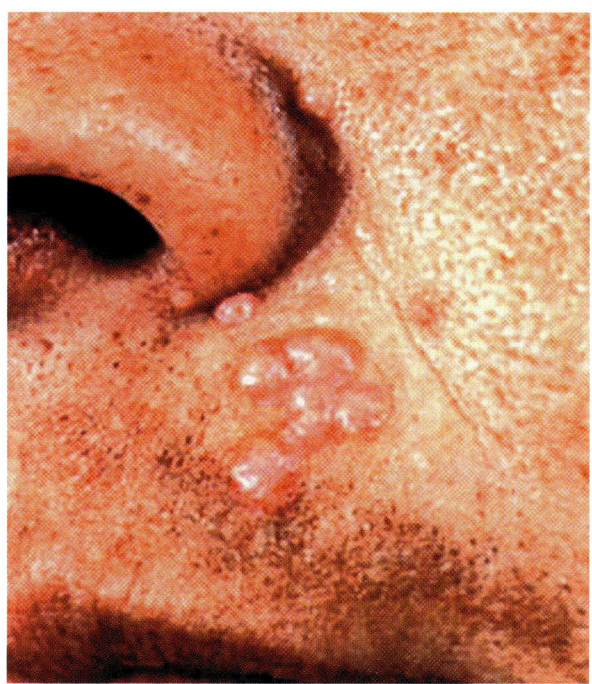

Figure 2-16

EPITHELIOMA ADENOIDES CYSTICUM (MULTIPLE TRICHOEPITHELIOMA) SYNDROME

Grouped, flesh-colored papules are seen in the facial skin.

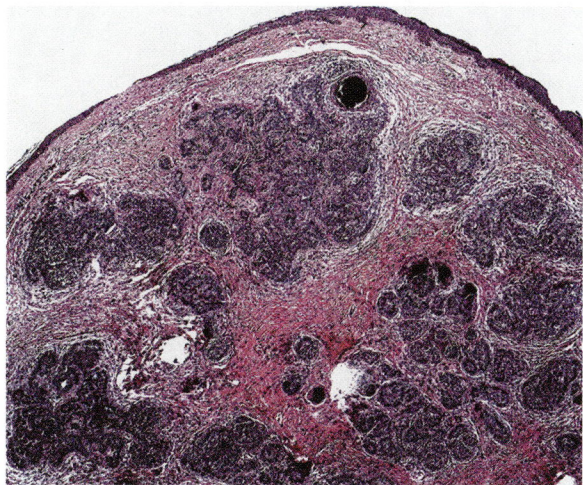

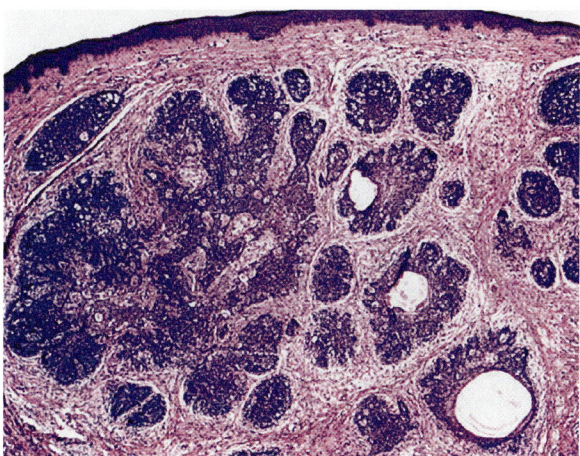

Figure 2-17

CLASSIC TRICHOEPITHELIOMA

Lobules of basaloid tumor cells are separated by collagenized stroma in the dermis.

in the facial skin, often appearing during childhood (76,89,95,96). It may attain an extremely large size in some instances, and also can arise in other body sites (81,85,100). The clinical distinction between this tumor and BCC may be extremely difficult, even histologically.

Multiple trichoepitheliomas are encountered in the *epithelioma adenoides cysticum (Brooke-Fordyce) syndrome,* an autosomal dominant condition (82,83). In this complex, the trichoepitheliomas are regionally numerous, with each tumor measuring less than 1 cm (fig. 2-16); skin fields outside the head and neck may be involved. Multiple trichoepitheliomas may coexist with multifocal cylindromas, spiradenomas, salivary glandular dermal analogue tumors (which resemble cylindromas), trichilemmomas, or BCCs (80,98). Systemic disorders associated with trichoepitheliomatosis include Rombo's syndrome (milia, hypotrichosis, atrophoderma, trichoepithelioma, BCC, and vasodilatation with cyanosis), systemic lupus erythematosus, and myasthenia gravis (73).

Pathologic Findings. Trichoepitheliomas, whether sporadic or syndromic, have a similar microscopic image. They demonstrate lobular dermal aggregates of uniform basaloid cells, separated by mature, collagenized, hypocellular matrix (fig. 2-17). The lobules often interconnect focally, and contain keratinous microcysts of variable sizes that are composed of cells with infundibular or isthmic differentiation (fig. 2-18). The dominant cell population is germinative in nature, and similar to that seen in nodulocystic or pilar-type BCC. The resemblance of these tumors to one another is even more striking if the trichoepithelioma also has retiform

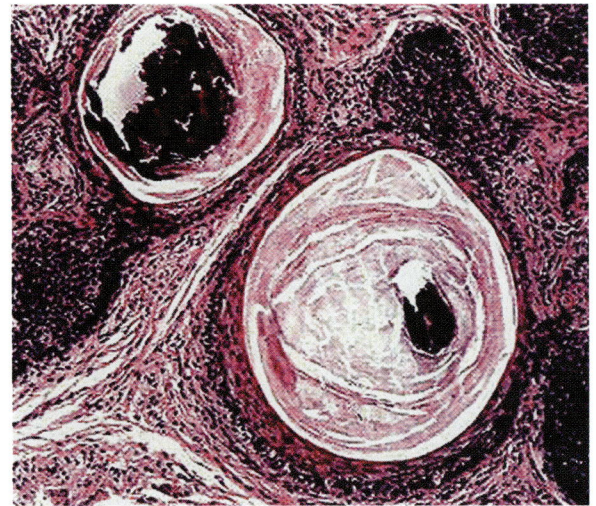
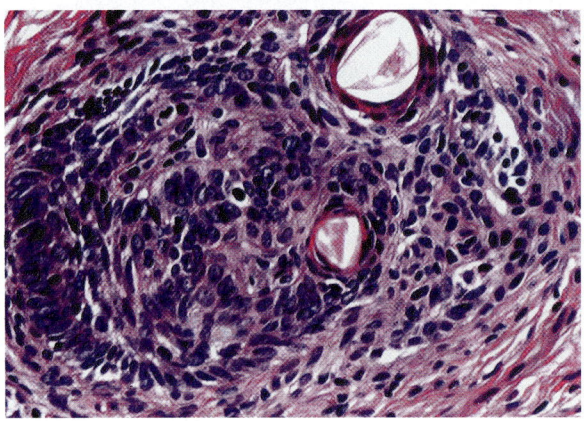

Figure 2-18

CLASSIC TRICHOEPITHELIOMA

Small, trichilemmal keratin-containing microcysts are present among the tumor cells.

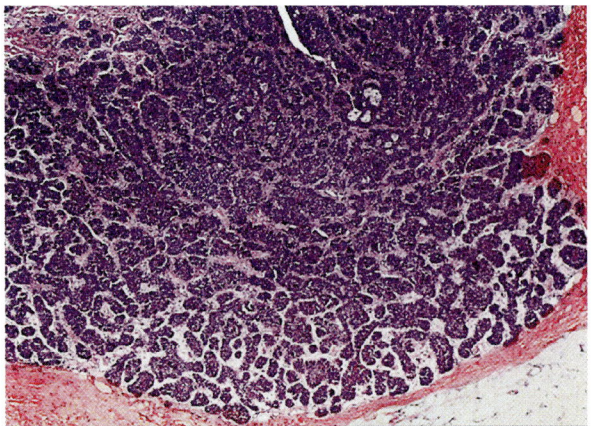
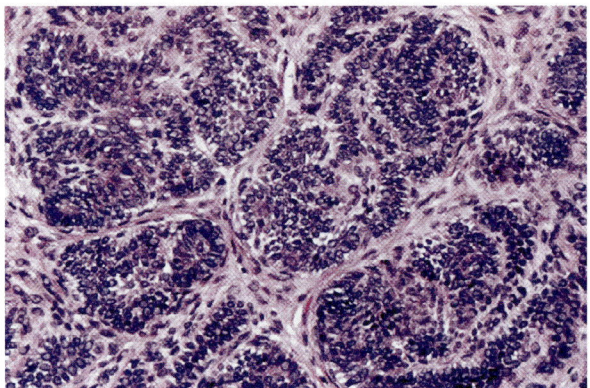

Figure 2-19

IMMATURE TRICHOEPITHELIOMA

Small groups of basaloid cells yield an organoid architectural pattern. Formation of trichilemmal keratin is absent.

or adenoid areas. Separating trichoepithelioma from BCC is especially troublesome if the former does not show obvious keratinous microcysts, but only solidly cellular basaloid cell groups; such lesions have been called "immature" trichoepitheliomas (fig. 2-19) (88). Rivet and colleagues (93) have described a variant with focal stromal atypia, resembling atypical fibroxanthoma.

Several features differentiate trichoepithelioma and BCC. These include a lack of fibromyxoid stroma in trichoepithelioma; nascent follicular papillae (papillary mesenchymal bodies) (78) in trichoepithelioma but not in BCC; and apoptotic foci in the presence of melanin in BCC. Despite these oft-cited differences, the authors suspect that both lesions are part of the same continuum. This view is not ours alone, and has support from both clinical (74, 75,84,86,94,101,103) and genetic observations. Trichoepitheliomas and multiple BCCs may be present in the same skin field (75,86,103); the genetic aspects of this concurrence are summarized below.

From a practical perspective, we advocate asking clinicians to remove trichoepithelioma completely whenever possible. If not feasible for cosmetic or other reasons, the tumor site should at least be surveilled regularly for possible tumor recurrence. The latter eventuality is by no means a certainty, because even in the construction that includes trichoepithelioma as a BCC variant, it appears to be a lesion with very low aggressivity; therefore, partial excision may be sufficient therapy in many cases.

Some investigators have used immunostains for bcl-2 protein and CD34 to distinguish trichoepithelioma from BCC (87,91,97). Some of those studies have cited an absence of bcl-2 protein in trichoepithelioma and its presence in BCC; conversely, CD34 is said to be apparent in the stroma adjacent to tumor cell groups in trichoepithelioma but not BCC. Our personal experience with these assertions has yielded inconsistent results (97), and we do not employ these immunostains in practice. In light of the foregoing comments on the probable relatedness of trichoepithelioma and BCC, one would not expect immunohistology to be effective in distinguishing between them.

Molecular genetic analyses have shown that syndromic trichoepithelioma is linked to genes with likely tumor-suppressor properties that reside on chromosomes 9p21 and 16q12-q13 (83,93a,103a). In contrast, and with particular relevance to the assumption that sporadic trichoepithelioma is a form of BCC, the latter two neoplasms share a loss of heterozygosity and chromosomal deletions at 9q22.3, the so-called Drosophila patched gene (77,90,99). This was shown by Matt et al. (90), using routinely processed clinical specimens and the polymerase chain reaction. Moreover, Hatta et al. (83a) have shown that overexpression of the Gli1 transcription factor is restricted to BCC and trichoepithelioma, among all basaloid skin tumors.

Differential Diagnosis. The histologic differential diagnosis of trichoepithelioma is basically that of basaloid skin tumors in general. Aside from BCC (72,92), additional considerations include cylindroma, spiradenoma, and other follicular lesions described in this section. Cylindroma and spiradenoma exhibit much more intercellular basement membrane material than that seen in trichoepithelioma; moreover, cylindroma features the formation of mucin-filled cylinders of cells, and spiradenoma shows an internal dispersion of mature lymphocytes and intratumoral lymphatic spaces. Follicular tumors other than trichoepithelioma generally manifest more advanced degrees of trichogenic differentiation or notable architectural dissimilarities (79,102).

Desmoplastic Trichoepithelioma

Clinical Features. *Desmoplastic trichoepithelioma,* also called *sclerosing epithelial hamartoma,* is a slow-growing, slightly umbilicated nodule or plaque in the skin of the central face in young or middle-aged women (105). A point of interest is whether this lesion is related biologically to classic trichoepithelioma (105,107,109,115). Desmoplastic trichoepithelioma is almost always unifocal, and has not been seen in patients with the Brooke-Fordyce syndrome or other systemic diseases (107,110).

Pathologic Findings. Microscopically, there are several dissimilarities between trichoepithelioma and desmoplastic trichoepithelioma. The latter is a disc-like dermal lesion, wider than it is deep. The lateral margins are sharply delimited. There are narrow linear or slightly branching cords of compact polygonal cells, without a truly basaloid component (fig. 2-20). An admixture of keratinous microcysts is common, and they may be filled with calcified material or show metaplastic ossification. These structures are connected to the linear tumor cell profiles (fig. 2-21). The stroma is densely collagenous and paucicellular, without fibromyxoid characteristics or retraction from the tumor cell nests. An association between desmoplastic trichoepithelioma and intradermal nevi or epidermoid cysts has been noted, leading some authors to suggest that they represent elements of combined hamartomas (106,111).

Immunohistochemical studies are helpful in making the distinction between desmoplastic trichoepithelioma and other differential diagnostic possibilities, principally morpheaform BCC and microcystic adnexal carcinoma. The latter lesions are also composed of narrow, slightly branching cords of epithelial cells, with or without dystrophic calcification, in a collagen-rich stroma (104). EMA is present in desmoplastic trichoepithelioma and microcystic adnexal carcinoma (114), but not BCC. In contrast, stromelysin-3, a metalloproteinase, is expressed by the stromal cells of morpheaform BCC and microcystic adnexal carcinoma, but is not seen in desmoplastic trichoepithelioma (113). Lastly, neuroendocrine cells are found mixed with the tumor cells of desmoplastic trichoepithelioma (104,108), but are absent in the other two neoplasms. Immunostains for chromogranin (fig. 2-22), neurofilament protein, synaptophysin, and cytokeratin (CK)20 may be employed to detect these elements and thereby

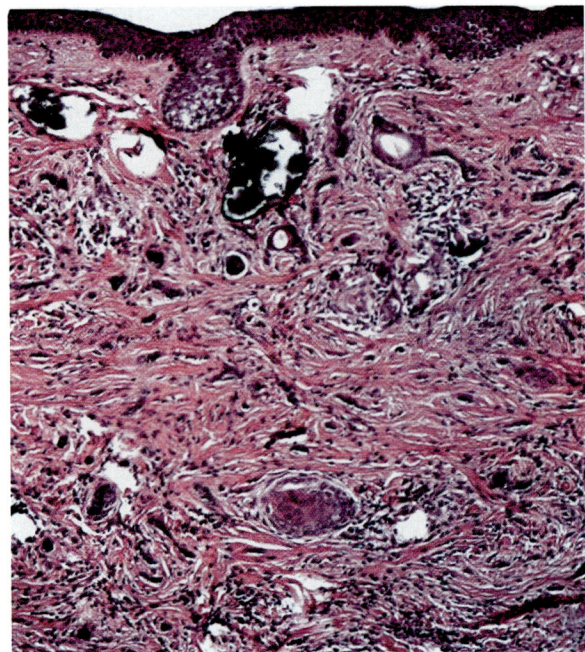

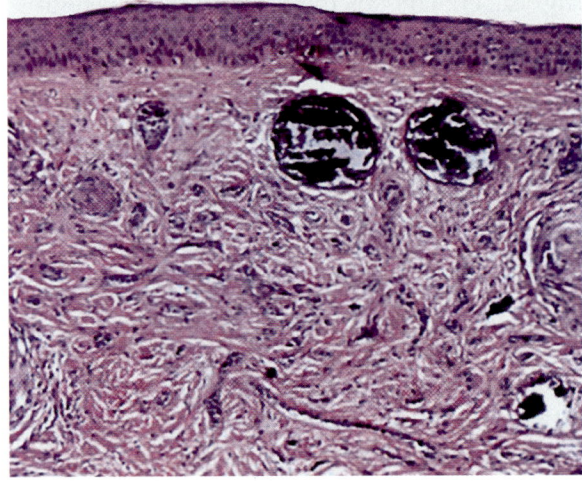

Figure 2-20

DESMOPLASTIC TRICHOEPITHELIOMA

Narrow cords of basaloid cells in the dermis are admixed with calcified microcysts. These tumors are generally confined to the upper reticular dermis.

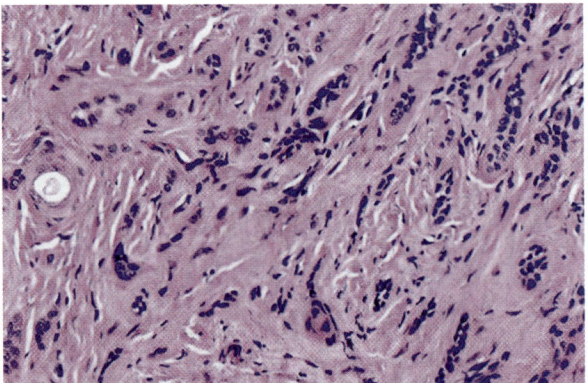

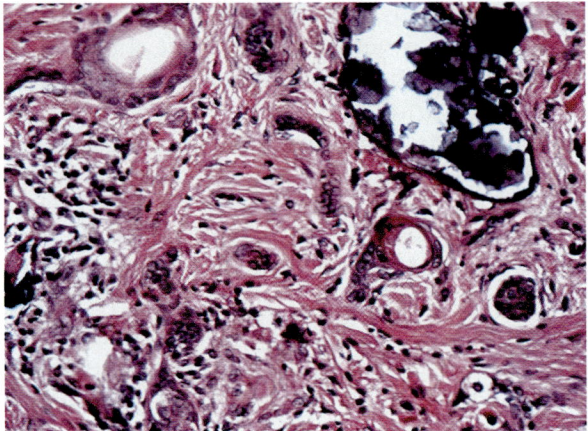

Figure 2-21

DESMOPLASTIC TRICHOEPITHELIOMA

The cells comprising the linear cords of desmoplastic trichoepithelioma are set in a densely collagenized stroma and connect to the calcified microcysts in the corium.

substantiate the diagnosis of desmoplastic trichoepithelioma.

Differential Diagnosis. It is useful to remember that BCCs of all types lack sharp circumscription and are composed of truly basaloid elements, whereas desmoplastic trichoepithelioma does not show such characteristics (112). Moreover, morpheaform BCC exhibits small areas in which the stroma is fibromyxoid and retracted, and it also contains larger cell groups than those seen in desmoplastic trichoepithelioma. Microcystic adnexal carcinoma features the presence of more tubular cell nests; if a large enough biopsy specimen is provided, microcystic adnexal carcinoma is seen to permeate deeply into the subjacent tissue, whereas desmoplastic trichoepithelioma has a limited, plate-like configuration.

Pilomatricoma

Clinical Features. *Pilomatricoma*, also known as *calcifying epithelioma of Malherbe*, *pilomatrixoma*, and *trichomatricoma*, is a peculiar tumor that is a caricature of matrical follicular differentiation. It occurs bimodally in patients under 25 or over 50 years of age, as a deep, slowly growing, cystic nodule on the head and

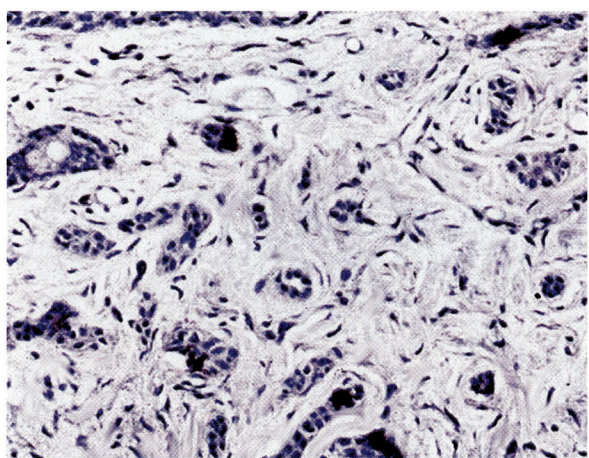

Figure 2-22

DESMOPLASTIC TRICHOEPITHELIOMA

Multifocal immunoreactivity for chromogranin A is apparent. The principal differential diagnostic alternative for this neoplasm, morpheaform basal cell carcinoma, is generally negative for that marker.

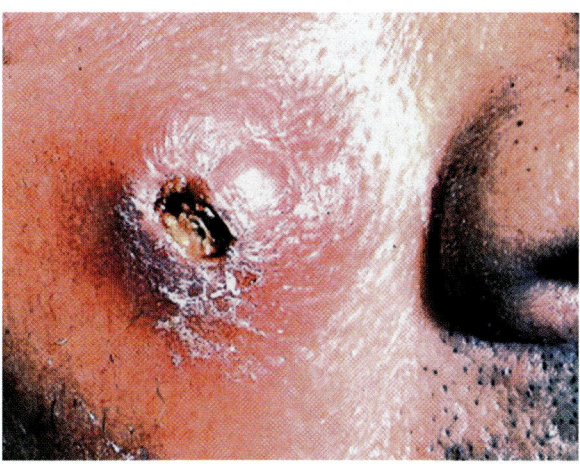

Figure 2-23

PILOMATRICOMA

Pilomatricoma in the skin of the cheek in a young man. The lesion is a nodular erythematous mass; the presence of a central epidermal defect in this case was caused by previous biopsy of the neoplasm.

neck (fig. 2-23). It also can arise in other anatomic sites, and may erode through the skin surface as well (116,118,121–124,128,129,131, 132,142,146,148). Multiple pilomatrical tumors may be seen in a familial setting in patients who also have myotonic dystrophy (Steinert's syndrome); there is also a well-documented association with anetoderma and a more questionable linkage to Turner's and Gardner's syndromes (127,132,141,143).

Because pilomatricoma is situated in the lower dermis and subcutis, it may simulate the appearance of an enlarged lymph node clinically. This possibility has resulted in some diagnostic misadventures in cases where fine needle aspiration biopsy was utilized to sample the lesion (147). The tumor cells of pilomatricoma are atypical-looking in such specimens (137,138, 144), and may be erroneously interpreted as reflecting the presence of metastatic carcinoma. Although a malignant counterpart of pilomatricoma is thought to exist (see below), there have been no convincing reports of carcinomatous transformation of benign tumors of this type. Accordingly, simple excision is usually sufficient for uncomplicated lesions.

Pathologic Findings. Some authors have suggested that pilomatricoma is initially a cystic dermal proliferation that is lined, in part, by both infundibular-type and germinative matrical cells (134). The latter have a basaloid appearance and are the most characteristic component of this neoplasm; they exhibit monotonous round nuclei, dark chromatin, small nucleoli, often-brisk mitotic activity, and cytoplasmic amphophilia (fig. 2-24). The peripheral basaloid cells phase into an intermediate zone in which nuclei assume a washed-out appearance and the cytoplasm becomes uniformly eosinophilic (ghost cells). Centrally, ghost cells are present to the exclusion of other elements (fig. 2-25). Dystrophic calcification may be apparent in that zone as well.

With time, the basaloid cells tend to be replaced by aggregates of ghost cells, calcifications, and foci of metaplastic ossification. Extravasated keratin often invokes a giant cell reaction in the adjacent soft tissue; indeed, these features may predominate in "ancient" pilomatricomas (134). The secondary heterotopic ossification may be prominent enough to produce an appearance like that of cutaneous osteoma, and intratumoral extramedullary hematopoiesis may be seen as well (133).

Microscopic variants of pilomatricoma include a *perforating* subtype, which is eliminated through the overlying epidermis (128); one could rightly assume that lesions that are linked to clinical anetoderma (132,136) represent an

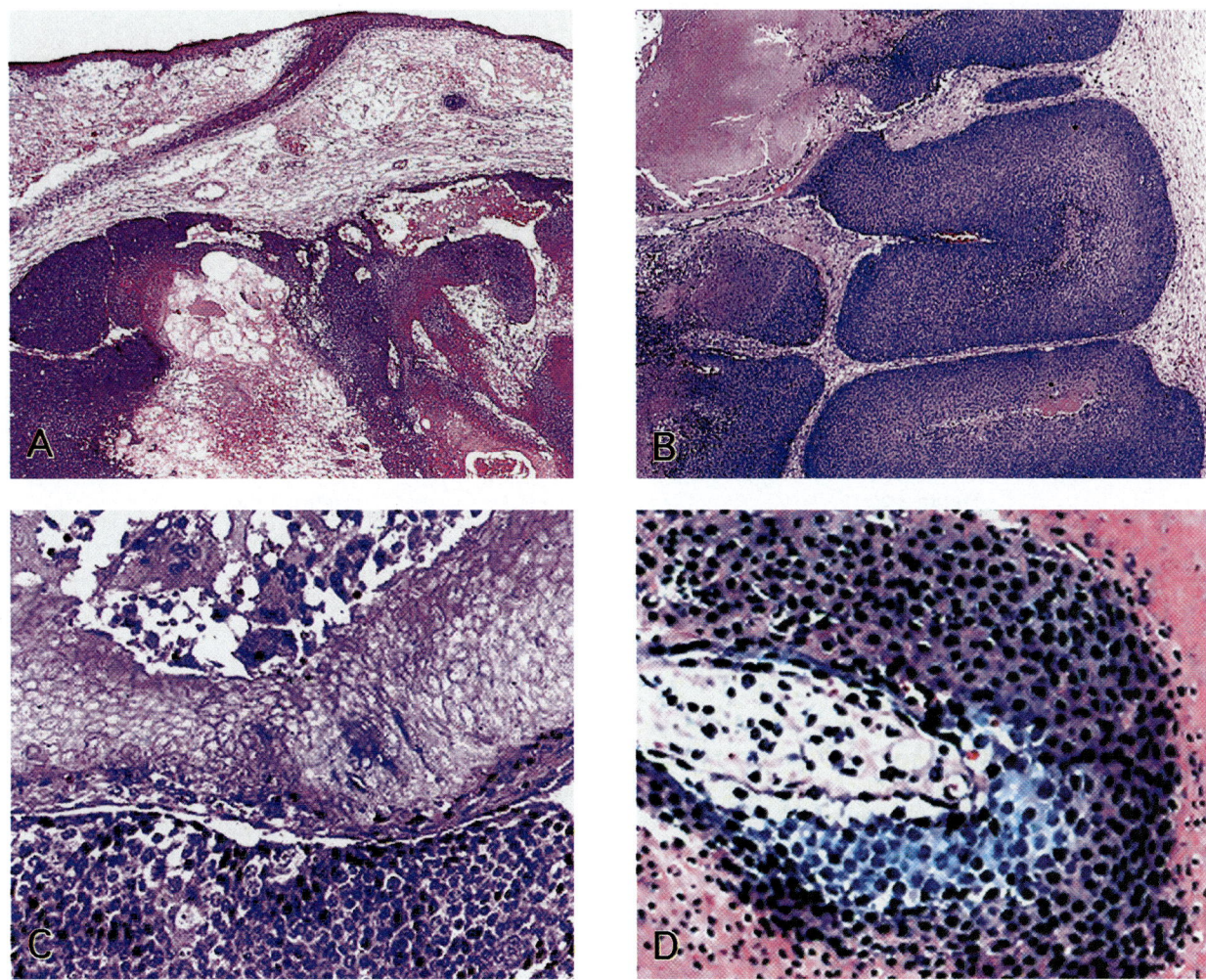

Figure 2-24

PILOMATRICOMA

Pilomatricoma is a potentially cystic lesion of the dermis that is composed of germinative basal cells in apposition to zones of ghost cell keratinization. The tumor cells often have small nucleoli and demonstrate brisk mitotic activity; these features have no untoward implications.

early stage of this subtype. Transformation of the tumor into an osteocalcific mass is the usual outcome for longstanding neoplasms of this type that are retained in situ. Another variant form of pilomatricoma is one in which budding groups of tumor cells infiltrate from the main tumor into the surrounding tissue and elicit a desmoplastic reaction (fig. 2-26). Lesions with this configuration are otherwise typical histologically, and may be considered as *atypical, invasive, proliferating,* or *aggressive pilomatricomas* (130,135,139, 140). They may recur locally, whereas that behavior is virtually unknown in ordinary lesions.

Finally, Carlson et al. (119) have described examples of pilomatrical neoplasms that demonstrated melanization of the tumor cells, similar to that seen in pigmented BCCs.

There have been case reports of occasional visceral carcinomas that superficially resemble pilomatricoma (125,126). We have not seen any examples of such lesions. To our knowledge, none of those documented in the literature has metastasized to the skin.

There have been reports linking pilomatricoma to mutations of the beta-catenin gene (120). Nevertheless, special evaluations of that moiety

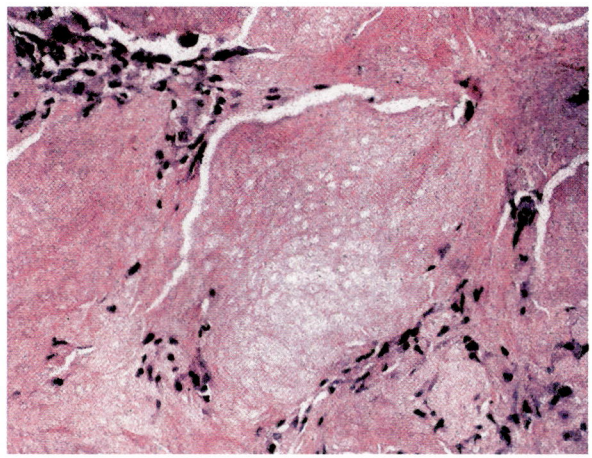

Figure 2-25

PILOMATRICOMA

Ghost cell keratinization is seen at the center of the mass.

are not necessary to establish the diagnosis, nor are cytometric assessments helpful in this regard (145). As mentioned earlier, the neoplastic cells in the fine-needle aspiration biopsy of pilomatricoma may be erroneously interpreted as a metastatic carcinoma. The presence of ghost, or shadow, cells in aspirate specimens should point to the proper diagnosis of pilomatricoma (137,138,144,147).

Differential Diagnosis. The differential diagnosis of pilomatricoma mainly centers on the unusual subtype of pilar BCC in which follicular matrical differentiation, complete with the presence of ghost cells, may be encountered (117). Overall, however, there are many cytologic and architectural differences between these neoplasms, and therefore their distinction should be straightforward.

Trichogerminoma

Clinical Features. In 1992, Sau et al. (149) described 14 cases of a rare tumor of the skin that they named *trichogerminoma*, because of the belief that it demonstrated germinative follicular differentiation. Patients with this neoplasm were between 16 and 73 years of age, with males predominating. The lesions were slow-growing deep-seated masses on the head and neck, trunk, or extremities, measuring up to 4 cm. All patients had a favorable clinical course, except for one whose tumor apparently underwent malignant transformation and metastasized distantly.

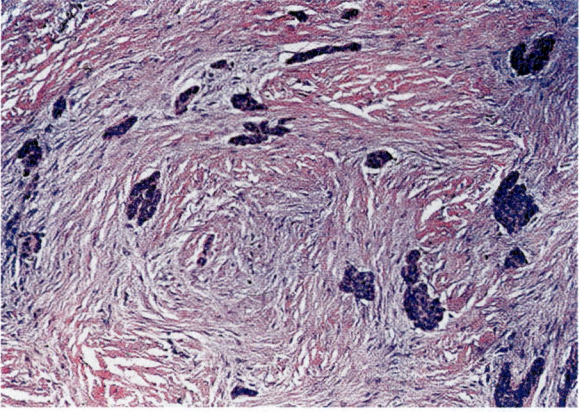

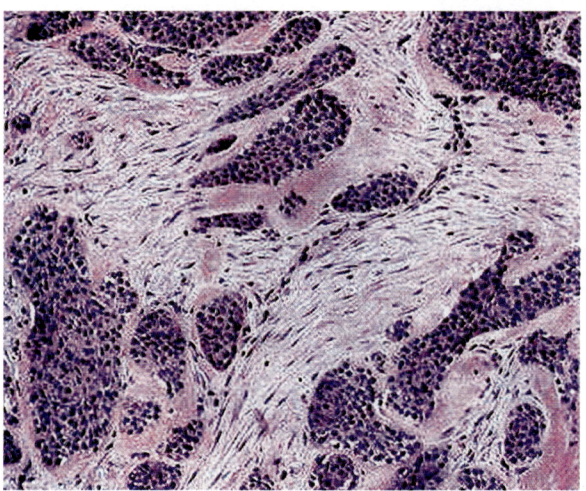

Figure 2-26

ATYPICAL (AGGRESSIVE) PILOMATRICOMA

There is irregular budding of basaloid cell nests into the surrounding dermis, which often acquires a desmoplastic character. These findings are associated with a risk of local recurrence.

Pathologic Findings. Trichogerminoma is a well-demarcated, cellular lesion that is centered in the deep corium. The tumor cells are basaloid and relatively uniform cytologically, with dispersed chromatin, small nucleoli, and mitotic activity. Cells are arranged in lobules, separated by a variably cellular collagenous stroma which may contain mucin focally. The most salient feature of trichogerminoma is the formation of cellular "balls," nodular aggregates that are internally concentric and peripherally condensed (fig. 2-27). Nuclear palisading also may be apparent, and the cell groups may be surrounded by PAS-positive membranes that resemble the vitreous layer of the outer root sheath. Keratinous

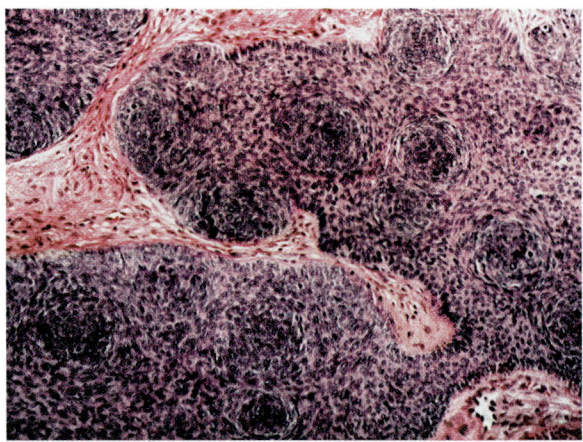

Figure 2-27

TRICHOGERMINOMA

Broad arborizing cords of basaloid cells contain concentric internal arrays or cellular "balls." The intervening stroma is fully collagenized.

microcysts can sometimes be seen within the cellular balls, as well as apoptotic foci, areas of clear cell change, abortive hair bulb–like structures, and divergent sebaceous differentiation.

Special studies have not as yet been performed on trichogerminoma. The potential diagnostic value of such evaluations, therefore, cannot be determined at this point.

Differential Diagnosis. Because of its variable microscopic features, trichogerminoma has a sizable differential diagnosis. It principally includes BCC, trichoepithelioma, and trichoblastoma (see below). Some skeptics may choose to classify this neoplasm as a subtype of pilar-type BCC, because of the general histologic image described above. For now, however, it would appear that the aggregate clinicopathologic profile of trichogerminoma justifies its existence as a distinct entity. The most important histologic element that distinguishes this tumor from other nosologic considerations is its constitution by cellular balls, as outlined above.

MIXED EPITHELIAL AND MESENCHYMAL FOLLICULAR PROLIFERATIONS

Two appendageal tumors are characterized by concurrent differentiation towards follicular epithelium and follicular mesenchyme. They are basaloid follicular hamartoma (included in this section as a "tumor" in the generic sense) and trichoblastoma.

Basaloid Follicular Hamartoma

Basaloid follicular hamartoma (BFH) is a pilar epithelial proliferation for which both malformative and neoplastic origins have been proposed. In light of its overall clinicopathologic characteristics, BFH is probably best regarded as a tumor-like lesion rather than a clonal disorder.

Clinical Features. As summarized by Ricks et al. (157), BFH may be seen in one of four clinical contexts: as a sporadic solitary papule; as a plaque in the skin of the scalp with associated alopecia; as grouped unilateral linear papules; and as generalized papular lesions in patients with evidence of systemic autoimmunity, including such conditions as myasthenia gravis and lupus erythematosus. Individual lesions measure from 1 to 5 mm in greatest dimension and are flesh colored. Patients of all ages may be affected; patients with multiple BFHs in early childhood generally belong to kindreds with autosomal dominant inheritance of the condition (150,151). An association with acrochordons and seborrheic keratoses has been suggested as well (150).

Pathologic Findings. BFH is typified by interanastomosing cords and strands of cytologically bland basaloid cells or compact polygonal cells, which produce a fenestrated image and are attached centrally to the basal epidermis or to hair follicles (152–155). There is little or no apoptosis among the lesional epithelial cells, and mitotic activity is likewise absent. No artifactual clefts are present in the adjacent stroma, nor is myxoid matrical change appreciated (figs. 2-28, 2-29). Structures resembling abortive follicular bulbs and primitive dermal papillae also have been reported in BFH (159).

As described below, the principal differential diagnostic consideration in cases of BFH is superficial multifocal BCC. Naeyaert et al. (154a) evaluated the immunophenotypes of BFH, multifocal BCC, trichoepithelioma, and other BCC variants. BFH and trichoepithelioma demonstrated circumferential labeling for CD34 around lesional epithelial cords, whereas BCCs did not. Moreover, BFH manifested a low proliferative (Ki-67) index, when compared with multifocal BCC and the other tumors in that study. To date, no gene-based or karyotypic comparisons between BFH and other skin lesions have been made.

Neoplastic and Pseudoneoplastic Lesions of the Hair Follicles

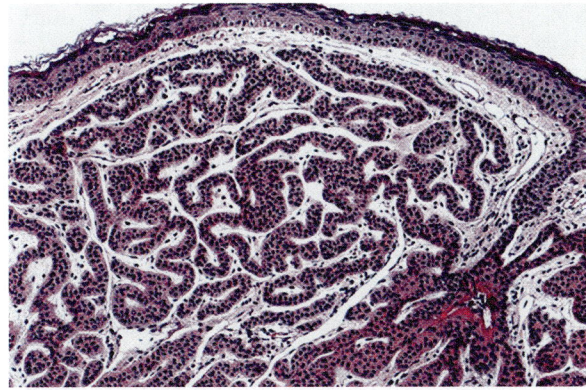

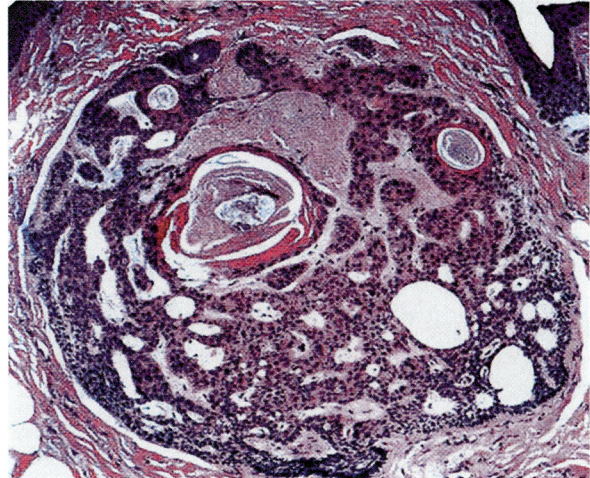

Figure 2-28

BASALOID FOLLICULAR HAMARTOMA

The tumor is characterized by interanastomosing cords of compact polyhedral cells. The surrounding stroma is fibrous.

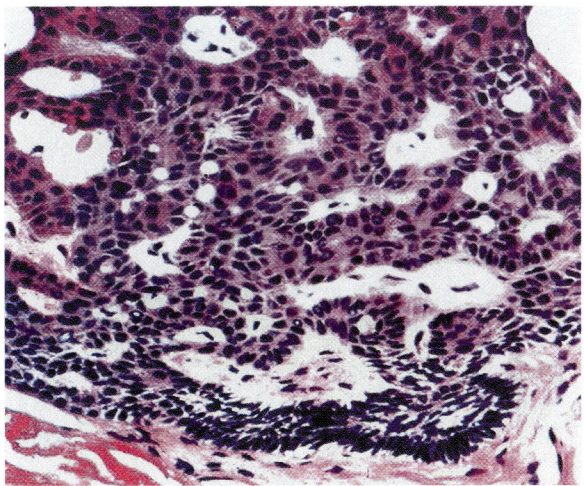

Figure 2-29

BASALOID FOLLICULAR HAMARTOMA

A lack of apoptosis and mitotic activity is seen in the lesional cells.

Differential Diagnosis. Multifocal BCC demonstrates central apoptosis within lesional clusters of basaloid cells, and mitoses are usually visible as well. Surrounding stromal collagen often is retracted away artifactually from the nests of basaloid cells, and mucomyxoid change is a common finding as well. Similar comments apply to infundibulocystic BCC, which may be multifocal and hereditary as well (156). None of these histologic changes is apparent in BFH. In our diagnostic practice, conventional trichoepithelioma is required to show much more of a nodular growth pattern than that seen in BFH, and structures resembling dermal papillae are more regularly seen in the former lesion. Nonetheless, Starink and colleagues (158) believe that BFH is a form of trichoepithelioma. The overall structure of BFH is similar to that of tumor of the follicular infundibulum; the latter, however, is composed of squamoid cells with more mature cytologic features and a greater volume of eosinophilic cytoplasm (150a).

Trichoblastoma

After the appearance of a text by Ackerman and colleagues on follicular tumors in 1993 (160), many pathologists have elected to follow their recommendation to use the term *trichoblastoma* in a relatively broad nosologic sense, to encompass several benign pilar tumors as well as lesions that would have been considered BCC variants in the past (162,164–168, 170–173,175,177,179,180,182,183). That is not the authors' preference, however. Headington's original description of trichoblastoma (also known as *trichogenic adnexal tumor*) (169) brought attention to two elements of that lesion: its relatively embryonic microscopic image, resembling that of developing hair, and other structural features which suggest an epithelial-stromal interaction to account for genesis. Depending upon which one of these is dominant, other terminological modifications such as *trichoblastic trichoblastoma* or *trichoblastic fibroma* (176) may be used as desired, although Wong and colleagues (181) have adopted a more generic approach to classification, preferring the

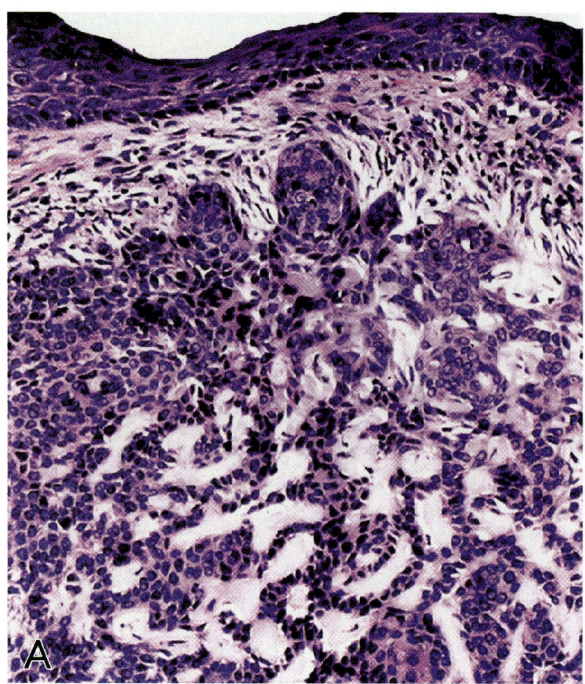
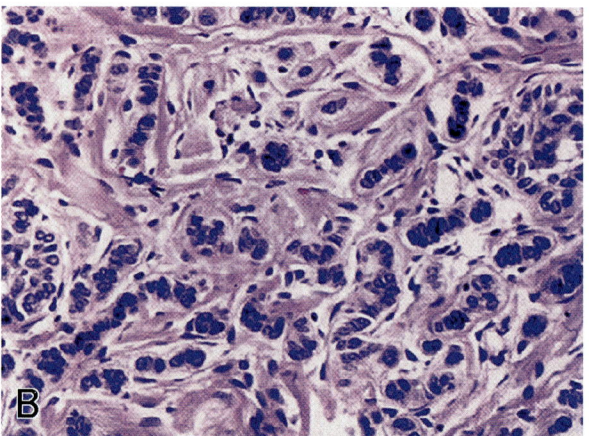
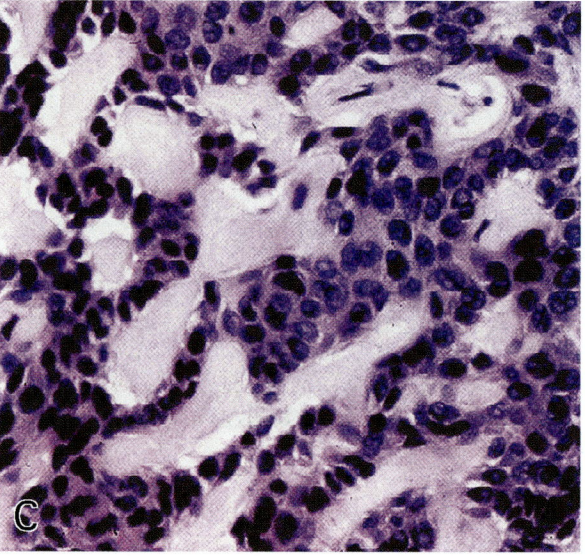

Figure 2-30

TRICHOBLASTOMA

A: A lacy network of basaloid cells in the dermis is separated by fibrohyaline stroma.

B: A more linear arrangement of the tumor cells and a more notably fibroblastic background are seen in this lesion, which may be termed trichoblastic fibroma by some observers.

C: The bland nature of the constituent tumor cells of trichoblastoma, with an absence of mitotic activity and apoptosis, is seen here.

all-encompassing term of *benign trichogenic tumor*. In our opinion, the basic term trichoblastoma is intended to denote a distinctive clinical and morphologic profile, and we believe that this narrow meaning should be retained. As such, trichoblastoma is a benign lesion that is adequately managed by simple excision.

Clinical Features. Trichoblastoma may arise at any topographic site, except the distal extremities. This tumor is typically a single, nondescript, dermal nodule, which may occasionally be deep seated. It measures less than 2 cm in most instances, but "giant" tumors have been described as well (174). There are no syndromes that are linked to these neoplasms.

Pathologic Findings. Microscopically, trichoblastoma is a basal cell lesion that is arranged in cords, sheets, or micronodules. The cord arrangement is the most common, in which profiles of two to three cells in thickness interanastomose and are separated by a cellular stroma (fig. 2-30). A hyaline membrane commonly invests the cellular cords, and rounded deposits of eosinophilic matrix may be present between them or in the adjacent dermis. Follicular differentiation is reflected by the presence of immature cell clusters that bud from the mass and are indented by stroma. This image resembles the primitive hair papilla and hair bulb; more mature foci may recapitulate hair root structures. Occasional tumors may demonstrate cellular melanization, as reported by Aloi and coworkers (161). A multinodular subtype with desmoplastic stroma was described by Chan et al. (163); this lesion exhibited foci of keratinization, mucomyxoid stroma, and foci of spindle cell change with infiltration of perineural spaces and pilar muscles. Despite these worrisome findings, the lesion failed to recur. Indeed, we do not recognize a malignant counterpart of trichoblastoma.

Given the doctrinaire definition of trichoblastoma, there are no special pathologic evaluations that contribute to its recognition. As cited above, virtually all of the studies which have appeared under the rubric of "trichoblastoma" in recent years concern lesions that we would classify under other diagnostic headings.

Differential Diagnosis. Depending on its particular image in an individual case, the differential diagnosis of trichoblastoma includes BCC of the nodulocystic and morpheaform types, trichogerminoma, cutaneous lymphadenoma (178), and basaloid follicular hamartoma (BFH) (162a). The last is the most challenging lesion to exclude because of its tendency for growth in single-file cords and because it has an interactive interface between the epithelium and stroma. Embryonic hair-like structures are not seen in BFH as they are in trichoblastoma. Cutaneous lymphadenoma shows a more nodular growth pattern than that of trichoblastoma and is composed of blander epithelial elements. Regularly dispersed mature lymphocytes are a necessary part of the image of lymphadenoma, but are not seen in trichoblastic tumors.

NEOPLASMS SHOWING DIFFERENTIATION TOWARDS FOLLICLE-RELATED MESENCHYME

Tumors exhibiting perifollicular stromal differentiation are rare. Furthermore, their clinical and histologic features are very similar. The lesions in this category are trichodiscoma, perifollicular fibroma, fibrofolliculoma, follicular myxoma, and pilar leiomyoma.

Trichodiscoma

The name *trichodiscoma* has been appended to a tumor that is presumed to show hair disc differentiation (189,192,194,195). Trichodiscoma is a receptor complex comprising nerve ends and fibrovascular stroma, and it is typically associated with overlying epidermal Merkel cells.

Clinical Features. Trichodiscoma is represented by a group of small, painless, nondescript dermal nodules, most often in the head and neck region, in patients of any age (189,192,194,195). The lesions may be grouped regionally or be seen as part of generalized trichodiscomatosis. This tumor may be associated with other follicular malformations or neoplasms, particularly Birt-Hogg-Dube syndrome (concurrent fibrofolliculomas, trichodiscomas, and acrochordons), which is an autosomal dominant condition (184–186, 188,191,196). De la Torre and coworkers (190) have suggested that the dermal tumors in Birt-Hogg-Dube complex are interrelated and reflect different faces of the same entity; however, that view is not universally accepted. Simple excision of trichodiscoma is curative.

Pathologic Findings. The diagnosis of trichodiscoma is based on the presence of a superficial "disc" of hypocellular fibrovascular tissue (fig. 2-31) that contains nerve twigs apparent only with special staining techniques. Mucin and elastin are also present in the stroma. The surface epithelium is thinned, and pilosebaceous units are usually seen at the periphery of the fibrovascular core. No special pathologic studies are required for the diagnosis of trichodiscoma.

Differential Diagnosis. The microscopic profile of this tumor is so characteristic that there is essentially no differential diagnosis for it. Indeed, that same statement applies to most of the other lesions discussed in this section. McCalmont et al. (193), however, have described peculiar fibromyxoid proliferations of the dermis that were thought to represent an early form of trichodiscoma, and Calonje and colleagues (187) likewise suggested that superficial angiomyxoma should be included in the differential diagnosis. Both of those lesions demonstrate much more stromal vascularity and myxoid matrical change than that seen in typical trichodiscoma, and angiomyxoma has a lobular rather than a disk-like configuration.

Perifollicular Fibroma

Perifollicular fibroma is another dermal fibroblastic proliferation, and the clinical features of this lesion are extremely superimposable with those of trichodiscoma (198–203). Perifollicular fibroma shows a vaguely nodular proliferation of bland, poorly cellular fibrous stroma, sometimes accompanied by mucin deposition, around hair follicles. It assumes a lamellar image and may be accompanied by fibrosis of the

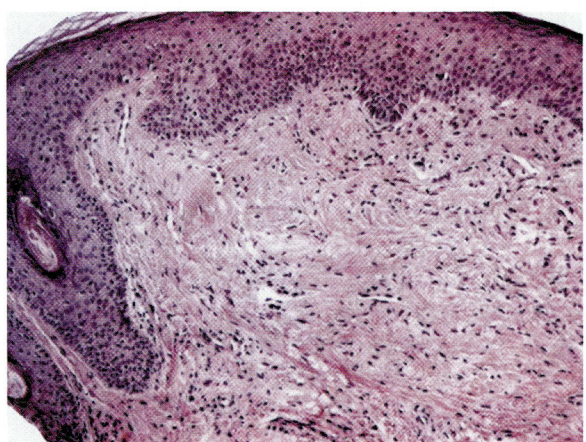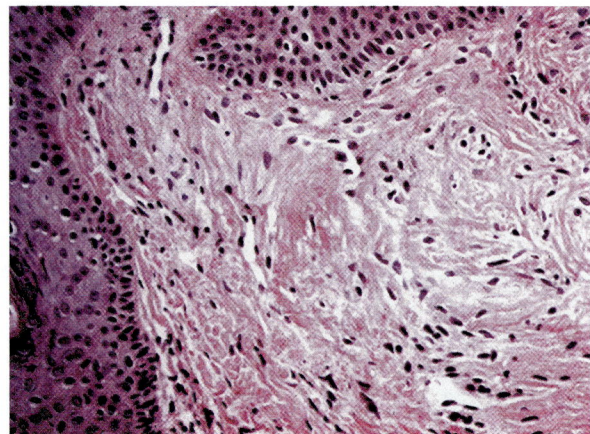

Figure 2-31

TRICHODISCOMA

Low- and high-power views show a disc of hypocellular fibrous tissue in apposition to a hair follicle. The lesion indents the follicular epithelium.

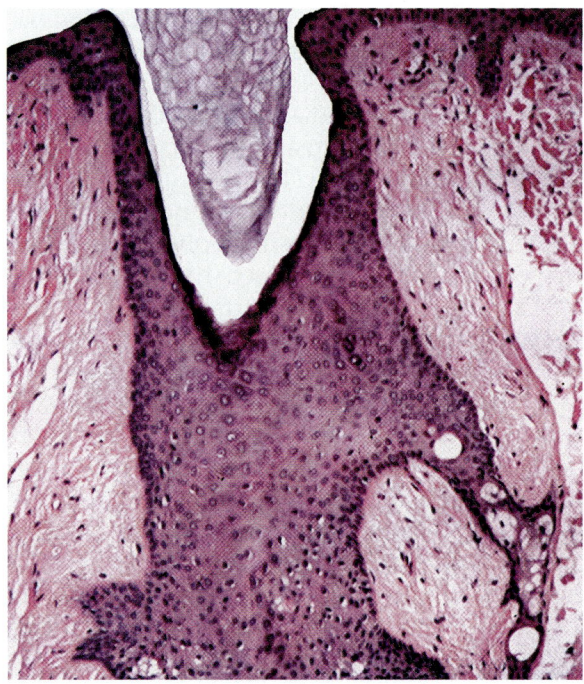

Figure 2-32

PERIFOLLICULAR FIBROMA

A fibroblastic and collagenized proliferation forms concentrically around a central hair follicle.

interfollicular dermis (fig. 2-32). No special studies are required for diagnosis.

The principal differential diagnostic considerations are the other lesions of the Birt-Hogg-Dube syndrome. This clinical complex is related to mutations in a gene locus on chromosome 17p11.2. It encodes a protein known as folliculin (200a,202a). Superficial angiomyxoma may be included, although the small size of perifollicular fibroma makes confusion of the two unlikely. Yet another tumor, known as storiform collagenoma, or sclerotic fibroma of the dermis (197), demonstrates a nodular, storiform proliferation of fibroblasts in a densely hyalinized and lamellated stroma. As such, its image differs substantially from that of perifollicular fibroma.

Fibrofolliculoma

Fibrofolliculoma resembles perifollicular fibroma clinically, but differs by being associated with central follicular dilatation and containing cords of epithelium that penetrate a laminated fibrous mantle around the affected hair follicle (fig. 2-33) (204,205,208). This image has been called an "epithelial net" (209). Fibrofolliculoma also may be linked to concurrent connective tissue nevi (203a). Junkins-Hopkins and Cooper (207) concluded that multiple lesions of this type may be associated with familial colonic polyposis and an increased risk of colorectal carcinoma (the Hornstein-Knickenberg syndrome [206]). These authors suggested that a former paradigm linking this visceral tumor to perifollicular fibroma was incorrect.

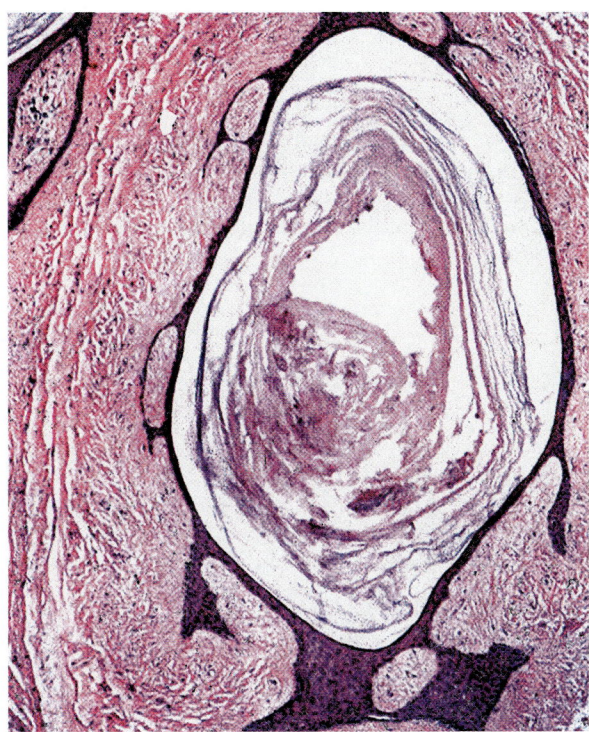

Figure 2-33

FIBROFOLLICULOMA

Fibrofolliculoma differs from perifollicular fibroma (see figure 2-32) only in demonstrating linear cords of epithelial cells that project outward from a dilated hair follicle.

Follicular Myxoma

Follicular myxoma is an uncommon lesion that is seen in adolescents and young adults. These patients may have other follicular tumors with germinative epithelial differentiation (210,211). The lesion is characterized by overtly myxoid stroma that surrounds a regionalized group of follicular units, which are often distorted and may interconnect. The overall image is that of a lobular proliferation (fig. 2-34). Branching capillaries are seen in the myxoid component, as are small groups of epithelial cells that sometimes show matrical features. Rare foci may be present in which primitive hair follicles or microcysts are formed. The epidermis often demonstrates papillomatous features. Lesions with similarity to follicular myxoma have been reported in patients with the NAME (nevi, atrial myxomas, myxoid neurofibromas [or cutaneous myxomas], ephelides) complex (212).

Pilar Leiomyoma

Cutaneous leiomyomas that are confined to the superficial dermis have been classified as pilar in origin. *Pilar leiomyomas* are usually single, nodular lesions that may be tender and generally measure under 1 cm (220,221,225); they are encountered at any age, and tend to favor the dorsal extremities (221) and genital skin (219). "Eruptive" tumors of this type, and others with a zosteriform pattern of growth, have been described (215,223).

Histologically, pilar leiomyoma shows fascicles of fusiform cells with generally bland nuclear chromatin and fibrillar eosinophilic cytoplasm (fig. 2-35), which are arranged in a whorling fashion. Tumor cells cut in cross section may exhibit perinuclear zones, and nuclear palisading, like that seen in some neural tumors, may be appreciated. Pilar leiomyomas are well demarcated and lack mitotic activity and necrosis. Nuclear pleomorphism is occasionally present, recalling the features of "symplastic" leiomyoma of the uterus (fig. 2-36) (218).

The relationship, if any, between epithelioid variants of pilar leiomyoma, in which tumor cells are polygonally shaped and arranged in sheets or groups, and cellular neurothekeoma has been questioned. Calonje et al. (214) offered the opinion that the two lesions were identical, but that contention is still being examined at the present time. For now, we prefer to regard these two tumors as separate entities.

The microscopic differential diagnosis of spindle cell pilar leiomyoma includes solitary myofibroma of the skin (217), cutaneous neurilemmoma (schwannoma) (213,222), and palisaded neuroma (216,222). The first of these three tumors lacks the whorled growth pattern of pure smooth muscle tumors, and instead shows micronodular arrays of bland spindle cells in a myxofibrous matrix. Myofibromas also commonly have a biphasic pattern of cell density, and they contain staghorn-shaped stromal blood vessels. Neural tumors may be difficult to distinguish from smooth muscle neoplasms in selected cases, and immunohistology may be necessary. Pilar leiomyomas are reactive for actin, desmin, or both, whereas benign neurogenic lesions are devoid of those markers; however, pilar leiomyomas commonly expresses S-100 protein, in common with neurogenic lesions (224).

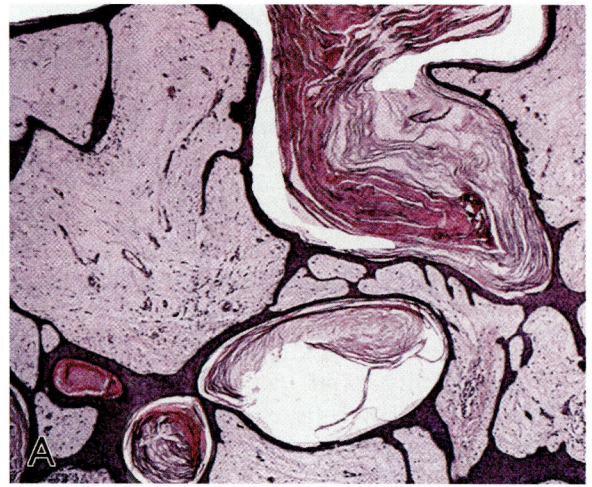

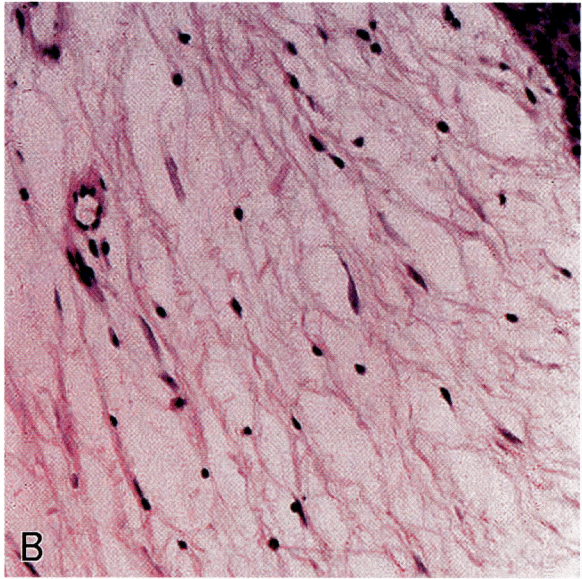

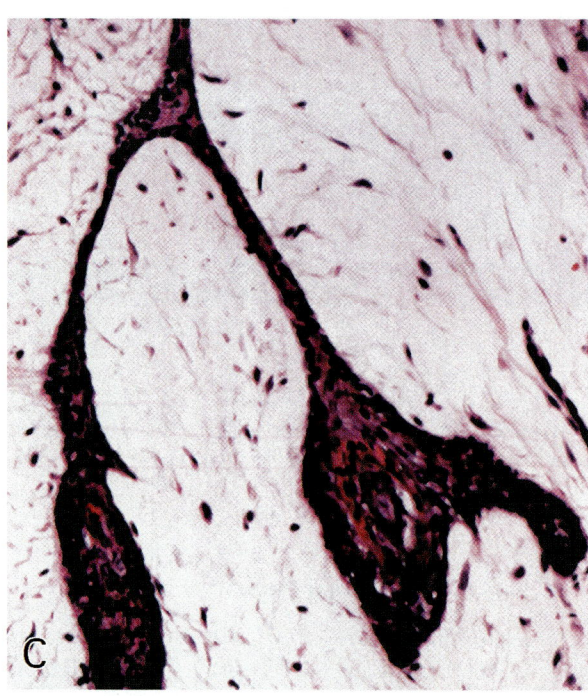

Figure 2-34

FOLLICULAR MYXOMA

A,B: Adjacent follicular units are interconnected and admixed with myxoedematous stroma.

C: Branching epithelial cords project outward from the follicles.

Epithelioid pilar leiomyoma may be confused with cellular neurothekeoma, melanocytic nevi, and histiocytomas of the skin. Again, immunohistology is the best means of distinguishing these entities; in our experience, epithelioid pilar leiomyoma is the only neoplasm just cited that labels for muscle-related markers.

MALIGNANT PILAR NEOPLASMS

Malignant follicular tumors are rare. This group of lesions commonly exhibits a spectrum of histologic features that does not lend itself easily to drawing clear parallels with non-neoplastic follicular epithelial differentiation. Therefore, many lesions in this general category demonstrate unexpected findings from a strict nosologic perspective.

Trichilemmal Carcinoma

Clinical Features. *Trichilemmal carcinoma* was initially described by Headington in 1976 (228a). In the past decade, several series have been published on this entity, making it clear that this is indeed a distinctive lesion (226,227,230,232,233). It is typically encountered in hair-bearing but actinically damaged skin: on the face, scalp, or ears. Patients are usually over 50 years of age. It usually presents as a single nodule or a plaque-like proliferation (fig. 2-37), although multiple lesions have also been observed concurrently

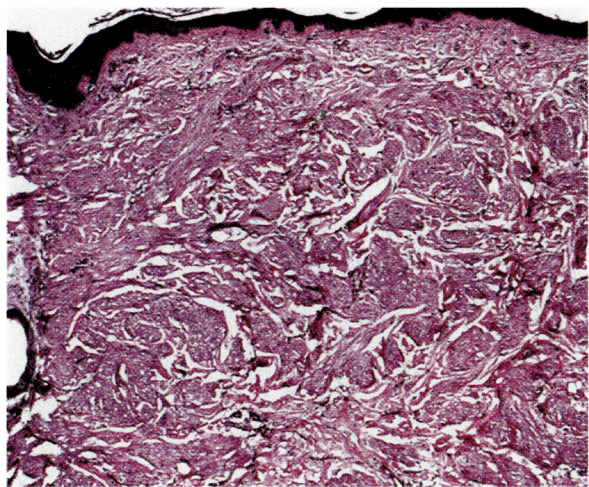

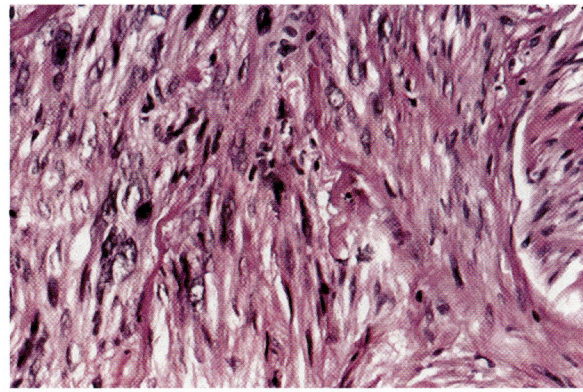

Figure 2-36

PILAR LEIOMYOMA

Nuclear atypia (in the absence of mitotic activity) may be seen in some examples of pilar leiomyoma, recalling the characteristics of "symplastic" uterine leiomyoma.

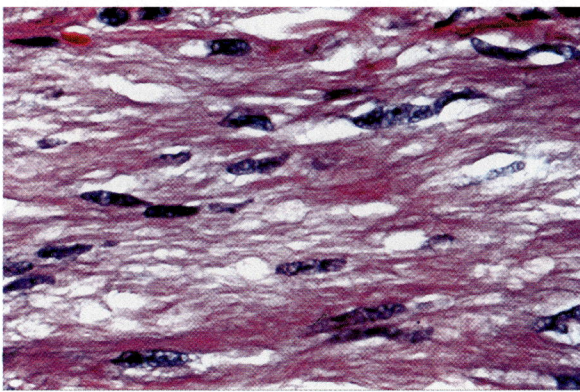

Figure 2-35

PILAR LEIOMYOMA

Top: A superficial, relatively well-circumscribed plate of spindle cell fascicles is seen in the dermis.

Bottom: The fascicles are composed of bland cells with fibrillary eosinophilic cytoplasm. This lesion often abuts a pilar unit and may rarely connect to the arrector pilorum muscles.

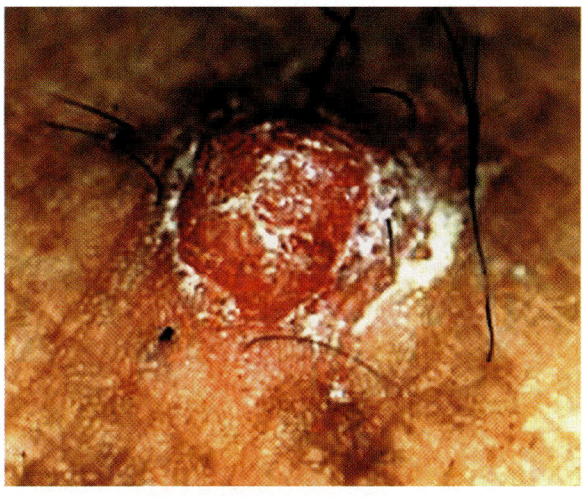

Figure 2-37

TRICHILEMMAL CARCINOMA

The tumor manifests as a nondescript reddish nodule in the facial skin of an elderly man.

(228). The lesion is whitish and hyperkeratotic, reddish and smooth-surfaced, or ulcerated; it generally measures less than 3 cm. This neoplasm is commonly interpreted as proliferative actinic keratosis, BCC, or squamous cell carcinoma by clinicians. There is no known linkage between trichilemmal carcinoma and Cowden's syndrome, and the former appears to arise de novo rather than by malignant transformation of a benign trichilemmoma. An association with burn scars has been described by Ko et al. (229).

Pathologic Findings. Histologically, trichilemmal carcinoma is a lobulated, follicle-centered lesion that may replace the sheath of one or several pilosebaceous units. This pattern of growth forms an image in which neoplastic cells replace not only several follicles but also the perifollicular epidermis, and are separated by normal surface epithelium (fig. 2-38). Invasive areas may involve the adjacent dermis irregularly (fig. 2-39), with surrounding chronic inflammation and desmoplasia. At least some of the tumor cells usually have PAS-positive, diastase-labile clear cytoplasm, and peripheral nuclear palisading may been seen in cellular lobules. Areas of trichilemmal keratinization are disposed irregularly throughout this neoplasm, which otherwise resembles squamous cell carcinoma cytologically and architecturally (fig. 2-40). Some cases exhibit pagetoid spread of the tumor cells in the adjacent epidermis (fig. 2-41) (232). Perineural or vascular infiltration also may be observed.

Differential Diagnosis. Because of its clear cell appearance, the differential diagnosis of trichilemmal carcinoma includes a number of alternatives. Virtually all other malignancies of the skin that may show a similar cellular composition (231) are included, such as hydropic BCC, clear cell squamous cell carcinoma, clear cell eccrine carcinoma, sebaceous carcinoma, "balloon cell" melanoma, and metastatic visceral clear cell adenocarcinoma. Attention to the aggregated histologic findings described above, together with clinical information regarding the duration of the lesion and its appearance, usually permits a confident diagnosis of trichilemmal carcinoma. PAS stains and selected immunostains may be needed, however. In particular, the application of antibodies to squamous-selective keratins (e.g., AE13 and AE14 [232]) can help exclude several

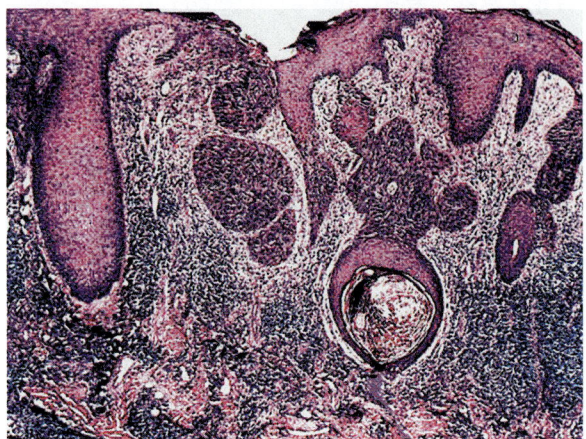

Figure 2-38

TRICHILEMMAL CARCINOMA

There is multifocal "skip" involvement of the surface epithelium, as well as the follicular epithelium.

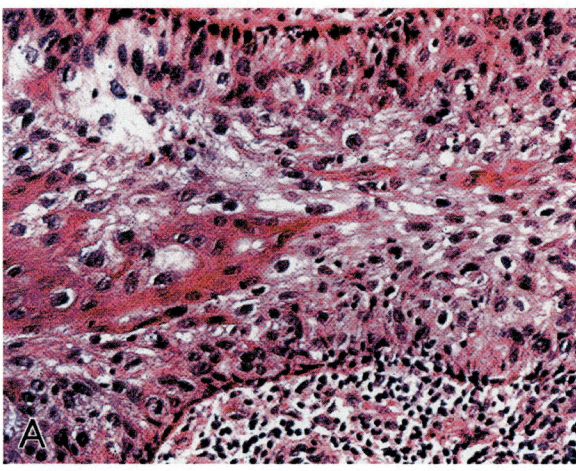

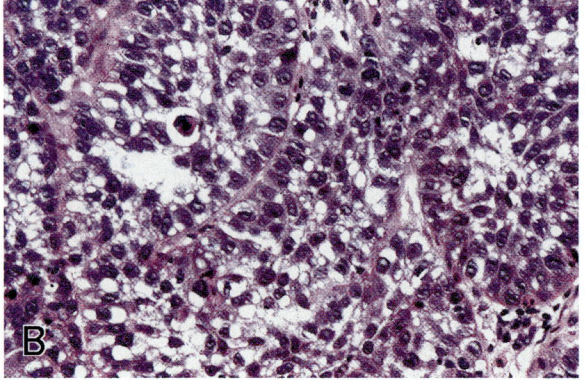

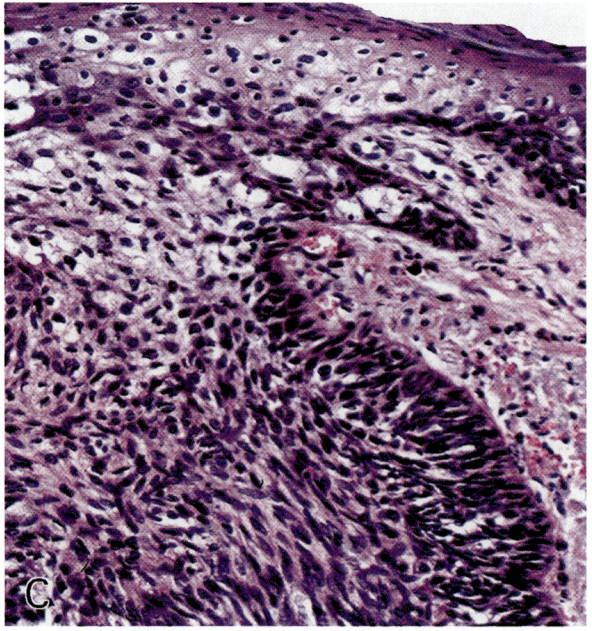

Figure 2-39

TRICHILEMMAL CARCINOMA

Foci of pilar-type keratinization, clear cell change, peripheral nuclear palisading, and necrosis are seen.

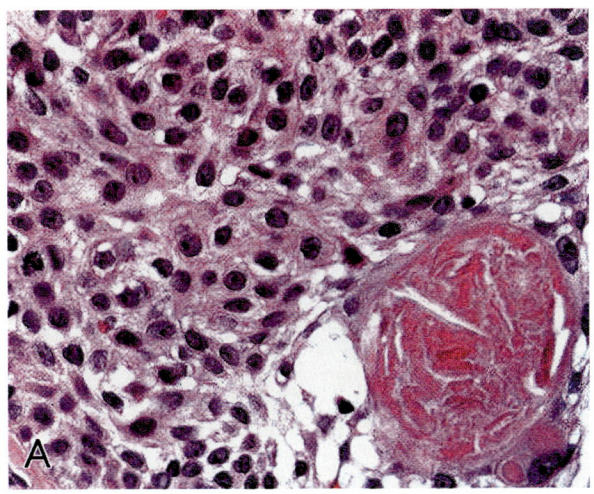

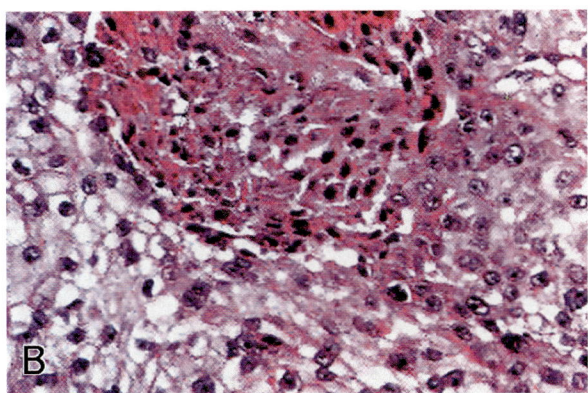

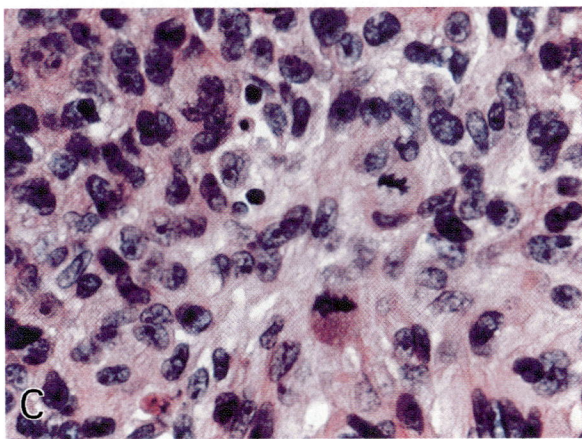

Figure 2-40

TRICHILEMMAL CARCINOMA

Trichilemmal keratinization (A,B) and overt nuclear atypia (C) in trichilemmal carcinoma.

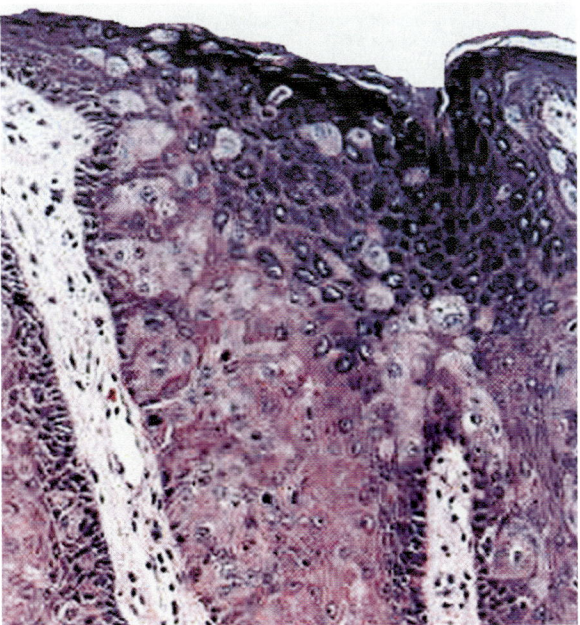

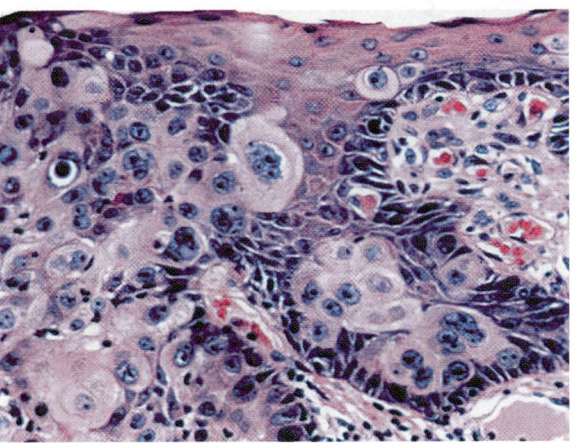

Figure 2-41

TRICHILEMMAL CARCINOMA

Pagetoid involvement of the epidermis in association with trichilemmal carcinoma.

of the lesions that simulate the appearance of trichilemmal carcinoma (fig. 2-42).

Malignant Proliferating Pilar Tumor

Clinical Features. The clinical profile of *malignant proliferating pilar tumor* (MPPT), also known as *malignant trichilemmal cyst, malignant pilar tumor, giant hair matrix tumor,* and *trichochlamydocarcinoma* (235,236,238a,239), is superimposable with that described above in connection with benign proliferating pilar tumor (BPPT). It appears

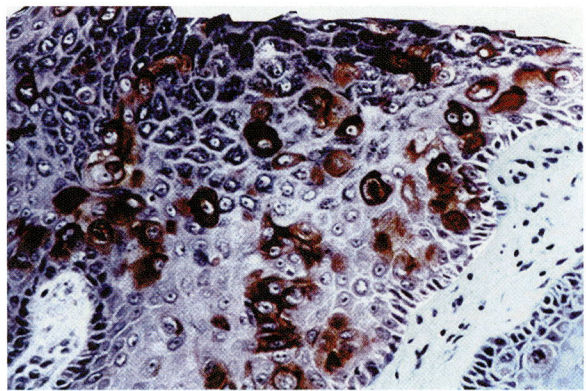

Figure 2-42

TRICHILEMMAL CARCINOMA

Immunoreactivity with AE13 (a pilar keratin-related monoclonal antibody) in a case of pagetoid trichilemmal carcinoma.

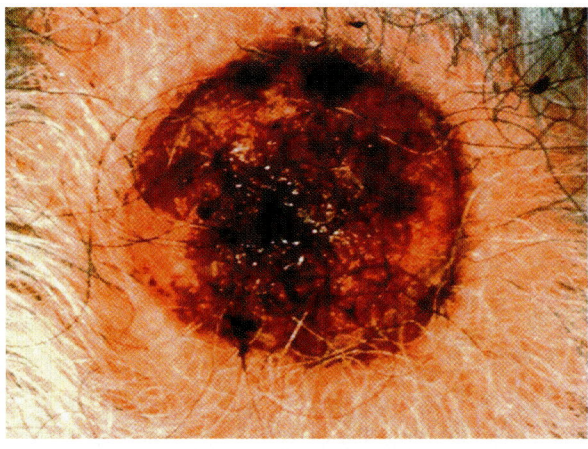

Figure 2-43

MALIGNANT PROLIFERATING PILAR TUMOR

Ulceration is seen in a scalp lesion.

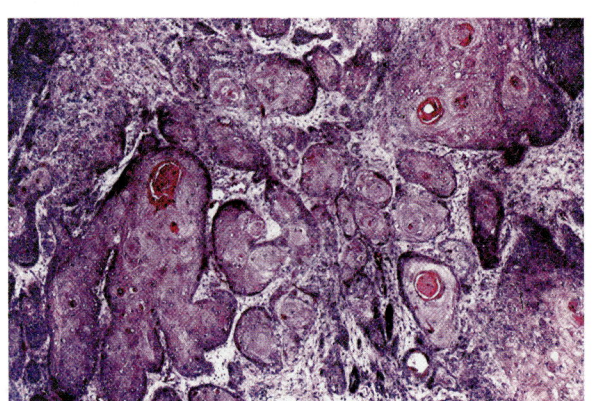
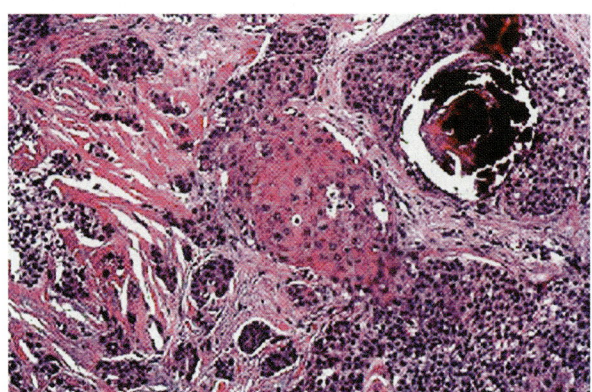

Figure 2-44

MALIGNANT PROLIFERATING PILAR TUMOR OF LOW-GRADE TYPE

Irregular invasion of the dermis and dystrophic calcification are present.

that some MPPTs arise by transformation of ordinary PPTs (234a,238). Rapid enlargement or ulceration of such lesions (fig. 2-43) is cause for concern that this eventuality has occurred.

Pathologic Findings. Brownstein and Arluk (40) concluded that BPPT shows a cytologic similarity to squamous cell carcinoma. Thus, as outlined previously, the growth pattern of such neoplasms has much greater significance in determining their biologic potentials.

There are two forms of MPPT, which demonstrate dissimilar behavior. The first, *low-grade MPPT*, is a close simulator of BPPT, except that its irregularly shaped and sized "buds" of neoplastic cells invade adjacent tissue (fig. 2-44). The remaining cytologic and architectural features of low-grade MPPT are basically the same as those of BPPT. *High-grade MPPT* loses the lobular growth of the benign variant and exhibits areas of geographic necrosis. The cytologic profile is poorly differentiated, with obvious nuclear pleomorphism (fig. 2-45), abnormal mitotic figures, and possible spindle cell change (234,237). Low-grade MPPTs only recur locally, but high-grade tumors have the ability to metastasize distantly (234).

Special studies play no particular role in the diagnosis or differential diagnosis of MPPT, and have been summarized above in reference to BPPT.

Differential Diagnosis. The main entity in the differential diagnosis of MPPT is squamous cell carcinoma, but high-grade MPPT also may resemble anaplastic ductal eccrine adenocarcinoma or metastatic carcinoma with squamous features. Unlike primary squamous carcinoma of the skin, MPPT lacks a connection with the epidermis, and contains areas of trichilemmal keratinization. Ductal eccrine carcinoma shows some foci of gland formation, unlike MPPT.

The separation of metastatic carcinoma and MPPT is best accomplished using clinical information. This typically indicates a solitary nature and relatively long duration of growth for MPPT, whereas metastatic lesions are usually multifocal and rapidly evolving. Furthermore, trichilemmal keratinization is not expected in metastatic carcinoma from the viscera.

Pilomatrix Carcinoma

Parallels can be drawn from the immediately preceding discussion of proliferating pilar tumors and the characteristics that influence their biologic potential to pilomatrical neoplasms. Invasive pilomatricoma differs from ordinary pilomatricoma by its irregular cellular growth into adjacent tissue, mirroring the pattern of low-grade MPPT (240,246,249a,250,252,253). *Pilomatrix carcinoma* shows zones of geographic necrosis, invasive growth, and cytologic anaplasia (241,244,245,247–249,254,255). The neoplastic cells exhibit high nuclear to cytoplasmic ratios, vesicular chromatin, and prominent nucleoli, and closely simulate the appearance of elements in lymphoepithelioma-like carcinomas (fig. 2-46). The additional presence of ghost or shadow cells, however, marks the tumor as matrical in nature.

Invasive pilomatricoma has the ability to recur locally, but does not metastasize (246,246a, 249a). In contrast, pilomatrix carcinoma may also involve regional lymph nodes or viscera (242,243,245,247,254,255).

Because of the singular microscopic appearance of pilomatrical lesions, their histologic recognition is generally not problematic. Small samples, however, may be confused with lymphoepithelioma-like carcinoma of the skin

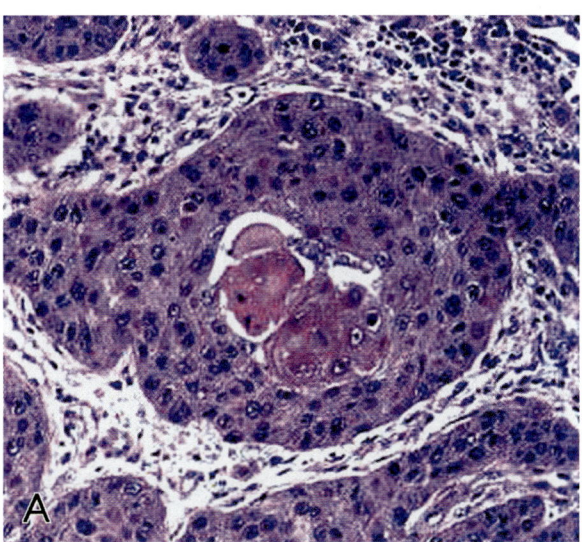
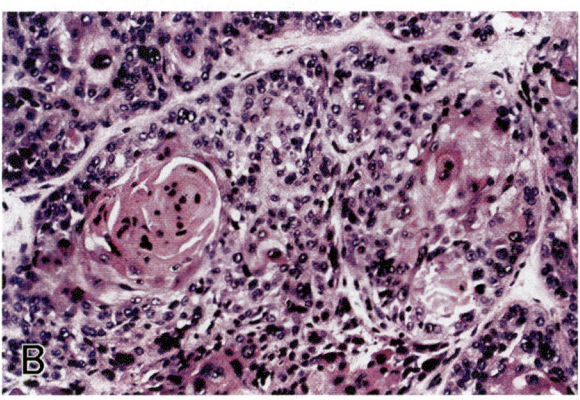
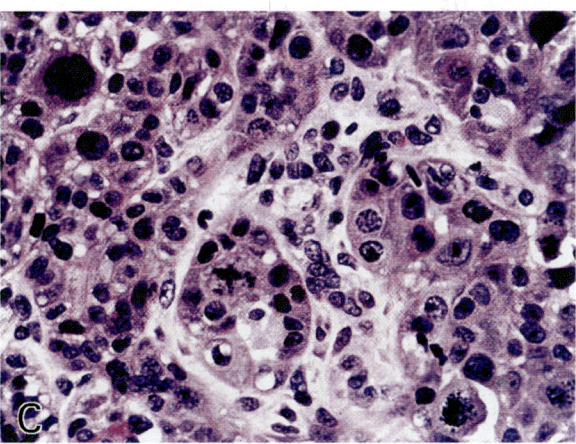

Figure 2-45

MALIGNANT PROLIFERATING PILAR TUMOR

There is obvious nuclear anaplasia with only small foci of pilar-type keratinization. The latter feature distinguishes this tumor from squamous cell carcinoma.

Figure 2-46
PILOMATRIX CARCINOMA

There is irregular and deep invasion of the dermis and subcutis by groups of tumor cells showing central ghost cell keratinization. The neoplastic cells are larger than the cells of ordinary pilomatricoma and have prominent nucleoli, resembling those of lymphoepithelioma-like carcinoma.

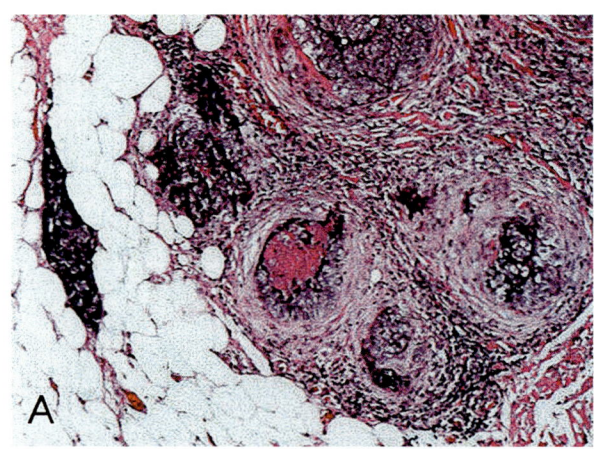

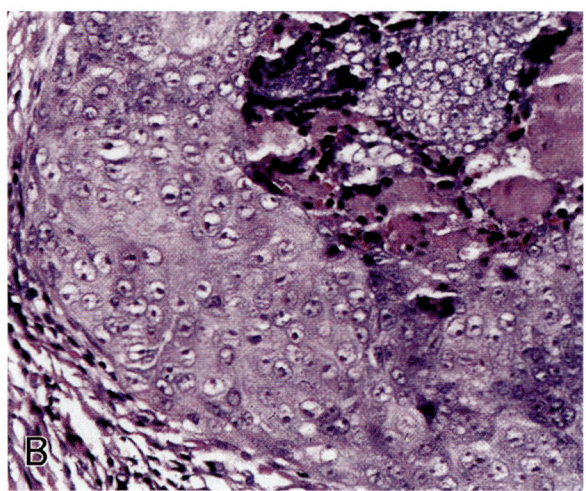

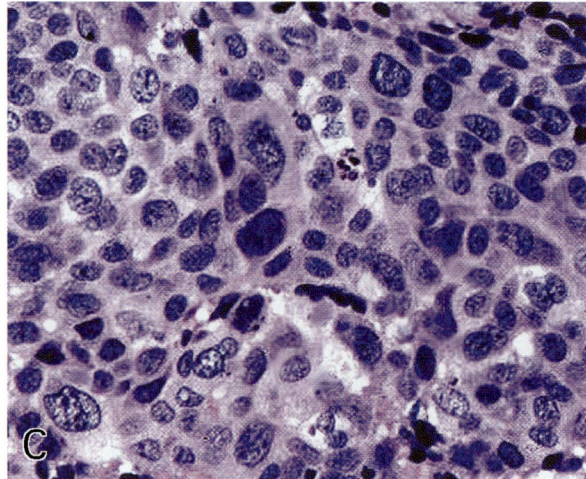

(251) or metastatic undifferentiated carcinoma. Clinical data are helpful in addressing the latter two possibilities, but there are no adjunctive methods that are effective in distinguishing pilomatrix carcinoma from these or other pilar lesions.

Adnexal Carcinomas with Mixed Differentiation

Pathologists who see a significant number of cutaneous appendage tumors encounter some that are not easily categorized nosologically. Sometimes, these exhibit differentiation along more than one adnexal pathway, and therefore potentially include combinations of tissue with sudoriferous, sebaceous, and pilar characteristics (257). We believe that the best diagnostic approach to these lesions is a descriptive one, using such descriptions as "adnexal carcinoma with mixed (or divergent) differentiation" rather than more complicated diagnostic terms (258).

Lymphoepithelioma-like carcinoma of skin may be a primitive member of this group of tumors. Several reports have described concurrent sweat glandular, follicular, or sebaceous differentiation in this neoplasm (256,259).

Pilar Leiomyosarcoma

The categorization of dermal leiomyosarcoma as a pilar tumor is admittedly hypothetical. This neoplasm is analogous architecturally and cytologically to pilar leiomyoma (see above), except that it is infiltrative and has discernible nuclear atypia and mitotic activity (260–262). S-100 protein is potentially seen in all pilar smooth muscle tumors, regardless of whether they are benign or malignant, and this marker is indeed shared by the non-neoplastic arrector pili muscles (262a). Dermal leiomyosarcoma is

Table 2-1

IMMUNOHISTOLOGIC DIFFERENTIAL DIAGNOSIS OF PILAR LEIOMYOSARCOMA

Tumor	VIM[a]	DES	MSA	CALD	PANK	P63	CD99	S-100P
Pilar leiomyosarcoma	+	+	+	+	0	0	0	+/−
Spindle cell (sarcomatoid) squamous cell carcinoma	+/−	0	0	0	+	+/−	0	0
Spindle cell (sarcomatoid) melanoma	+	0	0	0	0	0	+/−	+
Atypical fibroxanthoma	+	0	0	0	0	0	+	0

[a]VIM = vimentin; DES = desmin; MSA = muscle-specific actin; CALD = caldesmon; PANK = pankeratin; P63 = p63 protein; CD99 = MIC2 protein; S-100P = S-100 protein.

typically a borderline malignancy with some potential for local recurrence but only rare distant metastasis (262).

The differential diagnosis includes spindle cell squamous cell carcinoma, spindle cell melanoma, and atypical fibroxanthoma. Immunohistochemical analysis is the most useful method for separating these tumors (Table 2-1).

PSEUDONEOPLASTIC PROLIFERATIONS OF HAIR FOLLICLES AND FOLLICLE-RELATED MESENCHYME

Several other mass lesions of the skin contain follicular elements, and may be mistaken for true neoplasms. Some of these, such as basaloid follicular hamartoma, have already been discussed, somewhat arbitrarily, as neoplastic in the preceding material. Others are considered below.

Hair Follicle Nevus

Hair follicle nevus (congenital vellus hamartoma) has been defined clinicopathologically only relatively recently. In the past, these tumors were confused with trichofolliculomas, tumors of the follicular infundibulum, and basal follicular hamartomas, all of which are discussed elsewhere in this monograph.

Clinical Features. Nevi of the hair follicles are, as their name suggests, malformations rather than neoplasms. They are, therefore, most often encountered in young patients, with a predilection for the skin of the head and neck (264,265,274,276). An association with frontonasal dysplasia has been described (273). "Faun's tail," wherein misplaced tufts of hair are present in the presacral area, also likely represents a form of this disorder (269).

The lesion consists of multiple flesh-colored papules, that sometimes coalesce, and which are 1 to 5 mm in diameter. Hair follicle nevi may also be associated with alopecia of the lesional skin area instead of hypertrichosis, and may assume a linear disposition along Blaschko's lines (268). A distinction should be made between hair follicle nevus and "wooly hair nevus" or "curly hair nevus," (277,278), in which the hair shafts themselves are regionally coiled and aberrant, but in which there is little histologic abnormality in the associated skin.

Pathologic Findings. Biopsies of hair follicle nevi show a disorganized regional proliferation of miniature hair follicles in the dermis, associated with mature interfollicular collagen (fig. 2-47). The contents of the follicles approximate the size of vellus hairs, and the constituent epithelial cells are either basaloid or compact polyhedral keratinocytes, exhibiting similar levels of differentiation (264,265, 274,276). Basement membranes around the follicles are inconspicuous, as are intralesional adipocytes. Some debate has surrounded the question of a relationship between hair follicle nevus and accessory tragus (which contains microscopic cartilaginous components and mature fat cells) in the preauricular and lateral cervical skin (273). The latter lesion is a common component of the oculoauriculovertebral (Goldenhar's) syndrome (271). We consider both malformations to exist in a spectrum, but the existence of hair follicle nevus outside of the head and neck helps confirm its existence as a distinct entity.

Differential Diagnosis. Hair follicle nevus differs from trichofolliculoma in that the latter

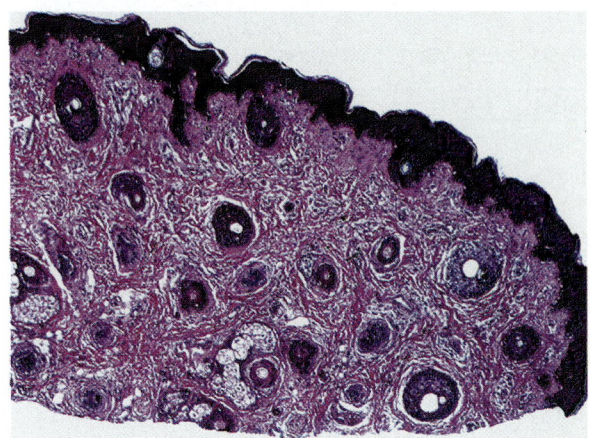 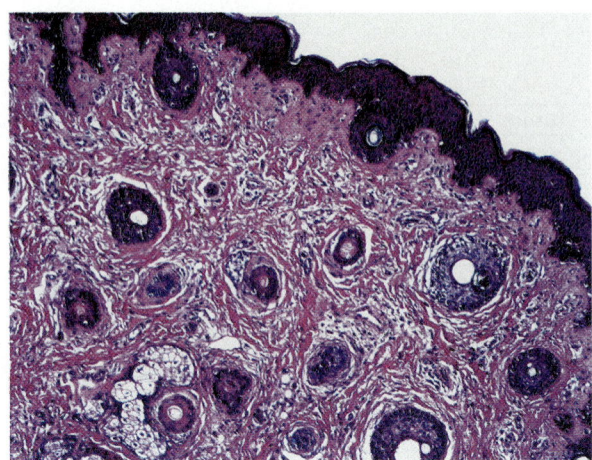

Figure 2-47

HAIR FOLLICLE NEVUS

This biopsy is from a small papule in the skin of the forehead of a child. It is histologically unremarkable at first glance, but the presence of several relatively immature hair follicles in the skin field calls the diagnosis of hair follicle nevus to mind.

shows a central "parent" follicle around which secondary follicles bud in a radial fashion (270). The hair shaft in the central ostium of trichofolliculoma is mature rather than vellus, and sebaceous glands are sometimes attached to the secondary structures as well. Vellus hair cysts have an obvious central cavity in which small hairs are contained, rather than individual hair follicles disposed throughout the corium as seen in follicular nevus (275). Basaloid follicular hamartoma (275a) and tumor of the follicular infundibulum (264a) demonstrate a latticework of basaloid or polygonal keratinocytic cords with a plate-like configuration, which is connected to the basal epidermis and enclosing fibrous stroma. Elgart and Patterson (267) have reported a complex malformative lesion, congenital midline hamartoma, in the central skin of the jaw, containing small hair follicles like those of hair follicle nevus, as well as sebaceous glands, eccrine sweat glands, arrector pili, adipose tissue, and skeletal muscle. Kroumpouzos et al. (272) documented an unusual constellation of bilateral linear porokeratosis overlying mature hair follicles and eccrine ostia, which they called systematized porokeratosis eccrine and hair follicle nevus. Despite such a partial sharing of terminology, the miniaturized follicles of follicular nevus were not seen in that lesion. Finally nevus comedonicus appears as multiple follicle-like inclusions in the corium, superficially imitating hair follicle nevus (266). Their contents, however, are keratinous rather than formed hair, and connections between the inclusions and the epidermal surface are typically present.

Linear Basal Cell Nevus

Clinical Features. *Linear basal cell nevus* (LBCN) is a zosteriform, papular, flesh-colored lesion that may be noted at any time of life, although it most often presents in young individuals (280). Comedones are typically, but not invariably, admixed in the abnormal skin field, and they also may be an integral part of the nevi themselves (282,284,285). Osteoma cutis, anodontia, and abnormal osseous mineralization have been reported in association with LBCN (279). The natural history of this proliferation is innocuous, in contrast to that of linear BCC or the nevoid BCC syndrome.

Pathologic Findings. The histologic image of LBCN is basically indistinguishable from that of ordinary BCC, except for the interposition of open or closed comedones throughout most of the lesions (280,282,284,285). Differentiation towards adnexal epithelial structures is common, particularly favoring pilar features (and explaining the inclusion of LBCN in this section); there may be multifocal connections of LBCN to the basal epidermis in a manner like that seen in

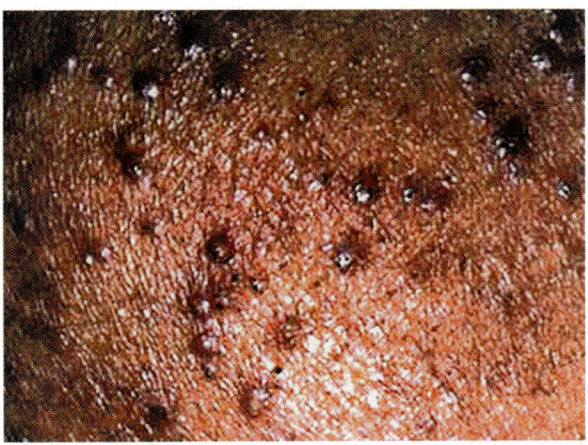

Figure 2-48

STEATOCYSTOMA MULTIPLEX

Grouped papulonodules in the skin of the trunk in a young man.

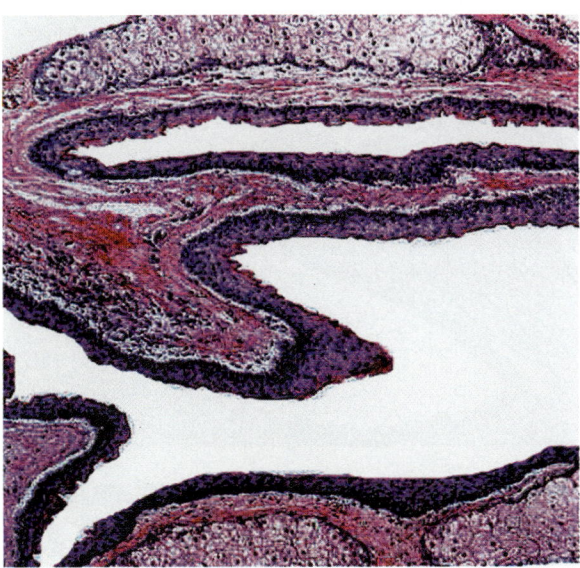

Figure 2-49

STEATOCYSTOMA

A central cyst cavity is mantled by an eosinophilic "cuticle" with attached sebaceous lobules.

superficial multifocal BCC. Occasionally, narrow interlocking cords of basal cells in LBCN enclose fibrous stroma, yielding a configuration resembling a miniature fibroepithelioma of Pinkus.

At this time, no adjuvant studies are applicable to the definitive identification of LBCN. Although this proliferation appears to be syndromic, chromosomal and genetic abnormalities that might be employed to recognize it are as yet undefined.

Differential Diagnosis. As evident in the foregoing discussion, the principal differential diagnostic consideration is nevoid BCC (281, 283). Comedones may coexist with syndrome-related or sporadic examples of BCC and therefore they are not particularly helpful in defining LBCN microscopically. Moreover, the histologic features of the latter are virtually superimposable with those of BCC. Only thorough integration of clinical and pathologic findings is effective in distinguishing the two.

Steatocystoma Multiplex and Simplex

Steatocystoma multiplex is an autosomal dominant disorder that features the appearance of cutaneous nodules in the genital area, axillae, shoulders and arms, and trunk; it usually first appears during adolescence (fig. 2-48) (288,289). An association exists between steatocystoma multiplex and eruptive vellus hair cysts, some forms of epidermoid inclusion cyst, and milia, such that some individuals may have all of these lesions concurrently (286,290,292,293).

Microscopically, cysts are seen in the corium. These communicate with the surface epithelium and are lined by squamoid cells showing trichilemmal-type keratinization, yielding a luminal "cuticle." Mature sebocytic nests are present in the cyst walls, and small pilosebaceous units may be attached (fig. 2-49). Confusion may arise over alternative interpretations of trichofolliculoma or sebaceous trichofolliculoma, but the overall architecture of those proliferations differs from that of steatocystoma on low-power microscopy.

Solitary, sporadic lesions with the appearance of steatocystoma multiplex are called *steatocystoma simplex* (287). These affect the oral mucosa as well as the skin (291).

Eruptive Vellus Hair Cyst

Eruptive vellus hair cysts are multiple, smooth, slate-colored papules in the skin of the trunk or face (294–296). Familial clusters have been described with autosomal dominant inheritance (297). These lesions are cystically dilated hair follicles that are mantled by flattened squamoid

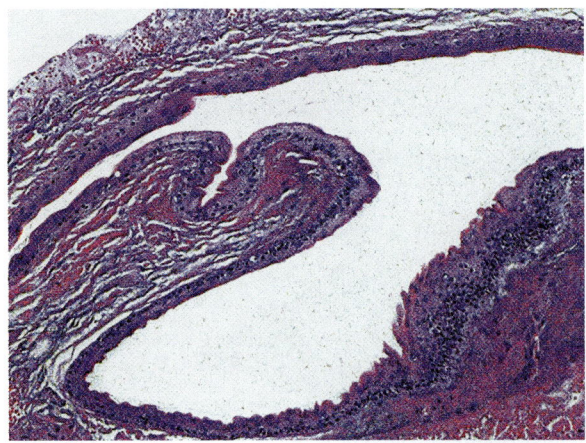

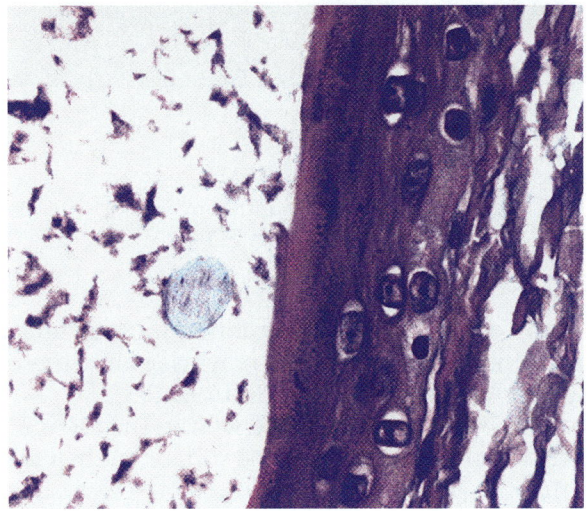

Figure 2-50

VELLUS HAIR CYST

The overall image of this lesion (top) is closely similar to that of steatocystoma, as shown in figure 2-49, except that sebaceous tissue is lacking and rare vellus hairs (bottom) are seen in the cyst cavity.

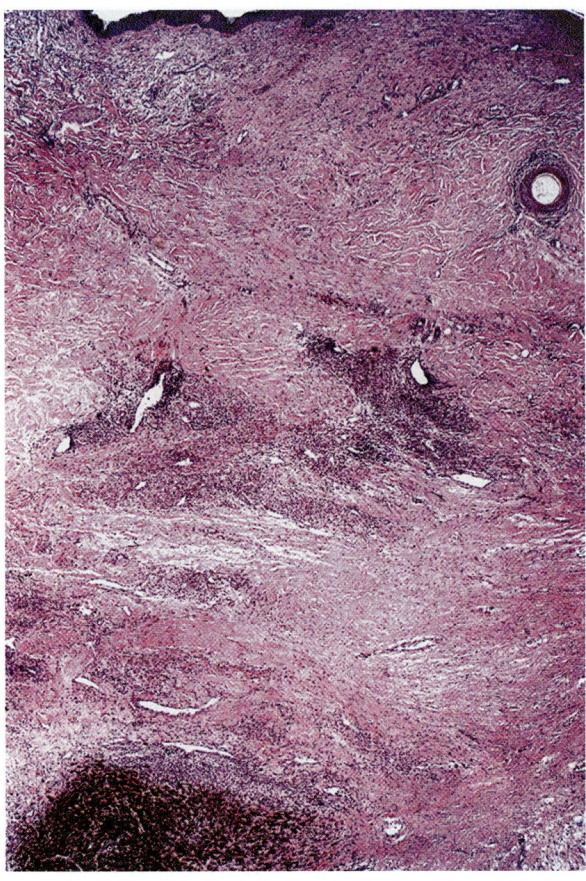

Figure 2-51

PILAR NEUROCRISTIC HAMARTOMA

A vaguely fascicular proliferation of stellate and fusiform cells forms in the dermis and subcutis. Some of the lesional cells are pigmented (bottom).

cells; the squamoid cells show either infundibular or trichilemmal keratinization. Other small follicles may be attached, and these are associated with minute vellus hairs (fig. 2-50); the latter structures may be surprisingly sparse. Lesions of steatocystoma multiplex, milia, or epidermoid inclusion cysts may be seen simultaneously in the same patient, and cysts with hybrid features of these lesions also may be encountered (298). The differential diagnosis centers on trichofolliculoma, but that tumor does not contain vellus hairs.

Neurofollicular and Pilar Neurocristic Hamartomas

There are two other mesenchymal proliferations in the dermis that are probably associated with the hair follicles: *neurofollicular hamartoma* (299,301) and *pilar neurocristic hamartoma* (300, 305,306). Neurofollicular hamartoma manifests as a single papule in the facial skin, and may arise at any age. This lesion has a microscopic kinship to both angiofibroma and neurofibroma, and exhibits an irregular proliferation of bland spindle cells, bounded laterally by hyperplastic hair follicles. This anatomic association has led to the conclusion that neurofollicular hamartoma is a malformation of nerve endings that are

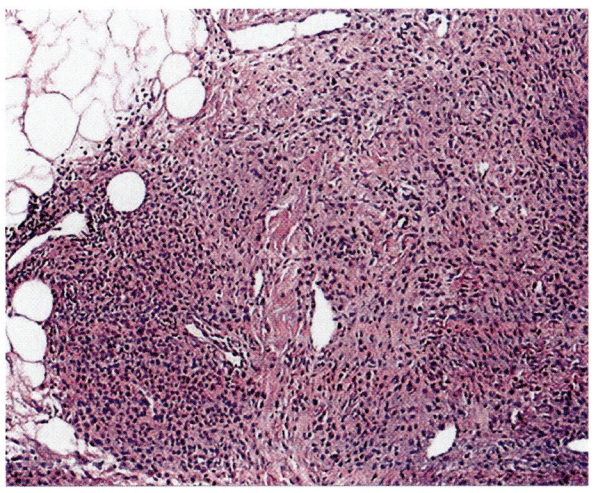

Figure 2-52

PILAR NEUROCRISTIC HAMARTOMA

The cytologic attributes of pilar neurocristic hamartoma are bland, and do not immediately suggest a neural or melanocytic lineage of differentiation.

related to the hair follicles. Sangueza and Requena (304) have suggested that the lesion may be related to trichodiscoma, as described above.

In contrast, pilar neurocristic hamartoma is a pigmented papule or plaque in the skin of the head and neck. It is composed of interdigitating fascicles of bland fusiform cells, some of which contain melanin pigment, and these are closely apposed to the hair follicles (figs. 2-51, 2-52). Some authors have described examples that were complicated by apparent transformation to malignant melanoma or related lesions (302,303), raising some doubt as to the "hamartomatous" nature of such proliferations.

REFERENCES

Tumor of the Follicular Infundibulum

1. Cribier B, Grosshans E. Tumor of the follicular infundibulum: a clinicopathologic study. J Am Acad Dermatol 1995;33:979–84.
2. Horn TD, Vennos EM, Bernstein BD, Cooper PH. Multiple tumors of follicular infundibulum with sweat duct differentiation. J Cutan Pathol 1995; 22:281–7.
3. Koch B, Rufli T. Tumor of the follicular infundibulum. Dermatologica 1991;183:68–9.
4. Mahalingam M, Bhawan J, Finn R, Stefanato CM. Tumor of the follicular infundibulum with sebaceous differentiation. J Cutan Pathol 2001;28: 314–7.
5. Mehregan AH. Tumor of follicular infundibulum. Dermatologica 1971;142:177–83.
6. Schirren CG, Maciejewski W. [Tumor of the follicular infundibulum. Study of determining follicular differentiation.] Pathologe 1996;17:440–5. (German.)
7. Trunnell TN, Waisman M. Tumor of the follicular infundibulum. Cutis 1979;24:317–18.
8. Verplancke P, Driessen L, Wynants P, Naeyaert JM. The Schopf-Schulz-Passarge syndrome. Dermatology 1998;196:463–6.

Pilar Sheath Acanthoma

9. Bhawan J. Pilar sheath acanthoma. A new benign follicular tumor. J Cutan Pathol 1979;6: 438–40.
10. Hurt MA. Pilar sheath acanthoma (lobular infundibuloisthmicoma). Am J Dermatopathol 1996;18:435.
11. Lee JY, Hirsch E. Pilar sheath acanthoma. Arch Dermatol 1987;123:569–70.
12. Mehregan AH, Brownstein MH. Pilar sheath acanthoma. Arch Dermatol 1978;114:1495–7.
13. Smolle J, Kerl H. [Pilar sheath acanthoma—a benign follicular hamartoma.] Dermatologica 1983;167:335–8. (German.)
14. Vakilzadeh F. [Pilar sheath acanthoma.] Hautarzt 1987;38:40–2. (German.)

Winer's Pore

15. Dudley K, Barr WG, Armin A, Massa MC. Nevus comedonicus in association with widespread, well-differentiated follicular tumors. J Am Acad Dermatol 1986;15:1123–7.
16. Steffen C. Winer's dilated pore: the infundibuloma. Am J Dermatopathol 2001;23:246–53.

Trichoadenoma

17. Cooper PH, Mills SE, Leonard DD, et al. Sclerosing sweat duct (syringomatous) carcinoma. Am J Surg Pathol 1985;9:422–33.
18. Kumar K, McGregor JC, Watson JD. Microcystic adnexal carcinoma: a report of three cases. J R Coll Surg Edinb 1998;43:412–4.
19. Manganaro AM, Will MJ, Bradley MD, Peckham S, Faulk-Eggleston J, Fish M. Benign keratotic squamous epithelial neoplasm of the palate: a unique lesion. Head Neck 1998;20:175–8.
20. Nikolowski W. [Trichoadenoma.] Z Hautkr 1978;53:87–90. (German.)
21. Rahbari H, Mehregan A, Pinkus H. Trichoadenoma of Nikolowski. J Cutan Pathol 1977;4:90–8.
22. Reibold R, Undeutsch W, Fleiner J. [Trichoadenoma of Nikolowski—review of four decades and seven new cases.] Hautarzt 1998;49:925–8. (German.)
23. Seifert G, Donath K, Jautzke G. Unusual choristoma of the parotid gland in a girl. A possible trichoadenoma. Virchows Arch 1999;434: 355–9.
24. Yamaguchi J, Takino C. A case of trichoadenoma arising in the buttock. J Dermatol 1992;19:503–6.

Trichilemmoma

25. Brownstein MH. Trichilemmoma. Benign follicular tumor or viral wart? Am J Dermatopathol 1980;2:229–31.
26. Brownstein MH, Mehregan AH, Bikowski JB, Lupulescu A, Patterson JC. The dermatopathology of Cowden's syndrome. Br J Dermatol 1979;100:667–3.
27. Brownstein MH, Shapiro L. Trichilemmoma. Analysis of 40 new cases. Arch Dermatol 1973; 107:866–9.
28. Chan P, White SW, Pierson DL, Rodman OG. Trichilemmoma. J Dermatol Surg Oncol 1979; 5:58–9.
29. Crowson AN, Magro CM. Basal cell carcinoma arising in association with desmoplastic trichilemmoma. Am J Dermatopathol 1996;18:43–8.
30. El-Shabrawi L, LeBoit PE. Basal cell carcinoma with thickened basement membrane: a variant that resembles some benign adnexal neoplasms. Am J Dermatopathol 1997;19:568–74.
31. Hidayat AA, Font RL. Trichilemmoma of eyelid and eyebrow. A clinicopathologic study of 31 cases. Arch Ophthalmol 1980;98:844–7.
32. Hunt SJ, Kilzer B, Santa Cruz DJ. Desmoplastic trichilemmoma: histologic variant resembling invasive carcinoma. J Cutan Pathol 1990;17:45–52.
33. Illueca C, Monteagudo C, Revert A, Llombart-Bosch A. Diagnostic value of CD34 immunostaining in desmoplastic trichilemmoma. J Cutan Pathol 1998;25:435–9.
34. Leonardi CL, Zhu WY, Kinsey WH, Penneys NS. Trichilemmomas are not associated with human papillomavirus DNA. J Cutan Pathol 1991;18: 193–7.
35. Massi D, Franchi A. Desmoplastic trichilemmoma: a case report with immunohistochemical characterization of the extracellular matrix components. Acta Derm Venereol 1997;77:347–9.
36. Mohlenbeck FW. [Trichilemmoma. A study of 100 cases.] Z Hautkr 1974;49:791–5. (German.)
37. Penneys NS, Mogollon RJ, Nadji M, Gould E. Papillomavirus common antigens. Papillomavirus antigen in verruca, benign papillomatous lesions, trichilemmoma, and bowenoid papulosis: an immunoperoxidase study. Arch Dermatol 1984;120:859–61.
38. Tellechea O, Reis JP, Baptista AP. Desmoplastic trichilemmoma. Am J Dermatopathol 1992;14: 107–14.

Benign Proliferating Pilar Tumor

39. Avinoach I, Zirkin HJ, Glezerman M. Proliferating trichilemmal tumor of the vulva. Case report and review of the literature. Int J Gynecol Pathol 1989;8:163–8.
40. Brownstein MH, Arluk DJ. Proliferating trichilemmal cyst: a simulant of squamous cell carcinoma. Cancer 1981;48:1207–14.
41. Burg G, Landthaler M. [Proliferating trichilemmal tumor.] Hautarzt 1988;39:117–9. (German.)
42. Christophers E, Spelberg H. [Proliferating tricholemmal cyst.] Hautarzt 1973;24:377–80. (German.)
43. Fernandez-Figueras MT, Casalots A, Puig L, Llatjos R, Ferrandiz C, Ariza A. Proliferating trichilemmal tumor: p53 immunoreactivity in association with p27Kip1 overexpression indicates a low-grade carcinoma profile. Histopathology 2001;38:454–7.
44. Gordon CJ. Proliferating trichilemmal cyst in an organoid nevus. Cutis 1991;48:49–52.
45. Hashimoto Y, Matsuo S, Iizuka H. A DNA-flow cytometric analysis of trichilemmal carcinoma, proliferating trichilemmal cyst and trichilemmal cyst. Acta Derm Venereol 1994;74:358–60.
46. Herrero J, Monteagudo C, Ruiz A, Llombart-Bosch A. Malignant proliferating trichilemmal tumors: an histopathological and immunohistochemical study of three cases with DNA ploidy and morphometric evaluation. Histopathology 1998;33:542–46.
47. Komuro Y, Takedai T, Tagawa K. Proliferating trichilemmal tumor on the dorsum of the hand. Ann Plast Surg 1995;34:657–9.

48. Laing V, Knipe RC, Flowers FP, Stoer CB, Ramos-Caro FA. Proliferating trichilemmal tumor: report of a case and review of the literature. J Dermatol Surg Oncol 1991;17:295–8.
49. Marcussen N. [Proliferating trichilemmal cyst. An important differential diagnosis from squamous cell carcinoma.] Ugeskr Laeger 1988;150: 484–7. (Danish.)
50. Naik R, Bharathi S, Bai BM. Proliferating trichilemmal tumours. Indian J Pathol Microbiol 1990;33:175–8.
51. Patterson JW. Infundibular and trichilemmal keratinization of a pilar tumor. Cutis 1985;36: 330–2.
52. Rahbari H, Mehregan AH. Development of proliferating trichilemmal cyst in organoid nevus. Presentation of two cases. J Am Acad Dermatol 1986;14:123–6.
53. Ramesh V, Iyengar B. Proliferating trichilemmal cysts over the vulva. Cutis 1990;45:187–9.
54. Rutty GN, Richman PI, Laing JH. Malignant change in trichilemmal cysts: a study of cell proliferation and DNA content. Histopathology 1992;21:465–8.
55. Sakamoto F, Ito M, Nakamura A, Sato Y. Proliferating trichilemmal cyst with apocrine-acrosyringeal and sebaceous differentiation. J Cutan Pathol 1991;18:137–41.
56. Sau P, Graham JH, Helwig EB. Proliferating epithelial cysts. Clinicopathological analysis of 96 cases. J Cutan Pathol 1995;22:394–406.
57. Sethi S, Singh UR. Proliferating trichilemmal cyst: report of two cases, one benign and the other malignant. J Dermatol 2002;29:214–20.
58. Shet T, Rege J, Naik L. Cytodiagnosis of simple and proliferating trichilemmal cysts. Acta Cytol 2001;45:582–8.
59. Sleater J, Beers B, Stefan M, Kilpatrick T, Hendricks J. Proliferating trichilemmal cyst. Report of four cases, two with nondiploid DNA content and increased proliferation index. Am J Dermatopathol 1993;15:423–8.
60. Takata M, Rehman I, Rees JL. A trichilemmal carcinoma arising from a proliferating trichilemmal cyst: the loss of the wild-type p53 is a critical event in malignant transformation. Hum Pathol 1998;29:193–5.
61. Urano Y, Oura H, Sakaki A, et al. Immunohistological analysis of P53 expression in human skin tumors. J Dermatol Sci 1992;4:69–75.
62. Vogelbruch M, Rutten A, Bocking A, Kapp A, Kiehl P. Differentiation between malignant and benign follicular adnexal tumors of the skin by DNA image cytometry. Br J Dermatol 2002;146: 238–43.

Trichofolliculoma and Pilomatricoma

63. Jacobson M, Ackerman AB. "Shadow" cells as clues to follicular differentiation. Am J Dermatopathol 1987;9:51–7.
64. MacMillan A, Roberts SO. Trichofolliculoma. Br J Dermatol 1971;85:491–2.
65. Mizutani H, Senga K, Ueda M. Trichofolliculoma of the upper lip: report of a case. Int J Oral Maxillofac Surg 1999;28:135–6.
66. Nomura M, Hata S. Sebaceous trichofolliculoma on scrotum and penis. Dermatologica 1990; 181:68–70.
67. Peterdy GA, Huettner PC, Rajaram V, Lind AC. Trichofolliculoma of the vulva associated with vulvar intraepithelial neoplasia: report of three cases and review of the literature. Int J Gynecol Pathol 2002;21:224–30.
68. Plewig G. Sebaceous trichofolliculoma. J Cutan Pathol 1980;7:394–403.
69. Schulz T, Hartschuh W. Folliculo-sebaceous cystic hamartoma is a trichofolliculoma at its very late stage. J Cutan Pathol 1998;25:354–64.
70. Schulz T, Hartschuh W. The trichofolliculoma undergoes changes corresponding to the regressing normal hair follicle in its cycle. J Cutan Pathol 1998;25:341–53.
71. Steffen C, Leaming DV. Trichofolliculoma of the upper eyelid. Cutis 1982;30:343–5.
72. Walsh N, Ackerman AB. Infundibulocystic basal cell carcinoma: a newly described variant. Mod Pathol 1990;3:599–608.

Trichoepithelioma

73. Akasaka T, Kon S, Mihm MC Jr. Multiple basaloid cell hamartoma with alopecia and autoimmune disease (systemic lupus erythematosus). J Dermatol 1996;23:821–4.
74. Aygun C, Blum JE. Trichoepithelioma 100 years later: a case report supporting the use of radiotherapy. Dermatology 1993;187:209–12.
75. Ayhan M, Adanali G, Senen D, Gorgu M, Erdogan B. Rarely seen cutaneous lesions in an elderly patient: malignant transformation of multiple trichoepithelioma. Ann Plast Surg 2001;47:98–9.
76. Bettencourt MS, Prieto VG, Shea CR. Trichoepithelioma: a 19-year clinicopathologic re-evaluation. J Cutan Pathol 1999;26:398–404.
77. Boni R, Fogt F, Vortmeyer AO, Tronic BS, Zhuang Z. Genetic analysis of a trichoepithelioma and associated basal cell carcinoma. Arch Dermatol 1998;134:1170–1.
78. Brooke JD, Fitzpatrick JE, Golitz LE. Papillary mesenchymal bodies: a histologic finding useful in differentiating trichoepithelioma from basal cell carcinomas. J Am Acad Dermatol 1989;21:523–8.

79. Brownstein MH. Basaloid follicular hamartoma: solitary and multiple types. J Am Acad Dermatol 1992;27(Pt 1):237–40.
80. Cecchi R, Crudeli F, Fedi E, Giomi A. [Multiple trichoepithelioma, cylindroma, eccrine spiradenoma present in the same family. Histologic and histopathogenetic considerations.] G Ital Dermatol Venereol 1985;120:149–52. (Italian.)
81. Cho D, Woodruff JD. Trichoepithelioma of the vulva. A report of two cases. J Reprod Med 1988;33:317–9.
82. D'Souza M, Garg BR, Ratnakar C, Agrawal K. Multiple trichoepitheliomas with rare features. J Dermatol 1994;21:582–5.
83. Harada H, Hashimoto K, Ko MS. The gene for multiple familial trichoepithelioma maps to chromosome 9p21. J Invest Dermatol 1996;107:41–3.
83a. Hatta N, Hirano T, Kimura T, et al. Molecular diagnosis of basal cell carcinoma and other basaloid cell neoplasms of the skin by the quantification of Gli1 transcript levels. J Cutan Pathol 2005;32:131–6.
84. Hunt SJ, Abell E. Malignant hair matrix tumor ("malignant trichoepithelioma") arising in the setting of multiple hereditary trichoepithelioma. Am J Dermatopathol 1991;13:275–81.
85. Jemec B, Lovgreen Nielsen P, Jemec GB, Balsev E. Giant solitary trichoepithelioma. Dermatol Online J 1999;5:1.
86. Johnson SC, Bennett RG. Occurrence of basal cell carcinoma among multiple trichoepitheliomas. J Am Acad Dermatol 1993;28:322–26.
87. Kirchmann TT, Prieto VG, Smoller BR. CD34 staining pattern distinguishes basal cell carcinoma from trichoepithelioma. Arch Dermatol 1994;130:589–92.
88. Long SA, Hurt MA, Santa Cruz DJ. Immature trichoepithelioma: report of six cases. J Cutan Pathol 1988;15:353–8.
89. Marrogi AJ, Wick MR, Dehner LP. Benign cutaneous adnexal tumors in childhood and young adults, excluding pilomatrixoma: review of 28 cases and literature. J Cutan Pathol 1991;18:20–7.
90. Matt D, Xin H, Vortmeyer AO, Zhuang Z, Burg G, Boni R. Sporadic trichoepithelioma demonstrates deletions at 9q22.3. Arch Dermatol 2000;136:657–60.
91. Poniecka AW, Alexis JB. An immunohistochemical study of basal cell carcinoma and tricho-epithelioma. Am J Dermatopathol 1999;21:332–6.
92. Requena L, Farina MC, Robledo M, et al. Multiple hereditary infundibulocystic basal cell carcinomas: a genodermatosis different from nevoid basal cell carcinoma syndrome. Arch Dermatol 1999;135:1227–35.
93. Rivet J, Rogez C, Wechsler J. Trichoepithelioma with "monster" stromal cells. J Cutan Pathol 2001;28:379–82.
93a Salhi A, Bornholdt D, Oeffner F, et al. Multiple familial trichoepithelioma caused by mutations in the cylindromatosis tumor suppressor gene. Cancer Res 2004;64:5113–7.
94. San Juan EB, Guana AL, Goldberg LH, Kolbusz RV, Orengo IF, Alford E. Aggressive trichoepithelioma versus keratotic basal cell carcinoma. Int J Dermatol 1993;32:728–30.
95. Simpson W, Garner A, Collin JR. Benign hair-follicle-derived tumors in the differential diagnosis of basal-cell carcinoma of the eyelids: a clinicopathological comparison. Br J Ophthalmol 1989;73:347–53.
96. Sternberg I, Buckman G, Levine MR, Sterin W. Trichoepithelioma. Ophthalmology 1986;93:531–3.
97. Swanson PE, Fitzpatrick MM, Ritter JH, Glusac EJ, Wick MR. Immunohistologic differential diagnosis of basal cell carcinoma, squamous cell carcinoma, and trichoepithelioma in small cutaneous biopsy specimens. J Cutan Pathol 1998;25:153–9.
98. Szepietowski JC, Wasik F, Szybejko-Machaj G, Bieniek A, Schwartz RA. Brooke-Spiegler syndrome. J Eur Acad Dermatol Venereol 2001;15:346–9.
99. Takata M, Quinn AG, Hashimoto K, Rees JL. Low frequency of loss of heterozygosity at the nevoid basal cell carcinoma locus and other selected loci in appendageal tumors. J Invest Dermatol 1996;106:1141–4.
100. Tatnall FM, Jones EW. Giant solitary trichoepitheliomas located in the perianal area: a report of three cases. Br J Dermatol 1986;115:91–9.
101. Wallace ML, Smoller BR. Trichoepithelioma with an adjacent basal cell carcinoma, transformation or collision? J Am Acad Dermatol 1997;37:343–5.
102. Wong TY, Suster S, Cheek RF, Mihm MC Jr. Benign cutaneous adnexal tumors with combined folliculosebaceous, apocrine, and eccrine differentiation. Clinicopathologic and immunohistochemical study of eight cases. Am J Dermatopathol 1996;18:124–36.
103. Yamamoto N, Gonda K. Multiple trichoepithelioma with basal cell carcinoma. Ann Plast Surg 1999;43:221–2.
103a. Zhang XJ, Liang YH, He PP, et al. Identification of the cylindromatosis tumor-suppressor gene responsible for multiple familial trichoepithelioma. J Invest Dermatol 2004;122:658–64.

Desmoplastic Trichoepithelioma

104. Abesamis-Cubillan E, El-Shabrawi-Caelen L, LeBoit PE. Merkel cells and sclerosing epithelial neoplasms. Am J Dermatopathol 2000;22: 311–5.
105. Brownstein MH, Shapiro L. Desmoplastic trichoepithelioma. Cancer 1977;40:2979–86.
106. Brownstein MH, Starink TM. Desmoplastic trichoepithelioma and intradermal nevus: a combined malformation. J Am Acad Dermatol 1987;17:489–92.
107. Dammert K, Kallioinen M. [Desmoplastic trichoepithelioma. Clinical aspects, histology, and differential diagnosis.] Hautarzt 1987;38: 603–6. (German.)
108. Hartschuh W, Schulz T. Merkel cells are integral constituents of desmoplastic trichoepithelioma: an immunohistochemical and electron microscopic study. J Cutan Pathol 1995;22: 413–21.
109. Imber MJ. Benign cutaneous lesions potential misdiagnosed as malignant neoplasms. Semin Diagn Pathol 1990;7:139–45.
110. Starink TM, Lane EB, Meijer CJ. Generalized trichoepitheliomas with alopecia and myasthenia gravis: clinicopathologic and immunohistochemical study and comparison with classic and desmoplastic trichoepithelioma. J Am Acad Dermatol 1986;15:1104–12.
111. Sumithra S, Jayaraman M, Yesudian P. Desmoplastic trichoepithelioma and multiple epidermal cysts. Int J Dermatol 1993;32:747–8.
112. Takei Y, Fukushiro S, Ackerman AB. Criteria for histologic differentiation of desmoplastic trichoepithelioma (sclerosing epithelial hamartoma) from morphea-like basal-cell carcinoma. Am J Dermatopathol 1985;7:207–21.
113. Thewes M, Worret WI, Engst R, Ring J. Stromelysin-3: a potent marker for histopathologic differentiation between desmoplastic trichoepithelioma and morphealike basal cell carcinoma. Am J Dermatopathol 1998;20:140–2.
114. Wick MR, Cooper PH, Swanson PE, Kaye VN, Sun TT. Microcystic adnexal carcinoma. An immunohistochemical comparison with other cutaneous appendage tumors. Arch Dermatol 1990;126:189–94.
115. Zuccati G, Massi D, Mastrolorenzo A, Urbano FG, Paoli S, Reali UM. Desmoplastic tricho-epithelioma. Australas J Dermatol 1998;39:273–4.

Pilomatricoma

116. Agarwal RP, Handler SD, Matthews MR, Carpentieri D. Pilomatrixoma of the head and neck in children. Otolaryngol Head Neck Surg 2001;125:510–5.
117. Ambrojo P, Aguilar A, Simon P, Requena L, Sanchez-Yus E. Basal cell carcinoma with matrical differentiation. Am J Dermatopathol 1992;14:293–7.
118. Behnke N, Schulte K, Ruzicka T, Megahed M. Pilomatricoma in elderly individuals. Dermatology 1998;197:391–3.
119. Carlson JA, Healy K, Slominski A, Mihm MC Jr. Melanocytic matricoma: a report of two cases of a new entity. Am J Dermatopathol 1999;21: 344–9.
120. Chan EF, Gat U, McNiff JM, Fuchs E. A common human skin tumour is caused by activating mutations in beta-catenin. Nat Genet 1999;21:410–3.
121. Danielson-Cohen A, Lin SJ, Hughes CA, An YH, Maddalozzo J. Head and neck pilomatrixoma in children. Arch Otolaryngol Head Neck Surg 2001;127:1481–3.
122. Darwish AH, Al-Halahema EK, Dhiman AK, Al-Khalifa KA. Clinicopathological study of pilomatricoma. Saudi Med J 2001;22:268–71.
123. Demircan M, Balik E. Pilomatricoma in children: a prospective study. Pediatr Dermatol 1997;14:430–2.
124. Diomedi-Camassei F, Francalanci P, Boldrini R, Spagnoli A, Lucchetti MC, Ferro F. Paratesticular pilomatricoma: a new location. Pediatr Surg Int 2001;17:652–3.
125. Fang J, Keh P, Katz L, Rao MS. Pilomatricoma-like endometrioid adenosquamous carcinoma of the ovary with neuroendocrine differentiation. Gynecol Oncol 1996;61:291–3.
126. Garcia-Escudero A, Navarro-Bustos G, Jurado-Escamez P, Rios-Martin J, Gonzalez-Campora R. Primary squamous cell carcinoma of the lung with pilomatricoma-like features. Histopathology 2002;40:201–2.
127. Geh JL, Moss AL. Multiple pilomatrixomata and myotonic dystrophy: a familial association. Br J Plast Surg 1999;52:143–5.
128. Honda Y, Oh-i T, Koga M, Tokuda Y. Perforating pilomatricoma: transepithelial elimination or not. J Dermatol 2002;29:100–3.
129. Imperiale A, Calabrese M, Monetti F, Zandrino F. Calcified pilomatrixoma of the breast: mammographic and sonographic findings. Eur Radiol 2001;11:2465–7.
130. Inglefield CJ, Muir IF, Gray ES. Aggressive pilomatricoma in childhood. Ann Plast Surg 1994; 33:656–8.
131. Ismail W, Pain S, al-Okati D, al Sewan M. Giant pilomatricoma simulating carcinoma of the male breast. Int J Clin Pract 2000;54:55–6.
132. Julian CG, Bowers PW. A clinical review of 209 pilomatricomas. J Am Acad Dermatol 1998;39: 191–5.

133. Kaddu S, Beham-Schmid C, Soyer HP, Hodl S, Beham A, Kerl H. Extramedullary hematopoiesis in pilomatricomas. Am J Dermatopathol 1995;17:126–30.
134. Kaddu S, Soyer HP, Hodl S, Kerl H. Morphological stages of pilomatricoma. Am J Dermatopathol 1996;18:333–8.
135. Kaddu S, Soyer HP, Wolf IH, Kerl H. Proliferating pilomatricoma. A histopathologic simulator of metrical carcinoma. J Cutan Pathol 1997;24:228–34.
136. Lee WS, Yoo MS, Ahn SK. Anetodermic cutaneous changes overlying pilomatricoma. Int J Dermatol 1995;34:144–5.
137. Lemos MM, Kindblom LG, Meis-Kindblom JM, Ryd W, Willen H. Fine-needle aspiration features of pilomatrixoma. Cancer 2001;93:252–6.
138. Ma KF, Tsui MS, Chan SK. Fine needle aspiration diagnosis of pilomatrixoma. A monomorphic population of basaloid cells with squamous differentiation, not to be mistaken for carcinoma. Acta Cytol 1991;35:570–4.
139. Marrogi AJ, Wick MR, Dehner LP. Pilomatrical neoplasms in children and young adults. Am J Dermatopathol 1992;14:87–94.
140. Masih S, Sorenson SM, Gentili A, Seeger LL. Atypical adult non-calcified pilomatricoma. Skeletal Radiol 2000;29:54–6.
141. Noguchi H, Kayashima K, Nishiyama S, Ono T. Two cases of pilomatrixoma in Turner's syndrome. Dermatology 1999;199:338–40.
142. Phyu KK, Bradley PJ. Pilomatrixoma in the parotid region. J Laryngol Otol 2001;115:1026–8.
143. Pujol RM, Casanova JM, Egido R, Pujol J, de Moragas JM. Multiple familial pilomatricomas: a cutaneous marker for Gardner syndrome? Pediatr Dermatol 1995;12:331–5.
144. Viero RM, Tani E, Skoog L. Fine needle aspiration (FNA) cytology of pilomatrixoma: report of 14 cases and review of the literature. Cytopathology 1999;10:263–9.
145. Vogelbruch M, Rutten A, Bocking A, Kapp A, Kiehl P. Differentiation between malignant and benign follicular adnexal tumors of the skin by DNA image cytometry. Br J Dermatol 2002;146:238–43.
146. Wells NJ, Blair GK, Magee JF, Whiteman DM. Pilomatrixoma: a common, benign childhood skin tumor. Can J Surg 1994;37:483–6.
147. Wong MP, Yuen ST, Collins RJ. Fine-needle aspiration biopsy of pilomatrixoma: still a diagnostic trap for the unwary. Diagn Cytopathol 1994;10:365–9.
148. Yoshimura Y, Obara S, Mikami T, Matsuda S. Calcifying epithelioma (pilomatrixoma) of the head and neck: analysis of 37 cases. Br J Oral Maxillofac Surg 1997;35:429–32.

Trichogerminoma
149. Sau P, Lupton GP, Graham JH. Trichogerminoma. Report of 14 cases. J Cutan Pathol 1992;19:357–65.

Basaloid Follicular Hamartoma
150. Brownstein MH. Basaloid follicular hamartoma: solitary and multiple types. J Am Acad Dermatol 1992;27:237–40.
150a. Cribier B, Grosshans E. Tumor of the follicular infundibulum: a clinicopathologic study. J Am Acad Dermatol 1995;33:979–84.
151. Girardi M, Federman GL, McNiff JM. Familial multiple basaloid follicular hamartomas: a report of two affected sisters. Pediatr Dermatol 1999;16:281–4.
152. Harman M, Inaloz HS, Akdeniz S, Inaloz SS, Aslan A. Congenital non-familial unilateral basaloid follicular hamartoma. J Eur Acad Dermatol Venereol 1999;13:210–3.
153. Kato N, Ueno H, Nakamura J. Localized basaloid follicular hamartoma. J Dermatol 1992;19:614–7.
154. Mehregan AH, Baker S. Basaloid follicular hamartoma: three cases with localized and systematized unilateral lesions. J Cutan Pathol 1985;12:55–65.
154a. Naeyaert JM, Pauwels C, Geerts ML, Verplancke P. CD-34 and Ki-67 staining patterns of basaloid follicular hamartoma are different from those in fibroepithelioma of Pinkus and other variants of basal cell carcinoma. J Cutan Pathol 2001;28:538–41.
155. Nelson BR, Johnson TM, Waldinger T, Gillard M, Lowe L. Basaloid follicular hamartoma: a histologic diagnosis with diverse clinical presentations. Arch Dermatol 1993;129:915–7.
156. Requena L, Farina MC, Robledo M, et al. Multiple hereditary infundibulocystic basal cell carcinomas: a genodermatosis different from nevoid basal cell carcinoma syndrome. Arch Dermatol 1999;135:1227–35.
157. Ricks M, Elston DM, Sartori CR. Multiple basaloid follicular hamartomas associated with acrochordons, seborrheic keratoses, and chondrosarcoma. Br J Dermatol 2002;146:1068–70.
158. Starink TM, Lane EB, Meijer CJ. Generalized trichoepitheliomas with alopecia and myasthenia gravis: clinicopathologic and immunohistochemical study and comparison with classic and desmoplastic trichoepithelioma. J Am Acad Dermatol 1986;15(Pt 2):1104–12.
159. Toyoda M, Kagoura M, Morohashi M. Solitary basaloid follicular hamartoma. J Dermatol 1998;25:434–7.

Trichoblastoma

160. Ackerman AB, Reddy VB, Soyer HP. Neoplasms with follicular differentiation. New York: Scribner; 1993.
161. Aloi F, Tomasini C, Pippione M. Pigmented trichoblastoma. Am J Dermatopathol 1992;14:345–9.
162. Betti R, Alessi E. Nodular trichoblastoma with adamantinoid features. Am J Dermatopathol 1996;18:192–5.
162a. Brownstein MH. Basaloid follicular hamartoma: solitary and multiple types. J Am Acad Dermatol 1992;27:237–40.
163. Chan JK, Ng CS, Tsang WY. Nodular desmoplastic variant of trichoblastoma. Am J Surg Pathol 1994;18:495–500.
164. Chang SN, Chung YL, Kim SC, Sim JY, Park WH. Trichoblastoma with sebaceous and sweat gland differentiation. Br J Dermatol 2001;144:1090–2.
165. Collina G, Eusebi V, Capella C, Rosai J. Merkel cell differentiation in trichoblastoma. Virchows Arch 1998;433:291–6.
166. Cowen EW, Helm KF, Billingsley EM. An unusually aggressive trichoblastoma. J Am Acad Dermatol 2000;42(Pt 2):374–7.
167. Cribier B, Scrivener Y, Grosshans E. Tumors arising in nevus sebaceus: a study of 596 cases. J Am Acad Dermatol 2000;42(Pt 1):263–8.
168. Graham BS, Barr RJ. Rippled-pattern sebaceous trichoblastoma. J Cutan Pathol 2000;27:455–9.
169. Headington JT. Differentiating neoplasms of hair germ. J Clin Pathol 1970;23:464–71.
170. Jaqueti G, Requena L, Sanchez-Yus E. Trichoblastoma is the most common neoplasm developed in nevus sebaceus of Jadassohn: a clinicopathologic study of a series of 155 cases. Am J Dermatopathol 2000;22:108–18.
171. Kaddu S, Schaeppi H, Kerl H, Soyer HP. Subcutaneous trichoblastoma. J Cutan Pathol 1999;26:490–6.
172. Kaddu S, Schappi H, Kerl H, Soyer HP. Trichoblastoma and sebaceoma in nevus sebaceus. Am J Dermatopathol 1999;21:552–6.
173. Misago N, Kodera H, Narisawa Y. Sebaceous carcinoma, trichoblastoma, and sebaceoma with features of trichoblastoma in nevus sebaceus. Am J Dermatopathol 2001;23:456–62.
174. Ogata T, Tanaka S, Goto T, et al. Giant trichoblastoma mimicking malignancy. Arch Orthop Trauma Surg 1999;119:225–7.
175. Regauer S, Beham-Schmid C, Okcu M, Hartner E, Mannweiler S. Trichoblastic carcinoma ("malignant trichoblastoma") with lymphatic and hematogenous metastases. Mod Pathol 2000;13:673–8.
176. Requena L, Requena I, Romero E, Sanchez M, Sanchez-Yus E. Trichogenic trichoblastoma. An unusual neoplasm of hair germ. Am J Dermatopathol 1990;12:175–81.
177. Rofagha R, Usmani AS, Vadmal M, Hessel AB, Pellegrini AE. Trichoblastic carcinoma: a report of two cases of a deeply infiltrative trichoblastic neoplasm. Dermatol Surg 2001;27:663–6.
178. Santa Cruz DJ, Barr RJ, Headington JT. Cutaneous lymphadenoma. Am J Surg Pathol 1991;15:101–10.
179. Schirren CG, Rutten A, Kaudewitz P, Diaz C, McClain S, Burgdorf WH. Trichoblastoma and basal cell carcinoma are neoplasms with follicular differentiation sharing the same profile of cytokeratin intermediate filaments. Am J Dermatopathol 1997;19:341–50.
180. Tronnier M. Clear cell trichoblastoma in association with a nevus sebaceus. Am J Dermatopathol 2001;23:143–5.
181. Wong TY, Reed JA, Suster S, Flynn SD, Mihm MC Jr. Benign trichogenic tumors: a report of two cases supporting a simplified nomenclature. Histopathology 1993;22:575–80.
182. Yamamoto O, Asahi M. Cytokeratin expression in trichoblastic fibroma (small nodular type trichoblastoma), trichoepithelioma, and basal cell carcinoma. Br J Dermatol 1999;140:8–16.
183. Yamamoto O, Hisaoka M, Yasuda H, Nishio D, Asahi M. A rippled-pattern trichoblastoma: an immunohistochemical study. J Cutan Pathol 2000;27:460–5.

Trichodiscoma

184. Alsina MM, Ferrando J, Bombi JA, Pou A, Torras H. [Multiple familial trichodiscoma.] Med Cutan Ibero Lat Am 1990;18:30–4. (Spanish.)
185. Balus L, Fazio M, Sacerdoti G, Morrone A, Marmo W. [Fibrofolliculoma, trichodiscoma, and acrochordon. The Birt-Hogg-Dube syndrome.] Ann Dermatol Venereol 1983;110:601–9. (French.)
186. Birt AR, Hogg GR, Dube WJ. Hereditary multiple fibrofolliculomas with trichodiscomas and acrochordons. Arch Dermatol 1977;113:1674–7.
187. Calonje E, Guerin D, McCormick D, Fletcher CD. Superficial angiomyxoma: clinicopathologic analysis of a series of distinctive but poorly-recognized cutaneous tumors with tendency for recurrence. Am J Surg Pathol 1999;23:910–7.
188. Camarasa JG, Calderon P, Moreno A. Familial multiple trichodiscomas. Acta Derm Venereol 1988;68:163–5.
189. Coskey RJ, Pinkus H. Trichodiscoma. Int J Dermatol 1976;15:600–1.

190. De la Torre C, Ocampo C, Doval IG, Losada A, Cruces MJ. Acrochordons are not a component of the Birt-Hogg-Dube syndrome: does this syndrome exist? Case reports and review of the literature. Am J Dermatopathol 1999;21:369–74.
191. Fujita WH, Barr RJ, Headley JL. Multiple fibrofolliculomas with trichodiscomas and acrochordons. Arch Dermatol 1981;117:32–5.
192. Grosshans E, Dungler T, Hanau D. [Pinkus' trichodiscoma (author's trans.).] Ann Dermatol Venereol 1981;108:837–46. (French.)
193. McCalmont CS, White WL, Jorizzo JL. Giant fibromyxoid tumors of the adventitial dermis. Forme fruste of trichodiscoma? Am J Dermatopathol 1991;13:403–9.
194. Mertens J, Schubert C. [Small papular tumors of the perifollicular and perivascular connective tissue of the head and neck area.] HNO 1991;39:266–70. (German.)
195. Pinkus H, Coskey R, Burgess GH. Trichodiscoma. A benign tumor related to haarscheibe (hair disk). J Invest Dermatol 1974;63:212–8.
196. Schulz T, Ebschner U, Harschuh W. Localized Birt-Hogg-Dube syndrome with prominent perivascular fibromas. Am J Dermatopathol 2001;23:149–53.

Perifollicular Fibroma

197. Chang SN, Chun SI, Moon TK, Park WH. Solitary sclerotic fibroma of the skin: degenerated sclerotic change of inflammatory conditions, especially folliculitis. Am J Dermatopathol 2000;22:22–5.
198. Cho S, Hahm JH. Perifollicular fibroma. J Eur Acad Dermatol Venereol 1999;13:46–9.
199. Foix C, Pichard JP, Civatte J, Belaich S. [Solitary acquired perifollicular fibroma.] Ann Dermatol Venereol 1978;105:963–4. (French.)
200. Freeman RG, Chernosky ME. Perifollicular fibroma. Arch Dermatol 1969;100:66–9.
200a. Kawasaki H, Sawamura D, Nakazawa H, Hattori N, Goto M, Sato-Matsumura KC, Akiyama M, Shimizu H: Detection of 1733insC mutations in an Asian family with Birt-Hogg-Dube syndrome. Br J Dermatol 2005;152:142–5.
201. McKenna DB, Barry-Walsh C, Leader M, Murphy GM. Multiple perifollicular fibromas. J Eur Acad Dermatol Venereol 1999;12:234–7.
202. Pinkus H. Perifollicular fibromas. Pure periadnexal adventitial tumors. Am J Dermatopathol 1979;1:341–2.
202a. Schmidt LS, Nickerson ML, Warren MB, et al. Germline BHD-mutation spectrum and phenotype analysis of a large cohort of families with Birt-Hogg-Dube syndrome. Am J Hum Genet 2005;76:1023–33.
203. Smith LR, Heaton CL. Perifollicular fibroma. Cutis 1979;23:354–55.

Fibrofolliculoma

203a. Coskey RJ, Pinkus H. Trichodiscoma. Int J Dermatol 1976;15:600–1.
204. Foucar K, Rosen T, Foucar E, Cochran RJ. Fibrofolliculoma: a clinicopathologic study. Cutis 1981;28:429–32.
205. Gartmann H. [Fibrofolliculoma.] Z Hautkr 1985;60:567–75. (German.)
206. Hornstein OP, Knickenberg M. Perifollicular fibromatosis cutis with polyps of the colon—a cutaneo-intestinal syndrome sui generis. Arch Dermatol Res 1975;253:161–75.
207. Junkins-Hopkins JM, Cooper PH. Multiple perifollicular fibromas: report of a case and analysis of the literature. J Cutan Pathol 1994;21:467–71.
208. Scully K, Bargman H, Assaad D. Solitary fibrofolliculoma. J Am Acad Dermatol 1984;11: 361–3.
209. Starink TM, Brownstein MH. Fibrofolliculoma: solitary and multiple types. J Am Acad Dermatol 1987;17:493–6.

Follicular Myxoma

210. Cohen C, Davis TS. Multiple trichogenic adnexal tumors. Am J Dermatopathol 1986;8:241–6.
211. Headington JT. Tumors of the hair follicle. A review. Am J Pathol 1976;85:479–514.
212. Nwokoro NA, Korytkowski MT, Rose S, et al. Spectrum of malignancy and premalignancy in Carney syndrome. Am J Med Genet 1997;31: 369–77.

Pilar Leiomyoma

213. Argenyi ZB. Recent developments in cutaneous neural neoplasms. J Cutan Pathol 1993;20: 97–108.
214. Calonje E, Wilson-Jones E, Smith NP, Fletcher CD. Cellular 'neurothekeoma': an epithelioid variant of pilar leiomyoma? Morphological and immunhistochemical analysis of a series. Histopathology 1992;20:397–404.
215. Dawn G, Handa S, Dos A, Kumar B. Bilateral symmetrical pilar leiomyomas on the breasts. Br J Dermatol 1995;133:331–2.
216. Dubovy SR, Clark BJ. Palisaded encapsulated neuroma (solitary circumscribed neuroma of skin) of the eyelid: report of two cases and review of the literature. Br J Ophthalmol 2001;85:949–51.
217. Guitart J, Ritter JH, Wick MR. Solitary cutaneous myofibromas in adults: report of six cases and discussion of differential diagnosis. J Cutan Pathol 1996;23:437–44.

218. Mahalingam M, Goldberg LJ. Atypical pilar leiomyoma: cutaneous counterpart of uterine symplastic leiomyoma? Am J Dermatopathol 2001;23:299–303.
219. Newman PL, Fletcher CD. Smooth muscle tumors of the external genitalia: clinicopathological analysis of a series. Histopathology 1991;18:523–9.
220. Orellana-Diaz O, Hernandez-Perez E. Leiomyoma cutis and leiomyosarcoma: a 10-year study and a short review. J Dermatol Surg Oncol 1983;9:283–7.
221. Raj S, Calonje E, Kraus M, Kavanagh G, Newman PL, Fletcher CD. Cutaneous pilar leiomyoma: clinicopathologic analysis of 53 lesions in 45 patients. Am J Dermatopathol 1997;19:2–9.
222. Requena L, Sangueza OP. Benign neoplasms with neural differentiation: a review. Am J Dermatopathol 1995;17:75–96.
223. Sahoo B, Radotra BD, Kaur I, Kumar B. Zosteriform pilar leiomyoma. J Dermatol 2001;28:759–61.
224. Swanson PE, Wick MR. Immunohistochemistry of cutaneous tumors. In: Leong AS, ed. Applied immunohistochemistry for the surgical pathologist. London: Arnold; 1993:270–308.
225. Yokoyama R, Hashimoto H, Daimaru Y, Enjoji M. Superficial leiomyomas. A clinicopathologic study of 34 cases. Acta Pathol Jpn 1987;37:1415–22.

Trichilemmal Carcinoma

226. Billingsley EM, Davidowski TA, Maloney ME. Trichilemmal carcinoma. J Am Acad Dermatol 1997;23:107–9.
227. Boscaino A, Terracciano LM, Donofrio V, Ferrara G, De Rosa G. Trichilemmal carcinoma: a study of seven cases. J Cutan Pathol 1992;19:94–9.
228. Chan KO, Lim IJ, Baladas HG, Tan WT. Multiple tumor presentation of trichilemmal carcinoma. Br J Plast Surg 1999;52:665–7.
228a. Headington JT. Tumors of the hair follicle. A review. Am J Pathol 1976;85:479–514.
229. Ko T, Tada H, Hatoko M, Muramatsu T, Shirai T. Trichilemmal carcinoma developing in a burn scar: a report of two cases. J Dermatol 1996;23:463–8.
230. Reis JP, Tellechea O, Cunha MF, Baptista AP. Trichilemmal carcinoma: review of 8 cases. J Cutan Pathol 1993;20:44–9.
231. Suster S. Clear cell tumors of the skin. Semin Diagn Pathol 1996;13:40–59.
232. Swanson PE, Marrogi AJ, Williams DJ, Cherwitz DL, Wick MR. Trichilemmal carcinoma: clinicopathologic study of 10 cases. J Cutan Pathol 1992;19:100–9.
233. Wong TY, Suster S. Tricholemmal carcinoma. A clinicopathologic study of 13 cases. Am J Dermatopathol 1994;16:463–73.

Malignant Proliferating Pilar Tumor

234. Amaral AL, Nascimento AG, Goellner JR. Proliferating pilar (trichilemmal) cyst. Report of two cases, one with carcinomatous transformation and one with distant metastases. Arch Pathol Lab Med 1984;108:808–10.
234a. Brownstein MH, Arluk DJ. Proliferating trichilemmal cyst: a simulant of squamous cell carcinoma. Cancer 1981;48:1207–14.
235. Jaworski R. Malignant trichilemmal cyst. Am J Dermatopathol 1988;10:276–7.
236. Mehregan AH, Lee KC. Malignant proliferating trichilemmal tumors—report of three cases. J Dermatol Surg Oncol 1987;13:1339–42.
237. Mori O, Hachisuka H, Sasai Y. Proliferating trichilemmal cyst with spindle cell carcinoma. Am J Dermatopathol 1990;12:479–84.
238. Saida T, Oohara K, Hori Y, Tsuchiya S. Development of a malignant proliferating trichilemmal cyst in a patient with multiple trichilemmal cysts. Dermatologica 1983;166:203–8.
238a. Sau P, Graham JH, Helwig EB. Proliferating epithelial cysts. Clinicopathological analysis of 96 cases. J Cutan Pathol 1995;22:394–406.
239. Weiss J, Heine M, Grimmel M, Jung EG. Malignant proliferating trichilemmal cyst. J Am Acad Dermatol 1995;32:870–3.

Pilomatrix Carcinoma

240. Arole G, Mosadomi A, Arain AH. Calcifying epithelioma of Malherbe (pilomatrixoma) of the cheek. J Oral Maxillofac Surg 1983;41:121–5.
241. Chen KT, Taylor DR Jr. Pilomatrix carcinoma. J Surg Oncol 1986;33:112–4.
242. De Galvez-Aranda MV, Herrera-Ceballos E, Sanchez-Sanchez P, Bosch-Garcia RJ, Matilla-Vicente A. Pilomatrix carcinoma with lymph node and pulmonary metastasis: report of a case arising on the knee. Am J Dermatopathol 2002;24:139–43.
243. Gould E, Kurzon R, Kowalczyk AP, Saldana M. Pilomatrix carcinoma with pulmonary metastasis. Report of a case. Cancer 1984;54:370–2.
244. Green DE, Sanusi ID, Fowler MR. Pilomatrix carcinoma. J Am Acad Dermatol 1987;17:264–70.
245. Hardisson D, Linares MD, Cuevas-Santos J, Contreras F. Pilomatrix carcinoma: a clinicopathologic study of six cases and review of the literature. Am J Dermatopathol 2001;23:394–401.
246. Kaddu S, Soyer HP, Cerroni L, Salmhofer W, Hodl S. Clinical and histopathologic spectrum of pilomatricomas in adults. Int J Dermatol 1994;33:705–8.

246a. Kaddu S, Soyer HP, Wolf IH, Kerl H. Proliferating pilomatricoma. A histopathologic simulator of metrical carcinoma. J Cutan Pathol 1997; 24:228–34.
247. Lineaweaver WC, Wang TN, LeBoit PE. Pilomatrix carcinoma. J Surg Oncol 1988;37:171–4.
248. Lopansri S, Mihm MC Jr. Pilomatrix carcinoma or calcifying epitheliocarcinoma of Malherbe: a case report and review of literature. Cancer 1980;45:2368–73.
249. Manivel C, Wick MR, Mukai K. Pilomatrix carcinoma: an immunohistochemical comparison with benign pilomatrixoma and other benign cutaneous lesions of pilar origin. J Cutan Pathol 1986;13:22–9.
249a. Marrogi AJ, Wick MR, Dehner LP. Pilomatrical neoplasms in children and young adults. Am J Dermatopathol 1992;14:87–94.
250. Nield DV, Saad MN, Ali MH. Aggressive pilomatrixoma in a child: a case report. Br J Plast Surg 1986;39:139–41.
251. Okamura JM, Barr RJ. Cutaneous lymphoepithelial neoplasms. Adv Dermatol 1997;12:277–94.
252. Rothman D, Kendall AB, Baldi A. Giant pilomatrixoma (Malherbe calcifying epithelioma). Arch Surg 1976;111:86–7.
253. Sasaki CT, Yue A, Enriques R. Giant calcifying epithelioma. Arch Otolaryngol 1976;102:753–5.
254. Sau P, Lupton GP, Graham JH. Pilomatrix carcinoma. Cancer 1993;71:2491–8.
255. Vico P, Rahier I, Ghanem G, Nagypal P, Deraemaecker R. Pilomatrix carcinoma. Eur J Surg Oncol 1997;23:370–1.

Adnexal Carcinomas with Mixed Differentiation

256. Foschini MP, Eusebi V. Divergent differentiation in endocrine and nonendocrine tumors of the skin. Semin Diagn Pathol 2000;17:162–8.
257. Nakhleh RE, Swanson PE, Wick MR. Cutaneous adnexal carcinomas with divergent differentiation. Am J Dermatopathol 1990;12:325–34.
258. Rahbari H, Mehregan AH. Pilary complex carcinoma: an adnexal carcinoma of the skin with differentiation towards the components of the pilary complex. J Dermatol 1993;20:630–7.
259. Wick MR, Swanson PE, LeBoit PE, Strickler JG, Cooper PH. Lymphoepithelioma-like carcinoma of the skin with adnexal differentiation. J Cutan Pathol 1991;18:93–102.

Pilar Leiomyosarcoma

260. Ikari Y, Tokuhashi I, Haramoto I, et al. Cutaneous leiomyosarcoma. J Dermatol 1992;19:99–104.
261. Suster S. Epithelioid leiomyosarcoma of the skin and subcutaneous tissue. Clinicopathologic, immunohistochemical, and ultrastructural study of five cases. Am J Surg Pathol 1994; 18:232–40.
262. Swanson PE, Stanley MW, Scheithauer BW, Wick MR. Primary cutaneous leiomyosarcoma. A histological and immunohistochemical study of 9 cases, with ultrastructural correlation. J Cutan Pathol 1988;15:129–41.
262a. Swanson PE, Wick MR. Immunohistochemistry of cutaneous tumors. In: Leong AS, ed. Applied immunohistochemistry for the surgical pathologist. London: Arnold; 1993:270–308.

Pseudoneoplastic Proliferations of Hair Follicles and Follicle-Related Mesenchyme

263. Ban M, Kamiya H, Yamada T, Kitajima Y. Hair follicle nevi and accessory tragi: variable quantity of adipose tissue in connective tissue framework. Pediatr Dermatol 1997;14:433–6.
264. Choi EH, Ahn SK, Lee SH, Bang D. Hair follicle nevus. Int J Dermatol 1992;31:578–1.
264a. Cribier B, Grosshans E. Tumor of the follicular infundibulum: a clinicopathologic study. J Am Acad Dermatol 1995;33:979–84.
265. Davis DA, Cohen PR. Hair follicle nevus: case report and review of the literature. Pediatr Dermatol 1996;13:135–8.
266. Dudley K, Barr WG, Armin A, Massa MC. Nevus comedonicus in association with widespread, well-differentiated follicular tumors. J Am Acad Dermatol 1986;15:1123–7.
267. Elgart GW, Patterson JW. Congenital midline hamartoma: case report with histochemical and immunohistochemical findings. Pediatr Dermatol 1990;7:199–201.
268. Germain M, Smith KJ. Hair follicle nevus in a distribution following Blaskho's lines. J Am Acad Dermatol 2002;46(5 Suppl):S125–7.
269. Hamm H. [Faun-tail nevus.] Hautarzt 1992;43:235–6. (German.)
270. Hunter GA, Donald GF. Trichofolliculoma. Australas J Dermatol 1966;8:216–8.
271. Jansen T, Romiti R, Altmeyer P. Accessory tragus: report of two cases and review of the literature. Pediatr Dermatol 2000;17:391–4.
272. Kroumpouzos G, Stefanato CM, Wilkel CS, Bogaars H, Bhawan J. Systematized porokeratotic eccrine and hair follicle nevus: report of a case and review of the literature. Br J Dermatol 1999;141:1092–6.
273. Kuwahara H, Lao LM, Kiyohara T, Kumakiri M, Igawa H. Hair follicle nevus occurring in frontonasal dysplasia: an electron microscopic observation. J Dermatol 2001;28:324–8.
274. Labandeira J, Peteiro C, Toribio J. Hair follicle nevus: case report and review. Am J Dermatopathol 1996;18:90–3.

275. Lee S, Kim JG. Eruptive vellus hair cyst. Clinical and histologic findings. Arch Dermatol 1979;115:744–6.
275a. Mehregan AH, Baker S. Basaloid follicular hamartoma: three cases with localized and systematized unilateral lesions. J Cutan Pathol 1985;12:55–65.
276. Pippione M, Aloi F, Depaoli MA. Hair-follicle nevus. Am J Dermatopathol 1984;6:245–7.
277. Reda AM, Rogers RS 3rd, Peters MS. Woolly hair nevus. J Am Acad Dermatol 1990;22:377–80.
278. Vignale RA, De Anda G. [Curly hair nevus.] Med Cutan Ibero Lat Amer 1983;11:167–70. (Spanish.)

Linear Basal Cell Nevus

279. Aloi F, Tomasini CF, Isaia G, Grazia-Bernengo M. Unilateral basal cell nevus associated with diffuse osteoma cutis, unilateral anodontia, and abnormal bone mineralization. J Am Acad Dermatol 1989;20(Pt 2):973–8.
280. Bleiberg J, Brodkin RH. Linear unilateral basal cell nevus with comedones. Arch Dermatol 1969;100:187–90.
281. Gorlin RJ. Nevoid basal cell carcinoma syndrome. Medicine 1987;66:98–113.
282. Guillemette J, Enjolras O, Lessana-Leibowitch M, Diner PA, Escande JP. [A little known unilateral skin disease: linear basal cell nevus.] Ann Dermatol Venereol 1989;116:902–4. (French.)
283. Gutierrez MM, Mora RG. Nevoid basal cell carcinoma syndrome. A review and case report of a patient with unilateral basal cell nevus syndrome. J Am Acad Dermatol 1986;15:1023–30.
284. Willis D, Rapini RP, Chernoskey ME. Linear basal cell nevus. Cutis 1990;46:493–4.
285. Zarour H, Grob JJ, Choux R, Collet-Villette AM, Bonerandi JJ. [Basal-cell and linear unilateral adnexal hamartoma (or linear unilateral basal-cell nevus).] Ann Dermatol Venereol 1992; 119:901–3. (French.)

Steatocystoma Multiplex and Simplex

286. Ahn SK, Chung J, Lee WS, Lee SH, Choi EH. Hybrid cysts showing alternate combination of eruptive vellus hair cyst, steatocystoma multiplex, and epidermoid cyst, and an association among the three conditions. Am J Dermatopathol 1996;18:645–9.
287. Brownstein MH. Steatocystoma simplex. A solitary steatocystoma. Arch Dermatol 1982;118:409–11.
288. Cho S, Chang SE, Choi JH, Sung KJ, Moon KC, Koh JK. Clinical and histologic features of 64 cases of steatocystoma multiplex. J Dermatol 2002;29:152–6.
289. Cole LA. Steatocystoma multiplex. Arch Dermatol 1976;112:1437–9.
290. Ohtake N, Kubota Y, Takayama O, Shimada S, Tamaki K. Relationship between steatocystoma multiplex and eruptive vellus hair cysts. J Am Acad Dermatol 1992;26:876–8.
291. Olsen DB, Mostofi RS, Lagrotteria LB. Steatocystoma simplex in the oral cavity: a previously undescribed condition. Oral Surg Oral Med Oral Pathol 1988;66:605–7.
292. Patrizi A, Neri I, Guerrini V, Costa AM, Passarini B. Persistent milia, steatocystoma multiplex and eruptive vellus hair cysts: variable expression of multiple pilosebaceous cysts within an affected family. Dermatology 1998;196:392–6.
293. Sanchez-Yus E, Aguilar-Martinez A, Cristobal-Gil MC, Urbina-Gonzalez F, Guerra-Rodriguez P. Eruptive vellus hair cyst and steatocystoma multiplex: two related conditions? J Cutan Pathol 1988;15:40–2.

Eruptive Vellus Hair Cysts

294. Esterly NB, Fretzin DF, Pinkus H. Eruptive vellus hair cysts. Arch Dermatol 1977;113:500–3.
295. Held JL, Andrew JE, Toback AC. Eruptive vellus hair cysts. Cutis 1987;40:259–60.
296. Lee S, Kim JG, Kang JS. Eruptive vellus hair cysts. Arch Dermatol 1984;120:1191–5.
297. Mayron R, Grimwood RE. Familial occurrence of eruptive vellus hair cysts. Pediatr Dermatol 1988;5:94–6.
298. Requena L, Sanchez Yus E. Follicular hybrid cysts. An expanded spectrum. Am J Dermatopathol 1991;13:228–33.

Neurofollicular and Pilar Neurocristic Hamartomas

299. Barr RJ, Goodman MM. Neurofollicular hamartoma: a light microscopic and immunohistochemical study. J Cutan Pathol 1989;16:336–41.
300. Mezebish D, Smith K, Williams J, Menon P, Crittenden J, Skelton H. Neurocristic cutaneous hamartoma: a distinctive dermal melanocytosis with an unknown malignant potential. Mod Pathol 1998;11:573–8.
301. Nova MP, Zung M, Halperin A. Neurofollicular hamartoma: a clinicopathological study. Am J Dermatopathol 1991;13:459–62.
302. Pathy AL, Helm TN, Elston D, Bergfeld WF, Tuthill RJ. Malignant melanoma arising in a blue nevus with features of pilar neurocristic hamartoma. J Cutan Pathol 1993;20:459–64.
303. Pearson JP, Weiss SW, Headington JT. Cutaneous malignant melanotic neurocristic tumors arising in neurocristic hamartomas. A melanocytic tumor morphologically and biologically distinct from common melanoma. Am J Surg Pathol 1996;20:665–77.

304. Sangueza OP, Requena L. Neurofollicular hamartoma. A new histogenetic interpretation. Am J Dermatopathol 1994;16:150–4.
305. Smith KJ, Mezebish D, Williams J, Elgart M, Skelton HG. The spectrum of neurocristic cutaneous hamartoma: clinicopathologic and immunohistochemical study of three cases. Ann Diagn Pathol 1998;2:213–23.
306. Tuthill RJ, Clark WH Jr, Levene A. Pilar neurocristic hamartoma: its relationship to blue nevus and equine melanotic disease. Arch Dermatol 1982;118:592–6.

SUPPLEMENTAL REFERENCES

Tumor of the Follicular Infundibulum

Cheng AC, Chang YL, Wu YY, Hu SL, Chuan MT. Multiple tumors of the follicular infundibulum. Dermatol Surg 2004;30;1246–8.

Trichoadenoma

Miller CJ, Ioffreda MD, Billingsley EM. Sebaceous carcinoma, basal cell carcinoma, trichoadenoma, trichoblastoma, and syringocystadenoma papilliferum arising within a nevus sebaceus. Dermatol Surg 2004;30(Pt 2):1546–9.

Trichilemmoma

Keskinbora KH, Buyukbabani N, Terzi N. Desmoplastic trichilemmoma: a rare tumor of the eyelid. Eur J Ophthalmol 2004;14:562–4.

Kurokawa I, Nishijima S, Kusumoto K, Senzaki H, Shikata N, Tsubura A. Trichilemmoma: an immunohistochemical study of cytokeratins. Br J Dermatol 2003;149:99–104.

Plumb SJ, Argenyi ZB, Stone MS, DeYoung BR. Cytokeratin 5/6 immunostaining in cutaneous adnexal neoplasms and metastatic adenocarcinoma. Am J Dermatopathol 2004;26:447–51.

Schweiger E, Spann CT, Weinberg JM, Ross B. A case of desmoplastic trichilemmoma of the lip treated with Mohs surgery. Dermatol Surg 2004;30:1062–4.

Proliferating Pilar Tumor

Folpe AL, Reisenauer AK, Mentzel T, Rutten A, Solomon AR. Proliferating trichilemmal tumors: clinicopathologic evaluation is a guide to biologic behavior. J Cutan Pathol 2003;30:492–8.

Ye J, Nappi O, Swanson PE, Patterson JW, Wick MR. Proliferating pilar tumors: a clinicopathologic study of 76 cases with a proposal for definition of benign and malignant variants. Am J Clin Pathol 2004;122:566–74.

Trichoepithelioma

Clarke J, Ioffreda M, Helm KF. Multiple familial trichoepitheliomas: a folliculosebaceous-apocrine genodermatosis. Am J Dermatopathol 2002;24:402–5.

Izikson L, Bhan A, Zembowicz A. Androgen receptor expression helps to differentiate basal cell carcinoma from benign trichoblastic tumors. Am J Dermatopathol 2005;27:91–95.

Lum CA, Binder SW. Proliferative characterization of basal-cell carcinoma and trichoepithelioma in small biopsy specimens. J Cutan Pathol 2004;31:550–4.

Minami Y, Uede K, Sagawa K, Kimura A, Tsuji T, Furukawa F. Immunohistochemical staining of cutaneous tumors with G-81, a monoclonal antibody to dermcidin. Br J Dermatol 2004;151:165–9.

Ozawa M, Aiba S, Kurosawa M, Tagami H. Ber-EP4 antigen is a marker for a cell population related to the secondary hair germ. Exp Dermatol 2004;13:401–5.

Uede K, Yamamoto Y, Furukawa F. Brooke-Spiegler syndrome associated with cylindroma, trichoepithelioma, spiradenoma, and syringoma. J Dermatol 2004;31:32–8.

Desmoplastic Trichoepithelioma

Matsuki T, Hayashi N, Mizushima J, Igarashi A, Kawashima M, Harada S. Two cases of desmoplastic trichoepithelioma. J Dermatol 2004;31:824–7.

Niimi Y, Kawana S. Desmoplastic trichoepithelioma: the association with compound nevus and ossification. Eur J Dermatol 2002;12:90–2.

Pilomatricoma

Doglioni C, Piccinin S, Demontis S, et al. Alterations of beta-catenin pathway in non-melanoma skin tumors: loss of alpha-ABC nuclear reactivity correlates with the presence of beta-catenin gene mutation. Am J Pathol 2003;163:2277–87.

Fetil E, Soyal MC, Menderes A, Lebe B, Gunes AT, Ozkan S. Bullous appearance of pilomatricoma. Dermatol Surg 2003;29:1066–7.

Greene RM, McGuff HS, Miller FR. Pilomatrixoma of the face: a benign skin appendage tumor mimicking squamous cell carcinoma. Otolaryngol Head Neck Surg 2004;130:483–5.

Haskell HD, Haynes HA, McKee PH, Redston M, Granter SR, Lazar AJ. Basal cell carcinoma with matrical differentiation: a case study with analysis of beta-catenin. J Cutan Pathol 2005;32:245–50.

Hassanein AM, Glanz SM. Beta-catenin expression in benign and malignant pilomatrix neoplasms. Br J Dermatol 2004;150:511–6.

Kizawa K, Toyoda M, Ito M, Morohashi M. Aberrantly differentiated cells in benign pilomatrixoma reflect the normal hair follicle: immunohistochemical analysis of Ca-binding S100A2, S100A3, and S100A6 proteins. Br J Dermatol 2005;152:314–20.

Kusama K, Katayama Yk, Oba K, et al. Expression of hard alpha-keratins in pilomatrixoma, craniopharyngioma, and calcifying odontogenic cyst. Am J Clin Pathol 2005;123:376–81.

Lan MY, Lan MC, Ho CY, Li WY, Lin CZ. Pilomatricoma of the head and neck: a retrospective review of 179 cases. Arch Otolaryngol Head Neck Surg 2003;129:1327–30.

Lemos LB, Brauchle RW. Pilomatrixoma: a diagnostic pitfall in fine-needle aspiration biopsies. A review from a small county hospital. Ann Diagn Pathol 2004;8:130–6.

Trichogerminoma

Kazakov DV, Kutzner H, Rutten A, Dummer R, Burg G, Kempf W. Trichogerminoma: a rare cutaneous adnexal tumor with differentiation toward the hair germ epithelium. Dermatology 2002;205:405–8.

Pozo L, Diaz-Cano SJ. Trichogerminoma: further evidence to support a specific follicular neoplasm. Histopathology 2005;46:108–10.

Trichodiscoma

Chartier M, Reed ML, Mandavilli S, Fung M, Grant-Kels JM, Murphy M. CD34-reactive trichodiscoma. J Cutan Pathol 2004;31:398–400.

Perifollicular Fibroma

Balfour E, Smoller BR. Exogenous trauma simulating perifollicular fibromas. Am J Dermatopathol 2005;27:42–4.

Fibrofolliculoma

Collins GL, Somach S, Morgan MB. Histomorphologic and immunophenotypic analysis of fibrofolliculomas and trichodiscomas in Birt-Hogg-Dube syndrome and sporadic disease. J Cutan Pathol 2002;29:529–33.

Vincent A, Farley M, Chan E, James WD. Birt-Hogg-Dube syndrome: a review of the literature and the differential diagnosis of firm facial papules. J Am Acad Dermatol 2003;49:698–705.

Pilar Leiomyoma

Garman ME, Blumberg MA, Ernst R, Raimer SS. Familial leiomyomatosis: a review and discussion of pathogenesis. Dermatology 2003;207:210–3.

Matthews JH, Pichardo RO, Hitchcock MG, Leshin B. Cutaneous leiomyoma with cytologic atypia, akin to uterine symplastic leiomyoma. Dermatol Surg 2004;30:1249–51.

Trichilemmal Carcinoma

Allee JE, Cotsarelis G, Solky B, Cook JL. Multiply recurrent trichilemmal carcinoma with perineural invasion and cytokeratin 17 positivity. Dermatol Surg 2003;29:886–9.

Garrett AB, Azmi FH, Ogburia KS. Trichilemmal carcinoma: a rare cutaneous malignancy: a report of two cases. Dermatol Surg 2004;30:113–5.

Pilomatrix Carcinoma

Bassarova A, Nesland JM, Sedloev T, Danielsen H, Christova S. Pilomatrix carcinoma with lymph node metastases. J Cutan Pathol 2004;31:330–5.

Petit T, Grossin M, Lefort E, Lamarche F, Henin D. [Pilomatrix carcinoma: histologic and immunohistochemical features. Two studies.] Ann Pathol 2003;23:50–4. (French.)

Schulz T. Pilomatrix carcinoma with metastasis. Am J Dermatopathol 2002;24:525.

Steatocystoma

Cunningham SC, Kao GF, Moore GW, Napolitano LM. Steatocystoma simplex. Surgery 2004;136:95–7.

Kaur T, Kanwar AJ. Steatocystoma multiplex in four successive generations. J Dermatol 2003;30:559–61.

Mortazavi H, Taheri A, Mansoori P, Kani ZA. Localized forms of steatocystoma multiplex: case report and review of the literature. Dermatol Online J 2005;11:22.

Yonekura K, Takeda K, Koura S, Kanzaki T. Giant steatocystoma simplex. J Dermatol 2005;32:209–310.

Eruptive Vellus Hair Cyst

Mieno H, Fujimoto N, Tajima S. Eruptive vellus hair cyst in patients with chronic renal failure. Dermatology 2004;208:67–9.

Pilar Neurocristic Hamartoma

Bevona C, Tannous Z, Tsao H. Dermal melanocytic proliferation with features of a plaque-type blue nevus and neurocristic hamartoma. J Am Acad Dermatol 2003;49:924–9.

3 TUMORS AND TUMOR-LIKE CONDITIONS WITH PREDOMINANTLY SEBACEOUS DIFFERENTIATION

Benign sebaceous proliferations are relatively common, but cutaneous neoplasms with sebaceous features are less so. This chapter presents the authors' nosologic and diagnostic approach to this group of lesions.

PSEUDONEOPLASTIC SEBACEOUS PROLIFERATIONS

Sebaceous Hyperplasia

Clinical Features. The most common sebaceous proliferation is that of hyperplasia, which usually is encountered in elderly persons. It presents as localized, yellow-tan, often umbilicated papules, typically on the face or eyelids, but also in the mammary areola, oral cavity, or genital skin (fig. 3-1); lesions may be confluent (11,19, 45,57,68,73,82,99).

Hyperplasia of the sebaceous glands may clinically imitate papulonodular basal cell carcinoma (BCC) and, rarely, assumes linear (zosteriform) or "giant" configurations (27,95). The Muir-Torre syndrome, in which sebaceous proliferations are linked to visceral malignancies (26,28), is not definably linked to sebaceous hyperplasia. There may be a causal association between sebaceous hyperplasia and the administration of immunosuppressive medications (20,54). "Premature" sebaceous hyperplasia is an autosomal dominant condition that begins early in life (9,99).

Pathologic Findings. Sebaceous hyperplasia is histologically defined (albeit somewhat arbitrarily) as the presence of four or more sebaceous lobules attached to the infundibulum of each hair follicle (fig. 3-2). Constituent cells are predominantly mature sebocytes, with compact nuclei and multivacuolated cytoplasm (fig. 3-3). A narrow cuff of basaloid cells is often present peripherally in some sebocytic clusters. The overlying epidermis may be thinned in exuberant cases, but is never ulcerated. No special studies are necessary to establish the diagnosis.

Differential Diagnosis. The principal differential diagnostic consideration is sebaceous adenoma. This condition, as defined below, merges at some point with localized hyperplasia, and there is no hard and fast division between the two lesions. Other considerations include sebaceous trichofolliculoma and folliculosebaceous cystic hamartoma (43), both of which feature the presence of a much more complicated pilar epithelial proliferation than that associated with sebaceous hyperplasia.

Nevus Sebaceus

Clinical Features. *Nevus sebaceus* (also known as *organoid nevus* and *Jadassohn's nevus*) is a hamartoma rather than a neoplasm. It is essentially confined to the head and neck, with most cases affecting the scalp (2,62); rarely, familial clustering may be observed (7,46). Nevus sebaceus is a yellow or tan plaque of several centimeters in greatest dimension, and its surface varies in

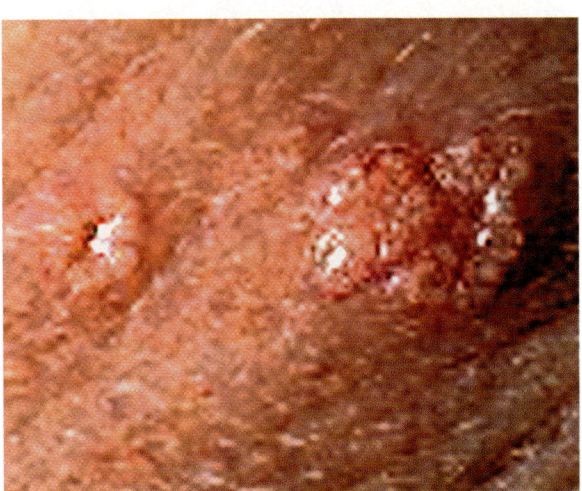

Figure 3-1
SEBACEOUS HYPERPLASIA
There are groups of slightly umbilicated, small, yellow-tan nodules on the facial skin.

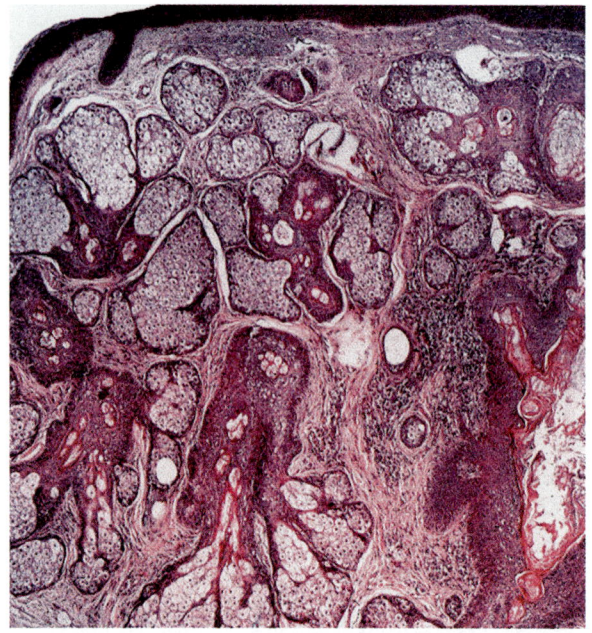

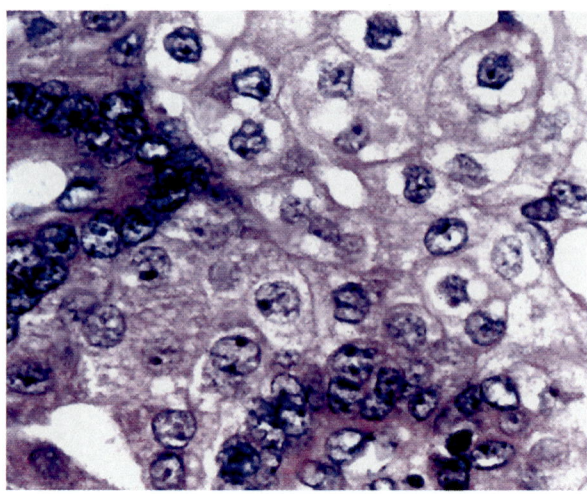

Figure 3-3

SEBACEOUS HYPERPLASIA

The sebocytes are fully mature.

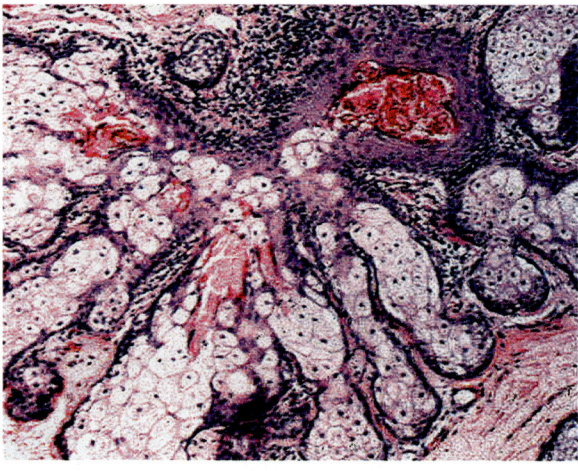

Figure 3-2

SEBACEOUS HYPERPLASIA

Pilosebaceous units have at least four sebaceous lobules per unit. The lobules are attached to a central follicular core.

texture from smooth to verrucoid (fig. 3-4). A linear multifocal configuration has also been reported (71,96). Hair is typically lacking within the lesion. No verifiable association exists with other developmental defects, and the clinical evolution of nevus sebaceus is usually uncomplicated (15). Occasionally, secondary neoplasms may develop in this lesion, including various surface epithelial, appendageal, and mesenchymal tumors (3,17,38,39,44,60,92,94). In our experience, BCC is the most frequent of these (39,94), but its biologic behavior is typically innocuous in this context. The latter comment reflects the difficulty that is often encountered in separating true BCC from basaloid pseudoepitheliomatous hyperplasias in this setting (88).

Pathologic Findings. The microscopic appearance of nevus sebaceus varies according to the anatomic location and the patient's age (2, 62). Lesions of the scalp and those in patients past puberty typically demonstrate marked acanthosis and surface papillation (fig. 3-5), such that the epidermal component may resemble seborrheic keratosis. In adolescents, the adnexal elements are more prominent, and are represented by sebaceous hyperplasia, apocrine proliferation and apocrine ductal dilatation, and variable proliferation of eccrine glands (figs. 3-6, 3-7). Hairs are usually vellus in nature, and hair follicles tend to be irregularly grouped within the lesion. Sebaceous gland attachments are abnormal as well, with some glands connecting directly to the epidermis and others to the base of hair follicles. The mesenchymal component of nevus sebaceus is aberrant as well, showing disorder in the orientation of dermal collagen bundles, variable dermal hypercellularity, and either an increase or decrease in the density of neurovascular structures. In light of these findings, the name *organoid nevus* seems particularly apropos.

Tumors and Tumor-Like Conditions with Sebaceous Differentiation

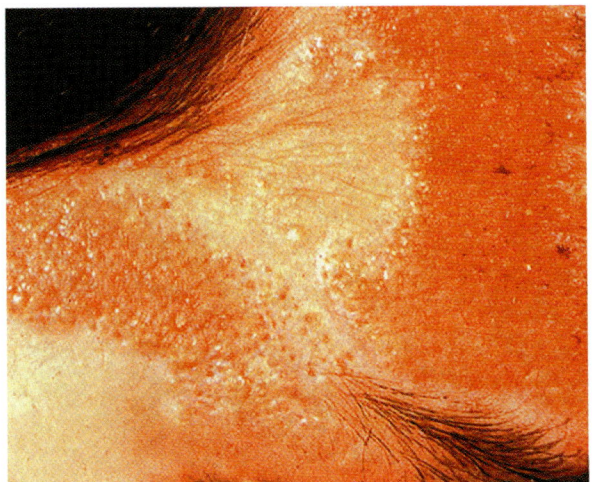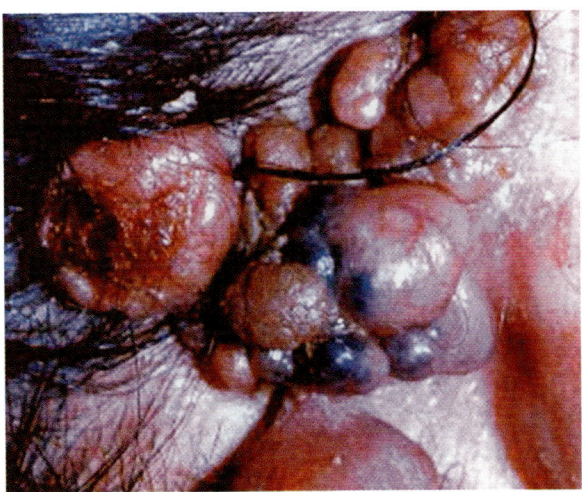

Figure 3-4
NEVUS SEBACEUS
Left: A yellow-tan plaque on the skin of the forehead.
Right: In another case, the lesion has a distinctly multinodular appearance and clinically simulates a neoplasm.

No special studies are necessary for a diagnosis of nevus sebaceus; however, it has recently been shown that the constituent tissues of this lesion manifest deletions in the *PTCH* gene, on chromosome 9q22.3 (104). This same locus is aberrant in cases of sporadic BCC, and may help to explain the frequency with which that tumor arises in nevus sebaceus.

Differential Diagnosis. In small biopsy specimens, particularly in the absence of a clinical history, the differential diagnosis is broad. It potentially includes surface epithelial lesions such as epidermal nevus, verruca, squamous cell carcinoma, and seborrheic keratosis. Other biopsies may present the image of uncomplicated nevus sebaceus. Also, secondary neoplasms in nevus sebaceus may dominate the picture, including BCC, squamous cell carcinoma, various adnexal tumors, smooth muscle neoplasms, and melanocytic nevi (3,15,17,38,39,44,60,92,94). The best method to avoid missing the diagnosis of nevus sebaceus is to bear in mind the relative rarity of the lesions just listed in young individuals, in whom nevus sebaceus is most common. A request for an excisional biopsy is best when this lesion is suspected in order to provide adequate diagnostic material as well as material to determine suitable treatment options.

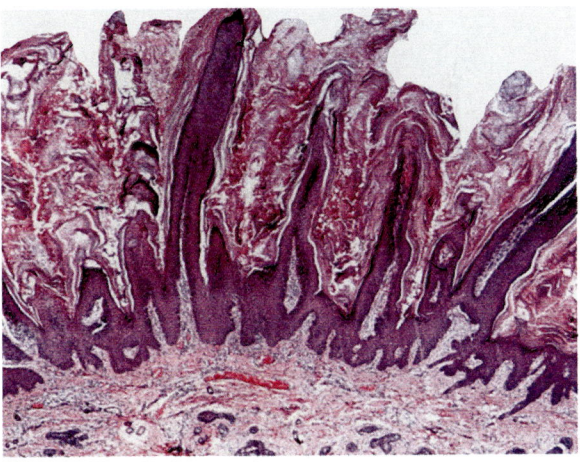

Figure 3-5
NEVUS SEBACEUS
This nevus sebaceus from an adult demonstrates marked surface epithelial papillomatosis.

BENIGN SEBACEOUS NEOPLASMS

Sebaceous Adenoma

Clinical Features. *Sebaceous adenoma* is a slowly enlarging, yellowish facial nodule in patients over 50 years of age (fig. 3-8); unusually, it may arise in the oral cavity, ear canal, or salivary gland as well (11,36,55,57,73,75). This neoplasm measures up to several centimeters in diameter.

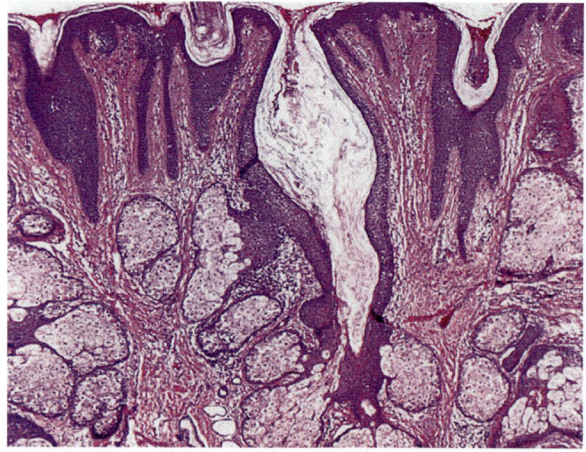

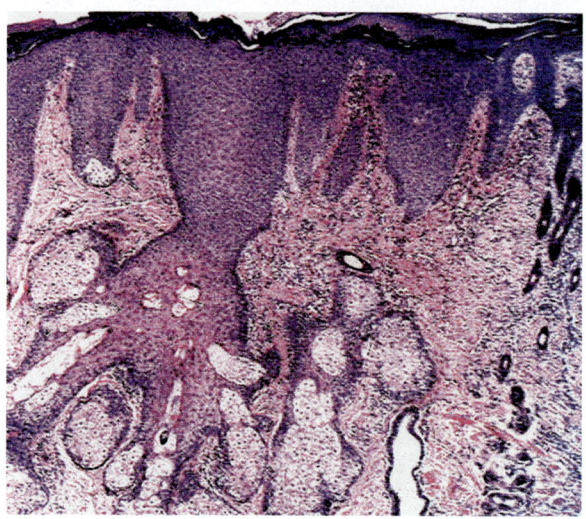

Figure 3-6

NEVUS SEBACEUS

These examples show "misplaced" sebaceous lobules, sebaceous hyperplasia, and a proliferation of sweat glands.

Clinical misinterpretation of sebaceous adenoma as BCC is common. It is associated with the Muir-Torre syndrome, together with visceral malignancies and well-differentiated cutaneous squamous cell tumors of the keratoacanthoma type (12,34,85). This clinical complex is caused by point mutations in various DNA mismatch repair genes, particularly *MSH-1*, *MSH-2*, and *MLH-1* (49). The internal neoplasms in patients with Muir-Torre syndrome are usually laryngeal, mammary, or gastrointestinal carcinoma, but others may be seen as well, including malignant lymphoma (12,21,34,49,85).

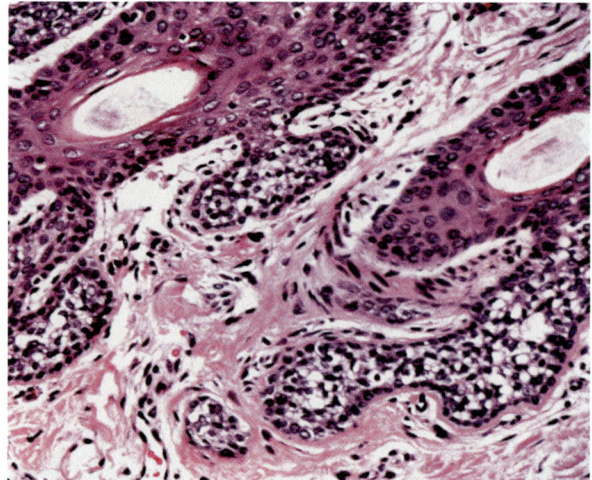

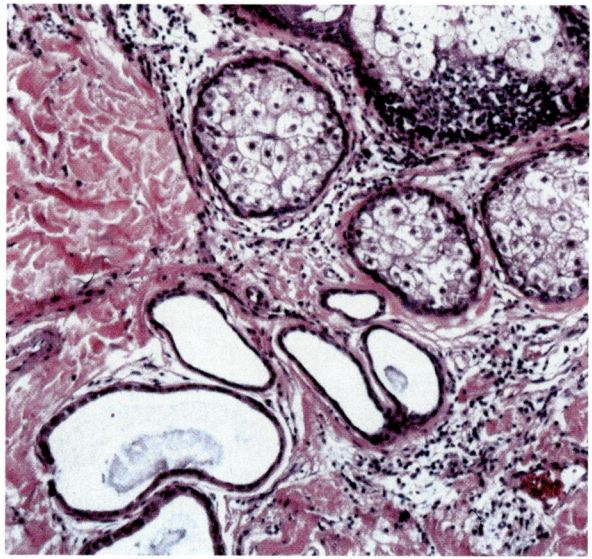

Figure 3-7

NEVUS SEBACEUS

Germinative hair follicles (top) and sweat gland proliferation (bottom) in nevus sebaceus.

Pathologic Findings. The histologic attributes of classic sebaceous adenoma are well-defined. There is a circumscribed proliferation of enlarged sebaceous lobules, made up of mature sebocytes (fig. 3-9). The tumor often thins the epidermis and occasionally abuts its base, and is surrounded by a fibrous pseudocapsule in some cases. The latter feature, as well as the presence of appendageal "collarettes," reflects the slow growth of sebaceous adenoma. The

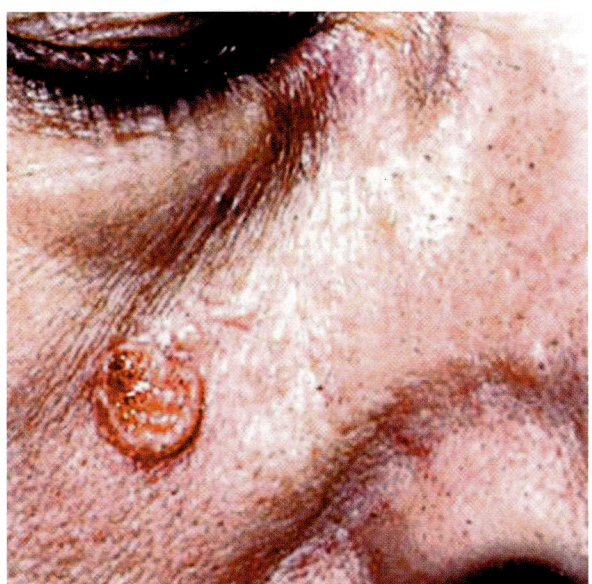

Figure 3-8

SEBACEOUS ADENOMA

A yellow-tan infraorbital nodule on the facial skin in an elderly man.

tumor cell lobules may exhibit focal duct-like differentiation and holocrine secretion, which potentially results in the formation of microcysts; lesions with this feature have been termed *sebocrine adenomas* (51,105). Small nucleoli may be present, but nuclear atypia and mitotic activity are absent (fig. 3-10).

"Variant" sebaceous adenomas in patients with Muir-Torre syndrome have histologic peculiarities (12). They are not as well demarcated from the adjacent dermis as are classic lesions, and some tumors include more basaloid, germinative epithelial cells at their periphery (fig. 3-11). There may be mild nuclear atypia and modest mitotic activity. Thus, Muir-Torre–type sebaceous adenoma may be similar morphologically to BCC with sebaceous differentiation (BCCSD) (basosebaceous epithelioma, sebaceous epithelioma) (22,80). The principal differences between these tumors are the presence of focally fibromyxoid stroma and epithelial-stromal "clefts" in BCCSD, as well as a basal cell population that accounts for more than 50 percent of the cellular total. Rutten et al. (81) also found that cystic change in cutaneous sebaceous tumors was more frequent in patients with Muir-Torre syndrome.

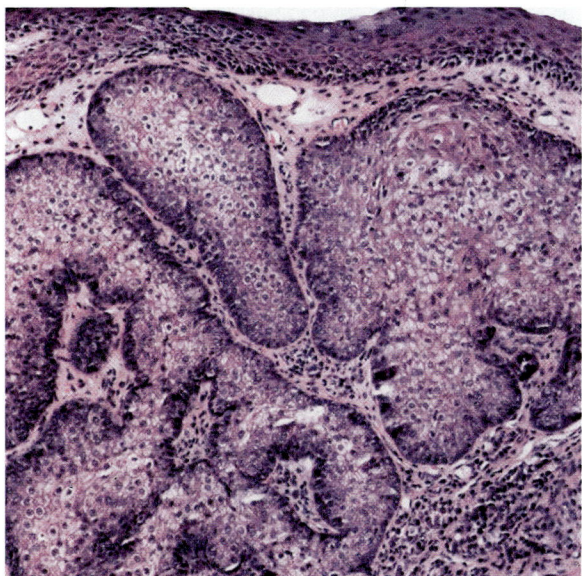

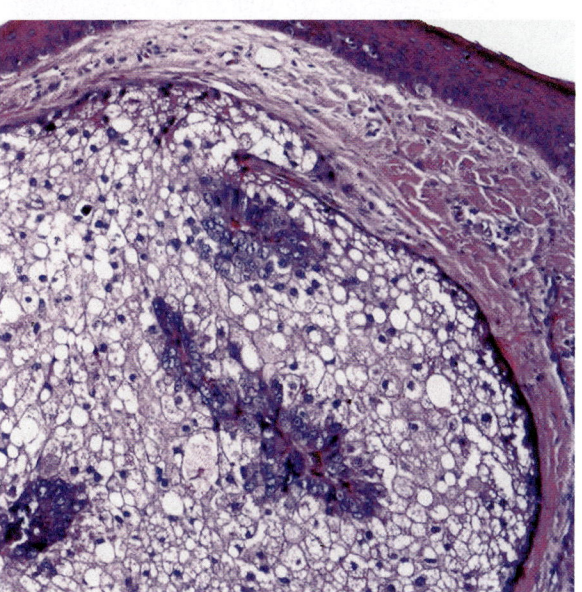

Figure 3-9

SEBACEOUS ADENOMA

Circumscribed lobules of mature sebocytes are seen in the dermis.

Sanchez-Yus et al. (83) have suggested that another term, *sebomatricoma*, be used to encompass all lesions containing basaloid elements. This is a tenable approach, with the caveat that examples of BCCSD would probably be included in the sebomatricoma group if it were embraced. It is wise to completely excise all sebaceous neoplasms composed of a mixture of well-differentiated sebocytes and germinative cells.

Special studies are not required for the diagnosis of sebaceous adenoma. Hassanein et al. (32), however, have suggested that immunostaining for Thomsen-Friedenreich antigen (TFA), a "cryptic" glycoprotein on epithelial cells, is capable of separating sebaceous carcinoma, which is TFA positive, from other tumors with sebaceous features. Moreover, Machin and colleagues (49) have proposed that immunoreactivity for the *MSH-2* and *MLH-1* gene products can be used to identify those sebaceous neoplasms that are associated with the Muir-Torre syndrome.

Differential Diagnosis. Other than BCCSD, the morphologic differential diagnosis centers on a distinction from other wholly or partially benign sebaceous tumors on one hand (73,79,103), and sebaceous carcinoma on the other (11,55,73, 80). Carcinomas demonstrate more cytologic atypia and infiltrative growth than do sebaceous adenomas; they are described subsequently.

Superficial Epithelioma with Sebaceous Differentiation

Superficial epithelioma with sebaceous differentiation (SESD) is a very rare sebaceous neoplasm. SESD has been reported as a slow-growing, smooth papule or an erythematous verrucoid nodule in the skin of the face, trunk, and proximal extremities, and it may be multiple (1,29,42, 79,98). As of yet, there is no proven association with the Muir-Torre syndrome or other systemic processes.

Histologically, there are similarities between SESD and other cutaneous neoplasms, including tumor of the follicular infundibulum, inverting follicular keratosis, and superficial BCC (50,55). SESD demonstrates interlocking "fenestrated" cords of compact polyhedral cells that

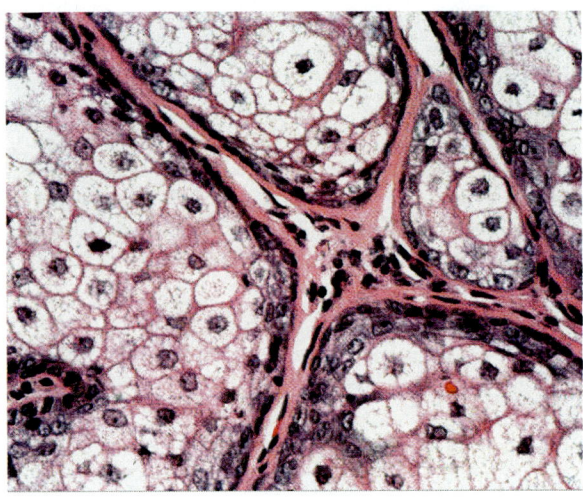

Figure 3-10

SEBACEOUS ADENOMA

Small nucleoli and a minor population of germinative basaloid cells are present.

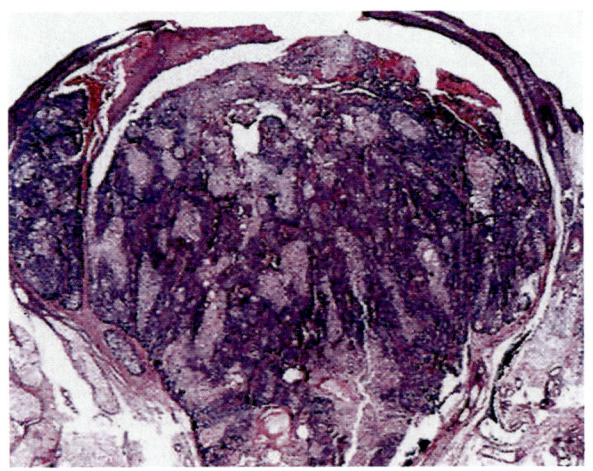 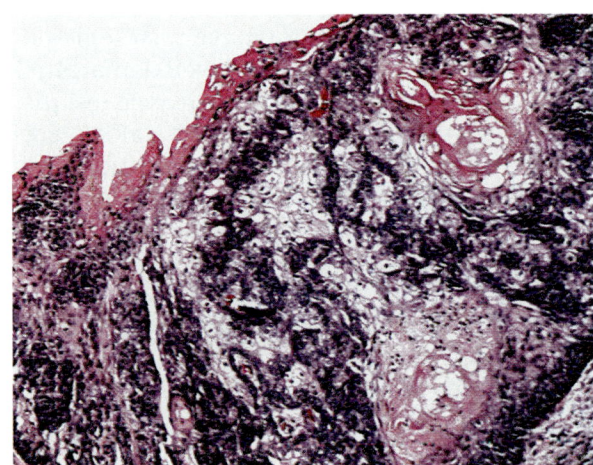

Figure 3-11

SEBACEOUS ADENOMA

Sebaceous adenomas seen in the context of Muir-Torre syndrome often have a greater constituency of basaloid cells, which are disposed towards the periphery of cellular lobules.

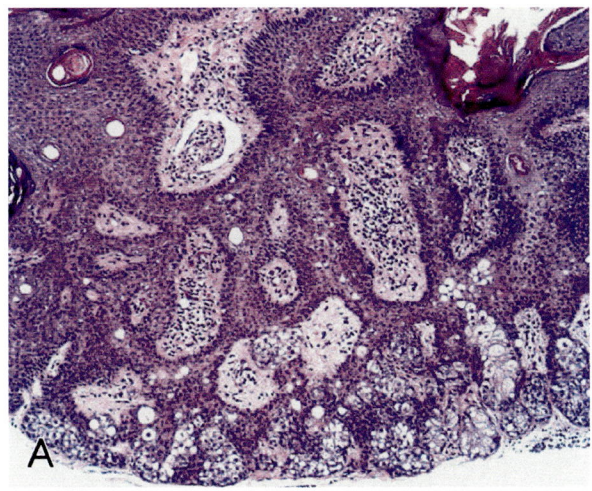
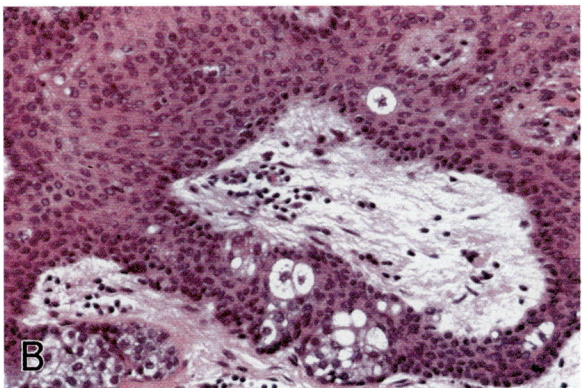
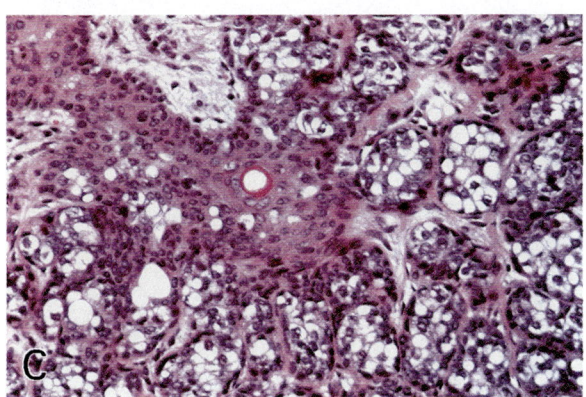

Figure 3-12

SUPERFICIAL EPITHELIOMA WITH SEBACEOUS DIFFERENTIATION

This lesion takes the form of a fenestrated congerie of keratinocytic plates that are connected to the epidermis. They are punctuated at the lesional base by randomly disposed nests of mature sebocytes.

are connected to the epidermal base over a limited span, giving the lesion a plate-like configuration in the superficial dermis. Peripheral palisading of nuclei also can be seen, but this finding is variable. Squamoid foci may likewise be observed, with the formation of cellular eddies, and duct-like spaces are apparent in the majority of cases. Those structures manifest the presence of an eosinophilic luminal cuticle, resembling that of the eccrine ducts. Mature sebaceous cells are present preferentially at the periphery of SESD, in small groups (fig. 3-12). Fibromyxoid change, stromal-epithelial clefts, apoptosis, mitoses, and stromal hypercellularity are all lacking. In aggregate, these attributes allow SESD to be separated reproducibly from other pilosebaceous neoplasms and from BCC. Sanchez-Yus et al. (84) have described a complex neoplasm featuring the conjoint presence of SESD with high-grade apocrine adenocarcinoma and immature trichoepithelioma. We regard that lesion as an adnexal carcinoma with divergent differentiation.

Sebaceoma

The tumor called *sebaceoma* by Troy and Ackerman (93) is a circumscribed, nodular dermal lesion which combines some of the microscopic features of classic sebaceous adenoma, classic trichoepithelioma, dermal duct tumor (intradermal poroma), and cylindroma. As such, it may have duct-like structures, basaloid cells, foci of trichilemmal-type keratinization, and sebocytic differentiation, in varying proportions (fig. 3-13) (58,93). Occasionally, Verocay body–like palisades of tumor cell nuclei or cribriform cellular arrangements are observed as well (59,66). Steffen (89) has suggested that an alternative term for sebaceoma should be *poorly differentiated sebaceous adenoma,* but this appellation has the disadvantage of joining a description usually associated with malignancies to a benign neoplasm. A more straightforward approach to such lesions is a descriptive one, as used by Wong et al. (103) and Apisarnthanarax and colleagues (5). This

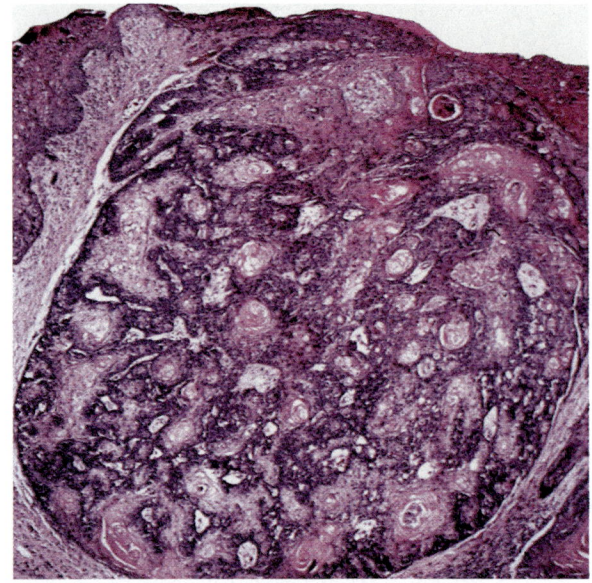

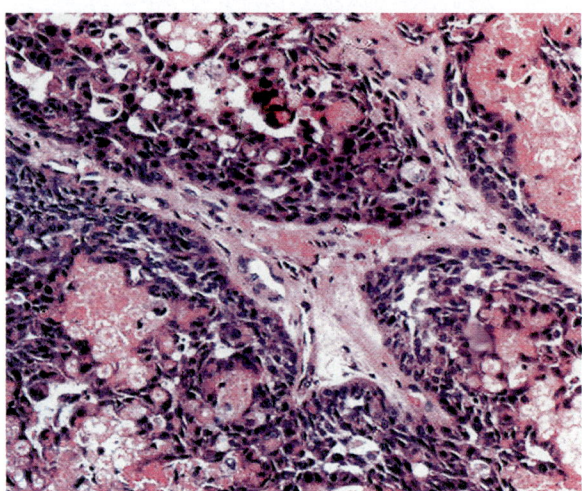

Figure 3-13

SEBACEOMA

The microscopic appearance of Muir-Torre–type sebaceous adenoma (see figure 3-11) is closely mirrored by this lesion, but with the additional presence of multifocal trichilemmal keratinization.

yields such terms as *benign adnexal neoplasm with divergent differentiation*. *Sebomatricoma* is also regarded as a synonym for sebaceoma by some authors (8). A connection between sebaceoma and the Muir-Torre syndrome probably exists (24), and it also may be a complicating lesion in nevus sebaceus (40).

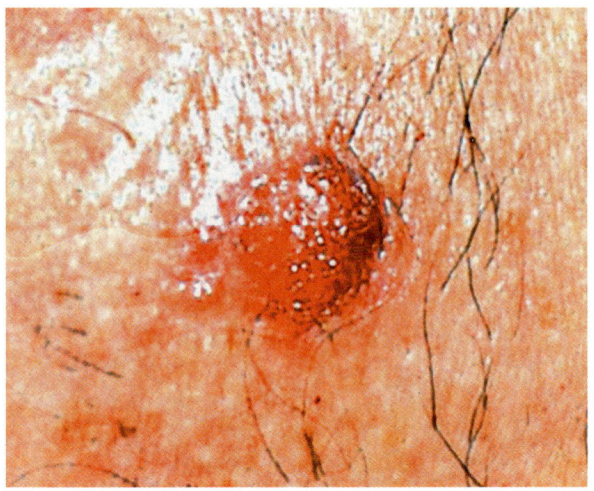

Figure 3-14

BASAL CELL CARCINOMA WITH SEBACEOUS DIFFERENTIATION

A nondescript nodule in the facial skin is indistinguishable from other forms of basal cell carcinoma (BCC).

BORDERLINE SEBACEOUS NEOPLASMS

Basal Cell Carcinoma with Sebaceous Differentiation

Basal cell carcinoma with sebaceous differentiation (BCCSD), also known as *sebaceous epithelioma* and *basosebaceous carcinoma*, is the only neoplasm of the skin with sebaceous differentiation that is appropriately termed a "borderline" malignancy (fig. 3-14), because it may recur locally but does not metastasize in the usual case (11,22,47,58,73,80). Although it is clinically comparable, this lesion shows several reproducible differences from other forms of BCC. As mentioned above, Sanchez-Yus et al. (83) have suggested that these dissimilarities justify the creation of another diagnostic category, that of sebomatricoma, to address the tumor in question. In our view, this term is unlikely to be accepted by clinical practitioners because it does not immediately suggest a predictable course of management. "Basal cell carcinoma with sebaceous differentiation," on the other hand, does.

The tumor cells of BCCSD are generally larger and contain more eosinophilic cytoplasm than those seen in conventional BCC (figs. 3-15–3-18). Moreover, the expected stroma of most other BCC variants, with fibromyxoid features and clefting around epithelial cell nests, is

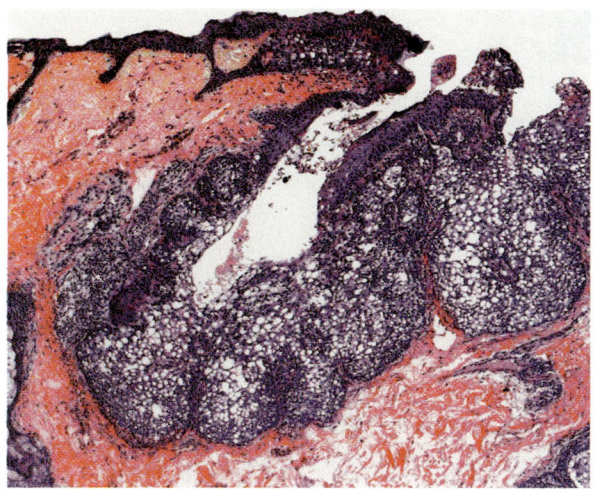

Figure 3-15

BASAL CELL CARCINOMA WITH SEBACEOUS DIFFERENTIATION

A bimodal cellular population of basaloid cells with fully mature sebocytes is seen.

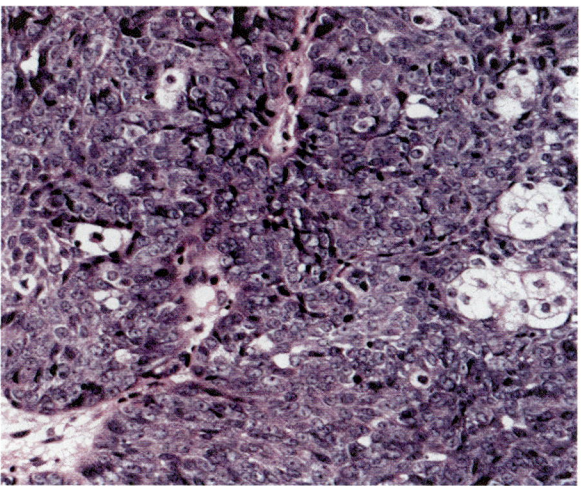

Figure 3-16

BASAL CELL CARCINOMA WITH SEBACEOUS DIFFERENTIATION

The juxtaposition of basaloid and sebocytic elements is clear.

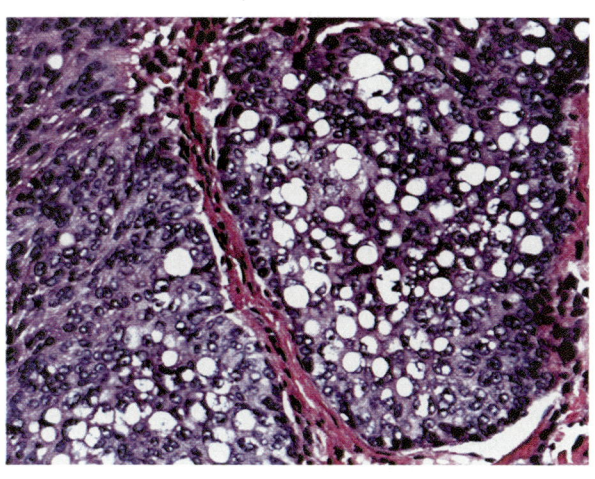

Figure 3-17

BASAL CELL CARCINOMA WITH SEBACEOUS DIFFERENTIATION

Sebocytes are disposed throughout tumor cell lobules or concentrated at their center.

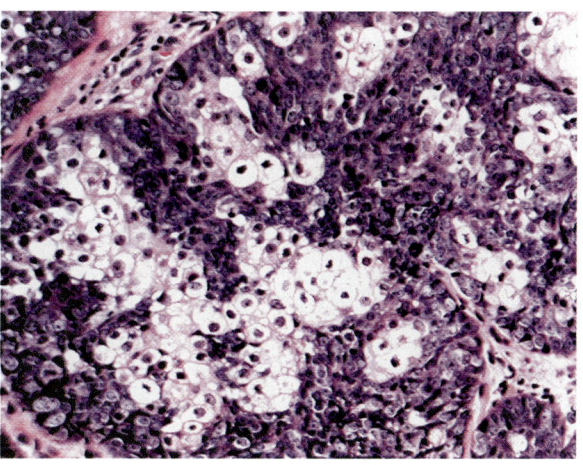

Figure 3-18

MATURE SEBOCYTIC DIFFERENTIATION IN BASAL CELL CARCINOMA WITH SEBACEOUS DIFFERENTIATION

This form of BCC does not demonstrate stromal-epithelial clefting or myxoid stromal changes, and tumor cells are somewhat larger than in other microscopic variants of this lesion.

inconstantly seen and poorly represented in BCCSD. Similarities between BCCSD and other BCCs include nuclear palisading, foci of basaloid cell growth with apoptosis, the ability for divergent differentiation into other appendageal tissues or squamous cells, and connection to the basal epidermis or dermal adnexa (fig. 3-19). The sebocytes in BCCSD are fully mature; they contrast sharply with the more "uncommitted" cells comprising the remainder of the tumor, and are typically clustered near the center of tumor cell lobules.

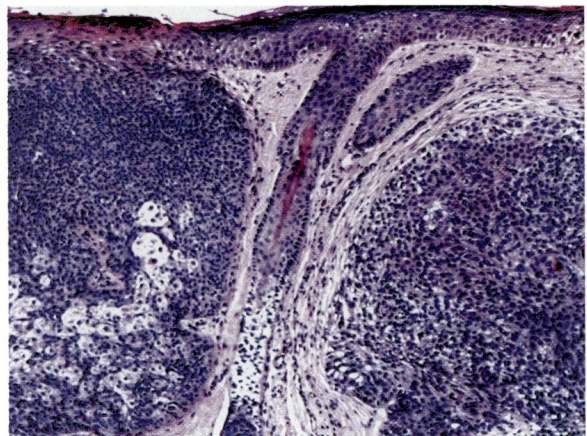

Figure 3-19

BASAL CELL CARCINOMA WITH SEBACEOUS DIFFERENTIATION

The lesion is connected to the surface epithelium as well as to dermal appendages.

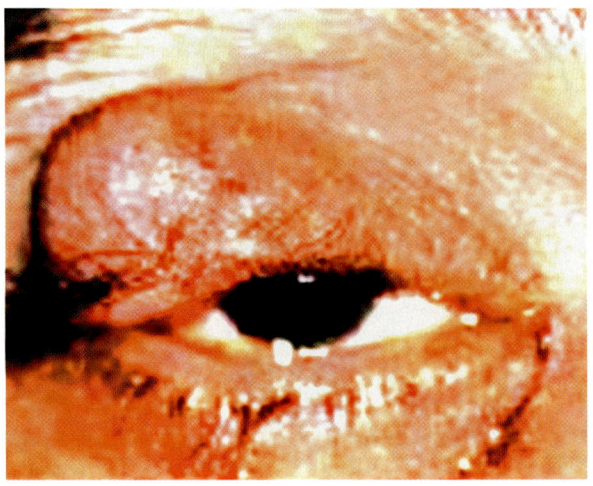

Figure 3-20

SEBACEOUS CARCINOMA OF THE OCULAR SKIN

The clinical appearance of a chalazion is simulated.

BCCSD is often confused with sebaceous adenoma on one hand and sebaceous carcinoma on the other, and is certainly more common than either of those neoplasms. The behavior of this tumor is also intermediate between that of those alternatives: BCCSD may recur but does not spread to distant sites. It is adequately treated by complete but conservative excision.

MALIGNANT SEBACEOUS NEOPLASMS

Sebaceous Carcinoma

Clinical Features. By historical convention, sebaceous carcinomas have been placed into two anatomic groups, *ocular* and *extraocular* (41, 53,64,70,72,78,100,106), because of an alleged dissimilarity in the behavior of the lesions in those two categories. Claims have been made suggesting that the ocular variant is associated with a more adverse prognosis (70); however, a critical review of the pertinent data does not support that contention. Both ocular and extraocular sebaceous carcinomas have a 30 to 40 percent risk for local tumor recurrence, 20 to 25 percent for distant metastases, and 10 to 20 percent for tumor-related mortality (4,41,53,61, 64,70,72,78,100,106). Thus, no constitutive biological difference appears to exist between them, except for the fact that a tumor origin in the eyelids or ocular adnexa is much more common than an extraocular location.

Sebaceous carcinoma usually arises in middle-aged or elderly patients, with a peak incidence in the fifth decade of life. For reasons that are unclear, tumors of the eyelids show a strong preference for Asian persons, and they may also follow radiotherapy (for such conditions as retinoblastoma) as second treatment-related malignancies (35). Ocular lesions present as painless masses of the lid margins or conjunctiva, and are commonly mistaken clinically for chalazions, blepharitis, or conjunctivitis (fig. 3-20) (23,30,102). Multifocality is seen in 5 to 10 percent of cases. Additional disorders that are potentially confused with sebaceous carcinomas clinically are cicatricial pemphigoid, BCC, and squamous cell carcinoma (102).

The majority of lesions arise in the head and neck, followed by the skin of the trunk, genitals, and extremities (25,37,41,53,64,70,72,78,100, 106). Rare examples arise in the oral cavity (48). They are nodular masses that may be painful or grow rapidly, and some are ulcerated (fig. 3-21). A proportion of patients have the Muir-Torre syndrome (87).

Pathologic Findings. True sebocytes, characterized by multivesicular, vacuolated, clear cytoplasm, are the hallmark of sebaceous neoplasms. As such, they must be distinguished from other cell types with cytoplasmic clarity, which are seen in cutaneous neoplasms with a variety of lineages (16,90).

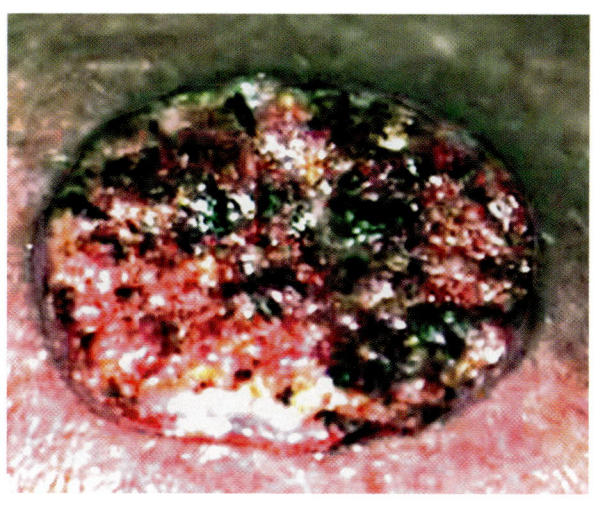

Figure 3-21

SEBACEOUS CARCINOMA OF THE FACIAL SKIN

This ulcerated nodule is clinically indistinguishable from squamous cell carcinoma.

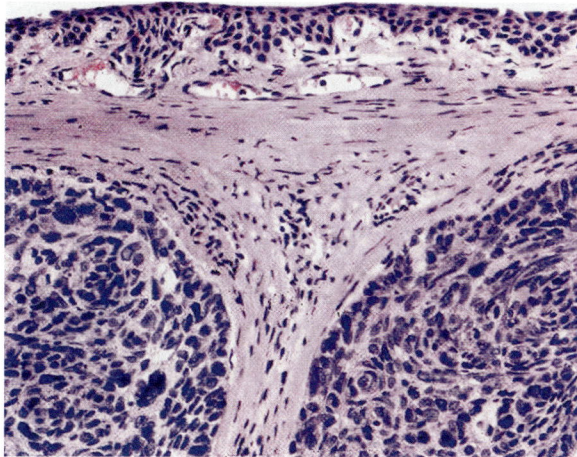

Figure 3-22

SEBACEOUS CARCINOMA

Lobules of neoplastic cells are seen in the dermis, without a desmoplastic or inflammatory host response.

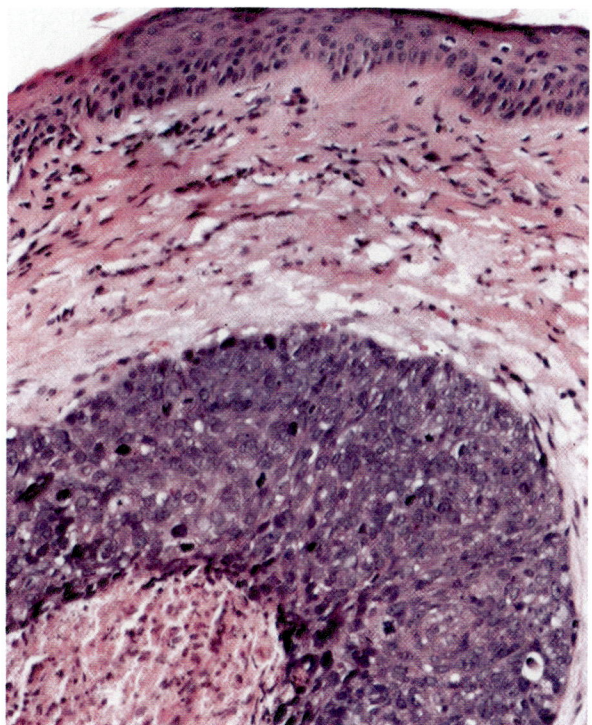

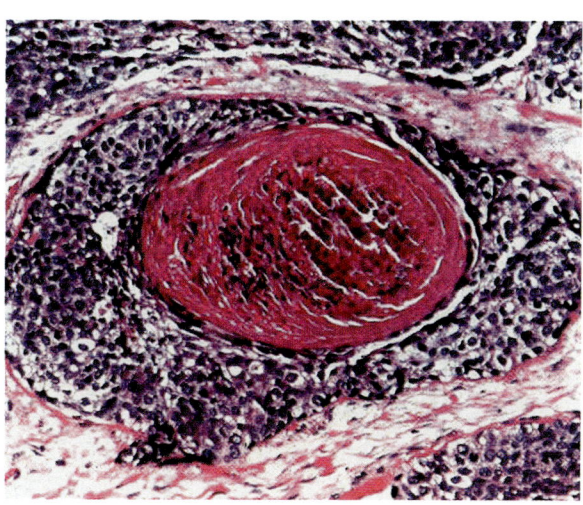

Figure 3-23

SEBACEOUS CARCINOMA

"Comedo"-type necrosis, as seen here, is apparent in the central aspects of tumor cell lobules in many sebaceous carcinomas.

Sebaceous carcinomas are organoid neoplasms that are composed of lobular groups of variably atypical polygonal cells in the dermis, with a fibrovascular stroma that is usually devoid of desmoplastic changes (fig. 3-22). Central aspects of the cellular nests may be necrotic, producing a "comedo" pattern (fig. 3-23). The constituent cells of well-differentiated lesions show abundant multivacuolated clear cytoplasm and oval vesicular nuclei, with distinct nucleoli (fig. 3-24) but few mitotic figures. In contrast, high-grade lesions contain more cytologically

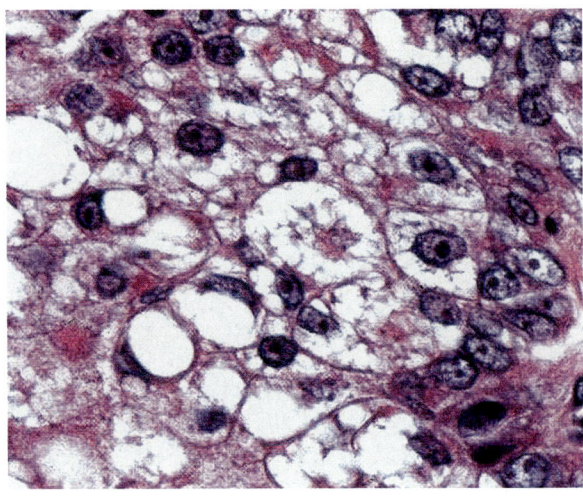

Figure 3-24

SEBACEOUS CARCINOMA

Well-differentiated sebaceous carcinoma shows a modestly increased nuclear to cytoplasmic ratio and discernible nucleoli.

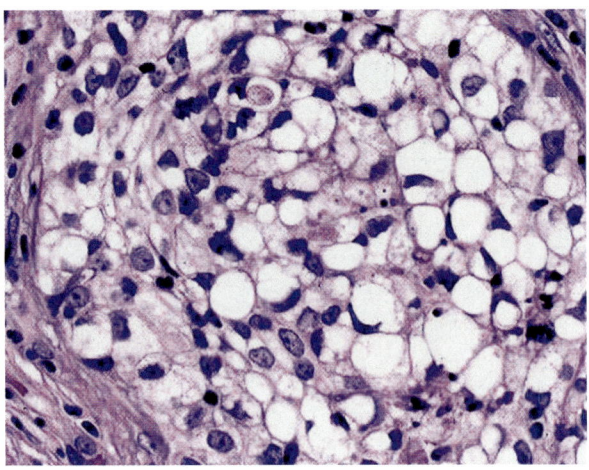

Figure 3-26

GRADE I SEBACEOUS CARCINOMA

Rounded, roughly equally sized lobules of tumor cells are present.

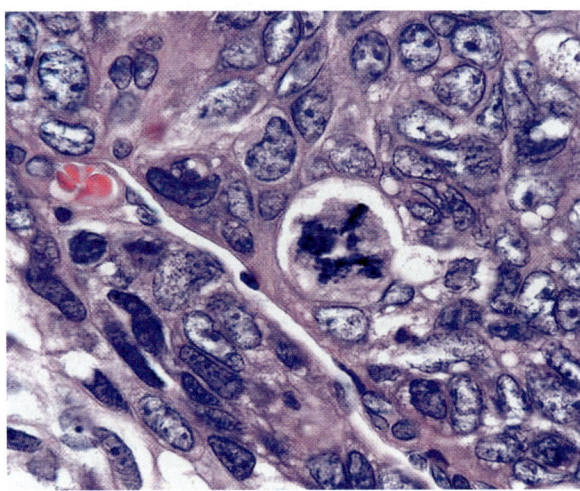

Figure 3-25

SEBACEOUS CARCINOMA

Obvious sebocytic differentiation is lacking in this example. Pathologically shaped mitotic figures are apparent.

nondescript cells with a high nuclear to cytoplasmic ratio, nuclear pleomorphism, nucleolar prominence, numerous mitoses (sometimes with pathologically shaped forms), and amphophilic or basophilic cytoplasm (fig. 3-25). Cytoplasmic vacuolization is not easily seen in these lesions, and may require the use of special histochemical stains, such as oil red-O or Sudan IV, to confirm its presence (101).

The grading of sebaceous carcinomas (into grades I through III) is predicated on tumor growth patterns rather than on the nuclear features of the tumor cells (76). Lesions composed of generally rounded, well-demarcated, roughly equal-sized cellular lobules are graded as I (fig. 3-26); those with an admixture of well-defined nests with infiltrative profiles or confluent cell groups are grade II. Grade III lesions demonstrate highly invasive cellular aggregates with irregular outlines or manifest a medullary sheet-like growth pattern (figs. 3-27, 3-28).

Regardless of grade, all sebaceous carcinomas share a possible association with carcinoma in situ (CIS), extramammary Paget's disease (EPD) of the sebaceous type, or both, in the surface epithelium overlying the tumor mass in the corium (fig. 3-29) (13,101). It is thought that EPD and CIS are marker lesions that reflect a neoplastic "field" defect in the skin, rather than direct precursors of, or extensions from, underlying sebaceous tumors. This opinion is supported by the existence of occasional cases in which only intraepithelial sebaceous carcinoma is present, with no subjacent tumor mass (33,52). Pathologists should consider the possibility of an underlying invasive oculocutaneous sebaceous

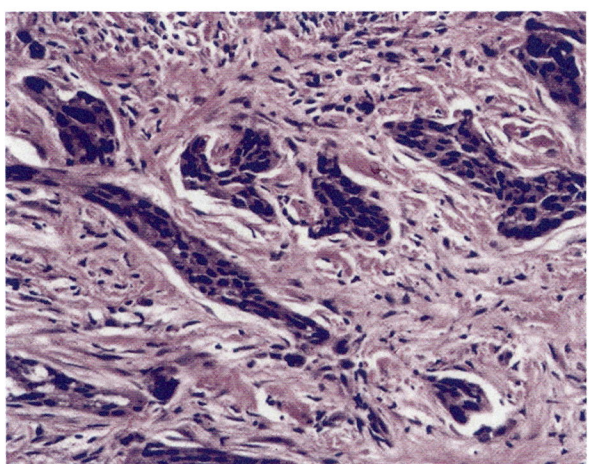

Figure 3-27

GRADE III SEBACEOUS CARCINOMA

There are narrow, infiltrative cords of tumor cells.

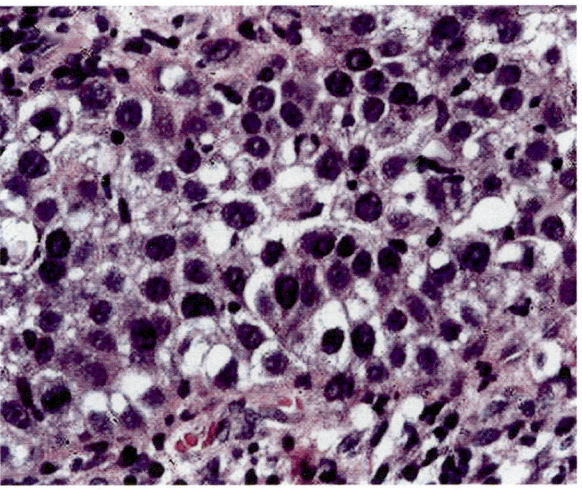

Figure 3-28

GRADE III SEBACEOUS CARCINOMA

A medullary (sheet-like) cellular growth pattern is evident.

carcinoma whenever EPD or CIS is seen in a conjunctival or eyelid biopsy. Outside of the ocular region, cases of EPD that lack epithelial mucin and immunohistologic markers of apocrine or enteric differentiation also may be associated with sebaceous carcinomas (65).

Particular histologic subtypes of sebaceous carcinomas merit special attention because they may cause diagnostic confusion with other skin tumors (101,102). *Basaloid sebaceous carcinoma* is composed of small cells with a limited amount of cytoplasm and common nuclear palisading at the periphery of tumor cell nests (fig. 3-30). Often, this variant has a grade III growth pattern, with highly atypical nuclear features and widely dispersed sebocytic elements that are difficult to identify as such. *Squamoid sebaceous carcinoma* exhibits prominent squamous metaplasia, often with keratin pearls. Another variant shows spindle cell change, yielding a sarcomatoid image (*sarcomatoid sebaceous carcinomas* [fig. 3-31]).

Sebaceous neoplasms, including sebaceous carcinomas, demonstrate immunoreactivity for epithelial membrane antigen (EMA) around each of the many vesicles comprising the vacuolated cytoplasm (86,91). This pattern is distinctive, even though EMA reactivity is shared with many other tumors of the skin. In addition, neoplastic sebocytes are potentially labeled for

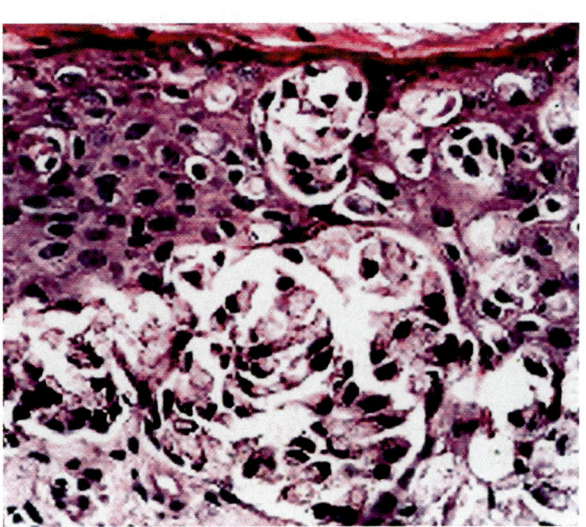

Figure 3-29

PAGETOID SEBACEOUS CARCINOMA

Pagetoid involvement of the overlying skin by tumor cells is seen in association with an extraocular sebaceous carcinoma.

androgen receptor protein (6) and human milk fat globule protein-2 (86). However, comparative studies of sufficient scope have not yet been performed to determine whether these markers are diagnostically helpful in excluding other clear cell malignancies. Other immunohistologic

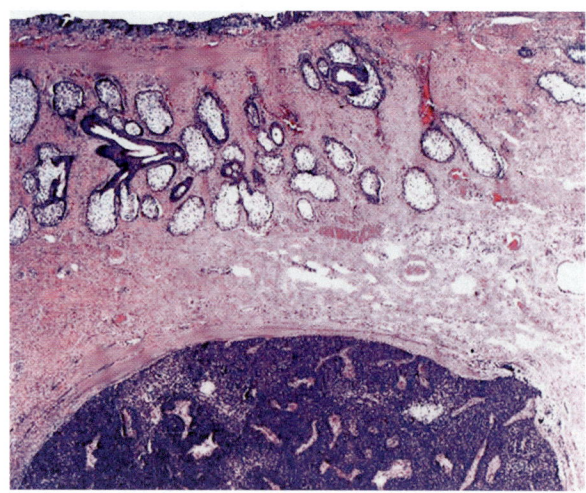 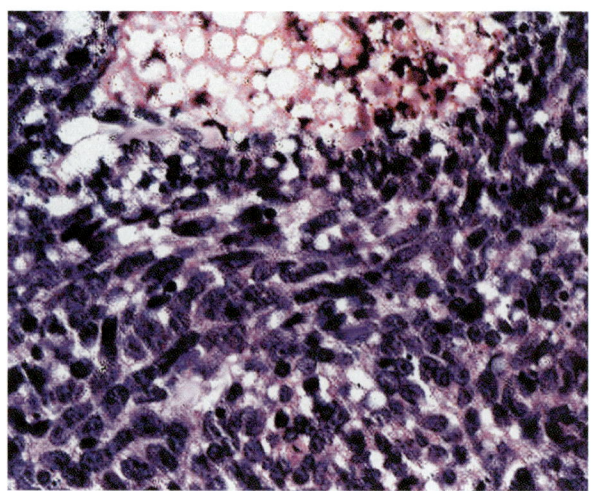

Figure 3-30

BASALOID SEBACEOUS CARCINOMA

The tumor cells resemble those of basaloid carcinomas of the viscera. Sebocytic differentiation is only rudimentary and widely dispersed among the neoplastic population. Contrast this image with those seen in figures 3-15 to 3-18.

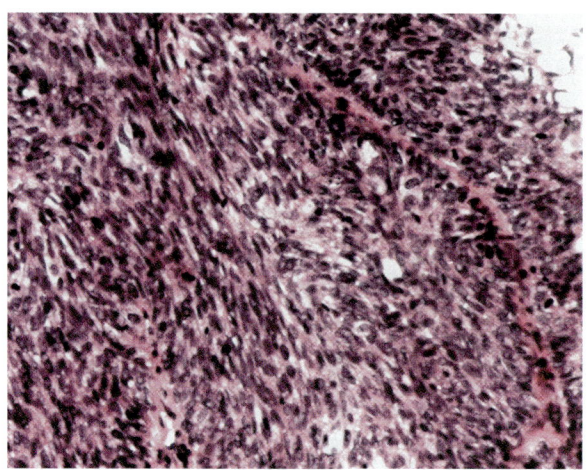

Figure 3-31

SARCOMATOID SEBACEOUS CARCINOMA

A spindle cell (sarcomatoid) growth pattern is present.

determinants that contribute to that process are discussed below. Immunoreactivity for various DNA mismatch repair gene products, particularly *MSH-2* and *MLH-1,* has correlated well with a syndromic relationship to the Muir-Torre complex (56).

Data are limited with regard to the prognosis of patients with sebaceous carcinoma. Immunoreactivity for mutant p53 protein (at a level of 10 percent or greater) and for proliferating cell nuclear antigen (at a level of 25 percent or greater) seems to be associated with an adverse outcome (31). Tumors that overexpress the c-erbB-2/HER-2/neu protein also appear to show similar biologic attributes (14,31). These findings are similar to those associated with breast and sweat gland carcinomas.

Differential Diagnosis. Predictably, the histopathologic differential diagnosis of sebaceous carcinoma is wide-ranging, including virtually all other malignant clear cell tumors of the skin. These have been summarized succinctly by Suster (90), and encompass such lesions as balloon cell melanoma, hydropic squamous carcinoma, clear cell BCC, clear cell eccrine adenocarcinoma, trichilemmal carcinoma, and metastatic and clear cell carcinomas from the viscera. The clear cell variant of atypical fibroxanthoma is another consideration (18). Except for the rare balloon cell melanoma, none of these tumors shows the distinctive pattern of vacuolization that is seen in sebaceous cells as defined above. Immunostains for EMA may be necessary to confirm the presence of multiple intracytoplasmic vesicles. Sebaceous carcinoma also lacks several specialized protein products that are often encountered in clear cell sweat gland tumors or metastatic visceral clear cell carcinomas. These include carcinoembryonic antigen (CEA), S-100 protein, gross cystic disease fluid protein-15 (GCDFP-15),

CA125, and CA19.9 (91). The desirability of searching for these markers is underscored by the knowledge that in rare instances sebaceous carcinoma may arise in the viscera (10,67,69,97), and could conceivably involve the skin only secondarily.

Basaloid sebaceous carcinoma can be separated from BCC at a cytologic level, because the nuclei of poorly differentiated sebaceous tumors are much more vesicular than those of BCC. In addition, the stroma of basaloid sebaceous carcinoma lacks fibromyxoid features, and the number of obvious sebocytes is extremely small. In contrast, BCCSD typically exhibits easily seen clusters of mature sebaceous cells. Both tumors can express the glycoprotein target for the BerEP4 antibody, but they are dissimilar in their labeling for EMA (86,91): sebaceous carcinoma is diffusely EMA reactive, whereas BCCSD is either completely EMA negative or manifests limited positivity only in areas of clear-cut sebocytic differentiation.

Squamoid sebaceous carcinoma should be separated diagnostically from ordinary squamous cell carcinoma. The presence of multivacuolated cells, a lack of continuity with the epidermis, and a dissimilarity in BerEP4 immunoreactivity (86) (sebaceous carcinoma is BerEP4 positive; squamous carcinoma is negative for that determinant) allows diagnosis.

Sarcomatoid sebaceous carcinoma can be recognized as epithelial in nature if small foci of ordinary carcinoma are interspersed throughout the lesion; otherwise, immunolabeling for keratin is necessary to exclude sarcoma from the differential diagnosis. Unfortunately, a specific diagnosis of sarcomatoid sebaceous carcinoma may not be feasible even with the use of special studies if vesiculated clear cells are entirely lacking, because the neoplastic spindle cells appear to lose their ability to show specialized features of differentiated sebocytes in this high-grade tumor variant.

A minor degree of divergent sebaceous differentiation is potentially a part of several other appendageal carcinoma morphotypes. These include such lesions as microcystic adnexal carcinoma (74), lymphoepithelioma-like carcinoma of the skin (77), and adnexal carcinoma with divergent differentiation (63), to name a few. A diagnosis of sebaceous carcinoma should be rendered only if the overall attributes of the lesion are appropriate for that interpretation.

REFERENCES

1. Akasaka T, Imamura Y, Tomichi N, Kon S. A case of superficial epithelioma with sebaceous differentiation. J Dermatol 1994;21:264–7.
2. Alessi E, Sala F. Nevus sebaceus. A clinicopathologic study of its evolution. Am J Dermatopathol 1986;8:27–31.
3. Alessi E, Wong SN, Advani HH, Ackerman AB. Nevus sebaceus is associated with unusual neoplasms. An atlas. Am J Dermatopathol 1988;10:116–27.
4. Antuna SA, Mendez JG, Cincunegui JA, Lopez-Fanjul JC. Metastatic lesion of the cervical spine secondary to an extraocular sebaceous carcinoma. Acta Orthop Belg 1996;62:229–32.
5. Apisarnthanarax P, Bovenmyer DA, Mehregan AH. Combined adnexal tumor of the skin. Arch Dermatol 1984;120:231–3.
6. Bayer-Garner IB, Givens V, Smoller B. Immunohistochemical staining for androgen receptors: a sensitive marker of sebaceous differentiation. Am J Dermatopathol 1999;21:426–31.
7. Benedetto L, Sood U, Blumenthal N, Madjar D, Sturman S, Hashimoto K. Familial nevus sebaceus. J Am Acad Dermatol 1990;23:130–2.
8. Biernat W, Biernat S. Ductal sebaceoma (sebomatricoma). Pol J Pathol 2000;51:55–7.
9. Boonchai W, Leenutaphong V. Familial presenile sebaceous gland hyperplasia. J Am Acad Dermatol 1997;36:120–2.
10. Borczuk AC, Sha KK, Hisler SE, Mann JM, Hajdu SI. Sebaceous carcinoma of the lung: histologic and immunohistochemical characterization of an unusual pulmonary neoplasm: report of a case and review of the literature. Am J Surg Pathol 2002;26:795–8.
11. Brownstein MH, Shapiro L. The pilosebaceous tumors. Int J Dermatol 1977;16:340–52.
12. Burgdorf WH, Pitha J, Fahmy A. Muir-Torre syndrome. Histologic spectrum of sebaceous proliferations. Am J Dermatopathol 1986;8:202–8.
13. Chao AN, Shields CL, Krema H, Shields JA. Outcome of patients with periocular sebaceous gland carcinoma with and without conjunctival intraepithelial invasion. Ophthalmology 2001;108:1877–83.

14. Cho KJ, Khang SK, Koh JS, Chung JH, Lee SS. Sebaceous carcinoma of the eyelids: frequent expression of c-erbB-2 oncoprotein. J Korean Med Sci 2000;15:545–50.
15. Chun K, Vazquez M, Sanchez JL. Nevus sebaceus: clinical outcome and considerations for prophylactic excision. Int J Dermatol 1995;34:538–41.
16. Civatte J. Clear-cell tumors of the skin: a histopathologic review. J Cutan Pathol 1984;11:165–75.
17. Cribier B, Scrivener Y, Grosshans E. Tumors arising in nevus sebaceus: a study of 596 cases. J Am Acad Dermatol 2000;42(Pt 1):263–8.
18. Crowson AN, Carlson-Sweet K, Macinnis C, et al. Clear cell atypical fibroxanthoma: a clinicopathologic study. J Cutan Pathol 2002;29:374–81.
19. Daley TD. Intraoral sebaceous hyperplasia. Diagnostic criteria. Oral Surg Oral Med Oral Pathol 1993;75:343–7.
20. De Berker DA, Taylor AE, Quinn AG, Simpson NB. Sebaceous hyperplasia in organ transplant recipients: shared aspects of hyperplastic and dysplastic processes? J Am Acad Dermatol 1996;35:696–9.
21. Descalzi ME, Rosenthal S. Sebaceous adenomas and keratoacanthomas in a patient with malignant lymphoma. A new form of Torre's syndrome. Cutis 1981;28:169–70.
22. Dinneen AM, Mehregan DR. Sebaceous epithelioma: a review of twenty-one cases. J Am Acad Dermatol 1996;34:47–50.
23. Dogru M, Matsuo H, Inoue M, Okubo K, Yamamoto M. Management of eyelid sebaceous carcinomas. Opthalmologica 1997;211:40–3.
24. Donati P. Solitary sebaceoma in Muir-Torre syndrome. Int J Dermatol 1996;35:601–2.
25. Escalonilla P, Grilli R, Canamero M, et al. Sebaceous carcinoma of the vulva. Am J Dermatopathol 1999;21:468–72.
26. Esche C, Kruse R, Lamberti C, et al. Muir-Torre syndrome: clinical features and molecular genetic analysis. Br J Dermatol 1997;136:913–7.
27. Fernandez N, Torres A. Hyperplasia of sebaceous glands in a linear pattern of papules. Report of four cases. Am J Dermatopathol 1984;6:237–43.
28. Finan MC, Connolly SM. Sebaceous gland tumors and systemic disease: a clinicopathologic analysis. Medicine 1984;63:232–42.
29. Friedman KJ, Boudreau S, Farmer ER. Superficial epithelioma with sebaceous differentiation. J Cutan Pathol 1987;14:193–7.
30. Gloor P, Ansari I, Sinard J. Sebaceous carcinoma presenting as a unilateral papillary conjunctivitis. Am J Ophthalmol 1999;127:458–9.
31. Hasebe T, Mukai K, Yamaguchi N, et al. Prognostic value of immunohistochemical staining for proliferating cell nuclear antigen, p53, and c-erbB-2 in sebaceous gland carcinoma and sweat gland carcinoma: comparison with histopathologic parameters. Mod Pathol 1994;7:37–43.
32. Hassanein AM, Al-Quran SZ, Kantor GR, Pauporte M, Telang GH, Spielvogel RL. Thomsen-Friedenreich (T) antigen: a possible tool for differentiating sebaceous carcinoma from its simulators. Appl Immunohistochem Mol Morphol 2001;9:250–4.
33. Honavar SG, Shields CL, Maus M, Shields JA, Demirci H, Eagle RC Jr. Primary intraepithelial sebaceous gland carcinoma of the palpebral conjunctiva. Arch Ophthalmol 2001;119:764–7.
34. Housholder MS, Zeligman I. Sebaceous neoplasms associated with visceral carcinomas. Arch Dermatol 1980;116:61–4.
35. Howrey RP, Lipham WJ, Schultz WH, et al. Sebaceous gland carcinoma: a subtle second malignancy following radiation therapy in patients with bilateral retinoblastoma. Cancer 1998;83:767–71.
36. Iezzi G, Rubini C, Fiorini M, Piattelli A. Sebaceous adenoma of the cheek. Oral Oncol 2002;38:111–3.
37. Jacobs DM, Sandles LG, LeBoit PE. Sebaceous carcinoma arising from Bowen's disease of the vulva. Arch Dermatol 1986;122:1191–3.
38. Jaqueti G, Requena L, Sanchez Yus E. Trichoblastoma is the most common neoplasm developed in nevus sebaceus of Jadassohn: a clinicopathologic study of a series of 155 cases. Am J Dermatopathol 2000;22:108–18.
39. Kaddu S, Schaeppi H, Kerl H, Soyer HP. Basaloid neoplasms in nevus sebaceus. J Cutan Pathol 2000;27:327–37.
40. Kaddu S, Schappi H, Kerl H, Soyer HP. Trichoblastoma and sebaceoma in nevus sebaceus. Am J Dermatopathol 1999;21:552–6.
41. Kato N, Sotodate A, Tomita Y. Zeis gland carcinoma. J Dermatol 1997;24:595–600.
42. Kato N, Ueno H. Superficial epithelioma with sebaceous differentiation. J Dermatol 1992;19:190–4.
43. Kimura T, Miyazawa H, Aoyagi T, Ackerman AB. Folliculosebaceous cystic hamartoma. A distinctive malformation of the skin. Am J Dermatopathol 1991;13:213–20.
44. Kopniczky Z, Kobor J, Mararz A, Vajtai L. Desmoplastic neuroepithelial tumor of infancy in the nevus sebaceus syndrome: report of a unique constellation and review of the literature. Pathol Res Pract 2001;197:279–84.
45. Kumar A, Kossard S. Band-like sebaceous hyperplasia over the penis. Australas J Dermatol 1999;40:47–8.
46. Laino L, Steensel MA, Innocenzi D, Camplone G. Familial occurrence of nevus sebaceus of Jadassohn: another cause of paradominant inheritance? Eur J Dermatol 2001;11:97–8.

47. Lasser A, Carter DM. Multiple basal cell epitheliomas with sebaceous differentiation. Arch Dermatol 1973;107:91–3.
48. Li TJ, Kitano M, Mukai H, Yamashita S. Oral sebaceous carcinoma: report of a case. J Oral Maxillofac Surg 1997;55:751–4.
49. Machin P, Catasus L, Pons C, et al. Microsatellite instability and immunostaining for MSH-2 and MLH-1 in cutaneous and internal tumors from patients with the Muir-Torre syndrome. J Cutan Pathol 2002;29:415–20.
50. Mahalingam M, Bhawan J, Finn R, Stefanato CM. Tumor of the follicular infundibulum with sebaceous differentiation. J Cutan Pathol 2001;28:314–7.
51. Mahalingam M, Byers HR. Intra-epidermal and intra-dermal sebocrine adenoma with cystic degeneration and hemorrhage. J Cutan Pathol 2000;27:472–5.
52. Margo CE, Grossniklaus HE. Intraepithelial sebaceous neoplasia without underlying invasive carcinoma. Surv Ophthalmol 1995;39:293–301.
53. Margo CE, Mulla ZD. Malignant tumors of the eyelid: a population-based study of non-basal cell and non-squamous cell malignant neoplasms. Arch Opthalmol 1998;116:195–8.
54. Marini M, Saponaro A, Remorino L, Lynch P, Magarinos G. Eruptive lesions in a patient with bone marrow transplantation. Int J Dermatol 2001;40:133–5.
55. Massa MC, Medenica M. Cutaneous adnexal tumors and cysts: a review. Part I. Tumors with hair follicular and sebaceous glandular differentiation and cysts related to different parts of the hair follicle. Pathol Annu 1985;20:189–233.
56. Mathiak M, Rutten A, Mangold E, et al. Loss of DNA mismatch repair proteins in skin tumors from patients with Muir-Torre syndrome and MSH2 or MLH1 germline mutations: establishment of immunohistochemical analysis as a screening test. Am J Surg Pathol 2002;26:338–43.
57. Mehregan AH, Rahbari H. Benign epithelial tumors of the skin. II. Benign sebaceous tumors. Cutis 1977;19:317–20.
58. Misago N, Mihara I, Ansai S, Narisawa Y. Sebaceoma and related neoplasms with sebaceous differentiation: a clinicopathologic study of 30 cases. Am J Dermatopathol 2002;24:294–304.
59. Misago N, Narisawa Y. Rippled-pattern sebaceoma. Am J Dermatopathol 2001;23:437–43.
60. Misago N, Narisawa Y. Tricholemmal carcinoma in continuity with trichoblastoma within nevus sebaceus. Am J Dermatopathol 2002;24:149–55.
61. Moreno C, Jacyk WK, Judd MJ, Requena L. Highly aggressive extraocular sebaceous carcinoma. Am J Dermatopathol 2001;23:450–5.
62. Morioka S. The natural history of nevus sebaceus. J Cutan Pathol 1985;12:200–13.
63. Nakhleh RE, Swanson PE, Wick MR. Cutaneous adnexal carcinomas with divergent differentiation. Am J Dermatopathol 1990;12:325–34.
64. Nelson BR, Hamlet KR, Gillard M, Railan D, Johnson TM. Sebaceous carcinoma. J Am Acad Dermatol 1995;33:1–15.
65. Nguyen GK, Mielke BW. Extraocular sebaceous carcinoma with intraepidermal (pagetoid) spread. Am J Dermatopathol 1987;9:364–5.
66. Nielsen TA, Maia-Cohen S, Hessel AB, Xie DL, Pellegrini AE. Sebaceous neoplasm with reticulated and cribriform features: a rare variant of sebaceoma. J Cutan Pathol 1998;25:233–5.
67. Ohara N, Taguchi K, Yamamoto M, Nagano T, Akagi T. Sebaceous carcinoma of the submandibular gland with high-grade malignancy: report of a case. Pathol Int 1998;48:287–91.
68. Ortiz-Rey JA, Martin-Jimenez A, Alvarez C, De La Fuente A. Sebaceous gland hyperplasia of the vulva. Obstet Gynecol 2002;99(Pt 2):919–21.
69. Papadopoulos AJ, Ahmed H, Pakarian FB, Caldwell CJ, McNicholas J, Raju KS. Sebaceous carcinoma arising within an ovarian cystic mature teratoma. Int J Gynecol Cancer 1995;5:76–9.
70. Pickford MA, Hogg FJ, Fallowfield ME, Webster MH. Sebaceous carcinoma of the periorbital and extraorbital regions. Br J Plast Surg 1995; 48:93–6.
71. Prayson RA, Kotagal P, Wyllie E, Bingaman W. Linear epidermal nevus and nevus sebaceus syndromes: a clinicopathologic study of 3 patients. Arch Pathol Lab Med 1999;123:301–5.
72. Pricolo VE, Rodil JV, Vezeridis MP. Extraorbital sebaceous carcinoma. Arch Surg 1985;120:853–5.
73. Prioleau PG, Santa Cruz DJ. Sebaceous gland neoplasia. J Cutan Pathol 1984;11:396–414.
74. Pujol RM, LeBoit PE, Su WP. Microcystic adnexal carcinoma with extensive sebaceous differentiation. Am J Dermatopathol 1997;19:358–62.
75. Raizada RM, Khan NU. Aural sebaceous adenomas. J Laryngol Otol 1986;100:1413–6.
76. Rao NA, Hidayat AA, McLean IW, Zimmerman LE. Sebaceous carcinomas of the ocular adnexa: a clinicopathologic study of 104 cases, with five-year follow-up data. Hum Pathol 1982;13:113–22.
77. Requena L, Sanchez Yus E, Jimenez E, Roo E. Lymphoepithelioma-like carcinoma of the skin: a light microscopic and immunohistochemical study. J Cutan Pathol 1994;21:541–8.
78. Roth JJ, Granick MS. Squamous cell and adnexal carcinomas of the skin. Clin Plast Surg 1997;24:687–703.
79. Rothko K, Farmer ER, Zeligman I. Superficial epithelioma with sebaceous differentiation. Arch Dermatol 1980;116:329–31.

80. Rulon DB, Helwig EB. Cutaneous sebaceous neoplasms. Cancer 1974;33:82–102.
81. Rutten A, Burgdorf WH, Hugel H, et al. Cystic sebaceous tumors as marker lesions for the Muir-Torre syndrome: a histopathologic and molecular genetic study. Am J Dermatopathol 1999;21:405–13.
82. Sanchez Yus E, Montull C, Valcayo A, Robledo A. Areolar sebaceous hyperplasia: a new entity? J Cutan Pathol 1988;15:62–3.
83. Sanchez Yus E, Requena L, Simon P, del Rio E. Sebomatricoma: a unifying term that encompasses all benign neoplasms with sebaceous differentiation. Am J Dermatopathol 1995;17;213–21.
84. Sanchez-Yus E, Requena L, Simon P, Sanchez M. Complex adnexal tumor of the primary epithelial germ with distinct patterns of superficial epithelioma with sebaceous differentiation, immature trichoepithelioma, and apocrine adenocarcinoma. Am J Dermatopathol 1992;14:245–52.
85. Schwartz RA, Goldberg DJ, Mahmood F, etc. The Muir-Torre syndrome: a disease of sebaceous and colonic neoplasms. Dermatologica 1989;178:23–8.
86. Sinard JH. Immunohistochemical distinction of ocular sebaceous carcinoma from basal cell and squamous cell carcinoma. Arch Ophthalmol 1999;117:776–83.
87. Southey MC, Young MA, Whitty J, et al. Molecular pathologic analysis enhances the diagnosis and management of Muir-Torre syndrome and gives insight into its underlying molecular pathogenesis. Am J Surg Pathol 2001;25:936–41.
88. Stashower ME, Smith K, Corbett D, Skelton HG. Basaloid/follicular hyperplasia overlying connective tissue/mesenchymal hamartomas simulating basal cell carcinomas. J Am Acad Dermatol 2001;45:886–91.
89. Steffen C. Neoplasms with sebaceous differentiation. In: Farmer ER, Hood AF, eds. Pathology of the skin, 2nd ed. New York: McGraw-Hill; 2000:1035–58.
90. Suster S. Clear-cell tumors of the skin. Semin Diagn Pathol 1996;13:40–59.
91. Swanson PE, Wick MR. Immunohistochemistry of cutaneous tumors. In: Leong AS, ed. Applied immunohistochemistry for the surgical pathologist. London: Edward Arnold; 1993:269–308.
92. Tronnier M. Clear cell trichoblastoma in association with a nevus sebaceus. Am J Dermatopathol 2001;23:143–5.
93. Troy JL, Ackerman AB. Sebaceoma. A distinctive benign neoplasm of adnexal epithelium differentiating toward sebaceous cells. Am J Dermatopathol 1984;6:7–13.
94. Turner CD, Shea CR, Rosoff PM. Basal cell carcinoma originating from a nevus sebaceus on the scalp of a 7-year-old boy. J Pediatr Hematol Oncol 2001;23:247–9.
95. Uchiyama N, Yamaji K, Shindo Y. Giant solitary sebaceous gland hyperplasia on the frontal region. Dermatologica 1990;181:60–1.
96. Van de Warrenburg BP, van Gulik S, Renier WO, Lammens M, Doelman JC. The linear nevus sebaceus syndrome. Clin Neurol Neurosurg 1998;100:126–32.
97. Varga Z, Kolb SA, Flury R, Burkhard R, Caduff R. Sebaceous carcinoma of the breast. Pathol Int 2000;50:63–6.
98. Vaughan TK, Sau P. Superfical epithelioma with sebaceous differentiation. J Am Acad Dermatol 1990;23(Pt 1):760–2.
99. Weisshaar E, Schramm M, Gollnick H. Familial nevoid sebaceous gland hyperplasia affecting three generations of a family. Eur J Dermatol 1999;9:621–3.
100. Wick MR, Goellner JR, Wolfe JT 3rd, Su WP. Adnexal carcinomas of the skin. II. Extraocular sebaceous carcinomas. Cancer 1985;56:1163–72.
101. Wolfe JT 3rd, Wick MR, Campbell RJ. Sebaceous carcinoma of the oculocutaneous adnexa and extraocular skin. In: Wick MR, ed. Pathology of unusual malignant cutaneous tumors. New York: Marcel Dekker; 1985:77–106.
102. Wolfe JT 3rd, Yeatts RP, Wick MR, Campbell RJ, Waller RR. Sebaceous carcinoma of the eyelid. Errors in clinical and pathologic diagnosis. Am J Surg Pathol 1984;8:597–606.
103. Wong TY, Suster S, Cheek RF, Mihm MC Jr. Benign cutaneous adnexal tumors with combined folliculosebaceous, apocrine, and eccrine differentiation. Clinicopathologic and immunohistochemical study of eight cases. Am J Dermatopathol 1996;18:124–36.
104. Xin H, Matt D, Qin JZ, Burg G, Boni R. The sebaceous nevus: a nevus with deletions of the PTCH gene. Cancer Res 1999;59:1834–6.
105. Zaim MT. Sebocrine adenoma. An adnexal adenoma with sebaceous and apocrine poroma-like differentiation. Am J Dermatopathol 1988;10:311–8.
106. Zurcher M, Hintschich CR, Garner A, Bunce C, Collin JR. Sebaceous carcinoma of the eyelid: a clinicopathological study. Br J Ophthalmol 1998;82:1049–55.

SUPPLEMENTAL REFERENCES

Sebaceous Hyperplasia

Bakaris S, Kiran H, Kiran G. Sebaceous gland hyperplasia of the vulva. Aust N Z J Obstet Gynaecol 2004;44:75–6.

Boschnakow A, May T, Assaf C, Tebbe B, Zouboulis CC. Cyclosporine A-induced sebaceous gland hyperplasia. B J Dermatol 2003;149:198–200.

Kaminagakura E, Andrade CR, Rangel AL, et al. Sebaceous adenoma of oral cavity: report of case and comparative proliferation study with sebaceous gland hyperplasia and Fordyce's granules. Oral Dis 2003;9:323–7.

Nevus Sebaceus

Chen W, Happle R. Phacomatosis pigmentovasculosebacea: an unusual case of phacomatosis multiplex. Eur J Dermatol 2003;13:231–3.

Dalle S, Skowron F, Balme B, Perrot H. Apocrine carcinoma developed in nevus sebaceus of Jadassohn. Eur J Dermatol 2003;13:487–9.

Diwan AH, Smith KJ, Brown R, Skelton HG. Mucoepidermoid carcinoma arising within nevus sebaceus of Jadassohn. J Cutan Pathol 2003;30:652–5.

Jang KS, Oh YH, Park CK, Paik SS. Nevus sebaceus with psammomatous calcified spherules in the apocrine glands. J Am Acad Dermatol 2005;52:724–5.

Margulis A, Bauer BS, Corcoran JF. Surgical management of the cutaneous manifestations of linear nevus sebaceus syndrome. Plast Reconstr Surg 2003;111:1043–50.

Miller CJ, Ioffreda MD, Billingsley EM. Sebaceous carcinoma, basal cell carcinoma, trichoadenoma, trichoblastoma, and syringocystadenoma papilliferum arising within a nevus sebaceus. Dermatol Surg 2004;30:1546–9.

Miyake H, Hara H, Shimojima H, Suzuki H. Follicular hybrid cyst (trichilemmal cyst and pilomatricoma) arising within a nevus sebaceus. Am J Dermatopathol 2004;26:390–3.

Munoz-Perez MA, Garcia-Hernandez MJ, Rios JJ, Camacho F. Sebaceus nevi: a clinicopathologic study. J Eur Acad Dermatol Venereol 2002;16:319–24.

Santibanez-Gallerani A, Marshall D, Duarte AM, Melnick SJ, Thaller S. Should nevus sebaceus of Jadassohn in children be excised? A study of 757 cases, and literature review. J Craniofac Surg 2003;14:658–60.

Tinschert S, Stein A, Goldner B, Dietel M, Happle R. Melorheostosis with ipsilateral nevus sebaceus (didymosis melorheosebacea). Eur J Dermatol 2003;13:21–4.

Zutt M, Strutz F, Happle R, et al. Schimmelpenning-Feuerstein-Mims syndrome with hypophosphatemic rickets. Dermatology 2003;207:72–6.

Sebaceous Adenoma

Abbott JJ, Hernandez-Rios P, Amirkhan RH, Hoang MP. Cystic sebaceous neoplasms in Muir-Torre syndrome. Arch Pathol Lab Med 2003;127:614–7.

Curry ML, Eng W, Lund K, Paek D, Cockerell CJ. Muir-Torre syndrome: role of the dermatopathologist in diagnosis. Am J Dermatopathol 2004;26:217–21.

Popnikolov NK, Gatalica Z, Colome-Grimmer MI, Sanchez RL. Loss of mismatch repair proteins in sebaceous gland tumors. J Cutan Pathol 2003;30:178–84.

Rishi K, Font RL. Sebaceous gland tumors of the eyelids and conjunctiva in the Muir-Torre syndrome: a clinicopathologic study of five cases and literature review. Ophthal Plast Reconstr Surg 2004;20:31–6.

Shields CL, Shields JA. Tumors of the conjunctiva and cornea. Surv Ophthalmol 2004;49:3–24.

Superficial Epithelioma with Sebaceous Differentiation

Lee MJ, Kim YC, Lew W. A case of superficial epithelioma with sebaceous differentiation. Yonsei Med J 2003;30:347–50.

Sebaceoma

Kazakov DV, Kutzner H, Rutten A, Mukensnabl P, Michal M. Carcinoid-like pattern in sebaceous neoplasms: another distinctive, previously unrecognized pattern in extraocular sebaceous carcinoma and sebaceoma. Am J Dermatopathol 2005;27:195–203.

Basal Cell Carcinoma with Sebaceous Differentiation

Hatta N, Hirano T, Kimura T, et al. Molecular diagnosis of basal cell carcinoma and other basaloid cell neoplasms of the skin by the quantification of Gli1 transcript levels. J Cutan Pathol 2005;32:131–6.

Kamiya M, Takeuchi Y, Katho M, Yokoo H, Sasaki A, Nakazato Y. Expression of p73 in normal skin and proliferative skin lesions. Pathol Int 2004;54:890–5.

Misago N, Suse T, Uemura T, Narisawa Y. Basal cell carcinoma with sebaceous differentiation. Am J Dermatopathol 2004;26:298–303.

Sebaceous Carcinoma

Ansai S, Mitsuhashi Y, Kondo S, Manabe M. Immunohistochemical differentiation of extraocular sebaceous carcinoma from other skin cancers. J Dermatol 2004;31:998–1008.

Bassetto F, Baraziol R, Sottosanti MV, Scarpa C, Montesco M. Biological behavior of the sebaceous carcinoma of the head. Dermatol Surg 2004;30:472–6.

Bogner PN, Su LD, Fullen DR. Cluster designation 5 staining of normal and non-lymphoid neoplastic skin. J Cutan Pathol 2005;32:50–4.

Hassanein AM. Sebaceous carcinoma and the T-antigen. Semin Cutan Med Surg 2004;23:62–72.

Lai TF, Huilgol SC, Selva D, James CL. Eyelid sebaceous carcinoma masquerading as in situ squamous cell carcinoma. Dermatol Surg 2004;30(Pt 1):222–5.

Li B, Li ND, Xu XL, et al. Telomerase expression in sebaceous carcinoma of the eyelid. Chin Med J 2004;117:445–8.

Ohara M, Sotozono C, Tsuchihashi Y, Kinoshita S. Ki-67 labeling index as a marker of malignancy in ocular surface neoplasms. Jpn J Ophthalmol 2004;48:524–9.

Shields JA, Demirci H, Marr BP, Eagle RC Jr, Shields CL. Sebaceous carcinoma of the ocular region: a review. Surv Ophthalmol 2005;50:103–22.

Shields JA, Demirci H, Marr BP, Eagle RC Jr, Shields CL. Sebaceous carcinoma of the eyelids: personal experience with 60 cases. Ophthalmology 2004;111:2151–7.

4 NEOPLASMS AND PSEUDONEOPLASTIC PROLIFERATIONS OF THE SWEAT GLANDS, AND PRIMARY NEUROENDOCRINE (MERKEL CELL) CARCINOMA

Cutaneous neoplasms that differentiate towards sweat gland units are uncommon in general pathology, but not in dermatopathology. The histologic diversity of these lesions, and the plethora of nosologic schemes that have been applied to them in the past, can be daunting. In this context, the pathologist needs to decide whether to adopt a stance of terminologic minimalism, using such diagnostic terms as "benign sweat gland neoplasm," or to embrace more eclectic nomenclature as applied to adnexal tumors. This chapter uses a classification system that is attuned as much as possible to concepts and terms that are commonly embraced in surgical pathology. Because of the relatively nondescript clinical features of many sweat gland tumors, these will not be covered in any detail except where they are distinctive and contribute meaningfully to the pathologic diagnosis. The topic of cutaneous adnexal neoplasia is broad and complicated; indeed, several entire textbooks have been devoted to it (1,25,61). Hence, the interested reader is referred to the reference sources cited above for additional information.

Merkel cell (neuroendocrine) carcinoma of the skin is included in this chapter. This inclusion may seem arbitrary, but some data do exist to support the classification of Merkel cell tumors as cutaneous adnexal neoplasms.

BENIGN ECCRINE SWEAT GLAND NEOPLASMS

Benign neoplasms that differentiate towards the eccrine unit are the most common cutaneous adnexal lesions. They may be found in virtually all skin fields, and are seen in both children and adults.

Eccrine Cylindroma

Clinical Features. Several sweat gland tumors are found consistently in the skin of the face, neck, and scalp. One of them, *eccrine cylindroma*, is a solitary sporadic nodule or a multifocal proliferation associated with the autosomal-dominant "turban tumor" (Ancell-Spiegler) complex (fig. 4-1) (8,13,18,50,60,64). The gene locus for familial cylindromatosis has been localized to chromosome 16q, and named *CYLD*. Patients with *CYLD* mutations may also develop multiple trichoepitheliomas (6a,28a,35a).

Pathologic Findings. Eccrine cylindroma demonstrates two cell populations: one that is compact and basaloid and the other having a polygonal character with more notable amphophilic cytoplasm. Nuclear chromatin is dispersed, nucleoli are inconspicuous, and mitotic activity is typically sparse. Two features enable its recognition on scanning microscopy: a "jigsaw puzzle" growth pattern, with angular cell nests that are molded to one another in a fibrous matrix (fig. 4-2), and deposits of eosinophilic, hyaline basement membrane material within the cellular clusters and immediately around them (fig. 4-3). Cylindroma often shows an irregular pattern of peripheral growth, with "buds" of tumor in the dermis or subcutis that are seemingly detached from the main mass. This finding has no particular prognostic significance and does not imply malignancy. Similarly, examples of cylindroma exhibiting mitotic activity behave innocuously if their nuclear characteristics and overall microscopic structure are characteristic (10). Truly malignant transformation of eccrine cylindroma features a distinctive histologic image, with obviously anaplastic tumor cells and a lack of organoid growth.

Cylindroma has been included as an eccrine neoplasm largely because of the authors' bias on that point. Others have considered it to represent an apocrine tumor.

Differential Diagnosis. The principal entity in the differential diagnosis of cylindroma is spiradenoma (see below).

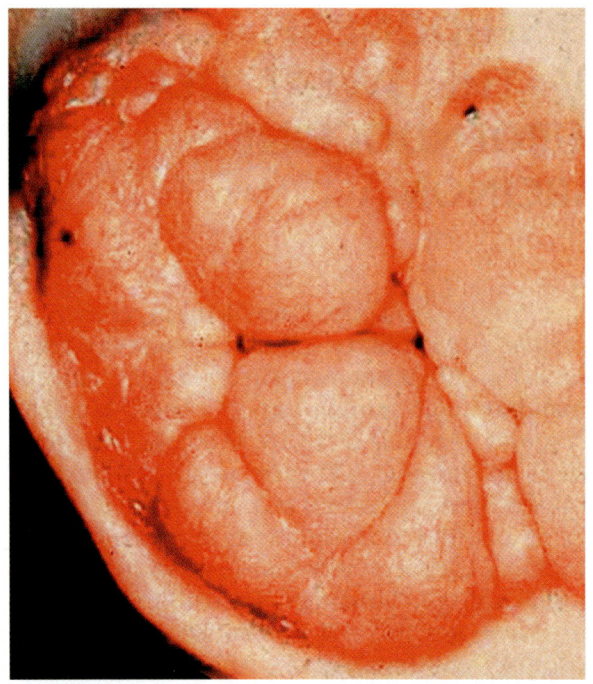

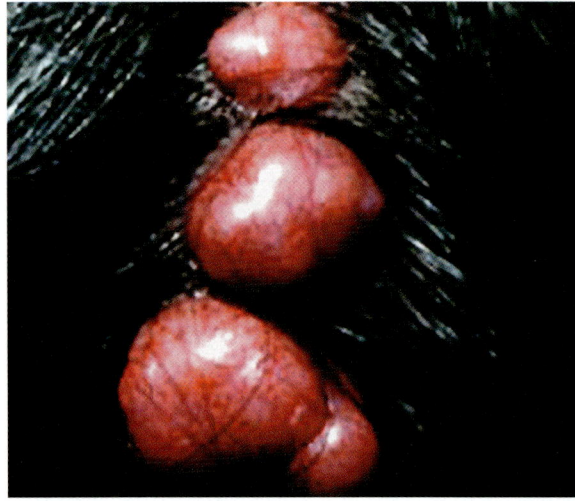

Figure 4-1

ECCRINE CYLINDROMA

Multiple cylindromas of the head and neck in a patient with the "turban tumor" syndrome.

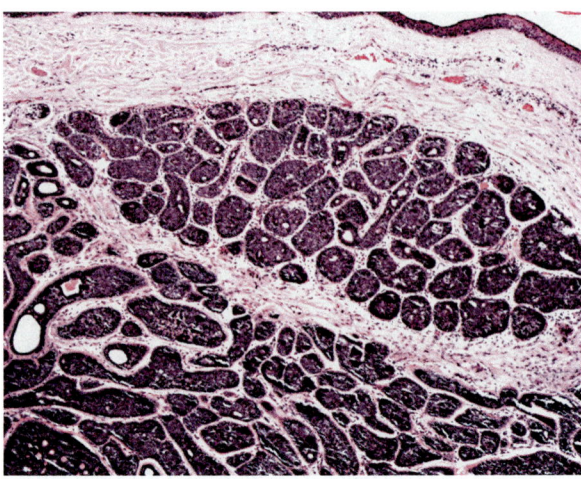

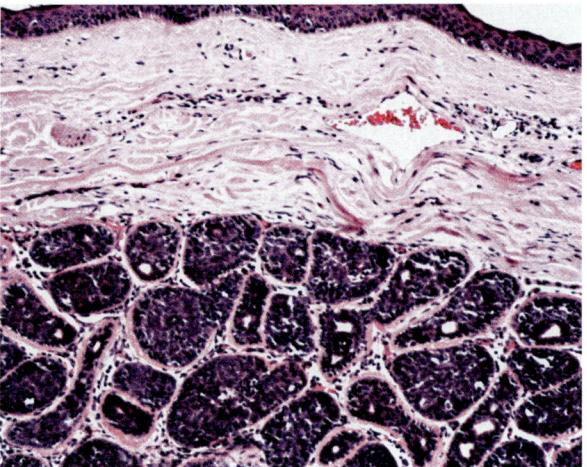

Figure 4-2

ECCRINE CYLINDROMA

Micronodular arrays of basaloid cells in the dermis mold to one another in a "jigsaw puzzle" pattern.

Eccrine Spiradenoma

Clinical Features. The clinical features of *eccrine spiradenoma* overlap largely with those of cylindroma (fig. 4-4), including a potential for multifocal regionalized growth.

Pathologic Findings. Eccrine spiradenoma differs only slightly in appearance from cylindroma. The former, however, generally lacks a jigsaw puzzle profile, and instead shows intratumoral vascular spaces that are often dilated and tend to be disposed towards the periphery of tumor cell clusters (fig. 4-5). These channels may contain lymphatic fluid, erythrocytes, or both, and may be so prominent that they give the lesion an appearance simulating that of a vascular neoplasm (35,36,51,58). Tumors such as this have been called *giant vascular spiradenomas* (12).

Other special attributes of spiradenoma include a diffuse intratumoral distribution of mature lymphocytes (fig. 4-6), as seen in thymomas, and the ability to present as a deep-seated tumor in the subcutaneous tissue (33).

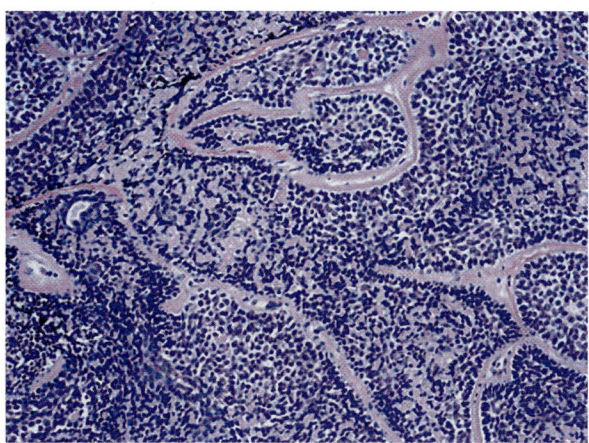 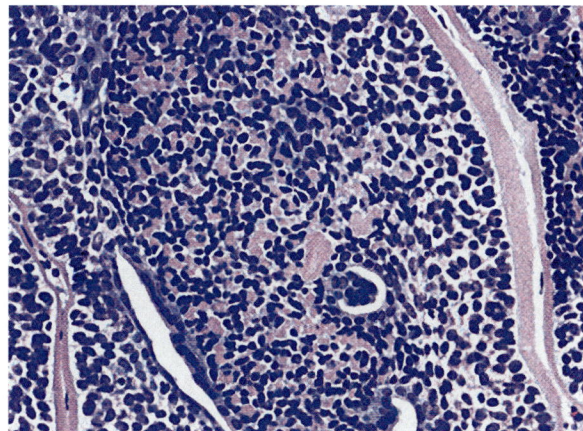

Figure 4-3

ECCRINE CYLINDROMA

Basement membrane material is deposited between and within tumor cell nests.

In some instances, it may be difficult to distinguish between cylindroma and spiradenoma microscopically; in fact, some patients with the Ancell-Spiegler syndrome also have multifocal spiradenomatosis (58).

Syringoma

Clinical Features. *Syringoma* is a benign eccrine proliferation that is probably malformative rather than neoplastic in most cases. This lesion commonly is multifocal, and is largely restricted to the upper face (fig. 4-7) and the genital skin (4,7,16,23,27,30,34,44,66). Solitary lesions do exist; they are nondescript papules and show no particular anatomic predilection (27).

Pathologic Findings. On scanning microscopy, syringoma has a well-demarcated periphery, and usually assumes a plate-like configuration in the corium. Small, comma-shaped cellular tubular aggregates, many of which have central lumens and luminal cuticles, are distributed in a fibrous stroma. The tubules are composed of one or two cuboidal cell layers, and eosinophilic secretions may be seen in them. The lesional cells are polygonal or flat, with eosinophilic or clear cytoplasm (4,27,44). Nuclei are compact, without nucleoli or mitotic figures. Syringomas lack nuclear atypia and permeative growth, and never extend into the subcutis (figs. 4-8, 4-9). Syringomas with clear cell features have been associated in some cases with diabetes mellitus (54a).

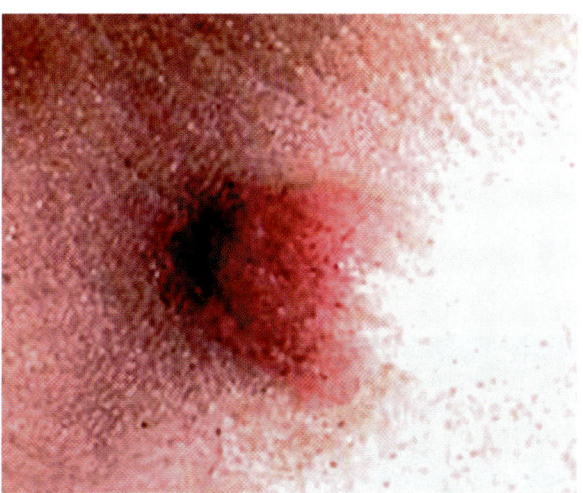

Figure 4-4

ECCRINE SPIRADENOMA

A nodular, reddish blue mass is seen in the skin of the neck.

Differential Diagnosis. A small superficial biopsy taken centrally in such a lesion may yield an image that simulates a type of appendageal malignancy (27), microcystic adnexal carcinoma, making excision mandatory in such circumstances if clinically feasible.

Eccrine Poroma

Clinical Features. *Eccrine poroma* is so named because it microscopically resembles elements

Nonmelanocytic Tumors of the Skin

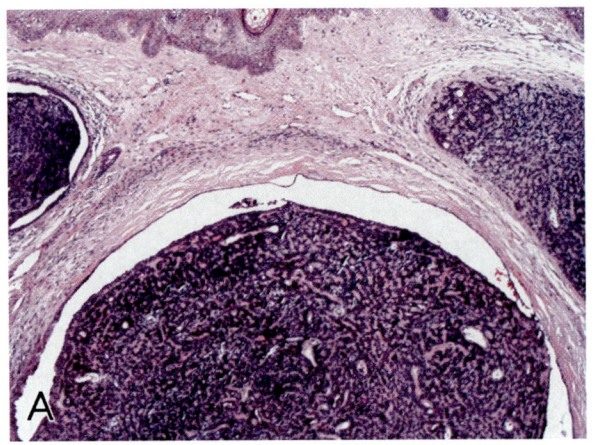
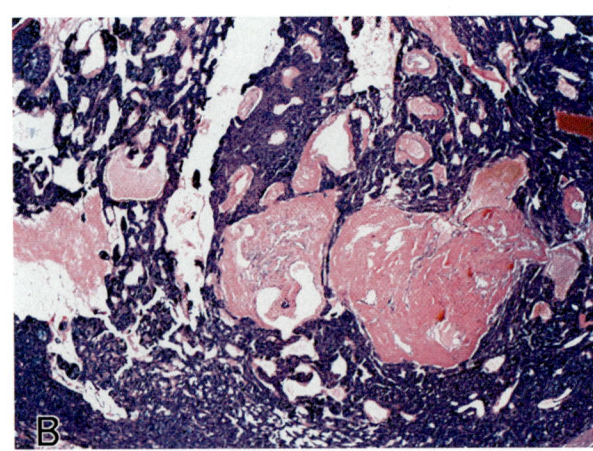
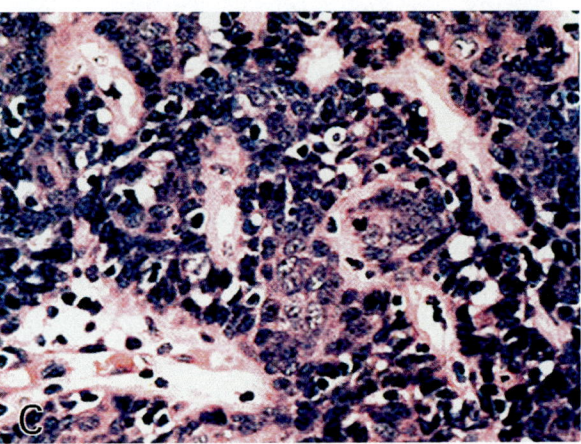

Figure 4-5

ECCRINE SPIRADENOMA

Prominent intratumoral lymphatic spaces and a basic composition by basaloid tumor cells are seen.

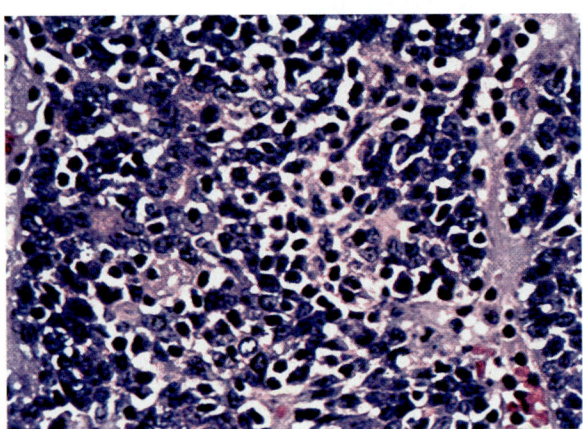
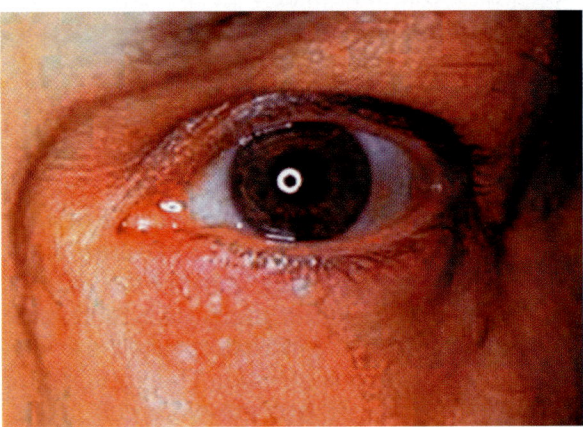

Figure 4-6

ECCRINE SPIRADENOMA

Spiradenoma typically contains numerous intralesional lymphocytes.

Figure 4-7

SYRINGOMA

There are multiple small papules in the infraorbital skin.

of the acrosyringeal-eccrine coil unit. This tumor typically is a papule or small nodule on the distal extremities, including the palms, soles, and digits (fig. 4-10), but can be located elsewhere as well (17,19,20,29,42,45,62). Patients of all ages develop poromas.

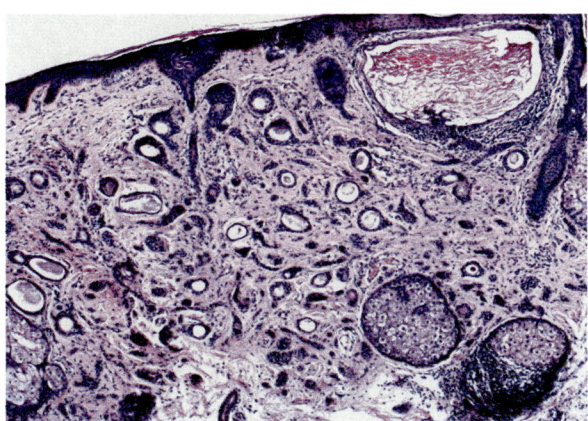 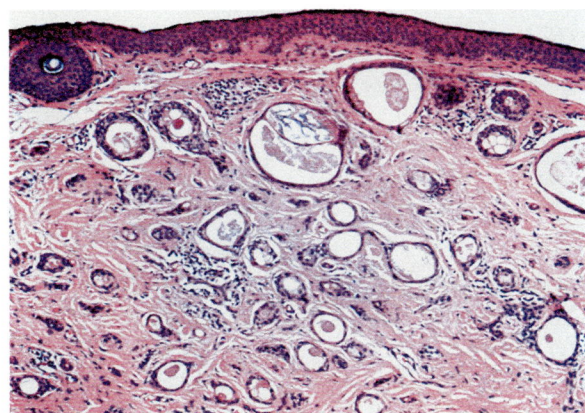

Figure 4-8

SYRINGOMA

This lesion is typified by a plate-like proliferation of small solid nests (often showing a "tadpole"-like configuration) and microcysts in the dermis.

Pathologic Findings. Histologically, the most consistent feature of eccrine poroma is the presence of intraepidermal "lakes" of small monotonous polygonal cells, which are sharply separated from adjacent keratinocytes. Nuclei are bland, with no nucleoli or mitoses, and the cytoplasm is amphophilic (17,19,29,45).

The form of poroma in which only an intraepidermal component is present is termed *hidroacanthoma simplex* (fig. 4-11) (39). When a dermal component predominates, with the formation of duct-like spaces inside the tumor cell nests, the lesion is known as *dermal duct tumor* (fig. 4-12) (3,28). These two represent poles in a continuum, and most poromas show both epidermal and dermal components (fig. 4-13). Variations in the prototypic image of this lesion are represented by focal squamous metaplasia, focal clear cell change, and extensive glandular lumen formation (45).

The usual features of this tumor are cytologic banality and monotony. Some examples show focal nuclear enlargement or the presence of nucleoli, with or without limited mitotic activity (45); nevertheless, if the overall pattern is that of an ordinary poroma, the tumors should not be labeled as malignant. True porocarcinomas exhibit infiltrative growth, and areas of spontaneous necrosis are also frequently seen. Poromatous tumors may also have an acanthotic or papillomatous surface. Rahbari (46) has suggested the term *syringoacanthoma* for those vari-

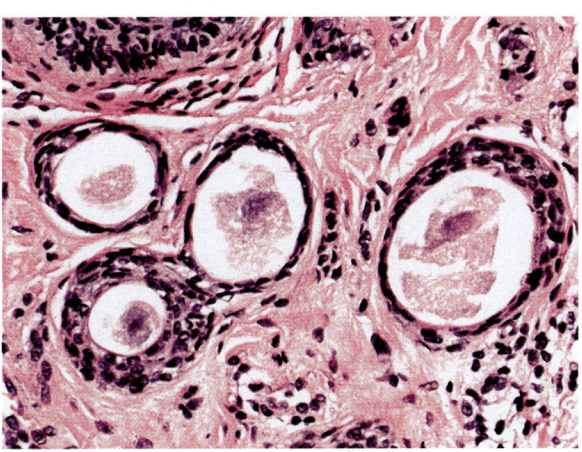

Figure 4-9

SYRINGOMA

The bland cytologic characteristics of syringoma are evident, together with a characteristic admixture of microcysts and solid cell nests.

ants, but we believe that they are basically poromas and label them as such.

Eccrine Syringofibroadenoma

Despite its name, *eccrine syringofibroadenoma* resembles poroma more than syringoma. This unique neoplasm features a complex interconnection of cellular cords in the dermis, with intraepidermal components. The surface epithelium is hyperplastic and may be overtly pseudoepitheliomatous; the dermal portion of

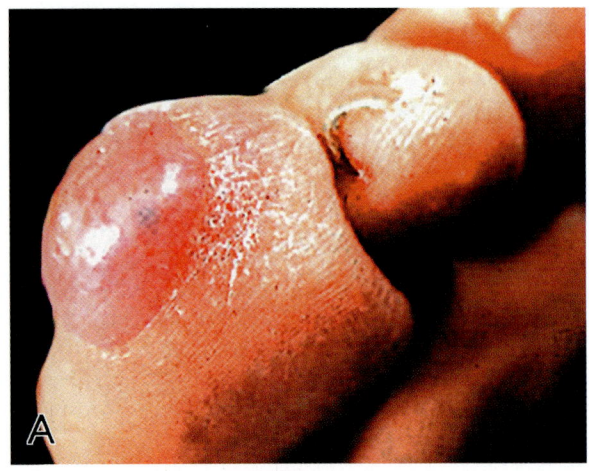
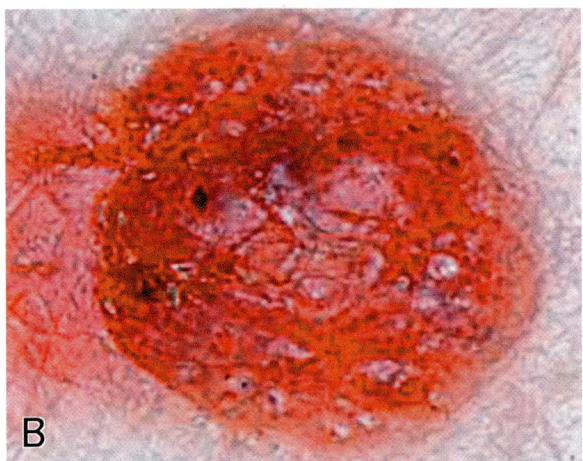
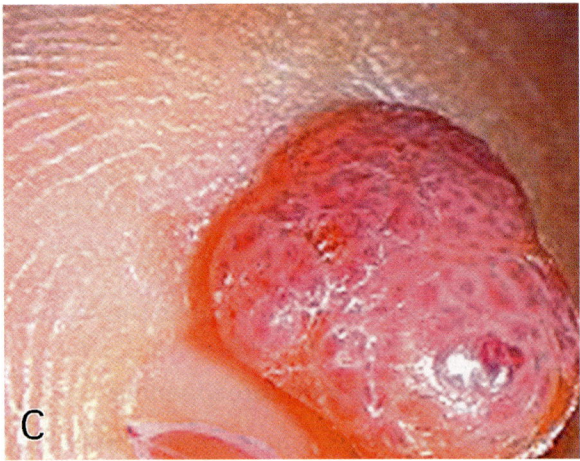

Figure 4-10

ECCRINE POROMA

Nodular red-pink lesions of the digits (A,C) and the palm (B).

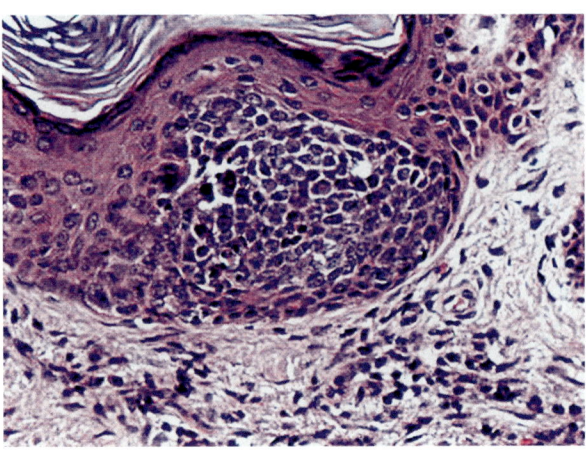

Figure 4-11

INTRAEPIDERMAL POROMA

Intraepidermal poroma is composed of bland basaloid cells that are sharply demarcated from the surrounding keratinocytes. This lesion is also known as hidroacanthoma simplex.

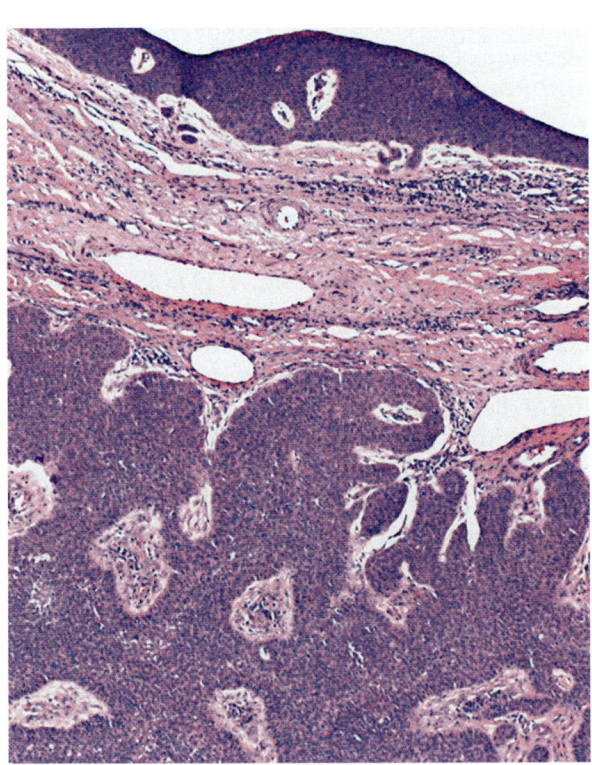

Figure 4-12

DERMAL DUCT TUMOR

This dermal tumor shows nests and tubular arrays of cells that are identical morphologically to those of conventional poroma. Although it is known as dermal duct tumor, this lesion is a variant of poroma and serial sections often demonstrate an intraepidermal component.

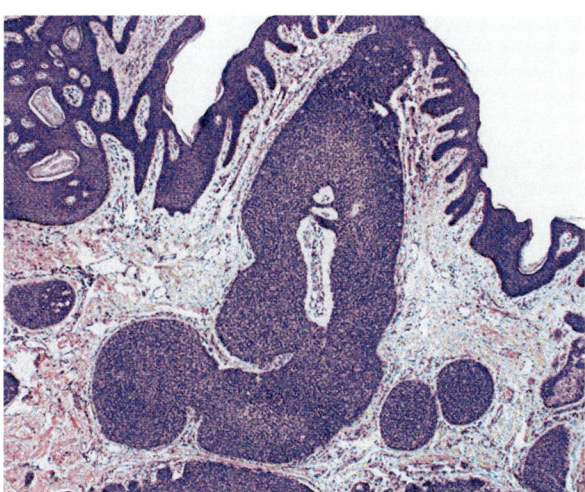
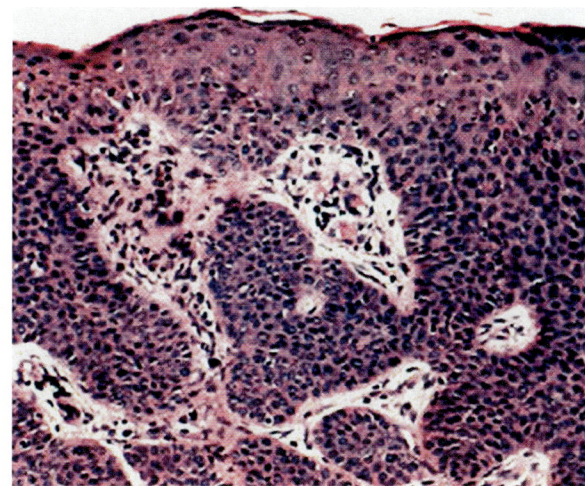

Figure 4-13

ECCRINE POROMA

Poroma is usually composed of nests of basaloid cells that penetrate the epidermis in a manner simulating the normal acrosyringium, but also involve the dermis.

the lesion has a fibroblastic and vascular stroma, and its epithelial portion is often squamoid but with small intercellular ductal lumens (fig. 4-14) (9,32). Thus, the overall appearance of syringofibroadenoma incorporates aspects of mammary fibroadenoma as well as fibroepithelioma of Pinkus (fibroepitheliomatous basal cell carcinoma). Weedon and Lewis (59) have used the alternate designation of *acrosyringeal nevus* for this proliferation.

The lesion is usually sharply circumscribed, without nuclear atypia or mitotic activity. The stroma of syringofibroadenoma is likely "induced" by the epithelial proliferation.

Papillary Eccrine Adenoma (Tubulopapillary Eccrine Hidradenoma)

Papillary eccrine adenoma is a nondescript dermal nodule, often located on the extremities. Non-Caucasian patients have been over-represented in some series.

Papillary eccrine adenoma is composed of uniform polyhedral cells that are arranged in multilayered dermal ductal profiles, subdivided by fibrovascular stroma. The tumor cells also mantle the peripheral aspects of dermal microcysts and form tubulopapillary complexes (figs. 4-15, 4-16) (2,6,11,47,49,57). The last of these characteristics explains the alternate designation of *tubulopapillary hidradenoma* suggested by Falck and Jordaan (15). Both eccrine and apocrine features may be present, and other synonyms, such as *tubular apocrine adenoma* (54), have been used, but eccrine differentiation is more common. Connections between the dermal cell nests and other cell nests in the epidermis may be observed focally, as expected in poromas (see above). Ductal spaces may contain luminal "cuticles," similar to those in syringomas.

The cytologic features of papillary eccrine adenoma are unremarkable: lack of nucleoli, no nuclear anaplasia, and no significant mitotic activity (fig. 4-17). The overall image is similar to that of localized, florid, mammary intraductal hyperplasia; however, the potential for recurrence attests to the neoplastic character of papillary eccrine adenoma.

Eccrine Acrospiroma (Solid and Cystic Hidradenoma, Nodular Eccrine Hidradenoma)

Eccrine acrospiroma, or *nodular hidradenoma*, is another type of eccrine adenoma. It is a solitary nodule without other discriminating clinical attributes (fig. 4-18). It may be seen in any skin field.

Acrospiroma has a nodular dermal growth pattern and a composition of monomorphous polygonal cells. This tumor often demonstrates microcystic changes, and may exhibit micropapillary and ductal differentiation (figs. 4-19,

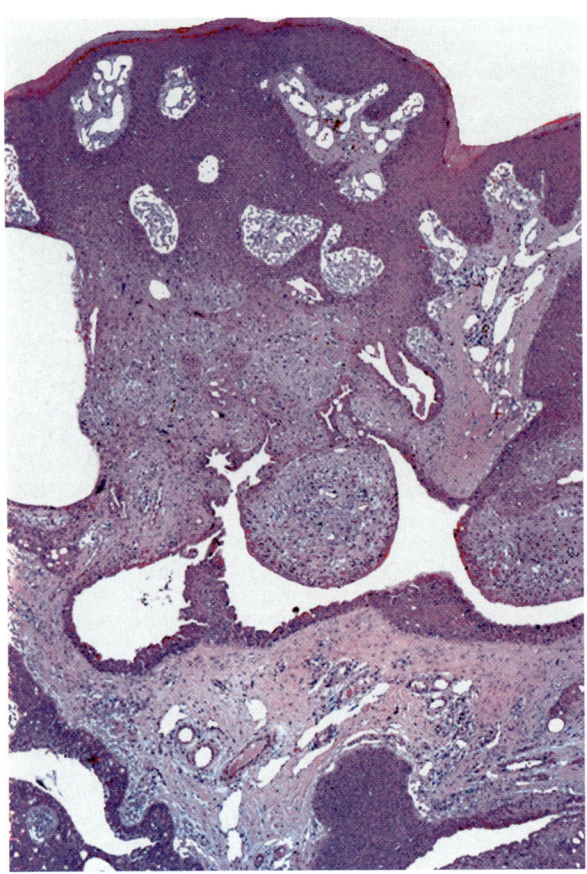

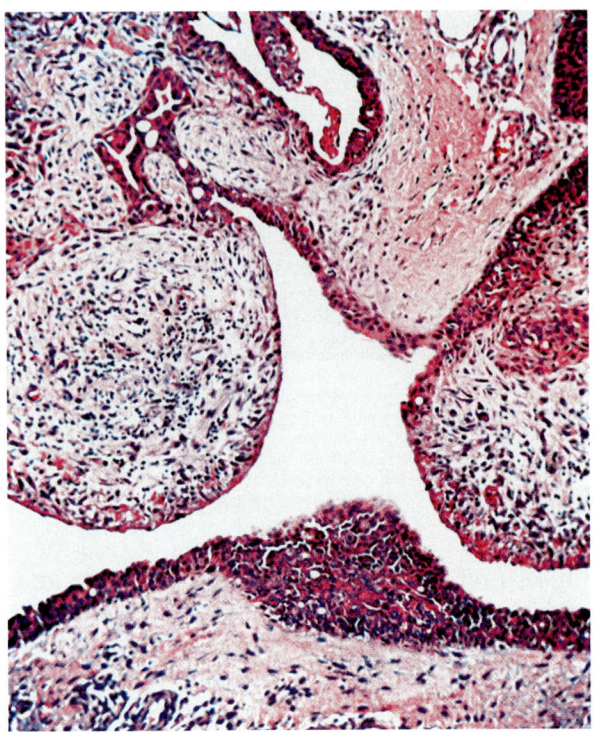

Figure 4-14

ECCRINE SYRINGOFIBROADENOMA

The peculiar interrelationship of epithelium and stroma simulates that seen in fibroadenoma of the breast.

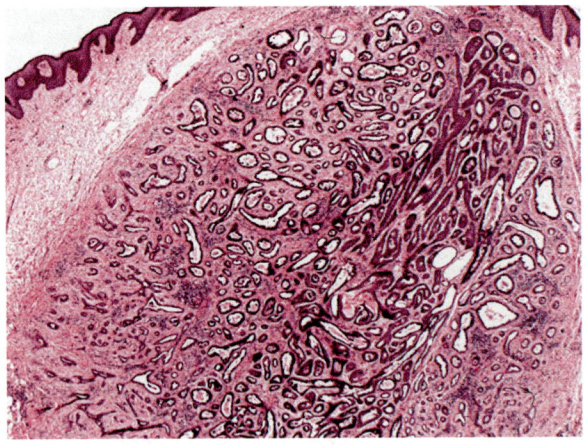

Figure 4-15

PAPILLARY ECCRINE ADENOMA

There is a relatively well-circumscribed proliferation of dermal tubules.

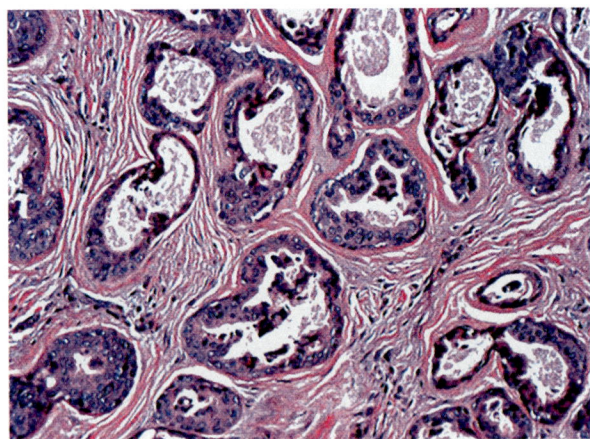

Figure 4-16

PAPILLARY ECCRINE ADENOMA

The tubules of papillary eccrine adenoma contain internal micropapillations, analogous to those seen in intraductal hyperplasia of the breast.

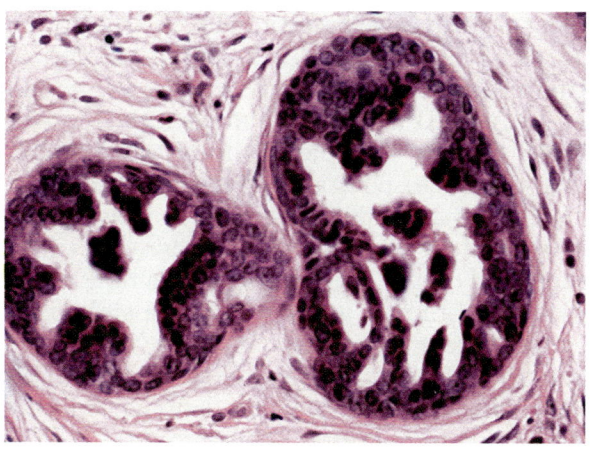

Figure 4-17

PAPILLARY ECCRINE ADENOMA

The bland cytologic characteristics and micropapillary features of papillary eccrine adenoma are shown here.

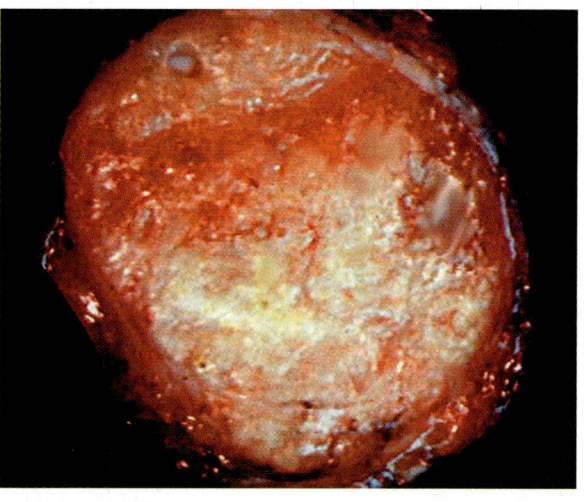

Figure 4-18

ECCRINE ACROSPIROMA

This surgically removed intact eccrine acrospiroma is a nondescript solid nodule from the dermis and subcutis.

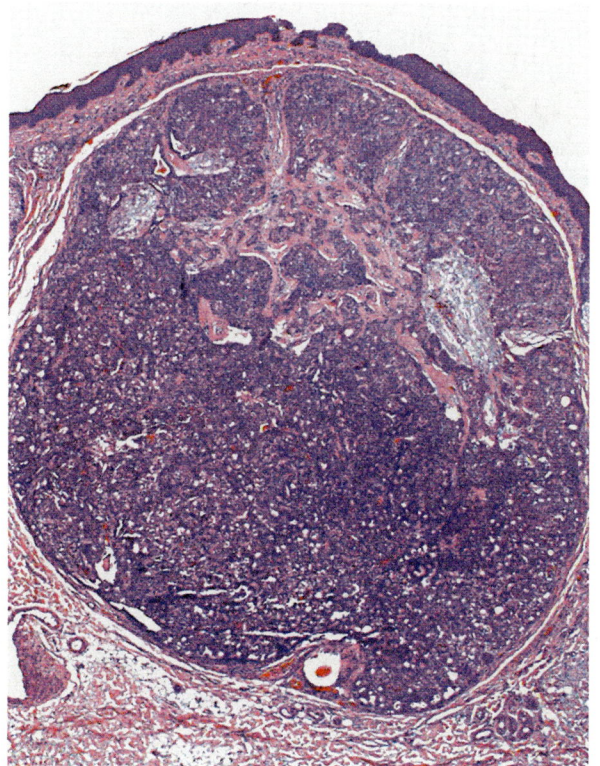
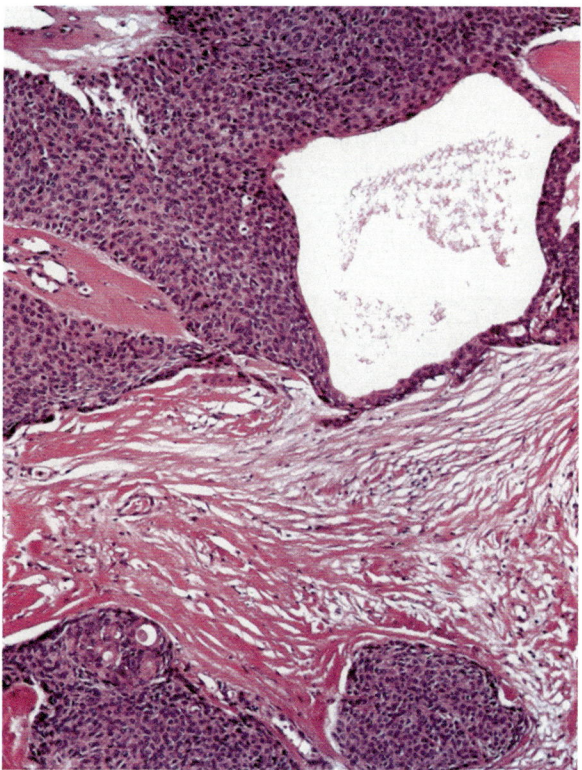

Figure 4-19

ECCRINE ACROSPIROMA

There is a solid, microcystic proliferation of bland epithelial cells in the dermis, with notable circumscription.

4-20) (24,31). Such characteristics led Winkelmann and Wolff (63) to use the designation, *solid and cystic hidradenoma*.

The peripheral aspects of these lesions demonstrate a "pushing" interface with the surrounding dermis, yielding a circumscribed profile. This is a crucial feature for assessing the biologic potential of acrospiromas, because even those that have bland cytologic features may recur if cords of neoplastic cells "bud" into the adjacent dermis (fig. 4-21). In the opinion of the authors, lesions with these attributes should be considered low-grade hidradenocarcinomas. Other features that predict untoward behavior in eccrine acrospiromas include broad zones of clear cell change, diffuse nuclear anaplasia, areas of geographic necrosis, and the presence of tumor giant cells (37). Conversely, squamous metaplasia is common and has no biologic significance. In fact, it was the characteristic used by Stanley and coworkers (53) to define the variant they called "epidermoid hidradenoma." Mitotic figures may sometimes be disturbingly numerous in acrospiromas (fig. 4-22), but, as observed by Cooper (10), they do not equate with malignancy. Focal connections between the dermal components and the epidermis are seen in roughly 50 percent of cases; this observation has resulted in the use of the term "acrospiroma" in reference to a spectrum of neoplasms including tubulopapillary hidradenomas, nodular hidradenomas, and poromas (14).

BENIGN APOCRINE SWEAT GLAND NEOPLASMS

Benign apocrine tumors are less common than eccrine adenomas. Their anatomic distribution is also more limited, principally centering on the head and neck, axilla, groin, and perineum.

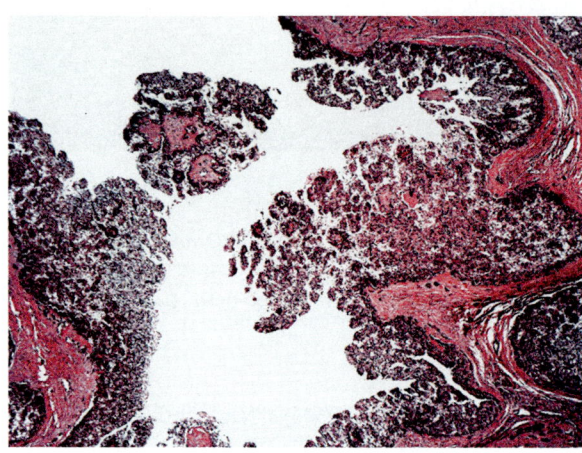

Figure 4-20

ECCRINE ACROSPIROMA

Micropapillary and cystic features are seen in this eccrine acrospiroma, accounting for the synonym of solid and cystic hidradenoma.

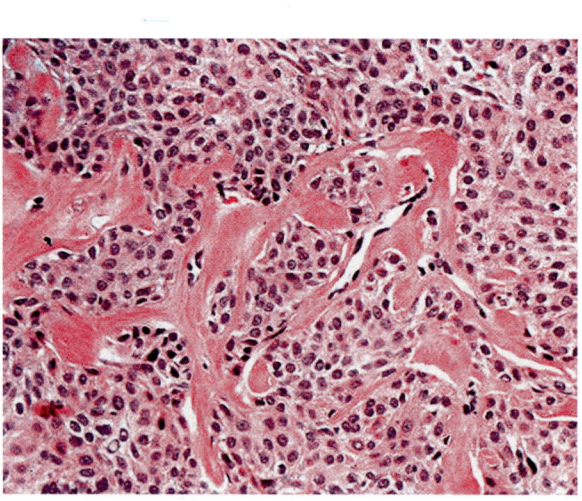
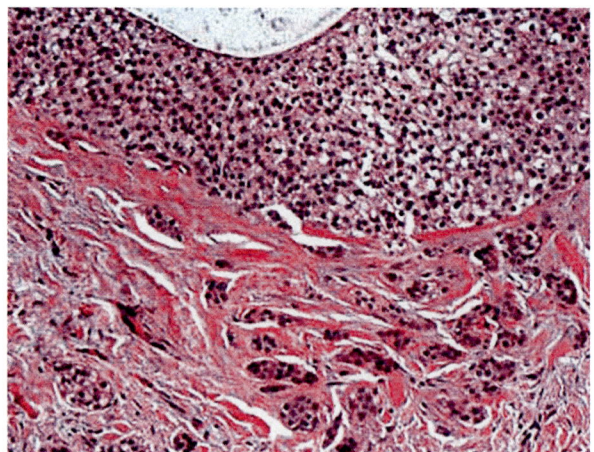

Figure 4-21

ECCRINE ACROSPIROMA

Small irregular epithelial nests "bud" into the surrounding dermis at the lesional periphery. Such a finding equates with a risk of local recurrence and justifies labeling the tumor as low-grade malignant.

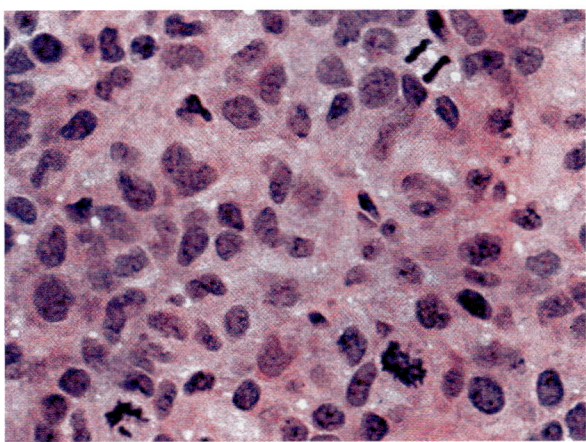

Figure 4-22

ECCRINE ACROSPIROMA

Numerous mitotic figures are present in this otherwise unremarkable acrospiroma. This finding has no biologic importance.

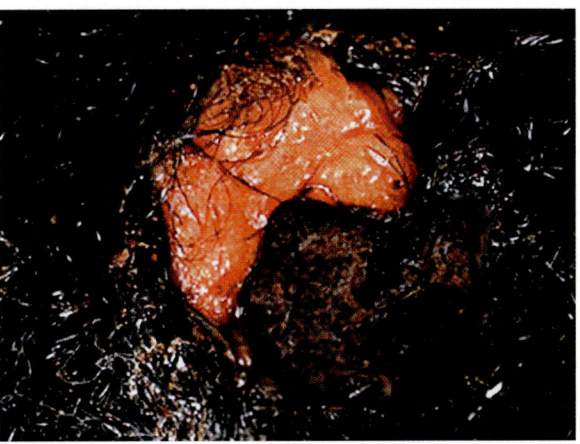

Figure 4-23

SYRINGOCYSTADENOMA PAPILLIFERUM

Syringocystadenoma papilliferum of the scalp appears as a friable reddish nodule.

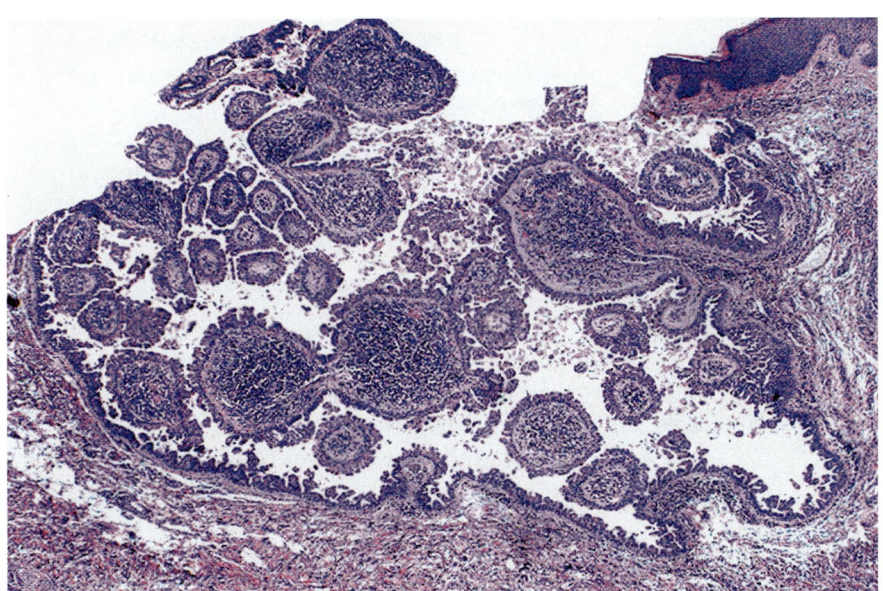

Figure 4-24

SYRINGOCYSTADENOMA PAPILLIFERUM

A micropapillary proliferation sits in a "dell" on the skin surface.

Syringocystadenoma Papilliferum

Clinical Features. *Syringocystadenoma papilliferum* is a distinctive, friable, nodular lesion that is usually encountered in the skin of the head and neck, particularly the scalp (fig. 4-23). It is one of several tumors that may be associated with nevus sebaceus of Jadassohn, but it most often represents a sporadic tumor (21,26,40,43).

Pathologic Findings. The histologic features are singular. The papillary lesion sits in a semicystic "dell" in the skin surface (fig. 4-24). At its interface with the epidermis, keratinocytes give way to aggregates of cuboidal or low columnar glandular cells that show apical decapitation "snouts." These also line micropapillary structures with fibrovascular cores, which are filled with plasmacytes and other chronic inflammatory cells (figs. 4-25, 4-26). Tubular structures are present at the base of the indentation in which the tumor sits; these are dispersed randomly in

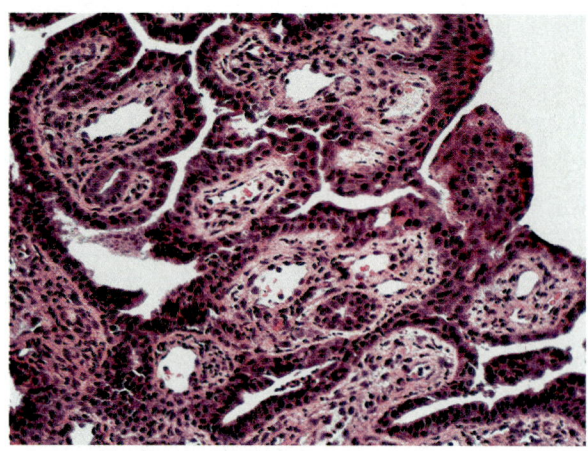

Figure 4-25

SYRINGOCYSTADENOMA PAPILLIFERUM

The micropapillary nature of syringocystadenoma papilliferum is evident.

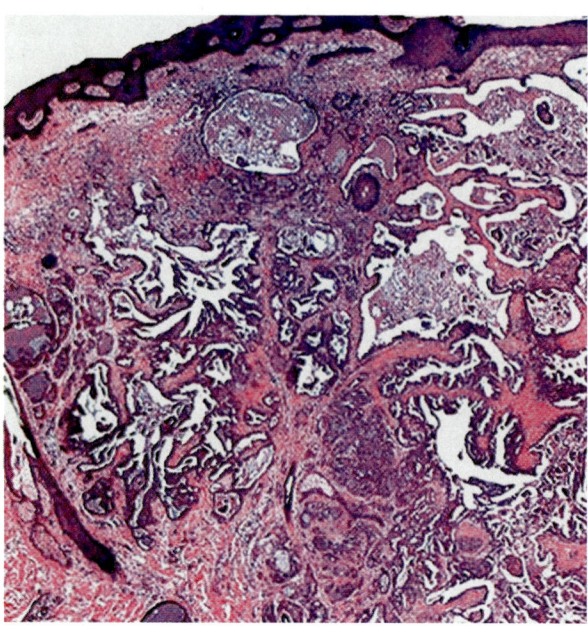

Figure 4-27

HIDRADENOMA PAPILLIFERUM

Intradermal epithelial tubules contain internal micropapillations.

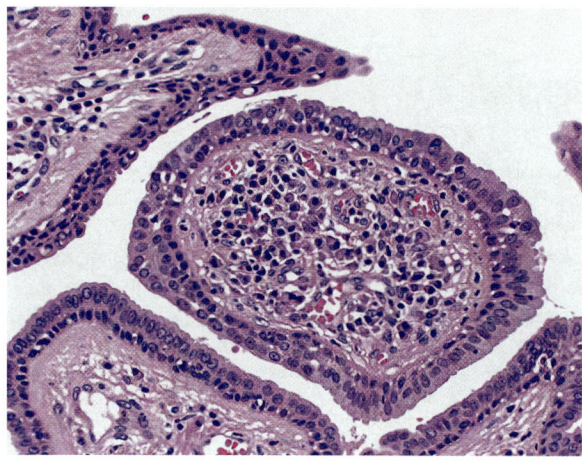

Figure 4-26

SYRINGOCYSTADENOMA PAPILLIFERUM

Plasma cells and other chronic inflammatory elements are usually numerous in the cores of the micropapillae.

the subjacent dermis, but the tumor has a circumscribed image on scanning microscopy. The tumor cells have compact oval nuclei and amphophilic to eosinophilic cytoplasm; mucinous metaplasia may sometimes be seen. Cytologic atypia is variable, but generally is absent or insignificant. Nonetheless, some tumors that have undergone trauma may show an alarming degree of nuclear pleomorphism and mitotic activity. Despite such findings, a well-documented case of malignant transformation in syringo- cystadenoma papilliferum has, in our opinion, not yet been described. Simple excision is adequate therapy.

Hidradenoma Papilliferum

Hidradenoma papilliferum is a nodular, reddish blue dermal tumor that is strictly restricted anatomically to the eyelids, axillae, and genitoperineal skin.

Hidradenoma papilliferum arises in the dermis and demonstrates a central cystic space into which micropapillary proliferations project. The lesion occurs almost exclusively in the genitoperineal skin in women (22,38,41,65); rarely, other examples have been seen elsewhere (48) and the tumor may uncommonly occur in males as well.

The basic configuration of the micropapillary elements is very similar to that seen in syringocystadenoma papilliferum, as described above (figs. 4-27, 4-28A–C). There are, however, more solid cellular foci in hidradenoma papilliferum, with more complex branching and interconnecting papillae; limited extracystic proliferation of tubular cell profiles may also be observed (fig. 4-28D) and no lymphoplasmacytic infiltrates are

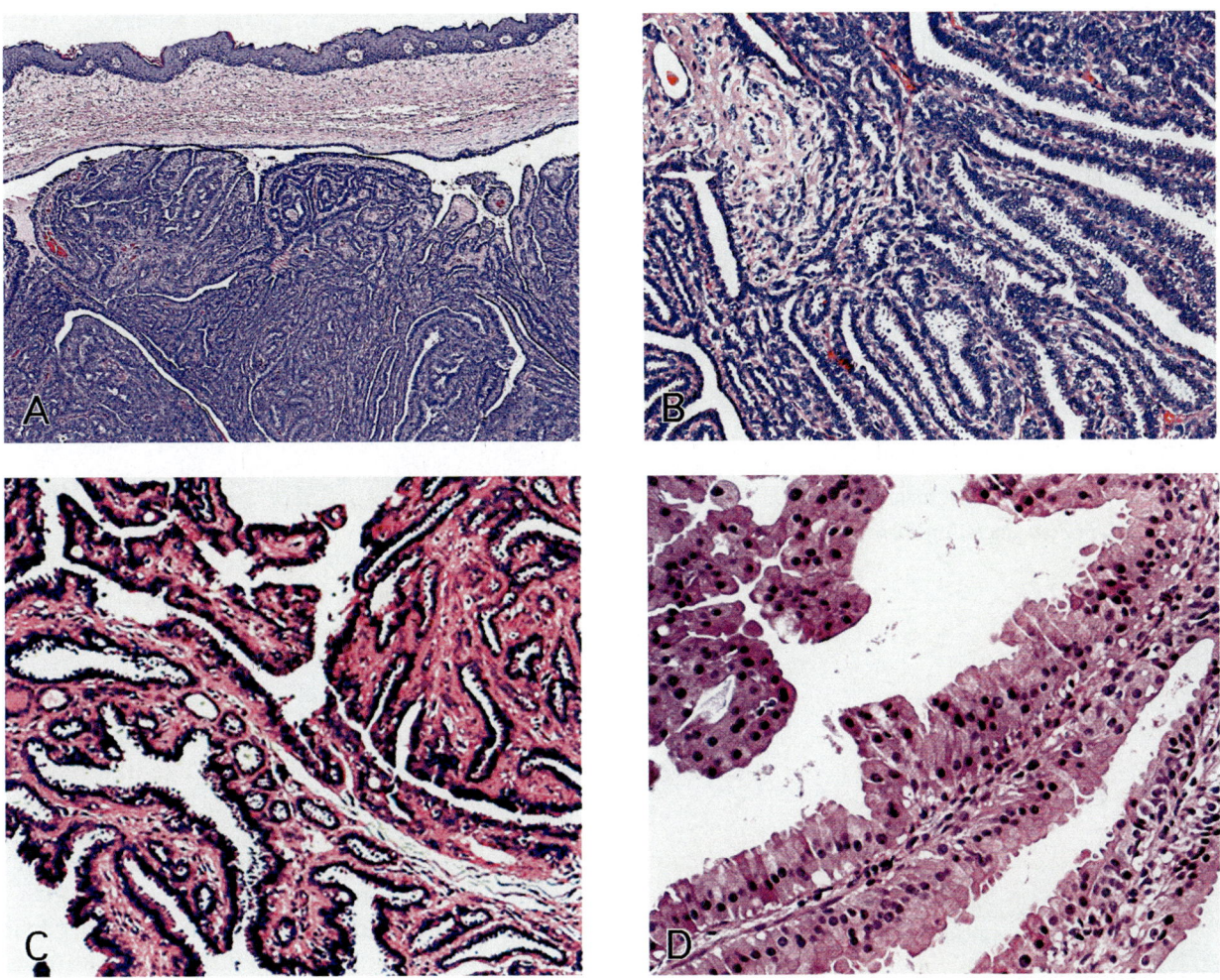

Figure 4-28

HIDRADENOMA PAPILLIFERUM

The micropapillary nature, apocrine "snouts," and limited extracystic growth are seen.

present in the micropapillae. As with syringocystadenoma papilliferum, the cytologic features of traumatized hidradenoma may be worrisome, and may result in the misdiagnosis of the lesion as an adenocarcinoma (52). This error may be circumvented by paying attention to the circumscribed low-power profile of hydradenoma, which typically equates with benignancy.

Tubular Apocrine Adenoma

Tubular apocrine adenoma is basically a synonym for the apocrine counterpart of papillary eccrine adenoma (tubulopapillary hidradenoma; see above), with regard to its clinical features and histologic structure (5,55,56). Occasional tumors have been described using this designation that more closely resemble apocrine versions of acrospiroma (fig. 4-29); such lesions may be labeled *apocrine hidradenomas*.

SWEAT GLAND TUMORS WITH MIXED DIFFERENTIATION

Benign Mixed Tumors of the Skin (Chondroid Syringoma)

Clinical Features. *Cutaneous mixed tumor* (CMT) is seen most often on the head and neck as a unexceptional dermal or subcutaneous nodule (fig. 4-30) (69–71). However, it may be sufficiently chondroid in some cases to have a

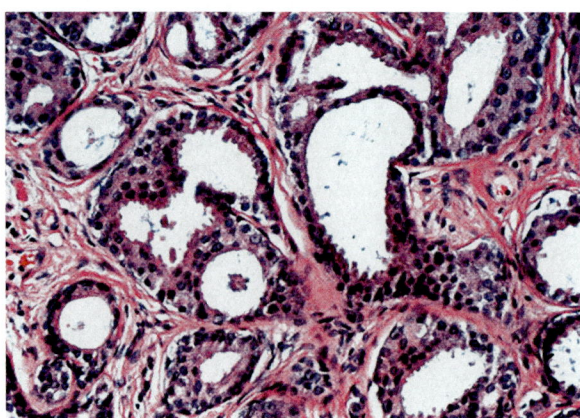

Figure 4-29

TUBULAR APOCRINE ADENOMA

Closely apposed ductal profiles of epithelial cells form luminal snouts.

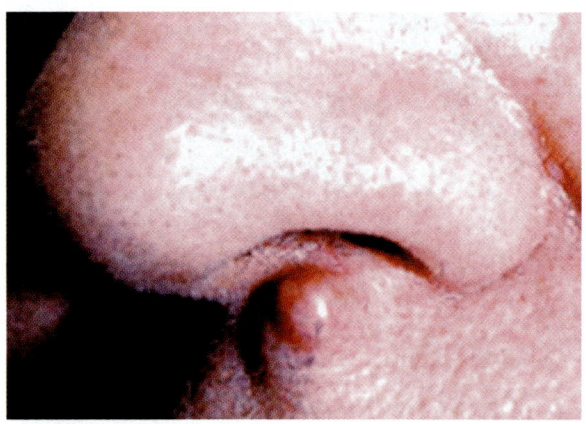
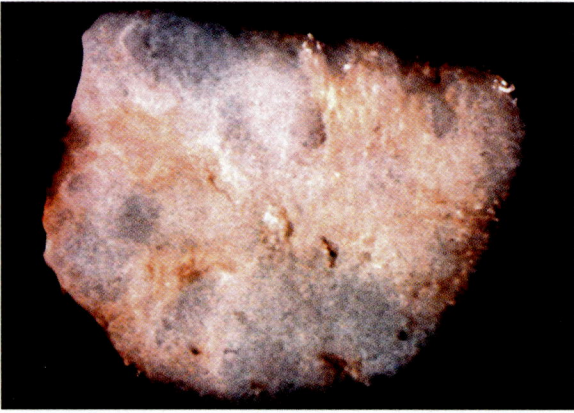

Figure 4-30

CUTANEOUS MIXED TUMOR

Top: The lesion is a firm nodule in the skin of the upper lip. Bottom: The cut surface of the lesion has a bluish white chondroid appearance.

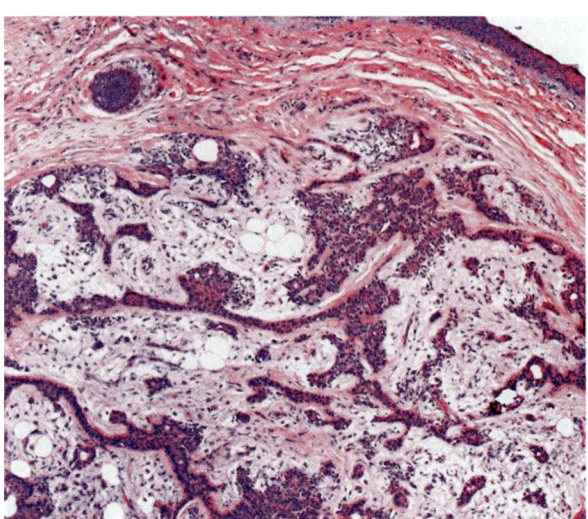

Figure 4-31

CUTANEOUS MIXED TUMOR

Interconnecting cords of lesional epithelial cells embrace mesenchymal-like tumor elements.

distinctly hard consistency on palpation. The potential for formation of a cartilage-like matrix accounts for the historical synonym, *chondroid syringoma*. We do not use this term because CMT is not universally chondroid and it has little clinicopathologic relationship to syringoma.

Pathologic Findings. As a tumor entity, CMT exemplifies a biologic paradigm that is common to many human tumors: the ability for a stem cell population to demonstrate divergent differentiation into dissimilar target tissues (75). Ultrastructural and immunohistochemical studies support the conclusion that all tumor cells in CMT are epithelial in nature (68,72,75,76), but some have acquired the ability for cartilage-like, fibroblastoid, myoid, myoepithelioid, adipocytic, or even osteogenic differentiation. Thus, the pathologist is confronted with a phenotype in which slightly branching tubules and clusters of epithelial cells with variable cytologic appearances (e.g., eccrine, apocrine, sebaceous, pilar, mucinous, simple glandular, or squamoid) are admixed with zones of matrical tissue with diverse mesenchymal images, sometimes all in the same individual lesion (figs. 4-31–4-33) (73,77). The name "mixed tumor" seems particularly apropos in light of these characteristics.

The cytologic characteristics of CMT are typically bland (fig. 4-34), but sometimes prominent

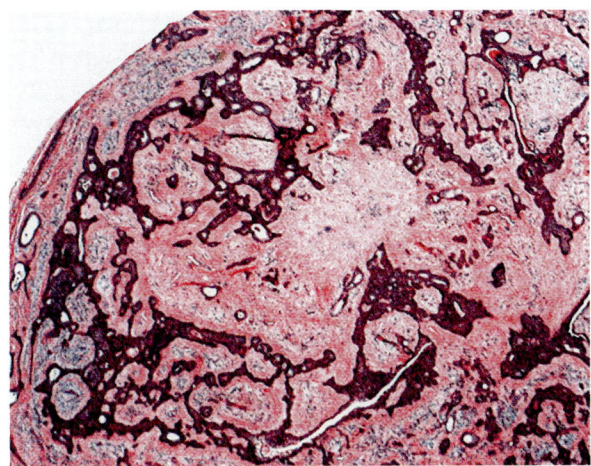

Figure 4-32

CUTANEOUS MIXED TUMOR

Epithelial cords with internal ductal lumens encompass mesenchymal-like neoplastic tissue.

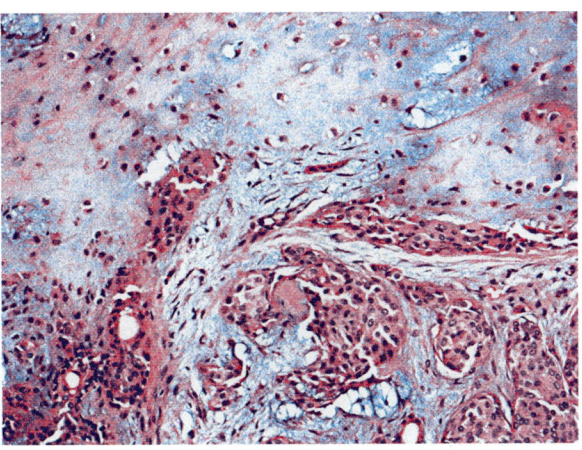

Figure 4-33

CUTANEOUS MIXED TUMOR

The mesenchymal-like elements are chondroid in nature in this example.

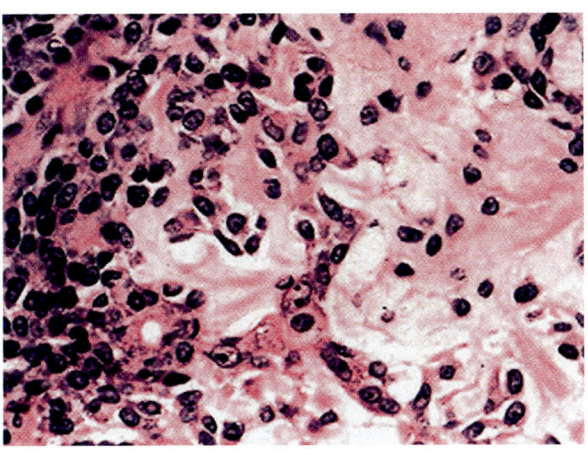

Figure 4-34

CUTANEOUS MIXED TUMOR

The cytologic features of cutaneous mixed tumor are bland.

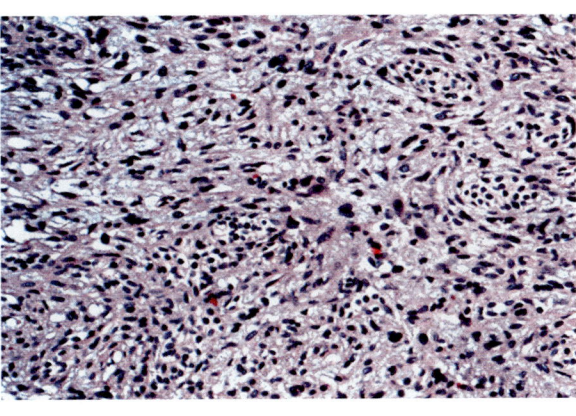

Figure 4-35

CUTANEOUS MIXED TUMOR

Extensive spindle cell change has led some observers to designate such lesions as myoepitheliomas of the skin.

nucleoli and mitotic activity can be seen in the overtly epithelial component. If the overall image is that of a well-circumscribed (but potentially multinodular) tumor, the atypical findings just mentioned are of no consequence. Similar comments apply to lesions with focally or globally dense spindle cell growth or clear cell change, some of which have been called *myoepithelioma* of the skin (fig. 4-35) (67).

Differential Diagnosis. The entities in the differential diagnosis include true chondroma, osteoma, or mesenchymal hamartoma of the skin. These are discussed elsewhere in this monograph.

Other Mixed Lineage Adnexal Tumors

Those observers with experience in examining appendageal skin tumors are accustomed to seeing lesions that are benign, but with more than one avenue of epithelial differentiation. Mixtures of eccrine and apocrine, sudoriferous and pilar, pilar and sebaceous, or sweat glandular and sebaceous tissues may be seen in such

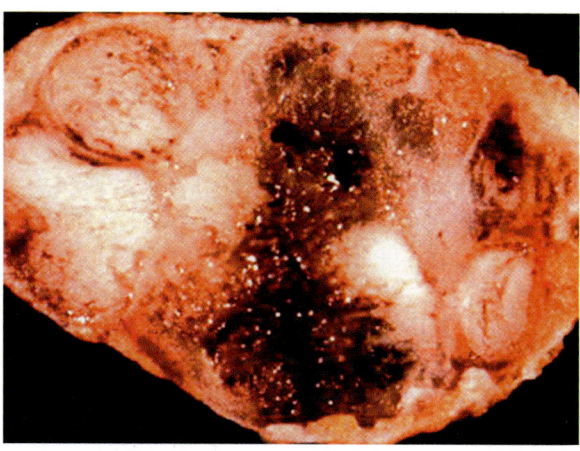

Figure 4-36

ECCRINE POROCARCINOMA OF THE FOOT

Internal hemorrhage and necrosis are seen in this surgical pathology specimen.

neoplasms. We prefer the generic labels of "adnexal adenoma with divergent differentiation" or "mixed sweat gland adenoma" (74) as appropriate diagnostic labels for these lesions. One can then provide their histologic details in a commentary, and offer opinions, if necessary, on which standard appendageal neoplasm is most closely related to them nosologically.

MALIGNANT SWEAT GLAND TUMORS

In the last several decades, there has been a good deal of revision in defining sweat gland carcinomas. Metastasis is no longer required as the only reliable marker of aggressiveness in adnexal skin tumors, because several histologic factors are known to be useful as prospective predictors of such behavior. The classification of carcinomas of the sweat glands can be approached in a broad way or by the use of detailed categories. Because differential diagnostic considerations vary in regard to the specific microscopic features of these tumors, we prefer to use relatively detailed but largely descriptive terms for these subtypes.

Eccrine Carcinomas

The best biologic model for understanding the scope of cutaneous eccrine malignancies is the spectrum of carcinoma morphotypes that are seen in the female breast (149). This similarity should be expected, because the mammary glands are a large and somewhat specialized form of the sudoriferous apparatus. It is, therefore, logical for pathologists to apply a nomenclatural system to sweat gland carcinomas which approximates that used for breast cancer.

Some malignant adnexal tumors have clinicopathologic features that attest to their primary nature in the skin, but others are morphologically indistinguishable from metastases to the integument from visceral neoplasms. These two major subgroups are considered below.

Eccrine Carcinomas that Are Histologically Definable as Primary Tumors

Eccrine Porocarcinoma. *Clinical Features.* Eccrine porocarcinoma is seen principally in acral skin sites, in adults, as a potentially ulcerated dermal nodule (fig. 4-36). Children are also occasionally affected.

Eccrine porocarcinoma is closely related to poroma. It differs from the latter by the presence of infiltrative, desmoplastic growth; tumor necrosis; cytologic anaplasia; extensive clear cell change; and perineural or vascular invasion (figs. 4-37, 4-38) (87,110,141,152,159, 168,172,178,193). Not all of these characteristics need be present to assign a diagnosis of malignancy, and infiltrative growth is usually a sufficient indicator.

Pathologic Findings. Invasive porocarcinoma has both acrosyringium-like and dermal components. A solely *intraepidermal* variant of this tumor has been recognized, which, in the past, was called "malignant hidroacanthoma simplex" (fig. 4-39, top) (79,124,145,146); it falls into the category of Borst-Jadassohn lesions. As such, it has a clonal, micronodular growth pattern, and is composed of atypical polygonal cells in the surface epithelium. The overall image is represented by nests of tumor cells that are sharply separated from the adjacent epidermis. It is often necessary to perform immunostains for such markers as carcinoembryonic antigen (CEA) or S-100 protein to recognize intraepidermal porocarcinoma, which is potentially reactive for either or both of these markers (174).

Differential Diagnosis. Other entities in the differential diagnosis (Bowen's disease, seborrheic keratosis, and melanoma in situ) have dissimilar immunophenotypes (114). Porocarcinoma, squamous cell carcinoma in situ, and seborrheic

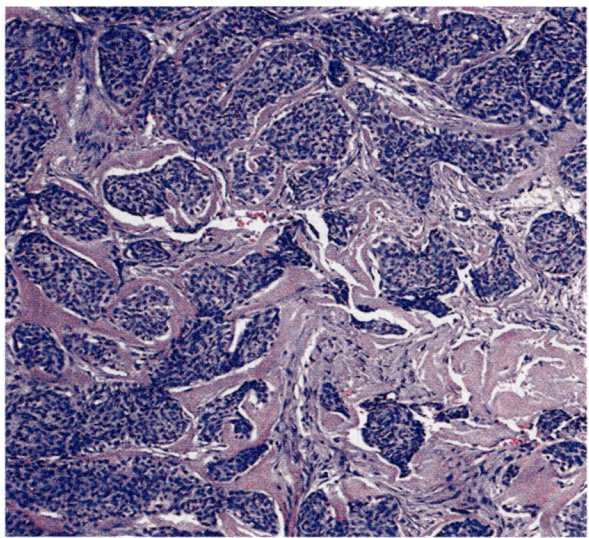

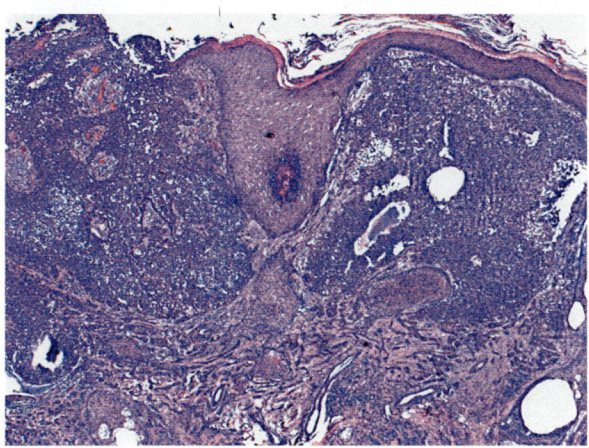

Figure 4-37

ECCRINE POROCARCINOMA

The epidermis is penetrated by cords of tumor cells which simulate the normal acrosyringia. The lesion is irregularly invasive in the dermis and shows cytologic atypia.

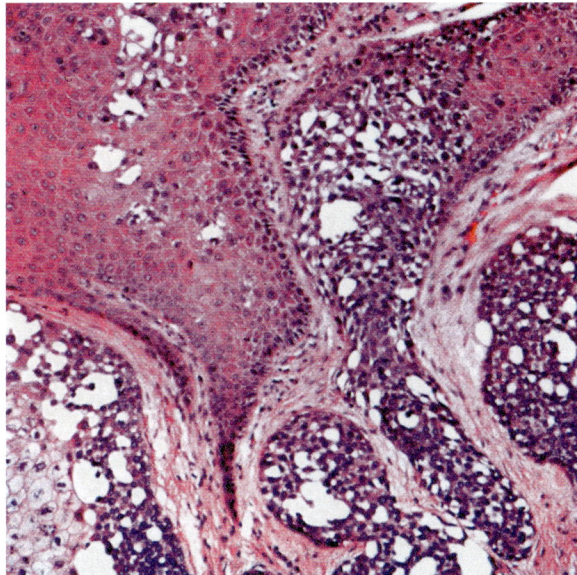

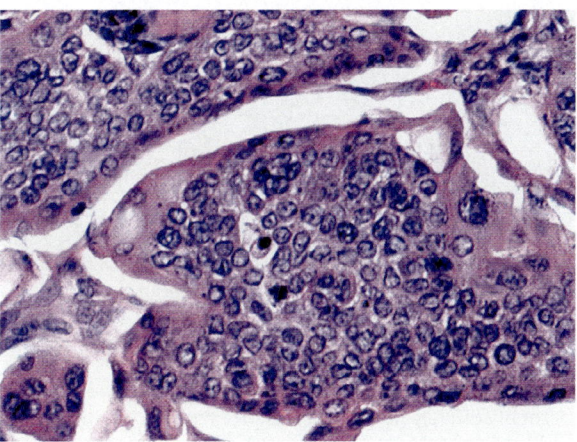

Figure 4-38

ECCRINE POROCARCINOMA

The architectural and cytologic atypia of eccrine porocarcinoma are shown.

keratosis are all positive for keratin, but only porocarcinoma demonstrates CEA, S-100 protein, or both. In contrast, melanoma is keratin negative. The scattering of single malignant cells throughout the epidermis, as seen in Paget's disease of the skin or amelanotic malignant melanoma, is not a feature of porocarcinoma. That is an important observation in cases of porocarcinoma where the neoplastic cells contain melanin (fig. 4-39, bottom), a well-recognized but rare capability of that tumor (115).

The particular microscopic features of eccrine porocarcinoma make the diagnosis of a primary skin tumor likely on pathologic grounds. It is true that examples of metastatic carcinoma in the skin demonstrate limited intraepidermal growth (135), but this phenomenon is rare.

Mucinous Eccrine Carcinoma. *Clinical Features.* Mucinous eccrine carcinoma (MEC) is a type of sweat gland carcinoma that has no benign counterpart. It is comparable histologically to mucinous (colloid) carcinoma of the breast or gastrointestinal tract. Therefore, when this tumor is seen in the skin, it often causes concern over the possibility of metastasis from one of these

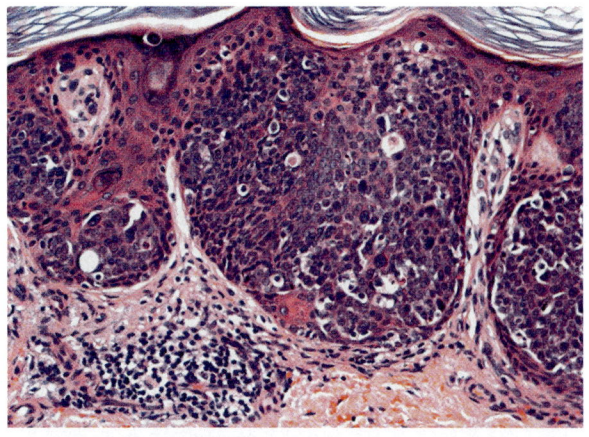

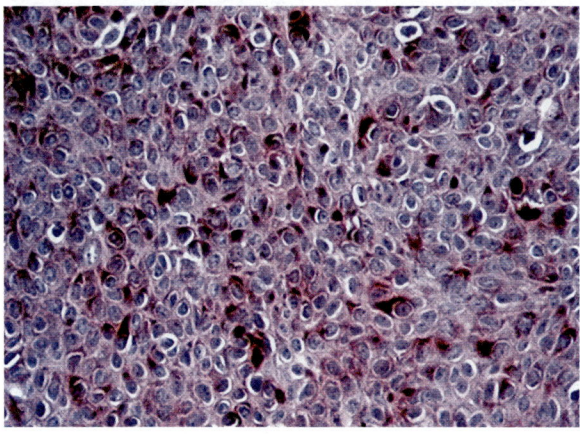

Figure 4-39

INTRAEPIDERMAL POROCARCINOMA

Top: There is marked nuclear anaplasia in an architecturally discrete intraepidermal proliferation of tumor cells.
Bottom: Melanin pigment is seen in another case.

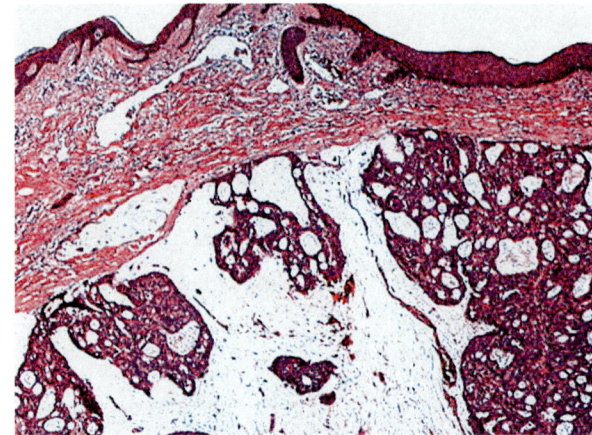

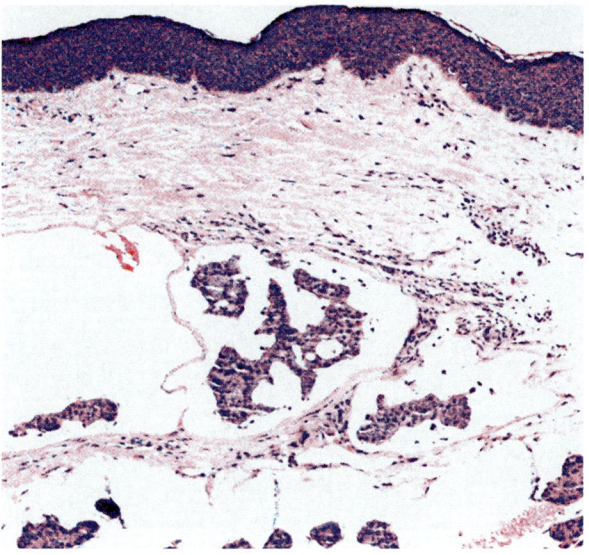

Figure 4-40

MUCINOUS ECCRINE CARCINOMA

Nests and tubules of relatively bland cuboidal tumor cells are suspended in abundant extracellular mucinous matrix.

lesions in the viscera. At a practical level, however, this is not a tenable possibility. Colloid carcinoma of the breast, stomach, or intestine does not involve the skin unless the patient has obvious and disseminated disease (158); i.e., these tumors lack the ability to selectively affect the dermis early in their development. The histologic image of MEC confidently diagnoses this cutaneous lesion as a primary neoplasm.

Pathologic Findings. MEC contains large, dermal, extracellular pools of epithelial mucin, in which rounded or irregular nests and slightly branching cords of polyhedral tumor cells are present (figs. 4-40, 4-41). The overall profile is infiltrative (107,109,112,126,142,150,156,163, 196). Nuclei are generally oval, with dispersed chromatin and small nucleoli; the cytoplasm is amphophilic or slightly eosinophilic and may be vacuolated. Mitotic figures are not numerous, and vascular or neural invasion is relatively uncommon. The mucin in MEC is strongly labeled by the mucicarmine or diastase-digested periodic acid–Schiff (PAS-D) method (fig. 4-42), but it is also decorated by the colloidal iron or Alcian blue techniques (142).

Differential Diagnosis. The most significant differential diagnostic consideration is a hypermyxoid cutaneous mixed tumor. The distinction between these lesions is usually made easily,

Neoplasms and Pseudoneoplastic Proliferations of the Sweat Glands

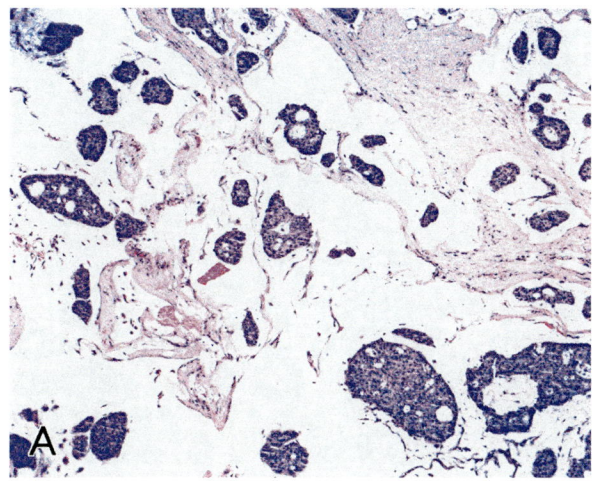
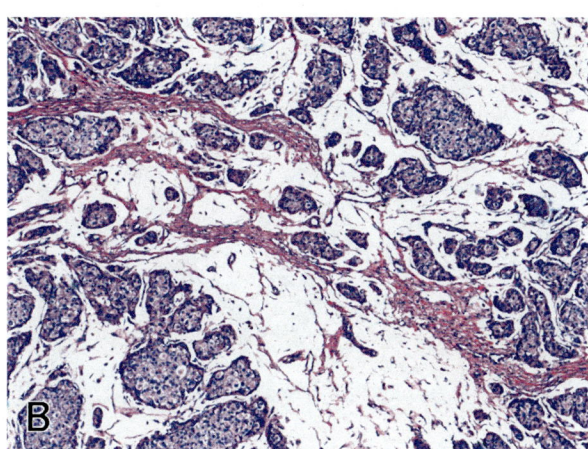
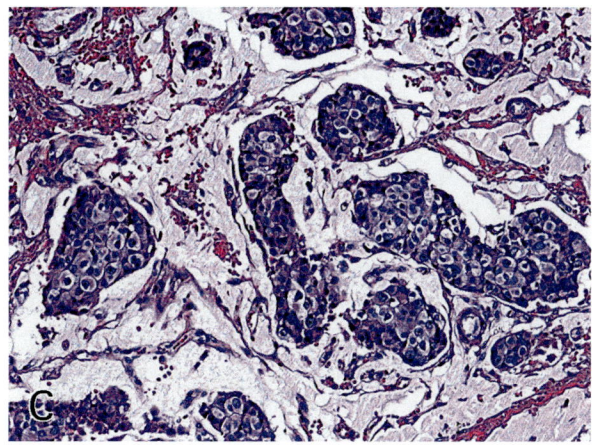

Figure 4-41
MUCINOUS ECCRINE CARCINOMA
Cords and nests of tumor cells are present within a richly mucinous stroma.

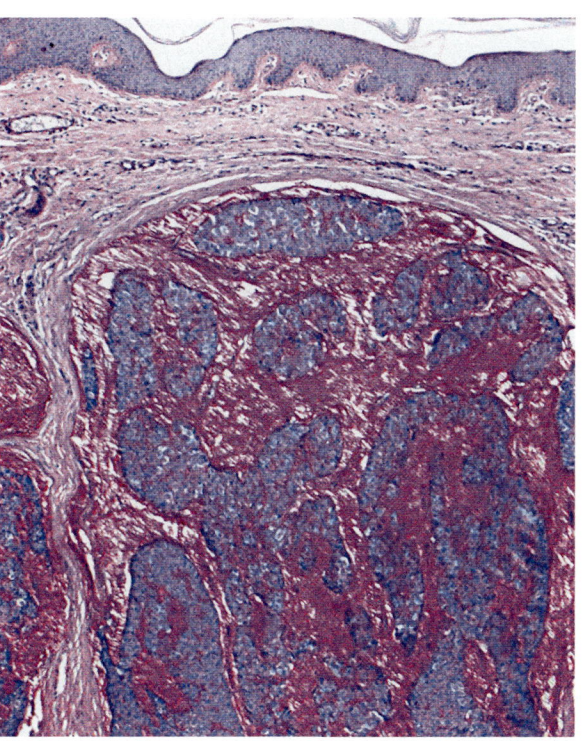

Figure 4-42
MUCINOUS ECCRINE CARCINOMA
The mucicarmine method labels the stroma.

because the mesenchymoid zones of mixed tumors contain fusiform stromal cells, contrasting with the acellular nature of mucin pools in MEC.

Adenoid Cystic Carcinoma of the Skin. *Clinical Features.* Adenoid cystic carcinoma (ACC) is a tumor type that is common to several organs and tissues, including the salivary glands, respiratory tract, breast, skin, uterine cervix, and prostate gland. In each of these locations, the usual evolution of the tumor is that of slow growth but with aggressive local behavior. Metastatic spread to other sites occurs late in the clinical course, if at all; therefore, for the pragmatic reasons cited in connection with MEC, ACC in the skin can reasonably be considered to represent a primary tumor whenever it is observed.

Pathologic Findings. This neoplasm is felt to show eccrine differentiation; it is composed of monomorphic basaloid cells arranged in tubules, elongated nests, and cords. Ductal lumens may be present, as may cylinders of lightly basophilic mucoid matrix. Another common finding is the deposition of linear profiles or globules

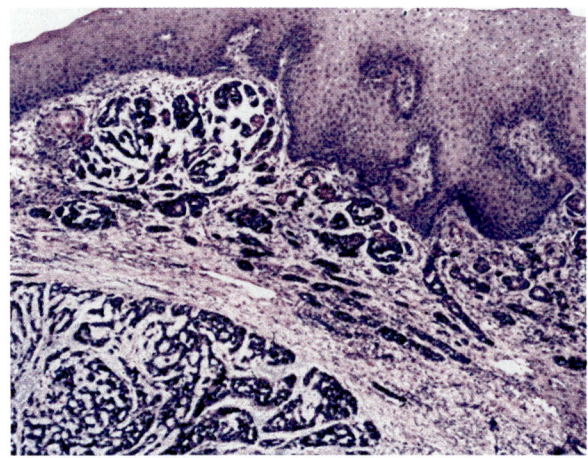

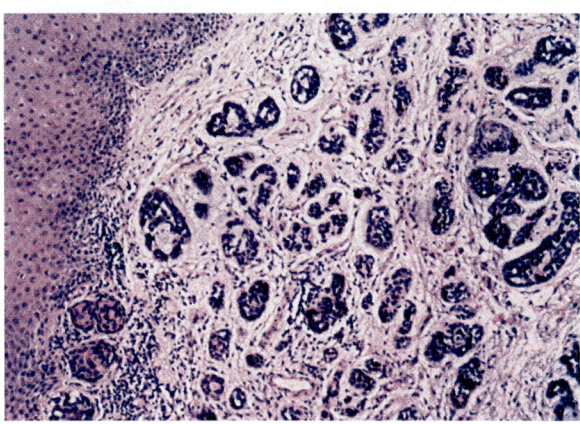

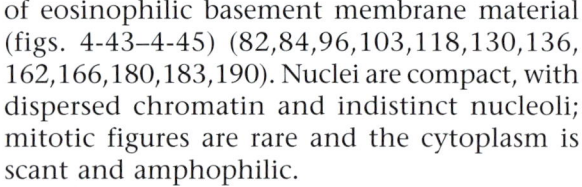

Figure 4-43

ADENOID CYSTIC CARCINOMA

Infiltrative cords, tubules, and lumen-forming profiles of compact and uniform polygonal cells are seen in the dermis.

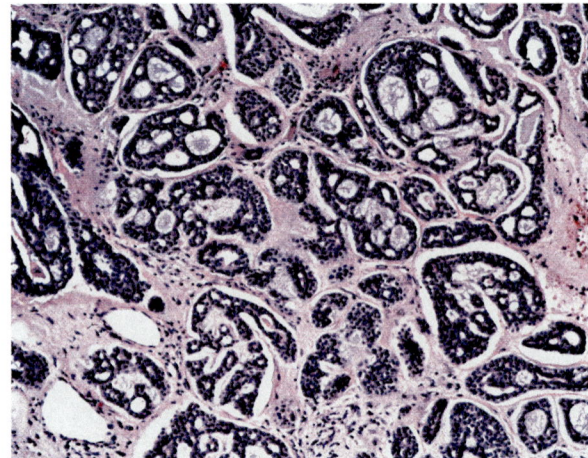

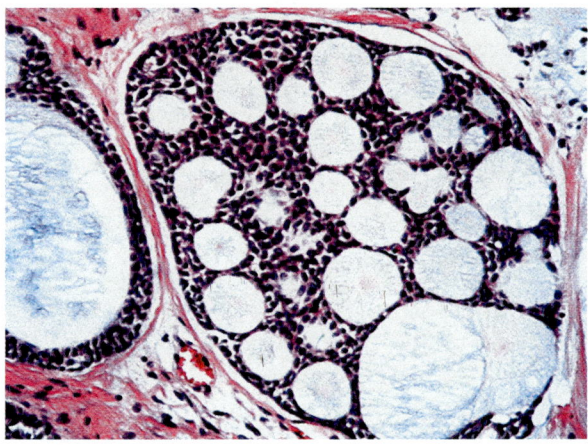

Figure 4-44

ADENOID CYSTIC CARCINOMA

The tubular and cribriform growth patterns of adenoid cystic carcinoma are shown here.

of eosinophilic basement membrane material (figs. 4-43–4-45) (82,84,96,103,118,130,136, 162,166,180,183,190). Nuclei are compact, with dispersed chromatin and indistinct nucleoli; mitotic figures are rare and the cytoplasm is scant and amphophilic.

Differential Diagnosis. The dermal stroma surrounding clusters of tumor cells in ACC lacks the retraction artifact and fibromyxoid alteration that is seen in adenoid basal cell carcinomas (BCC), which otherwise resembles the former tumor type (190). The growth pattern of both ACC and adenoid BCC is infiltrative, and involvement of vascular adventitia and perineural spaces is potentially seen in both. Points of difference include the regular presence of apoptotic cells in the center of tumor cell nests in adenoid BCC, as well as foci of en masse necrosis; neither of those features is seen in ACC. Furthermore, BCCs commonly exhibit multilinear differentiation (e.g., a mixture of adenoid and pilar-keratotic foci), and they may contain true melanin pigment. Such characteristics are again absent in ACC. Whenever it is needed, immunostaining is capable of distinguishing between these tumors: adenoid BCC is negative for epithelial membrane antigen (EMA), whereas ACC consistently expresses that glycoprotein (190). Conversely, ACC can be labeled for CD117 (122), but that determinant has not yet been studied in BCC of the skin.

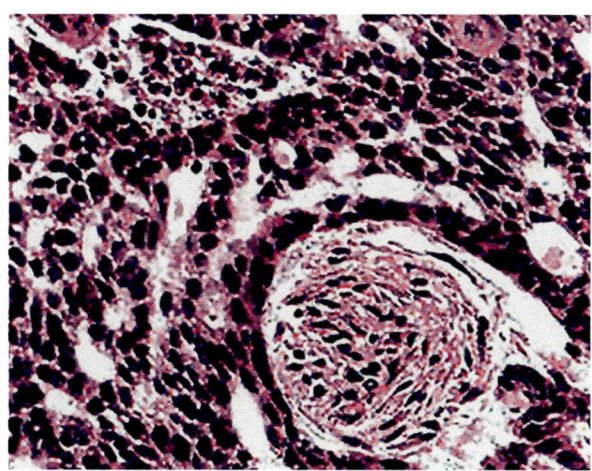

Figure 4-45

ADENOID CYSTIC CARCINOMA

Perineural invasion is common in adenoid cystic carcinoma of the skin.

Papillary Digital Eccrine Adenocarcinoma.
Clinical Features. A distinctive group of eccrine neoplasms is unique to the distal extremities, particularly the digits (125). These lesions were originally segregated into two groups, *aggressive digital papillary adenomas* and *aggressive digital papillary adenocarcinomas,* but current thinking suggests that they represent points in a continuum of universally malignant neoplasms. We prefer the more unifying term of *papillary digital eccrine adenocarcinoma* (PDEA). The features of PDEA are similar to those of invasive papillary large duct carcinoma of the female breast. However, because the latter lesion never involves the skin unless and until it metastasizes widely, a cutaneous tumor with the configuration of papillary adenocarcinoma is probably a primary tumor.

Pathologic Findings. PDEA features the formation of macropapillae projecting into large cystic spaces. Solid nests and tubules of polygonal cells regularly infiltrate the surrounding dermis and subcutis (figs. 4-46–4-49). The underlying bone may sometimes be involved (fig. 4-50). The nuclear characteristics are bimorphic: one subgroup of PDEAs (formerly called aggressive papillary digital "adenomas") shows dispersed chromatin, small or indistinct nucleoli, and limited mitotic activity (125,170), and are biologically low grade; the second variant (formerly aggres-

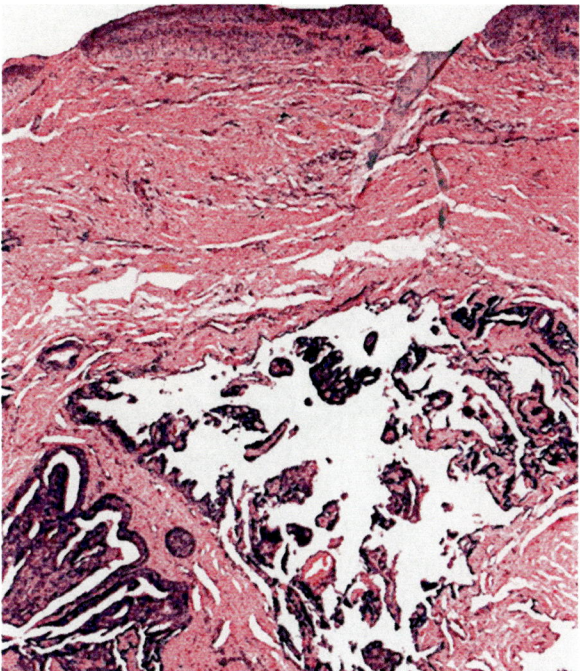
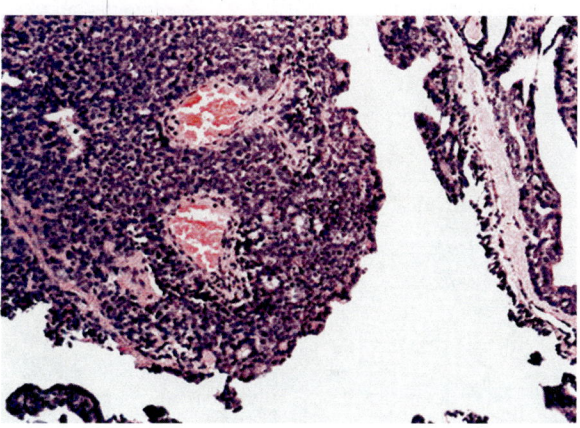

Figure 4-46

PAPILLARY DIGITAL ECCRINE ADENOCARCINOMA

Macropapillary profiles of tumor cells project into cystic spaces.

sive digital papillary "adenocarcinomas") shows greater cellularity, vesicular nuclei, prominent nucleoli, numerous mitotic figures, and foci of geographic necrosis (fig. 4-51) (125), and are high-grade tumors. Perineural and lymphatic invasion can be seen regardless of tumor grade, but, in our experience, only poorly differentiated tumors metastasize distantly. Squamous metaplasia and clear ovoid cells are seen more often in low-grade than high-grade PDEA (fig. 4-52).

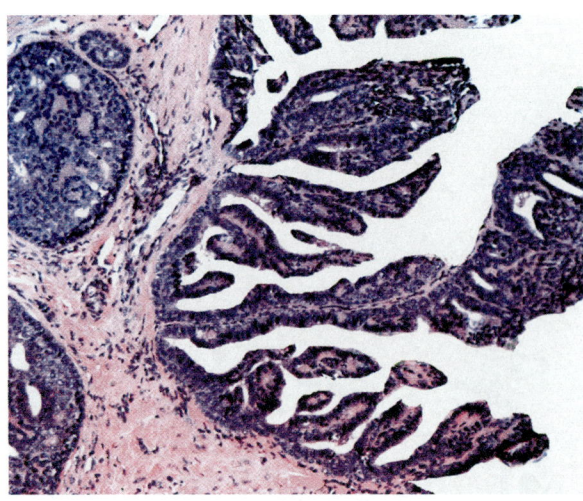

Figure 4-47

PAPILLARY DIGITAL ECCRINE ADENOCARCINOMA
The macropapillae resemble those seen in papillary carcinoma of the breast.

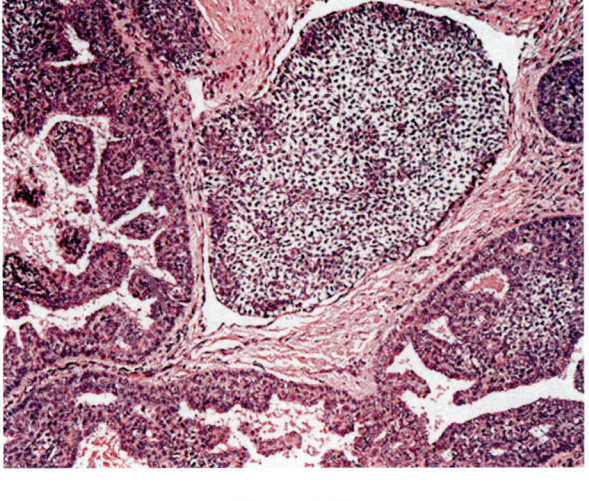

Figure 4-48

PAPILLARY DIGITAL ECCRINE ADENOCARCINOMA
Foci of solid cellular growth and clear cell change are present.

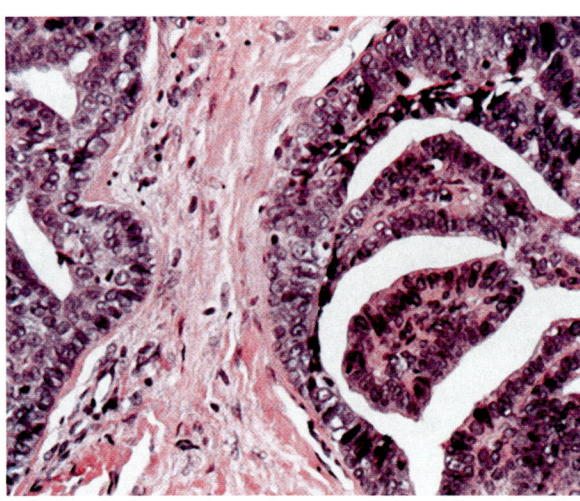

Figure 4-49

PAPILLARY DIGITAL ECCRINE ADENOCARCINOMA
Nuclei in low-grade papillary digital eccrine adenocarcinoma are relatively uniform in size and shape; necrosis and atypical mitoses are absent.

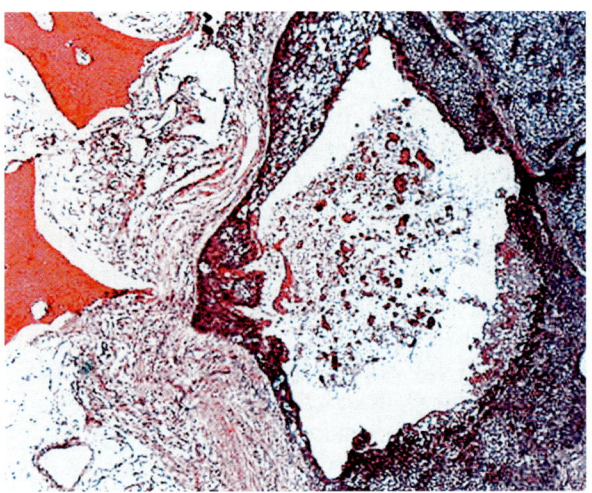

Figure 4-50

PAPILLARY DIGITAL ECCRINE ADENOCARCINOMA
All papillary digital eccrine adenocarcinomas may invade the subjacent bone of the fingers and toes, as shown here.

Differential Diagnosis. One plausible histologic differential diagnostic alternative to PDEA is hidradenoma papilliferum, but the latter lesion is never observed on the digits and a malignant form of it has never been documented convincingly. Despite having a name that is similar to that of PDEA, papillary eccrine adenoma forms micropapillae that project into tubular lumens (170) rather than containing macropapillae and cystic spaces. The comparative but dissimilar images of these two skin tumors correspond respectively to intraductal hyperplasia and papillary carcinoma of the breast.

Microcystic Adnexal Carcinoma (Sclerosing Sweat Duct Carcinoma). *Clinical Features.*

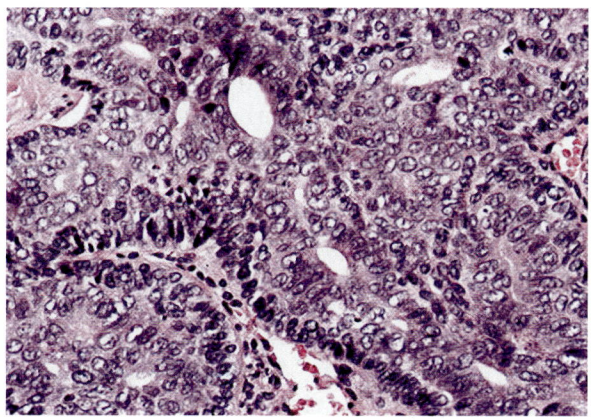

Figure 4-51

PAPILLARY DIGITAL ECCRINE ADENOCARCINOMA
High-grade papillary digital eccrine adenocarcinoma shows greater cellular density and more nuclear atypia than the low-grade form. Necrosis is also common.

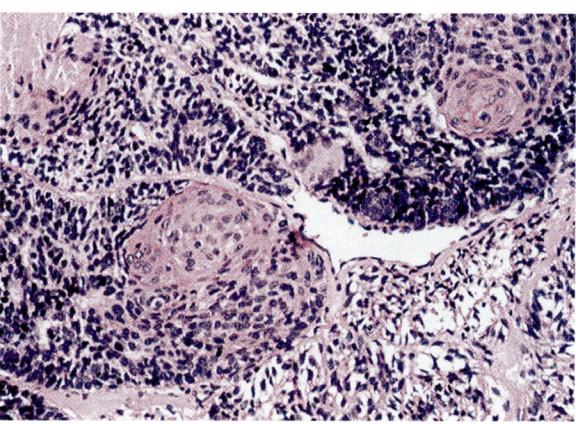

Figure 4-52

PAPILLARY DIGITAL ECCRINE ADENOCARCINOMA
Clear cell change, squamous metaplasia, and necrosis are present in this high-grade papillary digital eccrine adenocarcinoma.

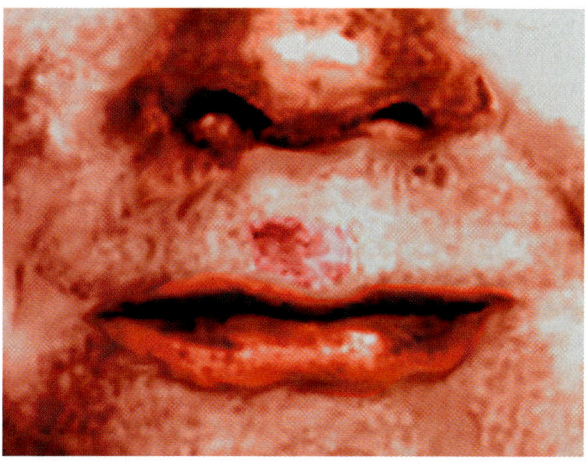

Figure 4-53

MICROCYSTIC ADNEXAL CARCINOMA
Microcystic adnexal carcinoma in the skin of the upper lip in an elderly woman is represented by an ill-defined reddish plaque.

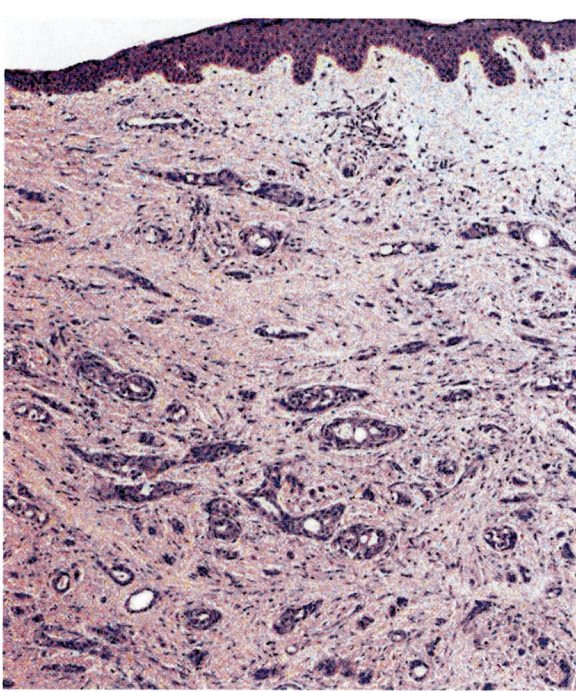

Figure 4-54

MICROCYSTIC ADNEXAL CARCINOMA
This microcystic adnexal carcinoma infiltrates throughout the whole dermis.

Microcystic adnexal carcinoma (MAC) is an unusual tumor of the skin that is encountered principally as a cutaneous plaque in middle-aged patients, usually women. The tumor shows a strong predilection for the facial skin (fig. 4-53).

Pathologic Findings. MAC demonstrates a bland syringoma-like profile, lacking nucleoli and mitotic activity, and infiltrates the dermis and subcutis randomly and often deeply (figs. 4-54, 4-55) (111). Tumors are occasionally punctuated by microcystic arrays containing pilar-type (trichilemmal) keratin (fig. 4-56, left). The name microcystic adnexal carcinoma was chosen to describe this lesion, and we believe that it has mixed eccrine and pilar differentiation (147,186). An alternate synonym, *sclerosing sweat duct carcinoma*, has also been used for a variant that lacks pilar microcysts (95,99); this subtype was termed *anaplastic syringoma* or *syringoid carcinoma* in the prior literature (fig. 4-56, right) (83,133).

Infiltration of perineural sheaths, vascular adventitia, and even subjacent muscle is common (fig. 4-57) (81,94,98,120,132,139,164,182). The neoplastic cells may focally form whorled, concentric dermal profiles. Luminal secretory material can be seen in the tubular cellular profiles (99). Clear cell change also has been described (161); this feature links MAC to low-grade clear cell carcinoma, as documented by Cooper and colleagues (100). Another variant shows a predominance of keratinous microcysts, simulating trichoadenoma of Nikolowsky (94), but it differs from the latter lesion in containing syringoid cell profiles and showing infiltrative growth. Occasional examples of MAC demonstrate sebaceous foci (fig. 4-58) as well as eccrine and pilar elements (132).

Differential Diagnosis. The differential diagnosis does not include metastatic carcinomas of visceral origin, which show more confined growth and cytologic anaplasia. Instead, other skin lesions that must be considered include conventional syringoma, desmoplastic trichoepithelioma, morpheaform BCC, trichoadenoma, and primary adenosquamous carcinoma of the skin.

Conventional syringoma and desmoplastic trichoepithelioma both are separable from MAC on clinical grounds. All three are usually facial lesions, but syringoma and desmoplastic trichoepithelioma are small, exquisitely circumscribed, and papulonodular, whereas MAC is ill-defined and plaque-like (91,99). Microscopically, the former lesions are broader than they are deep, with sharply defined peripheries. On the other hand, MAC extends to the base of biopsy specimens and "shades off" into the surrounding tissue (fig. 4-59) (91). Diagnostic

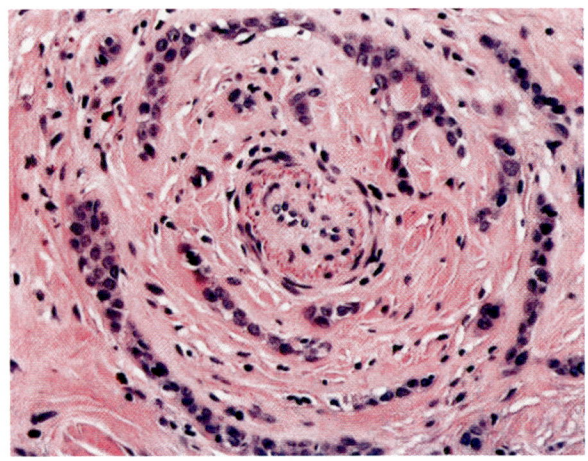

Figure 4-55
MICROCYSTIC ADNEXAL CARCINOMA
Profiles of tumor cells are in the deep dermis.

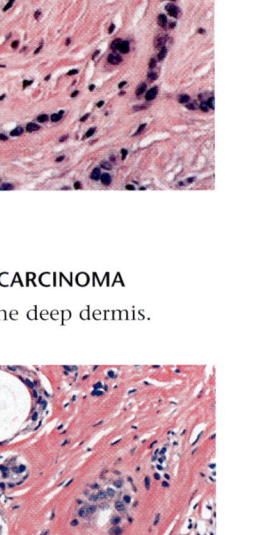
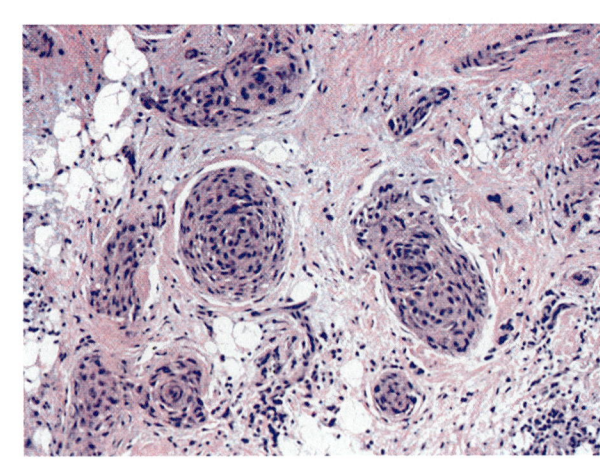

Figure 4-56
MICROCYSTIC ADNEXAL CARCINOMA
Left: Type I microcystic adnexal carcinoma is composed of microcystic structures that contain trichilemmal-type keratin.
Right: Type II microcystic adnexal carcinoma is principally composed of solid cellular cords and nests.

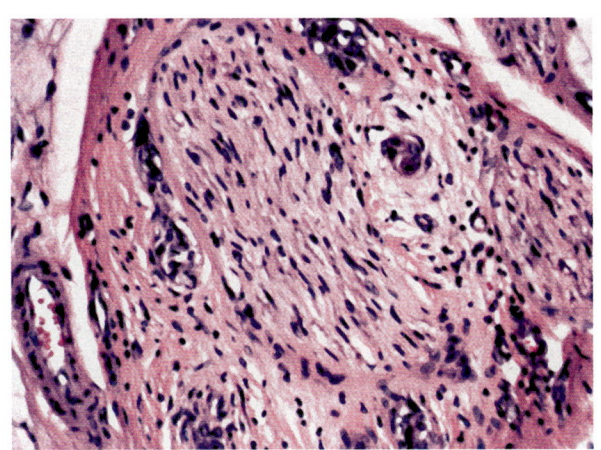

Figure 4-57

MICROCYSTIC ADNEXAL CARCINOMA

Infiltration of a perineural sheath is apparent.

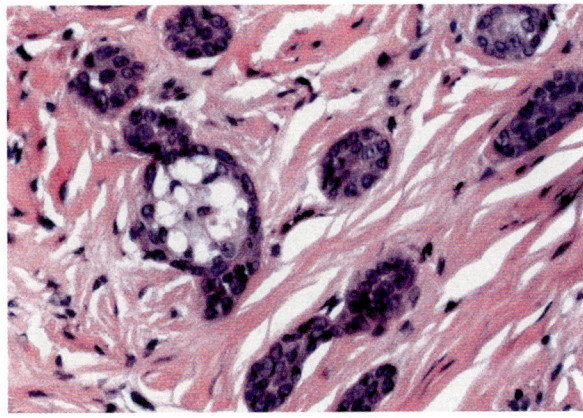

Figure 4-58

MICROCYSTIC ADNEXAL CARCINOMA

Sebaceous differentiation is evident in the tumor cell nests. (Courtesy of Dr. P. E. LeBoit, San Francisco, CA.)

equivocation is common (and even necessary) when faced with a shave biopsy containing a tumor that may represent MAC, in the absence of clinical data.

Morphea-like BCC contains more branched cellular nests, with no evidence of luminal differentiation. The stroma of BCC also shows characteristic "cleavage" away from tumor cell clusters (160), a feature not evident in MAC.

Primary Mucoepidermoid Carcinoma of the Skin. Mucoepidermoid carcinoma usually arises in the salivary glands or respiratory tree. These tumors have a well-differentiated histologic appearance (106,131,185), and are slow-growing in most instances, with only uncommon metastasis to distant sites. When the latter event occurs, it does so typically only after the primary neoplasm has been recognized and treated (80,143,154,171). In other words, patients with metastatic mucoepidermoid carcinoma of the skin are known to have a history of carcinoma.

Pathologic Findings. Microscopically, there are several differences between primary and secondary cutaneous mucoepidermoid carcinomas. The latter tumors are multinodular and have a sharp interface with the surrounding dermis or subcutis; primary neoplasms have indistinct borders and are often single nodules. An admixture of chronic inflammatory cells is frequently seen in primary cutaneous lesions but not in metastases.

Primary mucoepidermoid carcinomas are composed of polyhedral squamous cells admixed with

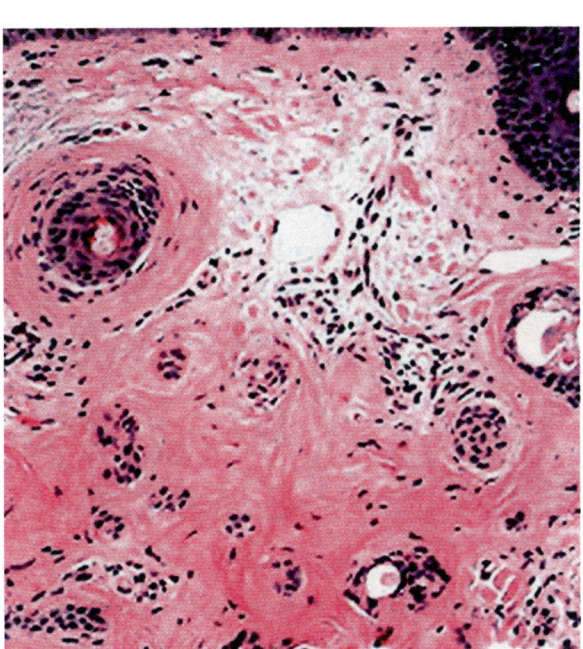

Figure 4-59

MICROCYSTIC ADNEXAL CARCINOMA

This shave biopsy demonstrates syringoid cell profiles that "shade off" at the inferior aspect of the specimen. A deeper biopsy demonstrated the diagnostic features of microcystic adnexal carcinoma in this case.

nondescript cuboidal tumor cells and mucin-forming cuboidal or low columnar elements (fig. 4-60) (106,131,185). Mucin-filled microcysts may be seen, as well as areas of clear cell change (154).

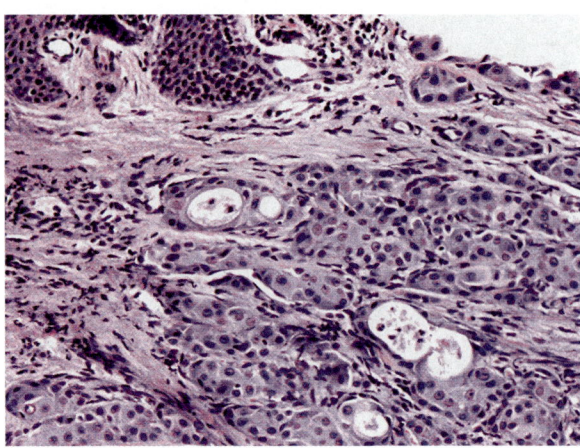 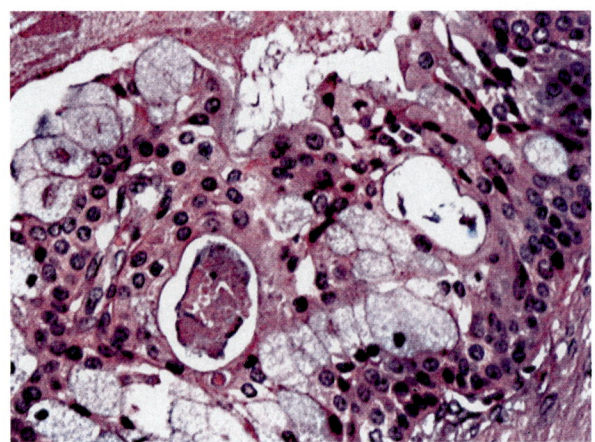

Figure 4-60

PRIMARY MUCOEPIDERMOID CARCINOMA

Left: Small mucinous microcysts are among the tumor cell nests in the dermis.
Right: Mucin-containing glandular cells are admixed with squamoid elements elsewhere in the lesion.

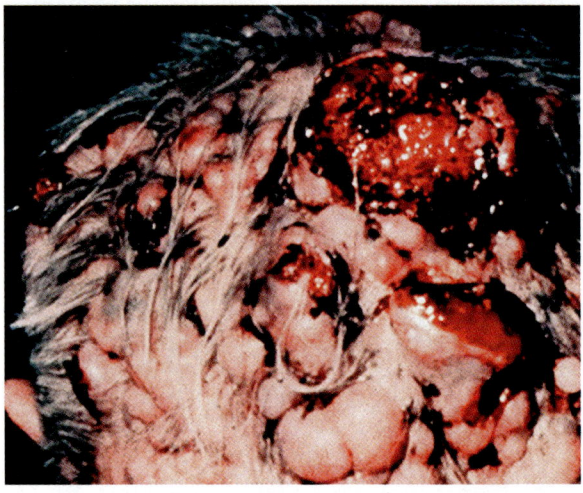

Figure 4-61

CARCINOMA EX DERMAL CYLINDROMA

Rapid growth and ulceration developed in one tumor nodule in the scalp of a patient with multiple cylindromas (turban tumor syndrome). The cylindroma proved to have undergone malignant transformation when examined microscopically.

The nuclear features are bland, with small inconspicuous nucleoli and dispersed chromatin; mitoses are rare. Usually, the tumor irregularly infiltrates the dermis, and perineural or lymphatic invasion may be present.

Differential Diagnosis. The microscopic attributes are so typical that the differential diagnosis is largely academic. It is conceivable that mucoepidermoid carcinoma is confused with the pseudoneoplastic-metaplastic proliferative lesions of sweat glands that are sometimes seen in response to chronic mechanical or pharmacologic insults (syringometaplasias); nevertheless, the latter processes rarely produce mass lesions.

Carcinoma Ex Dermal Cylindroma and Eccrine Spiradenoma. Despite the fact that they are slow-growing tumors, sweat gland carcinomas, in general, do not derive from preexisting adenomas. The only exceptions are carcinomas that evolve from "parent" cylindromas or spiradenomas (78,85,88,97,102,105,108,113, 134,140,155,179,181,191,195,197). Their presence is signaled by the rapid expansion of a previously indolent cutaneous nodule, with or without ulceration or pain (fig. 4-61). Pathologically, remnants of the "parent" lesion must be seen, along with a carcinomatous component, or confirmation must be available that a banal cylindroma or spiradenoma was removed previously from the same anatomic site where a sweat gland carcinoma is now present. Because of these requirements, it is beyond reason that one would diagnostically consider metastasis to the skin in this context.

Microscopically, remnants of the parent neoplasm have the typical appearance of cylindroma or spiradenoma. The malignant elements are usually undifferentiated, showing sheets or clusters of nondescript but highly

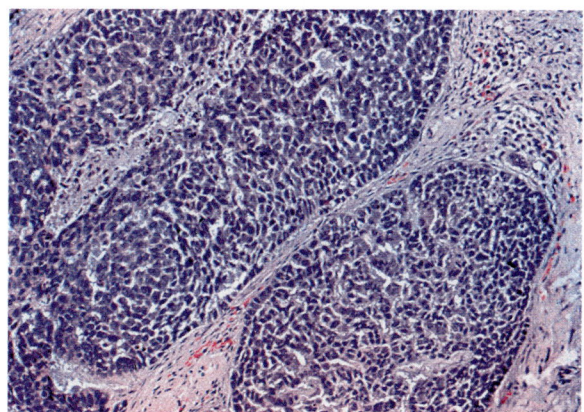

Figure 4-62

CARCINOMA EX DERMAL CYLINDROMA

The malignant portion of the tumor shown in the previous figure is depicted here. It does not resemble ordinary cylindroma.

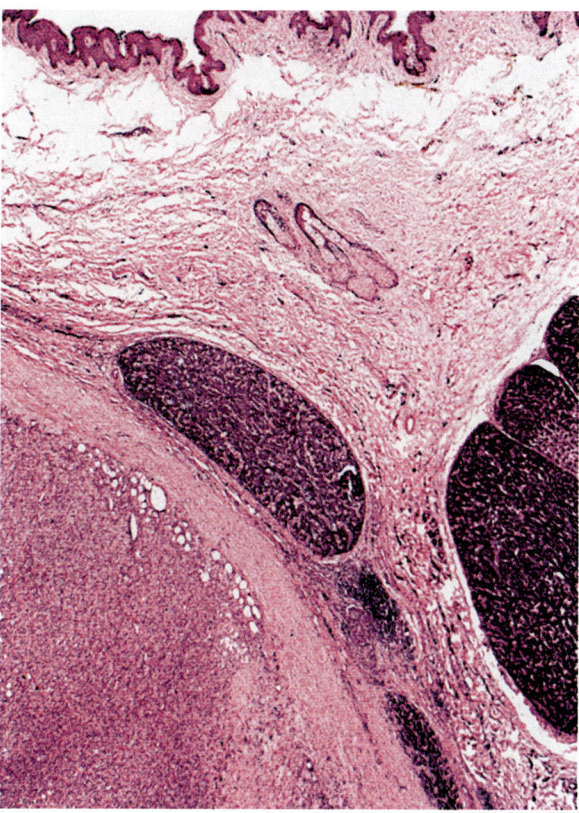

Figure 4-63

MALIGNANT TRANSFORMATION OF ECCRINE SPIRADENOMA

A new clone of tumor cells (lower left) is juxtaposed to the "parent" spiradenoma (right).

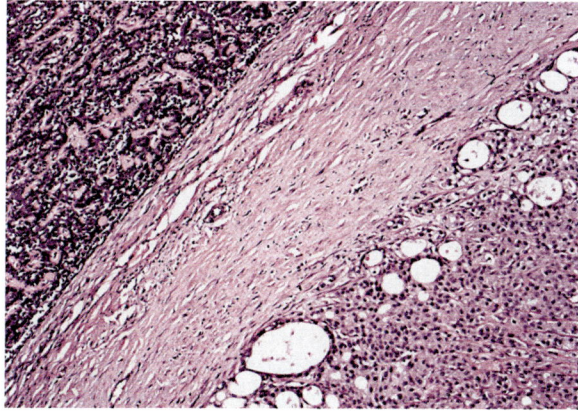

Figure 4-64

MALIGNANT TRANSFORMATION OF ECCRINE SPIRADENOMA

Another view of the tumor seen in figure 4-63 shows the sharp interface between the malignant (right) and benign (left) portions of the lesion.

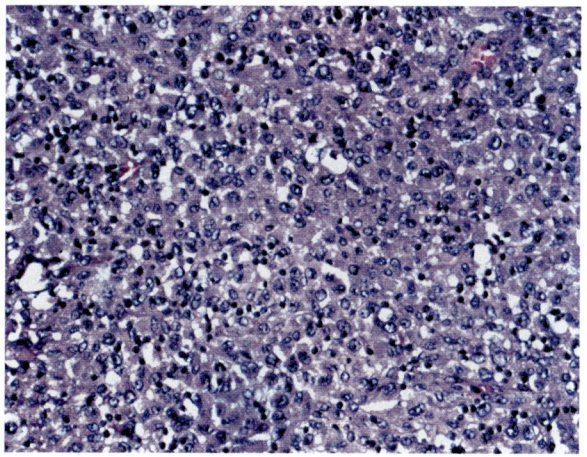

Figure 4-65

CARCINOMA EX ECCRINE SPIRADENOMA

This carcinoma ex eccrine spiradenoma has an undifferentiated image.

anaplastic epithelioid, stellate, or fusiform tumor cells with brisk mitotic activity (figs. 4-62–4-65) (88,134,191). Hence, the image of sarcomatoid carcinoma (carcinosarcoma) may be present (fig. 4-66) (140). Alternatively, more definable epithelial morphotypes may be present in carcinoma ex cylindroma or spiradenoma (108); these include squamous carcinoma, adenosquamous carcinoma, or pure adenocarcinoma, and various subtypes thereof

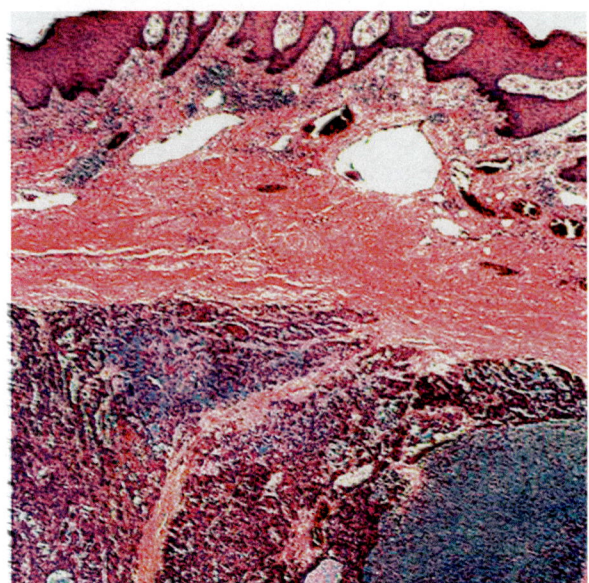

Figure 4-66

CARCINOMA EX ECCRINE SPIRADENOMA

This example of carcinoma ex eccrine spiradenoma shows divergent differentiation into chondroid-like tissue, yielding the image of sarcomatoid carcinoma.

(e.g., clear cell adenocarcinoma), all of which, in de novo form, would be differential diagnostic alternatives.

A behavioral peculiarity of carcinoma ex dermal cylindroma is reflected by an inexplicable disparity between the grade of the carcinomatous elements and the behavior of the neoplasm. Highly undifferentiated forms have been associated with a lack of metastasis and long-term disease-free survival (78,102,191).

Eccrine Carcinomas that Histologically Simulate Metastatic Tumors

There are other forms of eccrine carcinoma that closely simulate metastatic lesions, either because of uncertainties in the clinical picture or histologic appearance.

Ductal Eccrine Adenocarcinoma. *Clinical Features.* Ductal eccrine adenocarcinoma (DEA) is the most common of the eccrine carcinomas. It is most often seen on the head and neck or proximal extremities, as a solitary, slow-growing, clinically nondescript nodule that simulates the appearance of more ordinary forms of skin cancer (fig. 4-67).

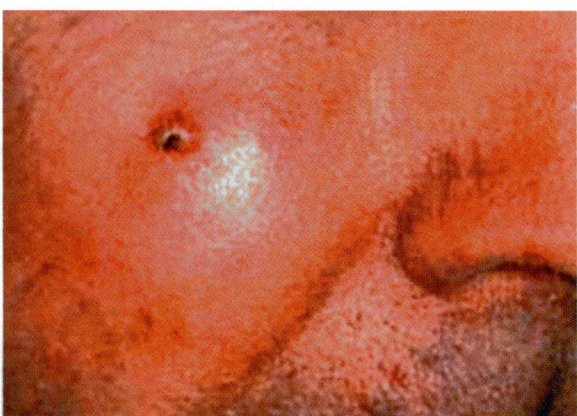

Figure 4-67

DUCTAL ECCRINE ADENOCARCINOMA OF THE CHEEK

A nondescript and ill-defined dermal nodule is indistinguishable from other more ordinary forms of skin cancer.

Pathologic Findings. DEA is composed of solid cords or tubules of obviously atypical polygonal cells that randomly permeate the dermis (fig. 4-68) (104,127,144,148,187). Focal ductal lumens are often seen, and entrapped eccrine ducts sometimes demonstrate the changes of carcinoma in situ (187). The stroma is variably desmoplastic and may contain chronic inflammatory cells (fig. 4-69). When the last two features are prominent, as they are in only a minority of cases, the primary nature of the neoplasm is certain, but their absence does not conversely equate with a diagnosis of metastatic disease. Nuclear chromatin is dense or vesicular, and prominent nucleoli are commonly present; mitotic activity is present but may be limited. The cytoplasm is usually amphophilic, and small intracytoplasmic vacuoles may be evident; sometimes, well-defined areas of overtly squamoid differentiation are seen, and a diagnosis of squamous cell carcinoma may be considered (fig. 4-70).

One variant of DEA that appears to be site-related is termed *ductal eccrine adenocarcinoma with fibromyxoid stroma* (DEAFS) (187). It is likely that this lesion was designated as malignant chondroid syringoma or syringoid carcinoma in the past. It shows a tendency to occur on the distal extremities (particularly the sole of the foot). DEAFS differs from usual DEA by its uniformly fibromyxoid stroma, which recalls one of the attributes of cutaneous mixed tumor (fig. 4-71). Other peculiarities of this tumor subtype are its

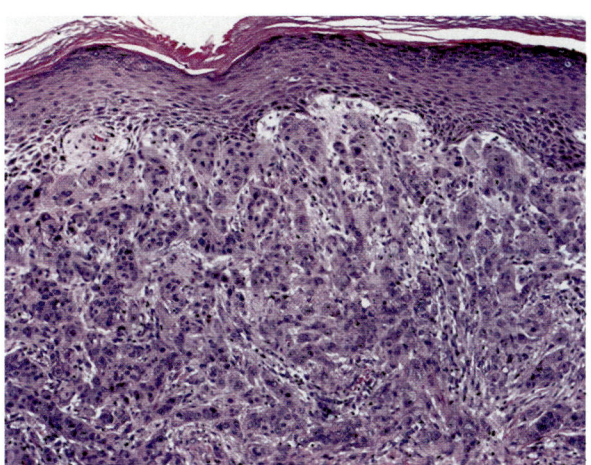 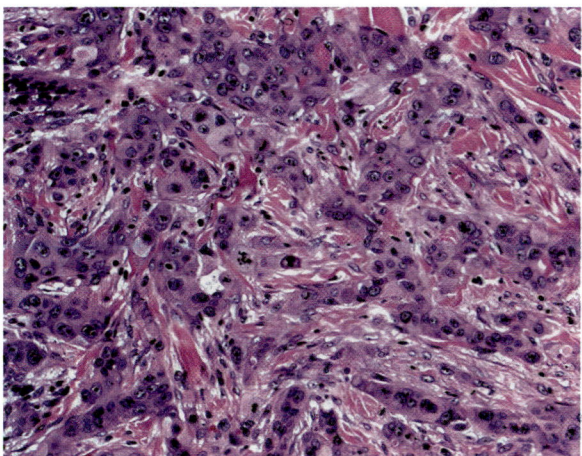

Figure 4-68

DUCTAL ECCRINE ADENOCARCINOMA

Ductal eccrine adenocarcinoma is composed of irregularly disposed and invasive nests and cords of tumor cells in the dermis. The overall image is remarkably similar to that of invasive ductal carcinoma of the breast.

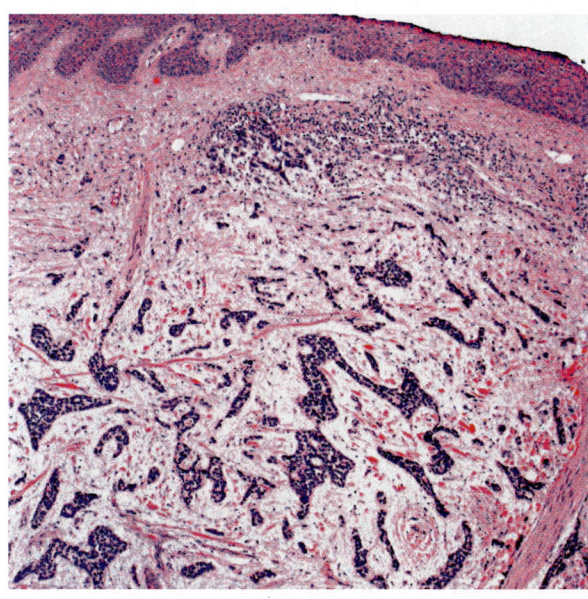 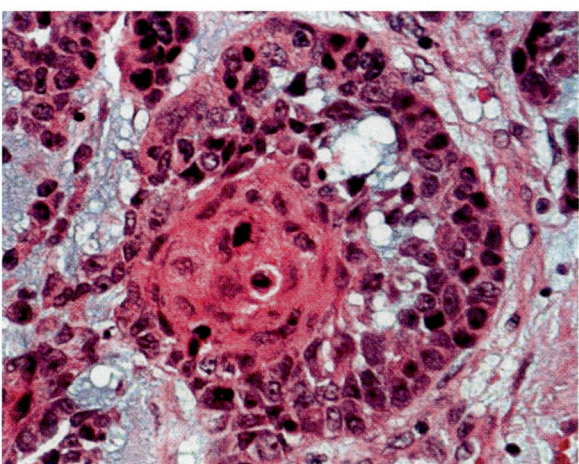

Figure 4-70

DUCTAL ECCRINE ADENOCARCINOMA

Squamoid foci are relatively common in ductal eccrine adenocarcinoma.

Figure 4-69

DUCTAL ECCRINE ADENOCARCINOMA

The stroma surrounding the invasive cords of tumor cells is fibroelastotic.

ability to communicate with the surface epithelium in a similar manner to that of poroma, and to be composed of compact, almost basaloid cells; indeed, a mistaken diagnosis of BCC may be made in such cases (fig. 4-72). When limited, artifactually distorted biopsy material is obtained, the latter problem can be addressed by performing immunostains for EMA. Virtually all forms of sweat gland carcinoma are EMA positive, whereas BCCs consistently lack that determinant (176).

Another form of DEA is one in which the tumor cells assume a fusiform or sarcomatoid configuration (fig. 4-73) (187). This feature may reflect the presence of myoepithelial differentiation. The spindle cells may further show

Nonmelanocytic Tumors of the Skin

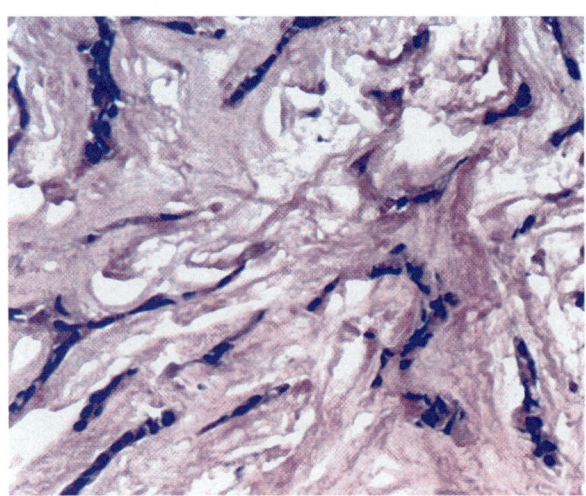

Figure 4-71

DUCTAL ECCRINE ADENOCARCINOMA

The stroma of some ductal eccrine carcinomas has a fibromyxoid character that has resulted in their being confused with mixed tumors in the past.

focally concentric growth, yielding tactoid-like structures, and they can blend imperceptibly with conventional epithelioid areas. Uncommon examples of DEA have been described in which there was a histologic admixture of mucoepidermoid carcinoma-like foci, as seen in some primary breast tumors as well (194). The metastatic risk for all DEA variants is approximately 40 percent.

Differential Diagnosis. Histologically, the features of DEC are comparable to those seen in conventional invasive ductal carcinoma of the breast, metastases of which, for obvious reasons, represent the principal differential diagnostic consideration (90). It is crucial to obtain a detailed clinical history of the skin lesion in question. DEA is virtually always a solitary, slow-growing mass that has been present for at least 6 months, and sometimes years, before the patient seeks medical attention. In contrast, metastases of mammary carcinoma are typically multifocal, occurring in "crops" and having a rapid clinical evolution (90,158). The reason for emphasizing the historical data is that the detailed pathologic features of ductal breast and eccrine carcinomas are identical; this synonymity even extends to the expression of estrogen and progesterone receptors by both tumors (175).

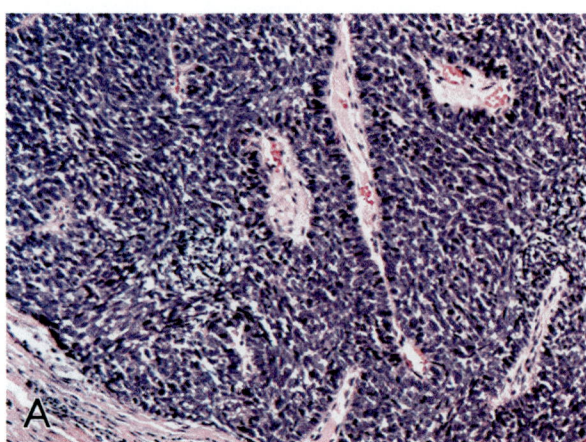

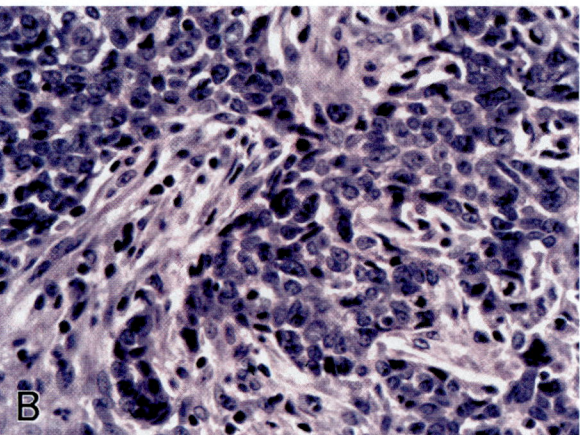

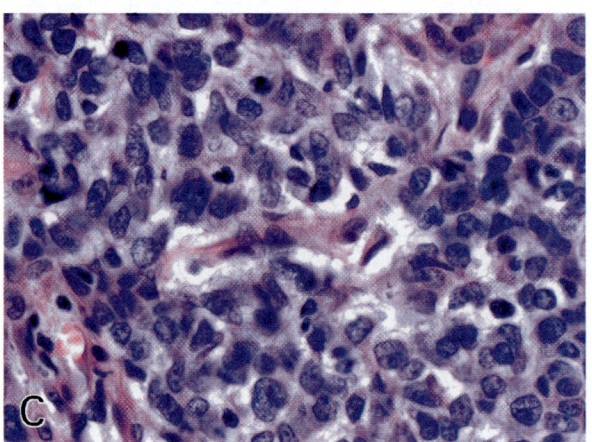

Figure 4-72

SMALL CELL (BASALOID) DUCTAL ECCRINE ADENOCARCINOMA

The neoplastic cells are arranged in indistinct dermal nests with little ductal differentiation. The overall image of this tumor variant may lead to confusion with such lesions as Merkel cell carcinoma.

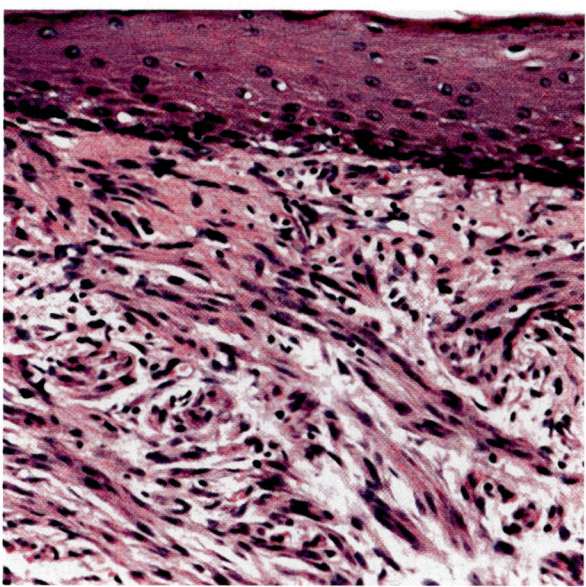

Figure 4-73

SARCOMATOID (SPINDLE CELL) CHANGE IN DUCTAL ECCRINE ADENOCARCINOMA

An exclusively spindle cell focus is seen here. Other areas of the mass showed the typical image for this tumor type.

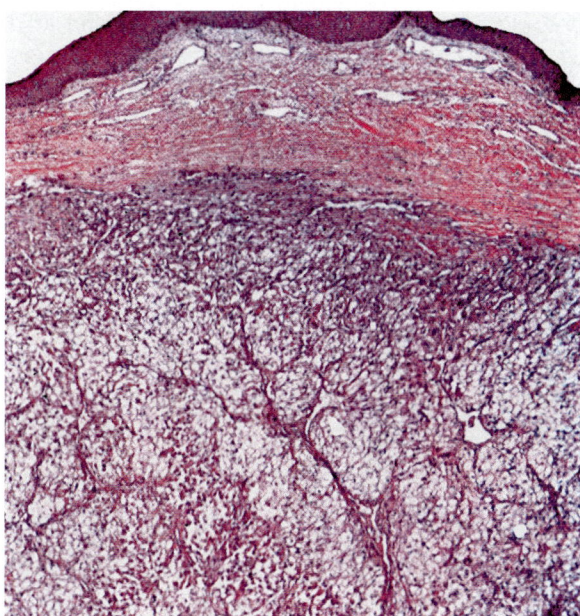

Figure 4-74

CLEAR CELL ECCRINE CARCINOMA

Nests and cords of polygonal tumor cells with lucent cytoplasm are dispersed irregularly throughout the dermis.

Carcinomas with the appearance of DEA may occur in the skin of the breast or the axillary mammary tails. The question arises under those circumstances as to whether the tumor is a sweat gland neoplasm or a carcinoma of the breast. By convention, we do not make the diagnosis of sweat gland carcinoma of any type in the skin of the breast, and we advise that such cases be managed as mammary parenchymal neoplasms.

Clear Cell Eccrine Carcinoma. *Clinical Features.* There are several eccrine neoplasms that have a potential for clear cell change: acrospiroma, MAC, poroma, and mixed tumors of the skin. One particular type of eccrine carcinoma is dominated by clear cells and derives its name from them; namely, *clear cell eccrine carcinoma* (CCEC) (173,192). This lesion is closely related clinicopathologically to malignant acrospiroma (hidradenocarcinoma) (92,101,117,119,128, 129,137,188), but its individual importance derives from a potential pathologic confusion with metastases of renal cell carcinoma and visceral clear cell malignancies (89). The most certain approach to excluding those possibilities is procurement of detailed clinical information on the solitary or multifocal nature of the lesion and its duration of growth. It should also be remembered that CCEC is most often seen in the skin of the head and neck, whereas clear-cell metastatic simulators show a predilection for the truncal surface.

Pathologic Findings. CCEC is a multilobulated dermal neoplasm that lacks connections to the epidermis, and shows a vague interface with the dermis and subcutis (fig. 4-74). Broad sheets or large clusters of polyhedral tumor cells with lucent cytoplasm are separated from one another by a fibrovascular stroma (fig. 4-75). Nuclei are compact, with evenly distributed chromatin and small nucleoli, or vesicular with prominent nucleoli (fig. 4-76). Mitotic activity is also heterogeneous from lesion to lesion. Geographic tumor necrosis and invasion of perineural or perivascular spaces are other potential findings (173,192).

Differential Diagnosis. The hobnail cell profiles and intercellular blood lakes, such as described in clear cell carcinoma of urogenital or renal origin, respectively, are not seen in CCEC (89,93,177). Immunostains for CEA and the CA125 glycoprotein are potentially helpful in the differential diagnosis. A positive CEA result favors CCEC because renal cell carcinoma and urogenital clear cell carcinoma are CEA negative. Carcinomas of the female genital tract express CA125 (and renal carcinomas may do so as well), whereas that marker is absent in CCEC.

Malignant Mixed Tumor of the Skin (Sarcomatoid Sweat Gland Carcinoma, "Carcinosarcoma"). The exceptionally rare neoplasm called malignant mixed tumor of the skin is not synonymous with carcinoma ex mixed tumor, as in the salivary glands. Almost all of the cutaneous lesions reported have been neoplasms that lacked any type of "parent" adenoma, and appeared to represent de novo sweat gland carcinomas with divergent mesenchymal-like differentiation (86,116,121,123, 138,151,153,157,165,169,184). An exception is the singular case reported by Sharvill (167), which is more aptly considered a "carcinoma ex cutaneous mixed tumor." In the usual "malignant mixed tumor," recognizable eccrine carcinoma morphotypes are admixed histologically with tissue foci resembling chondrosarcoma, osteosarcoma, rhabdomyosarcoma, fibrosarcoma, leiomyosarcoma, or undifferentiated sarcoma, all in the same lesion (fig. 4-77) (86,116,121,123,138,151,153,157,165,169,184).

Metastases to the skin from *"carcinosarcomas"* (more properly termed *sarcomatoid carcinomas*) of the kidney, lung, genital tract, and other sites (189) must be excluded through clinical investigation before a diagnosis of primary cutaneous malignancy can be assigned confidently in these circumstances. The biologic evolution of sarcomatoid sweat gland carcinomas is again paradoxical, since few have demonstrated aggressive behavior.

Apocrine Carcinomas

Apocrine carcinomas are divided into those that are histologically distinctive as primary lesions, and those that simulate metastases.

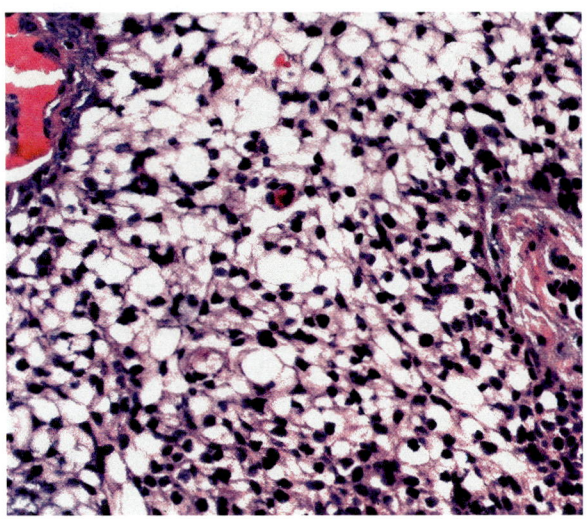

Figure 4-75
CLEAR CELL ECCRINE CARCINOMA
Nests of tumor cells efface the dermis.

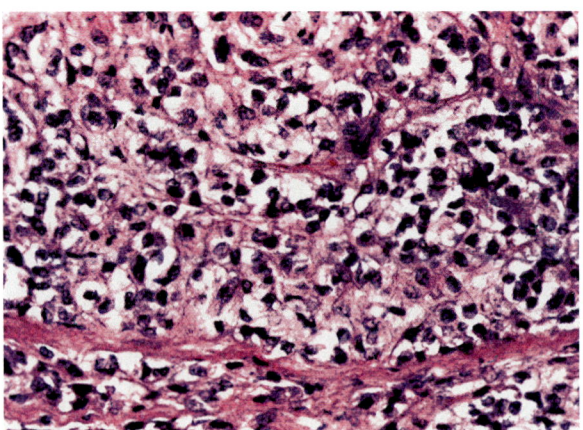
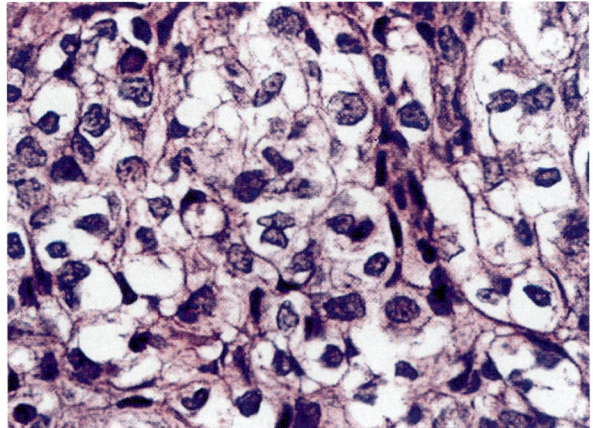

Figure 4-76
CLEAR CELL ECCRINE CARCINOMA
The tumor cells have discernible nucleoli and relatively high nuclear to cytoplasmic ratios.

Neoplasms and Pseudoneoplastic Proliferations of the Sweat Glands

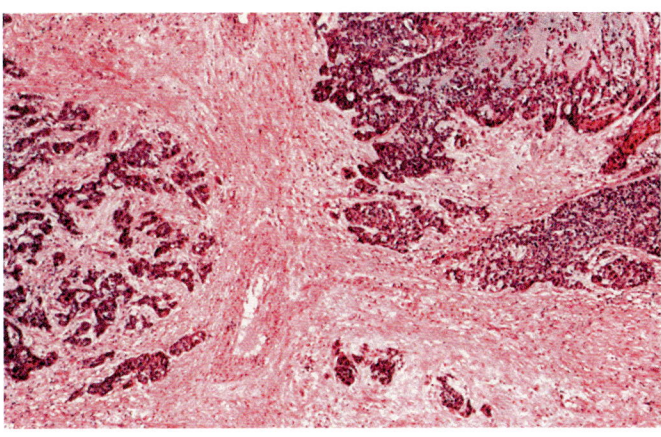 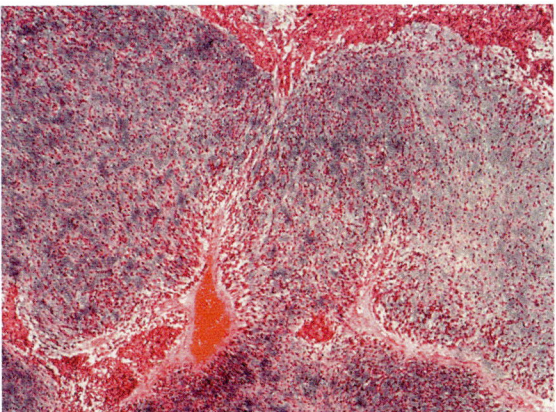

Figure 4-77

SARCOMATOID SWEAT GLAND CARCINOMA

This example of de novo sarcomatoid sweat gland carcinoma (carcinosarcoma) shows foci of chondroid differentiation within a lesion that otherwise resembles ductal eccrine adenocarcinoma.

Apocrine Carcinomas that Are Histologically Definable as Primary Tumors

Two forms of apocrine carcinoma are sufficiently distinctive that they are reliably diagnosed as primary lesions of the skin. These are ductopapillary apocrine carcinoma and the apocrine variant of mammary or extramammary cutaneous Paget's disease.

Ductopapillary Apocrine Carcinoma. Ductopapillary apocrine carcinoma (DPAC) is similar to papillary digital eccrine carcinoma (see above) histoarchitecturally, but DPAC is most often is encountered in the eyelids, axillae, and genitoperineal skin rather than the extremities (199,208,213,218,224,226,228,230,232).

Pathologic Findings. DPAC is recognizable as apocrine because the tumor cells have finely granular eosinophilic cytoplasm, with or without luminal intraglandular decapitation snouts (fig. 4-78). Nuclear atypia is easily appreciated and mitoses are present as well (230). DPAC shows irregular invasion of adjacent tissue (figs. 4-79, 4-80) and may involve perineural spaces or vascular adventitia.

Histochemical and immunohistochemical evaluations of this neoplasm help to define its lineage when morphologic features are less than definitive. The Prussian blue stain for iron is positive in approximately 40 to 50 percent of cases (a trait associated with apocrine differentiation in adnexal epithelium) (230), and im-

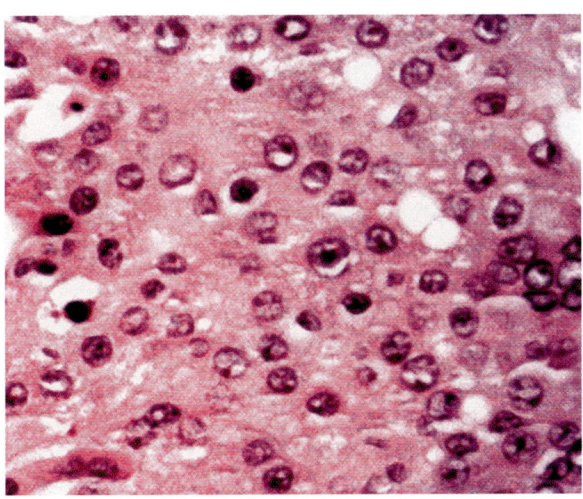

Figure 4-78

APOCRINE CARCINOMA

Eosinophilic granular cytoplasm typifies the cells of apocrine carcinomas.

munostains for gross cystic disease fluid protein-15 (GCDFP-15; an apocrine-selective protein) are uniformly positive.

Differential Diagnosis. The differential diagnosis of DPAC is limited. Papillary carcinoma of the breast may demonstrate apocrine attributes in some cases, but does not metastasize to the skin except in the context of systemic dissemination. Hidradenoma papilliferum has a superficial resemblance to DPAC, but it does not show the degree of nuclear atypia or

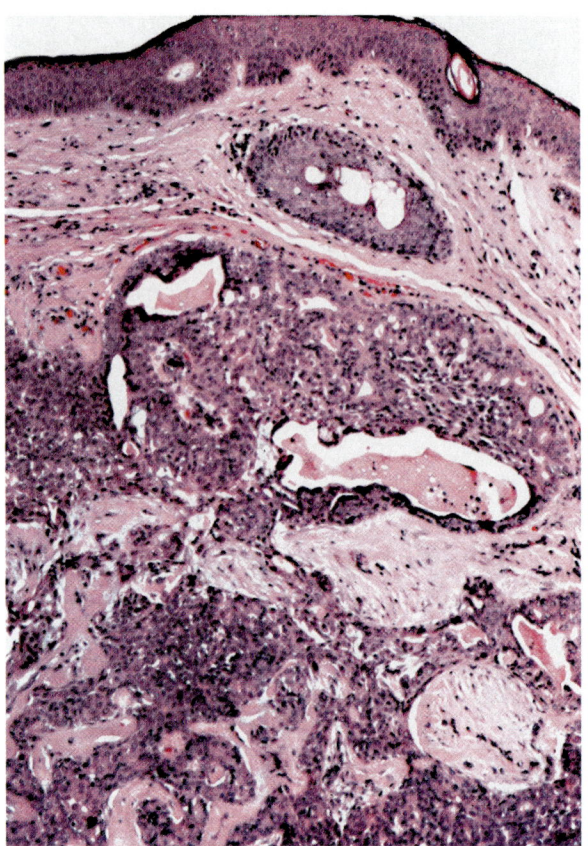

Figure 4-79

DUCTOPAPILLARY APOCRINE CARCINOMA

Nests of cells with internal papillations infiltrate the dermis deeply and irregularly.

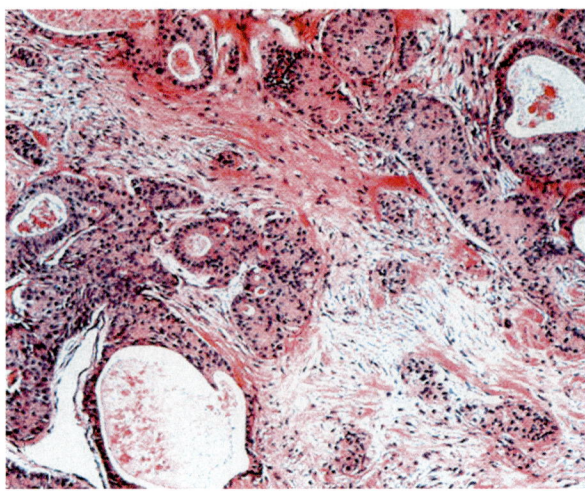

Figure 4-80

DUCTOPAPILLARY APOCRINE CARCINOMA

Irregular permeation of the dermis is apparent.

architectural complexity seen in carcinomas; infiltrative growth is also lacking. En masse necrosis and dystrophic calcification are additional potential features of DPAC that are not present in hidradenoma papilliferum.

Paget's Disease of the Skin, Apocrine Type. Conventional doctrine still teaches that mammary and extramammary Paget's disease of the skin represents two separate diseases, even though they are very similar clinically. On (fig. 4-81A) and outside (fig. 4-81B) the breasts, Paget's disease is an eczematoid, red, often pruritic lesion that is slowly evolving. *Mammary Paget's disease* (MPD) is said to reflect the migration of tumor cells into the epidermis from underlying carcinomas of the breast (201), whereas *extramammary Paget's disease* (EPD) is thought to originate within the epidermis, representing a proliferation of primitive native stem (basal) cells with the capacity for glandular differentiation (211). We have a somewhat iconoclastic view of this topic, and believe that both forms of pagetoid proliferation derive from intraepidermal stem cells. Perhaps the strongest support for this opinion comes from the observation that approximately 3 to 5 percent of MPD cases are not associated with an underlying carcinoma, despite exhaustive sampling of the breast (210,221). Thus, MPD and EPD are considered here as one disorder.

The classification of Paget's disease as a principally apocrine tumor is justified by the results of GCDFP-15 immunostains, which demonstrate positivity in the majority of both MPD and EPD lesions (217). Other cellular lineages are occasionally manifest in Paget's disease, including sebaceous, eccrine, and visceral enteric pathways.

Pathologic Findings. Microscopically, Paget's disease shows the presence of "foreign" epithelioid tumor cells within the epidermis (fig. 4-81C). The adjacent epidermis commonly exhibits hyperkeratosis and acanthosis. The tumor cells are dispersed singly or as small clusters throughout the surface epithelium (fig. 4-82); they are round to ovoid and have pale, amphophilic cytoplasm, which is sometimes vacuolated (fig. 4-83). The nuclei contain dispersed or vesicular chromatin, often with a discernible but small nucleolus; mitotic figures are sparse (204,212a,214,216,220,222).

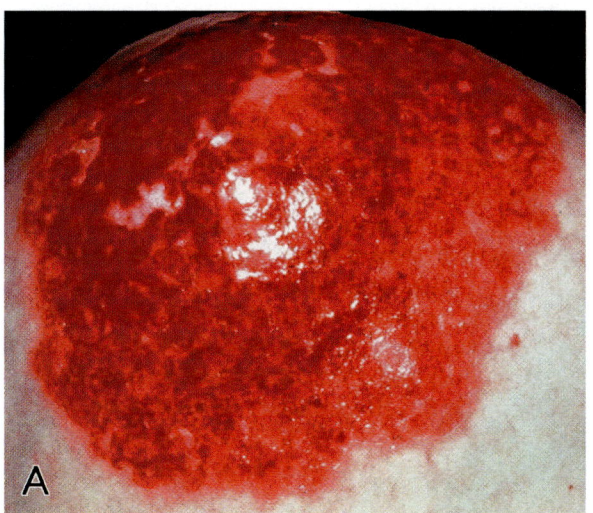
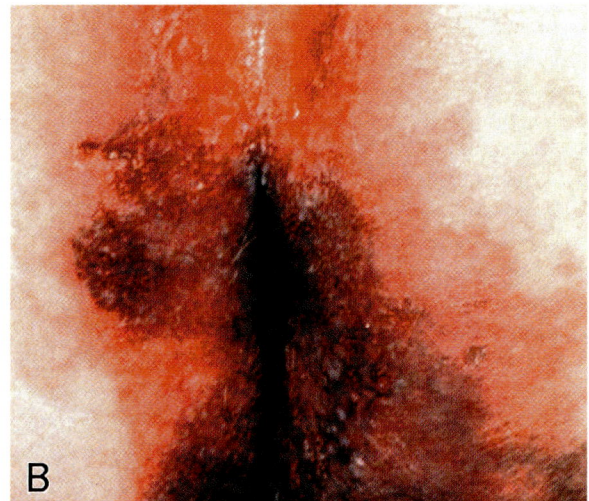
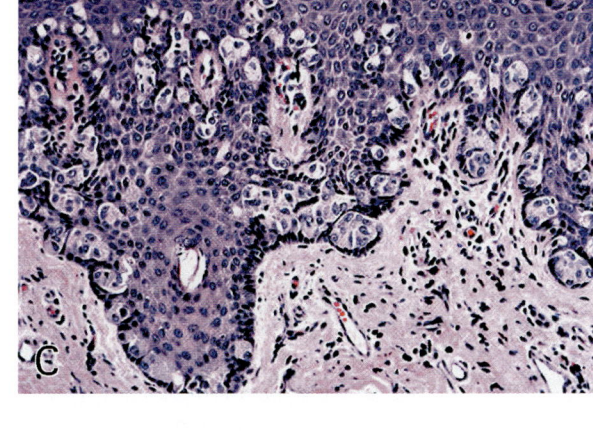

Figure 4-81

PAGET'S DISEASE

A: Mammary Paget's disease is represented by eczematoid bright red change in the skin around the nipple and areola.

B: Extramammary perianal Paget's disease shows similar macroscopic characteristics.

C: In both mammary and extramammary locations, the tumor cells of cutaneous Paget's disease are dispersed randomly throughout the epidermis in a "buckshot" fashion.

An anaplastic form of Paget's disease has been described (225). This subtype exhibits a marked variation in nuclear size, shape, and density, as well as the presence of anisocytosis. Another peculiarity of Paget's disease is caused by its potentially confluent growth in the basal epidermis. Because the tumor cells adhere to one another poorly, they often detach from one another. This phenomenon results in the formation of pseudobullae which can imitate the acantholysis that is associated with forms of pemphigus (fig. 4-84, left) (231). The tumor cells in MPD and EPD contain mucopolysaccharides that are positive with PAS-D, mucicarmine, and Alcian blue in 50 to 60 percent of cases (fig. 4-84, right). Invasion of the dermis is encountered in 1 to 5 percent of all EPD cases (fig. 4-85); when it is present, the lesion acquires metastatic potential (230a).

Differential Diagnosis. The differential diagnosis centers on superficial spreading amelanotic melanoma and bowenoid intraepidermal squamous carcinoma. Paget's cells may contain granules of melanin, which are produced by neighboring melanocytes and secondarily engulfed by the tumor cells. Hence, this may lead to diagnostic confusion with malignant melanoma. Conventional histochemistry can be helpful in confirming the diagnosis of Paget's disease because neither melanoma nor squamous carcinoma produces mucin. Immunostains are also beneficial diagnostically (205,206,212). Reactivity for CEA, GCDFP-15, or keratin type 7 confirms the diagnosis of Paget's disease in the narrow context under discussion here. Additional positivity for CA19.9 or keratin type 20 in genitoperineal disease should direct attention to the possibility of an associated adenocarcinoma in the rectum, urinary bladder, or endocervix (202,219,223, 227), because those markers reflect the presence of an enteric immunophenotype in EPD.

Nonmelanocytic Tumors of the Skin

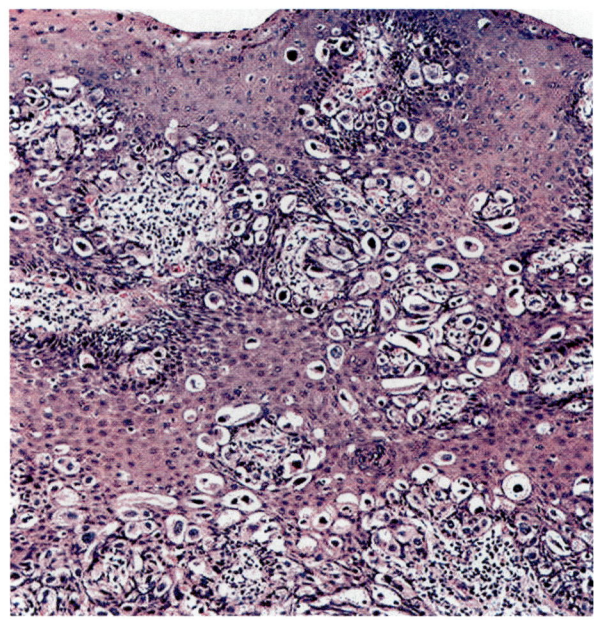

Figure 4-82

EXTRAMAMMARY PAGET'S DISEASE

Tumor cells are dispersed singly or in small groups throughout the epidermis.

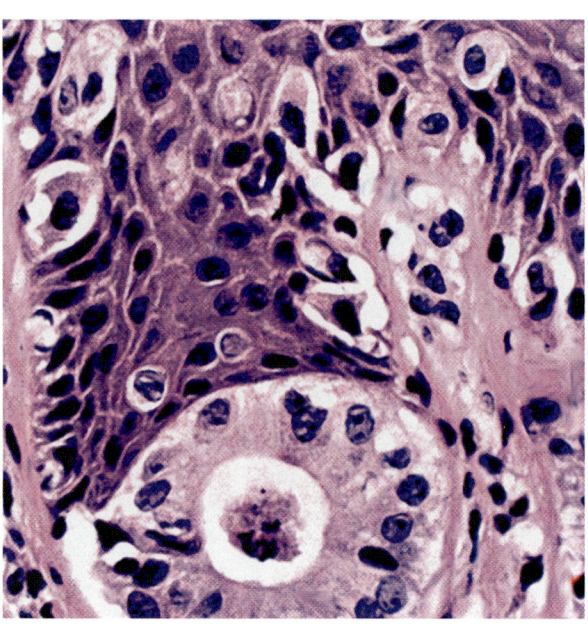

Figure 4-83

CUTANEOUS PAGET'S DISEASE

Focally, the tumor cell nests of cutaneous Paget's disease demonstrate lumen formation, indicating their glandular nature.

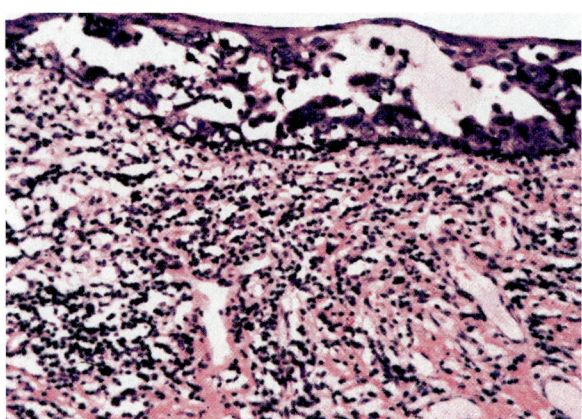

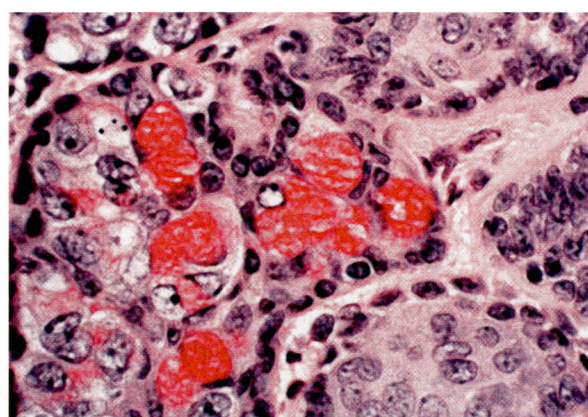

Figure 4-84

CUTANEOUS PAGET'S DISEASE

Left: Cutaneous Paget's disease may exhibit striking intraepidermal acantholysis, producing an image that superficially resembles that of pemphigus.

Right: Mucicarmine is positive in the tumor cells of Paget's disease in many cases.

Apocrine Carcinomas that May Histologically Simulate Metastases

There are basically two forms of apocrine carcinoma whose histologic features simulate those of metastatic tumors: ductal apocrine adenocarcinoma and primary signet ring cell carcinoma of the skin.

Ductal and Ductopapillary Apocrine Adenocarcinoma. As mentioned earlier in this chapter, the anatomic distribution of apocrine

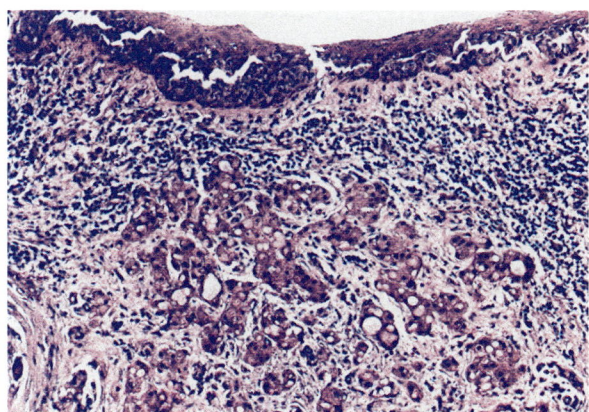
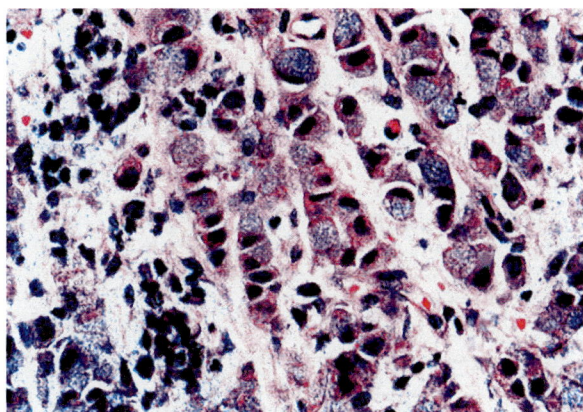

Figure 4-85

CUTANEOUS PAGET'S DISEASE

Invasion of the dermis is appreciated in 1 to 5 percent of cases of cutaneous Paget's disease, as seen here. The infiltrative component generally has the appearance of apocrine carcinoma.

tumors is relatively restricted. In addition to this topographic relatedness, there are many similarities between the histologic attributes of *ductal apocrine adenocarcinoma* (DAA) and *ductopapillary apocrine adenocarcinoma* (DPAC).

Pathologic Features. DAA and DPAC both contain irregular, randomly oriented proliferations of neoplastic ductal profiles in the dermis (fig. 4-86), with or without changes in entrapped sweat ducts, which simulate those of carcinoma in situ of the breast. Obvious cytologic atypia, mitotic activity, spontaneous necrosis, and infiltration of nerves and blood vessels are features common to both of these classes of apocrine gland carcinoma (fig. 4-87). The distinguishing features of DAA are much the same as those of DPAC; namely, the presence of decapitation secretion snouts and abundant, finely granular, eosinophilic cytoplasm (fig. 4-88). Histochemical and immunohistologic findings of DAA also mirror those of DPAC, as described above. The only real (but nonetheless important) difference between these tumor variants is the potential for papillary differentiation in DPAC.

Differential Diagnosis. The differential diagnosis centers on cutaneous metastases from those visceral adenocarcinomas that potentially feature a constitution of large "pink" cells: apocrine tumors of the breast and selected carcinomas of the lung, kidney, adrenal, and liver (203). Immunohistologic evaluation for GCDFP-15 reactivity is capable of narrowing the consider-

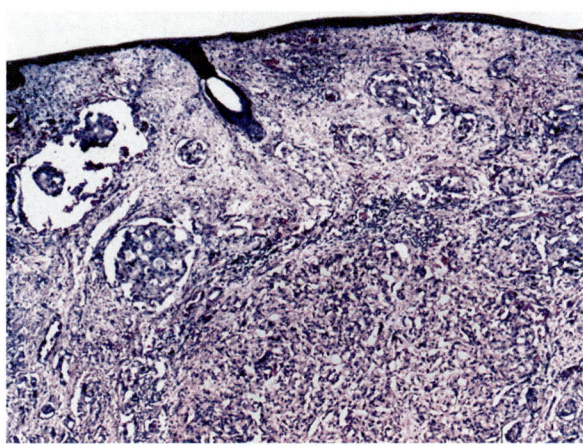

Figure 4-86

DUCTAL APOCRINE ADENOCARCINOMA

Ductal apocrine carcinoma is similar architecturally to ductal eccrine carcinoma, as shown here, but the cytologic details of these tumors differ.

ations to two tumor entities, DAA and apocrine carcinoma of the breast. Nevertheless, as with ductal eccrine adenocarcinoma, there are no reliable discriminators that can be applied by the pathologist to refine the diagnosis further. Hence, any patient with a carcinoma of the skin that shows an apocrine immunophenotype should have a thorough examination of the breasts, including mammography, before a diagnosis of DAA is made. Historical data concerning the duration of lesional growth and

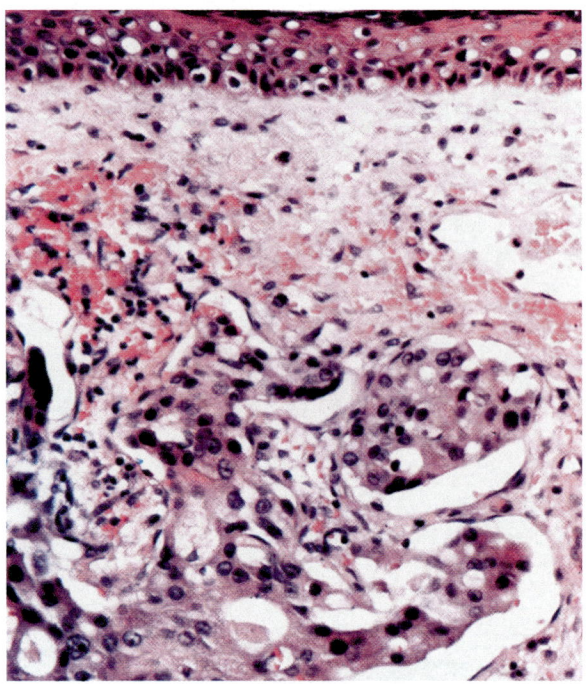

Figure 4-87

DUCTAL APOCRINE ADENOCARCINOMA

Striking vascular invasion is seen here. The tumor cells are plump, with relatively abundant granular eosinophilic cytoplasm.

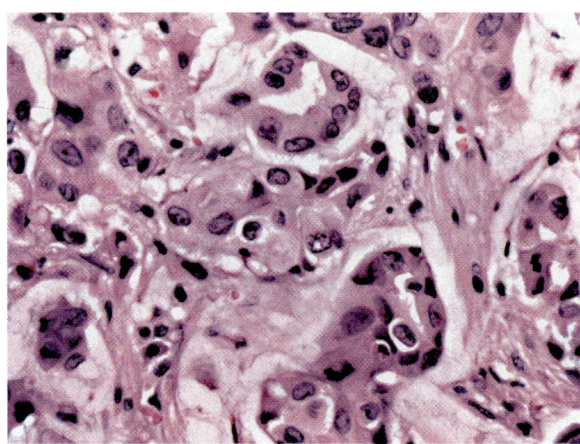

Figure 4-88

DUCTAL APOCRINE ADENOCARCINOMA

Vaguely defined decapitation snouts are present in the tumoral glands.

potential multifocality are also essential in this process, as outlined above in the section on ductal eccrine adenocarcinoma.

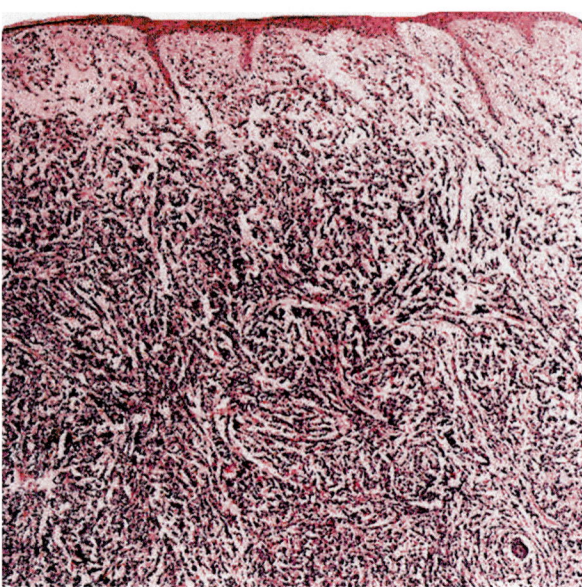

Figure 4-89

APOCRINE SIGNET RING CELL ADENOCARCINOMA OF THE EYELID

The dermis is effaced by linear arrays of tumor cells.

Primary Signet Ring Cell Adenocarcinoma. *Clinical Features.* Among all of the favored skin fields for apocrine neoplasia, the eyelid is virtually the only location in which primary signet ring cell adenocarcinoma (PSRCA) is seen. The lesion is nodular or plaque-like, and found in adults (209). This information is useful in narrowing the differential diagnostic considerations (see below), but metastasis still remains a possibility.

Pathologic Features. Small epithelioid cells grow randomly in the dermis, subcutis, or both. They are often arranged in single file or cords (figs. 4-89, 4-90), or in small clusters. Perineural invasion is apparent in only a few cases, but this finding is particularly important because it tends to support a primary origin in the skin. Vascular invasion may be seen as well. The individual neoplastic cells have round nuclei with dispersed chromatin and small nucleoli. They are displaced to the periphery of the cell by single cytoplasmic vacuoles that actually represent primitive lumens. Secretory material may be observed focally within such spaces. Necrosis is rare, and mitotic activity is usually surprisingly scant.

Differential Diagnosis. Because of the rarity of PSRCA, the differential diagnosis should favor

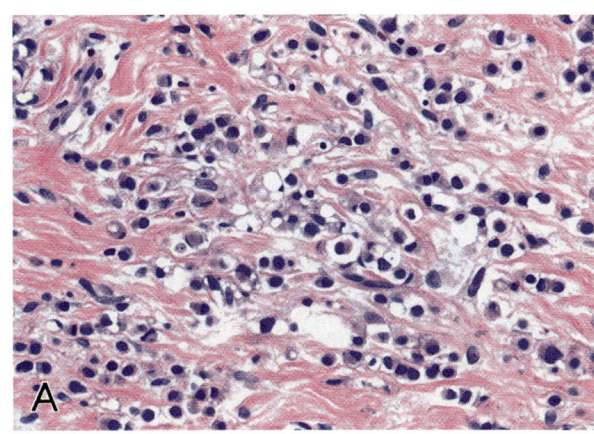
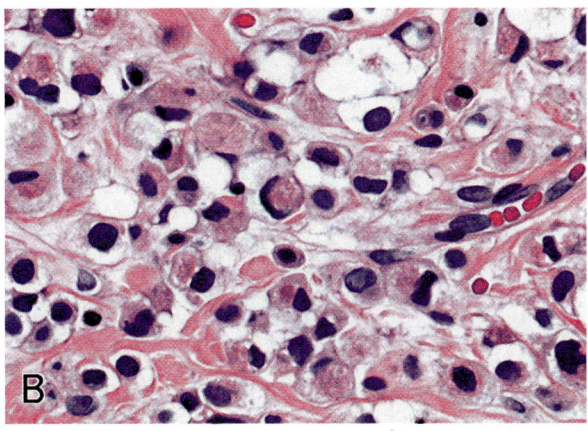
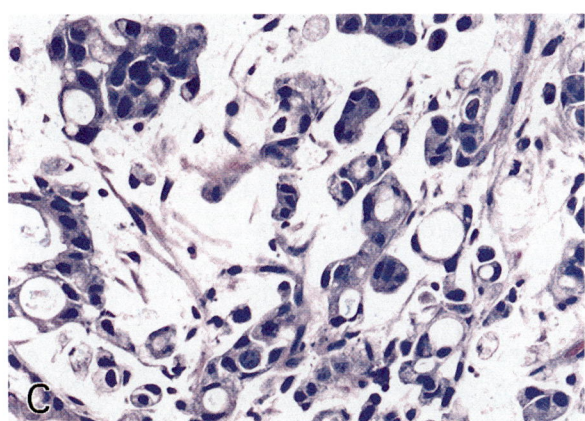

Figure 4-90

APOCRINE SIGNET RING CELL ADENOCARCINOMA

The tumor cells show internal cytoplasmic vacuoles and eccentric placement of nuclei.

metastasis when one is confronted with the microscopic image just cited. (The author [MRW] has seen only two cases in the past 10 years.) Several visceral organs have the capacity to harbor PSRCA, including the breasts, stomach, intestines, biliary tree, urinary tract, and female genitalia (198,207,215,229). Knowledge of the distribution of disease is helpful in diagnosis, because PSRCA is seemingly limited to the eyelid. In contrast, PSRCA of the abdominal and pelvic organs tend to metastasize to the skin of the trunk. Metastatic lobular carcinoma of the breast is capable of perfectly simulating the clinicopathologic attributes of PSRCA (207), including its immunophenotype. Thus, the history, as well as clinical and mammographic information, are paramount in securing a final interpretation.

ADNEXAL CARCINOMAS OF UNCERTAIN OR MIXED LINEAGE, WITH SWEAT GLANDULAR ELEMENTS

In selected malignant adnexal tumors, sudoriferous differentiation is histologically occult or exists simultaneously with obviously divergent appendageal elements. The two neoplasms in this group are lymphoepithelioma-like carcinoma of the skin and adnexal carcinoma with mixed differentiation.

Lymphoepithelioma-Like Carcinoma

In 1988, Swanson et al. (240) described several cutaneous tumors that apparently arose in the skin primarily, but which were identical microscopically to lymphoepithelioma-like carcinomas (LELCs) of the nasopharynx and other organ sites. Clinically, these lesions are nondescript, slow-growing nodules, most often seen in the skin of the head and neck in adults.

Microscopically, LELC of the skin is composed of syncytia or vague clusters of large epithelioid cells in the dermis, with vesicular nuclear chromatin, prominent nucleoli, and obvious mitoses (figs. 4-91, 4-92). Mature lymphocytes permeate the lesions diffusely, and surround them as well. Studies have shown that eccrine or pilar differentiation may be evident

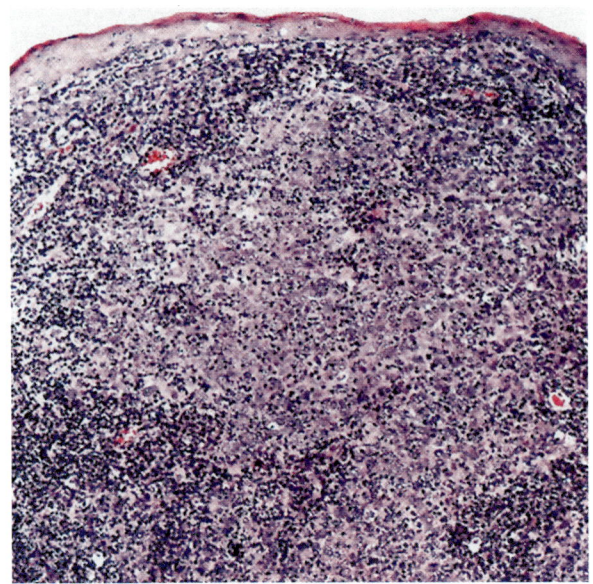

Figure 4-91

LYMPHOEPITHELIOMA-LIKE CARCINOMA

Vague lobules of undifferentiated polygonal cells, with numerous intralesional lymphocytes, are in the dermis.

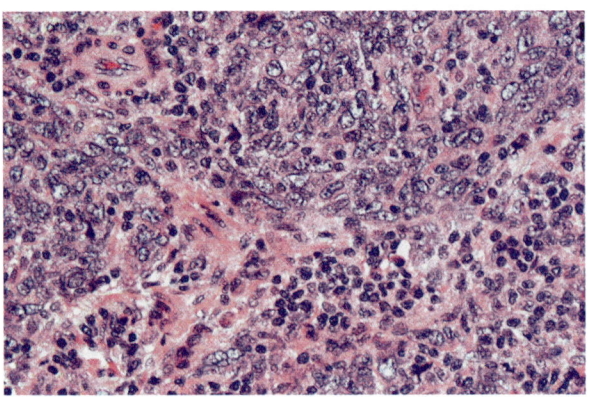

Figure 4-92

LYMPHOEPITHELIOMA-LIKE CARCINOMA

The intimate admixture of epithelial and lymphocytic cells is well demonstrated.

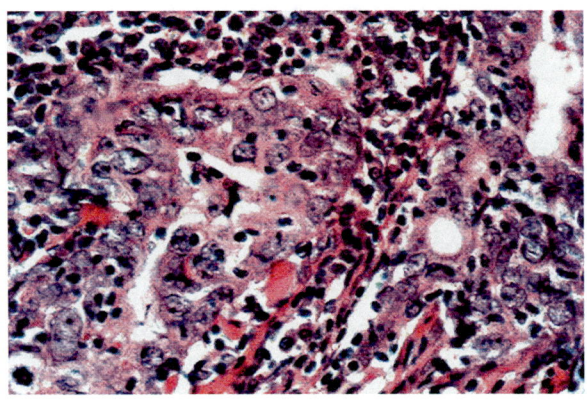

Figure 4-93

LYMPHOEPITHELIOMA-LIKE CARCINOMA

Primitive eccrine glandular differentiation.

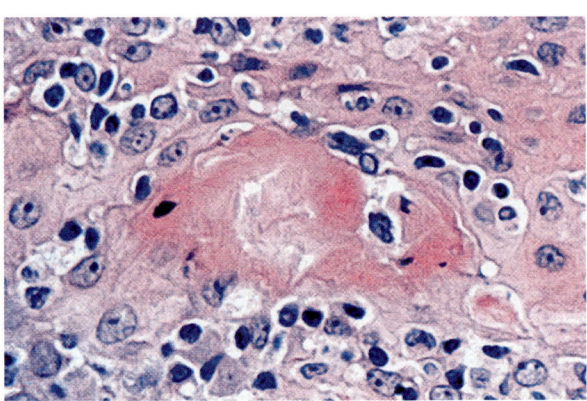

Figure 4-94

LYMPHOEPITHELIOMA-LIKE CARCINOMA

Focal trichilemmal-type pilar keratinization.

in LELC of the skin (figs. 4-93, 4-94), with the focal formation of intercellular ductal spaces or areas of trichilemmal-type keratinization (241). These features, together with the localization of most LELCs in the dermis, makes it likely that many tumors of this type are primitive appendageal neoplasms.

Although the histologic features of this tumor are those of a largely undifferentiated epithelial proliferation, its biologic behavior is indolent and few lesions have metastasized (233–235,237–239). Unlike LELCs of the nasopharynx, pharyngeal tonsil, salivary gland, and lung, similar tumors of the skin do not exhibit integration of genomic nucleic acid from the Epstein-Barr virus upon in situ hybridization or polymerase chain reaction studies (241). The latter finding may be helpful in excluding metastasis of an LELC to the skin, but such a lesion is extraordinarily rare.

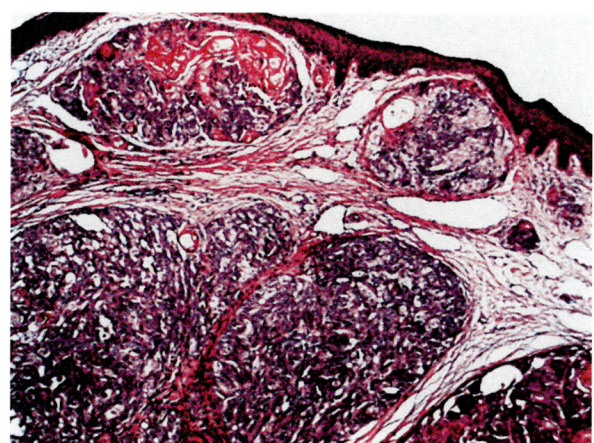
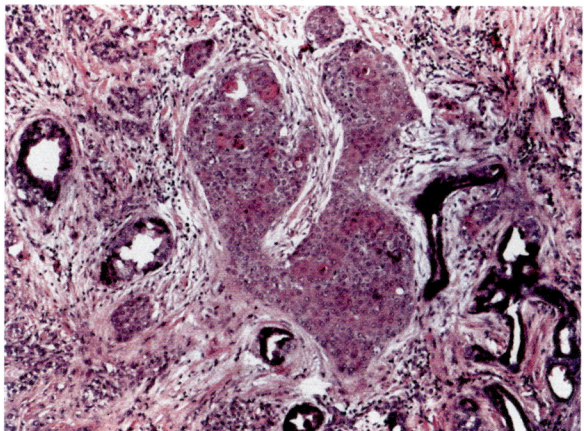

Figure 4-95

PRIMARY NEUROENDOCRINE CARCINOMA WITH MIXED DIFFERENTIATION

The lesions have an admixture of pilar, sebaceous, and glandular elements.

Adnexal Carcinoma with Mixed Differentiation

The examination of a meaningful number of cutaneous adnexal tumors cannot be done without realizing that some of them defy predefined nosologic schemes. Such tumors most often exhibit bilinear or even multilinear differentiation, showing mixtures of eccrine, apocrine, sebaceous, and pilar elements. This phenomenon has been cited above in reference to adenomas, and it applies to appendageal carcinomas as well. Several tumors have been documented that amalgamate the features of ductal eccrine carcinoma, porocarcinoma, ductal apocrine adenocarcinoma, sebaceous carcinoma, pilomatrix carcinoma, and malignant proliferating pilar tumors, all intimately admixed within the same mass (figs. 4-95–4-97) (236). The most appropriate diagnostic label for such lesions is simply the descriptive one of "adnexal carcinoma with mixed differentiation." Basic recognition of these tumors as malignant is accomplished by attention to the features that have been stressed repeatedly throughout this chapter: infiltrative growth, obvious cytologic anaplasia, spontaneous necrosis, and invasion of nerves or blood vessels. The behavior of these lesions has been indolent, and no fatalities have been ascribed to them as of this writing.

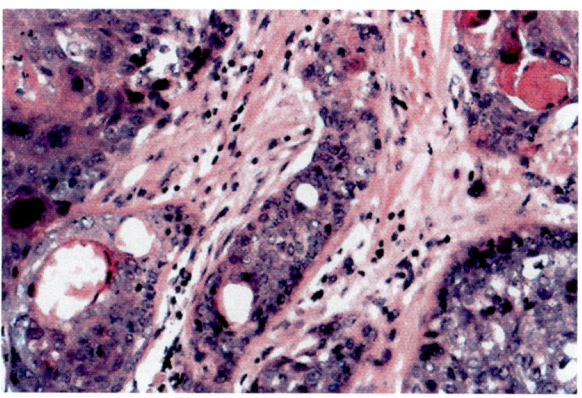

Figure 4-96

ADNEXAL CARCINOMA WITH MIXED DIFFERENTIATION

The presence of pilar-type keratinization in this otherwise glandular malignant neoplasm of the skin marks it as an adnexal carcinoma with mixed differentiation.

PRIMARY NEUROENDOCRINE (MERKEL CELL) CARCINOMA

Clinical Features. The lesion known as *trabecular carcinoma, primary neuroendocrine carcinoma, cutaneous apudoma,* or *Merkel cell carcinoma* (MCC) is a well-known small cell proliferation of the skin. Increasingly, this lesion has been classified as an appendageal cutaneous tumor, because normal skin demonstrates the presence of neuroendocrine cells in the outer hair sheath and in sweat ducts (273).

Nonmelanocytic Tumors of the Skin

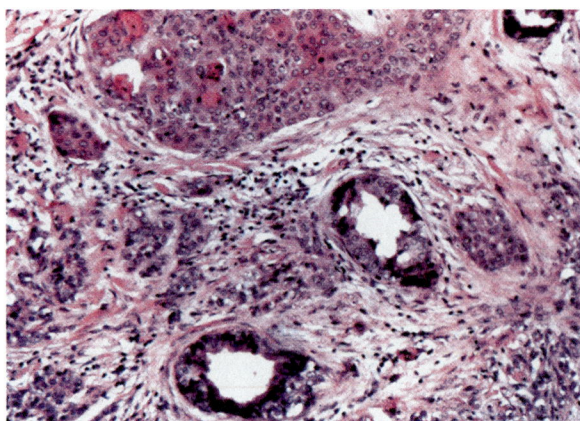
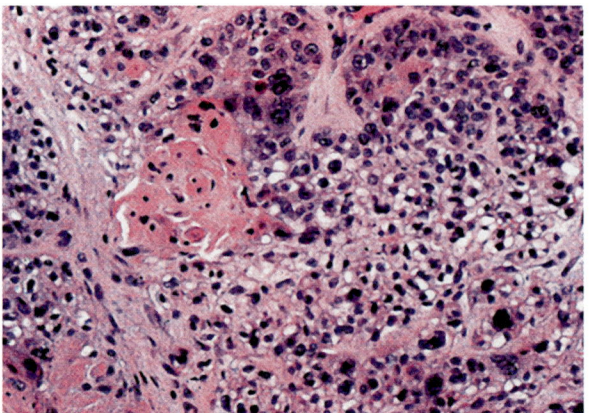

Figure 4-97

ADNEXAL CARCINOMA WITH MIXED DIFFERENTIATION
Glandular and pilar-type differentiation are seen in different fields of the same lesion.

MCC typically arises in the sun-exposed skin of elderly patients, particularly on the head and neck. Uncommon cases have been reported in adolescence and early adulthood, and in topographic areas that are usually covered by clothing. Only rare cases of MCC have been documented on mucosal surfaces other than the vulva (266). There appears to be no sex predilection for this lesion (242,243,246,247,250,256,262,263, 270,271,274–277,281,284,288,290).

The duration of growth of MCC varies before patients seek medical attention: from a few weeks to several years in some reports (247,256, 271,274,288,290). MCC assumes a diversity of macroscopic appearances. The most common is that of a nonulcerated, reddish violet, nodular dermal mass (fig. 4-98), but other forms grossly resemble fibrous papules, boils, epidermoid inclusion cysts, lymphoma cutis, or inflamed comedones (250,263,288). One reported multifocally recurrent lesion produced nodular and plaquelike violaceous lesions that were confused clinically with angiosarcoma (263). Tumor size varies from 2 to 3 mm to several centimeters in greatest dimension (263,285).

This neoplasm typically occurs as a single mass, but rare cases have demonstrated a multiplicity of lesions; these may appear either synchronously or metachronously (253,257,291). In the metachronous cases, a clinical similarity to cutaneous metastases from visceral tumors is remarkable. One spectacular case featured over 100 separate tumors; such a presentation would make one particularly skeptical of the primary nature of the cutaneous neoplastic process, but the patient in question survived for a prolonged period (289). Such prolonged survival would not be expected in individuals with metastatic cutaneous lesions, whose mean life span is less than 4 months after tumor presentation (285), which means that the diagnosis of primary, multifocal MCC is often made on a retrospective basis.

In roughly 10 percent of cases there is a history of squamous cell carcinoma in the same skin area as that harboring MCC (251,265). Accordingly, the favored clinical diagnosis for such patients is recurrent keratinocytic neoplasia. The macroscopic appearance of these lesions differs significantly, however, providing a clue to the error of such an assumption; squamous carcinomas are verrucoid or ulcerated, infiltrative, white-gray masses.

Rare examples of MCC have arisen in individuals with cutaneous dysplasia syndromes featuring hypohidrosis, dentoskeletal anomalies, basal cell carcinomas, and partial alopecia (291). We have observed one case occurring in association with a pituitary adenoma. This concurrence is interesting in that both neoplasms are neuroendocrine in nature; evaluation for the familial presence of other components of the multiple endocrine neoplasia syndrome are warranted in such instances. Nevertheless, a convincingly complete manifestation of these clinical tumor complexes has not been seen in connection with MCC to date.

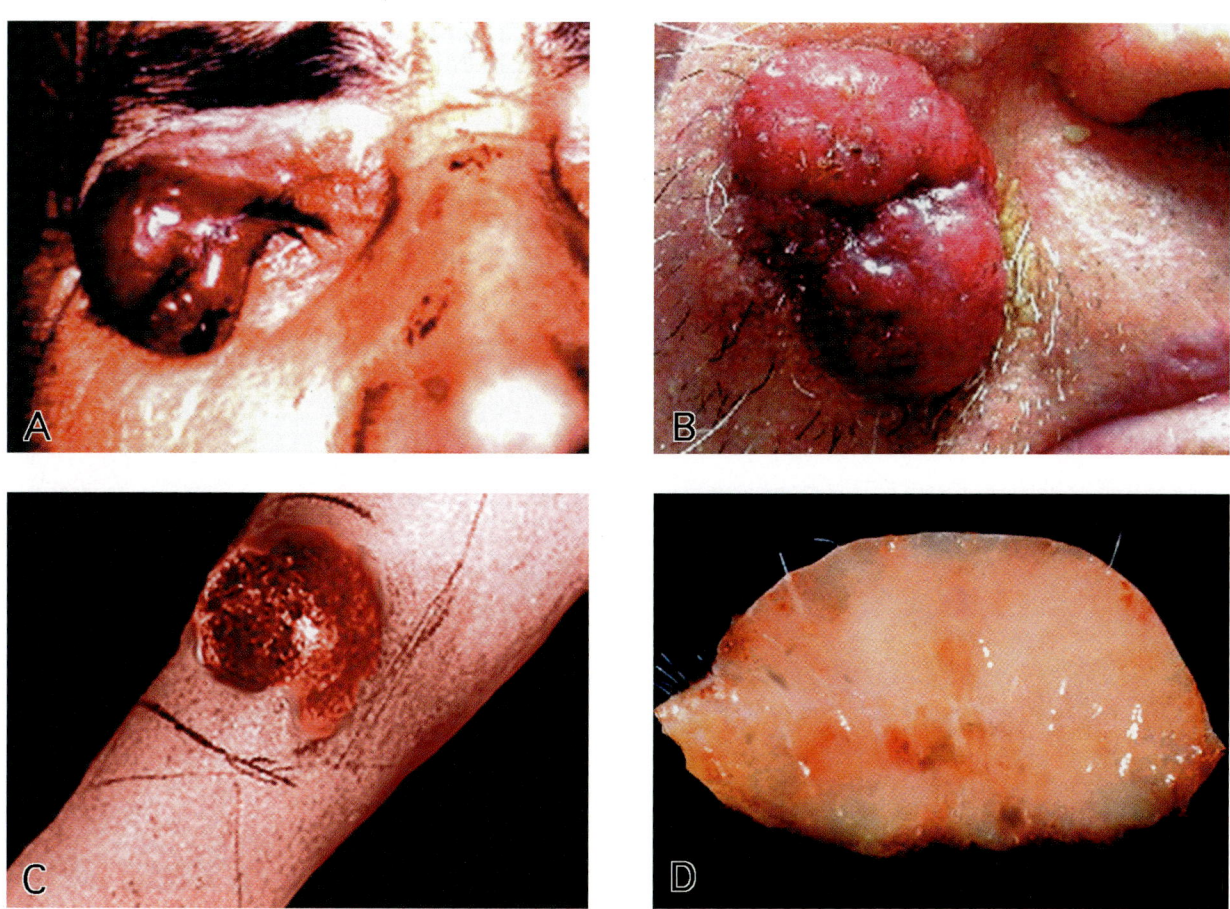

Figure 4-98

MERKEL CELL CARCINOMA

Nodular reddish masses are seen in the facial skin (A and B) and the skin of the leg (C). The cut surface of a resected lesion has a uniform white-gray appearance that resembles fish flesh (D).

There have been reports on the supposed existence of primary MCC of lymph nodes, presumably arising in epithelial neuroendocrine rests in such structures (248,249). In light of the fact that spontaneous regression of cutaneous tumors of this type may be observed (272), albeit rarely, we are unconvinced that a lymph node origin for MCC could ever be proven.

Pathologic Findings. The majority of MCCs are purely dermal in microscopic location and are separated from the overlying epidermis by a "grenz" zone (figs. 4-99, 4-100). They assume either a medullary (sheet-like) or trabecular and organoid growth pattern, with an ill-defined margin, and are composed of monotonous, small, round tumor cells (figs. 4-101, 4-102) (256a). These tumor cells possess oval nuclei with evenly distributed chromatin, inconspicuous nucleoli, and abundant mitotic activity (up to 20 mitotic figures per high-power [X400] field). The cytoplasm is typically scanty and amphophilic. The supporting stroma is delicate but richly vascular; indeed, dilated intratumoral venules and capillaries are thought to account for the reddish macroscopic color of most lesions (fig. 4-103) (258a). Infiltration of the underlying subcutis, with entrapment of adipocytes and vascular permeation, is observed in many cases (274,275).

Variations on this description include lesions composed of larger cells with more abundant cytoplasm, a subtype strongly resembling oat cell carcinoma of the lung (282,283), and another featuring the presence of randomly dispersed giant tumor cells, which may be multinucleated.

Merkel cell

The first of these appearances is similar to that of carcinoid tumors in other anatomic locations. In addition, some examples of MCC exhibit focal spindle cell change in the neoplastic cells or a myxoid quality of the intercellular matrix (277). Roughly 10 percent involve the epidermis focally and may simulate the histologic features of Pautrier's microabscesses in cutaneous T-cell lymphomas (263).

As mentioned above, MCC may be associated with squamous cell carcinoma or basal cell carcinoma in the same skin field (251). Some tumors assume a collision pattern, wherein intraepidermal squamous carcinoma or invasive squamous tumors are abruptly juxtaposed to the dermal small cell proliferation, while others demonstrate an admixture of malignant surface epithelial elements with the latter component (fig. 4-104) (247,251,276). Silva et al. (277), Gould et al. (252), and Walsh (287) have described foci of

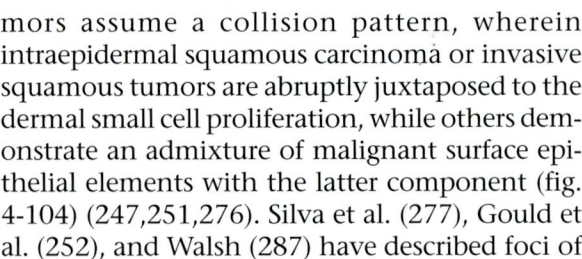

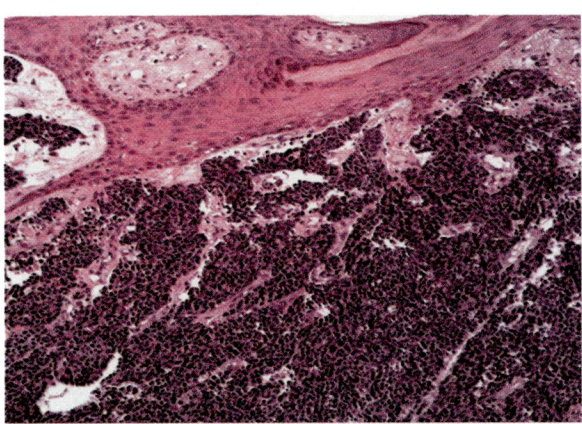

Figure 4-99

MERKEL CELL CARCINOMA

Scanning photomicrograph of Merkel cell carcinoma shows an ill-defined basaloid neoplasm in the dermis.

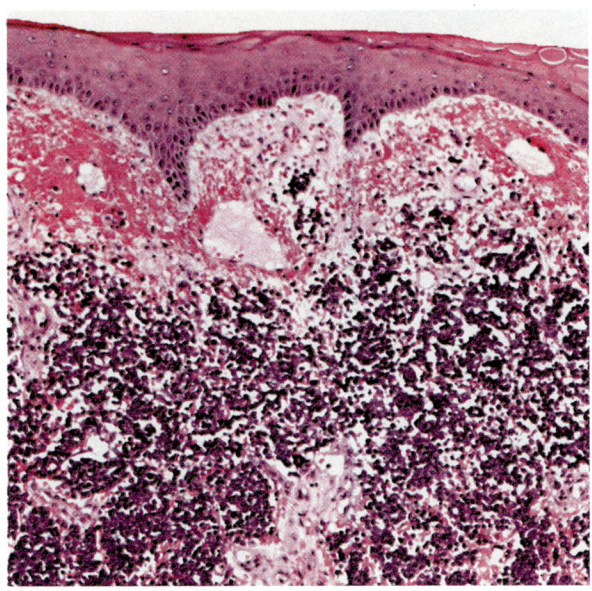

Figure 4-100

MERKEL CELL CARCINOMA

A "grenz" zone is clearly demonstrated between the epidermal basement membrane and the neoplasm.

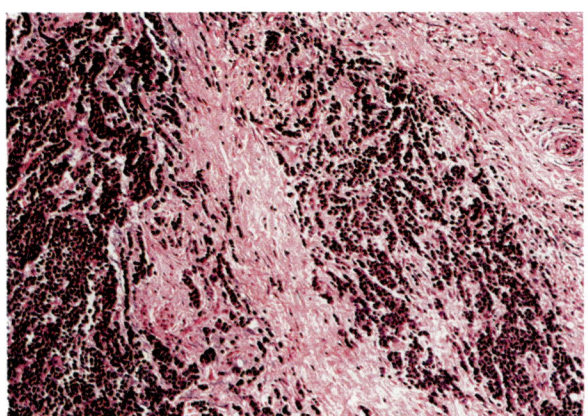 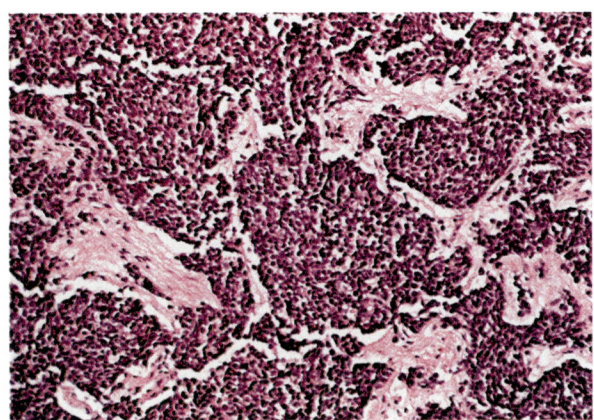

Figure 4-101

MERKEL CELL CARCINOMA

Trabecular growth (left) and organoid configurations (right) in Merkel cell carcinoma.

Neoplasms and Pseudoneoplastic Proliferations of the Sweat Glands

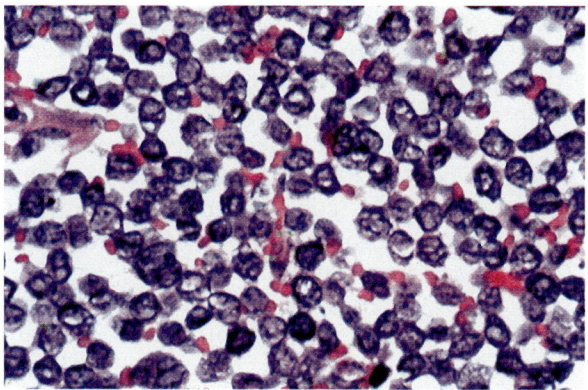

Figure 4-102

MERKEL CELL CARCINOMA

Cellular monotony, dispersed nuclear chromatin, and high nuclear to cytoplasmic ratios typify the cells of Merkel cell carcinoma.

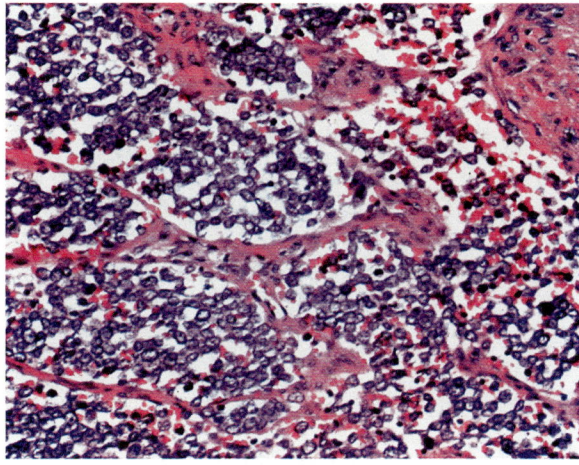

Figure 4-103

MERKEL CELL CARCINOMA

A fibrovascular stroma is often prominent in Merkel cell carcinoma and probably is responsible for its reddish clinical appearance.

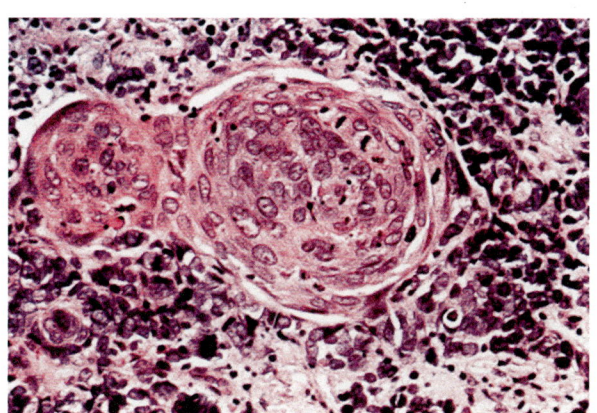
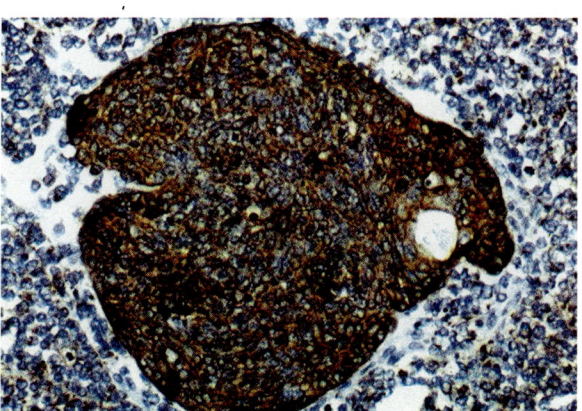

Figure 4-104

MERKEL CELL CARCINOMA

Left: Divergent squamous differentiation is apparent in the center.
Right: Immunostaining for keratin highlights a focus of divergent squamous differentiation.

divergent sudoriferous differentiation in these neoplasms. Melanin pigmentation has not been reported in MCC, and histologic detection of melanin excludes the diagnosis of MCC.

Regional coagulative necrosis is apparent in approximately 50 percent of MCCs, in a specific geographic pattern (263,277). Peritumoral lymphoplasmacytic inflammation varies considerably, but it may be prominent in rare cases. We have seen one example in which a superficial resemblance to medullary carcinoma of the breast was produced by lymphoid infiltrates in the tumor.

Special Studies. Ultrastructurally, MCC shows the generic electron microscopic attributes of any neuroendocrine carcinoma. These include macular-type intercellular junctional complexes, cytoplasmic dense-core granules measuring between 100 and 300 nm in diameter, and a tendency for intracellular intermediate filaments to be aggregated into whorls in a perinuclear location (274,276).

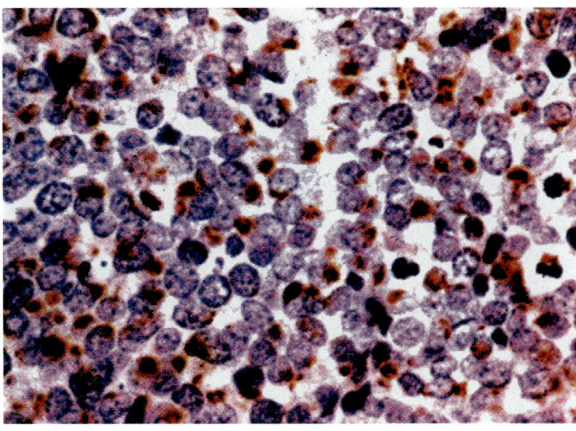

Figure 4-105

MERKEL CELL CARCINOMA

Typical perinuclear "dots" of keratin immunoreactivity in Merkel cell carcinoma. This finding simultaneously establishes the epithelial lineage and a neuroendocrine nature for this tumor.

The immunophenotypic characteristics of MCC mirror those of neuroendocrine carcinomas in other tissue sites. Keratin is uniformly expressed; neuroendocrine carcinomas may further demonstrate a unique pattern of reactivity for this intermediate filament protein, in the form of perinuclear globular staining of the cytoplasm (fig. 4-105) (254,258,286). This image is seen in approximately two thirds of all cases. Cytokeratin (CK) 20 is observed in approximately 85 percent of MCCs (267). CD45 is uniformly lacking, as are vimentin, muscle-specific actin, and desmin. Nearly all MCCs express neuron-specific enolase, and may be labeled for neurofilament protein, EMA, and the MOC-31 protein (259). The synthesis of chromogranin, CD99 (MIC-2), microtubule-associated protein-2, CD56, CD57, and neuropeptides such as somatostatin, calcitonin, corticotropin, pancreatic polypeptide, vasoactive intestinal polypeptide, and substance P, is also possible in MCCs, with variable frequency (259,261,267). Synaptophysin, a protein that is unique to neurons, neuroepithelial cells, and their neoplasms, is likewise detectable in one third of MCCs.

One notable difference between MCC and extracutaneous neuroendocrine carcinoma is the consistent absence in the former of CEA and thyroid transcription factor-1 (TTF1) (260,261, 268). Our practice has been to exclude a diagnosis of primary neuroendocrine skin cancer if either one of these determinants is detected immunohistochemically. Conversely, MCCs may label for CK20, as mentioned earlier, whereas visceral small cell carcinomas generally do not. Telomerase and CD117 (c-kit protein) are present in the majority of tumors, but these markers probably have more potential interest as possible targets for evaluation of therapy than as diagnostic determinants (279,280).

Differential Diagnosis. Because of the histologically undifferentiated small cell appearance of MCC, a considerable number of diagnostic considerations must be entertained before making a final interpretation. These principally include malignant lymphoma, neuroendocrine carcinomas metastatic to the skin, primary small cell squamous and eccrine carcinomas, small cell malignant melanoma, and peripheral neuroepithelioma/primitive neuroectodermal tumor. Immunohistologic analysis is probably the most productive method for separating these entities; expected immunophenotypes are shown in Table 4-1.

The Azzopardi phenomenon, the encrustation of intratumoral blood vessels by basophilic nucleic acid (fig. 4-106), is commonly observed by conventional microscopy in secondary small cell neuroendocrine carcinomas of the skin. We have never observed this feature in primary MCC.

Cytogenetic studies may also be useful. Primitive neuroectodermal tumors demonstrate a consistent t(11;22) chromosomal translocation, whereas preferential abnormalities in chromosome 1 are typical of MCC (278).

Treatment and Prognosis. MCCs should be regarded as aggressive neoplasms, with a relatively high risk of lethal behavior. A review of reported cases indicates that 40 percent of these tumors recur locally in the skin after surgical excision, and 75 percent of patients with at least one recurrence go on to develop regional lymph node or distant metastasis (247a). Visceral involvement (of the lungs, bones, brain, liver, and deep lymph nodes) has been observed in approximately 35 to 40 percent of patients, virtually all of whom die within an average of 6 months. An additional 5 percent of patients with MCC die of uncontrollable local recurrence (255,263,277).

Table 4-1

IMMUNOHISTOLOGIC DIFFERENTIAL DIAGNOSIS OF CUTANEOUS SMALL CELL MALIGNANCIES

Tumor	PAN-K[a]	CK20	CK5/6	p63	TTF1	CD99	CEA	S-100P	MEL-A	VIM	CD45
Merkel cell carcinoma	+	+	0	0	0	+/-	0	0	0	0	0
Metastatic neuroendocrine carcinoma (usually from the lung)	+	0	0	0	+	+/-	+/-	0	0	0	0
Small cell squamous carcinoma	+	0	+	+	0	0	0	0	0	+/-	0
Small cell eccrine carcinoma	+	0	0	0	0	0	+/-	+/-	0	+/-	0
Small cell melanoma	0	0	0	0	0	+/-	0	+	+	+	0
Primitive neuroectodermal tumor	+/-	0	0	0	0	+	0	0	0	+	0
Non-Hodgkin's lymphoma	0	0	0	0	0	+/-	0	0	0	+/-	+

[a]PAN-K = pankeratin; CK20 = cytokeratin type 20; CK5/6 = cytokeratin types 5 and 6; TTF1 = thyroid transcription factor-1; CEA = carcinoembryonic antigen; S-100P = S-100 protein; MEL-A = Melan-A/MART-1; VIM = vimentin.

Statistical analysis using the methods of Kaplan and Meier reveals an overall survival rate of 88 percent at 1 year, 72 percent at 2 years, and 55 percent at 5 years after diagnosis. Interestingly but inexplicably, female patients with MCC have a better survival rate than males (255).

Recommended treatment for this tumor is predicated on surgical extirpation, if at all possible; wide excision (like that utilized for malignant melanomas of similar size and depth of invasion) is recommended. In addition, it appears that MCC is a radiosensitive (but not radiocurable) lesion, and that response to therapeutic irradiation is related to overall tumor bulk (263). Accordingly, some authorities recommend that immediate postoperative radiotherapy should be administered to the tumor bed, regional lymphatic chains, and "in transit" tissue, particularly when lymphatic permeation by the primary neoplasm is present microscopically or the margin of excision is suboptimal (277). There is little agreement on the necessity of this measure. Silva et al. (277) have suggested that prophylactic regional lymphadenectomy should be performed if the primary neoplasm measures over 2 cm in greatest dimension and if mitotic activity averages more than 10 mitoses per high-power field. This guideline is based on the findings of Goepfert and coworkers (250), who reported topographically regional treatment failure in 75 percent of cases that had not been subjected to lymph node dissection.

The sentinel node biopsy technique (245,264, 269) has been applied in MCC cases. Mehrany et al. (264) have suggested that this method is effective in preventing short-term regional recurrence, but an effect on overall survival has not yet been determined with certainty.

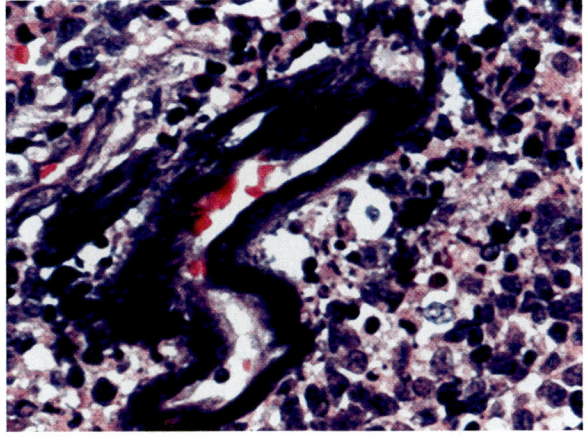

Figure 4-106

METASTATIC SMALL CELL PULMONARY CARCINOMA

The Azzopardi phenomenon is shown by intratumoral encrustation of blood vessels with basophilic nucleic acid. This finding is not observed in Merkel cell carcinoma.

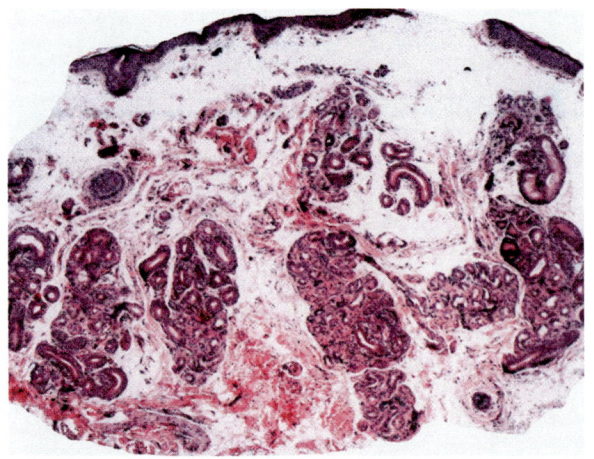 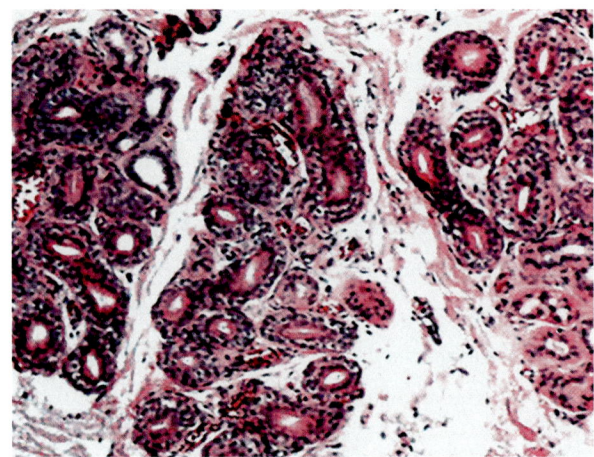

Figure 4-107

ECCRINE SWEAT GLAND NEVUS

A congerie of relatively immature eccrine coils is seen in the dermis.

PSEUDONEOPLASTIC LESIONS OF SWEAT GLANDS

Occasionally, the pathologist may be faced with biopsy specimens in which reactive proliferation of the sweat glands invokes a consideration of neoplastic disease. This is most often true when the clinical information is inadequate, but exceptions to that caveat do occur. Such pseudoneoplastic adnexal lesions are considered below.

Eccrine and Apocrine Nevi

Nevi, more aptly termed malformations, of the eccrine and apocrine apparatus are composed of cellular arrays that resemble embryonic sweat glands. They exhibit well-formed sudoriferous coils that are composed of compact polygonal cells, sometimes with a luminal cuticle. Each of the tubular aggregates is invested by a basement membrane, and small nerves may be seen in the lesions. The sweat gland units are slightly disordered architecturally, and they are more numerous than those found in mature skin (fig. 4-107) (292,295,298,299,304–308). This finding explains the common misinterpretation of such lesions as neoplasms, particularly as acrospiromas or syringomas. Nevertheless, sweat gland nevi do not show confluent cellular growth or "comma-tail" glandular configurations, as seen, respectively, in those tumors.

The lesion known as *eccrine angiomatous hamartoma* is a malformation that incorporates sweat glands and mesenchymal elements (293). It usually is seen in early childhood as a red, yellow, brownish, or tan papule or plaque on the arms or legs, and may be associated with localized sweating and pain on palpation. Eccrine angiomatous hamartoma differs slightly from uncomplicated adnexal nevi because it contains venular blood vessels and small nerve twigs between the nevoid sweat gland coils (fig. 4-108).

Syringometaplasia

Other lesions that resemble sweat gland nevi have been documented in patients with scarring forms of alopecia, in areas near keratoacanthomas, or in squamous cell carcinomas (303). Similar lesions may be seen in fibrosing dermatitides or adjacent to primary malignant tumors of the skin. Cutaneous syringoma-like proliferations, with the additional elements of acrosyringeal and eccrine ductal hyperplasia, and squamous or mucin-forming glandular cells, may arise after the use of oral nonsteroidal anti-inflammatory and antineoplastic drugs (figs. 4-109–4-112) (300,302). It is likely that these lesions are reactive or metaplastic in nature (syringometaplasia), reflecting a response to appendageal injury. They may regress after removal of the offending agent(s).

Neoplasms and Pseudoneoplastic Proliferations of the Sweat Glands

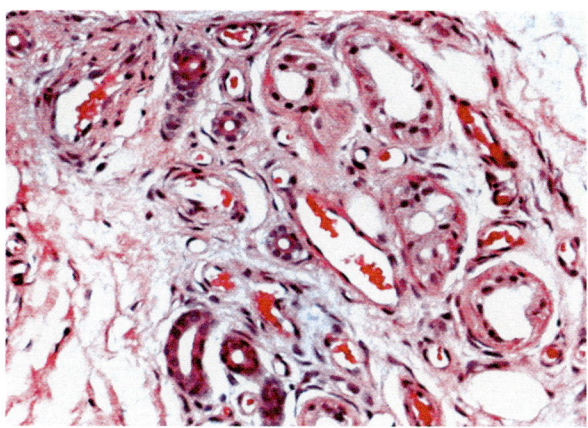

Figure 4-108

ECCRINE ANGIOMATOUS HAMARTOMA

This proliferation is similar to eccrine nevus, as depicted in the previous figure, but also contains lesional blood vessels and nerve twigs.

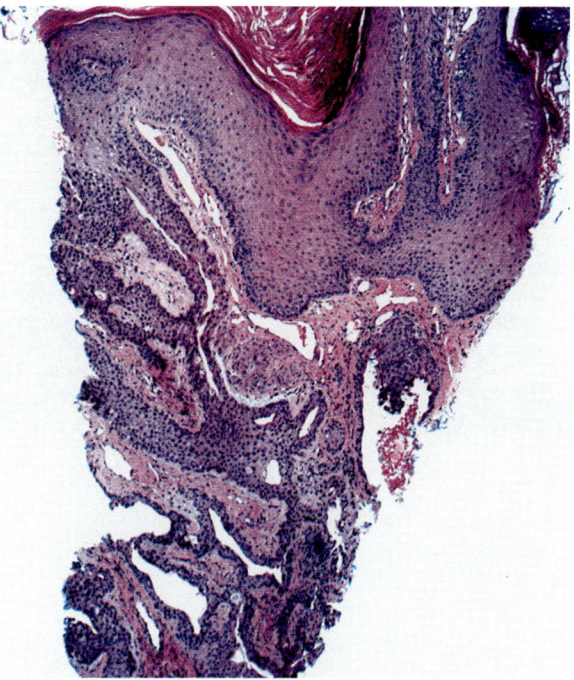

Figure 4-109

SYRINGOMETAPLASIA

Hyperplasia of the eccrine ducts and acrosyringium is seen.

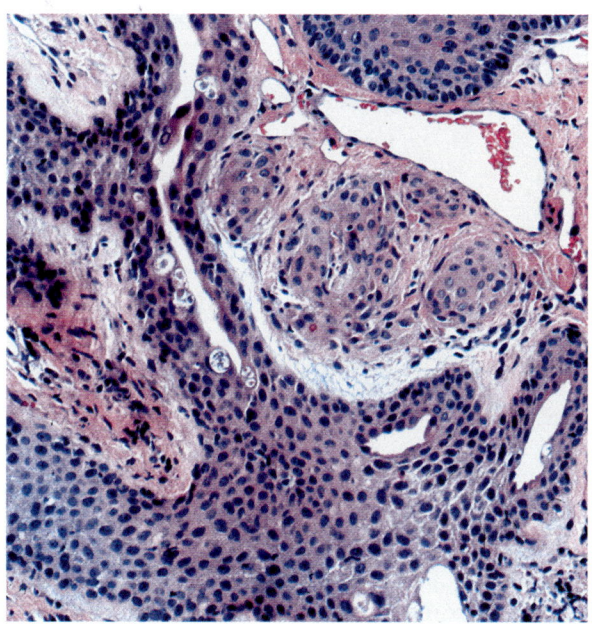

Figure 4-110

SYRINGOMETAPLASIA

Hyperplastic eccrine ducts are present.

Eccrine and Apocrine Hidrocystomas

Selected cystic lesions of the eccrine and apocrine sweat gland units, usually seen on the face of patients living in warm climates (fig. 4-113), have variously been described as neoplasms or reaction patterns. Most often, these are termed

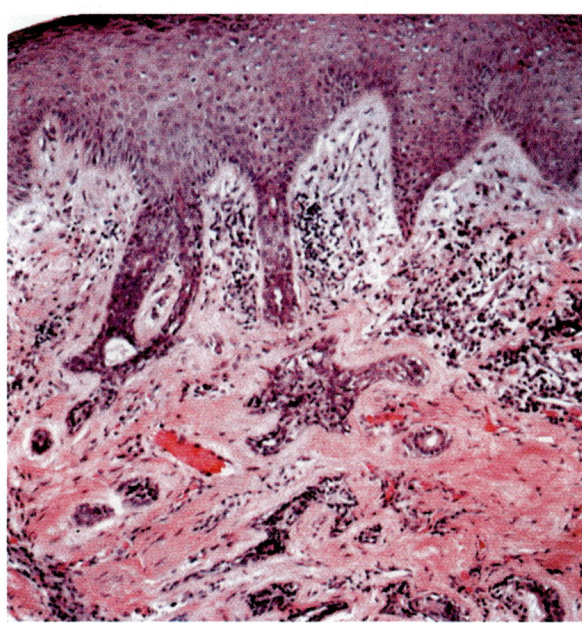

Figure 4-111

SYRINGOMETAPLASIA

Proliferation and squamoid changes in the eccrine ducts are seen.

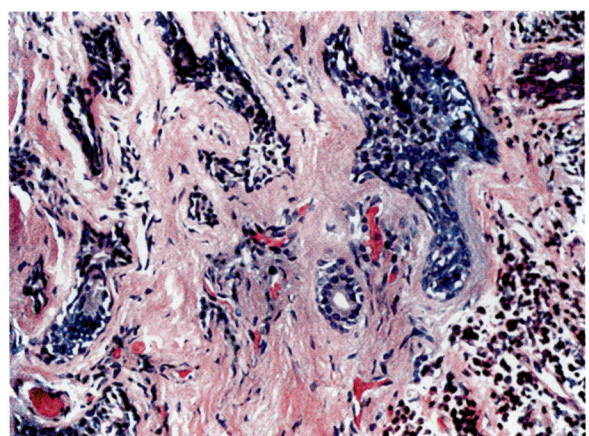

Figure 4-112

SYRINGOMETAPLASIA

The eccrine ducts are distorted and proliferative.

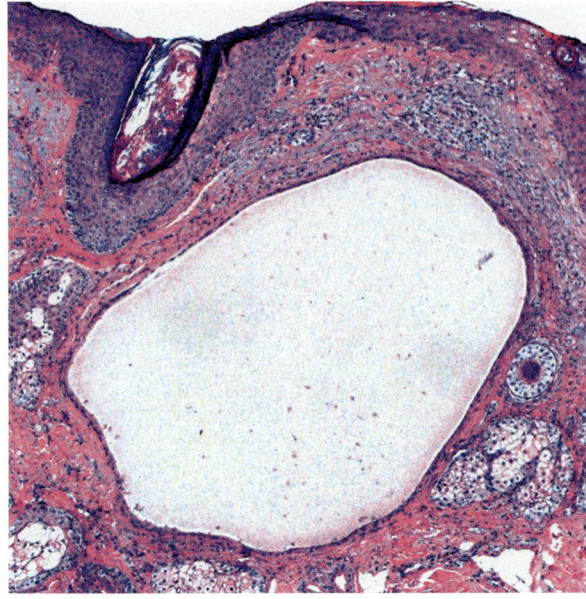

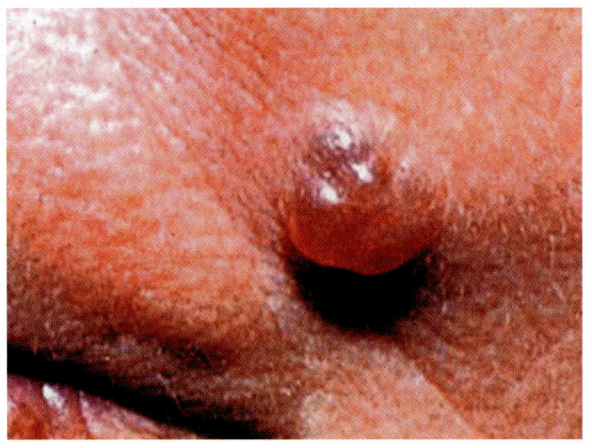

Figure 4-113

ECCRINE HIDROCYSTOMA

There is a thin-walled vesicular lesion in the skin of the cheek. The patient reported that the lesion grew in size during warm weather.

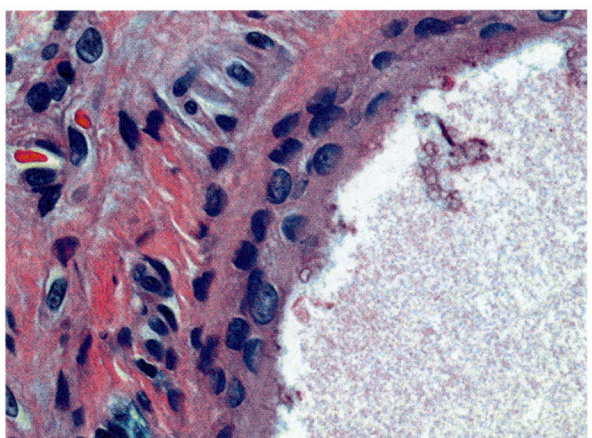

Figure 4-114

ECCRINE HIDROCYSTOMA

Eccrine hidrocystoma is characterized by cystic dilatation of the eccrine ducts, probably because of obstruction. The lining cells are indistinguishable from those of the normal sweat duct.

eccrine and apocrine hidrocystomas, and they are characterized by dilation of the sweat ducts and secondary architecturally bland proliferation of the ductal epithelium (fig. 4-114) (294,309,310). The latter phenomenon may produce micropapillary intraluminal cell profiles (as in so-called cystadenomas) (297,301). Apocrine hidrocystomas of the eyelid (fig. 4-115) have also been described as *Moll's gland cysts* in the ophthalmologic literature (296). It is likely that tumefactions in this general category are pseudoneoplastic in nature, and that they represent reactions to terminal sweat duct obstruction and inspissation of sweat glandular secretions.

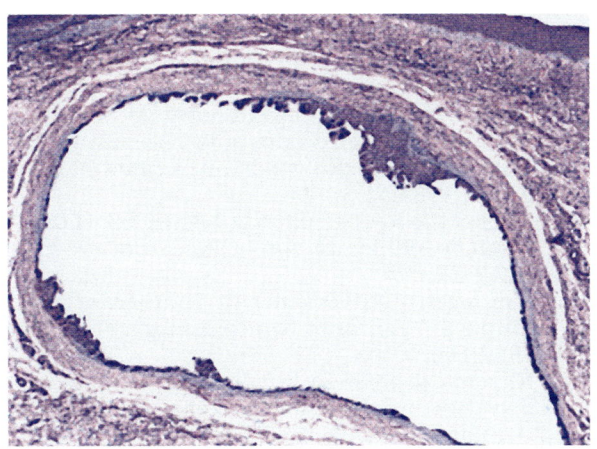 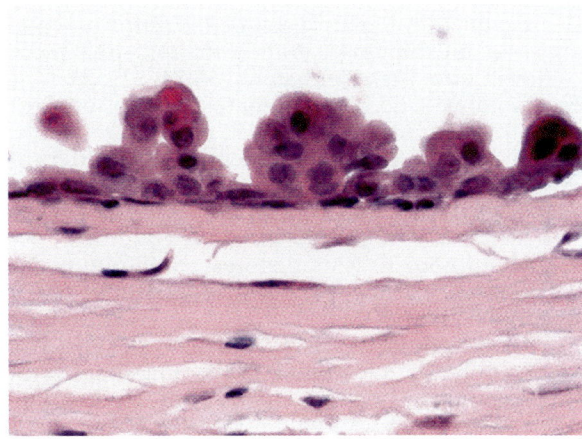

Figure 4-115

APOCRINE HIDROCYSTOMA OF THE EYELID

The configuration of this lesion is identical to that of eccrine hidrocystoma, except that the lining cells have apocrine cytologic features (right).

REFERENCES

Benign Eccrine and Apocrine Sweat Gland Neoplasms

1. Abenoza P, Ackerman AB. Neoplasms with eccrine differentiation. Philadelphia: Lea & Febiger; 1990.
2. Aloi F, Pich A. Papillary eccrine adenoma. A histopathological and immunohistochemical study. Dermatologica 1991;182:47–51.
3. Aloi FG, Pippione M. Dermal duct tumor. Appl Pathol 1986;4:175–8.
4. Ambrojo P, Requena Caballero L, Aguilar Martinez A, Sanchez Yus E, Furio V. Clear cell syringoma. Immunohistochemistry and electron microscopy study. Dermatologica 1989;178:164–6.
5. Ansai S, Watanabe S, Aso K. A case of tubular apocrine adenoma with syringocystadenoma papilliferum. J Cutan Pathol 1989;16:230–6.
6. Biernat W, Kordek R, Wozniak L. Papillary eccrine adenoma—a case of cutaneous sweat gland tumor with secretory and ductular differentiation. Pol J Pathol 1994;45:319–22.
6a. Bowen S, Gill M, Lee DA, et al. Mutations in the CYLD gene in Brooke-Spiegler syndrome, familial cylindromatosis, and multiple familial trichoepithelioma: lack of genotype-phenotype correlation. J Invest Dermatol 2005;124:919–20.
7. Brown SM, Freeman RG. Syringoma limited to the vulva. Arch Dermatol 1971;104:331.
8. Cecchi R, Crudeli F, Fedi E, Giomi A. [Multiple trichoepitheliomas, cylindromas, ecrine spiradenomas present in the same family. Histologic and histopathologenetic considerations.] G Ital Dermatol 1985;120:149–52. (Italian.)
9. Civatte J, Jeanmougin M, Barrandon Y, Jimenez de Franch A. [Mascaro's eccrine syringofibroadenoma. Discussion of a case.] Med Cutan Ibero Lat Am 1981;9:193–6. (Spanish.)
10. Cooper PH. Mitotic figures in sweat gland adenomas. J Cutan Pathol 1987;14:10–4.
11. Cooper PH, Frierson HF. Papillary eccrine adenoma. Arch Pathol Lab Med 1984;108:55–7.
12. Cotton DW, Slater DN, Rooney N, Goepel JR, Mills PM. Giant vascular eccrine spiradenomas: a report of two cases with histology, immunohistology, and electron microscopy. Histopathology 1986;10:1093–9.
13. Crain RC, Helwig EB. Dermal cylindroma (dermal eccrine cylindroma). Am J Clin Pathol 1961;35:504–5.
14. Cruz DJ. Sweat gland carcinoma: a comprehensive review. Semin Diagn Pathol 1987;4:38–74.
15. Falck VG, Jordaan HF. Papillary eccrine adenoma. A tubulopapillary hidradenoma with eccrine differentiation. Am J Dermatopathol 1986;8:64–72.
16. Feibelman CE, Maize JC. Clear-cell syringoma. A study by conventional and electron microscopy. Am J Dermatopathol 1984;6:139–50.
17. Freeman RG, Knox JM, Spiller WF. Eccrine poroma. Am J Clin Pathol 1961;36:444–50.
18. Goette DK, McConnell MA, Fowler VR. Cylindroma and eccrine spiradenoma coexistent in the same lesion. Arch Dermatol 1982;118:273–4.

19. Goldman P, Pinkus H, Rogin JR. Eccrine poroma; tumors exhibiting features of the epidermal sweat duct unit. Arch Dermatol 1956;74: 511–21.
20. Goldner R. Eccrine poromatosis. Arch Dermatol 1970;101:606–8.
21. Grund JL. Syringocystadenoma papilliferum and nevus sebaceus (Jadassohn) occurring as a single tumor; report of a case. AMA Arch Derm Syphilol 1952;65:340–7.
22. Hashimoto K. Hidradenoma papilliferum. An electron microscopic study. Acta Derm Venereol 1973;53:22–30.
23. Hashimoto K, DiBella RJ, Borsuk GM, Lever WF. Eruptive hidradenoma and syringoma. Histologic, histochemical, and electron microscopic studies. Arch Dermatol 1967;96:500–19.
24. Hashimoto K, DiBella RJ, Lever WF. Clear cell hidradenoma. Histological, histochemical, and electron microscopic studies. Arch Dermatol 1967;96:18–38.
25. Hashimoto K, Mehregan AH, Kumakiri M. Tumors of skin appendages. Boston: Butterworth; 1987.
26. Helwig EB, Hackney VC. Syringocystadenoma papilliferum; lesions with and without naevus sebaceous and basal cell carcinoma. AMA Arch Derm 1955;71:361–72.
27. Henner MS, Shapiro PE, Ritter JH, Leffell D, Wick MR. Solitary syringoma. Report of five cases and clinicopathologic comparison with microcystic adnexal carcinoma of the skin. Am J Dermatopathol 1995;17:465–70.
28. Hu CH, Marques AS, Winkelmann RK. Dermal duct tumor: a histochemical and electron microscopic study. Arch Dermatol 1978;114:1659–64.
28a. Hu G, Onder M, Gill M, et al. A novel missense mutation in CYLD in a family with Brooke-Spiegler syndrome. J Invest Dermatol 2003;121:732–4.
29. Hyman AB, Brownstein MH. Eccrine poroma. An analysis of forty-five new cases. Dermatologica 1969;138:29–38.
30. Isaacson D, Turner ML. Localized vulvar syringomas. J Am Acad Dermatol 1979;1:352–6.
31. Johnson BL Jr, Helwig EB. Eccrine acrospiroma. A clinicopathologic study. Cancer 1969;23:641–57.
32. Kanitakis J, Zambruno G, Euvrard S, Hermier C, Thivolet J. Eccrine syringofibroadenoma. Immunohistological study of a new case. Am J Dermatopathol 1987;9:37–40.
33. Kao GF, Laskin WB, Weiss SW. Eccrine spiradenoma occurring in infancy, mimicking a mesenchymal tumor. J Cutan Pathol 1990;17: 214–9.
34. Karam P, Benedetto AN. Syringomas: new approach to an old technique. Int J Dermatol 1996;35:219–20.
35. Kersting DW, Helwig EB. Eccrine spiradenoma. AMA Arch Dermatol 1956;73:199–227.
35a. Leonard N, Chaggar R, Jones C, Takahashi M, Nikitopoulou A, Lakhani SR. Loss of heterozygosity at cylindromatosis gene locus, CYLD, in sporadic skin adnexal tumors. J Clin Pathol 2001;54:689–92.
36. Mambo NC. Eccrine spiradenomas: clinical and pathologic study of 49 tumors. J Cutan Pathol 1983;10:312–20.
37. Mambo NC. The significance of atypical nuclear changes in benign eccrine acrospiromas: a clinical and pathological study of 18 cases. J Cutan Pathol 1984;11:35–44.
38. Meeker JH, Neubechker RD, Helwig EB. Hidradenoma papilliferum. Am J Clin Pathol 1962;37: 182–95.
39. Mehregan AH, Levson DN. Hidroacanthoma simplex. A report of two cases. Arch Dermatol 1969;100:303–5.
40. Niizuma K. Syringocystadenoma papilliferum: light and electron microscopic studies. Acta Dermatol Venereol 1976;56:327–36.
41. Novak E, Stevenson RR. Sweat gland tumors of the vulva, benign (hidradenoma) and malignant (adenocarcinoma). Am J Obstet Gynecol 1945; 50:641–59.
42. Palazzo J, Stenn KS, Wolf ER. Eccrine tubular poroma. Report of an unusual benign eccrine adnexal tumor. J Cutan Pathol 1987;14:365.
43. Pinkus H. Life history of naevus syringocystadenomatosus papilliferus. AMA Arch Derm Syphilol 1954;63:305–22.
44. Pruzan DL, Esterly NB, Prose NS. Eruptive syringoma. Arch Dermatol 1989;125:1119–20.
45. Pylyser K, De Wolf-Peeters C, Marien K. The histology of eccrine poroma: a study of 14 cases. Dermatologica 1983;167:243–9.
46. Rahbari H. Syringoacanthoma. Acanthotic lesion of the acrosyringium. Arch Dermatol 1984; 120:751–6.
47. Rulon DB, Helwig EB. Papillary eccrine adenoma. Arch Dermatol 1977;113:596–8.
48. Santa Cruz DJ, Prioleau PG, Smith ME. Hidradenoma papilliferum of the eyelid. Arch Dermatol 1981;117:55–6.
49. Sexton M, Maize JC. Papillary eccrine adenoma. A light microscopic and immunohistochemical study. J Am Acad Dermatol 1988;18:1114–20.
50. Sharma HS, Meorkamal MZ, Zainol H, Dharap AS. Eccrine cylindroma of the ear canal—report of a case. J Laryngol Otol 1994;108:706–9.
51. Shelley WB, Wood MG. A zosteriform network of spiradenomas. J Am Acad Dermatol 1980;2: 59–61.
52. Shenoy YM. Malignant perianal papillary hidradenoma. Arch Dermatol 1961;83:965–7.
53. Stanley RJ, Sanchez NP, Massa MC, Cooper AJ, Crotty CP, Winkelmann RK. Epidermoid hidradenoma. A clinicopathologic study. J Cutan Pathol 1982;9:293–302.
54. Tellechea O, Reis JP, Marques C, Baptista AP. Tubular apocrine adenoma with eccrine and apocrine immunophenotypes or papillary tubular adenoma? Am J Dermatopathol 1995;17: 499–505.

54a. Timpanidis PC, Lakhani SR, Groves RW. Progesterone receptor-positive syringoma associated with diabetes. J Am Acad Dermatol 2003; 48(Suppl 5):S103–4.
55. Toribio J, Zulaica A, Peteiro C. Tubular apocrine adenoma. J Cutan Pathol 1987;14:114–7.
56. Umbert P, Winkelmann RK. Tubular apocrine adenoma. J Cutan Pathol 1976;3:75–87.
57. Urmacher C, Lieberman PH. Papillary eccrine adenoma. Light-microscopic, histochemical, and immunohistochemical study. Am J Dermatopathol 1987;9:243–9.
58. Van der Putte SC. The pathogenesis of familial multiple cylindromas, trichoepitheliomas, milia, and spiradenomas. Am J Dermatopathol 1995;17:271–80.
59. Weedon D, Lewis J. Acrosyringeal nevus. J Cutan Pathol 1977;4:166–8.
60. Welch JP, Wells RS, Kerr CB. Ancell-Spiegler cylindromas (turban tumors) and Brooke-Fordyce trichoepitheliomas: evidence for a single genetic entity. J Med Genet 1968;5:29–35.
61. Wick MR, Swanson PE. Cutaneous adnexal tumors: a guide to pathologic diagnosis. Chicago: ASCP Press; 1991.
62. Wilkinson RD, Schopflocher P, Rozenfeld M. Hidrotic ectodermal dysplasia with diffuse eccrine poromatosis. Arch Dermatol 1977;113: 472–6.
63. Winkelmann RK, Wolff K. Solid-cystic hidradenoma of the skin. Clinical and histopathologic study. Arch Dermatol 1968;97:651–61.
64. Wollina U, Rulke D, Schaarschmidt H. Dermal cylindroma. Expression of intermediate filaments, epithelial and neuroectodermal antigens. Histol Histopathol 1992;7:575–82.
65. Woodworth H Jr, Dockerty MB, Wilson RB, Pratt JH. Papillary hidradenoma of the vulva: a clinicopathologic study of 69 cases. Am J Obstet Gynecol 1971;110:501–8.
66. Yesudian P, Thambiah A. Familial syringoma. Dermatologica 1975;150:32–5.

Sweat Gland Tumors with Mixed Differentiation

67. Efskind J, Eker R. Myo-epitheliomas of the skin. Acta Derm Venereol 1954:34:279–83.
68. Hara K. Mixed tumors of the skin: a histopathological, enzyme-histochemical, and immunohistochemical study. Histopathology 1995;26:145–52.
69. Hassab-El-Naby HM, Tam S, White WL, Ackerman AB. Mixed tumors of the skin: a histological and immunohistochemical study. Am J Dermatopathol 1989;11:413–28.
70. Headington JT. Mixed tumors of the skin: eccrine and apocrine types. Arch Dermatol 1961; 84:989–96.
71. Hernandez FJ. Mixed tumors of the skin of the salivary gland type: a light and electron microscopic study. J Invest Dermatol 1976;66:49–52.
72. Jaworski RC. The ultrastructure of chondroid syringoma (mixed tumor of the skin). Ultrastruct Pathol 1984;6:153–9.
73. Kunikane H, Ishikura H, Yamaguchi J, Yoshiki T, Itoh T, Aizawa M. Chondroid syringoma (mixed tumor of the skin). A clinicopathologic study of 13 cases. Acta Pathol Jpn 1987;37:615–25.
74. Letizia C, Marcheggiano A, De Toma G, Iannoni C, De Ciocchis A, Scavo D. Mixed type sweat gland adenoma: a case report. Ann Ital Med Int 1993;8:248–9.
75. Mills SE. Mixed tumor of the skin: a model of divergent differentiation. J Cutan Pathol 1984; 11:382–6.
76. Mohri S, Andoh S. An immunohistochemical study of mixed tumor of the skin. J Dermatol 1991;18:414–9.
77. Requena L, Sanchez Yus E, Santa Cruz DJ. Apocrine type of cutaneous mixed tumor with follicular and sebaceous differentiation. Am J Dermatopathol 1992;14:186–94.

Malignant Sweat Gland Tumors

78. Argenyi ZB, Nguyen AV, Balogh K, Sears JK, Whitaker DC. Malignant eccrine spiradenoma. A clinicopathologic study. Am J Dermatopathol 1990;12:335–43.
79. Bardach H. Hidroacanthoma simplex with in situ porocarcinoma. A case suggesting malignant transformation. J Cutan Pathol 1978;5:236–48.
80. Barsky SH, Martin SE, Matthews M, Gazdar A, Costa JC. "Low grade" mucoepidermoid carcinoma of the bronchus with "high grade" biological behavior. Cancer 1983;51:1505–9.
81. Batsakis JG, el-Naggar AK, Weber RS. Two perplexing skin tumors: microcystic adnexal carcinoma and keratoacanthoma. Ann Otol Rhinol Laryngol 1994;103:829–32.
82. Beck HG, Lechner W, Wunsch PH. [Adenoid cystic sweat gland cancer.] Hautarzt 1986; 37:405–9. (German.)
83. Berg JW, McDivitt RW. Pathology of sweat gland carcinomas. Pathol Annu 1968;3:123–44.
84. Boggio R. Adenoid cystic carcinoma of the scalp [letter]. Arch Dermatol 1975;111:793–4.
85. Bondeson L. Malignant dermal eccrine cylindroma. Acta Dermatol Venereol 1979;59:92–4.
86. Botha JB, Kahn LB. Aggressive chondroid syringoma. Report of a case in an unusual location and with local recurrence. Arch Dermatol 1978;114:954–5.
87. Bottles K, Sagebiel RW, McNutt NS, Jensen B, Deveney K. Malignant eccrine poroma. Case report and review of the literature. Cancer 1984;53:1579–85.
88. Bourland A, Clerens A, Sigart H. [Malignant cylindroma.] Dermatologica 1979;158:203–7. (French.)

89. Brownstein MH, Helwig EB. Metastatic tumors of the skin. Cancer 1972;29:1298–307.
90. Brownstein MH, Helwig EB. Patterns of cutaneous metastasis. Arch Dermatol 1972;105: 862–8.
91. Brownstein MH, Shapiro L. Desmoplastic trichoepithelioma. Cancer 1977;40:2979–86.
92. Chung CK, Heffernan AH. Clear cell hidradenoma with metastasis. Case report with a review of the literature. Plast Reconstr Surg 1971; 48:177–80.
93. Connor DH, Taylor HB, Helwig EB. Cutaneous metastases of renal cell carcinoma. Arch Pathol 1963;76:339–46.
94. Cooper PH. Carcinomas of sweat glands. Pathol Annu 1987;22(Pt 1):83–124.
95. Cooper PH. Sclerosing carcinomas of sweat ducts (microcystic adnexal carcinoma). Arch Dermatol 1986;122:261–4.
96. Cooper PH, Adelson GL, Holthaus WH. Primary cutaneous adenoid cystic carcinoma. Arch Dermatol 1984;120:774–7.
97. Cooper PH, Frierson HF Jr, Morrison AG. Malignant transformation of eccrine spiradenoma. Arch Dermatol 1985;121:1445–8.
98. Cooper PH, Mills SE. Microcystic adnexal carcinoma. J Am Acad Dermatol 1984;10:908–14.
99. Cooper PH, Mills SE, Leonard DD, et al. Sclerosing sweat duct (syringomatous) carcinoma. Am J Surg Pathol 1985;9:422–33.
100. Cooper PH, Robinson CR, Greer KE. Low-grade clear cell eccrine carcinoma. Arch Dermatol 1984;120:1076–8.
101. Czarnecki DB, Aarous I, Dowling JP, Lauritz B, Wallis P, Taft EH. Malignant clear cell hidradenoma: a case report. Acta Dermatol Venereol 1982;62:173–6.
102. Dabska M. Malignant transformation of eccrine spiradenoma. Pol Med J 1972;11:388–96.
103. Eckert F, Pfau A, Landthaler M. [Adenoid cystic sweat gland carcinoma: a clinicopathologic and immunohistochemical study.] Hautarzt 1994;45:318–23. (German).
104. el-Domeiri AA, Brasfield RD, Huvos AG, Strong EW. Sweat gland carcinoma: a clinico-pathologic study of 83 patients. Ann Surg 1971;173: 270–4.
105. Evans HL, Su D, Smith JL, Winkelmann RK. Carcinoma arising in eccrine spiradenoma. Cancer 1979;43:1881–4.
106. Friedman KJ. Low-grade primary cutaneous adenosquamous (mucoepidermoid) carcinoma. Report of a case and review of the literature. Am J Dermatopathol 1989;11:43–50.
107. Fukamizu H, Tomita K, Inoue K, Takigawa M. Primary mucinous carcinoma of the skin. J Dermatol Surg Oncol 1993;19:625–8.
108. Galadari E, Mehregan AH, Lee KC. Malignant transformation of eccrine tumors. J Cutan Pathol 1987;14:15–22.
109. Ghamande SA, Kasznica J, Griffiths CT, Finkler NJ, Hamid AM. Mucinous adenocarcinomas of the vulva. Gynecol Oncol 1995;57:117–20.
110. Goedde TA, Bumpers H, Fiscella J, Rao U, Karakousis CP. Eccrine porocarcinoma. J Surg Oncol 1994;55:261–4.
111. Goldstein DJ, Barr RJ, Santa Cruz DJ. Microcystic adnexal carcinoma: a distinct clinicopathologic entity. Cancer 1982;50:566–72.
112. Grossman JR, Izuno GT. Primary mucinous (adenocystic) carcinoma of the skin. Arch Dermatol 1974;110:274–6.
113. Grouls V, Iwaszkiewicz J, Berndt R. [Malignant dermal cylindroma.] Pathologe 1991;12:157–60. (German.)
114. Guldhammer B, Norgaard T. The differential diagnosis of intraepidermal malignant lesions using immunohistochemistry. Am J Dermatopathol 1986;8:295–301.
115. Hara K, Kamiya S. Pigmented eccrine porocarcinoma: a mimic of malignant melanoma. Histopathology 1995;27:86–8.
116. Harrist TJ, Aretz TH, Mihm MC Jr, Evans GW, Rodriguez FL. Cutaneous malignant mixed tumor. Arch Dermatol 1981;117:719–24.
117. Headington JT, Niederhuber JE, Beals TF. Malignant clear cell acrospiroma. Cancer 1978; 41:641–7.
118. Headington JT, Teears R, Niederhuber JE, Slinger RP. Primary adenoid cystic carcinoma of the skin. Arch Dermatol 1978;114:421–4.
119. Hernandez-Perez E, Cestoni-Parducci R. Nodular hidradenoma and hidradenocarcinoma. A 10-year review. J Am Acad Dermatol 1985;12:15–20.
120. Hesse RJ, Scharfenberg JC, Ratz JL, Griener E. Eyelid microcystic adnexal carcinoma. Arch Ophthalmol 1995;113:494–6.
121. Hilton JM, Blackwell JB. Metastasizing chondroid syringoma. J Pathol 1972;109:167–70.
122. Holst VA, Marshall CE, Moskaluk CA, Frierson HF Jr. KIT protein expression and analysis of c-kit gene mutation in adenoid cystic carcinoma. Mod Pathol 1999;12:956–60.
123. Ishimura E, Iwamoto H, Kobashi Y, Yamabe H, Ichijima K. Malignant chondroid syringoma. Report of a case with widespread metastasis and review of pertinent literature. Cancer 1983;52:1966–73.
124. Isikawa K. Malignant hidroacanthoma simplex. Arch Dermatol 1971;104:529–32.
125. Kao GF, Helwig EB, Graham JH. Aggressive digital papillary adenoma and adenocarcinoma. A clinicopathological study of 57 patients, with histochemical, immunopathological, and ultrastructural observations. J Cutan Pathol 1987;14:129–46.
126. Katoh N, Hirano S, Hosokawa Y, Miyashita A, Kishimoto S, Yasuno H. Mucinous carcinoma of the skin: report of a case with DNA cytofluorometric study. J Dermatol 1994;21:117–21.

127. Kay S, Hall WE. Sweat-gland carcinoma with proved metastases; report of a case. Cancer 1954;7:373–6.
128. Keasbey LE, Hadley GG. Clear cell hidradenoma: report of three cases with widespread metastases. Cancer 1954;7:934–52.
129. Kersting DW. Clear cell hidradenoma and hidradenocarcinoma. Arch Dermatol 1963;87:323–33.
130. Kuramoto Y, Tagami H. Primary adenoid cystic carcinoma masquerading as syringoma of the scalp. Am J Dermatopathol 1990;12:169–74.
131. Landman G, Farmer ER. Primary cutaneous mucoepidermoid carcinoma: report of a case. J Cutan Pathol 1991;18:56–9.
132. LeBoit PE, Sexton M. Microcystic adnexal carcinoma of the skin. A reappraisal of the differentiation and differential diagnosis of an underrecognized neoplasm. J Am Acad Dermatol 1993;29:609–18.
133. Lipper S, Peiper SC. Sweat gland carcinoma with syringomatous features: a light microscopic and ultrastructural study. Cancer 1979;44:157–63.
134. Lyon JB, Rouillard LM. Malignant degeneration of turban tumor of scalp. Trans St Johns Hosp Dermatol Soc 1961;46:74–7.
135. Manteaux A, Cohen PR, Rapini RP. Zosteriform and epidermotropic metastasis. Report of two cases. J Dermatol Surg Oncol 1992;18:97–100.
136. Matsumura T, Kumakiri M, Ohkaware A, Yoshida T. Adenoid cystic carcinoma of the skin—an immunohistochemical and ultrastructural study. J Dermatol 1993;20:164–70.
137. MacKenzie DH. A clear-cell hidradenocarcinoma with metastases. Cancer 1957;10:1021–3.
138. Matz R, McCully DJ, Stokes BA. Metastasizing chondroid syringoma: a case report. Pathology 1961;1:77–81.
139. McAlvany JP, Stonecipher MR, Leshin B, Prichard E, White W. Sclerosing sweat duct carcinoma in an 11 year old boy. J Dermatol Surg Oncol 1994;20:767–8.
140. McKee PH, Fletcher CD, Stavrinos P, Pambakian H. Carcinosarcoma arising in eccrine spiradenoma. A clinicopathologic and immunohistochemical study of two cases. Am J Dermatopathol 1990;12:335–43.
141. Mehregan AH, Hashimoto K, Rahbari H. Eccrine adenocarcinoma. A clinicopathologic study of 35 cases. Arch Dermatol 1983;119:104–14.
142. Mendoza S, Helwig EB. Mucinous (adenocystic) carcinoma of the skin. Arch Dermatol 1971;103:68–78.
143. Metcalf JS, Maize JC, Shaw EB. Bronchial mucoepidermoid carcinoma metastatic to skin. Report of a case and review of the literature. Cancer 1986;58:2556–9.
144. Miller WL. Sweat gland carcinoma. A clinicopathologic problem. Am J Clin Pathol 1967;47:767–80.
145. Miyashita M, Suzuki H. In situ porocarcinoma: a case with malignant expression in clear tumor cells. Int J Dermatol 1993;32:749–50.
146. Moreno A, Salvatella N, Guix M, Llistosella E, de Moragas JM. Malignant hidroacanthoma simplex. A light microscopic, ultrastructural, and immunohistochemical study of 2 cases. Dermatologica 1984;169:161–6.
147. Nickoloff BJ, Fleischmann HE, Carmel J, Wood CC, Roth RJ. Microcystic adnexal carcinoma. Immunohistologic observations suggesting dual (pilar and eccrine) differentiation. Arch Dermatol 1986;122:290–4.
148. Okada N, Ota J, Sato K, Kitano Y. Metastasizing sweat gland carcinoma. Report of a case. Arch Dermatol 1984;120:768–9.
149. Page DL, Anderson TJ, Sakamoto G. Infiltrating carcinoma: major histological types. In: Page DL, Anderson TJ, eds. Diagnostic histopathology of the breast. New York: Churchill Livingstone; 1987:193–295.
150. Pilgrim JP, Kloss SG, Wolfish PS, Heng MC. Primary mucinous carcinoma of the skin with metastases to the lymph nodes. Am J Dermatopathol 1985;7:461–9.
151. Pinto de Moraes H, Herrera GA, Mendonca AM, Estrela RR. Metastatic malignant mixed tumor of the skin. Ultrastructural and immunohistochemical characterization, histogenetic considerations, and comparison with benign mixed tumors of skin and salivary glands. Appl Pathol 1986;4:199–208.
152. Poiares Baptista A, Tellechea O, Reis JP, Cunha MF, Figueiredo P. [Eccrine porocarcinoma. A review of 24 cases.] Ann Dermatol Venereol 1993;120:107–15. (French.)
153. Redono C, Rocamora A, Villoria F, Garcia M. Malignant mixed tumor of the skin: malignant chondroid syringoma. Cancer 1982;49:1690–6.
154. Revercomb CH, Reitmeyer WJ, Pulitzer DR. Clear cell variant of mucoepidermoid carcinoma of the skin. J Am Acad Dermatol 1993;29:642–4.
155. Rockerbie N, Solomon AR, Woo TY, Beals TF, Ellis CN. Malignant dermal cylindroma in a patient with multiple dermal cylindromas, trichoepitheliomas, and bilateral dermal analogue tumors of the parotid gland. Am J Dermatopathol 1989;11:353–9.
156. Rodrigues MM, Lubowitz RM, Shannon GM. Mucinous (adenocystic) carcinoma of the eyelid. Arch Ophthalmol 1973;89:493–4.
157. Rosborough D. Malignant mixed tumors of the skin. Br J Surg 1963;50:697–9.
158. Rosen T. Cutaneous metastases. Med Clin North Am 1980;64:885–900.
159. Ryan JF, Darley CR, Pollock DJ. Malignant eccrine poroma: report of three cases. Clin Pathol 1986;39:1099–104.

160. Salasche SJ, Amonette RA. Morpheaform basal cell epitheliomas. A study of subclinical extensions in a series of 51 cases. J Dermatol Surg Oncol 1981;7:387–94.
161. Sanchez Yus ES, Requena Caballero L, Garcia-Salazar I, Coca-Menchero S. Clear cell syringoid eccrine carcinoma. Am J Dermatopathol 1987; 9:225–31.
162. Sanderson KV, Batten JC. Adenoid cystic carcinoma of the scalp with pulmonary metastases. Proc R Soc Med 1975;68:649–50.
163. Santz Cruz DJ, Meyers JH, Gnepp DR, Perez BM. Primary mucinous carcinoma of the skin. Br J Dermatol 1978;68:645–53.
164. Schipper JH, Holecek BU, Sievers KW. A tumor derived from Ebner's glands: microcystic adnexal carcinoma of the tongue. J Laryngol Otol 1995;109:1211–4.
165. Scott A, Metcalf JS. Cutaneous malignant mixed tumor. Report of a case and review of the literature. Am J Dermatopathol 1988;10:335–42.
166. Seab JA, Graham JH. Primary cutaneous adenoid cystic carcinoma. J Am Acad Dermatol 1987;17:113–8.
167. Sharvill DE. Mixed salivary-type tumour of the skin with malignant recurrence. Br J Dermatol 1962;74:103–4.
168. Shaw M, McKee PH, Lowe D, Black MM. Malignant eccrine poroma: a study of twenty-seven cases. Br J Dermatol 1982;107:675–80.
169. Shvili D, Rothem A. Fulminant metastasizing chondroid syringoma of the skin. Am J Dermatopathol 1986;8:321–5.
170. Smith KJ, Skelton HG, Holland TT. Recent advances and controversies concerning adnexal neoplasms. Dermatol Clin 1992;10:117–60.
171. Smoller BR, Narurkar V. Mucoepidermoid carcinoma metastatic to the skin. An histologic mimic of a primary sweat gland carcinoma. J Dermatol Surg Oncol 1992;18:365–8.
172. Snow SN, Reizner GT. Eccrine porocarcinoma of the face. J Am Acad Dermatol 1992;27:306–11.
173. Suster S. Clear cell tumors of the skin. Semin Diagn Pathol 1996;13:40–59.
174. Swanson PE, Cherwitz DL, Neumann MP, Wick MR. Eccrine sweat gland carcinoma: an histologic and immunohistochemical study of 32 cases. J Cutan Pathol 1987;14:65-86.
175. Swanson PE, Mazoujian G, Mills SE, Campbell RJ, Wick MR. Immunoreactivity for estrogen receptor protein in sweat gland tumors. Am J Surg Pathol 1991;15:835–41.
176. Swanson PE, Wick MR. Immunohistochemistry of cutaneous tumors. In: Leong AS, ed. Applied immunohistochemistry for the surgical pathologist. London: Edward Arnold; 1993: 269–308.
177. Tolia BM, Whitmore WF Jr. Solitary metastasis from renal cell carcinoma. J Urol 1975;114:836–8.
178. Turner JJ, Maxwell L, Bursle GA. Eccrine porocarcinoma: a case report with light microscopy and ultrastructure. Pathology 1982;14:469–75.
179. Urbanski SJ, From L, Abramowicz A, Joaquin A, Luk SC. Metamorphosis of dermal cylindroma: possible relation to malignant transformation. Case report of cutaneous cylindroma with direct intracranial invasion. J Am Acad Dermatol 1985;12(Pt 2):188–95.
180. van der Kwast TH, Vuzevski VD, Ramaekers F, Bousema MT, Van Joost T. Primary cutaneous adenoid cystic carcinoma: case report, immunohistochemistry, and review of the literature. Br J Dermatol 1988;118:567–77.
181. Varsa EW, Jordan SW. Fine needle aspiration cytology of malignant spiradenoma arising in congenital eccrine spiradenoma. Acta Cytol 1990;34:275–7.
182. Verdier-Sevrain S, Thomine E, Lauret P, Hemet J. [Syringomatous carcinoma: a propos of three cases with a review of the literature.] Ann Pathol 1995;15:280–4. (French.)
183. Wassef M, Thomas V, Deffrennes D, Saint-Guily JL. [Primary adenoid cystic carcinoma of the skin. Histologic and ultrastructural study of two cases localized in the external auditory canal.] Ann Pathol 1995;15:150–5. (French.)
184. Webb JN, Stott WG. Malignant chondroid syringoma of the thigh. Report of a case with electron microscopy of the tumor. J Pathol 1975; 116:43–6.
185. Wenig BL, Sciubba JJ, Goodman RS, Platt N. Primary cutaneous mucoepidermoid carcinoma of the anterior neck. Laryngoscope 1983;93:464–7.
186. Wick MR, Cooper PH, Swanson PE, Kaye VN, Sun TT. Microcystic adnexal carcinoma. An immunohistochemical comparison with other cutaneous appendage tumors. Arch Dermatol 1990;126:189–94.
187. Wick MR, Goellner JR, Wolfe JT 3rd, Su WP. Adnexal carcinomas of the skin. I. Eccrine carcinomas. Cancer 1985;56:1147–62.
188. Wick MR, Goellner JR, Wolfe JT 3rd, Su WP. Vulvar sweat gland carcinomas. Arch Pathol Lab Med 1985;109:43–7.
189. Wick MR, Swanson PE. Carcinosarcomas: current perspectives and a historical review of nosological concepts. Semin Diagn Pathol 1993;10:118–27.
190. Wick MR, Swanson PE. Primary adenoid cystic carcinoma of the skin. A clinical, histological, and immunocytochemical comparison with adenoid cystic carcinoma of salivary glands and adenoid basal cell carcinoma. Am J Dermatopathol 1986;8:2–13.
191. Wick MR, Swanson PE, Kaye VN, Pittelkow MR. Sweat gland carcinoma ex eccrine spiradenoma. Am J Dermatopathol 1987;9:90–8.
192. Wong TY, Suster S, Nogita T, Duncan LM, Dickersin RG, Mihm MC Jr. Clear cell eccrine carcinomas of the skin. A clinicopathologic study of nine patients. Cancer 1994;73:1631–43.

193. Yamamoto O, Haratake J, Yokoyama S, Imayama S, Asahi M. A histopathological and ultrastructural study of eccrine porocarcinoma with special reference to its subtypes. Virchows Arch A Pathol Anat Histopathol 1992;420:395–401.
194. Yamamoto O, Nakayama K, Asahi M. Sweat gland carcinoma with mucinous and infiltrating duct-like patterns. J Cutan Pathol 1992;19:334–9.
195. Yaremchuk MJ, Elias LS, Graham RR, Wilgis EF. Sweat gland carcinoma of the hand: two cases of malignant eccrine spiradenoma. J Hand Surg [Am] 1984;9:910–4.
196. Yeung KY, Stinson JC. Mucinous (adenocystic) carcinoma of sweat glands with widespread metastasis. Case report with ultrastructural study. Cancer 1977;39:2556–62.
197. Zamboni AC, Zamboni WA, Ross DS. Malignant eccrine spiradenoma of the hand. J Surg Oncol 1990;43:131–3.

Apocrine Carcinomas

198. Almagro UA. Primary signet-ring carcinoma of the colon. Cancer 1983;52:1453–7.
199. Aurora AL, Luxenberg MN. Case report of adenocarcinoma of glands of Moll. Am J Ophthalmol 1970;70:984–90.
200. Boehm F, Morris JM. Paget's disease and apocrine gland carcinoma of the vulva. Obstet Gynecol 1971;38:185–92.
201. Chaudary MA, Millis RR, Lane B, Miller NA. Paget's disease of the nipple: a ten year review including clinical, pathological, and immunohistochemical findings. Breast Cancer Res Treat 1986;8:139–46.
202. Degefu S, O'Quinn AG, Dhurandhar HN. Paget's disease of the vulva and urogenital malignancies: a case report and review of the literature. Gynecol Oncol 1986;25:347–54.
203. Gaffey MJ, Traweek ST, Mills SE, et al. Cytokeratin expression in adrenocortical neoplasia: an immunohistochemical and biochemical study with implications for the differential diagnosis of adrenocortical, hepatocellular, and renal cell carcinoma. Hum Pathol 1992;23:144–53.
204. Hart WR, Millman JB. Progression of intraepithelial Paget's disease of the vulva to invasive carcinoma. Cancer 1977;40:2333–7.
205. Helm KF, Goellner JR, Peters MS. Immunohistochemical stains in extramammary Paget's disease. Am J Dermatopathol 1992;14:402–7.
206. Hitchcock A, Topham S, Bell J, Gullick W, Elston CW, Ellis IO. Routine diagnosis of mammary Paget's disease. A modern approach. Am J Surg Pathol 1992;16:58–61.
207. Hood CI, Font RL, Zimmerman LE. Metastatic mammary carcinoma in the eyelid with histiocytoid appearance. Cancer 1973;31:793–800.
208. Horn RC Jr. Malignant papillary cystadenoma of sweat glands with metastases to the regional lymph nodes. Surgery 1944;16:348–55.
209. Jakobiec FA, Austin P, Iwamoto T, Trokel SL, Marquardt MD, Harrison W. Primary infiltrating signet ring carcinoma of the eyelids. Ophthalmology 1983;90:291–9.
210. Jones RE. Mammary Paget's disease without underlying carcinoma. Am J Dermatopathol 1985;7:361–5.
211. Jones RE Jr, Austin C, Ackerman AB. Extramammary Paget's disease. A critical reexamination. Am J Dermatopathol 1979;1:101–32.
212. Kariniemi AL, Ramaekers F, Lehto VP, Virtanen I. Paget cells express cytokeratins typical of glandular epithelia. Br J Dermatol 1985;112:179–83.
212a. King DT, Barr RJ. Syringometaplasia: mucinous and squamous variants. J Cutan Pathol 1979;6:284–91.
213. Kipkie GF, Haust MD. Carcinoma of apocrine glands; report of a case. AMA Arch Derm 1958;78:440–5.
214. Knauer WJ Jr, Whorton CM. Extramammary Paget's disease originating in Moll's glands of the lids. Trans Am Acad Ophthalmol Otolaryngol 1963;67:829–33.
215. Lauren P. The two histological main types of gastric carcinoma: diffuse and so-called intestinal type carcinoma. An attempt at histo-clinical classification. Acta Pathol Microbiol Scand 1965;64:31–49.
216. Lee SC, Roth LM, Ehrlich C, Hall JA. Extramammary Paget's disease of the vulva. A clinicopathologic study of 13 cases. Cancer 1977;39:2540–9.
217. Mazoujian G, Pinkus GS, Haagensen DE Jr. Extramammary Paget's disease—evidence for an apocrine origin. An immunoperoxidase study of gross cystic disease fluid protein-15. Am J Surg Pathol 1984;8:43–50.
218. McDonald JR. Apocrine sweat gland carcinoma of the vulva. Am J Clin Pathol 1941;11:890–7.
219. McKee PH, Hertogs KT. Endocervical adenocarcinoma and vulvar Paget's disease: a significant association. Br J Dermatol 1980;103:443–8.
220. Mitsudo S, Nakanishi I, Koss LG. Paget's disease of the penis and adjacent skin: its association with fatal sweat gland carcinoma. Arch Pathol Lab Med 1981;105:518–20.
221. Mori O, Hachisuka H, Nakano S, Maeyama Y, Sasai Y. A case of mammary Paget's disease without an underlying carcinoma: microscopic analysis of the DNA content in Paget cells. J Dermatol 1994;21:160–5.
222. Nadji M, Morales AR, Girtanner RE, Ziegels-Weissman J, Penneys NS. Paget's disease of the skin. A unifying concept of histogenesis. Cancer 1982;50:2203–6.
223. Ojeda VJ, Heenen PJ, Watson SH. Paget's disease of the groin associated with adenocarcinoma of the urinary bladder. J Cutan Pathol 1987;14:227–31.

224. Paties C, Taccagni GL, Papotti M, Valente G, Zangrandi A, Aloi F. Apocrine carcinoma of the skin. A clinicopathologic, immunocytochemical, and ultrastructural study. Cancer 1993;71: 375–81.
225. Rayne SC, Santa Cruz DJ. Anaplastic Paget's disease. Am J Surg Pathol 1992;16:1085–91.
226. Saigal RK, Khanna SD, Chandler J. Apocrine gland carcinoma in axilla. Indian J Dermatol 1971;37:177–80.
227. Takeshita K, Izumoi S, Ebuchi M, et al. A case of rectal carcinoma concomitant with pagetoid lesion in the perianal region—histopathological and electron microscopic observations. Gastroenterol Jpn 1978;13:85–95.
228. van der Putte SC, van Gorp LH. Adenocarcinoma of the mammary-like glands of the vulva: a concept unifying sweat gland carcinoma of the vulva, carcinoma of supernumerary mammary glands and extramammary Paget's disease. J Cutan Pathol 1994;21:157–63.
229. Vidmar D, Baxter DL Jr, Devaney K. Extensive dermal metastases from primary signet ring carcinoma of the urinary bladder. Cutis 1992;49:324–8.
230. Warkel RL, Helwig EB. Apocrine gland adenoma and adenocarcinoma of the axilla. Arch Dermatol 1978;114:198–203.
230a. Welch JP, Wells RS, Kerr CB. Ancell-Spiegler cylindromas (turban tumors) and Brooke-Fordyce trichoepitheliomas: evidence for a single genetic entity. J Med Genet 1968;5:29–35.
231. Wick MR, Coffin CM. Sweat gland and pilar carcinomas. In: Wick MR, ed. Pathology of unusual malignant cutaneous tumors. New York: Marcel Dekker; 1985:1–76.
232. Yamamoto O, Haratake J, Hisaoka M, Asahi M, Bhawan J. A unique case of apocrine carcinoma on the male pubic skin: histopathologic and ultrastructural observations. J Cutan Pathol 1993;20:378–83.

Lymphoepithelioma-Like Carcinomas/ Adnexal Carcinomas with Mixed Differentiation

233. Axelsen SM, Stamp IM. Lymphoepithelioma-like carcinoma of the vulvar region. Histopathology 1995;27:281–3.
234. Dozier SE, Jones TR, Nelson-Adesokan P, Hruza GJ. Lymphoepithelioma-like carcinoma of the skin treated by Mohs micrographic surgery. Dermatol Surg 1995;21:690–4.
235. Jimenez F, Clark RE, Buchanan MD, Kamino H. Lymphoepithelioma-like carcinoma of the skin treated with Mohs micrographic surgery in combination with immune staining for cytokeratins. J Am Acad Dermatol 1995;32(Pt 2):878–81.
236. Nakhleh RE, Swanson PE, Wick MR. Cutaneous adnexal carcinomas with mixed differentiation. Am J Dermatopathol 1990;12:325–34.
237. Ortiz-Frutos FJ, Zarco C, Gil R, Ballestin C, Iglesias L. Lymphoepithelioma-like carcinoma of the skin. Clin Exp Dermatol 1993;18:83–6.
238. Requena L, Sanchez Yus E, Jimenez E, Roo E. Lymphoepithelioma-like carcinoma of the skin: a light microscopic and immunohistochemical study. J Cutan Pathol 1994;21:541–8.
239. Robins P, Perez MI. Lymphoepithelioma-like carcinoma of the skin treated by Mohs micrographic surgery. J Am Acad Dermatol 1995;32(Pt 1):814–6.
240. Swanson SA, Cooper PH, Mills SE, Wick MR. Lymphoepithelioma-like carcinoma of the skin. Mod Pathol 1988;1:359–65.
241. Wick MR, Swanson PE, LeBoit PE, Strickler JG, Cooper PH. Lymphoepithelioma-like carcinoma of the skin with adnexal differentiation. J Cutan Pathol 1991;18:93–102.

Primary Neuroendocrine (Merkel Cell) Carcinoma

242. Alexiou G, Papadopoulou-Alexiou M, Karakousis CP. Primary neuroendocrine carcinoma of the skin (Merkel's cell carcinoma). J Surg Oncol 1984;27:31–4.
243. Arnulf C, Ettore F, Barety M, Abbes M, Duplay H. [Cutaneous apudoma. Apropos of a case and review of the literature.] Semin Hop 1983;59: 1453–7. (French.)
244. Balaton AJ, Capron F, Baviera EE, Meyrignac P, Vaury P, Vuong PN. Neuroendocrine carcinoma (Merkel cell tumor?) presenting as a subcutaneous tumor. An immunohistochemical and ultrastructural study of three cases. Pathol Res Pract 1989;184:211–6.
245. Blom A, Kolb F, Lumbroso J, et al. Significance of sentinel lymph node biopsy in Merkel cell sarcoma: analysis of 11 cases. Ann Dermatol Venereol 2003;130:417–22.
246. Bottles K, Lacey CG, Goldberg J, Lanner-Cusin K, Hom J, Miller TR. Merkel cell carcinoma of the vulva. Obstet Gynecol 1984;63(Suppl):61S–5.
247. Carpentier O, Carrotte-Lefebvre I, Patenotre P, Mirabel X, Delaporte E, Piette F. [Primitive cutaneous neuroendocrine carcinomas or Merkel's tumor. Clinical and therapeutic aspects in 22 patients.] Presse Med 2002;31:735–9. (French.)
247a. Efskind J, Eker R. Myo-epitheliomas of the skin. Acta Derm Venereol 1954:34:279–83.
248. Eusebi V, C.apella C, Cossu A, Rosai J. Neuroendocrine carcinoma within lymph nodes in the absence of a primary tumor, with special reference to Merkel cell carcinoma. Am J Surg Pathol 1992;16:658–66.
249. Fotia G, Barni R, Bellan C, Neri A. Lymph nodal Merkel cell carcinoma: primary or metastatic disease? A clinical case. Tumori 2002;88:424–6.
250. Goepfert H, Remmler D, Silva E, Wheeler B. Merkel cell carcinoma (endocrine carcinoma of the skin) of the head and neck. Arch Otolaryngol 1984;110:707–12.

251. Gomez LG, DiMaio S, Silva EG, Mackay B. Association between neuroendocrine (Merkel cell) carcinoma and squamous carcinoma of the skin. Am J Surg Pathol 1983;7:171–7.
252. Gould E, Albores-Saavedra J, Dubner B, Smith W, Payne CM. Eccrine and squamous differentiation in Merkel cell carcinoma: an immunohistochemical study. Am J Surg Pathol 1988;12:768–72.
253. Harrington M, Mitchell V, Curtin CT. Fine needle aspiration of two unusual tumors of the eyelid metastatic to preauricular lymph nodes. Acta Cytol 1983;27:560.
254. Heenan P, Cole JM, Spagnolo DV. Primary cutaneous neuroendocrine carcinoma (Merkel cell tumor). An adnexal epithelial neoplasm. Am J Dermatopathol 1990;12:7–16.
255. Hitchcock CL, Bland KI, Laney RG 3rd, Franzini D, Harris B, Copeland EM 3rd. Neuroendocrine (Merkel cell) carcinoma of the skin. Its natural history, diagnosis, and treatment. Ann Surg 1988;207:201–7.
256. Hohaus K, Kostler E, Schonlebe J, Klemm E, Wollina U. Merkel cell carcinoma—a retrospective analysis of 17 cases. J Eur Acad Dermatol Venereol 2003;17:20–4.
256a. Karam P, Benedetto AN. Syringomas: new approach to an old technique. Int J Dermatol 1996;35:219–20.
257. Katenkamp D, Watzig V. Multiple neuroendocrine carcinomas (so-called Merkel cell tumors) of the skin. Report on two cases with a unique clinical course. Virchows Arch A Pathol Anat Histopathol 1984;404:403–11.
258. Kuhajda FP, Olson JL, Mann RB. Merkel cell (small cell) carcinoma of the skin: immunohistochemical and ultrastructural demonstration of distinctive perinuclear cytokeratin aggregates and a possible association with B cell neoplasms. Histochem J 1986;18:239–44.
259. Kurokawa M, Nabeshima K, Akiyama Y, et al. CD56: a useful marker for diagnosing Merkel cell carcinoma. J Dermatol Sci 2003;31:219–24.
260. Lau SK, Luthringer DJ, Eisen RN. Thyroid transcription factor-1: a review. Appl Immunohistochem Mol Morphol 2002;10:97–102.
261. Leech SN, Kolar AJ, Barrett PD, Sinclair SA, Leonard N. Merkel cell carcinoma can be distinguished from metastatic small cell carcinoma using antibodies to cytokeratin 20 and thyroid transcription factor 1. J Clin Pathol 2001;54:727–9.
262. Luderschmidt C. [Neuroendocrine (Merkel cell?) carcinoma of the skin.] Z Hautkr 1987;62:290–302. (German.)
263. MacIntosh J, Wills EJ, Friedlander M. Merkel cell tumours. In: Williams CJ, Krikorian JG, Green MR, Raghavan D, eds. Textbook of uncommon cancer. New York: John Wiley & Sons Inc; 1988:913–23.
264. Mehrany K, Otley CC, Weenig RH, Phillips PK, Roenigk RK, Nguyen TH. A meta-analysis of the prognostic significance of sentinel lymph node status in Merkel cell carcinoma. Dermatol Surg 2002;28:113–7.
265. Merot Y, Mooy A. Merkel cell hyperplasia in hypertrophic varieties of actinic keratoses. Dermatologica 1989;178:189–93.
266. Mir R, Sciubba JJ, Bhuiya TA, Blomquist K, Zelig D, Friedman E. Merkel cell carcinoma arising in the oral mucosa. Oral Surg Oral Med Oral Pathol 1988;65:71–5.
267. Nicholson SA, McDermott MB, Swanson PE, Wick MR. CD99 and cytokeratin-20 in small-cell and basaloid tumors of the skin. Appl Immunohistochem Mol Morphol 2000;8:37–41.
268. Ordonez NG. Value of thyroid transcription factor-1 immunostaining in distinguishing small cell lung carcinomas from other small cell carcinomas. Am J Surg Pathol 2000;24:1217–23.
269. Pan D, Narayan D, Ariyan S. Merkel cell carcinoma: five case reports using sentinel lymph node biopsy and a review of 110 new cases. Plast Reconstr Surg 2002;110:1259–65.
270. Pollack SV, Goslen JB. Small-cell neuroepithelial tumor of the skin: a Merkel cell neoplasm? J Dermatol Surg Oncol 1982;8:116–22.
271. Quttainah A, Thoma A, Salama S. Clinical-pathological review of 14 cases of Merkel cell carcinoma. Can J Plast Surg 2002;10:196–202.
272. Sais G, Admella C, Soler T. Spontaneous regression in primary cutaneous neuroendocrine (Merkel cell) carcinoma: a rare immune phenomenon? J Eur Acad Dermatol Venereol 2002;16:82–3.
273. Santa Cruz DJ, Bauer EA. Merkel cells in the outer follicular sheath. Ultrastruct Pathol 1982;3:59–63.
274. Sibley RK, Dehner LP, Rosai J. Primary neuroendocrine (Merkel cell?) carcinoma of the skin. I. A clinicopathologic and ultrastructural study of 43 cases. Am J Surg Pathol 1985;9:95–108.
275. Sibley RK, Rosai J, Foucar E, Dehner L, Bosl G. Neuroendocrine (Merkel cell) carcinoma of the skin. A histologic and ultrastructural study of two cases. Am J Surg Pathol 1980;4:211–21.
276. Sidhu GS, Feiner H, Flotte TJ, Mullins JD, Schaefler K, Schultenover SJ. Merkel cell neoplasms. Histology, electron microscopy, biology, and histogenesis. Am J Dermatopathol 1980;2:101–19.
277. Silva EG, Mackay B, Goepfert H, Burgess MA, Fields RS. Endocrine carcinoma of the skin (Merkel cell carcinoma). Pathol Annu 1984;19:1–30.
278. Smith PD, Patterson JW. Merkel cell carcinoma (neuroendocrine carcinoma) of the skin. Am J Clin Pathol 2001;115(Suppl):S68–78.

279. Stoppler H, Stoppler MC, Kisiela M, et al. Telomerase activity of Merkel cell carcinomas and Merkel cell carcinoma-derived cell cultures. Arch Dermatol Res 2001;293:397–406.
280. Su LD, Fullen DR, Lowe L, Uherova P, Schnitzer B, Valdez R. CD117 (kit receptor) expression in Merkel cell carcinomas. Am J Dermatopathol 2002;24:289–93.
281. Tang CK, Toker C. Trabecular carcinoma of the skin: further clinicopathologic and ultrastructural study. Mt Sinai J Med 1979;46:516–23.
282. Tang CK, Toker C, Nedwich A, Zaman AN. Unusual cutaneous carcinoma with features of small cell (oat-cell-like) and squamous cell carcinomas. A variant of malignant Merkel cell neoplasm. Am J Dermatopathol 1982;4:537–48.
283. Taxy JB, Ettinger DS, Wharam MD. Primary small-cell carcinoma of the skin. Cancer 1980;46:2308–11.
284. Toker C. Trabecular carcinoma of the skin. Arch Dermatol 1972;105:107–10.
285. Tyring SK, Lee PC, Omura EF, Green LK, Merot Y. Recurrent and metastatic cutaneous neuroendocrine (Merkel cell) carcinoma mimicking angiosarcoma. Arch Dermatol 1987;123:1368–70.
285a. Van der Putte SC. The pathogenesis of familial multiple cylindromas, trichoepitheliomas, milia, and spiradenomas. Am J Dermatopathol 1995;17:271–80.
286. Visscher D, Cooper PH, Zarbo RJ, Crissman JD. Cutaneous neuroendocrine (Merkel cell) carcinoma: an immunophenotypic, clinicopathologic, and flow cytometric study. Modern Pathol 1989;2:331–8.
287. Walsh NM. Primary neuroendocrine (Merkel cell) carcinoma of the skin: morphologic diversity and implications thereof. Hum Pathol 2001;32:680–9.
288. Warner TF, Uno H, Hafez R, et al. Merkel cells and Merkel cell tumors. Ultrastructure, immunocytochemistry, and review of the literature. Cancer 1983;52:238–45.
289. Watzig V, Katenkamp D. [Disseminated neuroendocrine cancers of the skin—a cutaneous merkeliomatosis. Report of two cases.] Z Hautkr 1987;62:1105–12. (German.)
290. Wick MR, Goellner JR, Scheithauer BW, Thomas JR 3rd, Sanchez NP, Schroeter AL. Primary neuroendocrine carcinomas of the skin (Merkel cell tumors). A clinical, histologic, and ultrastructural study of thirteen cases. Am J Clin Pathol 1983;79:6–13.
291. Wick MR, Thomas JR 3rd, Scheithauer BW, Jackson IT. Multifocal Merkel's cell tumors associated with a cutaneous dysplasia syndrome. Arch Dermatol 1983;119:409–14.

Pseudoneoplastic Lesions of Sweat Glands

292. Ando K, Hashikawa Y, Nakashima M, Nakayama A, Ohashi M. Pure apocrine nevus. A study of light microscopic and immunohistochemical features of a rare tumor. Am J Dermatopathol 1991;13:71–6.
293. Challa VR, Jona J. Eccrine angiomatous hamartoma: a rare skin lesion with diverse histological features. Dermatologica 1977;155:206–9.
294. Farina MC, Pique E, Olivares M, Escalonilla P, Martin L, Requena L, Sarasa JL. Multiple hidrocystoma of the face: three cases. Clin Exp Dermatol 1995;20:323–7.
295. Goldstein N. Ephidrosis (local hyperhidrosis). Nevus sudoriferus. Arch Dermatol 1967;96:67–8.
296. Hashimoto K, Zagula-Mally ZW, Youngberg G, Leicht S. Electron microscopic studies of Moll's gland cyst. J Cutan Pathol 1987;14:23–6.
297. Hassan MO, Khan MA, Kruse TV. Apocrine cystadenoma. An ultrastructural study. Arch Dermatol 1979;115:194–200.
298. Imai S, Nitto H. Eccrine nevus with epidermal changes. Dermatologica 1983;166:84–8.
299. Kim JH, Hur H, Lee CW, Kim YT. Apocrine nevus. J Am Acad Dermatol 1988;18:579–81.
300. King DT, Barr RJ. Syringometaplasia: mucinous and squamous variants. J Cutan Pathol 1979;6:284–91.
301. Kruse TV, Khan MA, Hassan MO. Multiple apocrine cystadenomas. Br J Dermatol 1979;100:675–81.
302. Lerner TH, Barr RJ, Dolezal JF, Stagnone JJ. Syringosquamous hyperplasia and eccrine squamous syringometaplasia associated with benoxaprofen therapy. Arch Dermatol 1987;123:1202–4.
303. Mehregan AH. Proliferation of sweat ducts in certain diseases of the skin. Am J Dermatopathol 1981;3:27–31.
304. Mori O, Hachisuka H, Sasai Y. Apocrine nevus. Int J Dermatol 1993;32:448–9.
305. Neill JS, Park HK. Apocrine nevus: light microscopic, immunohistochemical, and ultrastructural studies of a case. J Cutan Pathol 1993;20:79–83.
306. Romer JC, Taira JW. Mucinous eccrine nevus. Cutis 1994;53:259–61.
307. Ruiz de Erenchun F, Vazquez-Doval FJ, Contreras Mejuto F, Quintanilla E. Localized unilateral hyperhidrosis: eccrine nevus. J Am Acad Dermatol 1992;27:115–6.
308. Schwartz RA, Rojas-Corona R, Lambert WC. The polymorphic apocrine nevus. A study of a unique tumor including carcinoembryonic antigen staining. J Surg Oncol 1984;26:183–6.
309. Shields JA, Eagle RC Jr, Shields CL, de Potter P, Markowitz G. Apocrine hidrocystoma of the eyelid. Arch Ophthalmol 1993;111:866–7.
310. Yasaka N, Iozumi K, Nashiro K, et al. Bilateral periorbital eccrine hidrocystoma. J Dermatol 1994;21:490–3.

SUPPLEMENTAL REFERENCES

Cylindroma

Albores-Saavedra J, Heard SC, McLaren B, Kamino H, Witkiewicz AK. Cylindroma (dermal analog tumor) of the breast: a comparison with cylindroma of the skin and adenoid cystic carcinoma of the breast. Am J Clin Pathol 2005;123:866–73.

De Francesco V, Frattasio A, Pillon B, et al. Carcinosarcoma arising in a patient with multiple cylindromas. Am J Dermatopathol 2005;27:21–6.

Kazakov DV, Soukup R, Mukensnabl P, Boudova L, Michal M. Brooke-Spiegler syndrome: report of a case with combined lesions containing cylindromatous, spiradenomatous, trichoblastomatous, and sebaceous differentiation. Am J Dermatopathol 2005;27:27–33.

Nonaka D, Rosai J, Spagnolo D, Fiaccavento S, Bisceglia M. Cylindroma of the breast of skin adnexal type: a study of 4 cases. Am J Surg Pathol 2004;28:1070–5.

Stoll C. Alembik Y, Wilk A, Grosshans E. Familial cylindromatosis. Genet Couns 2004;15:175–82.

Spiradenoma

Ter Poorten MC, Barrett K, Cook J. Familial eccrine spiradenoma: a case report and review of the literature. Dermatol Surg 2003;29:411–4.

Syringoma

Draznin M. Hereditary syringomas: a case report. Dermatol Online J 2004;10:19.

Hsiung SH. Eruptive syringoma. Dermatol Online J 2003;9:14.

Huang YH, Chuang YH, Kuo TT, Yang LC, Hong HS. Vulvar syringoma: a clinicopathologic and immunohistochemical study of 18 patients and results of treatment. J Am Acad Dermatol 2003;48:735–9.

Acrospiroma (Nodular Hidradenoma)

Perna AG, Smith MJ, Krishnan B, Reed JA. CD10 is expressed in cutaneous clear cell lesions of different histogenesis. J Cutan Pathol 2005;32:348–51.

Volmar KE, Cummings TJ, Wang WH, Creager AJ, Tyler DS, Xie HB. Clear cell hidradenoma: a mimic of metastatic clear cell tumors. Arch Pathol Lab Med 2005;129:e113–6.

Poroma

Elloumi-Jellouli A, Marrak H, Ben Ammar S, Ben Ayed M, Mokhtar I. [Pigmented eccrine poroma.] Ann Dermatol Venereol 2004;131:1023. (French.)

Lan CC, Yu HS, Wu CS, Tsai KB, Wen CH, Chen GS. Pigmented eccrine poroma with enhanced endothelin-1 expression: implications for mechanism of hyperpigmentation. Br J Dermatol 2005;152:1070–2.

Liu HN, Chang YT, Chen CC. Differentiation of hidroacanthoma simplex from clonal seborrheic keratosis—an immunohistochemical study. Am J Dermatopathol 2004:26:188–93.

Syringofibroadenoma

Clarke LE, Ioffreda M, Abt AB. Ecrine syringofibroadenoma arising in peristomal skin: a report of two cases. Int J Surg Pathol 2003;11:61–3.

Hu S, Bakshandeh H, Kerdel FA, Rongioletti F, Romanelli P. Eccrine syringofibroadenoma of clear cell variant: an immunohistochemical study. Am J Dermatopathol 2005;27:228–31.

Hidradenoma Papilliferum

Kazakov DV, Mikyskova I, Kutzner H, et al. Hidradenoma papilliferum with oxyphilic metaplasia: a clinicopathological study of 18 cases, including detection of human papillomavirus. Am J Dermatopathol 2005;27:102–10.

Nishie W, Sawamura D, Mayuzumi M, Takahashi S, Shimizu H. Hidradenoma papilliferum with mixed histopathologic features of syringocystadenoma papilliferum and anogenital mammary-like glands. J Cutan Pathol 2004;31;561–4.

Smith FB, Shemen LJ, Guerrieri C, Ismail SS. Hidradenoma papilliferum of nasal skin. Arch Pathol Lab Med 2003;127:E86–8.

Cutaneous Mixed Tumor

Adachi T, Oda Y, Sakamoto A, et al. Mixed tumor of deep soft tissue. Pathol Int 2003;53:35–9.

Mandeville JT, Roh JH, Woog JJ, et al. Cutaneous benign mixed tumor (chondroid syringoma) of the eyelid: clinical presentation and management. Ophthal Plast Reconstr Surg 2004;20:110–6.

Mentzel T, Requena L, Kaddu S, Soares de Aleida M, Sangueza OP, Kutzner H. Cutaneous myoepithelial neoplasms: clinicopathologic and immunohistochemical study of 20 cases suggesting a continuous spectrum ranging from benign mixed tumor of the skin to cutaneous myoepithelioma and myoepithelial carcinoma. J Cutan Pathol 2003;30:294–302.

Salama ME, Azam M, Ma CK, et al. Chondroid syringoma. Cytokeratin 20 immunolocalization of Merkel cells and reappraisal of apocrine folliculosebaceous differentiation. Arch Pathol Lab Med 2004;128:986–90.

Eccrine Sweat Gland Carcinomas

Akalin T, Sen S, Yuceturk A, Kandiloglu G. P53 expression in eccrine poroma and porocarcinoma. Am J Dermatopathol 2001;23:402–6.

Bjarke T, Ternesten-Bratel A, Hedblad M, Rausing A. Carcinoma and eccrine syringofibroadenoma: a report of five cases. J Cutan Pathol 2003;30:382–92.

Castro CY, Deavers M. Ductal carcinoma in-situ arising in mammary-like glands of the vulva. Int J Gynecol Pathol 2001;20:277–83.

Chang CH, Liao YL, Hong HS. Cutaneous metastasis from adenoid cystic carcinoma of the parotid gland. Dermatol Surg 2003;29:775–9.

Clement CI, Genge J, O'Donnell BA, Lochhead AG. Orbital and periorbital microcystic adnexal carcinoma. Ophthal Plast Reconstr Surg 2005;21:97–102.

Demarchi A, Bellis D, Nunziata R, Coverlizza S. [Aggressive digital papillary adenocarcinoma: a case report.] Pathologica 2003;95:447–51. (Italian.)

Doganay L, Bilgi S, Aygit C, Altaner S. Primary cutaneous adenoid cystic carcinoma with lung and lymph node metastases. J Eur Acad Dermatol Venereol 2004;18:383–5.

Duzova AN, Boztepe G, Sahin S, Gokoz A. Painful nodule on the scalp: a case of primary cutaneous adenoid cystic carcinoma. Acta Derm Venereol 2004;84:243–4.

Fischer S, Breuninger H, Metzler G, Hoffmann J. Microcystic adnexal carcinoma: an often-misdiagnosed, locally aggressive growing skin tumor. J Craniofac Surg 2005;16:53–8.

Gu LH, Ichiki Y, Kitajima Y. Aberrant expression of p16 and RB protein in eccrine porocarcinoma. J Cutan Pathol 2002;29:473–9.

Inaloz HS, Patel GK, Knight AG. An aggressive treatment for aggressive digital papillary adenocarcinoma. Cutis 2002;69:179–82.

Jih MH, Friedman PM, Kimyai-Asadi A, Goldberg LH. A rare case of fatal primary cutaneous mucinous carcinoma of the scalp with multiple in-transit and pulmonary metastases. J Am Acad Dermatol 2005;52(Suppl 1):S76–80.

Katane M, Akiyama M, Ohnishi T, Watanabe S, Matsuo I. Carcinomatous transformation of eccrine syringofibroadenoma. J Cutan Pathol 2003;30:211–4.

Kazakov DV, Suster S, Leboit PE, et al. Mucinous carcinoma of the skin, primary and secondary: a clinicopathologic study of 63 cases with emphasis on the morphologic spectrum of primary cutaneous forms: homologies with mucinous lesions in the breast. Am J Surg Pathol 2005;29:764–82.

Liegl B, Regauer S. Penile clear cell carcinoma: a report of 5 cases of a distinct entity. Am J Surg Pathol 2004;28:1513–7.

Locati LD, Quattrone P, Pizzi N, Fior A, Cantu G, Licitra L. Primary high-grade mucoepidermoid carcinoma of the minor salivary glands with cutaneous metastasis at diagnosis. Oral Oncol 2002;38:401–4.

Mirza I, Kloss R, Sieber SC. Malignant eccrine spiradenoma. Arch Pathol Lab Med 2002;126:591–4.

Mori O, Nakama T, Hashimoto T. Aggressive papillary digital adenocarcinoma arising on the right great toe. Eur J Dermatol 2002;12:491–4.

Perna C, Cuevas J, Jimenez-Heffernan JA, Hardisson D, Contreras F. Eccrine porocarcinoma (malignant eccrine poroma). Am J Surg Pathol 2002;26:272–4.

Plumb SJ, Argenyi ZB, Stone MS, DeYoung BR. Cytokeratin 5/6 immunostaining in cutaneous adnexal neoplasms and metastatic adenocarcinoma. Am J Dermatopathol 2004;26:447–51.

Qureshi HS, Salama ME, Chitale D, et al. Primary cutaneous mucinous carcinoma: presence of myoepithelial cells as a clue to the cutaneous origin. Am J Dermatopathol 2004;26:353–8.

Riedlinger WF, Hurley MY, Dehner LP, Lind AC. Mucoepidermoid carcinoma of the skin: a distinct entity from adenosquamous carcinoma: a case study with a review of the literature. Am J Surg Pathol 2005;29:131–5.

Rutten A, Requena L, Requena C. Clear-cell porocarcinoma in situ: a cytologic variant of porocarcinoma in situ. Am J Dermatopathol 2002;24:67–71.

Schroder U, Dries V, Klussmann JP, Wittekindt C, Eckel HE. Successful adjuvant tamoxifen therapy for estrogen receptor-positive metastasizing sweat gland adenocarcinoma: need for a clinical trial? Ann Otol Rhinol Laryngol 2004;113(Pt 1):242–4.

Stein JM, Ormsby A, Esclamado R, Bailin P. The effect of radiation therapy on microcystic adnexal carcinoma: a case report. Head Neck 2003;25:251–4.

Tran TA, Muller S, Chaudahri PJ, Carlson JA. Cutaneous carcinosarcoma: adnexal vs. epidermal types define high- and low-risk tumors. Results of a meta-analysis. J Cutan Pathol 2005;32:2–11.

Paget's Disease of the Skin

Bogner PN, Su LD, Fullen DR. Cluster designation 5 staining of normal and non-lymphoid neoplastic skin. J Cutan Pathol 2005;32:50–4.

Ewing T, Sawicki J, Ciaravino G, Rumore GJ. Microinvasive Paget's disease. Gynecol Oncol 2004;95:755–8.

Liegl B, Horn LC, Moinfar F. Androgen receptors are frequently expressed in mammary and extramammary Paget's disease. Mod Pathol 2005 May 13; [Epub ahead of print].

Reich O, Liegl B, Tamussino K, Regauer S. p185HER2 overexpression and HER2 oncogene amplification in recurrent vulvar Paget's disease. Mod Pathol 2005;18:354–7.

Salamanca J, Benito A, Garcia-Penalver C, Azorin D, Ballestin C, Rodriguez-Peralto JL. Paget's disease of the glans penis secondary to transitional cell carcinoma of the bladder: a report of two cases and review of the literature. J Cutan Pathol 2004;31:341–5.

Ueda Y, Enomoto T, Miyatake T, et al. Analysis of clonality and HPV infection in benign, hyperplastic, premalignant, and malignant lesions of the vulvar mucosa. Am J Clin Pathol 2004;122:266–74.

Willman JH, Golitz LE, Fitzpatrick JE. Vulvar clear cells of Toker: precursors of extramammary Paget's disease. Am J Dermatopathol 2005;27:185–8.

Yang CC, Lee JY, Wong TW. Depigmented extramammary Paget's disease. Br J Dermatol 2004;151:1049–53.

Yang WJ, Kim DS, Im YJ, et al. Extramammary Paget's disease of penis and scrotum. Urology 2005;65:972–5.

Zhang C, Zhang P, Sung CJ, Lawrence WD. Overexpression of p53 is correlated with stromal invasion in extramammary Paget's disease of the vulva. Hum Pathol 2003;34:880–5.

Primary Cutaneous Neuroendocrine (Merkel Cell) Carcinoma

Allen PJ, Bowne WB, Jaques DP, Brennan MF, Busam K, Coit DG. Merkel cell carcinoma: prognosis and treatment of patients from a single institution. J Clin Oncol 2005;23:2300–9.

Bickle K, Glass LF, Messina JL, Fenske NA, Siegrist K. Merkel cell carcinoma: a clinical, histopathologic, and immunohistochemical review. Semin Cutan Med Surg 2004;23:46–53.

Dong HY, Liu W, Cohen P, Mahle CE, Zhang W. B-cell specific activation protein encoded by the PAX-5 gene is commonly expressed in Merkel cell carcinoma and small cell carcinomas. Am J Surg Pathol 2005;29;687–92.

Eng TY, Naguib M, Fuller CD, Jones WE 3rd, Herman TS. Treatment of recurrent Merkel cell carcinoma: an analysis of 46 cases. Am J Clin Oncol 2004;27:576–83.

Feinmesser M, Halpern M, Kaganovsky E, et al. c-kit expression in primary and metastatic Merkel cell carcinoma. Am J Dermatopathol 2004;26:458–62.

Fernando-Figueras MT, Puig L, Musulen E, et al. Prognostic significance of p27Kip, p45Skp2, and Ki67 expression profiles in Merkel cell carcinoma, extracutaneous small cell carcinoma, and cutaneous squamous cell carcinoma. Histopathology 2005;46:614–21.

Ferringer T, Rogers HC, Metcalf JS. Merkel cell carcinoma in-situ. J Cutan Pathol 2005;32:162–5.

Koljonen V, Haglund C, Tukiainen E, Bohling T. Neuroendocrine differentiation in primary Merkel cell carcinoma—possible prognostic significance. Anticancer Res 2005;25:853–8.

Larramendy ML, Koljonen V, Bohling T, Tukiainen E, Knuutila S. Recurrent DNA copy number changes revealed by comparative genomic hybridization in primary Merkel cell carcinoma. Mod Pathol 2004;17:561–7.

Lehrer MS, Hershock D, Ming ME. Merkel cell carcinoma. Curr Treat Options Oncol 2004;5:195–9.

Llombart B, Monteagudo C, Lopez-Guerrero JA, et al. Clinicopathological and immunohistochemical analysis of 20 cases of Merkel cell carcinoma in search of prognostic markers. Histopathology 2005;46:622–34.

Mendenhall WM, Mendenhall CM, Mendenhall NP. Merkel cell carcinoma. Laryngoscope 2004;114:906–10.

Poulsen M. Merkel cell carcinoma of skin: diagnosis and management strategies. Drugs Aging 2005;22:219–29.

Rossi S, Orvieto E, Furlanetto A, Laurino L, Ninfo V, Dei Tos AP. Utility of immunohistochemical detection of FLI-1 expression in round cell and vascular neoplasms using a monoclonal antibody. Mod Pathol 2004;17:547–52.

Suarez C, Rodrigo JP, Ferlito A, Devaney KO, Rinaldo A. Merkel cell carcinoma of the head and neck. Oral Oncol 2004;40:773–9.

van der Heijden HF, Heijdra YF. Extrapulmonary small cell carcinoma. South Med J 2005;98:345–9.

Yang DT, Holden JA, Florell SR. CD117, CK20, TTF-1, and DNA topoisomerase II-alpha antigen expression in small cell tumors. J Cutan Pathol 2004;31:254–61.

Pseudoneoplastic Sweat Gland Lesions

Baysse L, Boralevi F, Lepreux S, et al. [Eccrine squamous syringometaplasia and cytomegalovirus infection.] Rev Med Interne 2003;24:394–8. (French.)

Jiang J, Petronic-Rosic V, Hoag J, Shea CR. Eccrine mucinous metaplasia associated with an apocrine cystadenoma. J Cutan Pathol 2005;32:307–9.

Ozdal PC, Callejo SA, Codere F, Burnier MN Jr. Benign ocular adnexal tumors of apocrine, eccrine, or hair follicle origin. Can J Ophthalmol 2003;38:357–63.

Penas PF, Jones-Caballero M, Aragues M, Fernandez-Herrera J, Fraga J, Garcia-Diez A. Sclerodermatous graft-vs-host disease: clinical and pathologic study of 17 patients. Arch Dermatol 2002;138:924–34.

5 METASTATIC NEOPLASMS

Metastatic tumors in the skin usually pose little or no diagnostic difficulty for pathologists, because their clinical attributes have already been interpreted by dermatologists as those of secondary cutaneous malignancies. There are instances, however, where that rule does not hold true, and those typically involve solitary "messenger" metastases from visceral adenocarcinomas. Metastatic glandular tumors are most likely to be confused with primary adnexal neoplasms of the skin because both principally involve the dermis and may demonstrate considerable histologic similarity.

Because fewer than 1 in 1,000 malignant cutaneous tumors display appendageal differentiation (87), pathologists should be appropriately reluctant to render a diagnosis of primary adnexal skin carcinoma. The experience of the authors certainly reflects these statistics: in the consultation cases we have received, nonadnexal neoplasms of the skin are much more often observed than malignant appendage tumors, by a factor of 10 to 1, despite the fact that many specimens are sent with a tentative interpretation that favors the latter diagnosis.

As stated above, these misinterpreted lesions are often metastases from visceral tumors, which have been missed in the excitement of encountering a potentially rare case, such as an adnexal carcinoma. In particular, the admonition that sweat gland carcinoma is largely a diagnosis of exclusion is forgotten in many cases, with consequent inattention to the possibility of occult internal neoplasia. This error is a serious one, in light of the horrible prognosis attending cutaneous metastases: almost all patients with such lesions die from their primary tumors within 6 months of diagnosis (52,53,84). Also, unfamiliarity with the many potential images of such "banal" primary tumors as basal cell carcinoma, squamous cell carcinoma, and malignant melanoma of the skin, accounts for some diagnostic misadventures in which they are mistaken for metastases.

VISCERAL CARCINOMAS THAT INVOLVE THE SKIN

Clinical Features

There are many carcinomas that arise in internal organs and are capable of dissemination to secondary cutaneous sites. In fact, a review of the literature reveals that virtually all visceral malignant neoplasms have such potential (2–5,7–10,13–16,21,22,25,29,32,34,35,41,44–47,51,52,55,57,59,64,65,68,69,73,74,79,83,85,86,88,89,93). At autopsy, up to 4 percent of patients with noncutaneous epithelial malignant neoplasms have skin involvement (1,30,58,84). Cancers of the breast, lung, gastrointestinal tract, and oropharynx are most commonly implicated, in respective order (1,58). Accordingly, adenocarcinomas are more frequently observed as cutaneous metastases than neoplasms with squamous or transitional cell differentiation (10).

Because cutaneous metastasis is usually observed in the context of widespread disease when the primary site of growth has already been well documented (68), one must analyze visceral neoplasms from another perspective to gain insights on those that most commonly simulate primary cutaneous carcinomas. Lookingbill et al. (53) studied visceral neoplasms with the unusual capacity for "herald metastasis," wherein skin involvement is the initial manifestation of an internal malignant growth. They found that the most frequent sites of origin were the lung, kidney, stomach, and internal female genitals, and other studies have reached similar conclusions (10,68). Fortunately, in light of the microscopic similarities between sweat gland carcinomas and breast cancer, the mammary glands relatively rarely give rise to distant cutaneous metastases in the absence of obvious primary disease (11).

The clinical history given by the patient is often the most valuable piece of information in this context, provided it is reliable. Sweat gland carcinomas are solitary masses in almost all cases and

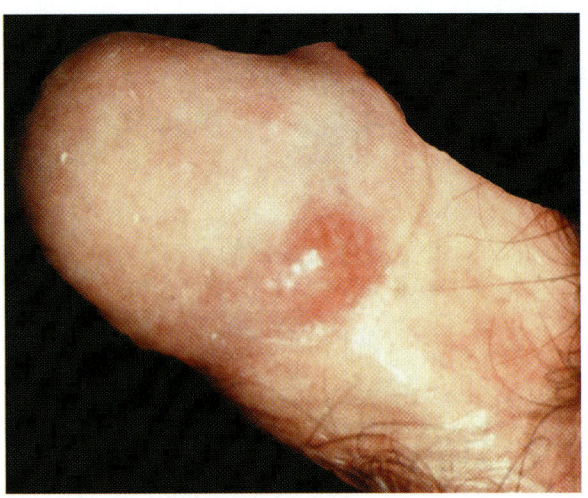

Figure 5-1

SOLITARY METASTASIS OF PROSTATIC ADENOCARCINOMA IN THE CORONA OF THE PENIS

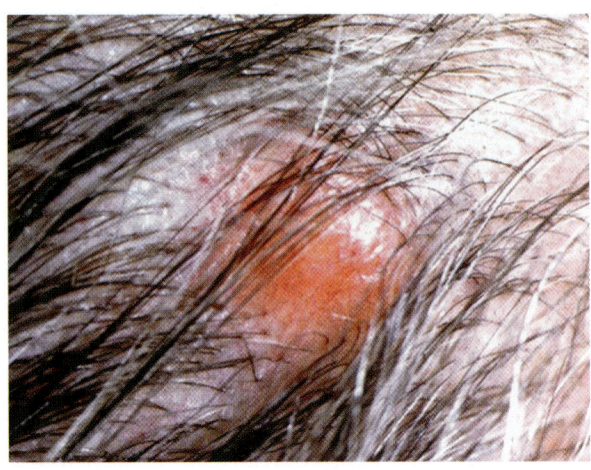

Figure 5-2

SOLITARY METASTASIS OF ADENOCARCINOMA OF THE LUNG IN THE SKIN OF THE SCALP

have been present for at least 6 months, gradually enlarging over time. In contrast, metastatic tumors are rapidly growing lesions, even when solitary (68). Even though only one secondary skin lesion may be noted initially (figs. 5-1, 5-2) (10,11,45,59,68,76,78,86), the usual evolution of such cases is typified by the appearance of several additional tumors within a short time after presentation (11,68).

The topography of these lesions may also be important. Metastatic carcinomas tend to display a regional preference for certain skin areas that are close to the underlying organ of origin (11,68). For example, lung and breast cancers often involve the skin of the chest or back, whereas those in the rectum and internal genitalia typically spread to the genitoperineal skin (2,8,11,16,33,46,53,56,75,80,90). These descriptions are valid generalizations, but carcinomas that commonly demonstrate angioinvasion (such as those in the kidney and lung) may also present at sites that are distant from the primary neoplasm (10). Furthermore, there are peculiar dermatologic presentations of metastases that are strongly linked to origin from a particular internal organ. The association of carcinoma en cuirasse (ligneous cutaneous change produced by intradermal metastases in the skin of the thorax, resembling armor plate), carcinoma erysipelatoides (intralymphatic cutaneous tumor spread, resembling the brawny red appearance of cellulitis), and scarring alopecia with breast cancer (figs. 5-3, 5-4) (19,37,43,49,64,67,80) and the relationship of "Sister Mary Joseph" nodules of the umbilicus to malignant neoplasms of the alimentary tract (fig. 5-5) (17,18,28,38,59,61,63,72,79,96) serve as illustrations of this point.

Other idiosyncratic presentations of metastatic carcinoma are notable. Breast carcinoma may involve the nasal skin selectively, producing erythema and enlargement that has been termed "clown nose" (77). Grouped, vesicular, epidermotropic tumor nodules may resemble the clinical appearance of shingles (fig. 5-6) (54), and this image can be seen with a number of different tumor types. Metastatic lesions that imitate the changes of elephantiasis (39), pyogenic granuloma (34), condyloma acuminatum (88), and cutaneous vasculitis (62) have been documented. In addition, like some other cutaneous diseases such as sarcoidosis, dermal metastases have a tendency to "home" to prior scars or other defects in the skin, including fields of prior irradiation (24). Lastly, selected anatomic locations are so unusually affected by metastatic disease that they have special clinical associations; for example, subungual metastases on the digits of the hands usually derive from carcinomas of the lung, genitourinary tract, and breast, in that order of likelihood (20).

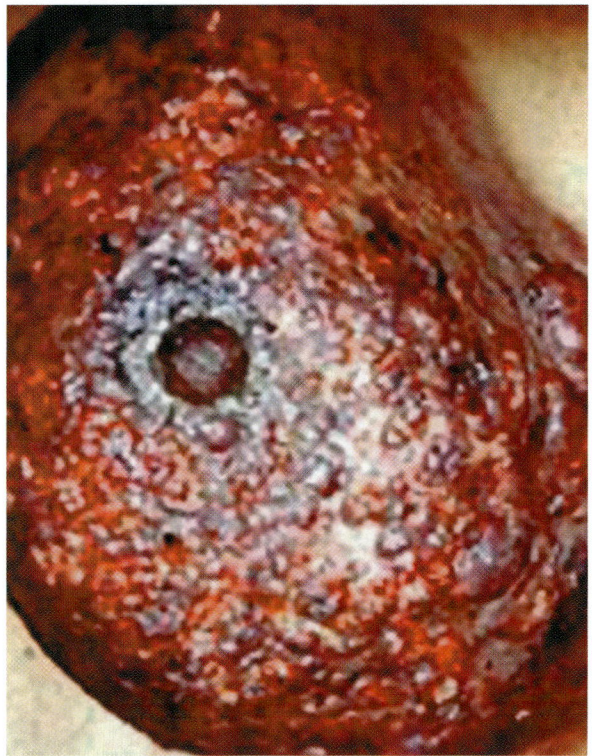

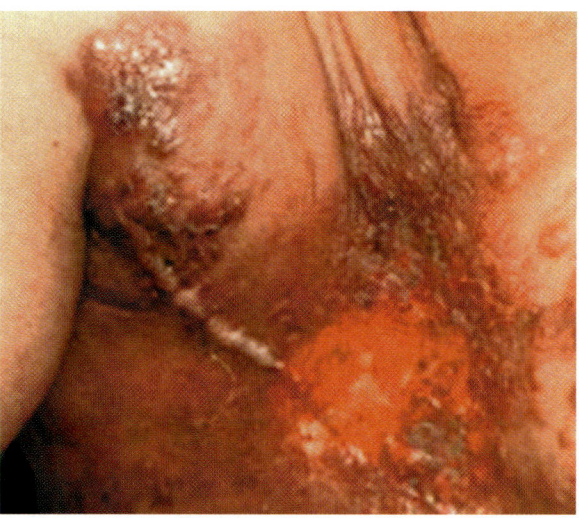

Figure 5-3

METASTATIC CARCINOMA

Left: The intensely erythematous change in the skin of the breast is produced by metastatic, intralymphatic mammary adenocarcinoma.

Above: Wood-hard thickening in the skin of the chest wall is associated with recurrent breast carcinoma.

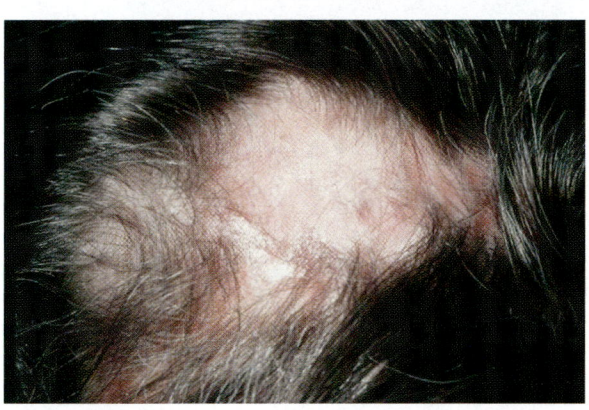

Figure 5-4

SCARRING ALOPECIA NEOPLASTICA

This lesion is related to metastatic breast carcinoma in the scalp.

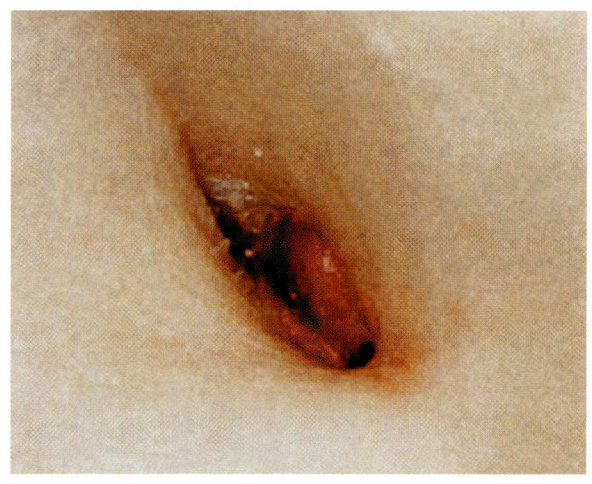

Figure 5-5

"SISTER MARY JOSEPH" NODULE

Metastatic gastric carcinoma is present in the peri-umbilical skin.

Pathologic Findings

Selected morphologic features may be used as potential diagnostic aids. Metastatic carcinomas in the skin often manifest a disorganized pattern of growth, with extensive dissection of dermal collagen bundles by the tumor cells (fig. 5-7). Single neoplastic cells are commonly scattered throughout the corium in such cases; aside from signet ring sweat gland carcinomas, cellular arrangement in single file is distinctly unusual in primary skin tumors and should sway diagnostic opinion toward that of metastasis. Renal cell carcinomas tend to exhibit

Nonmelanocytic Tumors of the Skin

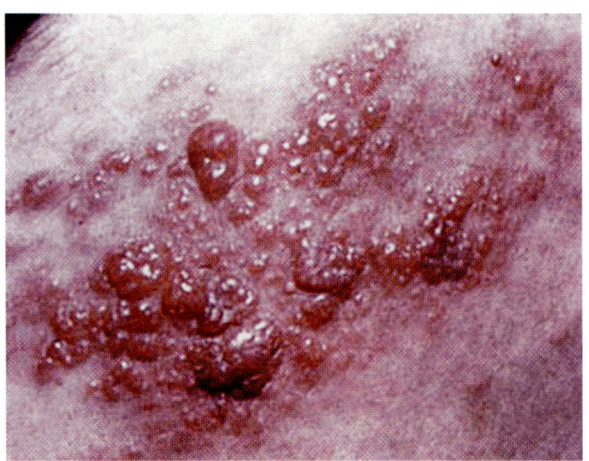

Figure 5-6

ZOSTERIFORM METASTASIS OF LUNG CARCINOMA

The lesion simulates the clinical appearance of shingles.

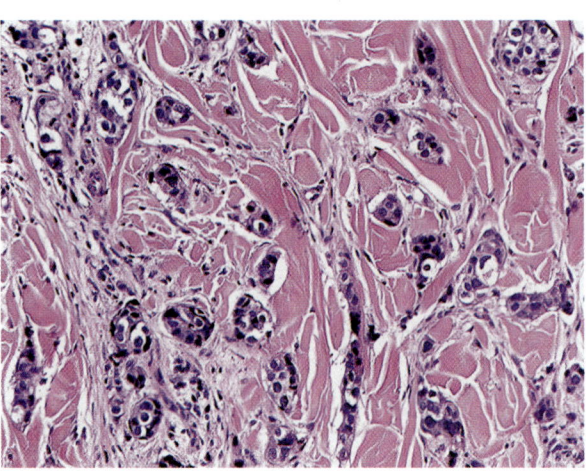

Figure 5-7

METASTATIC ADENOCARCINOMA OF THE BREAST

There is disorganized and dissecting intradermal growth.

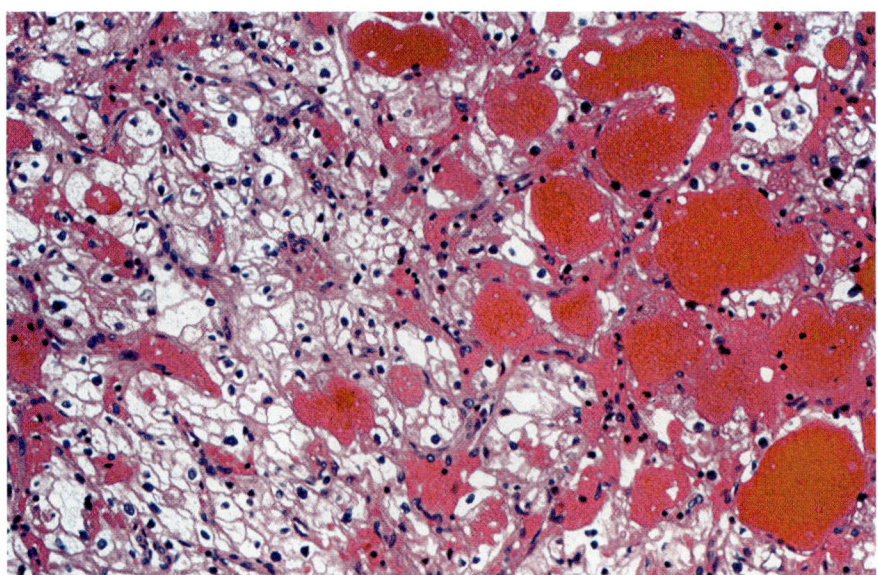

Figure 5-8

METASTATIC CLEAR CELL RENAL CELL CARCINOMA

Typical intratumoral hemorrhage is seen.

intratumoral hemorrhage into the lumens of neoplastic tubules (fig. 5-8) (10), but this feature is not shared by primary cutaneous carcinomas. Overt intracellular mucigenesis is not typical of most sweat gland carcinomas, as visualized with the hematoxylin and eosin stain, with mucinous and mucoepidermoid carcinomas being distinctive exceptions. Obviously, this feature would again favor a metastatic tumor as the correct interpretation.

Specific Visceral Sources of Cutaneous Metastasis

Carcinomas of the Lung. All of the four major types of pulmonary carcinoma (squamous, glandular, large cell undifferentiated, and small cell neuroendocrine) have been reported to involve the skin secondarily (2,10,16,29,58,76,84,94). Of these, small cell cancers do so most often (10,29,94). The principal diagnostic alternative in these cases is Merkel cell carcinoma,

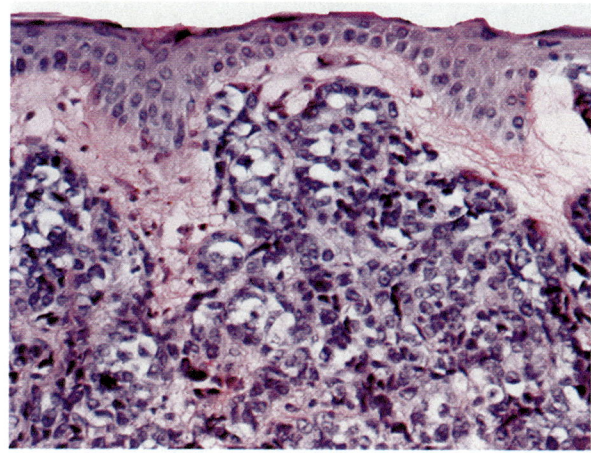

Figure 5-9

METASTATIC ADENOCARCINOMA OF THE LUNG

There is a histologic resemblance to primary ductal eccrine adenocarcinoma.

as discussed in chapter 4. Immunostains for carcinoembryonic antigen, cytokeratin (CK) 20, and thyroid transcription factor-1 (TTF1) may assist in separating these lesions from one another (50,82), but thorough clinical evaluation of the lungs is still recommended in all instances.

Of the remaining lung cancer histotypes, metastatic moderately differentiated adenocarcinoma is most often mistaken for sweat gland carcinoma (10). In some cases, the cytologic appearance is similar to that of some adnexal lesions, with a relatively organized growth pattern in the skin (fig. 5-9). These factors make a definitive diagnosis extremely difficult by conventional morphologic studies.

Immunohistochemical analyses are potentially helpful in such circumstances. Although reactivity for carcinoembryonic antigen and S-100 protein is shared by both tumors (91), TTF1 is unique to lung tumors in this particular setting. Electron microscopic findings may be contributory if tumor cells are found to contain lysosomes with complex substructures; these inclusions are common in adenocarcinomas of the lung but are not observed in sweat gland tumors.

Only rare examples of primary carcinoma of the skin demonstrate the degree of cytologic atypia and architectural disorganization that is seen in large cell undifferentiated or poorly differentiated lung cancer (fig. 5-10). Specialized pathologic studies are of limited use in these cases.

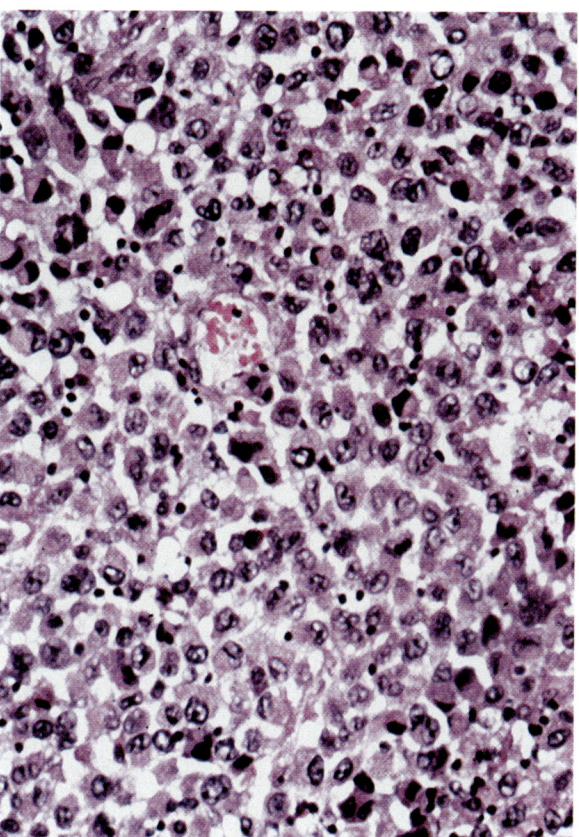

Figure 5-10

METASTASIS OF LARGE CELL UNDIFFERENTIATED LUNG CARCINOMA

This dermal metastasis of large cell undifferentiated lung carcinoma could be confused with several forms of primary undifferentiated cutaneous neoplasia.

Renal Cell Carcinoma. Metastatic clear cell renal cell carcinoma involving the skin can sometimes be suspected on the basis of routine microscopy, as mentioned above. Even those cases of renal cell carcinoma that lack intralesional hemorrhage may still be separable from other clear cell cutaneous tumors. Clear cell eccrine hidradenocarcinoma does not contain appreciable cytoplasmic lipid on staining with the oil red-O or Sudan IV method unlike renal cell carcinoma (10). In addition, clear cell hidradenocarcinoma is often reactive for carcinoembryonic antigen or S-100 protein, differing from the immunophenotype of renal cell carcinoma (57,81,82,91). Ultrastructural analysis commonly demonstrates the presence of cytoplasmic tonofibrils in primary cutaneous carcinomas

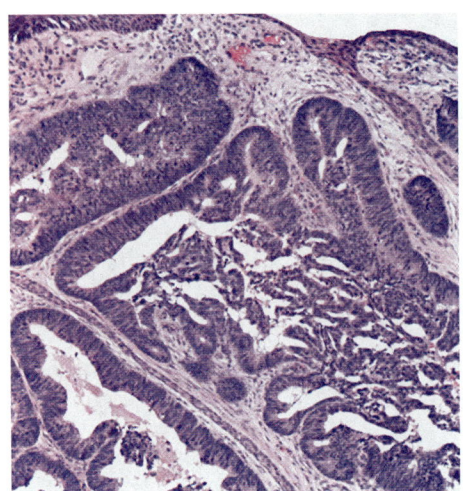 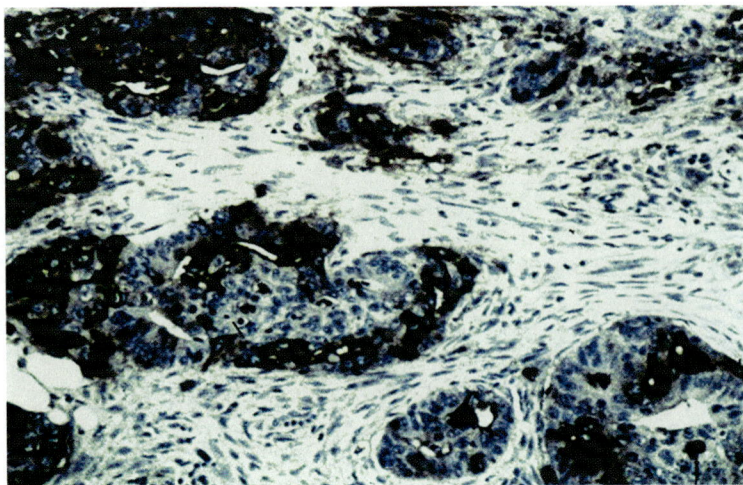

Figure 5-11

METASTATIC COLORECTAL ADENOCARCINOMA IN THE SKIN OF THE ABDOMEN

Left: The characteristic basally-oriented nuclei in the tumor cells and intraglandular necrosis (bottom) are seen.
Right: Immunoreactivity for CA19.9 antigen.

that are composed of clear cells, whereas renal cell carcinoma lacks such structures (6,83).

Sebaceous carcinoma is distinguished from renal neoplasms by its lack of glycogen, as revealed by the periodic acid–Schiff (PAS) stain (71,74,86). Also, sebaceous tumors have finely vacuolated cytoplasm, as opposed to the uniformly lucent appearance of neoplastic cells in most renal cell carcinomas. Electron microscopy reveals intracellular tonofilaments in the majority of sebaceous carcinomas (93). Finally, associated pagetoid change in the epidermis, which is observed in some cases of sebaceous neoplasia (72), is not present in metastatic carcinomas.

Gastrointestinal Carcinoma. Typical colorectal carcinoma has a distinctive cytologic and architectural appearance that is unlike that of sweat gland carcinoma. The former neoplasm typically shows a columnar cell constituency, basally oriented nuclei, and discernible intracellular mucin production (fig. 5-11). Moreover, immunohistochemical studies reveal reactivity for the CA19.9 antigen and villin in a significant proportion of metastatic intestinal cancers, contrasted with their absence in primary neoplasms of the skin (82). This discriminant is important, in view of the shared positivity for carcinoembryonic antigen in these two tumor groups (81,82,91). Electron microscopy reveals the presence of microvillous "core rootlets" and a "terminal web" of cytoplasmic intermediate filaments in intestinal cancers (fig. 5-12) (40), but not in sweat gland carcinoma (92).

Another subset of alimentary tract malignant neoplasm, signet-ring cell carcinoma, may be identified in the skin in many instances. These neoplasms arise in the stomach and colon, and their cutaneous metastases bear a striking resemblance to primary apocrine signet ring cell tumors (10). Immunostains for gross cystic disease fluid protein-15 are usually positive in apocrine neoplasms but not in gastrointestinal tumors (82).

Ovarian Carcinomas. Ovarian carcinomas of all histologic types have been implicated in "precocious" cutaneous metastases (10,80,89). Those that have such potential are usually poorly differentiated and do not manifest the papillary or hobnail appearance that is commonly associated with malignant surface epithelial tumors of the female gonads. Instead, solid sheets of anaplastic cells characterize metastasizing ovarian carcinomas, with or without lumen formation or clear cell (mesonephroid) features (fig. 5-13). The presence of psammoma bodies (fig. 5-14) is an important microscopic finding in these lesions, because these are never seen in primary cutaneous tumors (10).

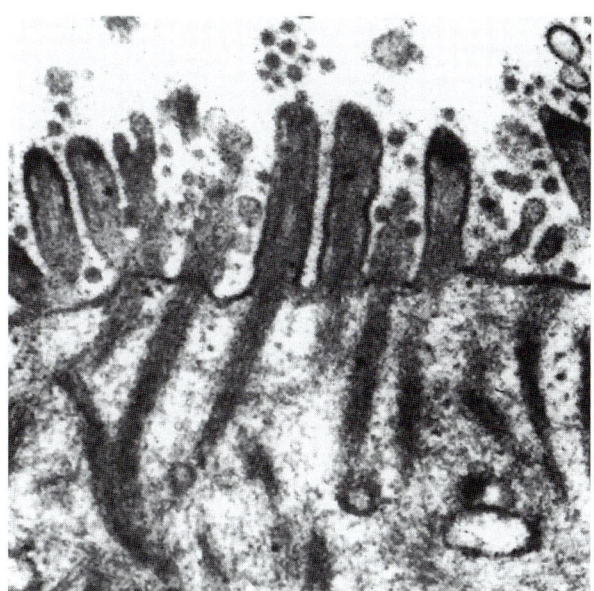

Figure 5-12

COLORECTAL ADENOCARCINOMA

The typical "terminal web" of microfilaments is associated with plasmalemmal microvilli.

Attention to the details of the clinical presentation is diagnostically helpful in these cases. Most primary carcinomas of the skin have well-defined topographic predilections and usually arise in the sun-exposed extremities or head and neck. In contrast, metastases of ovarian carcinomas demonstrate a regional preference for the flanks, the lower abdomen, and the external genital skin (11,80). Unfortunately, apocrine ductopapillary carcinoma also favors the external genital skin, making its separation from secondary gonadal tumors potentially problematic on anatomic grounds alone. Indeed, we have observed individual cases in which the distinction of a metastatic ovarian neoplasm from primary sweat gland carcinoma was extremely challenging. Immunohistochemical studies are capable of yielding discriminating information in this context. As a general group, ovarian carcinomas express the CA125 antigen and lack carcinoembryonic antigen, whereas histologically similar primary cutaneous carcinomas show the reverse of that profile (34,39,57).

Breast Carcinomas. Carcinomas of the breast only uncommonly become clinically evident through cutaneous metastasis. Nonetheless, the striking histologic similarity between sweat

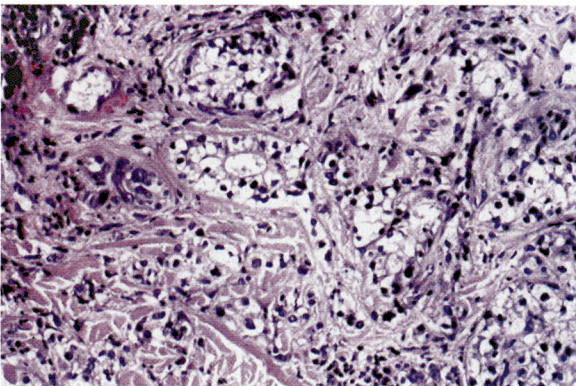
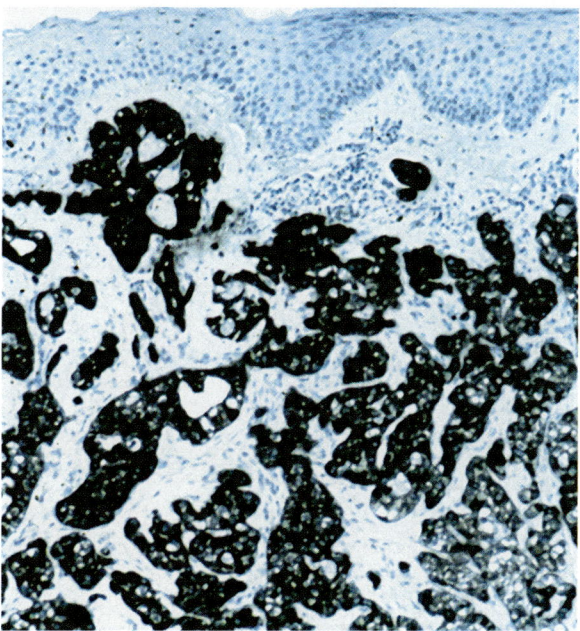

Figure 5-13

METASTATIC CLEAR CELL OVARIAN CARCINOMA

Top: Metastatic clear cell ovarian carcinoma in the skin of the flank.

Bottom: Immunoreactivity for CA125 in metastatic intradermal clear cell ovarian carcinoma.

gland carcinoma and ductal or papillary breast cancer (fig. 5-15) often makes the pathologist wary of trusting that generalization too implicitly. Thorough clinical assessment of the breasts, by careful physical examination and mammography, is the only reliable method for excluding the rare possibility of occult mammary cancer. This dogmatic statement stems from the observation that sweat gland carcinomas of the skin are potentially analogous to

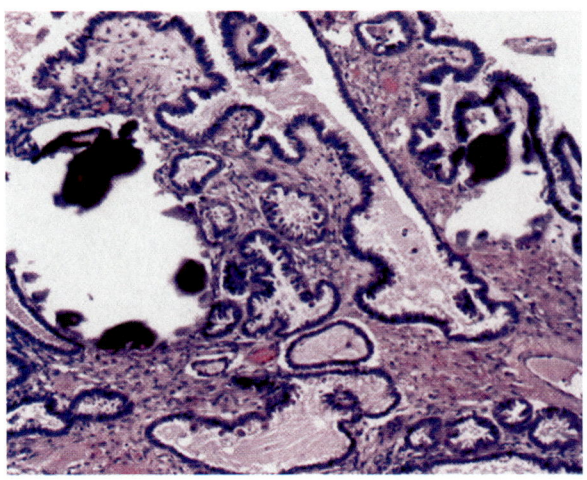

Figure 5-14

METASTASIS OF SEROUS OVARIAN CARCINOMA IN THE SKIN

Psammoma bodies are present.

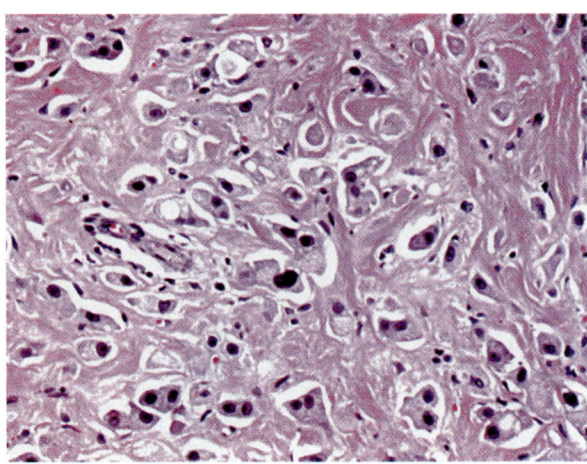

Figure 5-16

METASTATIC HISTIOCYTOID BREAST CARCINOMA IN THE SKIN OF THE EYELID

This tumor simulates primary cutaneous apocrine signet ring cell carcinoma.

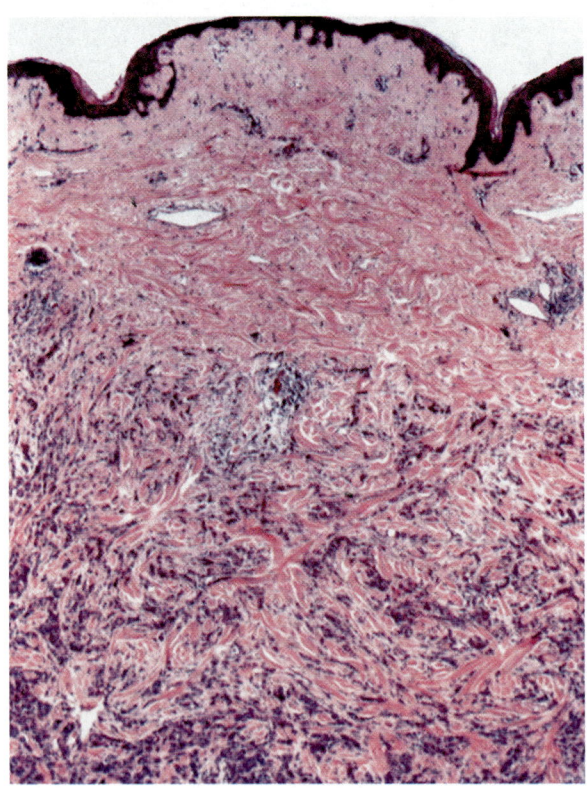

Figure 5-15

METASTATIC INTRADERMAL DUCTAL CARCINOMA OF THE BREAST

There is a histologic resemblance to primary sweat gland carcinoma.

metastatic malignant breast neoplasms in every way, including the expression of gross cystic disease fluid protein-15 (55,91,95) and S-100 protein (91). Hormonal receptor proteins also may be seen in both tumors (82).

One particular variant of breast cancer does seem to metastasize distantly with relative frequency, in the absence of overt primary disease. This is the histiocytoid form of lobular carcinoma, which mimics signet ring carcinoma of sweat gland origin (fig. 5-16) (41). Because secondary involvement of the skin by the former lesion favors the eyelids (41), its similarity to signet ring apocrine carcinoma is particularly striking.

Salivary Gland Tumors. The presentation of salivary glandular carcinomas through metastasis to the skin is virtually unknown. Common malignant lesions of the salivary glands, such as adenoid cystic, mucoepidermoid, and acinic cell carcinomas, virtually never manifest such behavior (12). A solitary report has been made of a malignant mixed tumor of the parotid that metastasized to the scalp as the first sign of disease (32). Closer analysis of that report, however, revealed that the patient had a resected salivary gland tumor 35 years previously. Hence, the history would have raised at least some doubt as to the primary nature of his cutaneous tumor.

This point is germane to diagnosing malignant mixed tumor of eccrine origin, which is

Table 5-1
SQUAMOUS CELL CARCINOMA VARIANTS THAT ARE POTENTIALLY CONFUSED WITH METASTASES
Acantholytic (Adenoid) Squamous Cell Carcinoma
Clear Cell (Hydropic) Squamous Cell Carcinoma
Squamous Cell Carcinoma with Mucinous Metaplasia

Table 5-2
BASAL CELL CARCINOMA VARIANTS THAT ARE POTENTIALLY CONFUSED WITH METASTASES
Adenoid (Pseudoglandular) Basal Cell Carcinoma
Basal Cell Carcinoma with Divergent Sweat Glandular Differentiation (Eccrine Epithelioma, Apocrine Epithelioma)
Signet Ring Cell Basal Cell Carcinoma
Clear Cell Basal Cell Carcinoma

otherwise identical histologically to malignant pleomorphic adenoma of the parotid gland (27, 31,85). Secondary deposits of carcinosarcomas of the female genitals and other organs could theoretically simulate sarcomatoid primary cutaneous tumors microscopically; however, to the best of our knowledge, these extracutaneous tumors have not been reported to involve the skin through selective and solitary metastasis.

Immunohistochemistry in the Determination of Primary Site

As mentioned throughout the foregoing discussion, immunohistologic analysis is the most expeditious means to address the probable origin of a metastatic carcinoma in the skin, in the absence of a known primary neoplasm. Further discussion of this subject is beyond the scope of this treatise, and can be found in other publications that are devoted to diagnostic immunohistology (for a representative citational listing see reference 23). An overall approach to the topic is represented by the algorithm in figure 5-17, which includes the principal antibody reagents that are needed in this area of anatomic pathology.

PRIMARY NONADNEXAL EPITHELIAL SKIN TUMORS THAT MAY RESEMBLE METASTATIC LESIONS

The diagnostic separation of selected primary nonadnexal epithelial tumors of the skin from metastatic carcinomas can be problematic in selected cases. The former are predominantly variants of squamous cell carcinoma and basal cell carcinoma. They are listed in Tables 5-1 and 5-2, and readers are referred to other portions of this monograph for more detailed descriptions of the tumors in question. Again, it should be remembered that primary lesions of the skin are slow-growing, whereas metastatic neoplasms evolve rapidly. That single point is probably the most discriminatory in the differential diagnostic process.

OTHER METASTATIC NEOPLASMS

Sarcomas of various viscera may also involve the skin metastatically, but this is a rare event. Generally, only those secondary lesions that simulate primary mesenchymal tumors of the dermis pose potential diagnostic problems on theoretical grounds; these principally include metastatic leiomyosarcomas, fibrohistiocytic neoplasms, and vascular sarcomas. We have never seen a tumor that was given genuine consideration as a possible primary cutaneous sarcoma, but which proved to be metastatic. Thus, this situation may be more hypothetical than real in actual practice.

Malignant melanoma is, by far, the nonepithelial tumor that most frequently metastasizes to the skin (excluding hematopoietic proliferations, which are conceptually regarded as systemic ab initio and therefore incapable of true metastasis). Readers are referred to the excellent Fascicle in this series by Elder and Murphy on melanocytic tumors (26), for a complete discussion of their clinicopathologic features.

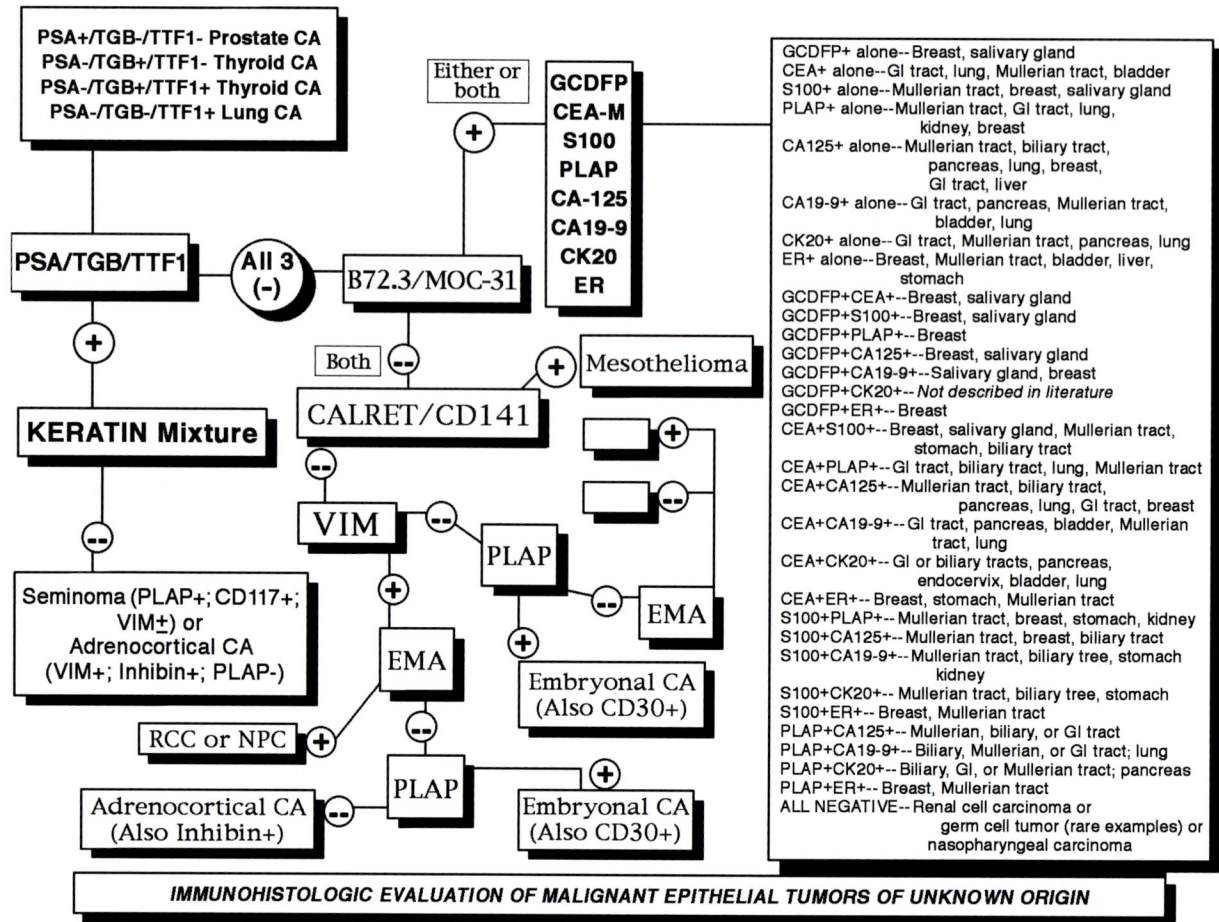

Figure 5-17

ALGORITHM FOR ADJUNCTIVE IMMUNOHISTOLOGIC DIAGNOSIS OF METASTATIC CARCINOMAS IN THE SKIN

PSA = prostate-specific antigen; TGB = thyroglobulin; TTF1 = thyroid transcription factor-1; CA = carcinoma; GCDFP = gross cystic disease fluid protein-15; CEA-M = carcinoembryonic antigen (detected by monoclonal antibodies); S100 = S-100 protein; PLAP = placental alkaline phosphatase; CK20 = cytokeratin 20; ER = estrogen receptor protein; CALRET = calretinin; VIM = vimentin; EMA = epithelial membrane antigen; NPC = nasopharyngeal carcinoma; HCC = hepatocellular carcinoma; RCC = renal cell carcinoma; ACC = adrenocortical carcinoma; GI = gastrointestinal.

REFERENCES

1. Abrams HL, Spiro R, Goldstein N. Metastases in carcinoma: analysis of 1000 autopsied cases. Cancer 1950;3:74–85.
2. Ask-Upmark E. On the location of malignant metastases, with special regard to the behavior of the primary malignant tumors of the lung. Acta Pathol Microbiol Scand 1932;9:239–48.
3. Atkinson RC. Skin metastases from bladder tumors. J Urol 1942;48:350–6.
4. Auty RM. Dermal metastases from a follicular carcinoma of the thyroid. Arch Dermatol 1977;113:675–6.
5. Batres E, Knox JM, Wolf JE Jr. Metastatic renal cell carcinoma resembling a pyogenic granuloma. Arch Dermatol 1978;114:1082–3.
6. Bennington JL, Beckwith JB. Tumors of the kidney. Atlas of Tumor Pathology, 2nd Series, Fascicle 12. Washington, DC: Armed Forces Institute of Pathology; 1975:93–199.

7. Bischoff AJ, Fishkin BG. Carcinoma of the urinary bladder with cutaneous metastasis: report of 4 cases. J Urol 1956;75:701–10.
8. Bluefarb SM, Wallk S, Gecht M. Carcinoma of the prostate with zosteriform cutaneous lesions. AMA Arch Derm 1957;76:402–7.
9. Brody HJ, Stallings WP, Fine RM, Someren A. Carcinoid in an umbilical nodule. Arch Dermatol 1978;114:570–2.
10. Brownstein MH, Helwig EB. Metastatic tumors of the skin. Cancer 1972;29:1298–307.
11. Brownstein MH, Helwig EB. Patterns of cutaneous metastasis. Arch Dermatol 1972;105:862–8.
12. Cameron J. Tumors of salivary tissue. J Clin Pathol 1961;14:232–45.
13. Camiel MR, Aron BS, Alexander LL. Metastases to palm, sole, nailbed, nose, face, and scalp from an unsuspected carcinoma of the lung. Cancer 1969;23:214–20.
14. Carabelli A. [Cutaneous metastasis of clear-cell renal carcinoma.] G Ital Dermatol Venereol 1986;121:427–9. (Italian.)
15. Chakraborty AK, Reddy AN, Grosberg JS. Pancreatic carcinoma with dissemination to umbilicus and skin. Arch Dermatol 1977;113:838–9.
16. Charache H. Bronchogenic carcinoma with subcutaneous metastases. Am J Cancer 1939;37:431–4.
17. Chatterjee SN, Bauer HM. Umbilical metastasis from carcinoma of the pancreas. Arch Dermatol 1980;116:954–5.
18. Clements AB. Metastatic carcinoma of the umbilicus. J Am Med Assoc 1952;150:556–9.
19. Cohen I, Levy E, Schreiber H. Alopecia neoplastica due to breast carcinoma. Arch Dermatol 1961;84:490–2.
20. Cohen PR. Metastatic tumors to the nail unit: subungual metastases. Dermatol Surg 2001;27:280–93.
21. Connor DH, Taylor HB, Helwig EB. Cutaneous metastases of renal cell carcinoma. Arch Pathol 1963;76:339–46.
22. Criep LH, Miller HI. Carcinoma of the stomach with metastases to the skin. J Lab Clin Med 1935;55:895–916.
23. DeYoung BR, Wick MR. Immunohistologic evaluation of metastatic carcinomas of unknown origin: an algorithmic approach. Semin Diagn Pathol 2000;17:184–93.
24. Diehl LF, Hurwitz MA, Johnson SA, Butler WM, Taylor HG. Skin metastases confined to a field of previous irradiation. Report of two cases and review of the literature. Cancer 1984;53:1864–8.
25. Edelstein JM. Pancreatic carcinoma with unusual metastasis to the skin and subcutaneous tissue simulating cellulitis. N Engl J Med 1950;242:779–81.
26. Elder DE, Murphy GF. Melanocytic tumors of the skin. Atlas of Tumor Pathology, 2nd Series Fascicle 2. Washington, DC: Armed Forces Institute of Pathology; 1991.
27. Fine G, Marshall R. Malignant mixed tumors of parotid gland. Am J Surg 1961;102:86–9.
28. Flynn VT, Spurrett BR. Sister Joseph's nodule. Med J Aust 1969;1:728–30.
29. Fox JL, Berman B, Prioleau PG. Skin metastasis from small-cell carcinoma of the lung. J Dermatol Surg Oncol 1983;9:451–4.
30. Gates O. Cutaneous metastases of malignant disease. Am J Cancer 1937;30:718–30.
31. Gerughty RM, Scofield HH, Brown FM, Hennigar GR. Malignant mixed tumors of salivary gland origin. Cancer 1969;24:471–86.
32. Giltman L. Alderete M, Minkowitz S. Malignant mixed tumor of the parotid presenting as a scalp nodule: a case report. Hum Pathol 1977;8:706–9.
33. Gottlieb J, Schermer DR. Cutaneous metastases from carcinoma of the colon. JAMA 1970;213:2083.
34. Hager CM, Cohen PR. Cutaneous lesions of metastatic visceral malignancy mimicking pyogenic granuloma. Cancer Invest 1999;17:385–90.
35. Hamer HG, Nourse MH. Cutaneous metastasis from carcinoma of bladder. J Urol 1951;65:850–2.
36. Hamilton D. Cutaneous metastases from a follicular thyroid carcinoma. J Dermatol Surg Oncol 1980;6:116–7.
37. Hazelrigg DE, Rudolph AH. Inflammatory metastatic carcinoma. Carcinoma erysipelatoides. Arch Dermatol 1977;113:69–70.
38. Head JR. Cancer of the umbilicus secondary to cancer of the cecum. Surg Gynecol Obstet 1926;42:356–8.
39. Heidenheim M, Hansen U, Andersen J. Elephantiasis-like cutaneous metastases from signet-ring cell carcinoma of the stomach. Cutis 1989;44:455–8.
40. Hickey WF, Seiler MW. Ultrastructural markers of colonic adenocarcinoma. Cancer 1981;47:140–5.
41. Hood CI, Font RL, Zimmennan LE. Metastatic mammary carcinoma in the eyelid with histiocytoid appearance. Cancer 1973;31:793–800.
42. Horiguchi Y, Takahasi C, Imamura S. Cutaneous metastases from papillary carcinoma of the thyroid gland. Report of two cases. J Am Acad Dermatol 1984;10:988–92.
43. Ingram JT. Carcinoma erysipelatoides and carcinoma telangiectaticum. Arch Dermatol 1938;77:227–31.

44. Kabawat SE, Bast RC, Welch WR, Knapp RC, Colvin RB. Immunopathologic characterization of a monoclonal antibody that recognizes common surface antigens of human ovarian tumors of serous, endometrial, and clear-cell types. Am J Clin Pathol 1983;79:98–104.
45. Kahn JA, Sinhamohapatra SB, Schneider AF. Hepatoma presenting as a skin metastasis. Arch Dermatol 1971;104:299–300.
46. Katske FA, Waisman J, Lupu AN. Cutaneous and subcutaneous metastases from carcinoma of prostate. Urology 1982;19:373–6.
47. Keane J, Fretzin DF, Jao W, Shapiro CM. Bronchial carcinoid metastatic to skin. Light and electron microscopic findings. J Cutan Pathol 1980;7:43–9.
48. Landow RK, Rhoades DW, Bauer M. Cutaneous metastases. Report of two cases of prostatic cancer. Cutis 1980;26:399–401, 409.
49. Lee BJ, Tannenbaum NE. Inflammatory carcinoma of the breast. Surg Gynecol Obstet 1924;39:580–95.
50. Leech SN, Kolar AJ, Barrett PD, Sinclair SA, Leonard N. Merkel cell carcinoma can be distinguished from metastatic small cell carcinoma using antibodies to cytokeratin 20 and thyroid transcription factor 1. J Clin Pathol 2001;54:727–9.
51. Lombardi LE, Parsons L. Carcinoma of the umbilicus metastatic from carcinoma of the stomach. Ann Intern Med 1945;65:386–8.
52. Lookingbill DP, Spangler N, Helm KF. Cutaneous metastases in patients with metastatic carcinoma: a retrospective study of 4020 patients. J Am Acad Dermatol 1993;29(Pt 1):228–36.
53. Lookingbill DP, Spangler N, Sexton FM. Skin involvement as the presenting sign of internal carcinoma. A retrospective study of 7316 cancer patients. J Am Acad Dermatol 1990;22:19–26.
54. Manteaux A, Cohen PR, Rapini RP. Zosteriform and epidermotropic metastasis. Report of two cases. J Dermatol Surg Oncol 1992;18:97–100.
55. Mazoujian G, Pinkus GS, Davis S, Haagensen DE Jr. Immunohistochemistry of a gross cystic disease fluid protein (GCDFP-15) of the breast. A marker of apocrien epithelium and breast carcinomas with apocrine features. Am J Pathol 1983:110:105–12.
56. McBurney RP, Kirklin JW, Woolner LB. Metastasizing bronchial adenomas. Surg Gynecol Obstet 1953;96:482–92.
57. Medeiros LJ, Michie SA, Johnson DE, Warnke RA, Weiss LM. An immunoperoxidase study of renal cell carcinomas: correlation with nuclear grade, cell type, and histologic pattern. Hum Pathol 1988;19:980–7.
58. Mehregan AH. Metastatic carcinoma to the skin. Dermatologica 1961;123:311–25.
59. Melicow MM. Classification of renal neoplasms: a clinical and pathological study based on 199 cases. J Urol 1944;51:331–85.
60. Norman JL, Cunningham PI, Cleveland BR. Skin and subcutaneous metastases from gastrointestinal carcinoid tumors. Arch Surg 1971;103:767–9.
61. O'Leary JL, O'Leary JA. Carcinoma of the umbilicus. Am J Obstet Gynecol 1964;89:136–7.
62. Pickard C, Callen JP, Blumenreich M. Metastatic carcinoma of the breast. An unusual presentation mimicking cutaneous vasculitis. Cancer 1987;59:1184–6.
63. Powell FC, Cooper AJ, Massa MC, Goellner JR, Su WP. Sister Mary Joseph's nodule: a clinical and histologic study. J Am Acad Dermatol 1984;10:610–5.
64. Rasch C. Carcinoma erysipelatoides. Br J Dermatol 1931;43:351–4.
65. Reingold IM, Escovitz WE. Metastastic cutaneous carcinoid. Report of a case of functioning malignant bronchial carcinoid. Arch Dermatol 1960;82:971–5.
66. Reingold IM, Smith BR. Cutaneous metastases from hepatomas. Arch Dermatol 1978;114:1045–6.
67. Reuter MJ, Nomland R. Inflammatory cutaneous metastatic carcinoma. Wis Med J 1941;41:196–201.
68. Rosen T. Cutaneous metastases. Med Clin North Am 1980;64:885–900.
69. Rosenthal AL, Lever WF. Involvement of the skin in renal carcinoma; report of two cases with review of the literature. AMA Arch Derm 1957;76:96–103.
70. Rudner EJ, Lentz C, Brown J. Bronchial carcinoid tumor with skin metastases. Arch Dermatol 1965;92:73–5.
71. Rulon DB, Helwig EB. Cutaneous sebaceous neoplasms. Cancer 1974;33:82–102.
72. Russell WG, Page DL, Hough AJ, Rogers LW. Sebaceous carcinoma of Meibomian gland origin. The diagnostic importance of pagetoid spread of neoplastic cells. Am J Clin Pathol 1980;73:504–11.
73. Samitz MH. Umbilical metastasis from carcinoma of the stomach. Sister Joseph's nodule. Arch Dermatol 1975;111:1478–9.
74. Scorer CG. Cutaneous metastases from renal neoplasms. Br J Urol 1951;23:250–9.
75. Scott LS, Head MA, Mack WS. Cutaneous metastases from tumors of the bladder, urethra, and penis. Br J Urol 1954;26:382–400.
76. Simpson SL. Primary carcinoma of the lung. Q J Med 1929;22:413–49.

77. Soyer HP, Cerroni L, Smolle J, Kerl H. ["Clown nose"—skin metastasis of breast cancer.] Z Hautkr 1990;65:929–31. (German.)
78. Stack BH. Bronchial carcinoma presenting with a solitary skin metastasis. Br J Dis Chest 1964;58:131–4.
79. Steck WD, Helwig EB. Tumors of the umbilicus. Cancer 1965;18:907–15.
80. Su WPD, Powell FC, Goellner JR. Malignant tumors metastatic to the skin. In: Wick MR, ed. Pathology of unusual malignant cutaneous tumors. New York: Marcel Dekker; 1985:357–97.
81. Swanson PE, Cherwitz DL, Neumann MP, Wick MR. Eccrine sweat gland carcinoma: an histologic and immunohistochemical study of 32 cases. J Cutan Pathol 1987;14:65–86.
82. Swanson PE, Wick MR. Immunohistochemistry of cutaneous tumors. In: Leong AS, ed. Applied immunohistochemistry for the surgical pathologist. London: Edward Arnold; 1993:269–308.
83. Tannenbaum M. Ultrastructural pathology of human renal cell tumors. Pathol Annu 1971;6:249–77.
84. Tharakaram S. Metastases to the skin. Int J Dermatol 1988;27:240–2.
85. Thomas WH, Coppola ED. Distant metastasis from mixed tumors of the salivary glands. Am J Surg 1965;109:724–30.
86. Tolia BM, Whitmore WF Jr. Solitary metastasis from renal cell carcinoma. J Urol 1975;114:836–8.
87. Tulenko JF, Conway H. An analysis of sweat gland tumors. Surg Gynecol Obstet 1965;121:343–8.
88. Uemura Y, Ohtsuki Y, Sonobe H, et al. [Perianal skin metastasis in a case of lung cancer.] Gan No Rinsho 1988;34:1054–6. (Japanese.)
89. Urbach E, Waldow I, Stamm C. Diffuse cutaneous metastatic lesions from an ovarian carcinoma. Arch Dermatol 1941;43:962–70.
90. White JW Jr. Evaluating cancer metastatic to the skin. Geriatrics 1985;40:67–73.
91. Wick MR. Immunohistochemistry in the diagnosis of solid malignant tumors. In: Jeannette JC, ed. Diagnostic immunohistology. Boca Raton, Fla: CRC Press Inc; 1988.
92. Wick MR, Goellner JR, Wolfe JT 3rd, Su WP. Adnexal carcinomas of the skin. I. Eccrine carcinomas. Cancer 1985;56:1147–62.
93. Wick MR, Goellner JR, Wolfe JT 3rd, Su WP. Adnexal carcinomas of the skin. II. Extraocular sebaceous carcinoma. Cancer 1985;56:1163–72.
94. Wick MR, Millns JL, Sibley RK, Pittelkow MR, Winkelmann RK. Secondary neuroendocrine carcinomas of the skin. An immunohistochemical comparison with primary neuroendocrine carcinoma of the skin ("Merkel cell" carcinoma). J Am Acad Dermatol 1985;13:134–42.
95. Wick MR, Ockner DM, Mills SE, Ritter JH, Swanson PE. Homologous carcinomas of the breasts, skin, and salivary glands. A histologic and immunohistochemical comparison of ductal mammary carcinoma, ductal sweat gland carcinoma, and salivary duct carcinoma. Am J Clin Pathol 1998;109:75–84.
96. Zeligman I, Schwilm A. Umbilical metastasis from carcinoma of the colon. Arch Dermatol 1974;110:911–2.

SUPPLEMENTAL REFERENCES

Alwaheeb S, Ghazarian D, Boerner SL, Asa SL. Cutaneous manifestations of thyroid cancer: a report of four cases and review of the literature. J Clin Pathol 2004;57:435–58.

Aygit AC, Top H, Cakir B, Yalcn O. Salivary duct carcinoma of the parotid gland metastasizing to the skin: a case report and review of the literature. Am J Dermatopathol 2005;27:48–50.

Barry Delongchamps N, Peyromaure M, Debre B, Zerbib M. [Renal cancer presenting as an isolated cutaneous metastasis.] Prog Urol 2004;14:538–9. (French.)

Bayer-Garner IB, Kozovska ME, Schwartz MR, Reed JA. Carcinoma with thymus-like differentiation arising in the dermis of the head and neck. J Cutan Pathol 2004;31:625–9.

Chang CH, Liao YL, Hong HS. Cutaneous metastasis from adenoid cystic carcinoma of the parotid gland. Dermatol Surg 2003;29:775–9.

Kanitakis J, Chouvet B, Claudy A, Scoazec JY. Immunoreactivity of hepatocyte paraffin 1 monoclonal antibody in cutaneous metastatic tumors. Am J Clin Pathol 2004;122:85–9.

Kazakov DV, Suster S, Leboit PE, et al. Mucinous carcinoma of the skin, primary, and secondary: a clinicopathologic study of 63 cases with emphasis on the morphologic spectrum of primary cutaneous forms: homologies with mucinous lesions in the breast. Am J Surg Pathol 2005;29:764–82.

Langner C, Ratschek M, Rehak P, Schips L, Ziguner R. CD10 is a diagnostic and prognostic marker in renal malignancies. Histopathology 2004;45:460–7.

LeSueur BW, Abraham RJ, DiCaudo DJ, O'Connor WJ. Zosteriform skin metastases. Int J Dermatol 2004;43:126–8.

Locati LD, Quattrone P, Pizzi N, Fior A, Cantu G, Licitra L. Primary high-grade mucoepidermoid carcinoma of the minor salivary glands with cutaneous metastasis at diagnosis. Oral Oncol 2002;38:401–4.

Mueller TJ, Wu H, Greenberg RE, et al. Cutaneous metastases from genitourinary malignancies. Urology 2004;63:1021–6.

Nakamura H, Shimizu T, Kodama K, Shimizu H. Metastasis of lung cancer to the finger: a report of two cases. Int J Dermatol 2005;44:47–9.

Perna AG, Smith MJ, Krishnan B, Reed JA. CD10 is expressed in cutaneous clear cell lesions of different histogenesis. J Cutan Pathol 2005;32:348–51.

Pomara G, Pastina I, Simone M, Casale P, Marchetti G, Francesca F. Penile metastasis from primary transitional cell carcinoma of the renal pelvis: first manifestation of systemic spread. BMC Cancer 2004;4:90.

Prabhudesai SG, Pramesh CS, Jambhekar NA, Pathak KA, Sanghvi VD. Epidermotropic cutaneous metastases from hypopharyngeal carcinoma. J Otolaryngol 2004;33;198–200.

Preetha R, Kavishwar VS, Butle P. Cutaneous metastasis from silent renal cell carcinoma. J Postgrad Med 2004;50:287–8.

Saeed S, Keehn CA, Morgan MB. Cutaneous metastasis: a clinical, pathological, and immunohistochemical appraisal. J Cutan Pathol 2004;31:419–30.

Volmar KE, Cummings TJ, Wang WH, Creager AJ, Tyler DS, Xie HB. Clear cell hidradenoma: a mimic of metastatic clear cell tumors. Arch Pathol Lab Med 2005;129:e113–6.

Zuetenhorst JM, Taal BG. Metastatic carcinoid tumors: a clinical review. Oncologist 2005;10:123–31.

6 FIBROUS TISSUE TUMORS

A wide variety of tumors have been traditionally classified as fibrohistiocytic in origin. As knowledge of cellular biology has increased, it has become apparent that this is a heterogeneous group of disorders that includes tumors comprised of various types of fibroblasts and myofibroblasts, including dermal dendrocytes and hemopoietic progenitor cells. The diagnostic features of these disparate lesions are considered in this chapter. The pathologic features of cutaneous fibrous tissue tumors overlap with those of soft tissue tumors. While some duplication with other works in this series of Fascicles is unavoidable, we attempt to emphasize those aspects of fibrohistiocytic tumors that are of particular importance to dermatopathology.

BENIGN FIBROUS TISSUE TUMORS

Fibroepithelial Polyps

Clinical Features. *Fibroepithelial polyps* (also called *acrochordons*, *skin tags*, or, in the case of larger, more fleshy lesions, *soft fibromas*) are sessile to pedunculated outgrowths of skin that may be present almost anywhere on the cutaneous surface. They are particularly concentrated around the eyelids or in flexural areas such as the neck, axillae, and groin. They may be flesh colored or hyperpigmented, smooth or verrucous. When a lesion becomes twisted about its pedicle, inflammation, tenderness, or necrosis may ensue. An increase in the number of lesions often accompanies weight gain.

An association between cutaneous fibroepithelial polyps and colonic polyps was proposed in earlier studies (112). The preponderance of evidence seems to indicate that these cutaneous lesions are not markers or risk factors for colorectal polyps (23,41,66,125,159,165). Cutaneous fibroepithelial polyps have also been regarded as components of the dominantly inherited Birt-Hogg-Dube syndrome, along with trichodiscomas, fibrofolliculomas, colonic polyps, and renal cell carcinoma. A recent study has suggested, however, that the "acrochordon-like" lesions in this syndrome are actually polypoid variants of trichodiscomas and fibrofolliculomas and not simple fibroepithelial polyps (43).

The need for submitting fibroepithelial polyps for histologic examination has been questioned in clinical dermatology. This remains a reasonable subject for debate, but one study indicates a very low prevalence of malignancy in lesions clinically diagnosed as fibroepithelial polyps, and zero prevalence among lesions clinically diagnosed by dermatologists.

Pathologic Findings. The fibroepithelial polyp consists of an epidermal lining about a connective tissue stalk (fig. 6-1). More sessile variants also occur. The epidermis may be thinned, particularly when associated with larger soft fibromas, but varying degrees of acanthosis and papillomatosis also occur, which may be verrucous or seborrheic keratosis-like. Collagen is loosely organized, and dilated capillaries may be present. Nevus cells are sometimes encountered. Soft fibromas may have fat in the central portion of the lesion, in

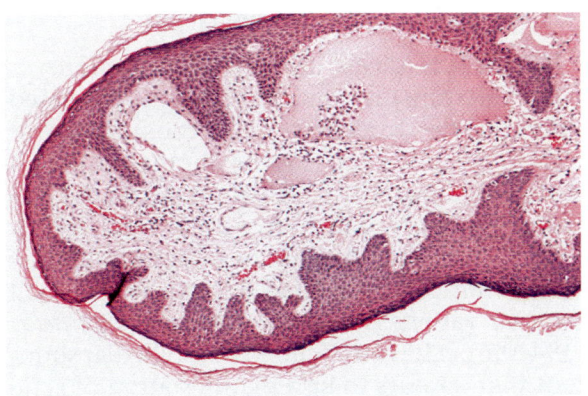

Figure 6-1

FIBROEPITHELIAL POLYP

This lesion shows a smooth-surfaced epidermal lining about a connective tissue stalk. Vasodilatation is present.

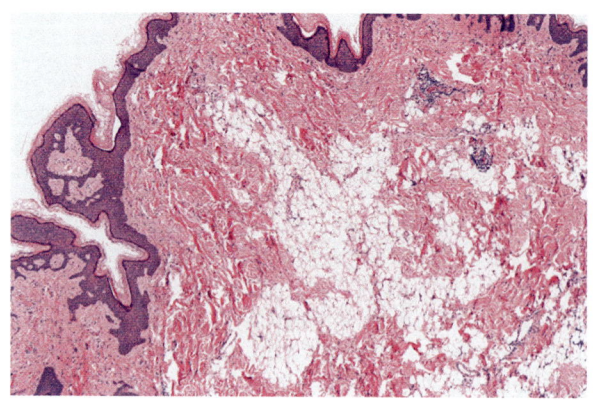

Figure 6-2

SOFT FIBROMA

There are aggregates of lipocytes in the superficial portion of the lesion.

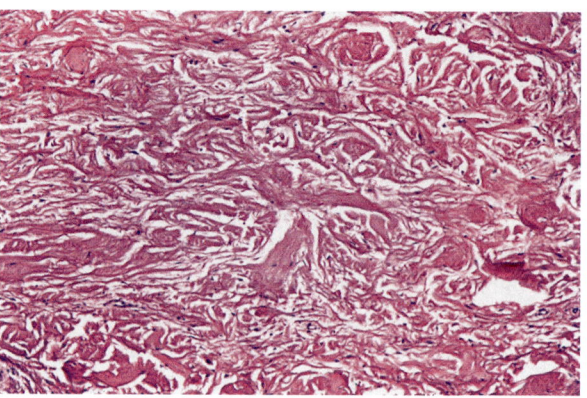

Figure 6-3

CONNECTIVE TISSUE NEVUS

The dermis is composed of thickened, interwoven collagen bundles.

amounts similar to those of nevus lipomatosus (fig. 6-2). Elastic fibers are normal both in quantity and morphology (3). Irritated, traumatized, or twisted lesions show varying degrees of inflammation, vascular engorgement, connective tissue degeneration, and necrosis.

Findings rarely reported in lesions with clinical features of fibroepithelial polyps include basal cell carcinoma (80) or pleomorphic spindled or stellate cells constituting the cutaneous pseudosarcomatous polyp (231). Findings such as these, although uncommon, support the argument that fibroepithelial polyps should be submitted for microscopic study; certainly this is true for clinically atypical lesions.

Connective Tissue Nevus

Clinical Features. The *connective tissue nevus* is a hamartoma in which collagen is increased in amount or thickness, while the quantity of elastic tissue fibers may be increased (*nevus elasticus*), apparently normal, or decreased (*nevus anelasticus*). Clinically, these nevi are elevated, indurated papules or nodules that may be disseminated or organized in plaques. A small papular variety is termed *papular elastorrhexis* (194,196). It has an acquired perifollicular simulant that appears to be a manifestation of acne scarring (232). Usually connective tissue nevi are unassociated with epithelial abnormalities, but the coexistence of these lesions with epidermal nevus or Becker's nevus has been reported (50,81). Connective tissue nevi can occur in sporadic fashion, without involvement of other organ systems, but they can also be inherited as an autosomal dominant trait (216). A variant of connective tissue nevus occurs in association with osteopoikilosis (sclerotic foci and stippled densities in long, round, and flat bones) and is termed the *Buschke-Ollendorff syndrome*. Despite some dispute in the literature, we believe that the shagreen patch of tuberous sclerosis should also be considered a variant of connective tissue nevus.

Pathologic Findings. There are usually increased numbers of thickened collagen bundles, either in a compact configuration, resembling morphea, or in a more complex interwoven pattern (fig. 6-3). With special staining, elastic fibers can be demonstrated to be increased in number and density, normal in appearance, or decreased, fragmented, or virtually absent (fig. 6-4). In papular elastorrhexis and papular acne scars, collagen appears normal or attenuated, while elastic fibers are decreased in number, fragmented, or both (194,232). Elastic fibers are also usually decreased in the shagreen patches of tuberous sclerosis (104).

Differential Diagnosis. The major challenge of these lesions is to recognize that *any* abnormality is present, since in many cases the findings on hematoxylin and eosin (H&E)-stained sections are subtle. It is well known that the appearance of dermal connective tissue can be significantly influenced by both the tissue handling and the quality of staining, while at the

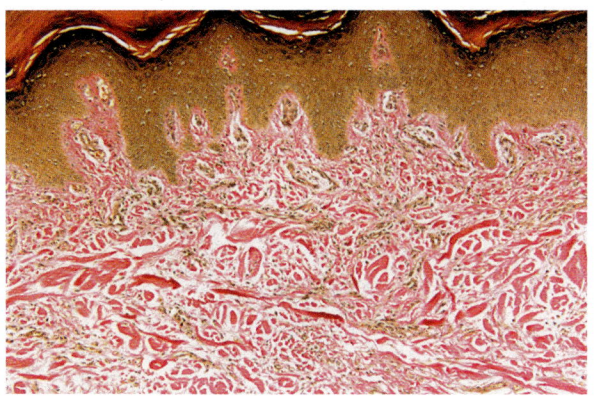

Figure 6-4

CONNECTIVE TISSUE NEVUS

The Verhoeff-van Gieson stain shows an absence of elastic fibers.

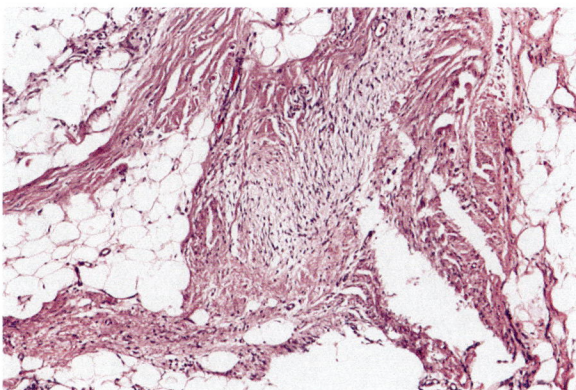

Figure 6-5

FIBROUS HAMARTOMA OF INFANCY

The three elements that comprise this lesion can be observed: fibrous trabeculae, mature adipose tissue, and (in the central portion of the figure) immature, rounded to spindled cells within a mucinous matrix.

same time, comparative thickening of dermal collagen can normally be expected in truncal skin or overlying large joints. For these reasons, clinical correlation is essential for accurate diagnosis. Elastic tissue stains can be helpful for those cases in which elastic fibers are either quantitatively or qualitatively altered.

Fibrous Hamartoma of Infancy

Clinical Features. *Fibrous hamartoma of infancy* was first reported by Reye in 1956, under the term "subdermal fibromatous tumors in infancy," although previous examples may have been described by Stout and Allen (162). Enzinger (47) gave the lesion its present name in 1965. These tumors typically are present at birth or arise during the first 12 months of life. They are most common in boys. Fibrous hamartomas are almost always solitary subcutaneous nodules, ranging from 2.5 to 15.0 cm in greatest diameter. Their location is usually truncal, with the highest percentage arising in the axillary region. Occurrence in the arm or wrist is common. Other reported locations include the face or scalp, foot, and pharynx (162). Fibrous hamartoma of infancy appears to remain stable after a period of initial growth, and excision is typically curative.

Pathologic Findings. These lesions have three main components: fibrous trabeculae that are composed of thick collagen bundles with bland-appearing spindled cells; mature adipose tissue; and aggregates of small rounded to spindled cells of immature appearance within mucinous (hyaluronic acid) matrices (fig. 6-5). The latter are often termed primitive mesenchymal cells (47,162,208). The mesenchymal cells are often present at the borders of fibrous trabeculae or around vessels (1). These three elements form a characteristic organoid arrangement and are regularly present, although one or two of the features may predominate. The changes are sufficiently characteristic that even diagnosis by fine-needle aspiration is possible (92). Both the small mesenchymal cells and the cells in trabeculae are vimentin positive; cells within trabeculae only may be actin and desmin positive (55,69). Electron microscopy confirms that constituent cells have the morphologic characteristics of fibroblasts and myofibroblasts (68,147).

Differential Diagnosis. The unique combination of the above three microscopic features makes this entity among the most readily diagnosable of the fibrous tissue tumors, but shallow biopsies, or lesions that have one predominating feature, may create diagnostic confusion. Entities that can occasionally be confused with fibrous hamartoma of infancy include forms of fibromatosis, particularly infantile fibromatosis, deep fibrous histiocytoma, infantile fibrosarcoma, embryonal rhabdomyosarcoma, calcifying aponeurotic fibroma, and fibrolipoma. Keys to the correct diagnosis include the subcutaneous location of the tumor, the organoid

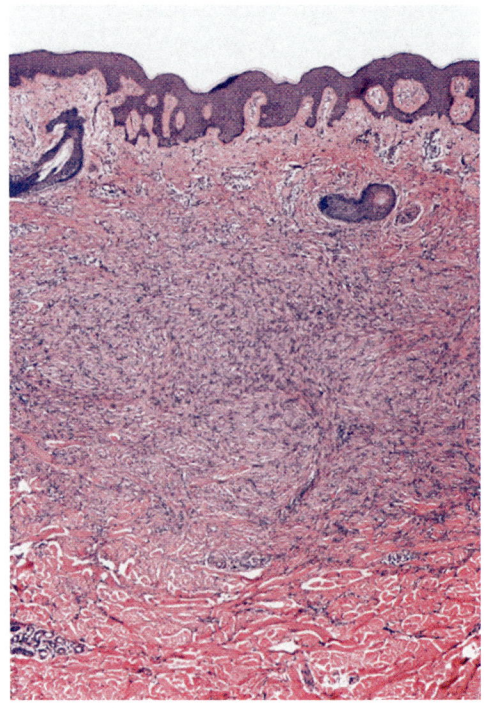
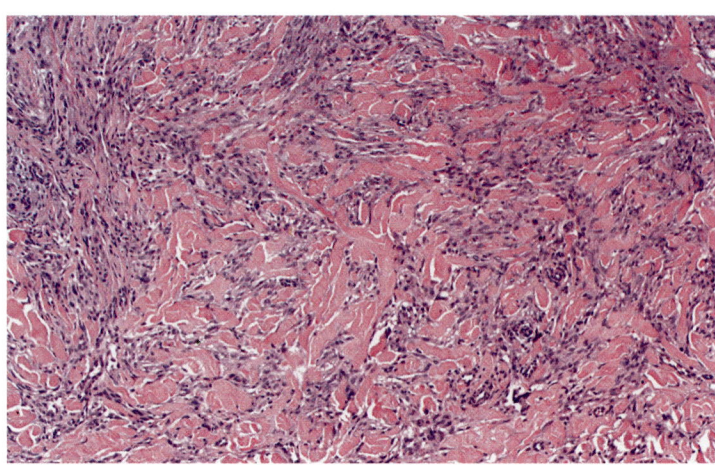

Figure 6-6

DERMATOFIBROMA

Left: Mid-dermal proliferation of spindled cells with overlying acanthosis.

Above: High-power view shows fibroblasts forming "curlicue" arrangements. In this example, collagen bundles are thickened and eosinophilic.

arrangement of its key elements, and the lack of cytologic atypia.

Dermatofibroma

Clinical Features. *Dermatofibroma* (also termed *cutaneous fibrous histiocytoma*) is among the most common cutaneous tumors and is generally among the most clinically recognizable. The microscopic features are usually also typical, but there are numerous histopathologic variations that at times can create substantial diagnostic difficulty.

Dermatofibromas are firm, round to oval papules or small nodules that are usually elevated but may be slightly depressed. Colors range from tan to yellow to reddish brown. These firm lesions show the Fitzpatrick sign: grasping a lesion between the thumb and forefinger results in depression of the lesion, with puckering of the normal skin around it. Lesions are often present on the lower legs, and are also commonly encountered on the upper arms and sides of the trunk, although other locations have been reported. They can be solitary or multiple. Multiple lesions have been reported in patients with lupus erythematosus, human immunodeficiency virus (HIV) infection (118,123,150,201), and myasthenia gravis (9), although some of these patients were also receiving corticosteroids or other immunosuppressive therapies at the time of presentation (9,118). Lesions improve or virtually disappear after cryotherapy or incisional surgery, and recurrences are uncommon.

There is continuing debate about the neoplastic versus reactive nature of these lesions (25). The frequent history of onset following trauma, such as after an arthropod bite, as well as the microscopic changes, suggest a reparative process. On the other hand, recent genetic and cytogenetic studies provide evidence that dermatofibroma may be a clonal disease and therefore represents a neoplastic condition (31,218).

Pathologic Findings. Dermatofibromas feature varying combinations of fibroblasts and histiocytes (macrophages), small vessels, and collagen, usually centered in the dermis. Typically on low-power microscopic examination, there is a lens-shaped zone of intradermal involvement, the long axis of which parallels the surface epidermis (fig. 6-6, left). This zone often has a faintly bluish cast in H&E-stained sections. There are proliferations of fibroblasts and macrophages in varying proportions, with small groups of fibroblasts in a matted, storiform, or "curlicue" arrangement (fig. 6-6, above). In some lesions, newly formed, slightly bluish-staining

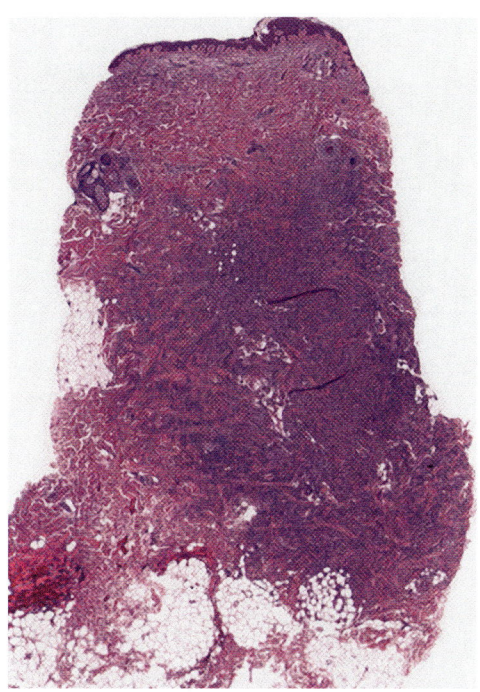
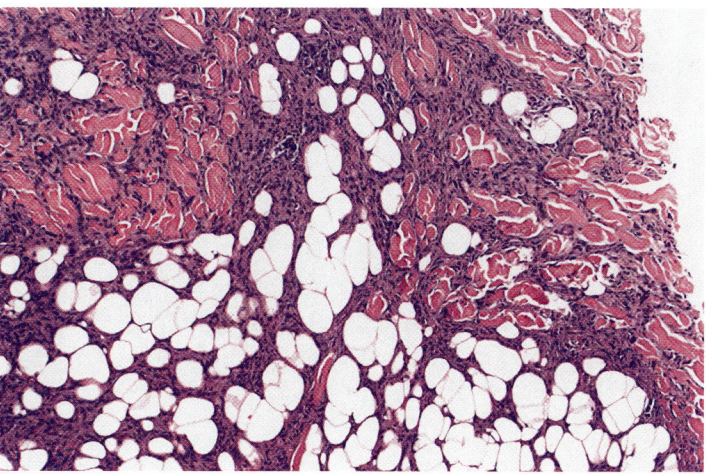

Figure 6-7

DEEP PENETRATING DERMATOFIBROMA

There is predominant involvement of the deep dermis and subcutis.
Left: Low-power view.
Above: High-power view showing "vertical" infiltration of the subcutis.

collagen forms the scaffold for the cellular component, while in others the collagen bundles are thickened and intensely eosinophilic (fig. 6-6, above). At the periphery of the lesion, spindled cells tend to surround cross-sectional profiles of mature collagen, a phenomenon sometimes termed collagen entrapment. Scattered small vessels are also present. These spindle cell aggregates are often separated from the overlying epidermis by a zone of uninvolved connective tissue. Lesions may also be relatively well demarcated at the base, although extension along the subcutaneous septa also occurs. Lesions with deep subcutaneous permeation have been termed *deep penetrating dermatofibromas* (fig. 6-7) (111, 228). There is often an associated inflammatory infiltrate at the base of the lesion.

The overlying epidermis is typically acanthotic, with exaggerated, somewhat lentiginous budding, but often with flattening of the rete ridges, a feature that can be diagnostically useful, especially when superficially shaved biopsies are submitted for evaluation (fig. 6-6, left). These changes may be accompanied by basilar hypermelanosis. Epidermal changes may be minimal or absent in deeper variants of dermatofibroma. On the other hand, the cellular and connective tissue changes may encroach upon the epidermis, with resultant effacement of the rete ridge pattern and apparent thinning of the epidermis. Nevertheless, adequately sampled specimens often show that the flattened overlying or immediately adjacent epidermis is of greater thickness than the normal epidermis at the periphery of the lesion. The epidermal changes have been linked to stromal induction, a process whereby altered connective tissue induces epidermis to proliferate, much in the way the dermal hair papilla induces normal follicular development. Occasionally, this induction process may be associated with the formation of mature hair follicles or sebaceous glands, or there may be basal cell hyperplasia that closely resembles basal cell carcinoma (fig. 6-8, right). Erosion, ulceration, or scale crusting may be observed, often secondary to lesional trauma.

Several microscopic variations of dermatofibroma are encountered. Some lesions can be lipidized *(lipidized dermatofibromas)*, with a prominent component of foamy macrophages, often associated with extravasated erythrocytes and hemosiderin deposition (fig. 6-9, left). In these lesions, characteristic Touton-like giant cells are often present and can be useful diagnostic clues. Like the classic Touton giant cell, these cells possess a central core of eosinophilic cytoplasm, multiple nuclei arrayed at the periphery, and a surrounding layer of lipid. They

Nonmelanocytic Tumors of the Skin

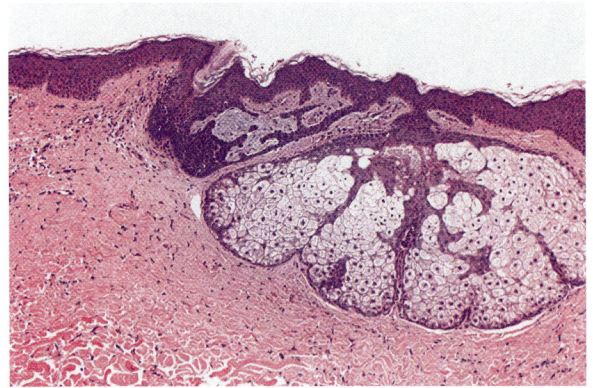 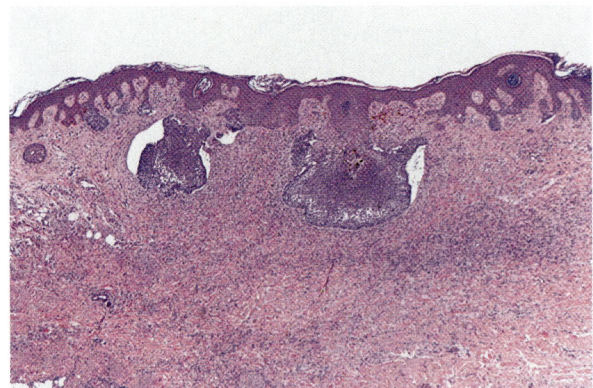

Figure 6-8

DERMATOFIBROMA

Stromal induction can result in the formation of sebaceous lobules (left) or foci of basal cell hyperplasia resembling basal cell carcinoma (right).

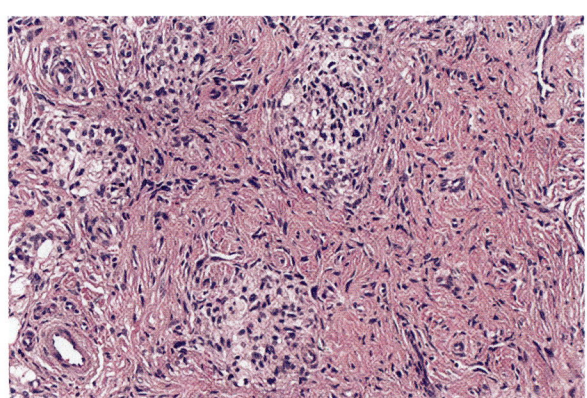 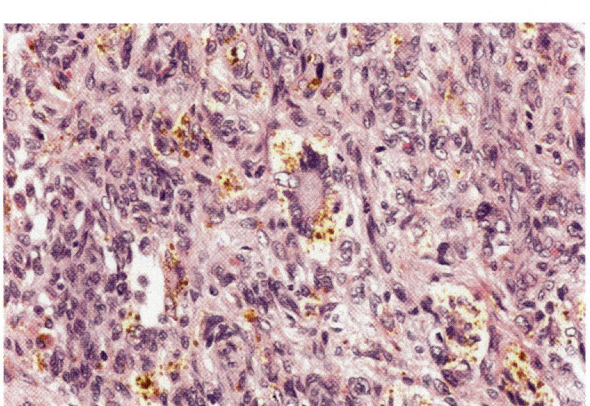

Figure 6-9

LIPIDIZED DERMATOFIBROMA

Left: Aggregates of pale-staining foamy macrophages can be identified.
Right: A Touton-like giant cell is seen. Hemosiderin pigment is seen within the outer lipid layer.

also exhibit angulated profiles, nuclear clumping, and granules of hemosiderin within the lipid layer (fig. 6-9, right).

The degree of cellularity can vary widely. Highly cellular lesions, appropriately termed *cellular dermatofibromas,* feature numerous rounded to fusiform cells with little intervening collagen (fig. 6-10). A variant composed of sharply circumscribed aggregates of larger, epithelioid cells has been termed *epithelioid cell histiocytoma* (fig. 6-11) (64,95,141). More fibrotic variants show relatively sparse cellularity, closely resembling the *sclerotic fibroma* described by Rapini and Golitz (172) and others (see below) or show *keloid-like changes* (105). The cutaneous *aneurysmal fibrous histiocytoma* combines features of lipidized, hemosiderin-containing dermatofibromas with large, blood-filled spaces that are not lined by endothelium (fig. 6-12) (188). These large blood-filled spaces explain the clinical findings of rapid growth, pain, and blue-black appearance.

Lymphocytes occasionally permeate the tumor, producing an appearance analogous to halo nevus. Clinical halos can form around either traditional dermatofibromas (15) or those with eczematous qualities (the so-called Meyerson phenomenon) (58). Dermatofibromas can have an atrophic appearance (179), which may

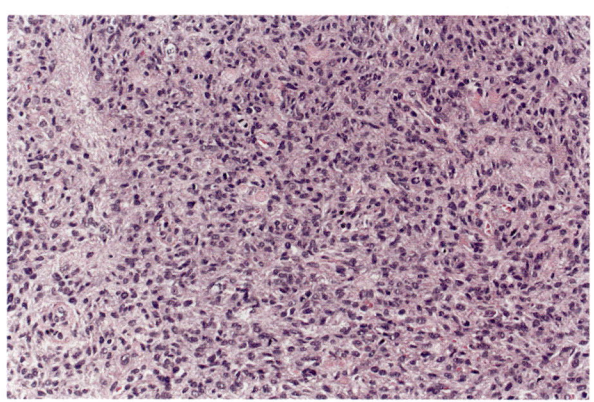
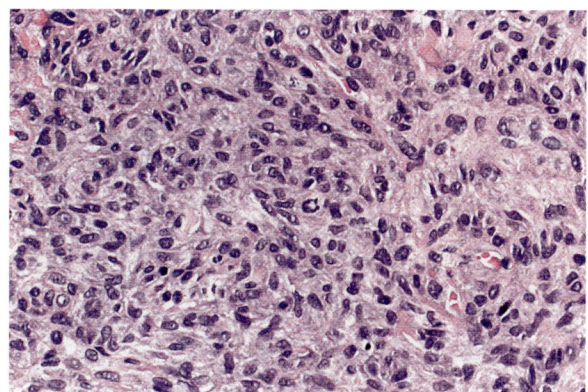

Figure 6-10

CELLULAR DERMATOFIBROMA

Left: There are numerous rounded to spindled cells, with little intervening collagen.
Right: A mitotic figure is present in the central portion of the field.

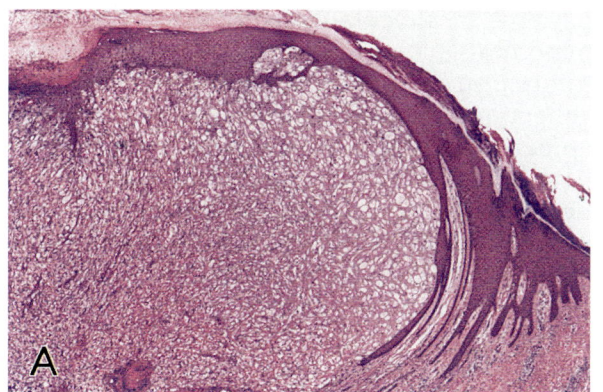
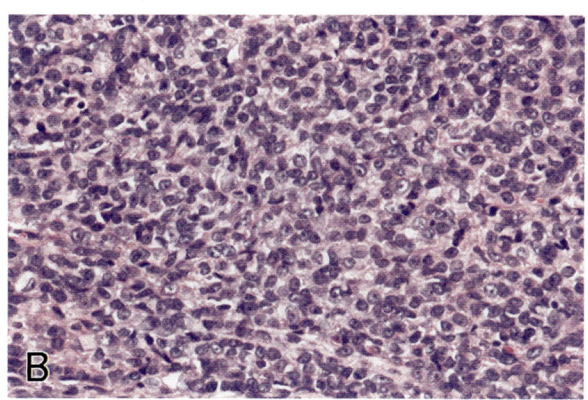
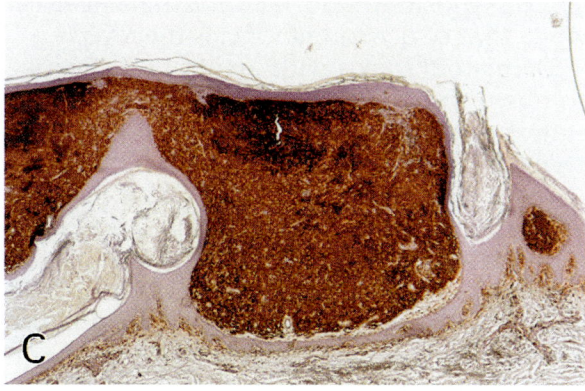

Figure 6-11

EPITHELIOID CELL HISTIOCYTOMA

A: A sharply circumscribed aggregate of tumor cells is surrounded by adjacent epidermis in a "ball in claw" manner.
B: The epithelioid appearance of constituent cells is seen.
C: These cells are strongly factor XIIIa positive, a feature of most other forms of dermatofibroma.

in part be due to elastophagocytosis by proliferating cells (103). A rare *granular cell* variant of dermatofibroma also occurs (210). Unlike conventional granular cell tumor (granular cell schwannoma), cells are S-100 protein negative and variably factor XIIIa positive (239).

Cytologic atypia can occur in dermatofibromas and create considerable diagnostic confusion. The atypia may present in the form of mononucleated or multinucleated, sometimes xanthomatized, cells with large, bizarre, and/or hyperchromatic nuclei (fig. 6-13) (116,215).

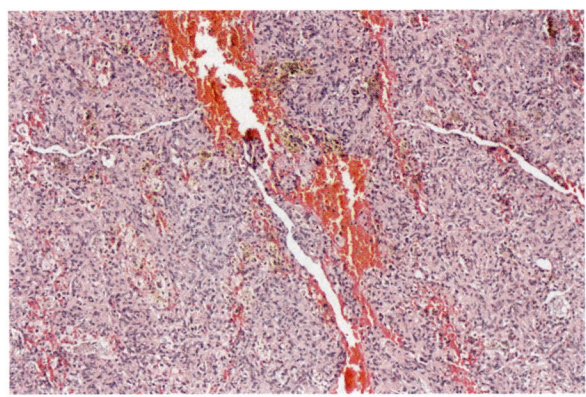

Figure 6-12

ANEURYSMAL FIBROUS HISTIOCYTOMA

There is a blood-filled space and hemosiderin deposition.

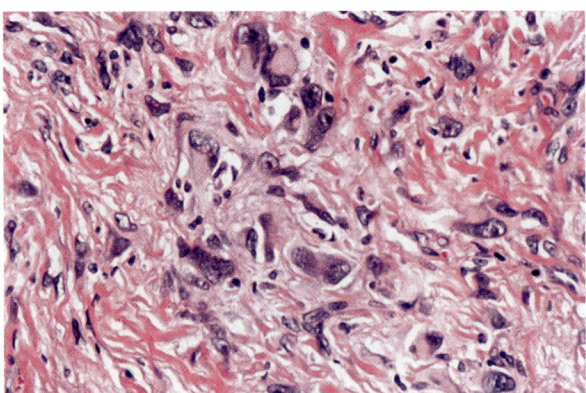

Figure 6-13

DERMATOFIBROMA WITH ATYPIA

There are scattered, large cells with coarse chromatin and prominent nucleoli.

Mitotic figures may also be identified. The overall configuration is that of a dermatofibroma, however, and experience indicates an absence of biologically aggressive behavior among such lesions. Mitotic figures can be present in dermatofibromas with or without other evidence of cytologic atypia; they are particularly likely to be encountered in cellular, lipidized, and traditional dermatofibromas (fig. 6-10, right). In our experience, up to 3 mitoses per 10 high-power fields seems to be within the acceptable range for dermatofibromas, but we have seen several cellular dermatofibromas that possess up to 12 mitoses per 10 high-power fields.

Immunohistochemically, positivity for factor XIIIa antigen is a characteristic, although not pathognomonic, feature of most dermatofibromas. The aneurysmal variant may not express this antigen (26). Staining for macrophage markers, such as CD68, may also occur. Myofibroblastic differentiation is demonstrated by the presence of elongated spindle cells that stain for smooth muscle actin (242), a feature that may create confusion with leiomyoma.

Differential Diagnosis. The resemblance of dermatofibroma to dermatofibrosarcoma protuberans (see below) can be striking, particularly in cellular or deep penetrating variants or where "cartwheel" arrangements of nuclei are observed. In contrast to dermatofibroma, dermatofibrosarcoma protuberans tends to be larger or multinodular, and typically lacks overlying epidermal hyperplasia. The patterns of subcutaneous infiltration of dermatofibrosarcoma protuberans include lace-like infiltration of fat lobules or horizontally arrayed collections of spindled cells that parallel the epidermal surface. Dermatofibromas tend to have either bulbous, "pushing" margins or "vertical" subcutaneous infiltration along the septa (96). Polarizable collagen can usually be demonstrated within the substance of the tumor in dermatofibroma but is absent in dermatofibrosarcoma protuberans (10). Immunohistochemistry is also helpful, as the characteristic profile of dermatofibrosarcoma protuberans is CD34 positive and factor XIIIa negative, while that of dermatofibroma is the reverse.

Dermatofibromas with atypical cells can be confused with atypical fibroxanthoma, and it is almost certain that some of the past reports of atypical fibroxanthoma on the extremities of younger persons are actually examples of lipidized dermatofibromas with atypia. Small size, presence of typical overlying epidermal changes, cell arrangements consistent with dermatofibroma, and absence of atypical mitoses all favor dermatofibroma (116). Immunohistochemistry is of limited value in differentiation: significant percentages of both tumors are factor XIIIa positive.

Dermatofibromas with myofibroblastic differentiation may be confused with cutaneous leiomyoma, particularly piloleiomyoma. In addition to architectural features (see Dermatomyofibroma, below), dermatofibromas (unlike most leiomyomas) are typically desmin negative.

Dermatofibromas can resemble melanocytic tumors. Sparsely or nonpigmented blue nevi (19) and desmoplastic (sclerotic) nevi (73) can closely mimic dermatofibroma, and can even feature overlying epidermal hyperplasia. They differ by showing occasional sparse melanin pigmentation, identifiable with the Fontana stain, and positive immunohistochemical staining for S-100 protein and (variably) for Melan-A or HMB45 (19,73). Epithelioid cell histiocytoma closely resembles the intradermal variant of Spitz's nevus. Careful evaluation of multiple sections for junctional involvement can help to exclude a subtle compound Spitz's nevus. As a further argument against a melanocytic tumor, the cells of epithelioid cell histiocytoma are S-100 protein and HMB45 negative and are often factor XIIIa positive (fig. 6-11C) (64,141).

Sclerotic fibroma (see below) is regarded by many as a unique entity, but there is an opinion that at least some of these lesions may represent sclerotic variants of dermatofibroma (30, 167). Since dermatofibroma can resemble basal cell carcinoma clinically, a superficial shave biopsy of a lesion showing basal cell hyperplasia could easily be interpreted as a superficial basal cell carcinoma. Knowledge that the basal cell changes are associated with a dermatofibroma is useful, since such lesions are likely to have a limited potential for biologic aggressiveness.

Dermatomyofibroma

Clinical Features. This entity was first reported by Kamino et al. in 1992 (98), accompanied by an editorial by Cooper that reported an additional case (36). Since then, a number of other reports have appeared in the literature. The lesion presents as a plaque, measuring 1 to 2 cm in diameter, most commonly located on the neck, shoulder, and upper trunk. Young adults and children are most often affected.

Pathologic Findings. The lesion consists of interlacing fascicles of spindled cells that generally parallel the slightly hyperplastic surface epidermis. The spindled cells are concentrated in the reticular dermis and extend into the superficial subcutis (fig. 6-14). The cells are separated by thin collagen bundles, and are surrounded by a reticulin meshwork; elastic fibers are preserved (35, 98). Cytologic atypia is not a feature, and mitoses are absent or rare (36,98). The cells of dermato-

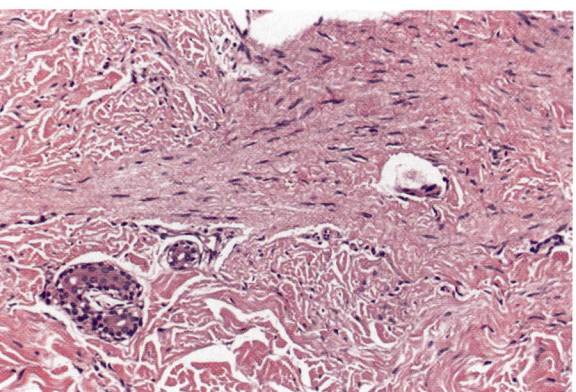

Figure 6-14

DERMATOMYOFIBROMA

Horizontally aligned fascicles of spindled cells are in the reticular dermis. These cells have the characteristics of myofibroblasts.

myofibroma are smooth muscle actin positive but muscle-specific actin and desmin negative; factor XIIIa-positive cells are also present.

Differential Diagnosis. These lesions have a distinctive microscopic appearance that is not typical for dermatofibroma, although the differential diagnosis may include that lesion as well as localized fibromatosis, other myofibroblastic tumors, plaque-type dermatofibrosarcoma protuberans (142), leiomyoma, or hypertrophic scar (35).

Angiofibroma and Related Lesions

Angiofibroma is widely considered to represent a family of acral lesions, each of which is characterized by dermal fibrosis and varying degrees of vasodilatation and/or vascular proliferation. The entities that comprise this family include *fibrous papule of the face, pearly penile papule, digital fibrokeratoma, angiofibroma of tuberous sclerosis* (historically but erroneously termed *adenoma sebaceum*), and *familial myxovascular fibroma*. Occasionally, sporadic lesions with microscopic features of angiofibroma do not clearly fit into one of these categories.

Clinical Features. Fibrous papule of the face was first delineated by Graham et al. in 1965 (67). It is typically a solitary, firm, dome-shaped lesion on the nose or adjacent portions of the face. It is often flesh colored, but may be red or focally pigmented. Pearly penile papules are tiny (1 to 3 mm in diameter) white lesions that tend to be

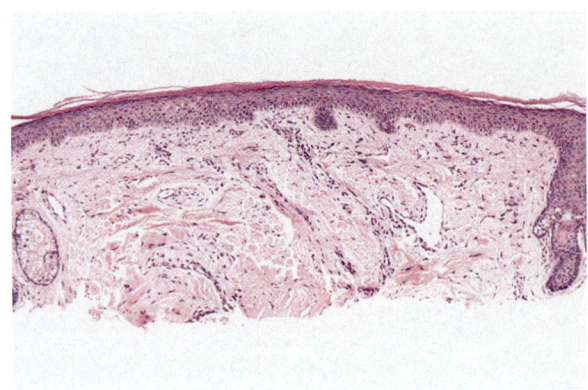 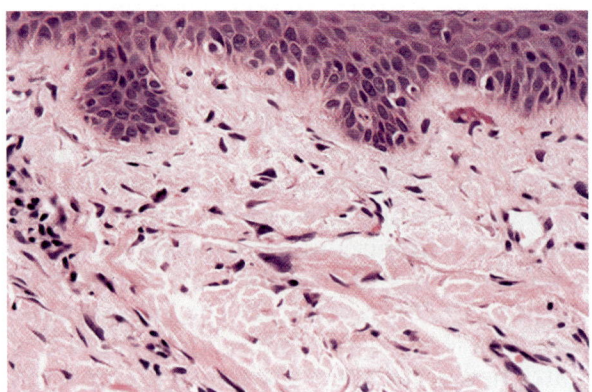

Figure 6-15
FIBROUS PAPULE OF THE FACE
Left: Low-power view shows a gently dome-shaped papule with vasodilatation, fibrosis, and scattered spindled cells.
Right: High-power view shows scattered stellate cells in the superficial dermis. There is a slight degree of junctional melanocytic hyperplasia.

arranged in a linear fashion around the coronal margin. They are fairly common among young adult males, more so among the uncircumcised (175,206), and are often confused with warts. The digital fibrokeratoma is a dome-shaped to pedunculated nodule that occurs most commonly on the hands and fingers, feet and toes of adults (11). It is generally believed that the periungual and subungual tumors once described as garlic clove fibromas, seen in both patients with tuberous sclerosis and in otherwise normal individuals, are actually examples of digital fibrokeratoma (102,121). The lesions are firm and variably hyperkeratotic, and often feature collarettes of scale at their bases. They respond to simple excision. The angiofibromas associated with tuberous sclerosis are typically reddish brown papules that are distributed symmetrically over the nasolabial folds, cheeks, and chin. Larger lesions may be asymmetrically distributed over the face and scalp. Familial myxovascular fibroma is a rare, heritable disorder in which multiple wart-like lesions develop over the fingers and hands.

Pathologic Findings. Fibrous papule of the face often has a gently dome-shaped low-power profile (fig. 6-15, left). Dermal fibrosis is associated with vasodilatation. There is a scattering of variably enlarged, angulated or stellate cells in the superficial dermis. There may also be a degree of overlying junctional melanocytic hyperplasia (fig. 6-15, right). The latter two findings, plus the occasional presence of unequivocal nevus cells, have led some authors to suspect that fibrous papules are effete melanocytic nevi (137). This has generally not been borne out by ultrastructural (170,189) or immunohistochemical (153) studies, which indicate a predominance of factor XIIIa-positive fibroblasts. Cerio et al. (29) found S-100 protein positivity among the cells in a few of their cases, suggesting that a minority of lesions could be involuted nevi (29). One reported case showed CD34 positivity among deep dermal, spindle-shaped cells (202).

Pearly penile papules also display dense connective tissue, dilated vessels, and plump fibroblasts (fig. 6-16) (2,94). Polymerase chain reaction (PCR) studies have failed to demonstrate human papillomavirus DNA in these lesions (51).

Digital fibrokeratomas show hyperkeratosis and acanthosis (fig. 6-17, left). The dermis is composed of thick intermingled collagen bundles that tend to be oriented perpendicularly to the overlying epidermis, and small blood vessels are prominent. These changes place this lesion within the broad family of angiofibromas (fig. 6-17, right).

Microscopically, the angiofibromas that occur in tuberous sclerosis, and those that are not otherwise classifiable, show three major changes: sclerosis of dermal connective tissue; small vessel dilatation, proliferation, or both; and scattered large, stellate fibroblasts or multinucleated cells. In older lesions or in large angiofibromas, concentric perifollicular fibrosis results in compressed, atrophic follicular units (fig. 6-18). Vasodilatation may be inconspicuous, particularly in larger lesions. The fibroblasts have a glial appearance; although they clearly express the fibroblast marker, factor XIIIa (153), in one study, cultured stromal cells from angiofibroma expressed glial fibrillary acidic protein (100). Elastic tissue is reported to be absent in angiofibromas.

Only a few cases of the rare familial myxovascular fibroma have been reported. These lesions feature hyperkeratosis, acanthosis, fibrosis, and vascular proliferation, changes also seen in digital fibrokeratoma, but in addition, mucin deposition is prominent (38,164).

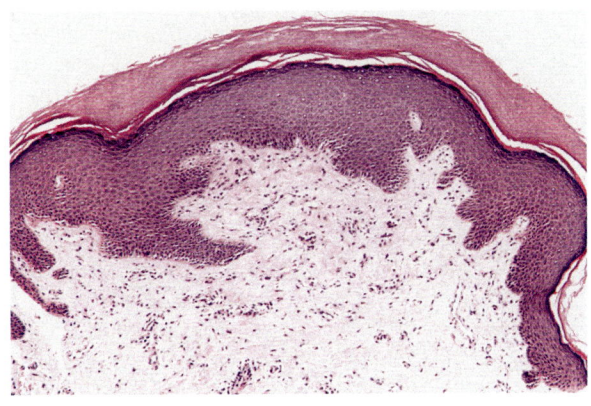

Figure 6-16
PEARLY PENILE PAPULE
Dense connective tissue, scattered fibroblasts, and slightly dilated blood vessels are observed.

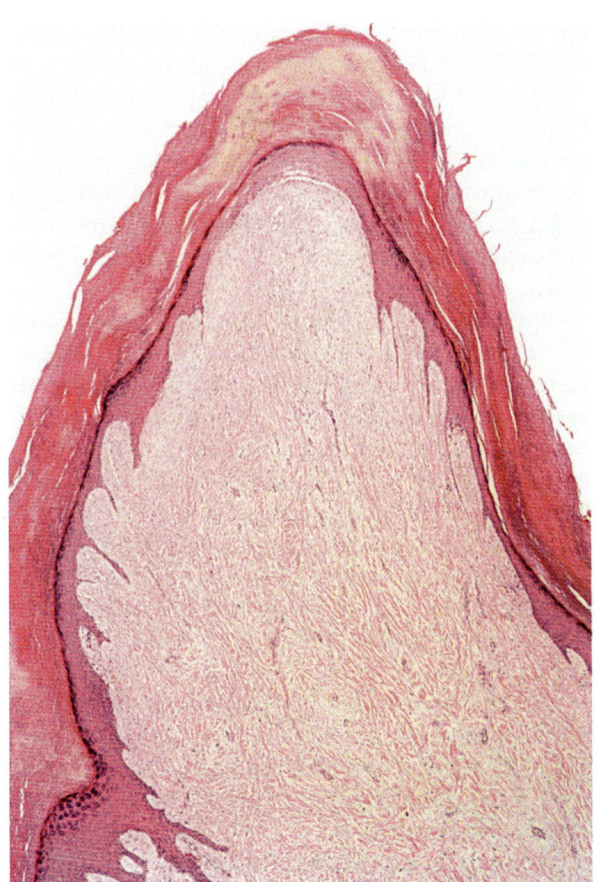
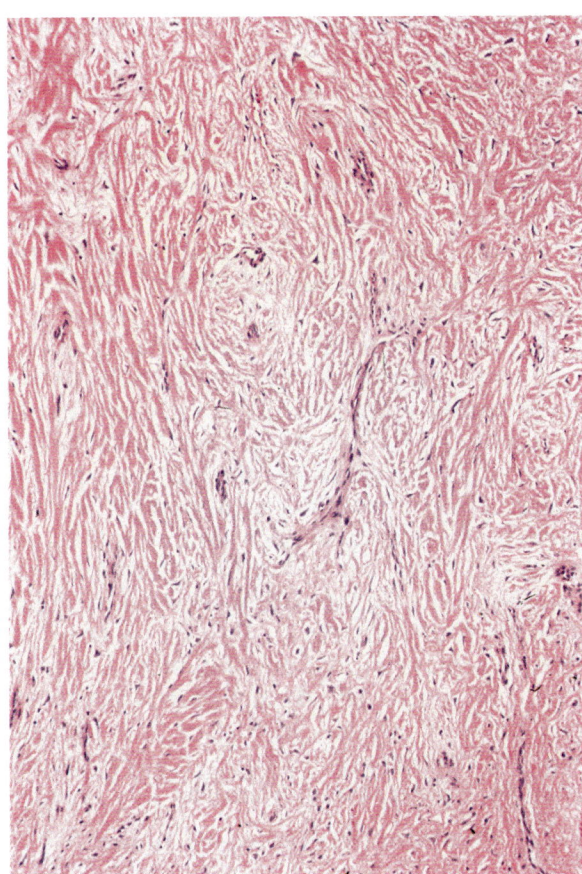

Figure 6-17
DIGITAL FIBROKERATOMA
Left: This elongated papule shows hyperkeratosis and acanthosis.
Right: Within the dermis, collagen bundles are oriented perpendicularly to the surface epidermis. Scattered small blood vessels are seen.

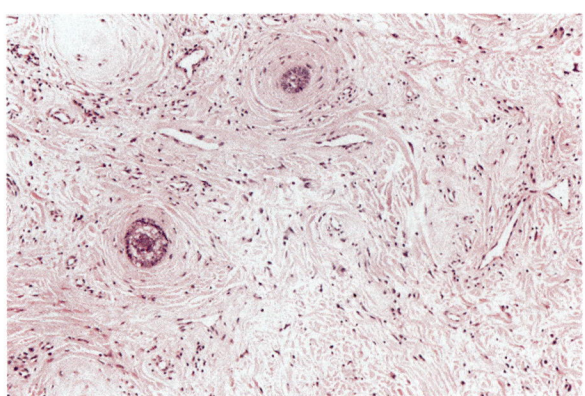

Figure 6-18

ANGIOFIBROMA

This older lesion shows concentric perifollicular fibrosis with atrophic-appearing follicular units.

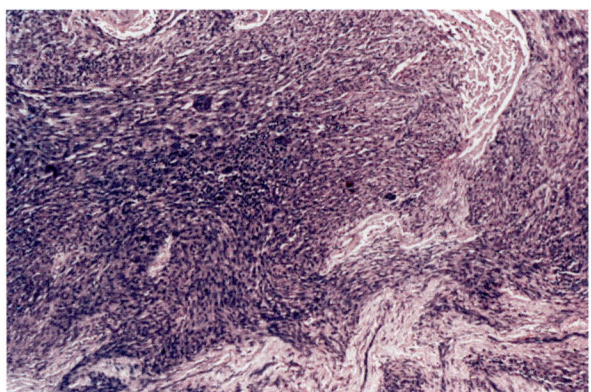

Figure 6-19

PLEXIFORM FIBROHISTIOCYTIC TUMOR

The fibroblast-like cells are in a plexiform arrangement and multinucleated giant cells are present.

Differential Diagnosis. Angiofibromas and their variants are relatively distinctive. Larger lesions have features in common with connective tissue nevi, and these may in fact be closely related entities. For digital fibrokeratoma, the chief differential diagnostic consideration is supernumerary digit (rudimentary polydactyly), which can closely resemble digital fibrokeratoma clinically as well as microscopically. However, supernumerary digits occur at the base of the fifth finger, are present at birth, may be bilateral, and show prominent nerve bundles in the deep dermis, with a configuration comparable to neuromas of other types. These are believed to occur as the result of autoamputation of a true accessory digit (200). In support of this concept, we have actually seen an example of an accesssory digit that was surmounted by a neuroma with the features of supernumerary digit. The myxoid changes in lesions of familial myxovascular fibroma may resemble forms of focal mucinosis. The correct diagnosis can be facilitated by a family history of such lesions, and by the presence of other microscopic changes typical of angiofibromas.

Plexiform Fibrohistiocytic Tumor

Clinical Features. This rare tumor was first reported by Enzinger and Zhang in 1988 (48). It is a slow-growing lesion that most often occurs in children or young adults, with a particular female predominance. It is located most often on the upper extremities, especially the wrists and hands (176) but also on the trunk (7,238); rarely, other sites are involved, such as the foot (230). The majority of patients have a favorable outcome following excision, but up to one third of lesions recur, and metastases have been reported to regional lymph nodes and lungs (48,176,185). For this reason, *plexiform fibrohistiocytic tumor* is generally regarded as a low-grade malignancy.

Pathologic Findings. Microscopically, this tumor is a poorly demarcated dermal or subcutaneous mass, composed of multinodular or plexiform arrangements of histiocytes and fibroblast-like cells, and multinucleated osteoclast-like giant cells (fig. 6-19). Epithelioid cells and osteoclast-like giant cells tend to be arranged in the central portions of the plexiform aggregates or nodules (238). Cytologic atypia is minimal. There may be up to 3 mitotic figures per 10 high-power fields, but atypical mitoses are uncommon (176).

Immunohistochemical studies are consistent in demonstrating staining for alpha-subunit actin (particularly in the fibroblast-like cells) and for CD68 (particularly in the histiocytic and osteoclast-like giant cells) (7,176,238). These results, together with ultrastructural studies (7), suggest that the plexiform fibrohistiocytic tumor is at least in part a lesion composed of myofibroblasts. Positivity has also been demonstrated for alpha-1-antitrypsin, alpha-1-antichymotrypsin, and vimentin. In one study, all nine tumors examined had a diploid DNA content (176). There appears to be no direct correlation between the clinical and microscopic features of a given lesion and its ultimate biologic behavior (48,176).

Differential Diagnosis. The differential diagnosis includes cutaneous fibrous histiocytoma (dermatofibroma), plexiform neurofibroma, fibromatosis, and a variety of giant cell tumors, both benign and malignant. In most instances, however, the clinical, microscopic, and immunohistochemical features are sufficiently distinctive to allow an accurate diagnosis.

Superficial Acral Fibromyxoma

Clinical Features. In 2001, Fetsch et al. (52) reported a series of 37 cases of a soft tissue tumor occurring in acral sites, which they termed *superficial acral fibromyxoma*. These are solitary lesions that show a male predominance and occur within a wide age range, with a mean incidence in the fifth decade. This lesion presents as a solitary mass on the fingers, toes, or palms; many cases involve the nail regions. They respond well to complete excision, but recurrences are reported, particularly following incomplete removal.

Pathologic Findings. The lesions are dermal or subcutaneous proliferations of spindled to stellate cells in loosely organized fascicular arrangements. The stroma may be fibrotic or myxoid, and mast cells accompany the process. A significant degree of cytologic atypia is not observed, and mitotic figures are sparse (fig. 6-20). Multinucleated cells have been noted (52). The cells comprising the lesion are positive for CD34, epithelial membrane antigen, and CD99. They are negative for cytokeratin and smooth muscle or melanocytic markers, although weak S-100 protein positivity was reported in one case (52).

Differential Diagnosis. In contrast to superficial acral fibromyxoma, fibrokeratomas show thick connective tissue, sparse cellularity, and prominence of vessels; mucinous changes are not typically present. Familial myxovascular fibromas have mucinous changes, but lack the cytologic features of superficial acral fibromyxoma and present as multiple wart-like papules. Baran and Perrin (8) recently described a lesion, designated *subungual perineurioma*, that had diffuse CD34 positivity. A possible relationship between this tumor and the superficial acral fibromyxoma remains to be determined.

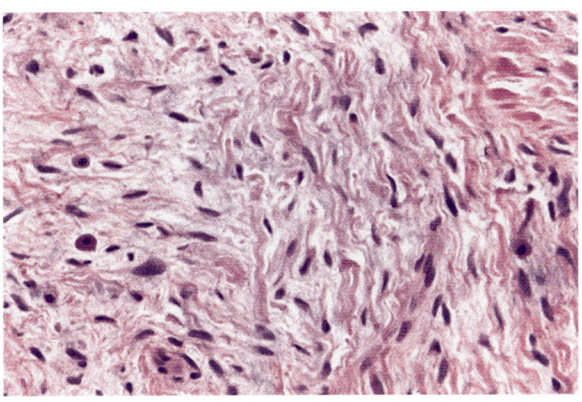

Figure 6-20

SUPERFICIAL ACRAL FIBROMYXOMA

Spindled cells in loosely organized fascicles are present within a myxoid stroma. Several mast cells can be identified. (Courtesy of J. H. Meyerle, CPT, MC, USAR, Washington, DC.)

Pleomorphic Fibroma

Clinical Features. First delineated as a clinicopathologic entity by Kamino et al. in 1989 (97), *pleomorphic fibromas* are polypoid or dome-shaped lesions that may arise on the trunk, extremities, face, or scalp of adults. Unusual locations have included the subungual region (79), eyelid (187), and tendon sheath (109). Pleomorphic cells with similar characteristics have been identified in an odontogenic fibroma (71). Despite the microscopic findings of markedly atypical cells that give this lesion its name, these are nonaggressive tumors that respond to local excision and apparently only recur if incompletely excised (97).

Pathologic Findings. Pleomorphic fibromas are relatively acellular lesions, composed of dense collagen and vessels with varying degrees of dilatation (79,187). Mucin deposition has been prominent in several cases (79,145). Scattered spindled cells with markedly pleomorphic, hyperchromatic nuclei and occasional mitotic figures can be observed (fig. 6-21) (4,79,97). These cells are consistently vimentin positive and are variably positive for actin and factor XIIIa (59,97,187). The results of CD34 staining are controversial, as some authors have not demonstrated positivity (59), while others have noted strong immunoreactivity of pleomorphic cells for this antigen (79,183). Results are less convincing with other histiocytic markers, but

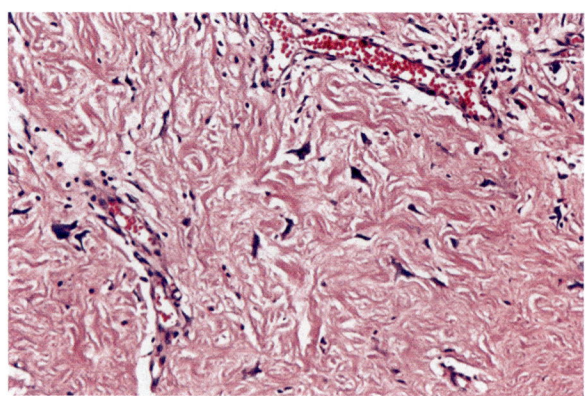 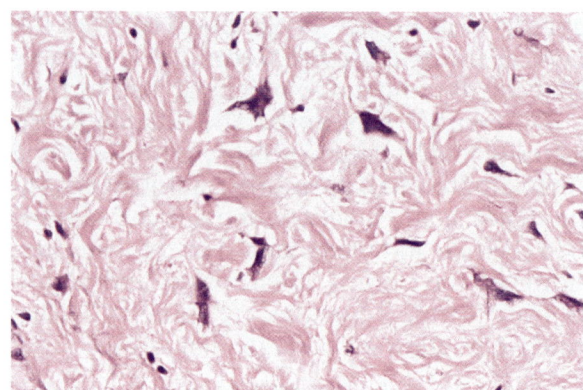

Figure 6-21

PLEOMORPHIC FIBROMA

Left: Scattered pleomorphic spindled cells and dense collagen are seen.
Right: Higher-power view of another case, in which pleomorphic cells are present within a myxoid stroma.

negativity for S-100 protein has been repeatedly observed (59,79,183). The configuration of these lesions has suggested to some authors that they may represent variants of the sclerotic fibroma (see below) (59,134), and we have observed several examples that would otherwise qualify as fibrous papule of the nose.

Differential Diagnosis. The presence of markedly pleomorphic cells within a relatively acellular, collagenous lesion is distinctive, and reminiscent of other clinically benign, cytologically malignant mesenchymal tumors, including pleomorphic lipomas and leiomyomas (97). Microscopically, these lesions are not often confused with atypical dermatofibromas (dermatofibromas with "monster cells"). In the occasional problem case, immunohistochemistry may be of some help, as pleomorphic fibroma cells may be CD34 positive and are Ki-M1p negative, whereas the reverse is true of the atypical cells in dermatofibromas (183).

Sclerotic Fibroma

Clinical Features. This distinctive fibrous tissue tumor received its first in-depth microscopic description in 1985, in connection with the multiple fibromas that occur in Cowden's syndrome (213). In 1989, Rapini and Golitz (172) reported solitary lesions with identical microscopic features in 11 patients who did not have Cowden's disease. It is now well recognized that this tumor can arise in both of these clinical settings (120,177).

Sclerotic fibromas are firm, flesh-colored to white papules, typically measuring less than 1 cm in diameter. They are particularly common on the extremities or head and neck, but may also occur on the trunk. A variant of sclerotic fibroma associated with the tendon sheath has been reported (223), and there is also a report of a *sclerotic lipoma* (240). These lesions are usually cured by local excision (229), but recurrence has been reported (34).

Pathologic Findings. Sclerotic fibroma is a circumscribed but not encapsulated, dome-shaped papule or nodule, often with an attenuated overlying epidermis (fig. 6-22, left). It consists of thick, whorled bundles of laminated collagen separated by cleft-like spaces that may contain mucin. This configuration has been described as having a "plywood-like" appearance (fig. 6-22, right) (172,213). Elastic fibers are absent. Lesions are typically hypocellular, containing only a few spindled to stellate cells, but occasionally more cellular areas containing multinucleated cells are identified (82). As previously pointed out, lesions have also been reported with pleomorphic cells resembling those of pleomorphic fibroma (59,134).

The cells of sclerotic fibroma are regularly vimentin positive and occasionally express factor XIIIa or smooth muscle actin (the latter indicative of myofibroblastic differentiation). CD34 positivity has also been detected among cells at the lower border of some lesions (229). The constituent cells are S-100 protein and neuron-

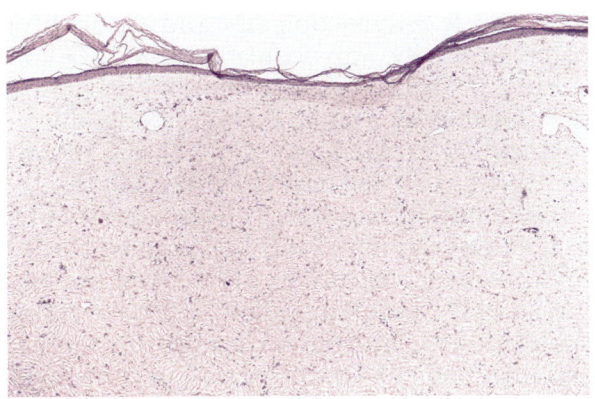 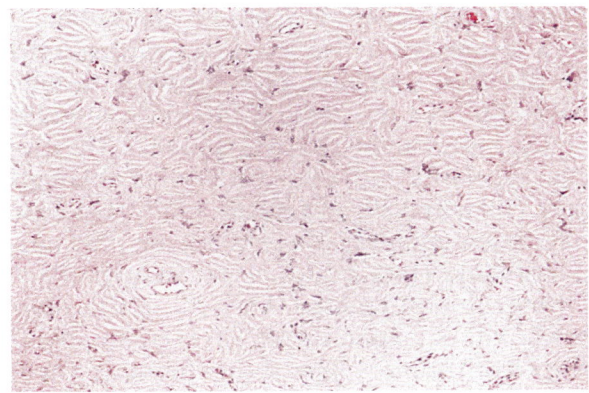

Figure 6-22

SCLEROTIC FIBROMA

Left: Dome-shaped nodule with attenuated epidermis.
Right: The lesion is composed of thick, whorled, collagen bundles producing a "plywood-like" appearance.

specific enolase negative (156). In one report of recurrent sclerotic fibroma, it was noted that over a period of time, cellularity diminished and the plywood-like appearance became more prominent (34). This report, together with findings linking sclerotic fibroma changes with dermatofibromas (fig. 6-23) or foci of folliculitis (30,167), has suggested to some that sclerotic fibroma represents a late, inert, or senescent change that can develop in more proliferative lesions. Immunohistochemical studies, however, have shown positive staining of cell nuclei for proliferative markers (136), as well as evidence of a procollagen peptide that normally indicates recent collagen synthesis (204). These studies seem to indicate that the sclerotic fibroma is an actively proliferating neoplasm.

Differential Diagnosis. The plywood-like microscopic appearance of these lesions is distinctive, and should ordinarily make diagnosis of sclerotic fibroma a simple matter. Similar features can occasionally be encountered in dermatofibroma or pleomorphic fibroma, lesions that some would argue have a close relationship with sclerotic fibroma. Additional diagnostic considerations include two uncommon neural tumors: sclerotic perineurioma (53) and pacinian neurofibroma (180), which has also been termed fibrolamellar nerve sheath tumor (174). Sclerotic perineurioma features dense connective tissue but also epithelioid and spindled cells in trabecular or whorled arrangements; these cells are epithelial membrane antigen positive,

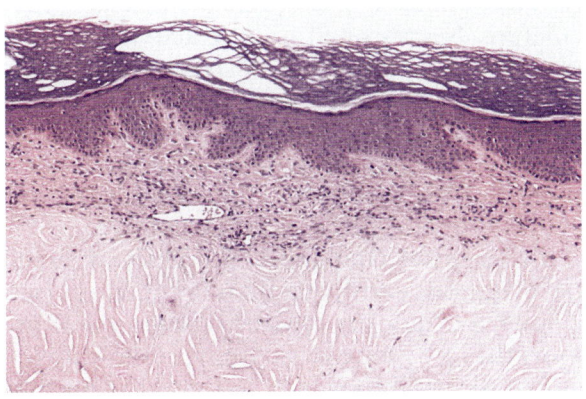

Figure 6-23

DERMATOFIBROMA WITH CHANGES OF SCLEROTIC FIBROMA

as is typical for cells of the perineurium (53). Pacinian neurofibroma, or fibrolamellar nerve sheath tumor, is said to closely resemble sclerotic fibroma but may feature increased amounts of mucin, scattered cells with small nuclei, some of which can be S-100 protein positive, and occasional pigmented dendritic melanocytes (174).

Collagenous Fibroma (Desmoplastic Fibroblastoma)

Clinical Features. This recently described tumor is predominantly within the province of soft tissue pathologists, but is discussed here because it can involve the subcutaneous tissues and skeletal muscle (144,154). *Collagenous* *fibroma,* also called *desmoplastic fibroblastoma,* typically arises as a painless, slow-growing mass on the neck, shoulders, or extremities. Lesions have also been reported on the forehead (225) and as a mass in the parotid gland (87). The median age of incidence is around 50 years, although both children (129) and elderly adults (144,233) have been reported. There is a male predominance (144). There is rarely if ever recurrence following complete excision. A genetic relationship to fibroma of tendon sheath has been proposed, since both tumors may show the same chromosomal rearrangement at 11q12 (195).

Pathologic Findings. Microscopically, the tumor is relatively well demarcated, although focal infiltration of adjacent tissues, including skeletal muscle, is often observed (77). Scattered stellate to spindled cells are present within a fibrous to fibromyxoid stroma, with sparse vasculature. Necrosis and mitotic activity are not observed. Calcification and metaplastic bone formation are unusual features (77). The constituent cells are vimentin and often smooth muscle actin positive. Faint S-100 protein positivity has been reported, but tumor cells are cytokeratin and CD34 negative (154).

Differential Diagnosis. The chief differential diagnostic consideration is fibromatosis (see below), a diagnostic category comprised of tumors that are prone to recurrence following local excision. Fibromatosis lesions are typically more cellular, with distinctly fascicular arrangements of cells, and show greater degrees of peripheral infiltration (57).

Postoperative Spindle Cell Nodule

Clinical Features. This unusual spindle cell proliferative lesion is well known to occur in the prostate and urinary bladder following surgical trauma (84,237). Similar lesions, arising under similar circumstances, have been observed in the buccal mucosa (243), vulva (132, 227), and skin of the face and scalp (227).

Pathologic Findings. These nodules are comprised of cytologically bland spindled cells (fig. 6-24), which, however, display brisk mitotic activity (132,227). Varying degrees of vascular proliferation, hemorrhage, and inflammation are present. The spindled cells are vimentin, actin, and desmin positive, indicating the presence of myofibroblasts. This lesion has much in common, both microscopically and (probably) pathogenetically, with nodular fasciitis (227), and should probably be regarded as one of the pseudosarcomas, a group that includes proliferative fasciitis, proliferative myositis, and myositis ossificans as well as nodular fasciitis (5).

Differential Diagnosis. Postoperative spindle cell nodules can mistakenly be identified as leiomyosarcomas, but a history of preceding trauma, the generally bland appearance of proliferating spindled cells, and the accompanying stromal and inflammatory changes should usually permit a correct diagnosis.

Inflammatory Pseudotumor

Clinical Features. *Inflammatory pseudotumor* is a lesion well known to occur in a variety of organ systems, including the lung (113) and urinary bladder (237), but it has also recently been reported in skin (86,236). It bears some microscopic resemblance to the postoperative spindle cell nodule, but it is not known to be a post-traumatic phenomenon and tends to occur in a younger age group. Cutaneous examples have thus far been reported on the neck and extremities (86,236). These are typically solitary lesions that respond to complete excision.

Pathologic Findings. Lesions are well circumscribed, and feature polymorphous inflammatory infiltrates composed of lymphocytes, plasma cells, neutrophils, eosinophils, zones of fibrosis, and, in one case, multinucleated cells resembling Reed-Sternberg cells (236). Hurt and Santa Cruz (86) observed a zonation phenomenon in their cases, with a peripheral rim of lymphocytes and plasma cells, and a central area of fibrosis containing mononucleated cells, neutrophils, and eosinophils (fig. 6-25); this arrangement mimicked the appearance of lymph node. These authors suggest an eventual transition from inflammatory to sclerotic lesions. Descriptions of inflammatory pseudotumors from other organs emphasize the presence of spindled cells which possess basophilic cytoplasm and can be plump or strap-like (resembling rhabdomyoblasts) (20,155). Scattered mitoses may be present, although atypical mitotic figures are not observed. The stroma can be mucinous, and the degree of vascularity can vary from case to case (86). Spindled cells have the immunohistochemical characteristics of fibroblasts or myofibroblasts

Fibrous Tissue Tumors

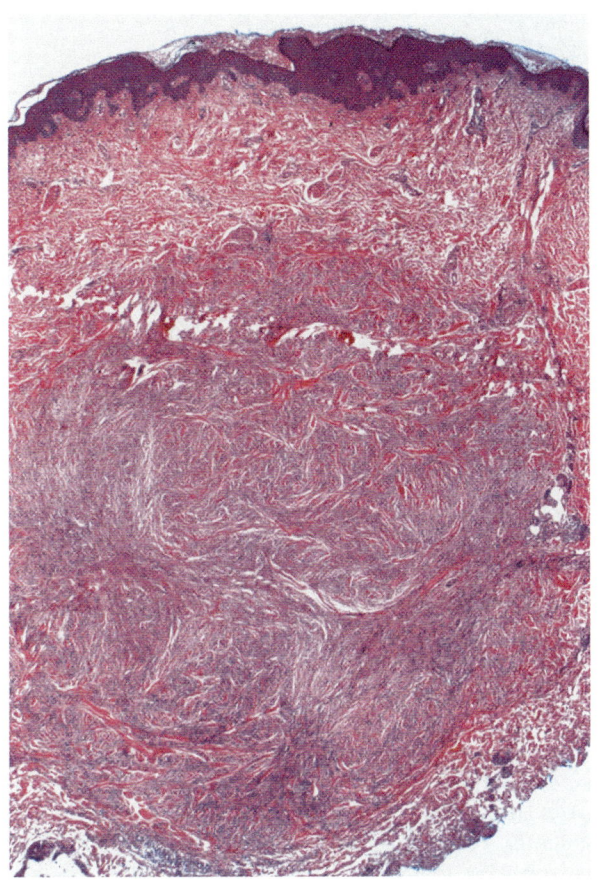 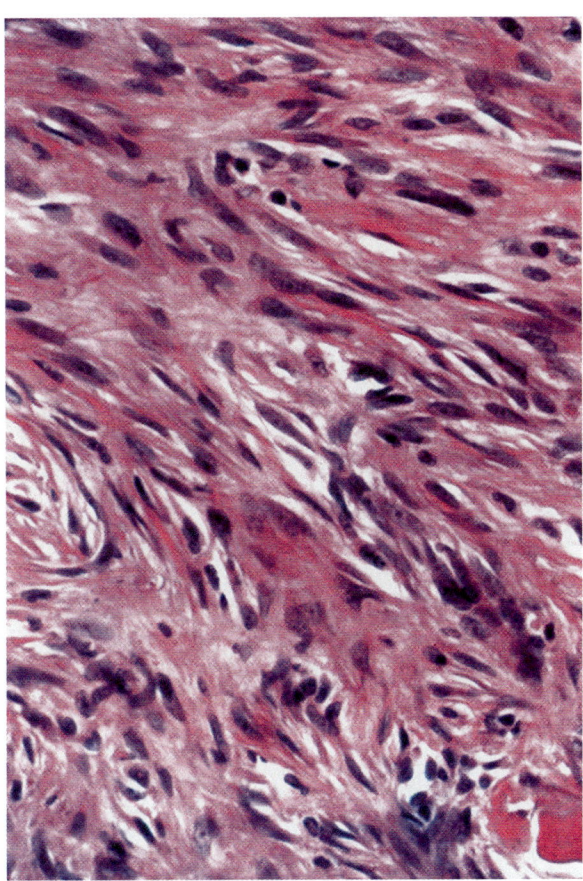

Figure 6-24

POSTOPERATIVE SPINDLE CELL NODULE

Left: Low-power view.
Right: High-power view. The nodule consists of plump but cytologically bland spindled cells.

(181). The Reed-Sternberg–like cells described by Yang (236) are vimentin positive and negative for actin, desmin, and histiocytic markers.

Another lesion that is closely related, if not identical, is the *pseudosarcomatous fibromyxoid tumor* that has occurred in the bladder, prostate, and spermatic cord (181). To date, no cutaneous lesion with this specific designation has been reported.

Differential Diagnosis. As with postoperative spindle cell nodule, inflammatory pseudotumor must be distinguished from malignant mesenchymal tumors, including leiomyosarcoma and malignant fibrous histiocytoma. In contrast to most sarcomas, the nuclei of the spindled cells of inflammatory pseudotumor are p53 negative (113). We have also encountered several examples of desmoplastic malignant melanoma with sufficient inflammation to closely mimic inflammatory pseudotumor; therefore, panels of special stains should ideally include antibodies to S-100 protein and other melanocytic markers.

Keloid

Clinical Features. *Keloids* are among the most familiar of cutaneous tumors. There may be a familial predisposition to these lesions (151), and black individuals are much more likely to develop them than whites (160). Keloids are firm, smooth nodules that may be flesh colored or livid in appearance. They typically develop in areas that have been subjected to injury, but they extend beyond the confines

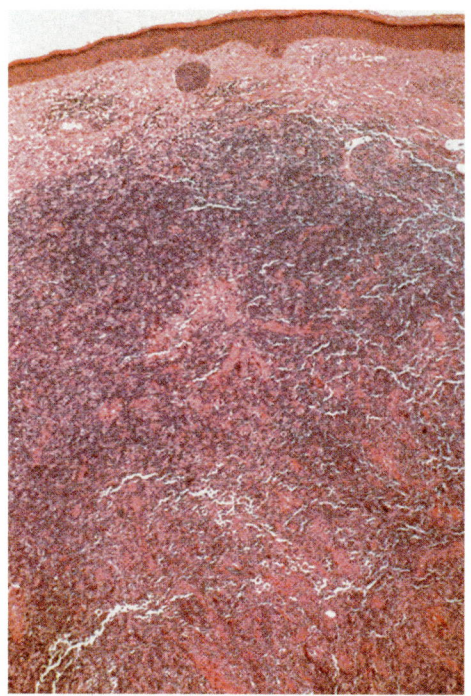
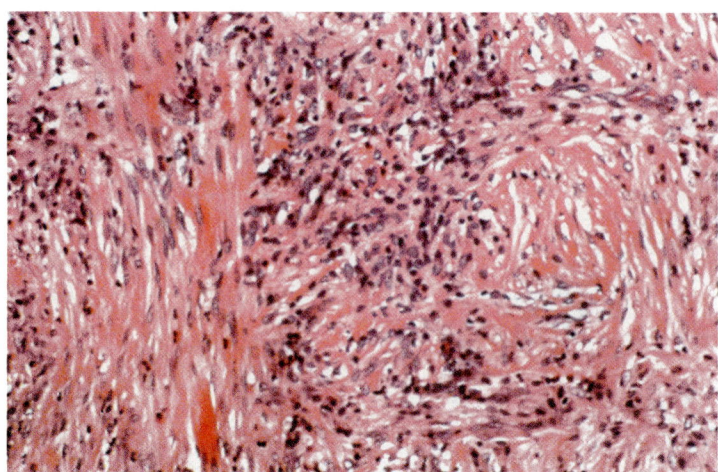

Figure 6-25

INFLAMMATORY PSEUDOTUMOR

Left: Low-power view shows a degree of circumscription and central fibrosis.

Above: High-power view of the central portion of the lesion shows fibrosis and inflammatory cells.

of the original wound, a feature that usually permits distinction from hypertrophic scars. They can arise in any cutaneous site. A particularly common one is the earlobe, where keloids develop secondary to ear piercing. Keloids of varying sizes also occur over the posterior neck and scalp as a consequence of chronic deep folliculitis; this condition is termed *acne keloidalis* or *folliculitis keloidalis nuchae*. Keloids also develop in an apparently spontaneous fashion. This phenomenon can occur on the trunk or over large joints, where growth spurts or unseen inflammatory events such as ruptured cysts or deep folliculitis may play a role in their development. Spontaneous keloid formation has been reported in association with the Rubinstein-Taybe syndrome, which consists of short stature, mental retardation, small cranium, beaked nose, strabismus, and other anomalies (106).

Pathologic Findings. Keloids are composed of whorled arrangements of thick, compact collagen, often with a "smudged" or hyalinized appearance (fig. 6-26) (119). The overlying epidermis may be normal or thinned. Fibroblasts may be numerous, particularly in early lesions, while more mature lesions appear less cellular. A suppurative variant of keloid has been reported (161). Changes consistent with corticosteroid injection (224) are commonly encountered in keloids, reflecting prior attempts to shrink or soften the lesions; these consist of islands of pale, somewhat frothy material surrounded by inflammatory cells. Sometimes, granulomatous inflammation lines these foci, mimicking a palisading, necrobiotic granuloma (fig. 6-27).

There has been considerable interest in the metabolic state and capabilities of keloidal fibroblasts, since they are likely keys to understanding the evolution and persistence of these lesions. In early or active keloids, myofibroblasts are prominent (93). An intimate relationship between mast cells and the myofibroblasts of active keloids has been observed (115), suggesting a role for mast cells and their mediators in pathogenesis. In situ hybridization studies have demonstrated high levels of procollagen mRNA when compared to control fibroblasts, consistent with increased levels of collagen production in keloid fibroblasts (24,114,205). Keloidal fibroblasts are actively proliferating cells, as can be determined in tissue sections through increased numbers of nucleolar organizer regions (60), and in "wounding" experiments in tissue culture, where these cells show increased incorporation of tritiated thymidine

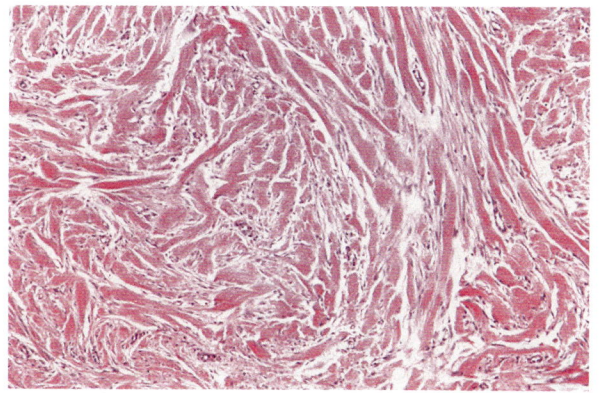

Figure 6-26
KELOID
There are thick, "smudged" collagen bundles in whorled arrangements.

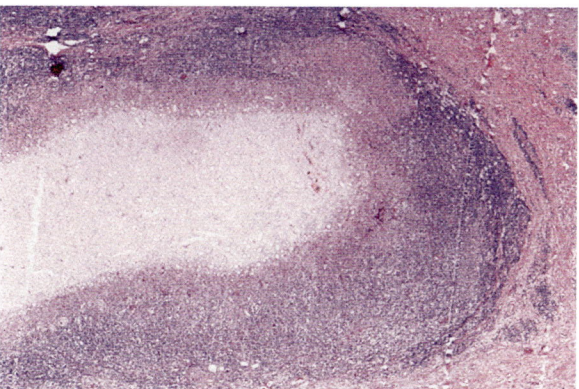

Figure 6-27
CORTICOSTEROID INJECTION CHANGES IN A KELOID
Pale, frothy material is surrounded by granulomatous inflammation in a palisaded arrangement.

and autoradiographic labeling when compared to normal fibroblasts (24). Keloidal fibroblasts demonstrate increased levels of platelet-derived growth factor (PDGF)-alpha receptors, and therefore not unexpectedly show enhanced responses to PDGF in chemotactic and mitogenic assays (72). Finally, apoptosis may be another important determinant in the development and evolution of keloids, since p53 and bcl-2 expression in "younger," hypercellular areas appears to favor increased proliferation and decreased cell death (107).

Differential Diagnosis. Keloids are sufficiently distinctive that microscopic diagnosis is seldom a problem. Dermal foci resembling keloid can occasionally be observed in other fibrotic or sclerosing conditions, including morphea and dermatofibroma (105). These conditions are often excluded by clinical data or by selected microscopic features (e.g., appendageal atrophy, dermal/subcutaneous inflammation in morphea; curlicue cellular arrangements or xanthomatization in dermatofibromas).

Occasionally, small foci resembling keloid formation can be identified in otherwise ordinary-appearing dermal scars. Hypertrophic scars differ clinically from keloids in that: 1) they do not extend beyond the bounds of the original wound; 2) they tend to regress over time; and 3) they are more amenable to surgical revision. Microscopically, hypertrophic scars tend to lack the thick, densely packed, hyalinized collagen bundles of keloid. Instead, they are more likely to have nodular structures composed of vessels, fibroblasts, and fine collagen. In one recent study, only the nodular structures of hypertrophic scars contained alpha-smooth muscle actin–expressing myofibroblasts (46).

Elastofibroma Dorsi

Clinical Features. *Elastofibroma dorsi* is a slow-growing soft tissue tumor that usually occurs in the subscapular region of elderly adults, as a result of which there can be pain or limited range of motion of the arm. Although considered a rare tumor, autopsy and radiographic studies reveal a surprisingly high prevalence among older individuals (21,214). Bilateral tumors have been reported on a number of occasions and may be more common than generally recognized (14,152). Despite its predominance among the elderly, elastofibroma has been diagnosed in a child (44). In addition, tumors with microscopic features similar to elastofibroma have been reported in the foot (138), sigmoid colon (184), and limbic conjunctiva (83). Computerized tomographic and magnetic resonance imagery studies show a heterogeneous soft tissue mass with a characteristic layered appearance (21,152).

Pathologic Findings. Microscopic findings include the presence of dense collagen, variable numbers of fibroblasts, and aggregates of mature lipocytes. The unique feature of this tumor, however, is the presence of thick, eosinophilic globules and fibers that sometimes show beaded or wavy contours (fig. 6-28, left). These structures

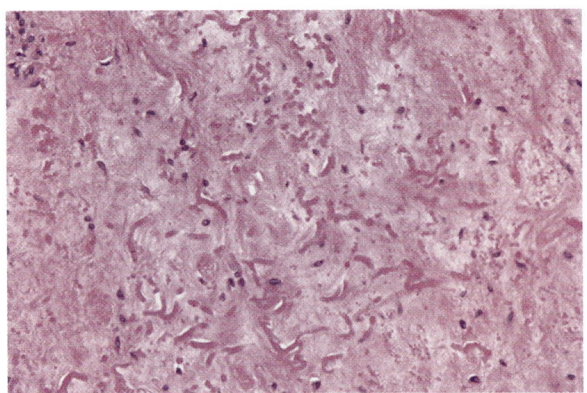 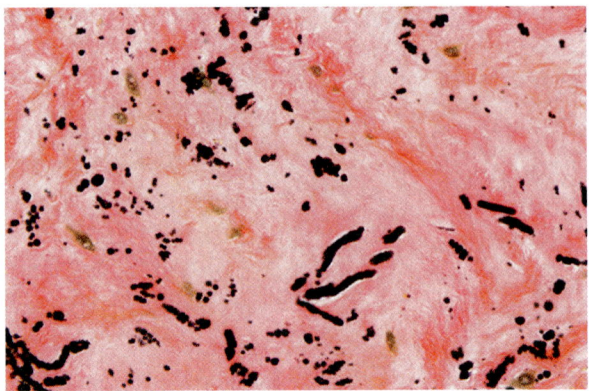

Figure 6-28

ELASTOFIBROMA DORSI

Left: Thick eosinophilic globules and fibers can be identified in hematoxylin and eosin (H&E)–stained sections.
Right: These structures have the characteristics of elastic tissue, and stain black with the Verhoeff-van Gieson stain.

stain as elastic fibers, and therefore appear black with the Verhoeff-van Gieson stain (fig. 6-28, right). Although there was initially some thought that these may represent degenerated collagen fibers, ultrastructural studies show that they indeed have characteristics of elastic tissue and are actively secreted by fibroblasts (45). Immunohistochemical staining in one case showed S-100 protein positivity among fibroblast-like cells (128). There exists the usual question regarding the identity of this lesion as a reactive versus a neoplastic process (133), but the locations and histories of these tumors suggest a possible role for chronic, repetitive trauma in their development (83,152,184).

Differential Diagnosis. The major differential diagnostic issue revolves around the possibility of sarcoma in a patient with an undiagnosed subscapular soft tissue tumor. However, the clinical history of a slow-growing mass in this location is typical, and the presumptive diagnosis can be aided by radiographic findings (21) and characteristic findings on fine-needle aspiration cytology (149). With incisional biopsy or tumor resection, the microscopic features are diagnostic.

Giant Cell Tumor of Tendon Sheath

Clinical Features. The *giant cell tumor of tendon sheath*, also termed *localized nodular tenosynovitis*, is located most commonly on the fingers, hands, and wrists. Similar lesions also occur about large joints such as the ankle and knee (182,217). This tumor is closely related to a more diffuse process involving the joint space and occasionally other soft tissues, known as *pigmented villonodular synovitis* (157,171). Lesions occurring on the distal extremities are firm subcutaneous tumors, ranging from 1 to 3 cm in diameter. They typically extend to the synovium of the adjacent joint space, explaining in part the significant recurrence rate following attempted local excision (182). They may also involve the overlying dermis (12,101).

Pathologic Findings. Giant cell tumors have a lobulated contour and are surrounded by dense connective tissue. Cellular areas contain numerous histiocytes (macrophages) with variably foamy cytoplasm and hemosiderin deposits (fig. 6-29, left). Less cellular areas consist of thickened collagen fibers and scattered fibroblasts. Lesions located near large joints are more apt to show large slit-like or pseudovascular spaces lined by synovial cells (182,217). The distinctive multinucleated giant cells feature eosinophilic, smudged cytoplasm and nuclei that tend to be clumped or in a haphazard array (fig. 6-29, right) (12,171). These characteristic features can also be seen in fine-needle aspiration preparations (222). These giant cells morphologically resemble osteoclasts, and this relationship is further supported by their possession of similar phenotypic characteristics. As is true of osteoclasts, the giant cells of giant cell tumor of tendon sheath strongly express

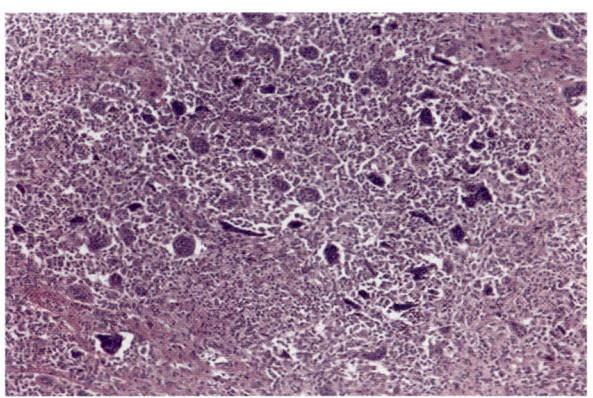 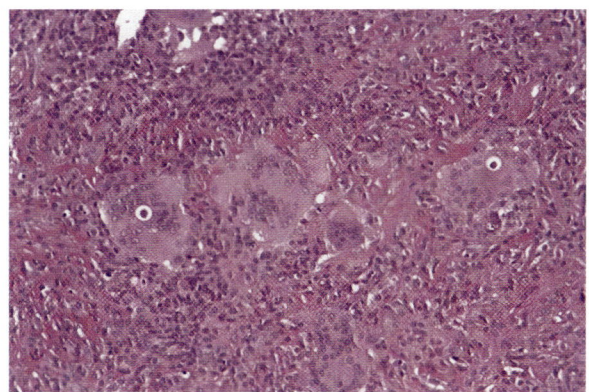

Figure 6-29

GIANT CELL TUMOR OF TENDON SHEATH

Left: There are numerous histiocytes (macrophages) and multinucleated giant cells.
Right: Detail of the multinucleated giant cells.

acid phosphatase, lack alkaline phosphatase (235), possess the vitronectin receptor alpha V beta 3 integrin, and express the mRNA for the calcitonin receptor (42). In addition, spindled cells and mononucleated cells as well as giant cells express a variety of macrophage markers (130,148,197). In particular, the giant cells have been reported to stain for alpha-1-antitrypsin; alpha-1-antichymotrypsin; lysozyme; ferritin (148); human leukocyte antigens (HLA) A, B, C, and DR; leukocyte common antigen (235); CD68; HAM56; and MAC387 (130).

Differential Diagnosis. The combination of clinical and microscopic features makes the diagnosis of giant cell tumor of tendon sheath relatively straightforward. Some controversy surrounds the possible existence of a *malignant giant cell tumor of tendon sheath*. Several such cases have been reported (28,203), one arising from a preexisting aggressive giant cell tumor that had been present over a 20-year period (28), and distant metastases have occurred. This is particularly troubling in view of the widely held concept that giant cell tumor of tendon sheath is a reactive rather than a neoplastic process (12). That view is supported to some extent by a recent study by Vogrincic and O'Connell (221) showing that this tumor lacks clonality. The issue is certainly not resolved, but the possibility exists that lesions that have been termed "malignant giant cell tumor of tendon sheath" actually represent other soft tissue tumors that feature giant cells, such as malignant fibrous histiocytoma.

Peripheral Giant Cell Granuloma (Giant Cell Epulis)

Clinical Features. *Peripheral giant cell granuloma*, or *giant cell epulis*, is a solitary tumor of the gingival or alveolar process. Most current authors avoid the term epulis, a nonspecific designation for any tumor or tumor-like process involving the gingiva, and seem to prefer the term peripheral giant cell granuloma, which links this lesion to the histologically indistinguishable central giant cell granuloma that involves the jaw.

This tumor occurs over a wide age range: it is common among children and young adults (6), but older, edentulous patients develop it as well (61). It presents as a sessile or pedunculated, dark red nodule, and may be ulcerated. The underlying bone may be uninvolved or show erosions with "peripheral cuffing" (199). Complete excision is curative. The precise explanation for its origin is unclear, but it is widely considered to represent a proliferative response to mechanical injury or infection.

Pathologic Findings. Peripheral giant cell granuloma is well circumscribed and features large numbers of fibroblast-like cells in a delicate fibrillar connective tissue stroma that contains numerous vessels, sometimes with hemorrhage and hemosiderin deposition. Mitoses are sparse to absent. The characteristic multinucleated giant cells feature eosinophilic cytoplasm and numerous nuclei in irregular arrangements.

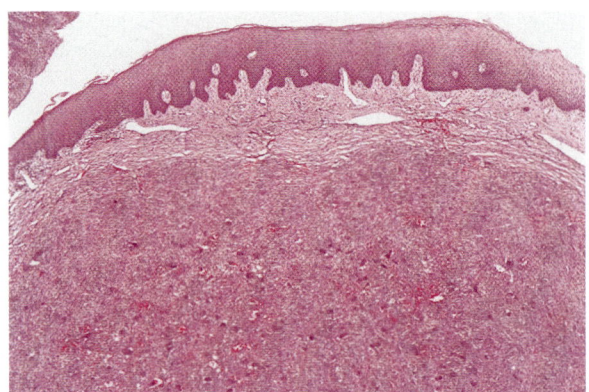 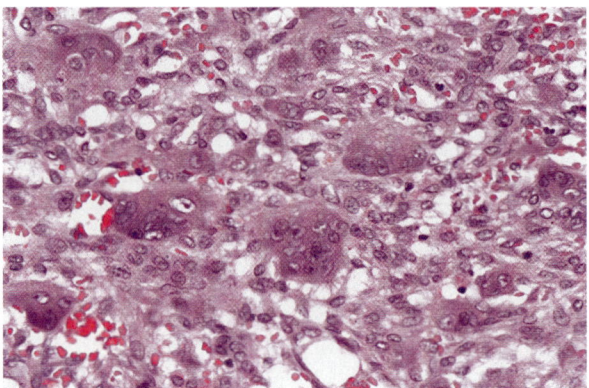

Figure 6-30

PERIPHERAL GIANT CELL GRANULOMA

Left: Low-power view of a gingival nodule.
Right: The lesion consists of fibroblast-like cells and characteristic multinucleated giant cells. The latter resemble osteoclasts and the cells of giant cell tumor of tendon sheath.

The giant cells resemble those of giant cell tumor of tendon sheath and are also similar in appearance to osteoclasts (fig. 6-30). Although there has been some debate about the origin of these cells, their ultrastructural characteristics (190), activities in relation to bone, response to calcitonin (hormonal), and reactions with monoclonal antibodies all suggest that the giant cells are essentially osteoclasts (54). The microscopic features are characteristic, particularly when encountered in a lesion in this anatomic location.

Fibroma of Tendon Sheath

Clinical Features. *Fibroma of tendon sheath* clinically resembles giant cell tumor of tendon sheath in that it is a painless, slow-growing mass that frequently involves the fingers and hands, particularly the volar surfaces (37,91). Lesions have also been reported in the foot, knee, and tibial region. The median age of incidence is early in the fourth decade of life, with occurrence both in infants and the elderly (78,168). Reported complications include limited range of motion (91), carpal tunnel syndrome (49), and median nerve neuropathy (17). Bony erosion can be detected on radiographic study (122). Fibromas of tendon sheath are treated by excision, but are prone to recur (37). In a recently reported chromosomal analysis of one lesion, a 2;11 translocation was detected, suggesting that fibroma of tendon sheath may be a neoplastic rather than a reactive process (40).

Pathologic Findings. Fibromas of tendon sheath consist of dense collagenous tissue, with variable numbers of spindled or stellate cells (fig. 6-31A). Slit-like spaces are also present (fig. 6-31B) (37), particularly at the periphery of tumors (126), and these are identified in some reports as vascular channels (85,126). Foamy macrophages are not observed, and multinucleated giant cells are rare (85,130). Cooper (37) noted "pseudopods" or small foci of tumor in the surrounding connective tissue (fig. 6-31C), one possible explanation for the tendency of these lesions to recur. Areas resembling nodular fasciitis have also been described; lesions with the latter feature are best considered variants of nodular fasciitis rather than true fibromas of tendon sheath (168). Ultrastructural studies have repeatedly shown that the constituent cells are fibroblasts and myofibroblasts (126,168), and these cells may be positive for smooth muscle actin (78,130).

Differential Diagnosis. The close clinical resemblance between giant cell tumor of tendon sheath and fibroma of tendon sheath, and the rare presence of giant cells in the latter, suggest that these two tumors are related. They may simply represent different stages in the evolution of a single lesion (fibroma of tendon sheath presumably representing a later developmental stage). This concept is supported by histologic studies that have shown transitional forms between the two (191), and by immunohistochemical studies showing evidence of

Fibrous Tissue Tumors

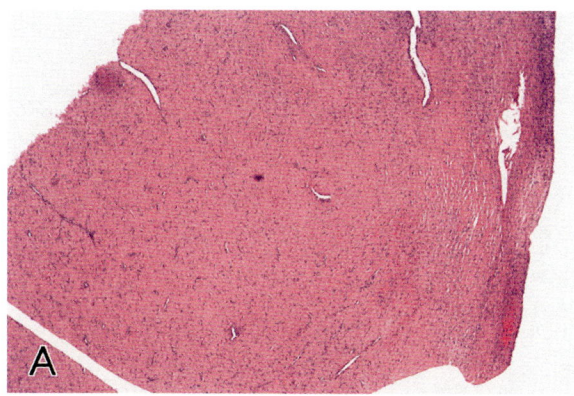
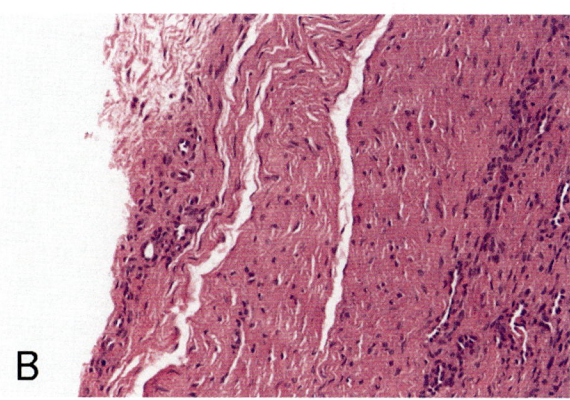
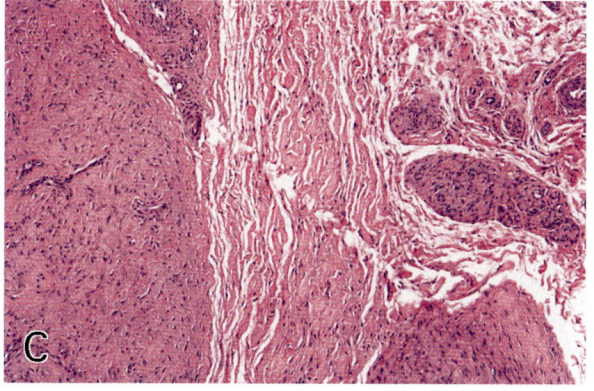

Figure 6-31

FIBROMA OF TENDON SHEATH

A: Dense collagenous tissue is scattered with spindled or stellate cells.
B: Slit-like spaces at the periphery of a tumor.
C: "Pseudopod" formation provides a possible explanation for recurrences.

macrophagic and myofibroblastic differentiation in both tumors (130).

Fibromatosis

Clinical Features. *Fibromatosis* includes a group of proliferative fibrous tissue lesions that share the features of bland cytology (although sometimes with pronounced cellularity), locally infiltrative growth, and a proneness to recurrence. For the most part, this category of tumor resides within the province of soft tissue pathology, but the relatively superficial, subcutaneous extension of some lesions makes it relevant to dermatopathology practice. Forms of fibromatosis that are likely to be encountered by the dermatologist include *palmar fibromatosis* (producing *Dupuytren's contracture*), *plantar fibromatosis (Ledderhose's disease)*, *penile fibromatosis (Peyronie's disease)*, *knuckle pads* or, less commonly, *pachydermodactyly,* and occasionally *abdominal* or *extra-abdominal desmoid tumors.* An association among the first four lesions has been reported. Palmar fibromatosis shows an increased association with epilepsy and diabetes mellitus, and desmoid tumors have a well-known link with Gardner's syndrome.

The various forms of fibromatosis are associated with induration or the development of a mass lesion. They may induce other specific symptoms and signs depending upon the location: flexion contractures with palmar fibromatosis or difficulties with urination or intercourse with Peyronie's disease. Lesions otherwise do not cause symptoms, although they may be painful; this is particularly true of intra-abdominal desmoid tumors.

Pathologic Findings. Fibromatoses show proliferations of fibroblasts in interconnecting fascicles, associated with pronounced collagen production. The nuclei have bland characteristics, and mitoses are uncommon (fig. 6-32). The lesions infiltrate adjacent connective tissue and may appear to "entrap" skeletal muscle fibers (fig. 6-33). One immunohistochemical study of extra-abdominal fibromatosis showed that tumor cells were positive for alpha-smooth muscle actin, factor XIIIa, CD34, and vimentin (193). The presence of myofibroblasts in these tumors

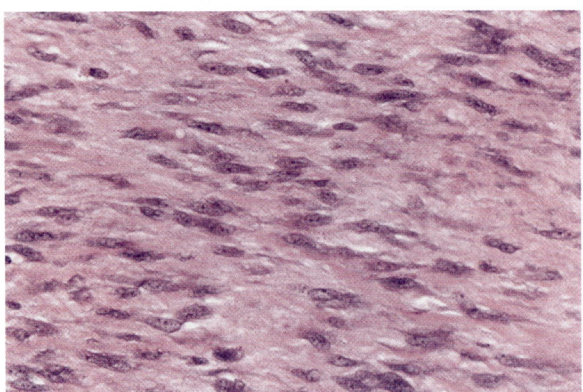

Figure 6-32
PALMAR FIBROMATOSIS
High-power view of fibroblasts and collagenous stroma. The nuclei have a relatively bland appearance.

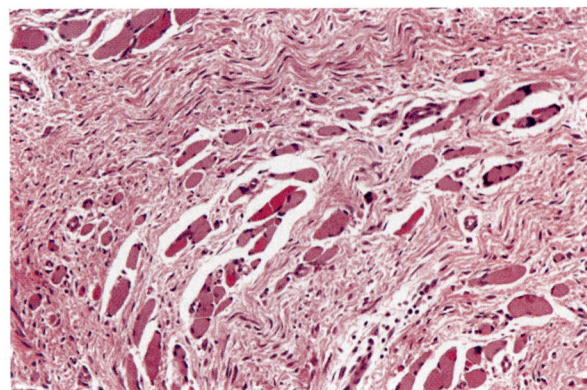

Figure 6-33
FIBROMATOSIS
Cells at the margins of this tumor infiltrate and appear to "entrap" skeletal muscle fibers.

has also been confirmed ultrastructurally (65). Our own studies of varying forms of fibromatosis seem to show sparse to absent factor XIIIa staining, although this antigen is more strikingly expressed in infantile fibromatosis. Studies by Li et al. (117) have shown that desmoid fibromatosis is a clonal, and therefore presumably a neoplastic, process. Recent studies have also shown that angiogenesis-associated cytokines, common accompaniments of healing wounds and invasive tumors, are also expressed in the desmoid tumor (146).

Differential Diagnosis. The chief considerations in the differential diagnosis are scar, as a reaction to injury, or fibrosarcoma. In addition to the history, scar would be favored by the detection of other evidence of injury, such as hemorrhage or hemosiderin deposition. Fibrosarcoma shows an irregular growth pattern and increased mitotic activity.

Recurrent Infantile Digital Fibroma

Clinical Features. *Infantile digital fibromas* usually present as solitary or multiple firm nodules on the fingers and toes. As the name indicates, these lesions develop in infancy or in the first 3 years of life. Similar lesions, however, have occurred in other locations, such as the arm (169), and a tumor with identical microscopic features has been reported in nondigital locations in adults (220). Recurrences are common but not invariable, and spontaneous regression may occur after several years (226); for this reason, there has been a trend towards less aggressive surgical management of these lesions.

Pathologic Findings. Microscopically, the tumor is composed of thick, intersecting collagen bundles and spindled cells with the appearance of fibroblasts. The distinctive feature of these cells is the presence of paranuclear, cytoplasmic inclusion bodies which approximate the size of erythrocytes but are more variable in diameter. They are eosinophilic with H&E, red with Masson trichrome, and purple with phosphotungstic acid–hematoxylin (PTAH) stains, and they are actin and vimentin positive (fig. 6-34) (220). Ultrastructural studies have shown that these inclusions consist of bundles of microfilaments containing dense bodies. More typical arrangements of microfilaments are also visualized elsewhere in the cytoplasm. These findings indicate that most of the constituent cells are myofibroblasts (18,89,220), and for this reason, *infantile digital myofibroblastoma* has been proposed as a preferable name for the tumor (18).

Differential Diagnosis. The characteristic clinical presentation and cytoplasmic inclusions make infantile digital fibroma unique, although it resembles some forms of fibromatosis.

Myofibroma

Clinical Features. *Myofibroma* is the preferred term for a group of solitary or generalized soft tissue tumors that may be located in the skin and subcutis, or within skeletal muscle, bone, and viscera. Cases formerly labeled *congenital*

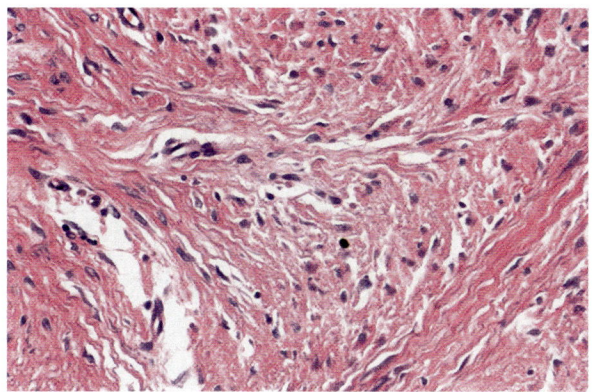 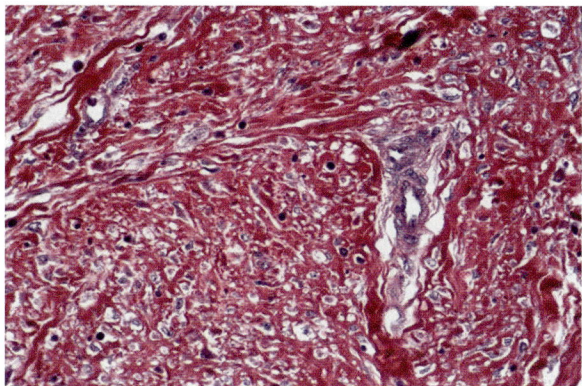

Figure 6-34

RECURRENT INFANTILE DIGITAL FIBROMA

Left: The tumor consists of thick, intersecting collagen bundles. The cytoplasm of some constituent spindled cells contains paranuclear inclusions. Several examples can be seen in the mid-portion of the figure.

Right: The inclusions stain purple with phosphotungstic acid–hematoxylin (PTAH).

(generalized) fibromatosis apparently represent examples of this entity (211). The best known version of this tumor consists of nodules that are present at birth or in early childhood. A favorable outcome is typical for patients with solitary, superficial lesions, although recurrences are not unusual (32,212). On the other hand, death can occur in patients with multiple visceral involvement (32,211). Among those with solitary or superficial lesions, and for some individuals with generalized lesions, spontaneous involution may occur (32,207,211,212). A soft tissue myofibroma with identical histopathologic features has been described in adults (39,70,178).

Pathologic Findings. Lesions are well circumscribed but not encapsulated, and generally consist of two components (fig. 6-35A). The first includes proliferations of plump spindled cells with the appearance of myofibroblasts, arranged in short fascicles (32,207). The stroma may be somewhat mucinous (fig. 6-35B). The second component is more vascular and features numerous polygonal to small spindled cells with hyperchromatic nuclei; these areas often resemble hemangiopericytoma (fig. 6-35C) (127,143,219,241). Monophasic variants of myofibroma have been reported that feature only one of these components (241). Requena et al. (178) have identified four histopathologic patterns in their series of adult cases that appear to correlate with increasing lesional age: vascular, nodular or cellular, multinodular or biphasic, and leiomyoma-like or fascicular types (178). The close resemblance of some lesions to hemangiopericytoma has led a number of authors to conclude that infantile myofibromatosis and hemangiopericytoma are histogenetically related (143,219).

Several findings indicate the myofibroblastic nature of the tumor cells. The intracellular fibrils stain with PTAH. Immunopositivity for alpha-smooth muscle actin and vimentin is characteristic (13,39,76,207). Ultrastructural findings include microfilaments, dense bodies, and incomplete basal laminae (76). Staining for desmin is usually negative. Massive apoptosis has been observed in some examples and has been proposed as a mechanism for spontaneous regression of these tumors (56).

Differential Diagnosis. The differential diagnosis for myofibromas (in addition to the possibly related hemangiopericytoma) includes leiomyoma, forms of fibrous histiocytoma, neurothekeoma, and other tumors that may contain myofibroblasts, such as dermatomyofibroma and nodular fasciitis (70). The biphasic lesions of myofibroma have characteristic features, but older lesions or those with a predominance of spindle cell fascicles can closely mimic leiomyoma or other myofibroblastic lesions. Myofibromas lack the "tissue culture" appearance of nodular fasciitis, the epidermal hyperplasia that accompanies traditional dermatofibromas, or the multilobulated, compartmentalized configuration of the myxoid variant of

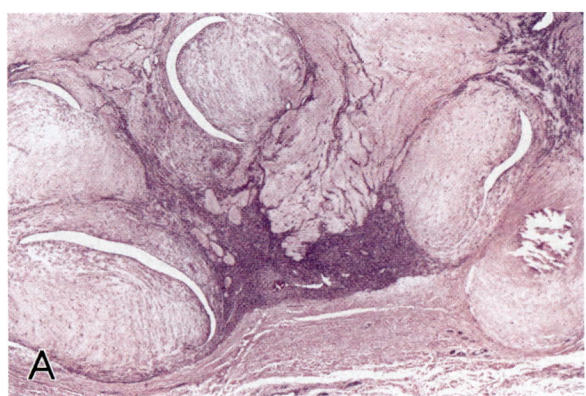
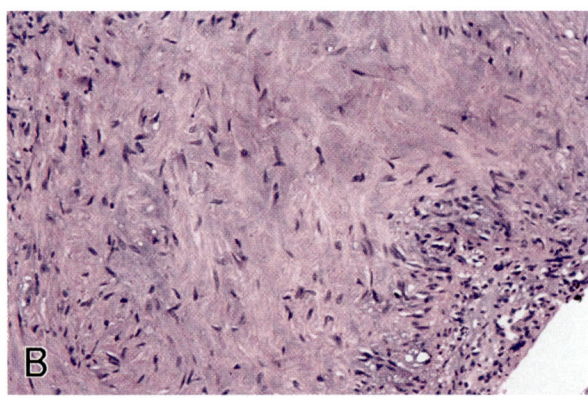
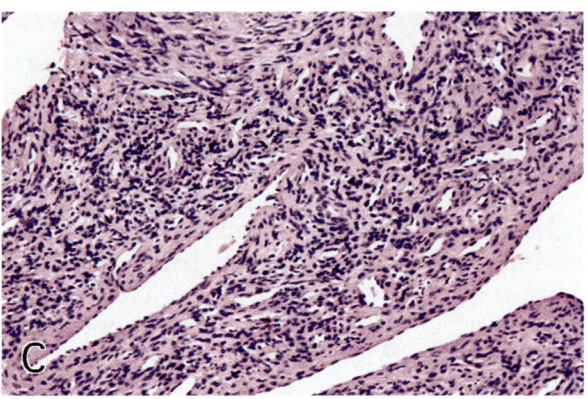
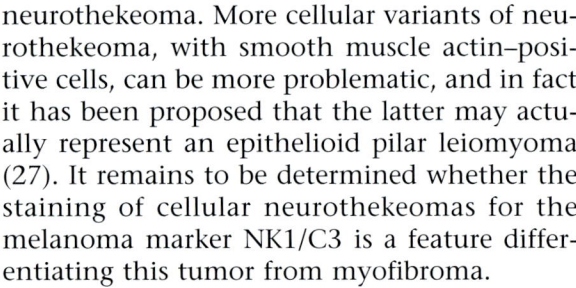

Figure 6-35

MYOFIBROMA

A: The biphasic nature of this tumor is evident in this low-power view.

B: One component consists of plump spindled cells within a somewhat mucinous stroma.

C: The second component consists of small polygonal to spindled cells and vessels, resembling hemangiopericytoma.

neurothekeoma. More cellular variants of neurothekeoma, with smooth muscle actin–positive cells, can be more problematic, and in fact it has been proposed that the latter may actually represent an epithelioid pilar leiomyoma (27). It remains to be determined whether the staining of cellular neurothekeomas for the melanoma marker NK1/C3 is a feature differentiating this tumor from myofibroma.

Juvenile Hyaline Fibromatosis

Clinical Features. *Juvenile hyaline fibromatosis* was first described at the end of the 19th century, but it is still considered extremely rare. The familial incidence and frequent consanguinity indicate a recessive inheritance. Numerous cutaneous nodules develop, particularly over the scalp, face, nose, ears, back, and extremities, beginning in the first few years of life. These lesions range from small, pearly papules to large, deforming (although painless) nodules (131). Other major manifestations include joint contractures and gingival hyperplasia. Muscle weakness (124) and osteolytic lesions (192) have been described.

A closely related condition, perhaps a variant of the disease, is *infantile systemic hyalinosis*. This consists of stiff skin, painful joint contractures, cutaneous papules and nodules, gingival hyperplasia, diarrhea, and failure to thrive (62,63). The nodular skin lesions are excised for cosmetic reasons or for functional improvement.

Pathologic Findings. Microscopic features include spindled cells, arranged singly and in cords, within an amorphous, eosinophilic (hyaline) matrix (fig. 6-36). Shrinkage artifact may produce clear spaces around these cells, creating a chondroid appearance. The cells are vimentin positive and alpha-smooth muscle actin and S-100 protein negative; they have the ultrastructural characteristics of fibroblasts (90,198).

Extensive investigations have been performed on the hyaline material. Electron microscopic studies demonstrate that it has a granular-fibrillar appearance (88), fills structures within fibroblasts, and is released into the extracellular space (198). The hyaline material is composed of glycosaminoglycans and type VI and, to a lesser extent, type I collagens, and lacks type III collagen (22,99,124). The glycosaminoglycans are

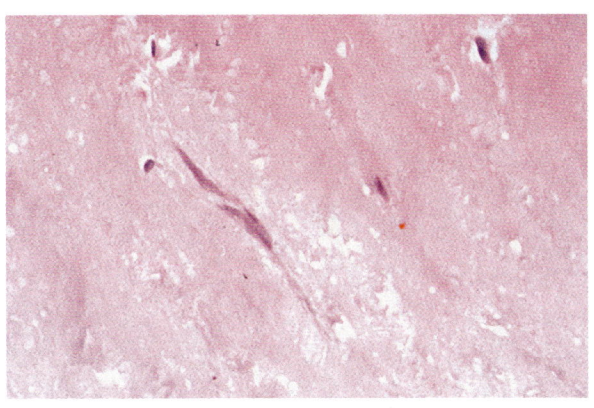

Figure 6-36

JUVENILE HYALINE FIBROMATOSIS

Spindled cells are present within an amorphous, eosinophilic matrix.

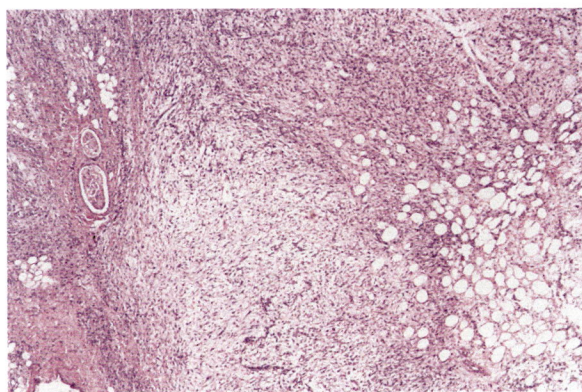

Figure 6-37

NODULAR FASCIITIS

This lesion involves the deep subcutis.

predominantly chondroitin sulfates A and C and dermatan sulfate, with lesser amounts of hyaluronate (90,99,135).

Differential Diagnosis. The cutaneous lesions of juvenile hyaline fibromatosis clinically resemble those of myofibromatosis, neurofibromatosis, multiple cylindromas, and some mucopolysaccharidoses, but other clinical features (gingival hyperplasia, joint contractures), and the microscopic findings of fibroblasts within a hyaline matrix, make juvenile hyaline fibromatosis unique.

Lipoid proteinosis is another recessively inherited disorder characterized by cutaneous papules and nodules (with tongue and vocal cord involvement) and by deposition of amorphous, hyaline material in the dermis. However, large deforming nodules and joint contractures, as seen in juvenile hyaline fibromatosis, are not typical, and the amorphous material consists of glycoprotein and hyaluronic acid. In addition, lesions of lipoid proteinosis are characterized by reduplication of basement membrane material and by a lack of proliferative fibroblasts.

Nodular Fasciitis

Clinical Features. *Nodular fasciitis* is a common tumor of superficial soft tissues, first described as such by Konwaler in 1955 (104a). It most commonly presents as a rapidly growing subcutaneous mass on the arm or forearm of a young adult. These lesions, however, can also arise on the head and neck, trunk, and lower extremities. Well-documented cases have been described in locations such as the orbital region (139,173), nasal cavity (74), and vulva (158). The incidence of nodular fasciitis drops off significantly beyond the age of 50 years, whereas related lesions, such as proliferative fasciitis, proliferative myositis, and intravascular fasciitis, tend to occur in an older age group (33,186). Lesions usually do not cause symptoms, although slight tenderness is sometimes reported; medical intervention is usually prompted by their rapid growth. Lesions may regress either spontaneously or following incomplete excision, and traditional excisional surgery is curative. In fact, recurrence of nodular fasciitis is sufficiently rare that such an event should prompt a review of the original diagnosis (16).

A clinical variant of this tumor is termed *cranial fasciitis*. This is a subcutaneous tumor of the scalp that arises in infants and children, and is capable of eroding the outer table of the skull or extending through the inner table and attaching to the dura mater (110). As is true of other examples of nodular fasciitis, cranial fasciitis pursues a benign clinical course, and is cured by excision, with or without curettage of the underlying bone (110,163).

Pathologic Findings. Typically, as the term implies, nodular fasciitis attaches to fascia and may extend into skeletal muscle or into the subcutis (fig. 6-37). Intradermal examples have been reported (108,166), and one of our cases of cranial fasciitis showed substantial dermal

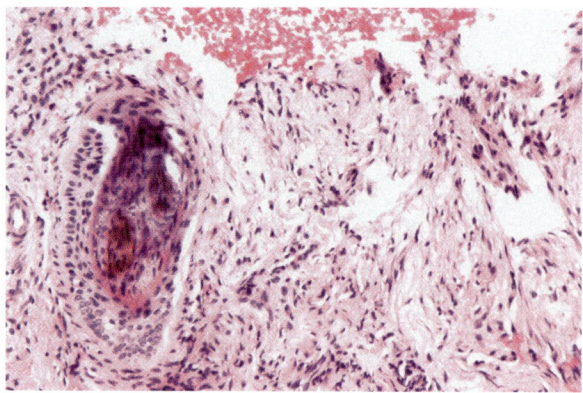

Figure 6-38

CRANIAL FASCIITIS

Spindled cells extend into the dermis and surround a follicular unit.

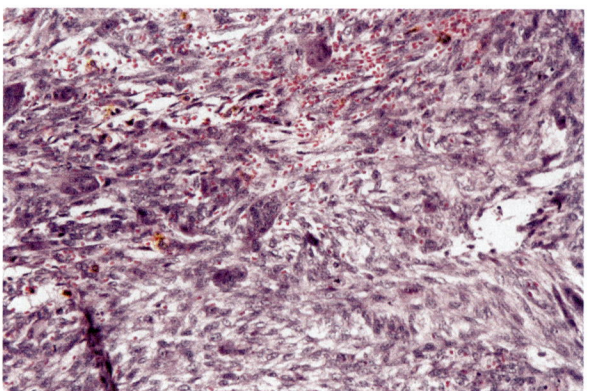

Figure 6-40

NODULAR FASCIITIS

At the periphery of this lesion are extravasated erythrocytes, a few inflammatory cells, and scattered multinucleated cells.

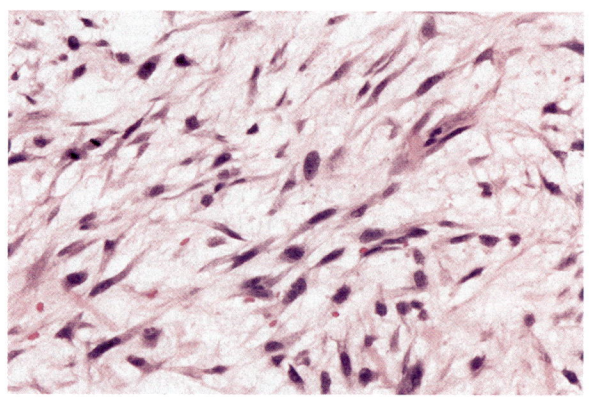

Figure 6-39

NODULAR FASCIITIS

The tumor is composed of elongated spindled cells that have a "tissue culture-like" appearance.

involvement (fig. 6-38) (163). It may be that some, if not all, of the latter cases could be designated postoperative/post-traumatic spindle cell nodules of the skin (227).

The lesion consists of large, elongated spindled cells that are often described as having a "tissue culture–like" appearance (fig. 6-39). The spindled cells are associated with a variably mucinous and vascular stroma, and erythrocyte extravasation may be prominent. Small, stellate to spindled multinucleated cells may be present (fig. 6-40). Mitoses are expected, but atypical mitotic figures are not seen. Osseous or cartilaginous metaplasia is sometimes observed (16,110). An inflammatory infiltrate often accompanies the process and tends to be concentrated at the periphery of the lesion (140). Older lesions are characterized by greater collagenization of the stroma (209).

Immunohistochemically, the cells comprising the tumor are positive for vimentin, alpha-1-antichymotrypsin, smooth muscle actin, and muscle-specific actin; desmin positivity has been reported (75,163). These results tend to confirm the ultrastructural findings in tumor cells (microfilaments with focal condensations, basal lamina–like material, desmosomes, pinocytotic vesicles) that indicate the presence of myofibroblasts (163,234).

Among the related lesions mentioned above (proliferative fasciitis, proliferative myositis, and intravascular fasciitis), special mention should be made of proliferative fasciitis. This lesion closely resembles nodular fasciitis clinically, with the exception of a somewhat older age of incidence, and since it can definitely involve the subcutis, it does fall within the purview of the dermatopathologist. Microscopically, in addition to other features of nodular fasciitis, it possesses bizarre basophilic giant cells that resemble ganglion cells. Nevertheless, these lesions respond well to local excision (33).

Differential Diagnosis. Nodular fasciitis must be distinguished from fibrosarcoma and malignant fibrous histiocytoma. In addition to its characteristic superficial location and rapid

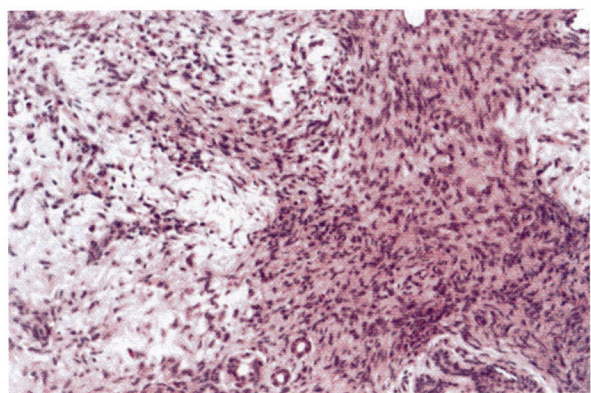 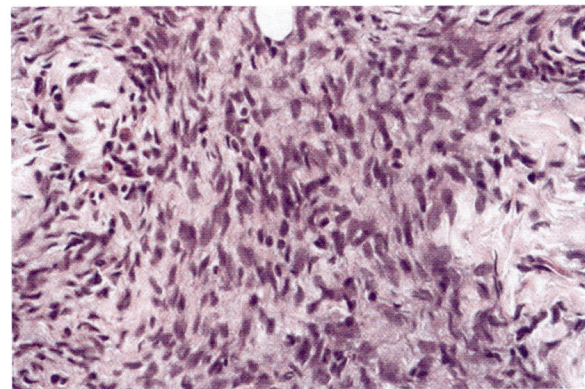

Figure 6-41

SOLITARY FIBROUS TUMOR

Left: Spindled cells are arranged in short fascicles or in a "patternless pattern."
Right: The constituent spindled cells have a generally bland appearance.

growth, nodular fasciitis lacks the dense cellularity, herring-bone pattern, and marked mitotic activity expected in fibrosarcoma or the marked pleomorphism of malignant fibrous histiocytoma. The interconnecting fascicles of bland-appearing fibroblasts, dense collagen, and pronounced skeletal muscle infiltration associated with forms of fibromatosis help to distinguish this group of lesions from nodular fasciitis. Deep fibrous histiocytomas can often be distinguished by whorled or "curlicue" arrangements of cells, dense collagen, and sometimes by the presence of hemosiderin, lipid-containing macrophages, and Touton-like giant cells.

FIBROUS TISSUE TUMORS OF INTERMEDIATE MALIGNANCY

Solitary Fibrous Tumor

Clinical Features. *Solitary fibrous tumor* was first reported by Klemperer and Rabin in 1931 (313). It has been well known to surgical pathologists as a tumor of the pleura or peritoneum that must be distinguished from mesothelioma. In recent years it has been reported in a variety other organs, including the orbit, oral mucosa, soft tissue, and skin, and therefore may be encountered by dermatopathologists. Skin lesions have presented as nodules in the head and neck region (264,297,336), which may become painful (264). Most patients with solitary fibrous tumor, both in skin and elsewhere, are middle-aged to older adults, but we have observed one case in an infant. Large pleural lesions may produce pulmonary symptoms or hypertrophic osteoarthropathy (278), and hypoglycemia occurs in a few cases as the result of secretion of insulin-like growth factors (290). These symptoms have not been reported in patients with cutaneous lesions.

Classically, the solitary fibrous tumor is benign, responding well to excision or wedge resection in the case of pleural tumors. Recurrence or metastasis can occur, however, particularly among those tumors with malignant histopathologic features. One study suggests that similar aggressive behavior can be expected among atypical extrathoracic tumors (364). Of the few cases thus far reported in skin, one occipital lesion invaded the underlying calvaria, but responded to local excision with no recurrence in 6 months of follow-up (264).

Pathologic Findings. Solitary fibrous tumors are well circumscribed (257,258,264) and found in the dermis and subcutis. They are composed of spindled cells that are best known for forming a "patternless pattern" (297), although the cells may also be arranged in short fascicles or storiform configurations (fig. 6-41, left) (264). Cellular areas are interspersed with zones of thick, hyalinized collagen or, occasionally, with myxoid foci (257,258,297,336). Vessels may be numerous, and may take on "staghorn" contours, thereby mimicking hemangiopericytoma (258,264,297,336). Mast cells are not frequent in solitary fibrous tumors (264). The constituent spindled cells usually have a bland appearance (fig. 6-41, right), and mitotic figures are rare. Malignant variants do occur, although they have not yet been reported in skin. These tumors feature increased cellularity, pleomorphism, and mitotic activity. Greater than 4 mitoses per 10 high-power fields has been used as a criterion to define malignant solitary fibrous tumors (370).

Immunohistochemical staining regularly shows CD34 expression by spindled cells, and this feature has come to represent part of the definition of solitary fibrous tumor (258,264, 297,336). Vimentin is also usually positive (258). Staining for bcl-2 protein is also frequently observed (279). Interspersed dermal dendritic cells are factor XIIIa positive (264). Staining for desmin is usually negative, and negative results are obtained when staining for cytokeratins and epithelial membrane antigen (264). Electron microscopy shows cells with fibroblastic and myofibroblastic features (257).

Differential Diagnosis. The differential diagnosis includes a variety of spindle cell neoplasms. Hemangiopericytoma shares with solitary fibrous tumor both a similar morphology and immunohistochemistry, suggesting that these could be variants of the same entity (264). The type of spindled cells, however, as well as their arrangement in solitary fibrous tumor differ from those of classic hemangiopericytoma. In contrast to solitary fibrous tumor, hemangiopericytomas lack hyalinized collagen and do contain mast cells (264). Dermatofibromas (fibrous histiocytomas) often feature epidermal hyperplasia and xanthomatization, and CD34 expression is typically either absent or focal. Dermatofibrosarcoma protuberans is poorly circumscribed, usually has a distinctive storiform pattern, and lacks either thick, hyalinized collagen or prominent vasculature. The cells of monophasic synovial sarcoma express cytokeratins and epithelial membrane antigen, in contrast to solitary fibrous tumor. Spindle cell lipoma is potentially a close mimic of solitary fibrous tumor, as has been discussed in recently published correspondence (354). Features of spindle cell lipoma that differ from those of solitary fibrous tumor include overwhelming occurrence in middle-aged to elderly men, location on the posterior neck or shoulder, interspersed mature lipocytes, and numerous mast cells (354).

Dermatofibrosarcoma Protuberans

Clinical Features. *Dermatofibrosarcoma protuberans* (DFSP) is widely regarded as a subcutaneous fibrous tissue tumor of intermediate malignancy because of its slow but relentless growth, tissue infiltration, tendency to recur, and uncommon but well-documented ability to metastasize. It most commonly presents as an indurated plaque with one or more cutaneous nodules. These nodules represent a "tip of the iceberg" phenomenon, as they are accompanied by often extensive subcutaneous growth. An atrophic variant has also been described (376).

Lesions most commonly arise on the trunk or proximal extremities, but they also develop on the scalp, neck, face, and distal extremities. They occur most often in young to middle-aged adults, but children may be affected. The tumor has a male predominance, but this is not sufficiently striking to be diagnostically useful. Vulvar involvement has repeatedly been described, and accelerated growth of DFSP during pregnancy is a known phenomenon (341).

Metastasis has been estimated to occur in 3 percent of cases (253), in which case there may be involvement of lymph nodes or hematogenous dissemination, especially to the lungs (308). Treatment traditionally consists of wide local excision, but as mentioned, recurrences are frequent. Considerable therapeutic success (with lower recurrence rates) has been obtained with the use of micrographic surgery (293,340).

Pathologic Findings. DFSPs have characteristic patterns of subcutaneous infiltration, including growth within septa and between lipocytes in a honeycomb configuration or in a horizontally layered arrangement, parallel to the epidermal surface (fig. 6-42, left) (309,376). Lateral extension of tumor beyond the dermal component may be extensive, and later in the development of a lesion, fascia and muscle may be infiltrated. This growth pattern explains the difficulty of obtaining tumor-free margins in many cases. The overlying epidermis may be normal, thinned, or ulcerated, but acanthosis can also occur; the latter change appears to be inversely related to the proximity of the spindle cell proliferation to the epidermis (262).

DFSP is characterized by a dense proliferation of spindled cells, notable for their monotony, that tend to form storiform or "cartwheel"

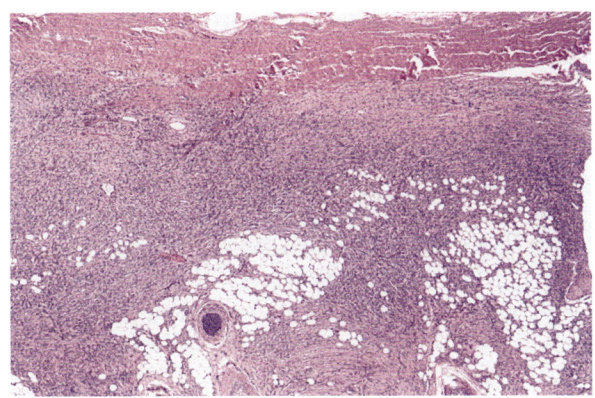
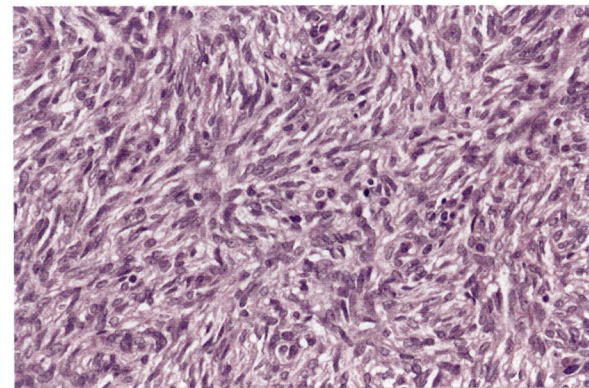

Figure 6-42

DERMATOFIBROSARCOMA PROTUBERANS

Left: Horizontally layered tumor in the subcutis.
Right: Slender tumor cells form a "cartwheel" arrangement.

arrangements (360). The constituent cells are slender, with tapered nuclei that, at most, are only moderately enlarged (fig. 6-42, right). Occasional mitoses are present, but they tend not to be numerous, and atypical forms are not usually observed. These changes are sufficiently characteristic to permit diagnosis by fine-needle aspiration cytology in appropriate circumstances (283). Polarizable collagen is not present within the stroma of these tumors (247). Myxoid changes can be present and are sometimes extensive (fig. 6-43). Our experience and that of numerous other investigators has been that myxoid change is most often seen in recurrent tumors (254,338,349), but such changes can apparently also be encountered in primary tumors (285). Replacement of tumor cells by fibrotic tissue has been described, and this may represent a kind of regression phenomenon (272).

Although monotony of the cellular proliferation is usually the hallmark of DFSP, other findings can occasionally be encountered, including multinucleated giant cells, areas resembling giant cell fibroblastoma, hypercellular zones (353), and myoid or myofibroblastic differentiation (259,332,346). The latter changes have been observed in examples of the tumor showing fibrosarcoma-like areas (see below). In the cases reported by Sanz-Trelles et al. (346), the smooth muscle proliferation may have originated in vessel walls and was at times sufficiently extensive to form nodules resembling leiomyoma. The relationship between DFSP and giant cell fibro-

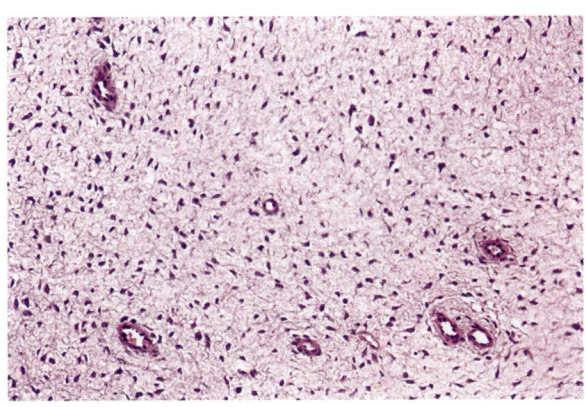

Figure 6-43

DERMATOFIBROSARCOMA PROTUBERANS

Myxoid changes are shown here, although other areas were more typical for this tumor. This was a recurrent lesion.

blastoma and the Bednar tumor (pigmented dermatofibrosarcoma protuberans) is considered in the sections pertaining to those disorders.

It is important to examine the lesion for the presence of fibrosarcoma-like areas. These foci are characterized by a fascicular arrangement of tumor cells that are larger and more atypical than those ordinarily seen in DFSP (fig. 6-44). There is ample evidence in the literature that lesions with these changes are prone to local recurrence and metastasis (273,302,335,349). There has been a recent report of a *fibrosarcomatous DFSP with giant rosettes* (373). These rosettes resemble those of another tumor that has been

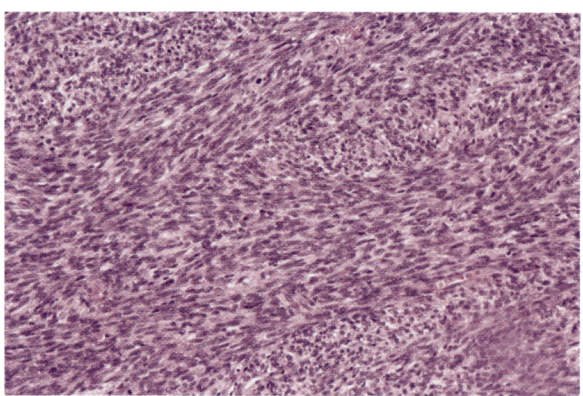

Figure 6-44

DERMATOFIBROSARCOMA PROTUBERANS

The fibrosarcoma-like area shows larger tumor cells than those seen in figure 6-42, in a fascicular arrangement.

designated hyalinizing spindle cell tumor with giant rosettes (316), which may in turn be closely related to the low-grade fibromyxoid sarcoma (see below) (288). There has also been one report of progression of DFSP to malignant fibrous histiocytoma (333).

The immunohistochemical hallmark of DFSP is the CD34 positivity that is almost always (although not invariably) present among tumor cells (303). Factor XIIIa has been reported to be positive in some cases (294), but not in others (303,376). Its occasional presence has been suggested to represent dermal dendrocytes entrapped by the tumor (294). In the case of DFSP with giant rosettes, the latter structures are also CD34 positive (373). Smooth muscle markers, such as smooth muscle actin and muscle-specific actin, are positive in those cases showing myoid or myofibroblastic differentiation (259,332).

Expression of mutant p53 protein has been identified in DFSP (270,302,347), and overexpression of this protein has been identified in examples of the tumor with fibrosarcoma areas (302). The Mib-1 labeling index (a proliferation marker measuring Ki-67 antigen expression) is higher in DFSP than in dermatofibroma, and is higher still in recurrent tumors (347). There does not appear to be a correlation between Mib-1 staining and mutant p53 expression (270,347). Fusion of the *COL1A1* (collagen) gene to the *PDGFβ* (platelet-derived growth factor-beta chain) gene has been repeatedly described and is considered a characteristic genetic marker of DFSP (331).

Differential Diagnosis. A frequent differential diagnostic consideration is dermatofibroma, and particularly the deep variant that is sometimes termed deep penetrating dermatofibroma. These lesions may demonstrate increased cellularity and a somewhat storiform arrangement of tumor cells. Dermatofibromas most often show a degree of overlying acanthosis that is usually lacking in DFSP. Acanthosis is sometimes identified in the latter tumor, but it has a different character than that of dermatofibroma, as elongation of rete ridges and a lack of basilar hypermelanosis are more often encountered in DFSP (262). Hemorrhage, lipidization, hemosiderin deposition, and formation of Touton-like giant cells are characteristic of dermatofibroma and can be diagnostic when present. The subcutaneous growth pattern for dermatofibroma is different from that of DFSP, in that dermatofibromas tend to show vertical growth along septa or smooth, bulging protrusions into the subcutis, rather than the honeycomb or horizontally layered configuration of DFSP (309,371,376). Polarizable collagen is usually identifiable in dermatofibromas but not in the stroma of DFSP (247). Immunohistochemical staining provides another means of differentiation, since in contrast to most dermatofibromas, DFSPs are CD34 positive and factor XIIIa negative. However, it should be recognized that CD34 staining is sometimes present in dermatofibromas, and cells within DFSP may express factor XIIIa (294,303). Mutant p53 protein is often observed in DFSP (270), particularly in lesions with fibrosarcoma-like areas (302) or those with aneuploidy and elevated proliferative activity as assessed by Mib-1 staining (347). Mib-1 staining may be comparable in primary DFSP and dermatofibroma, but a higher Mib-1 labeling index is associated with recurrent DFSP (347).

Incomplete sampling of DFSP with myoid differentiation may lead to an erroneous diagnosis of myofibroma (259). Similar sampling errors could lead to diagnoses of fibrosarcoma or, less commonly, malignant fibrous histiocytoma, but on the other hand, the finding of areas with these features in a DFSP should raise concern that one is dealing with a sarcoma with metastatic potential. In contrast to DFSP, neurofibromas feature scattered small cells with buckled or "S-shaped" nuclei, associated nerve elements, and S-100 protein positivity. The myxoid variant of DFSP resembles other myxoid tumors, including myxoid liposarcoma, but its superficial location, lack of lipoblasts, and S-100 protein negativity argue against the latter possibility. In addition, a history of recurrent tumor should raise the possibility of DFSP, and a review of previous biopsy material and careful search for more characteristic cellular, storiform foci will often lead to the correct diagnosis.

Bednar's Tumor (Pigmented Dermatofibrosarcoma Protuberans)

Clinical Features. First reported by Bednar in 1957 (250) as pigmented storiform neurofibroma, the tumor that bears his name is now widely regarded as a pigmented variant of DFSP, since except for the pigment cell component, it has nearly identical clinical and histopathologic features. *Bednar's tumor* represents up to 5 percent of total DFSP cases (256,275,286,344). As might be expected, it has a similar age of incidence, with most cases occurring during the third and fourth decades of life. These tumors also develop in infancy and childhood (306, 321). One paper suggested that the lesions occur predominantly in black individuals (275). Like DFSP, Bednar's tumor most commonly arises on the trunk, with the remainder of cases about equally distributed among upper and lower extremities and head and neck (275). One study suggested that the recurrence rate for these tumors is somewhat lower than for other DFSPs (274); nevertheless, recurrences have been reported, including one tumor that recurred after 23 years (326). Although uncommon, metastases and death have occurred (256,337). The usual treatment is wide local excision.

Pathologic Findings. As is true of DFSP, Bednar's tumor may have an exophytic, multinodular appearance but diffusely infiltrates the deep dermis and subcutis. It is composed of spindled cells that form storiform or cartwheel-like arrangements. In addition, there are scattered dendritic cells that contain melanin pigment (fig. 6-45). These typically comprise about 1 to 5 percent of the total tumor cell population in a lesion (256). Fibrosarcoma-like areas can be identified and have been associated with metastasizing lesions (256,337).

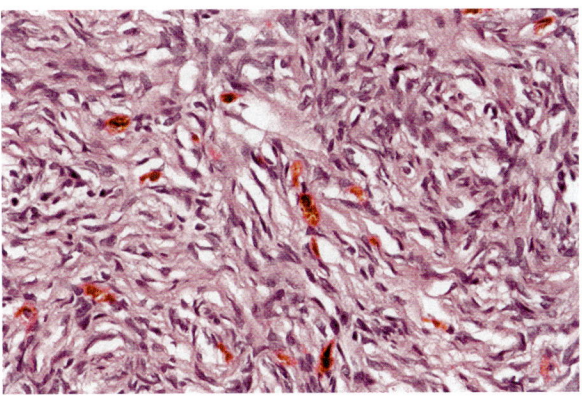

Figure 6-45

BEDNAR'S TUMOR

There are spindled cells in a storiform arrangement as well as scattered, pigment-containing dendritic cells.

Immunohistochemical staining shows that, as is the case in DFSP, the predominating spindled cells are CD34 positive (276,307,314,326). They are also vimentin positive but are negative for S-100 protein, HMB45, and neuron-specific enolase (307,314). The pigmented dendritic cells are positive for S-100 protein, vimentin, and neuron-specific enolase (307,314,327) and in one study were HMB45 negative (274). Kagoura et al. (307) found a population of factor XIIIa-positive cells around the melanin-containing cells.

Ultrastructurally, the features of the predominating cells are those of fibroblasts (274,275). The pigmented cells contain mainly stage IV but also stage II melanosomes (274,275,307) and are invested by basement membrane material (275,327). These findings have led to the conclusion that the pigmented cells are probably non-neoplastic melanocytes, and that a Bednar tumor is most likely not a tumor of neuroectodermal differentiation (274,286). The source of the melanocytic component of the tumor is still in doubt, although origin from the overlying epidermis has been suggested (286).

Differential Diagnosis. A Bednar tumor with heavy pigmentation may be confused with cellular blue nevus, but the former tumor is more storiform, more infiltrative, and not prone to forming cellular islands, and the nonpigmented component is CD34 positive and S-100 protein negative. A true pigmented neurofibroma also exists, but unlike Bednar's tumor it is less

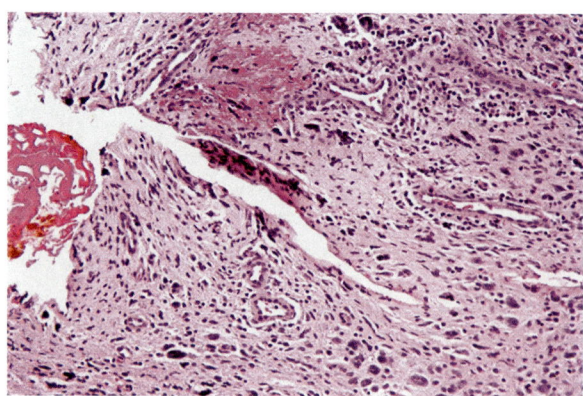
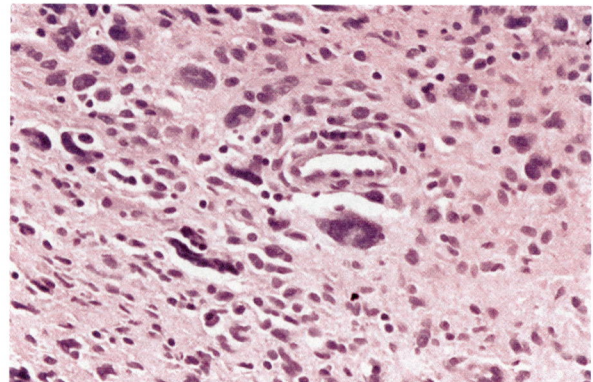

Figure 6-46

GIANT CELL FIBROBLASTOMA

Left: Sinusoidal spaces are surrounded by spindled cells and multinucleated giant cells.

Right: High-power view shows "multinucleated" cells. On ultrastructural study, these cells actually possess single, multilobated nuclei.

storiform, more apt to have prominent nerve elements, shows a lesser degree of CD34 positivity, and displays diffuse S-100 protein–positive Schwann cells (282).

Giant Cell Fibroblastoma

Clinical Features. Another tumor that is widely regarded as a variant of DFSP is *giant cell fibroblastoma*, first described by Shmookler in 1982 (351). This tumor arises mostly in children under the age of 5 years, but it is reported infrequently in adults. There is a male predominance among patients. It presents as a painless mass in the dermis and subcutis, mainly in the thigh, inguinal region, or chest. Recurrences are frequent, but metastases of pure examples of the tumor have not been reported (351).

Pathologic Findings. There are proliferations of spindled cells, of varying density, that in some areas resemble DFSP. Other areas may be less cellular, with a myxoid or hyaline stroma (351). However, the most characteristic features are sinusoidal (angiectoid) spaces lined by spindled cells and mononucleated or "multinucleated" giant cells (fig. 6-46) (248,271,351,353). On ultrastructural examination, the multinucleated cells in reality are multilobated single nuclei (351). Immunohistochemical studies show that tumor cells are CD34 and vimentin positive (271,298,369). They are negative for desmin, myoglobin, S-100 protein, neurofilaments, factor VIII, and for *Ulex europaeus* binding (284).

A relationship between giant cell fibroblastoma and DFSP has long been suspected, and in fact this tumor has been considered to be a juvenile variant of DFSP (351). Over the years, evidence has accumulated that lends strong support to this relationship. In addition to the CD34 positivity that these tumors share (369), there are reports of DFSP with foci of giant cell fibroblastoma (fig. 6-47) (251,298,353), and of giant cell fibroblastoma with DFSP areas (310,324). In addition, DFSP has recurred as a giant cell fibroblastoma (265), and giant cell fibroblastoma has recurred as DFSP (269,298). The association of these two tumors is well documented but not necessarily common, as indicated by studies such as that of Connelly and Evans (263), in which 75 DFSPs failed to reveal any areas of giant cell fibroblastoma. Both tumors have demonstrated cytogenetic abnormalities involving chromosomes 17 and 22, resulting in fusion of the *COL1A1* and *PDGFβ* genes (266,366). The occurrence of foci resembling giant cell fibroblastoma in other tumors, such as giant cell angiofibroma (356) and hemangiopericytoma (310), suggests that this change may reflect a peculiar host response to tumor rather than a specific clinicopathologic entity (310).

Differential Diagnosis. The distinctive features of giant cell fibroblastoma, particularly the sinusoidal spaces lined by giant cells, together with CD34 positivity, usually allow an accurate diagnosis. Reports of foci of giant cell

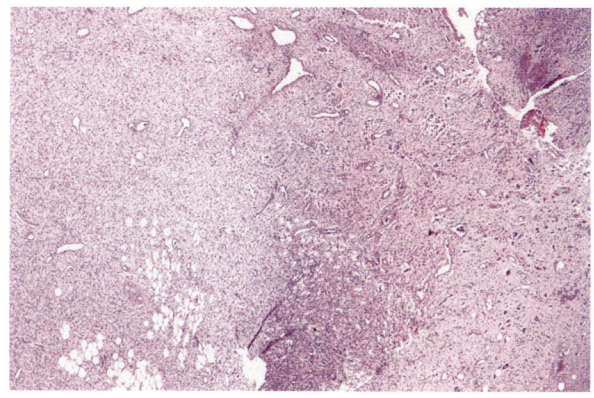

Figure 6-47

DERMATOFIBROSARCOMA PROTUBERANS WITH FOCUS OF GIANT CELL FIBROBLASTOMA

DFSP occupies the left side of the figure. There is a focus of giant cell fibroblastoma on the right.

fibroblastoma in other lesions, such as giant cell angiofibroma and hemangiopericytoma, indicate that these changes are found, rarely, in other tumors. The combination of the characteristic histopathologic features and relatively superficial location of giant cell fibroblastoma should permit distinction from soft tissue sarcomas such as myxoid liposarcoma or malignant fibrous histiocytoma.

Aggressive Angiomyxoma, Superficial Angiomyxoma, and Angiomyofibroblastoma

These entities are considered as a group because they may have overlapping clinical, morphologic, and immunohistochemical features (367,368), although typical examples of each do have distinguishing characteristics that tend to correlate with biologic behavior.

Clinical Features. *Aggressive angiomyxoma* was first reported as such in 1983 by Steeper and Rosai (359). It is best known as a tumor of the genital and perineal region of women (359), but examples have also been reported in men, in whom they often present as scrotal lesions (304). This is a slow-growing, infiltrative tumor that is difficult to excise completely and has a notoriously high recurrence rate (359), although metastasis is rarely reported (352).

Although *superficial angiomyxomas* may also arise in the genital region (281), they demonstrate a much more widespread anatomic distribution, with most examples presenting as papules, nodules, or polypoid lesions on the trunk, extremities, or head and neck (245,249, 260). There is a male predominance, and recurrences are much less common than is the case for their aggressive counterparts.

Angiomyofibroblastoma was delineated as an entity in 1992 by Fletcher et al. (287). These lesions typically present as vulvar masses that are often mistaken for Bartholin cysts (287,291, 365). Cases involving the scrotum have also been reported in men (355,374). Angiomyofibroblastoma is typically described as a well-circumscribed tumor that generally does not recur following excision (287,291,317).

Pathologic Findings. In aggressive angiomyxoma, widely scattered spindled to stellate cells are present within a loose myxoid stroma (fig. 6-48A), with focal abundance of collagen fibrils. There is a prominent vascular component composed of thick-walled, hyalinized vessels (fig. 6-48B). Cytologic atypia is minimal and mitotic activity is typically low (259). Bundles of cells with smooth muscle features may be identified, particularly adjacent to vessels (fig. 6-48C) (296). The stromal cells are vimentin positive; in several studies, they have also been found to express desmin and smooth muscle actin (296,357). Ultrastructural studies have shown cells with features of fibroblasts, smooth muscle cells, and myofibroblasts (357, 359). The stromal cells of aggressive angiomyxoma are estrogen receptor and progesterone receptor positive, although positivity is also seen among stromal cells in fibroepithelial polyps, smooth muscle tumors, nerve sheath tumors, and normal vulvar skin (322).

Superficial angiomyxomas are poorly circumscribed or multinodular, with at least focally lobular outlines (260). Scattered spindled cells and small blood vessels are present within a myxoid stroma (fig. 6-49). Cellularity is variable, and occasional multinucleated giant cells are identified (249), but cytologic atypia is minimal and mitotic figures are rare (260). A mixed inflammatory infiltrate with a neutrophilic component is also present (260). In about 20 to 30 percent of cases, an epithelial component is present, consisting of epidermal (infundibular) cysts, narrow epithelial strands, or basilar buds (245,260). Immunohistochemical studies have shown that stromal cells are vimentin and, at

Figure 6-48

AGGRESSIVE ANGIOMYXOMA

A: Widely scattered spindled cells are within a loose myxoid stroma.
B: Vascular component of the tumor.
C: Adjacent to vessels are bundles of cells resembling smooth muscle.

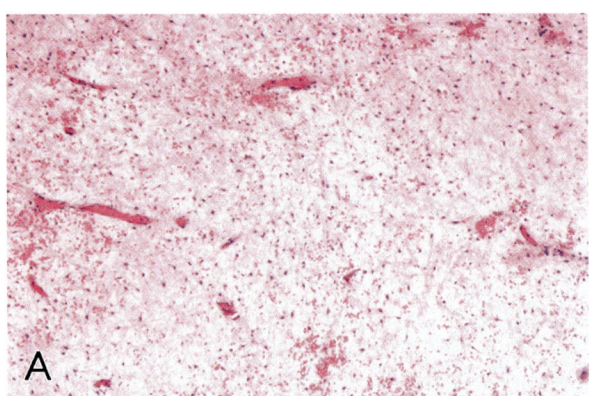

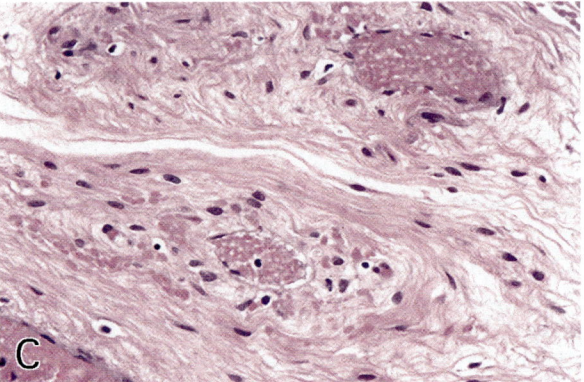

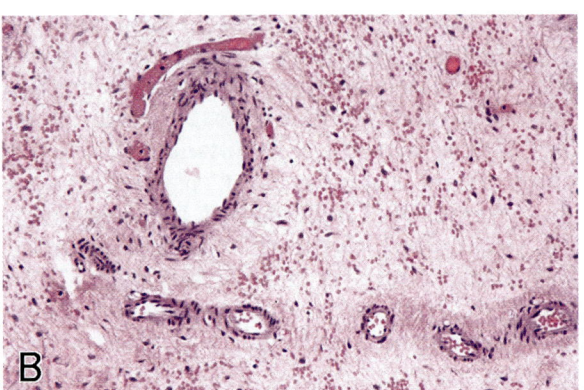

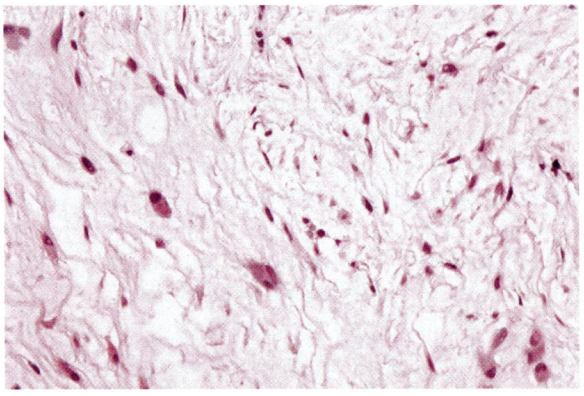

Figure 6-49

SUPERFICIAL ANGIOMYXOMA

Scattered spindled cells are present within a myxoid stroma. A few larger cells can also be seen, including one binucleate cell.

least focally, CD34 positive, but are S-100 protein, cytokeratin, and desmin negative (245,249, 260,281,368). Staining for smooth muscle actin has been negative in most studies (249,260, 368), however, Fetsch et al. (281) demonstrated muscle-specific actin and smooth muscle actin positivity in a number of cases; factor XIIIa was positive in about half of the cases. Staining for estrogen and progesterone receptors was negative in the one study that investigated this issue (281). Fibroblasts are identified on ultrastructural examination of these tumors (245).

Angiomyofibroblastomas are usually described as well-circumscribed lesions. They feature alternating hypercellular and hypocellular areas, and abundant, thin-walled blood vessels. The cells comprising the tumor are spindled, ovoid, or epithelioid, and tend to be arranged in clusters or concentrated around the blood vessels (fig. 6-50A), although they are also loosely scattered within hypocellular areas (287,291,301,317,330, 334). An adipose component is often identified within the tumor (291,317,330). Cytologic atypia is minimal, and mitotic activity is low (fig. 6-50B) (287,330). Numerous immunohistochemical studies have been performed. Tumor cells commonly express vimentin and desmin (287, 317,330), and there are reports of positivity for CD34 (317,330,348). Actin positivity is less common (317), and staining for S-100 protein and

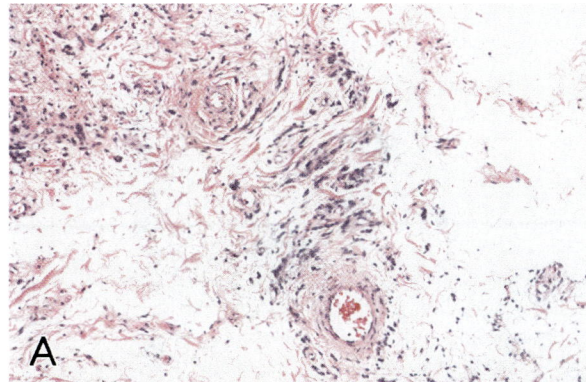
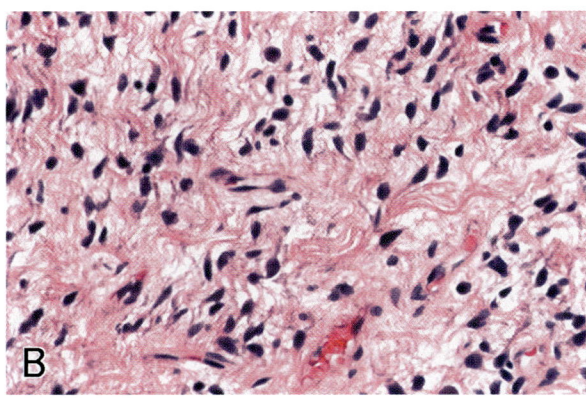
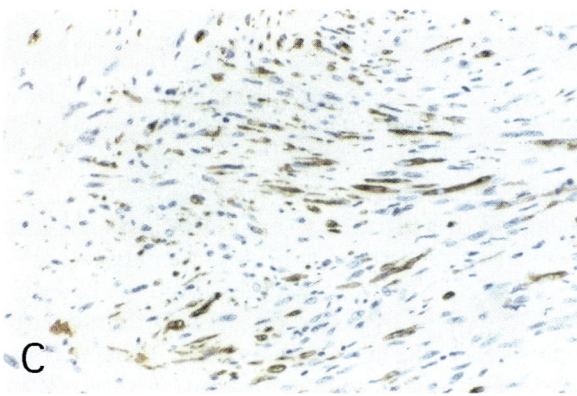

Figure 6-50

ANGIOMYOFIBROBLASTOMA

A: This view shows hypocellular and hypercellular areas. Cells comprising the tumor are clustered or concentrated around blood vessels.

B: The constituent cells are spindled to ovoid and display minimal cytologic atypia.

C: The tumor cells are estrogen receptor positive.

cytokeratin is negative. The cells are estrogen receptor and progesterone receptor positive (fig. 6-50C) (317,334,348,355). On DNA analysis, tumors have been both diploid and aneuploid (291,348), and in a study of one case, Ki-67 labeling was less than 1 percent (348). Electron microscopy has shown evidence of myoid or myofibroblastic differentiation (287,301,330,334).

Differential Diagnosis. It is apparent from the foregoing that there are significant similarities among these three tumors (368). In particular, it has been repeatedly suggested that aggressive angiomyxoma and angiomyofibroblastoma are closely related, perhaps representing parts of a spectrum of myoid or myofibroblastic tumors (296,334,355,357,374). Superficial angiomyxomas can often be distinguished from the other two lesions because of their frequent occurrence outside of the genital/perineal region, their multinodularity, the abundance of mucin and low cellularity, and the absence of a perivascular arrangement of stromal cells (368). In addition, the association with epithelial proliferations in up to 30 percent of cases is distinctive. The histopathologic differential diagnosis for superficial angiomyxoma, therefore, often includes cutaneous lesions that combine mucin deposition with epithelial proliferation, such as trichogenic myxoma, trichodiscoma, and myxoid perifollicular fibromas, in addition to traditional focal mucinosis (245,260).

Despite a probable histogenetic relationship, there is value in distinguishing angiomyofibroblastoma from aggressive angiomyxoma, since the incidence of recurrence is much less in the former lesion. In contrast to aggressive angiomyxoma, angiomyofibroblastoma shows better circumscription, greater cellularity, increased numbers of vessels without hyalinization, plump stromal cells that tend to surround vessels, and minimal mucin deposition (287,368). The overlapping immunohistochemical profiles of these two tumors suggests that this approach is of limited value in terms of differential diagnosis. A report of CD44 expression in an aggressive angiomyxoma and weak expression of this antigen in angiomyofibroblastoma is intriguing, however, since this hyaluronate receptor may facilitate migration of neoplastic cells, and therefore explain in part the more

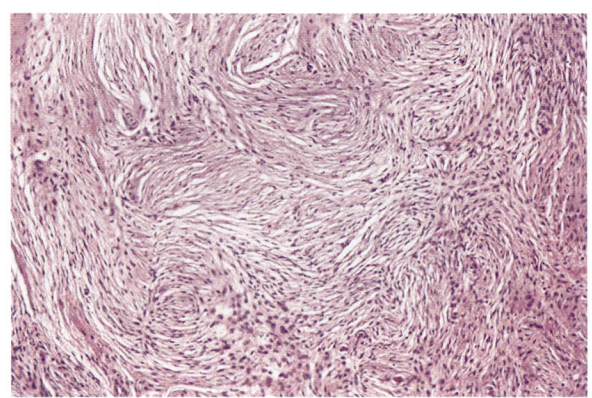 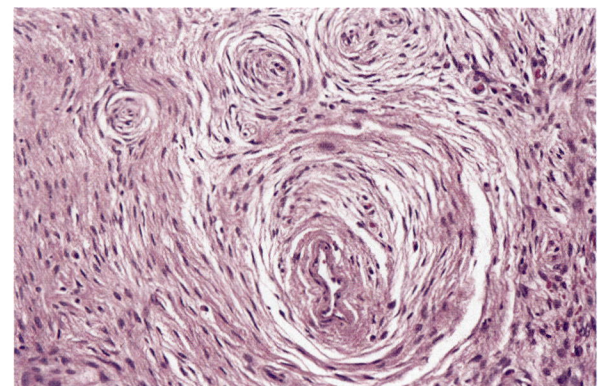

Figure 6-51
LOW-GRADE FIBROMYXOID SARCOMA
Left: Slender spindled cells are arranged in a storiform fashion.
Right: In this view, spindled cells are observed to form cuffs around vessels.

aggressive biologic behavior of angiomyxoma (255). Further studies to evaluate CD44 expression in these tumors would be worthwhile.

Aggressive angiomyxoma should also be differentiated from other myxoid soft tissue tumors. Myxoid leiomyomas differ in that they possess interlacing smooth muscle cells (328) that are desmin and actin positive, and have a less prominent vascular component. Careful review of the morphology and immunohistochemistry should permit distinction from soft tissue sarcomas such as myxoid liposarcoma and myxoid malignant fibrous histiocytoma.

Low-Grade Fibromyxoid Sarcoma

Clinical Features. *Low-grade fibromyxoid sarcoma* (LGFMS) is a rare tumor of deep soft tissues that may involve the subcutis. It arises most commonly in young adults, and is seen on the trunk (especially the axilla and chest wall) and lower extremities. Tumors have also been reported on the arm, neck, groin, small bowel mesentery, and retroperitoneum (279, 295,350,375). Recurrences are frequent, and there may be metastasis, particularly to lung (279) and bone (350). Although metastasis and death do occur, relatively long survival periods are possible even in the face of recurrent or metastatic disease (279). Wide local excision is the usual treatment; this has sometimes been supplemented by radiation therapy (350).

Pathologic Findings: LGFMS is composed of foci of myxoid and fibrous tissue with a sweeping, whorled growth pattern (279,329,375). The cells comprising the tumor are slender and spindled, sometimes arranged in storiform (fig. 6-51, left) or linear fashion, or forming cuffs around vessels (fig. 6-51, right) (279,329). These cells usually lack significant pleomorphism and mitotic activity is low, although a greater degree of pleomorphism may be noted in recurrent tumors (279). The vascularity of these tumors is variable, but there may be numerous delicate capillaries, either within myxoid foci or scattered throughout the tumor (279,350).

With immunohistochemical staining, the stromal cells are most consistently positive for vimentin (292,295,329,362), and there are sporadic reports of positivity for CD34 (329), actin, and desmin (292,295). Tumor cells are typically negative for epithelial, neural, histiocytic, melanocytic, or vascular markers (292,329,362). Ultrastructurally, the cells have the characteristics of fibroblasts (295,318,362). One reported case showed a diploid DNA content with S-phase fraction of 6.6 percent (292), while another demonstrated DNA tetraploidy and high proliferative activity as indicated by Ki-67 staining (350). A ring chromosome was detected in a case of LGFMS, a feature previously described in other low-grade malignancies of soft tissue and bone (323).

LGFMS may be closely related to another tumor that has been designated *hyalinizing spindle cell tumor with giant rosettes* (316). As is true of LGFMS, the latter tumor occurs in soft tissues of the trunk and lower extremities in young to middle-aged adults, and consists of bland spindled cells in a myxoid or hyalinized stroma. In addition, it features large rosette-like structures that contain a central collagen core and a rim of rounded cells with different immunohistochemical characteristics (S-100 protein, neuron-specific enolase, and leu-22 positive). As additional evidence of a link between these tumors, rosettes can occasionally be encountered in otherwise typical LGFMS (288), and a case of metastasizing LGFMS has been reported in which the pulmonary metastasis had the features of hyalinizing spindle cell tumor with giant rosettes (323). A small percentage of both tumors show nuclear enlargement, hyperchromasia, necrosis, and mitotic activity, and both can metastasize, although the evidence thus far does not indicate that the presence of atypical histologic foci necessarily portends an adverse outcome in the short term (288).

Differential Diagnosis. The combination of clinical, histopathologic, and immunohistochemical features usually allows distinction of LGFMS from other cutaneous or soft tissue tumors (295,329). In particular, adequate sampling should permit differentiation from myxomas or other myxoid sarcomas, a potential pitfall with techniques such as fine-needle aspiration cytology (318). CD34-positive examples could also be confused with myxoid DFSP, although the latter tumor lacks the distinctive perivascular cuffing of slender spindled cells.

Atypical Fibroxanthoma

Clinical Features. First described by Helwig in 1963 (299), *atypical fibroxanthoma* (AFX) is a cutaneous mesenchymal tumor that histopathologically closely resembles the more aggressive soft tissue tumor, malignant fibrous histiocytoma. AFX typically arises in the sun-exposed skin of the head and neck region in elderly individuals. Development on the trunk or extremities is uncommon. We have seen only a few such cases, one of which arose on the arm in the repeatedly blistered and scarred skin of an adult patient with recessive dystrophic epidermolysis bullosa. It was once believed that AFX had a bimodal distribution, with a second peak incidence in younger patients who had lesions on the extremities. Occurrence of AFX in young patients is rare, however, in the absence of unusual predisposing factors, such as xeroderma pigmentosum (one of the authors reported such a case on the face of a 3-year-old [342]). It is likely that most cases reported on the extremities of young persons are actually atypical variants of dermatofibroma (fibrous histiocytoma).

AFX frequently presents as an elevated, sometimes ulcerated nodule. It may have a reddened, raw, eroded surface, and at times may be almost polypoid, thereby resembling pyogenic granuloma (lobular capillary hemangioma). Basal or squamous cell carcinomas are frequently considered in the clinical differential diagnosis, particularly because of the clinical setting in sun-exposed skin of elderly patients.

AFX responds well to excisional surgery, and despite its often markedly pleomorphic microscopic appearance, recurrence is uncommon and metastases are rare. Nevertheless, metastasis of AFX has been reported on a number of occasions (289,300,305,311), usually to lymph nodes and, in the case of head and neck lesions, particularly to the region of the parotid gland (300). Several reports of metastasis involved patients who had developed a lesion in an area of radiation therapy (305), or who had coexistent lymphoma (311). According to Helwig and May (300), warning signs of potentially aggressive behavior include diminished host resistance (i.e., immune compromise), deep invasion, recurrence, tumor necrosis, and vascular invasion. We have had experience with one AFX that lacked any of these features and was completely excised, but later metastasized to the lung. MOHS micrographic surgery has been proposed as a means of reducing recurrences while conserving normal tissue (267).

The overwhelmingly frequent occurrence of AFX in sun-exposed areas of the head and neck has suggested a role for ultraviolet (UV) light in the production of these tumors. This is supported by a study by Dei Tos et al. (268) showing frequent UV-induced *p53* mutations in AFX, involving cytosine bases and all but one occurring at dipyrimidine sites.

Pathologic Findings. AFX is usually a highly cellular tumor. There is an extensive intradermal proliferation of spindled to polygonal cells that often contact the overlying epidermis or the ulcerated surface of the lesion, and yet actual origination from the epidermis cannot be

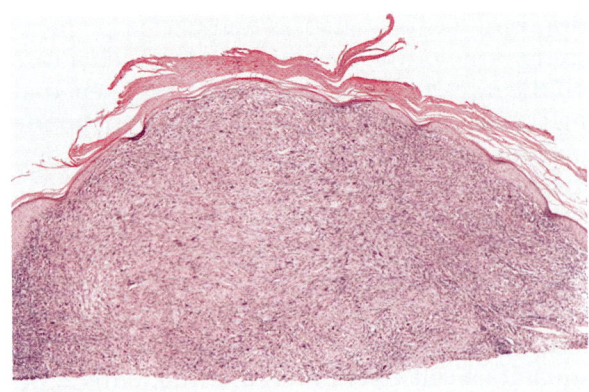

Figure 6-52

ATYPICAL FIBROXANTHOMA

The dome-shaped cutaneous nodule lacks evidence of origination in the overlying epidermis.

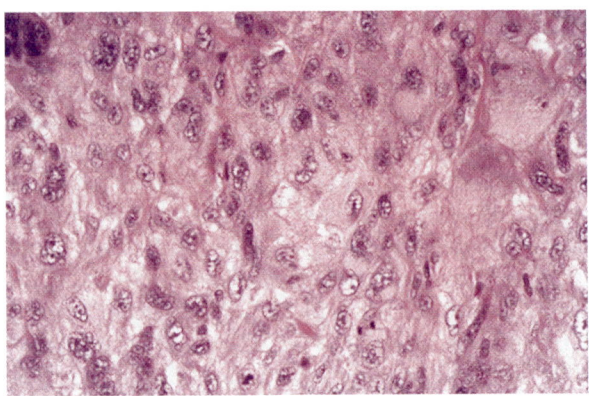

Figure 6-53

ATYPICAL FIBROXANTHOMA

The cells often possess vacuolated, foamy cytoplasm.

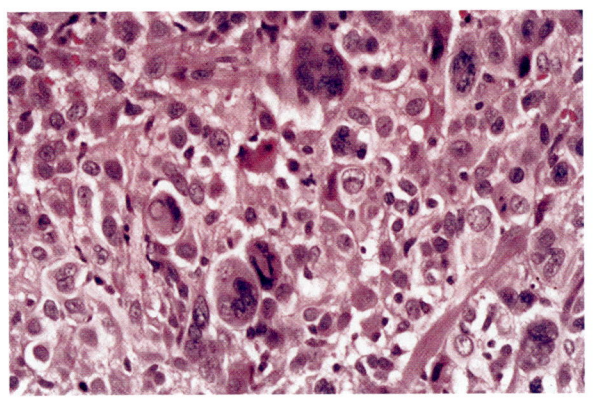

Figure 6-54

ATYPICAL FIBROXANTHOMA

There is marked pleomorphism of tumor cells.

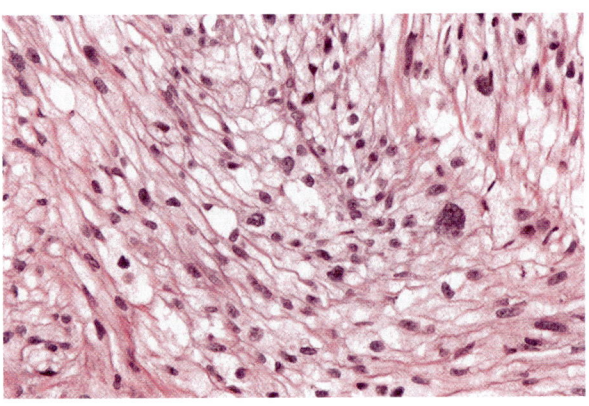

Figure 6-55

ATYPICAL FIBROXANTHOMA

This is an example of the clear cell variant of the tumor.

demonstrated (fig. 6-52). Spindled cells are often arranged in fascicles. The constituent cells may have vacuolated, foamy cytoplasm (fig. 6-53). Large, atypical multinucleated giant cells are sometimes present (315). The nuclei of these various cells are markedly pleomorphic and hyperchromatic (fig. 6-54), and mitotic figures, including atypical forms, are readily identified (252). A *myxoid form* of AFX has been described (276), and we have seen at least one example of an *angiomatoid variant* that raised initial concerns about angiosarcoma. The nonpleomorphic but mitotically active *spindle cell variant* of the tumor differs significantly from the usual appearance of AFX and can create diagnostic difficulties because of its resemblance to other malignant spindle cell tumors (261). Other variants include *clear cell AFX* (fig. 6-55) (343,345) and *AFX with osteoclast-like giant cells* (fig. 6-56) (312,361,363).

With immunohistochemical methods, the tumor cells of AFX are regularly vimentin positive, and occasionally also express alpha-smooth muscle actin or muscle-specific actin (261,319,320). Positivity has also been reported for the monocyte-macrophage marker CD68, alpha-1-antitrypsin and alpha-1-antichymotrypsin, factor XIIIa, and NKI/C3, which though known as a melanoma marker does show cross reactivity with other neoplasms (320). The osteoclast-

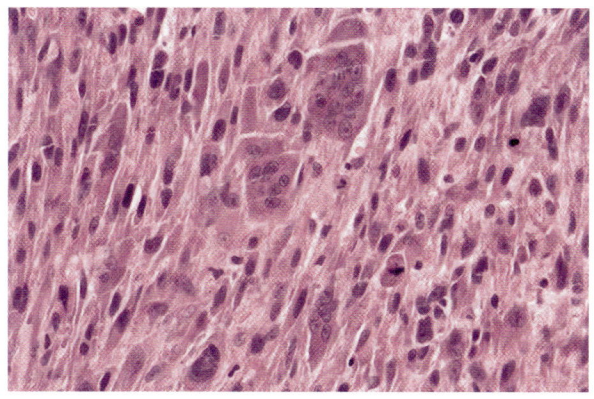

Figure 6-56

ATYPICAL FIBROXANTHOMA WITH OSTEOCLAST-LIKE GIANT CELLS

like giant cells are CD68 positive (361). Tumor cells are typically negative for cytokeratins, S-100 protein, HMB45, and desmin (261,320,345). The cells of a given lesion may fail to stain with any of these antibodies, so that in some cases the diagnosis becomes one of exclusion. Ultrastructural studies have described cells with the characteristics of fibroblasts or histiocytes (macrophages) (244,246,345).

Differential Diagnosis. The clinicopathologic features of AFX are relatively unique, but the differential diagnosis includes malignant melanoma, especially of the spindle cell or desmoplastic type, and spindle cell squamous cell carcinoma. An absence of junctional nesting argues against melanoma, although unquestionably some desmoplastic melanomas also lack junctional changes. Immunohistochemistry is usually decisive, as the cells of AFX are S-100 protein and HMB45 negative.

Spindle cell squamous cell carcinoma (SC-SCC) can be easily confused with AFX, and in fact, prior to the advent of immunohistochemistry there was some thought that AFX might represent a variant of SC-SCC. Unequivocal evidence of an epidermal origination is not always present in SC-SCC, and differentiation from AFX then requires immunohistochemistry or electron microscopy, since the cells of SC-SCC are cytokeratin positive and possess desmosomes and tonofilaments (280,358). There is evidence that squamous cell carcinomas are capable of undergoing metaplasia to a tumor with mesenchymal characteristics (358), and conceivably AFX could represent a completely dedifferentiated example of this phenomenon.

Leiomyosarcoma can be confused with AFX, particularly with the nonpleomorphic variant, but the latter tumor is desmin negative and shows only focal actin positivity (261).

The morphologic and immunohistochemical resemblance of AFX to malignant fibrous histiocytoma (MFH) has suggested to many that AFX represents a superficial variant of that soft tissue sarcoma, its more favorable prognosis being related to its small size, earlier detection, and amenability to complete excision (252). Reports of metastasizing AFX lend further support to this relationship. Several papers have reported in-depth comparisons of the two tumors using DNA analysis and measures of proliferative activity. Worrell et al. (372) found that 13 of their 14 cases of AFX were diploid by flow cytometric analysis, while the literature has indicated that most cases of MFH are aneuploid. Michie et al. (325), using an image analysis method, concluded that AFX and MFH are indistinguishable by DNA content analysis. Oshiro et al. (339) also demonstrated considerable overlap of the two tumors in terms of proliferative activity and p53 positivity, and they noted an aneuploid pattern in only 42 percent of their cases of MFH. Thus, at the present time, the weight of scientific evidence favors a close relationship between AFX and MFH.

MALIGNANT FIBROUS TISSUE TUMORS

Malignant Fibrous Histiocytoma

Clinical Features. *Malignant fibrous histiocytoma* (MFH) usually arises in deep soft tissues, including muscle, fascia, and retroperitoneum, and therefore does not commonly fall within the purview of dermatopathologists (with the exception of the tumor many consider to be its superficial variant, atypical fibroxanthoma [AFX]). These tumors, however, may extend into the subcutis (395,418) or on occasion be confined to the subcutis (390,408,415,418). MFH has also been reported to arise in burn scars (377,417).

MFH most commonly arises in middle-aged and older adults, although occurrence in children has been reported (408). There is a relatively high incidence of recurrence and metastasis, the latter most often involving lung, bone,

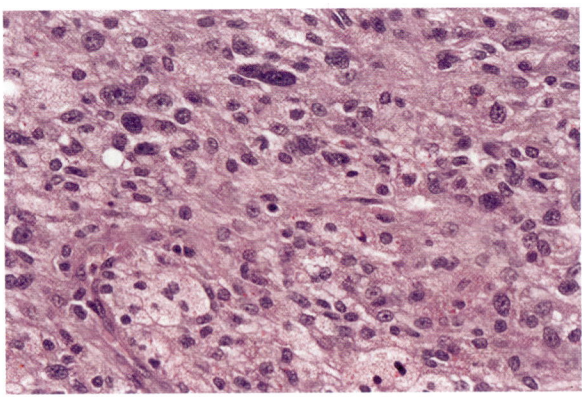

Figure 6-57

MALIGNANT FIBROUS HISTIOCYTOMA

Pleomorphic tumor cells and xanthoma cells are evident.

and liver. Prognosis varies depending upon the depth and size of tumor, and possibly also tumor grade. Small, superficial tumors tend to have lower metastatic rates and patients have better survival rates (418). Treatment involves combinations of excision, radiation therapy, and, in some cases, forms of adjuvant therapy (422).

Pathologic Findings. MFH is a highly cellular and pleomorphic tumor, featuring fascicles of spindled cells in storiform arrangements, polygonal cells with markedly atypical nuclei, and numerous mitotic figures, some with bizarre configurations. Xanthoma cells and inflammatory elements are also noted, and collagen production is slight (fig. 6-57). This description pertains to the common *storiform-pleomorphic type*, but there are other variants, including *inflammatory* (418), *myxoid* (415,419), *angiomatoid* (383), and *giant cell* (378) types. Immunohistochemical studies are performed mainly to exclude other soft tissue tumors. The tumor cells are vimentin positive (379), and although they may sometimes express histiocytic markers such as alpha-1-antitrypsin or HLA-DR, there is strong evidence that these cells are not of monocyte/macrophage lineage (380,421). The cells of MFH have the ultrastructural characteristics of fibroblasts (389).

Differential Diagnosis. Careful assessment of morphologic features on well-sampled specimens, along with immunohistochemistry and electron microscopy, help in distinguishing MFH from other soft tissue sarcomas or poorly differentiated carcinomas. One study has indicated that expression of LN-2 (CD74) is typical of MFH but usually not observed in AFX, thereby suggesting a possible means of distinguishing these tumors (396).

Epithelioid Sarcoma

Clinical Features. *Epithelioid sarcoma* is a tumor of disputed histogenesis that commonly occurs on the extremities of young adults. It is important to dermatologists and dermatopathologists because epithelioid sarcoma is a biologically aggressive tumor that not only arises in the dermis but can also be a clinical and histopathologic mimic of several inflammatory dermatoses.

This slow-growing tumor arises most commonly in young adults; however, it can develop in children (391) as well as older adults. Despite a predominance of lesions on the hands, forearms, lower legs, and feet, epithelioid sarcoma also occurs on proximal extremities or the trunk (388). Both penile (381,403) and vulvar (416) involvement have been reported. Patients may present with multifocal disease (414). Superficial lesions may resemble infectious diseases, such as sporotrichosis (406) or granuloma annulare, either of the perforating or nonperforating varieties (399,409). Penile lesions can mimic the features of Peyronie's disease (381,403). Deeper lesions present as subcutaneous nodules or areas of induration.

Epithelioid sarcoma shows a tendency to local recurrence, regional lymph node involvement, and distant metastasis, particularly to the lungs (405,407,414). The 5-year survival rate is about 70 percent (392,407,414). Adverse prognostic factors include large tumor size, tumor deep to the fascia, prominent tumor necrosis, vascular invasion, and local recurrence following initial excision (392,405,414). The treatment includes wide local excision or amputation, depending upon the clinical circumstances.

Pathologic Findings. Epithelioid sarcoma is characterized by the formation of nodules within the dermis or subcutaneous tissues. There may be central foci of necrosis surrounded by palisades of cells (fig. 6-58) (404). Cell types include polygonal cells with prominent, deeply eosinophilic cytoplasm (fig. 6-59, top) and spindled cells that form storiform arrangements (fig. 6-59, bottom) (405). These two

Fibrous Tissue Tumors

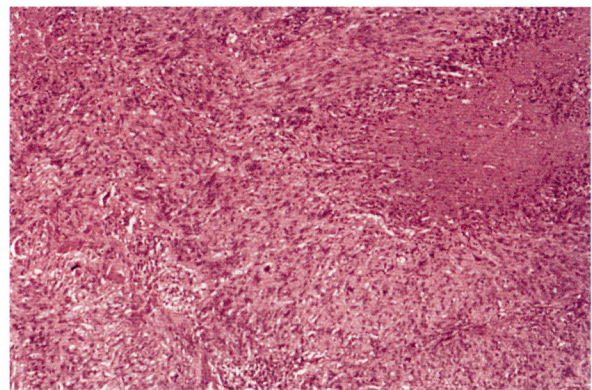

Figure 6-58

EPITHELIOID SARCOMA

A zone of necrosis is surrounded by palisades of cells.

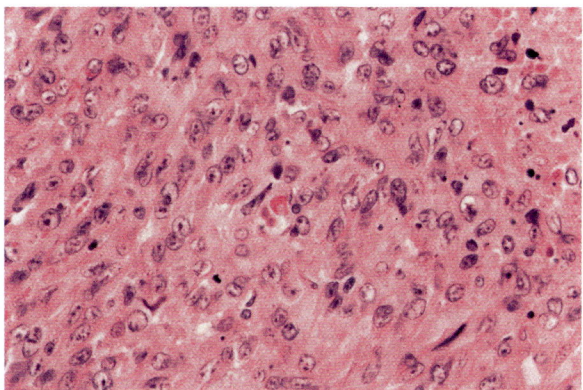

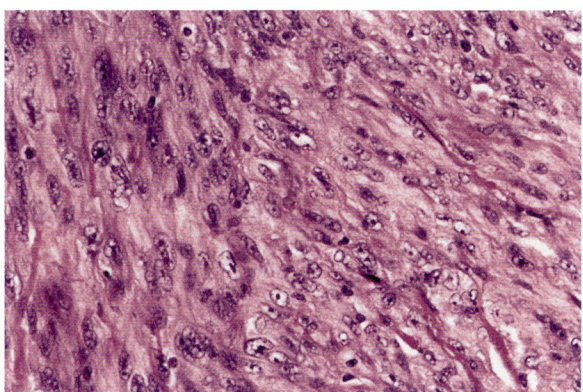

Figure 6-59

EPITHELIOID SARCOMA

Top: Polygonal cells with eosinophilic cytoplasm.
Bottom: Another example featuring a prominent spindle cell component.

cell types merge imperceptibly with one another, and therefore these tumors lack a clearcut biphasic appearance. Several variant forms have been described, including *angiomatoid, large cell/rhabdoid,* and *fibroma-like types* (401). Superficial lesions may ulcerate, while deep tumors show a tendency to grow along tendons and fascial planes; the latter finding is particularly characteristic of recurrent tumors (405). Admixtures of tumor cells with lymphocytes can be observed, and this may represent an immune-mediated defense against the tumor (400).

The cells of epithelioid sarcoma are positive for vimentin, epithelial membrane antigen, and cytokeratin. A significant proportion of tumors are also CD34 and muscle-specific actin positive (381,401). Tumor cells are S-100 protein negative. A few may focally express CD31, an endothelial cell marker, but staining for factor VIII–associated antigen is negative (401). Ultrastructurally, undifferentiated mesenchymal cells and cells with epithelial differentiation are observed (400). Large aggregates of intermediate filaments may be identified in the cytoplasm of eosinophilic, epithelioid tumor cells (402). A variety of cytogenetic anomalies has been detected in epithelioid sarcoma (384,394,400,411).

Differential Diagnosis. A major problem in the differential diagnosis is the confusion of superficial forms of epithelioid sarcoma with inflammatory processes, especially necrobiotic granulomas such as granuloma annulare. Careful attention to the cells comprising the lesion is worthwhile, since those of epithelioid sarcoma have an atypical, immature appearance and often deeply staining eosinophilic cytoplasm. Immunohistochemistry can also be of great help, since, unlike the cells of necrobiotic granulomas, the tumor cells of epithelioid sarcoma are cytokeratin and epithelial membrane antigen positive. Conversely, only the cells of necrobiotic granulomas stain for leukocyte common antigen (420). The distinctive configuration and staining pattern of these lesions helps in separating epithelioid sarcoma from other soft tissue sarcomas and malignant melanoma. The CD34 staining that is sometimes demonstrable in epithelioid sarcoma has been proposed as a means of distinguishing this lesion from metastatic carcinoma or from malignant rhabdoid tumor (401). See the next section for differentiation from synovial sarcoma.

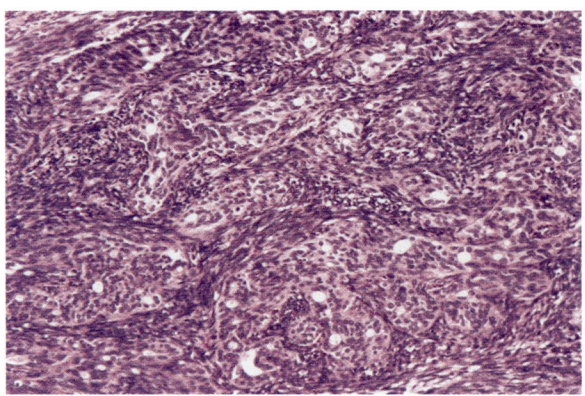

Figure 6-60

SYNOVIAL SARCOMA

This biphasic type shows spindled cells and nests of epithelial cells.

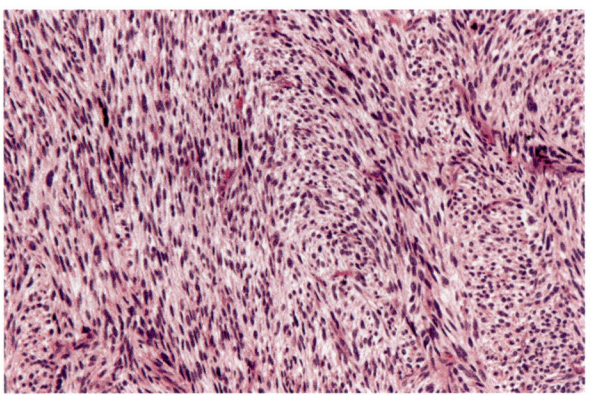

Figure 6-61

FIBROSARCOMA

Atypical spindled cells are arranged in a "herringbone" configuration.

Synovial Sarcoma

Clinical Features. *Synovial sarcoma* is a deep soft tissue tumor that only rarely involves the skin. Despite the name, these tumors are not clearly derived from or related to synovium, and they do not usually arise from joint or tendon (382,385). Synovial sarcoma develops most commonly in the extremities of young adults; the leg is a particularly common location. Lesions arising in the hands and feet may involve the dermis (386), and a case has been reported that involved the dermis and superficial subcutis of the knee region (387). Wide excision is the usual treatment (393), but recurrences are common and metastasis occurs, particularly to lungs and lymph nodes. The 5-year survival rate is 40 to 60 percent (393,413). Clinical factors that portend an adverse prognosis include short duration of symptoms, large size of primary tumor, and local recurrence (398,413).

Pathologic Findings. Synovial sarcoma consists of two components: interdigitating fascicles of spindled cells, and nests and cords of epithelial cells (fig. 6-60) (382,385,393). Transitions between the two cell types can be observed (382). This biphasic appearance is the classic presentation of synovial sarcoma, but monophasic variants also occur, particularly of the spindle cell type, although there may be rare examples of a monophasic epithelial synovial sarcoma. Myxoid changes or hemangiopericytoma-like areas are sometimes observed in these tumors. Both the epithelial and spindled elements are cytokeratin and epithelial membrane antigen positive, and the spindled cells are also vimentin positive. Spindled cells tend to express simple keratins, while epithelial cells, in addition, express more complex keratins (397). Synovial sarcomas may be S-100 protein positive but are CD34 negative (385). Histopathologic features that are of adverse prognostic significance include a high mitotic rate, low numbers of mast cells, and an elevated proliferating cell nuclear antigen labeling index (393,398).

Differential Diagnosis. Synovial sarcomas must be differentiated from other spindle cell sarcomas and occasionally from adnexal or metastatic carcinomas. A microscopic resemblance to epithelioid sarcoma is also possible, and the staining reactions of the two tumors are similar. Differences include their usual clinical locations (epithelioid sarcoma is more likely to involve the forearm and hand and to show dermal involvement), cell arrangements (epithelioid sarcoma features nodular aggregates of tumor cells with central zones of necrosis), and the deeply eosinophilic cytoplasm characteristic of the polygonal cells of epithelioid sarcoma.

Fibrosarcoma

Clinical Features. *Fibrosarcoma* is a soft tissue tumor that is diagnosed with diminishing frequency because of the establishment of criteria for other entities that display overlapping microscopic features (such as malignant fibrous histiocytoma, fibromatosis, and dermatofibrosarcoma protuberans). This has been made possible, in part, by the increasing availability of immunohistochemical staining. Fibrosarcoma is a poorly circumscribed tumor that arises in fascia, muscle, and other deep tissues in a variety of body sites. Subcutaneous involvement and ulceration have been reported (412). There are local recurrences and metastases, and survival rates vary, depending in part upon the histologic grade of the tumor (410).

Pathologic Findings. There is usually a dense proliferation of spindled cells arranged in fascicles with a "herringbone" configuration (fig. 6-61). A fine reticulin meshwork surrounds the tumor cells, which are vimentin positive but fail to stain consistently with other markers. This feature may help in the differentiation from other spindle cell sarcomas.

Differential Diagnosis. Fibrosarcoma lacks the pleomorphism usually encountered in malignant fibrous histiocytoma. Unlike fibrosarcoma, dermatofibrosarcoma protuberans has a more superficial (dermal) location and usually displays a "cartwheel" arrangement of tumor cells. Dermatopathologists should be aware of the development of fibrosarcoma-like areas in the latter, as the presence of such foci may portend more aggressive biologic behavior than is usually the case for that tumor (see above).

REFERENCES

Benign Fibrous Tissue Tumors

1. Aberer E, Mainitz M, Entacher U, Gebhart W. Fibrous hamartoma of infancy—infantile subcutaneous myofibroblastoma. Dermatologica 1988;176:46–51.
2. Ackerman AB, Kronberg R. Pearly penile papules. Acral angiofibromas. Arch Dermatol 1973;108:673–5.
3. Adams BB, Mutasim DF. Elastic tissue in fibroepithelial polyps. Am J Dermatopathol 1999;21:446–8.
4. Ahn SK, Won JH, Lee SH, Lee WS, Choi SI. Pleomorphic fibroma on the scalp. Dermatology 1995;191:245–8.
5. Allen PW, Allen LJ. Perce the permissive pathologist: a cautionary tale of one who misdiagnosed a pseudosarcoma, killed the patient and was found out. Aust N Z J Surg 1994;64:273–4.
6. Andersen L, Fejerskov O, Philipsen HP. Oral giant cell granulomas. A clinical and histological study of 129 new cases. Acta Pathol Microbiol Scand [A] 1973;81:606–16.
7. Angervall L, Kindblom LG, Lindholm K, Eriksson S. Plexiform fibrohistiocytic tumor. Report of a case involving preoperative aspiration cytology and immunohistochemical and ultrastructural analysis of surgical specimens. Pathol Res Pract 1992;188:350–6; discussion 356–9.
8. Baran R, Perrin C. Subungual perineurioma: a peculiar location. Br J Dermatol 2002;146:125–8.
9. Bargman HB, Fefferman I. Multiple dermatofibromas in a patient with myasthenia gravis treated with prednisone and cyclophosphamide. J Am Acad Dermatol 1986;14(Pt 2):351–2.
10. Barr RJ, Young EM Jr, King DF. Non-polarizable collagen in dermatofibrosarcoma protuberans: a useful diagnostic aid. J Cutan Pathol 1986;13:339–46.
11. Bart RS, Andrade R, Kopf AW, Leider M. Acquired digital fibrokeratomas. Arch Dermatol 1968;97:120–9.
12. Bastian BC, Kuchler A, Brocker EB. [Benign giant cell tumor of the tendon sheath. A differential diagnosis of cutaneous tumors near the joint.] Hautarzt 1994;45:385–8. (German.)
13. Bellman B, Wooming G, Landsman L, Penneys N, Schachner LA. Infantile myofibromatosis: a case report. Pediatr Dermatol 1991;8:306–9.
14. Bennett KG, Organ CH Jr, Cook S, Pitha J. Bilateral elastofibroma dorsi. Surgery 1988;103:605–7.
15. Berman A. Halo around a histiocytoma. Arch Dermatol 1978;114:1717–8.
16. Bernstein KE, Lattes R. Nodular (pseudosarcomatous) fasciitis, a nonrecurrent lesion: clinicopathologic study of 134 cases. Cancer 1982;49:1668–78.
17. Bertolotto M, Rosenberg I, Parodi RC, et al. Case report: fibroma of tendon sheath in the distal forearm with associated median nerve neuropathy: US, CT and MR appearances. Clin Radiol 1996;51:370–2.

18. Bhawan J, Bacchetta C, Joris I, Majno G. A myofibroblastic tumor. Infantile digital fibroma (recurrent digital fibrous tumor of childhood). Am J Pathol 1979;94:19–36.
19. Bhawan J, Cao SL. Amelanotic blue nevus: a variant of blue nevus. Am J Dermatopathol 1999;21:225–8.
20. Bisceglia M, Fusilli S, Zaffarano L, Fiorentino F, Tardio B. [Inflammatory pseudotumor of the breast. Report of a case and review of the literature.] Pathologica 1995;87:59–64. (Italian.)
21. Brandser EA, Goree JC, El-Khoury GY. Elastofibroma dorsi: prevalence in an elderly patient population as revealed by CT. AJR Am J Roentgenol 1998;171:977–80.
22. Breier F, Fang-Kircher S, Wolff K, Jurecka W. Juvenile hyaline fibromatosis: impaired collagen metabolism in human skin fibroblasts. Arch Dis Child 1997;77:436–40.
23. Brendler SJ, Watson RD, Katon RM, Parsons ME, Howatt JL. Skin tags are not a risk factor for colorectal polyps. J Clin Gastroenterol 1989;11:299–302.
24. Calderon M, Lawrence WT, Banes AJ. Increased proliferation in keloid fibroblasts wounded in vitro. J Surg Res 1996;61:343–7.
25. Calonje E. Is cutaneous benign fibrous histiocytoma (dermatofibroma) a reactive inflammatory process or a neoplasm? Histopathology 2000;37:278–80.
26. Calonje E, Fletcher CD. Aneurysmal benign fibrous histiocytoma: clinicopathological analysis of 40 cases of a tumour frequently misdiagnosed as a vascular neoplasm. Histopathology 1995;26:323–31.
27. Calonje E, Wilson-Jones E, Smith NP, Fletcher CD. Cellular 'neurothekeoma': an epithelioid variant of pilar leiomyoma? Morphological and immunohistochemical analysis of a series. Histopathology 1992;20:397–404.
28. Castens HP, Howell RS. Maglignant giant cell tumor of tendon sheath. Virchows Arch A Pathol Pathol Anat Histol 1979;382:237–43.
29. Cerio R, Rao BK, Spaull J, Jones EW. An immunohistochemical study of fibrous papule of the nose: 25 cases. J Cutan Pathol 1989;16:194–8.
30. Chang SN, Chun SI, Moon TK, Park WH. Solitary sclerotic fibroma of the skin: degenerated sclerotic change of inflammatory conditions, especially folliculitis. Am J Dermatopathol 2000;22:22–5.
31. Chen TC, Kuo T, Chan HL. Dermatofibroma is a clonal proliferative disease. J Cutan Pathol 2000;27:36–9.
32. Chung EB, Enzinger FM. Infantile myofibromatosis. Cancer 1981;48:1807–18.
33. Chung EB, Enzinger FM. Proliferative fasciitis. Cancer 1975;36:1450–8.
34. Cohen PR, Tschen JA, Abaya-Blas R, Cochran RJ. Recurrent sclerotic fibroma of the skin. Am J Dermatopathol 1999;21:571–4.
35. Colome MI, Sanchez RL. Dermatomyofibroma: report of two cases. J Cutan Pathol 1994;21:371–6.
36. Cooper PH. Dermatomyofibroma: a case of fibromatosis revisited. J Cutan Pathol 1992;19:81–2.
37. Cooper PH. Fibroma of tendon sheath. J Am Acad Dermatol 1984;11(Pt 1):625–8.
38. Coskey RJ, Mehregan AH, Lupulescu AP. Multiple vascular fibromas and myxoid fibromas of the fingers. A histologic and ultrastructural study. J Am Acad Dermatol 1980;2:425–31.
39. Daimaru Y, Hashimoto H, Enjoji M. Myofibromatosis in adults (adult counterpart of infantile myofibromatosis). Am J Surg Pathol 1989;13:859–65.
40. Dal Cin P, Sciot R, De Smet L, Van den Berghe H. Translocation 2;11 in a fibroma of tendon sheath. Histopathology 1998;32:433–5.
41. Dalton AD, Coghill SB. No association between skin tags and colorectal adenomas. Lancet 1985;1:1332–3.
42. Darling JM, Goldring SR, Harada Y, Handel ML, Glowacki J, Gravallese EM. Multinucleated cells in pigmented villonodular synovitis and giant cell tumor of tendon sheath express features of osteoclasts. Am J Pathol 1997;150:1383–93.
43. De la Torre C, Ocampo C, Doval IG, Losada A, Cruces MJ. Acrochordons are not a component of the Birt-Hogg-Dube syndrome: does this syndrome exist? Case reports and review of the literature. Am J Dermatopathol 1999;21:369–74.
44. Devaney D, Livesley P, Shaw D. Elastofibroma dorsi: MRI diagnosis in a young girl. Pediatr Radiol 1995;25:282–3.
45. Dixon AY, Lee SH. An ultrastructural study of elastofibromas. Hum Pathol 1980;11:257–62.
46. Ehrlich HP, Desmouliere A, Diegelmann RF, et al. Morphological and immunochemical differences between keloid and hypertrophic scar. Am J Pathol 1994;145:105–13.
47. Enzinger FM. Fibrous hamartoma of infancy. Cancer 1965;18:241–8.
48. Enzinger FM, Zhang RY. Plexiform fibrohistiocytic tumor presenting in children and young adults. An analysis of 65 cases. Am J Surg Pathol 1988;12:818–26.
49. Evangelisti S, Reale VF. Fibroma of tendon sheath as a cause of carpal tunnel syndrome. J Hand Surg [Am] 1992;17:1026–7.
50. Fenske NA, Donelan PA. Becker's nevus coexistent with connective-tissue nevus. Arch Dermatol 1984;120:1347–50.

51. Ferenczy A, Richart RM, Wright TC. Pearly penile papules: absence of human papillomavirus DNA by the polymerase chain reaction. Obstet Gynecol 1991;78:118–22.
52. Fetsch JF, Laskin WB, Miettinen M. Superficial acral fibromyxoma: a clinicopathologic and immunohistochemical analysis of 37 cases of a distinctive soft tissue tumor with a predilection for the fingers and toes. Hum Pathol 2001; 32:704–14.
53. Fetsch JF, Miettinen M. Sclerosing perineurioma: a clinicopathologic study of 19 cases of a distinctive soft tissue lesion with a predilection for the fingers and palms of young adults. Am J Surg Pathol 1997;21:1433–42.
54. Flanagan AM, Nui B, Tinkler SM, Horton MA, Williams DM, Chambers TJ. The multinucleate cells in giant cell granulomas of the jaw are osteoclasts. Cancer 1988;62:1139–45.
55. Fletcher CD, Powell G, van Noorden S, McKee PH. Fibrous hamartoma of infancy: a histochemical and immunohistochemical study. Histopathology 1988;12:65–74.
56. Fukasawa Y, Ishikura H, Takada A, et al. Massive apoptosis in infantile myofibromatosis. A putative mechanism of tumor regression. Am J Pathol 1994;144:480–5.
57. Fukunaga M, Ushigome S. Collagenous fibroma (desmoplastic fibroblastoma): a distinctive fibroblastic soft tissue tumor. Adv Anat Pathol 1999;6:275–80.
58. Gallais V, Lacour JP, Perrin C, Halioua B, Ortonne JP. [Halo eczema around a histiocytofibroma: the Meyerson phenomenon.] Ann Dermatol Venereol 1993;120:617–20. (French.)
59. Garcia-Doval I, Casas L, Toribio J. Pleomorphic fibroma of the skin, a form of sclerotic fibroma: an immunohistochemical study. Clin Exp Dermatol 1998;23:22–4.
60. Ghazizadeh M, Miyata N, Sasaki Y, Arai K, Aihara K. Silver-stained nucleolar organizer regions in hypertrophic and keloid scars. Am J Dermatopathol 1997;19:468–72.
61. Giansanti JS, Waldron CA. Peripheral giant cell granuloma: review of 720 cases. J Oral Surg 1969;27:787–91.
62. Glover MT, Lake BD, Atherton DJ. Clinical, histologic, and ultrastructural findings in two cases of infantile systemic hyalinosis. Pediatr Dermatol 1992;9:255–8.
63. Glover MT, Lake BD, Atherton DJ. Infantile systemic hyalinosis: newly recognized disorder of collagen? Pediatrics 1991;87:228–34.
64. Glusac EJ, Barr RJ, Everett MA, Pitha J, Santa Cruz DJ. Epithelioid cell histiocytoma. A report of 10 cases including a new cellular variant. Am J Surg Pathol 1994;18:583–90.
65. Goellner JR, Soule EH. Desmoid tumors. An ultrastructural study of eight cases. Hum Pathol 1980;11:43–50.
66. Gould BE, Ellison RC, Greene HL, Bernhard JD. Lack of association between skin tags and colon polyps in a primary care setting. Arch Intern Med 1988;148:1799–800.
67. Graham JH, Sanders JB, Johnson WC, Helwig EB. Fibrous papule of the nose: a clinicopathological study. J Invest Dermatol 1965;45:194–203.
68. Greco MA, Schinella RA, Vuletin JC. Fibrous hamartoma of infancy: an ultrastructural study. Hum Pathol 1984;15:717–23.
69. Groisman G, Kerner H. A case of fibrous hamartoma of infancy in the scrotum including immunohistochemical findings. J Urol 1990;144 (Pt 1):340–1.
70. Guitart J, Ritter JH, Wick MR. Solitary cutaneous myofibromas in adults: report of six cases and discussion of differential diagnosis. J Cutan Pathol 1996;23:437–44.
71. Gunhan O, Gurbuzer B, Gardner DG, Demiriz M, Finci R. A central odontogenic fibroma exhibiting pleomorphic fibroblasts and numerous calcifications. Br J Oral Maxillofac Surg 1991;29:42–3.
72. Haisa M, Okochi H, Grotendorst GR. Elevated levels of PDGF alpha receptors in keloid fibroblasts contribute to an enhanced response to PDGF. J Invest Dermatol 1994;103:560–3.
73. Harris GR, Shea CR, Horenstein MG, Reed JA, Burchette JL Jr, Prieto VG. Desmoplastic (sclerotic) nevus: an underrecognized entity that resembles dermatofibroma and desmoplastic melanoma. Am J Surg Pathol 1999;23:786–94.
74. Harrison HC, Motbey J, Kan AE, de Silva M. Nodular fasciitis of the nose in a child. Int J Pediatr Otorhinolaryngol 1995;33:257–64.
75. Hasegawa T, Hirose T, Kudo E, Abe J, Hizawa K. Cytoskeletal characteristics of myofibroblasts in benign neoplastic and reactive fibroblastic lesions. Virchows Arch A Pathol Anat Histopathol 1990;416:375–82.
76. Hasegawa T, Hirose T, Seki K, Hizawa K, Okada J, Nakanishi H. Solitary infantile myofibromatosis of bone. An immunohistochemical and ultrastructural study. Am J Surg Pathol 1993;17:308–13.
77. Hasegawa T, Shimoda T, Hirohashi S, Hizawa K, Sano T. Collagenous fibroma (desmoplastic fibroblastoma): report of four cases and review of the literature. Arch Pathol Lab Med 1998;122:455–60.

78. Hashimoto H, Tsuneyoshi M, Daimaru Y, Ushijima M, Enjoji M. Fibroma of tendon sheath: a tumor of myofibroblasts. A clinicopathologic study of 18 cases. Acta Pathol Jpn 1985;35:1099–107.
79. Hassanein A, Telang G, Benedetto E, Spielvogel R. Subungual myxoid pleomorphic fibroma. Am J Dermatopathol 1998;20:502–5.
80. Hayes AG, Berry AD 3rd. Basal cell carcinoma arising in a fibroepithelial polyp. J Am Acad Dermatol 1993;28:493–5.
81. Herbst VP, Kauh YC, Luscombe HA. Connective tissue nevus masquerading as a localized linear epidermal nevus. J Am Acad Dermatol 1987;16(Pt 2):264–6.
82. Herrera Sanchez M, Suanez Fernandez R, del Cerro Heredero M, Rueda Gomez-Calcerrada M, Vigaray Conde J, Sanchez Yus E. Sclerotic fibroma. Dermatology 1998;196:429–30.
83. Hsu JK, Cavanagh HD, Green WR. An unusual case of elastofibroma oculi. Cornea 1997;16:112–9.
84. Huang WL, Ro JY, Grignon DJ, Swanson D, Ordonez NG, Ayala AG. Postoperative spindle cell nodule of the prostate and bladder. J Urol 1990;143:824–6.
85. Humphreys S, McKee PH, Fletcher CD. Fibroma of tendon sheath: a clinicopathologic study. J Cutan Pathol 1986;13:331–8.
86. Hurt MA, Santa Cruz DJ. Cutaneous inflammatory pseudotumor. Lesions resembling "inflammatory pseudotumors" or "plasma cell granulomas" of extracutaneous sites. Am J Surg Pathol 1990;14:764–73.
87. Ide F, Shimoyama T, Horie N, Tanaka H. Collagenous fibroma (desmoplastic fibroblastoma) presenting as a parotid mass. J Oral Pathol Med 1999;28:465–8.
88. Ishikawa H, Maeda H, Takamatsu H, Saito Y. Systemic hyalinosis (juvenile hyaline fibromatosis). Ultrastructure of the hyaline with particular reference to the cross-banded structure. Arch Dermatol Res 1979;265:195–206.
89. Iwasaki H, Kikuchi M, Mori R, et al. Infantile digital fibromatosis. Ultrastructural, histochemical, and tissue culture observations. Cancer 1980;46:2238–47.
90. Iwata S, Horiuchi R, Maeda H, Ishikawa H. Systemic hyalinosis or juvenile hyaline fibromatosis. Ultrastructural and biochemical study of cultured skin fibroblasts. Arch Dermatol Res 1980;267:115–21.
91. Jablokow VR, Kathuria S. Fibroma of tendon sheath. J Surg Oncol 1982;19:90–2.
92. Jadusingh IH. Fine needle aspiration cytology of fibrous hamartoma of infancy. Acta Cytol 1997;41(Suppl):1391–3.
93. James WD, Besanceney CD, Odom RB. The ultrastructure of a keloid. J Am Acad Dermatol 1980;3:50–7.
94. Johnson BL, Baxter DL. Pearly penile papules. Arch Dermatol 1964;90:166–7.
95. Jones EW, Cerio R, Smith NP. Epithelioid cell histiocytoma: a new entity. Br J Dermatol 1989;120:185–95.
96. Kamino H, Jacobson M. Dermatofibroma extending into the subcutaneous tissue. Differential diagnosis from dermatofibrosarcoma protuberans. Am J Surg Pathol 1990;14:1156–64.
97. Kamino H, Lee JY, Berke A. Pleomorphic fibroma of the skin: a benign neoplasm with cytologic atypia. A clinicopathologic study of eight cases. Am J Surg Pathol 1989;13:107–13.
98. Kamino H, Reddy VB, Gero M, Greco MA. Dermatomyofibroma. A benign cutaneous, plaque-like proliferation of fibroblasts and myofibroblasts in young adults. J Cutan Pathol 1992;19:85–93.
99. Katagiri K, Takasaki S, Fujiwara S, Kayashima K, Ono T, Shinkai H. Purification and structural analysis of extracellular matrix of a skin tumor from a patient with juvenile hyaline fibromatosis. J Dermatol Sci 1996;13:37–48.
100. Kato M, Katsumoto T, Ohno K, Kato S, Herz F, Takeshita K. Expression of glial fibrillary acidic protein (GFAP) by cultured angiofibroma stroma cells from patients with tuberous sclerosis. Neuropathol Appl Neurobiol 1992;18:559–65.
101. King DT, Millman AJ, Gurevitch AW, Hirose FM. Giant cell tumor of the tendon sheath involving skin. Arch Dermatol 1978;114:944–6.
102. Kint A, Baran R. Histopathologic study of Koenen tumors. Are they different from acquired digital fibrokeratoma? J Am Acad Dermatol 1988;18(Pt 1):369–72.
103. Kiyohara T, Kumakiri M, Kobayashi H, Ohkawara A, Lao LM. Atrophic dermatofibroma. Elastophago-cytosis by the tumor cells. J Cutan Pathol 2000;27:312–5.
104. Kobayasi T, Wolf-Jurgensen P, Danielsen L. Ultrastructure of shagreen patch. Acta Derm Venereol 1973;53:275–8.
104a. Konwaler BE, Keasbey L, Kaplan L. Subcutaneous pseudosarcomatous fibromatosis (fasciitis). Am J Clin Pathol 1955;25:241–52.
105. Kuo TT, Hu S, Chan HL. Keloidal dermatofibroma: report of 10 cases of a new variant. Am J Surg Pathol 1998;22:564–8.
106. Kurwa AR. Rubinstein-Taybi syndrome and spontaneous keloids. Clin Exp Dermatol 1979;4:251–4.

107. Ladin DA, Hou Z, Patel D, et al. p53 and apoptosis alterations in keloids and keloid fibroblasts. Wound Repair Regen 1998;6:28–37.
108. Lai FM, Lam WY. Nodular fasciitis of the dermis. J Cutan Pathol 1993;20:66–9.
109. Lamovec J, Bracko M, Voncina D. Pleomorphic fibroma of tendon sheath. Am J Surg Pathol 1991;15:1202–5.
110. Lauer DH, Enzinger FM. Cranial fasciitis of childhood. Cancer 1980;45:401–6.
111. Laughlin CL, Carrington PR. Deep penetrating dermatofibroma. Dermatol Surg 1998;24:592–4.
112. Leavitt J, Klein I, Kendricks F, Gavaler J, VanThiel DH. Skin tags: a cutaneous marker for colonic polyps. Ann Intern Med 1983;98:928–30.
113. Ledet SC, Brown RW, Cagle PT. p53 immunostaining in the differentiation of inflammatory pseudotumor from sarcoma involving the lung. Mod Pathol 1995;8:282–6.
114. Lee KS, Song JY, Suh MH. Collagen mRNA expression detected by in situ hybridization in keloid tissue. J Dermatol Sci 1991;2:316–23.
115. Lee YS, Vijayasingam S. Mast cells and myofibroblasts in keloid: a light microscopic, immunohistochemical and ultrastructural study. Ann Acad Med Singapore 1995;24:902–5.
116. Leyva WH, Santa Cruz DJ. Atypical cutaneous fibrous histiocytoma. Am J Dermatopathol 1986;8:467–71.
117. Li M, Cordon-Cardo C, Gerald WL, Rosai J. Desmoid fibromatosis is a clonal process. Hum Pathol 1996;27:939–43.
118. Lin RY, Landsman L, Krey PR, Lambert WC. Multiple dermatofibromas and systemic lupus erythematosus. Cutis 1986;37:45–7, 9.
119. Linares HA, Kischer CW, Dobrkovsky M, Larson DL. The histiotypic organization of the hypertrophic scar in humans. J Invest Dermatol 1972;59:323–31.
120. Lo WL, Wong CK. Solitary sclerotic fibroma. J Cutan Pathol 1990;17:269–73.
121. LoBuono P, Jothikumar T, Kornblee L. Acquired digital fibrokeratoma. Cutis 1979;24:50–1.
122. Lourie JA, Lwin KY, Woods CG. Case report 734. Fibroma of tendon sheath eroding 3rd metatarsal bone. Skeletal Radiol 1992;21:273–5.
123. Lu I, Cohen PR, Grossman ME. Multiple dermatofibromas in a woman with HIV infection and systemic lupus erythematosus. J Am Acad Dermatol 1995;32(Pt 2):901–3.
124. Lubec B, Steinert I, Breier F, Jurecka W, Pillwein K, Fang-Kircher S. Skin collagen defects in a patient with juvenile hyaline fibromatosis. Arch Dis Child 1995;73:246–8.
125. Luk GD. Colonic polyps and acrochordons (skin tags) do not correlate in familial colonic polyposis kindreds. Ann Intern Med 1986;104:209–10.
126. Lundgren LG, Kindblom LG. Fibroma of tendon sheath. A light and electron-microscopic study of 6 cases. Acta Pathol Microbiol Immunol Scand [A] 1984;92:401–9.
127. Magid MS, Campbell WG Jr, Ngadiman S, Godwin TA, Ward R. Infantile myofibromatosis with hemangiopericytoma-like features of the tongue: a case study including ultrastructure. Pediatr Pathol Lab Med 1997;17:303–13.
128. Magro G, Giannone G, Carrubba G, Belfiore G, Grasso S. S-100 protein expression in a case of elastofibroma dorsi. Pathologica 1995;87:528–30.
129. Magro G, Venti C. Childhood desmoplastic fibroblastoma (collagenous fibroma) with a 12-year follow-up. Pediatr Dev Pathol 1999;2:62–4.
130. Maluf HM, DeYoung BR, Swanson PE, Wick MR. Fibroma and giant cell tumor of tendon sheath: a comparative histological and immunohistological study. Mod Pathol 1995;8:155–9.
131. Mancini GM, Stojanov L, Willemsen R, et al. Juvenile hyaline fibromatosis: clinical heterogeneity in three patients. Dermatology 1999;198:18–25.
132. Manson CM, Hirsch PJ, Coyne JD. Post-operative spindle cell nodule of the vulva. Histopathology 1995;26:571–4.
133. Marin ML, Perzin KH, Markowitz AM. Elastofibroma dorsi: benign chest wall tumor. J Thorac Cardiovasc Surg 1989;98:234–8.
134. Martin-Lopez R, Feal-Cortizas C, Fraga J. Pleomorphic sclerotic fibroma. Dermatology 1999;198:69–72.
135. Mayer-da-Silva A, Poiares-Baptista A, Guerra Rodrigo F, Teresa-Lopes M. Juvenile hyaline fibromatosis. A histologic and histochemical study. Arch Pathol Lab Med 1988;112:928–31.
136. McCalmont TH. Sclerotic fibroma: a fossil no longer. J Cutan Pathol 1994;21:82–5.
137. McGibbon DH, Jones EW. Fibrous papule of the face (nose). Fibrosing nevocytic nevus. Am J Dermatopathol 1979;1:345–8.
138. McPherson FC, Norman LS, Truitt CA, Morgan MB. Elastofibroma of the foot: uncommon presentation: a case report and review of the literature. Foot Ankle Int 2000;21:775–7.
139. Meffert JJ, Kennard CD, Davis TL, Quinn BD. Intradermal nodular fasciitis presenting as an eyelid mass. Int J Dermatol 1996;35:548–52.
140. Mehregan AH. Nodular fasciitis. Arch Dermatol 1966;93:204–10.
141. Mehregan AH, Mehregan DR, Broecker A. Epithelioid cell histiocytoma. A clinicopathologic and immunohistochemical study of eight cases. J Am Acad Dermatol 1992;26(Pt 1):243–6.

142. Mentzel T, Calonje E, Fletcher CD. Dermatomyofibroma: additional observations on a distinctive cutaneous myofibroblastic tumour with emphasis on differential diagnosis. Br J Dermatol 1993;129:69–73.
143. Mentzel T, Calonje E, Nascimento AG, Fletcher CD. Infantile hemangiopericytoma versus infantile myofibromatosis. Study of a series suggesting a continuous spectrum of infantile myofibroblastic lesions. Am J Surg Pathol 1994; 18:922–30.
144. Miettinen M, Fetsch JF. Collagenous fibroma (desmoplastic fibroblastoma): a clinicopathologic analysis of 63 cases of a distinctive soft tissue lesion with stellate-shaped fibroblasts. Hum Pathol 1998;29:676–82.
145. Miliauskas JR. Myxoid cutaneous pleomorphic fibroma. Histopathology 1994;24:179–81.
146. Mills BG, Frausto A, Brien E. Cytokines associated with the pathophysiology of aggressive fibromatosis. J Orthop Res 2000;18:655–62.
147. Mitchell ML, di Sant'Agnese PA, Gerber JE. Fibrous hamartoma of infancy. Hum Pathol 1982;13:586–8.
148. Mizuno K, Ishikura H, Aizawa M. Giant cell tumor of tendon sheath. An immunohistochemical study of 28 cases. Acta Pathol Jpn 1986;36: 1487–94.
149. Mojica WD, Kuntzman T. Elastofibroma dorsi: elaboration of cytologic features and review of its pathogenesis. Diagn Cytopathol 2000;23: 393–6.
150. Murphy SC, Lowitt MH, Kao GF. Multiple eruptive dermatofibromas in an HIV-positive man. Dermatology 1995;190:309–12.
151. Murray JC, Pollack SV, Pinnell SR. Keloids: a review. J Am Acad Dermatol 1981;4:461–70.
152. Naylor MF, Nascimento AG, Sherrick AD, McLeod RA. Elastofibroma dorsi: radiologic findings in 12 patients. AJR Am J Roentgenol 1996;167:683–7.
153. Nemeth AJ, Penneys NS. Factor XIIIa is expressed by fibroblasts in fibrovascular tumors [see comments]. J Cutan Pathol 1989;16:266–71.
154. Nielsen GP, O'Connell JX, Dickersin GR, Rosenberg AE. Collagenous fibroma (desmoplastic fibroblastoma): a report of seven cases. Mod Pathol 1996;9:781–5.
155. Nochomovitz LE, Orenstein JM. Inflammatory pseudotumor of the urinary bladder—possible relationship to nodular fasciitis. Two case reports, cytologic observations, and ultrastructural observations. Am J Surg Pathol 1985;9:366–73.
156. Nogita T, Akiyoshi E, Kawashima M. Sclerotic fibromas of the skin. J Dermatol 1991;18:472–4.
157. O'Connell JX, Fanburg JC, Rosenberg AE. Giant cell tumor of tendon sheath and pigmented villonodular synovitis: immunophenotype suggests a synovial cell origin. Hum Pathol 1995;26: 771–5.
158. O'Connell JX, Young RH, Nielsen GP, Rosenberg AE, Bainbridge TC, Clement PB. Nodular fasciitis of the vulva: a study of six cases and literature review. Int J Gynecol Pathol 1997;16:117–23.
159. Ochsendorf FR, Leopolder-Ochsendorf A, Holtermuller KH, Milbradt R. [Soft skin fibromas: study of their importance and diagnostic significance for colonic neoplasms.] Hautarzt 1990;41:207–11. (German.)
160. Onwukwe MF. Classification of keloids. J Dermatol Surg Oncol 1978;4:534–6.
161. Onwukwe MF. The suppurative keloid. J Dermatol Surg Oncol 1978;4:333–5.
162. Paller AS, Gonzalez-Crussi F, Sherman JO. Fibrous hamartoma of infancy. Eight additional cases and a review of the literature. Arch Dermatol 1989;125:88–91.
163. Patterson JW, Moran SL, Konerding H. Cranial fasciitis. Arch Dermatol 1989;125:674–8.
164. Peterson JL, Read SI, Rodman OG. Familial myxovascular fibromas. J Am Acad Dermatol 1982;6(Pt 1):470–2.
165. Piette AM, Meduri B, Fritsch J, Fermanian J, Piette JC, Chapman A. Do skin tags constitute a marker for colonic polyps? A prospective study of 100 asymptomatic patients and metaanalysis of the literature. Gastroenterology 1988;95: 1127–9.
166. Price SK, Kahn LB, Saxe N. Dermal and intravascular fasciitis. Unusual variants of nodular fasciitis. Am J Dermatopathol 1993;15:539–43.
167. Pujol RM, de Castro F, Schroeter AL, Su WP. Solitary sclerotic fibroma of the skin: a sclerotic dermatofibroma? Am J Dermatopathol 1996;18: 620–4.
168. Pulitzer DR, Martin PC, Reed RJ. Fibroma of tendon sheath. A clinicopathologic study of 32 cases. Am J Surg Pathol 1989;13:472–9.
169. Purdy LJ, Colby TV. Infantile digital fibromatosis occurring outside the digit. Am J Surg Pathol 1984;8:787–90.
170. Ragaz A, Berezowsky V. Fibrous papule of the face. A study of five cases by electron microscopy. Am J Dermatopathol 1979;1:353–6.
171. Rao AS, Vigorita VJ. Pigmented villonodular synovitis (giant-cell tumor of the tendon sheath and synovial membrane). A review of eighty-one cases. J Bone Joint Surg Am 1984;66:76–94.
172. Rapini RP, Golitz LE. Sclerotic fibromas of the skin. J Am Acad Dermatol 1989;20(Pt 1):266-71.

173. Recchia FM, Buckley EG, Townshend LM, Klintworth GK. Nodular fasciitis of the orbital rim in a pediatric patient. J Pediatr Ophthalmol Strabismus 1997;34:316–8.
174. Reed RJ, Argenyi Z. Tumors of neural tissue. In: Elder D, Elenitsas R, Jaworsky C, Johnson B Jr, eds. Lever's histopathology of the skin, 8th ed. Philadelphia: Lippincott-Raven; 1997:995–6.
175. Rehbein HM. Pearly penile papules: incidence. Cutis 1977;19:54–7.
176. Remstein ED, Arndt CA, Nascimento AG. Plexiform fibrohistiocytic tumor: clinicopathologic analysis of 22 cases. Am J Surg Pathol 1999;23:662–70.
177. Requena L, Gutierrez J, Sanchez Yus E. Multiple sclerotic fibromas of the skin. A cutaneous marker of Cowden's disease. J Cutan Pathol 1992;19:346–51.
178. Requena L, Kutzner H, Hugel H, Rutten A, Furio V. Cutaneous adult myofibroma: a vascular neoplasm. J Cutan Pathol 1996;23:445–57.
179. Requena L, Reichel M. The atrophic dermatofibroma: a delled dermatofibroma. J Dermatol 1995;22:334–9.
180. Requena L, Sangueza OP. Benign neoplasms with neural differentiation: a review. Am J Dermatopathol 1995;17:75–96.
181. Ro JY, Ayala AG, Ordonez NG, Swanson DA, Babaian RJ. Pseudosarcomatous fibromyxoid tumor of the urinary bladder. Am J Clin Pathol 1986;86:583–90.
182. Rodrigues C, Desai S, Chinoy R. Giant cell tumor of the tendon sheath: a retrospective study of 28 cases. J Surg Oncol 1998;68:100–3.
183. Rudolph P, Schubert C, Zelger BG, Zelger B, Parwaresch R. Differential expression of CD34 and Ki-M1p in pleomorphic fibroma and dermatofibroma with monster cells. Am J Dermatopathol 1999;21:414–9.
184. Sakatani T, Shomori K, Adachi H, Hosoda A, Ito H. Elastofibroma of the sigmoid colon. Pathol Res Pract 2000;196:205–7.
185. Salomao DR, Nascimento AG. Plexiform fibrohistiocytic tumor with systemic metastases: a case report. Am J Surg Pathol 1997;21:469–76.
186. Samaratunga H, Searle J, O'Loughlin B. Nodular fasciitis and related pseudosarcomatous lesions of soft tissues. Aust N Z J Surg 1996;66:22–5.
187. Sandinha T, Lee WR, Reid R. Pleomorphic fibroma of the eyelid. Graefes Arch Clin Exp Ophthalmol 1998;236:333–8.
188. Santa Cruz DJ, Kyriakos M. Aneurysmal ("angiomatoid") fibrous histiocytoma of the skin. Cancer 1981;47:2053–61.
189. Santa Cruz DJ, Prioleau PG. Fibrous papule of the face. An electron-microscopic study of two cases. Am J Dermatopathol 1979;1:349–52.
190. Sapp JP. Ultrastructure and histogenesis of peripheral giant cell reparative granuloma of the jaws. Cancer 1972;30:1119–29.
191. Satti MB. Tendon sheath tumours: a pathological study of the relationship between giant cell tumour and fibroma of tendon sheath. Histopathology 1992;20:213–20.
192. Schaller M, Stengel-Rutkowski S, Sollberg S, Kind P. [Juvenile hyaline fibromatosis.] Hautarzt 1997;48:253–7. (German.)
193. Schirren CG, Schirren H, Gyzicki-Nienhaus B, Kind P. [Extra-abdominal fibromatosis. An immunohistochemical analysis.] Hautarzt 1993;44:789–94. (German.)
194. Schirren H, Schirren CG, Stolz W, Kind P, Plewig G. Papular elastorrhexis: a variant of dermatofibrosis lenticularis disseminata (Buschke-Ollendorff syndrome)? Dermatology 1994;189:368–72.
195. Sciot R, Samson I, van den Berghe H, Van Damme B, Dal Cin P. Collagenous fibroma (desmoplastic fibroblastoma): genetic link with fibroma of tendon sheath? Mod Pathol 1999;12:565–8.
196. Sears JK, Stone MS, Argenyi Z. Papular elastorrhexis: a variant of connective tissue nevus. Case reports and review of the literature. J Am Acad Dermatol 1988;19(Pt 2):409–14.
197. Seki K, Hirose T, Hasegawa T, Hizawa K. Giant cell tumor of tendon sheath. An immunohistochemical observation on the characteristics and the capacity of proliferation of tumor cells. Zentralbl Pathol 1993;139:287–94.
198. Senzaki H, Kiyozuka Y, Uemura Y, Shikata N, Ueda S, Tsubura A. Juvenile hyaline fibromatosis: a report of two unrelated adult sibling cases and a literature review. Pathol Int 1998;48:230–6.
199. Shafer WG, Hine MK, Levy BM. Benign and malignant tumors of the oral cavity. In: Shafer WG, Hine MK, Levy BM, eds. A textbook of oral pathology, 4th ed. Philadelphia: W.B. Saunders; 1983;144–6.
200. Shapiro L, Juhlin EA, Brownstein MH. "Rudimentary polydactyly": an amputation neuroma. Arch Dermatol 1973;108:223–5.
201. Sharata H, Hashimoto K, Fernandez-Madrid F. Multiple hyperpigmented nodules. Multiple dermatofibromas in a patient with systemic lupus erythematosus (SLE). Arch Dermatol 1994;130:650–1, 653.
202. Shea CR, Salob S, Reed JA, Lugo J, McNutt NS. CD34-reactive fibrous papule of the nose. J Am Acad Dermatol 1996;35(Pt 2):342–5.
203. Shinjo K, Miyake N, Takahashi Y. Malignant giant cell tumor of the tendon sheath: an autopsy report and review of the literature. Jpn J Clin Oncol 1993;23:317–24.

204. Shitabata PK, Crouch EC, Fitzgibbon JF, Swanson PE, Adesokan PN, Wick MR. Cutaneous sclerotic fibroma. Immunohistochemical evidence of a fibroblastic neoplasm with ongoing type I collagen synthesis. Am J Dermatopathol 1995;17:339–43.
205. Sollberg S, Peltonen J, Uitto J. Combined use of in situ hybridization and unlabeled antibody peroxidase anti-peroxidase methods: simultaneous detection of type I procollagen mRNAs and factor VIII-related antigen epitopes in keloid tissue. Lab Invest 1991;64:125–9.
206. Sonnex C, Dockerty WG. Pearly penile papules: a common cause of concern. Int J STD AIDS 1999;10:726–7.
207. Sonoda T, Itami S, Seguchi S, Kurata S, Takayasu S. Infantile myofibromatosis: report of two cases. J Dermatol 1994;21:508–13.
208. Sotelo-Avila C, Bale PM. Subdermal fibrous hamartoma of infancy: pathology of 40 cases and differential diagnosis. Pediatr Pathol 1994; 14:39–52.
209. Soule EH. Proliferative (nodular) fasciitis. Arch Pathol 1962;73:437–44.
210. Soyer HP, Metze D, Kerl H. Granular cell dermatofibroma. Am J Dermatopathol 1997;19:168–73.
211. Spraker MK, Stack C, Esterly NB. Congenital generalized fibromatosis: a review of the literature and report of a case associated with porencephaly, hemiatrophy, and cutis marmorata telangiectatica congenita. J Am Acad Dermatol 1984;10(Pt 2):365–71.
212. Stanford D, Rogers M. Dermatological presentations of infantile myofibromatosis: a review of 27 cases. Australas J Dermatol 2000;41:156–61.
213. Starink TM, Meijer CJ, Brownstein MH. The cutaneous pathology of Cowden's disease: new findings. J Cutan Pathol 1985;12:83–93.
214. Stejskal J, Kubena M, Povysilova V. [Elastofibroma dorsi.] Cesk Patol 1982;18:165–9. (Czech.)
215. Tamada S, Ackerman AB. Dermatofibroma with monster cells. Am J Dermatopathol 1987;9:380–7.
216. Uitto J, Santa-Cruz DJ, Eisen AZ. Familial cutaneous collagenoma: genetic studies on a family. Br J Dermatol 1979;101:185–95.
217. Ushijima M, Hashimoto H, Tsuneyoshi M, Enjoji M. Giant cell tumor of the tendon sheath (nodular tenosynovitis). A study of 207 cases to compare the large joint group with the common digit group. Cancer 1986;57:875–84.
218. Vanni R, Fletcher CD, Sciot R, et al. Cytogenetic evidence of clonality in cutaneous benign fibrous histiocytomas: a report of the CHAMP study group. Histopathology 2000;37:212–7.
219. Variend S, Bax NM, van Gorp J. Are infantile myofibromatosis, congenital fibrosarcoma and congenital haemangiopericytoma histogenetically related? Histopathology 1995;26:57–62.
220. Viale G, Doglioni C, Iuzzolino P, et al. Infantile digital fibromatosis-like tumour (inclusion body fibromatosis) of adulthood: report of two cases with ultrastructural and immunocytochemical findings. Histopathology 1988;12:415–24.
221. Vogrincic GS, O'Connell JX, Gilks CB. Giant cell tumor of tendon sheath is a polyclonal cellular proliferation. Hum Pathol 1997;28:815–9.
222. Wakely PE Jr, Frable WJ. Fine-needle aspiration biopsy cytology of giant-cell tumor of tendon sheath. Am J Clin Pathol 1994;102:87–90.
223. Watanabe T, Sasaki T, Ogata F, Okochi H, Furue M. Sclerotic fibroma of tendon sheath. Dermatology 1997;195:563–5.
224. Weedon D, Gutteridge BH, Hockly RG, Emmett AJ. Unusual cutaneous reactions to injections of corticosteroids. Am J Dermatopathol 1982;4:199–203.
225. Weisberg NK, DiCaudo DJ, Meland NB. Collagenous fibroma (desmoplastic fibroblastoma). J Am Acad Dermatol 1999;41(Pt 2):292–4.
226. Werther K, Seiersen M. [Recurrent infantile digital fibromatosis.] Ugeskr Laeger 1997;159:4656–7. (Danish.)
227. Wick MR, Mills SE, Ritter JH, Lind AC. Postoperative/posttraumatic spindle cell nodule of the skin: the dermal analogue of nodular fasciitis. Am J Dermatopathol 1999;21:220–4.
228. Wick MR, Ritter JH, Lind AC, Swanson PE. The pathological distinction between "deep penetrating" dermatofibroma and dermatofibrosarcoma protuberans. Semin Cutan Med Surg 1999;18:91–8.
229. Wilk M, Kaiser HW, Steen KH, Kreysel HW. [Sclerotic fibroma.] Hautarzt 1995;46:413–6. (German.)
230. Wilkin MM, Lane JW. Plexiform fibrohistiocytic tumor of the foot. J Foot Ankle Surg 1999;38:135–8.
231. Williams BT, Barr RJ, Barrett TL, Everett MA, Lin F. Cutaneous pseudosarcomatous polyp: a histological and immunohistochemical study. J Cutan Pathol 1996;23:189–93.
232. Wilson BB, Dent CH, Cooper PH. Papular acne scars. A common cutaneous finding. Arch Dermatol 1990;126:797–800.
233. Wilson C, Summerall J, Lubin J, Mesko TW. Collagenous fibroma (desmoplastic fibroblastoma): a unique presentation as a goiter in an 88-year-old man. Ann Diagn Pathol 2000;4:165–9.

234. Wirman JA. Nodular fasciitis, a lesion of myofibroblasts: an ultrastructural study. Cancer 1976;38:2378–89.
235. Wood GS, Beckstead JH, Medeiros LJ, Kempson RL, Warnke RA. The cells of giant cell tumor of tendon sheath resemble osteoclasts. Am J Surg Pathol 1988;12:444–52.
236. Yang M. Cutaneous inflammatory pseudotumor: a case report with immunohistochemical and ultrastructural studies. Pathology 1993; 25:405–9.
237. Young RH. Spindle cell lesions of the urinary bladder. Histol Histopathol 1990;5:505–12.
238. Zelger B, Weinlich G, Steiner H, Zelger BG, Egarter-Vigl E. Dermal and subcutaneous variants of plexiform fibrohistiocytic tumor. Am J Surg Pathol 1997;21:235–41.
239. Zelger BG, Steiner H, Kutzner H, Rutten A, Zelger B. Granular cell dermatofibroma. Histopathology 1997;31:258–62.
240. Zelger BG, Zelger B, Steiner H, Rutten A. Sclerotic lipoma: lipomas simulating sclerotic fibroma. Histopathology 1997;31:174–81.
241. Zelger BW, Calonje E, Sepp N, Fink FM, Zelger BG, Schmid KW. Monophasic cellular variant of infantile myofibromatosis. An unusual histopathologic pattern in two siblings. Am J Dermatopathol 1995;17:131–8.
242. Zelger BW, Zelger BG, Rappersberger K. Prominent myofibroblastic differentiation. A pitfall in the diagnosis of dermatofibroma. Am J Dermatopathol 1997;19:138–46.
243. Zellers RA, Bicket WJ, Parker MG. Posttraumatic spindle cell nodule of the buccal mucosa. Report of a case. Oral Surg Oral Med Oral Pathol 1992;74:212–5.

Fibrous Tissue Tumors of Intermediate Malignancy

244. Alguacil-Garcia A, Unni KK, Goellner JR, Winkelmann RK. Atypical fibroxanthoma of the skin: an ultrastructural study of two cases. Cancer 1977;40:1471–80.
245. Allen PW, Dymock RB, MacCormac LB. Superficial angiomyxomas with and without epithelial components. Report of 30 tumors in 28 patients. Am J Surg Pathol 1988;12:519–30.
246. Barr RJ, Wuerker RB, Graham JH. Ultrastructure of atypical fibroxanthoma. Cancer 1977; 40:736–43.
247. Barr RJ, Young EM Jr, King DF. Non-polarizable collagen in dermatofibrosarcoma protuberans: a useful diagnostic aid. J Cutan Pathol 1986;13: 339–46.
248. Barr RJ, Young EM, Liao SY. Giant cell fibroblastoma: an immunohistochemical study. J Cutan Pathol 1986;13:301–7.
249. Bedlow AJ, Sampson SA, Holden CA. Congenital superficial angiomyxoma. Clin Exp Dermatol 1997;22:237–9.
250. Bednar B. Storiform neurofibromas of the skin, pigmented and nonpigmented. Cancer 1957;10:368–76.
251. Beham A, Fletcher CD. Dermatofibrosarcoma protuberans with areas resembling giant cell fibroblastoma: report of two cases. Histopathology 1990;17:165–7.
252. Bell D. Atypical fibroxanthoma and malignant fibrous histiocytoma. Am J Dermatopathol 1979;1:185.
253. Berbis P, Devant O, Echinard C, Le Treut YP, Dor AM, Privat Y. [Metastatic Darier-Ferrand dermato-fibrosarcoma. Review of the literature apropos of a case.] Ann Dermatol Venereol 1987;114:1217–27. (French.)
254. Betti R, Inselvini E, Crosti C. Unusual features of primary dermatofibrosarcoma protuberans and its myxoid recurrence. J Cutan Pathol 1996; 23:283–7.
255. Bigotti G, Coli A, Gasbarri A, Castagnola D, Madonna V, Bartolazzi A. Angiomyofibroblastoma and aggressive angiomyxoma: two benign mesenchymal neoplasms of the female genital tract. An immunohistochemical study. Pathol Res Pract 1999;195:39–44.
256. Bisceglia M, Vairo M, Calonje E, Fletcher CD. [Pigmented fibrosarcomatous dermatofibrosarcoma protuberans (Bednar tumor). 3 case reports, analogy with the "conventional" type and review of the literature.] Pathologica 1997; 89:264–73. (Italian.)
257. Briselli M, Mark EJ, Dickersin GR. Solitary fibrous tumors of the pleura: eight new cases and review of 360 cases in the literature. Cancer 1981;47:2678–89.
258. Brunnemann RB, Ro JY, Ordonez NG, Mooney J, El-Naggar AK, Ayala AG. Extrapleural solitary fibrous tumor: a clinicopathologic study of 24 cases. Mod Pathol 1999;12:1034–42.
259. Calonje E, Fletcher CD. Myoid differentiation in dermatofibrosarcoma protuberans and its fibrosarcomatous variant: clinicopathologic analysis of 5 cases. J Cutan Pathol 1996;23:30–6.
260. Calonje E, Guerin D, McCormick D, Fletcher CD. Superficial angiomyxoma: clinicopathologic analysis of a series of distinctive but poorly recognized cutaneous tumors with tendency for recurrence. Am J Surg Pathol 1999;23:910–7.
261. Calonje E, Wadden C, Wilson-Jones E, Fletcher CD. Spindle-cell non-pleomorphic atypical fibroxanthoma: analysis of a series and delineation of a distinctive variant. Histopathology 1993;22:247–54.

262. Carlson JA, Slominski A, Heasley D, Mihm MC Jr, Toda S. Dermatofibrosarcoma protuberans can induce epidermal hyperplasia that is inversely related to its proximity to the epidermis. Am J Dermatopathol 1998;20:428–30.
263. Connelly JH, Evans HL. Dermatofibrosarcoma protuberans. A clinicopathologic review with emphasis on fibrosarcomatous areas. Am J Surg Pathol 1992;16:921–5.
264. Cowper SE, Kilpatrick T, Proper S, Morgan MB. Solitary fibrous tumor of the skin. Am J Dermatopathol 1999;21:213–9.
265. Coyne J, Kaftan SM, Craig RD. Dermatofibrosarcoma protuberans recurring as a giant cell fibroblastoma. Histopathology 1992;21:184–7.
266. Craver RD, Correa H, Kao YS, Van Brunt T, Golladay ES. Aggressive giant cell fibroblastoma with a balanced 17;22 translocation. Cancer Genet Cytogenet 1995;80:20–2.
267. Davis JL, Randle HW, Zalla MJ, Roenigk RK, Brodland DG. A comparison of Mohs micrographic surgery and wide excision for the treatment of atypical fibroxanthoma. Dermatol Surg 1997;23:105–10.
268. Dei Tos AP, Maestro R, Doglioni C, et al. Ultraviolet-induced p53 mutations in atypical fibroxanthoma. Am J Pathol 1994;145:11–7.
269. Denoux Y, Busson A, de Ranieri J, Contesso G, Lemerle J, Mandard AM. [Recurrence of giant-cell fibroblastoma as dermatofibrosarcoma protuberans in the adult.] Ann Pathol 1996;16:457–9. (French.)
270. Diaz-Cascajo C, Bastida-Inarrea J, Borrego L, Carretero-Hernandez G. Comparison of p53 expression in dermatofibrosarcoma protuberans and dermatofibroma: lack of correlation with proliferation rate. J Cutan Pathol 1995;22:304–9.
271. Diaz-Cascajo C, Borrego L, Bastida-Inarrea J, Borghi S. Giant cell fibroblastoma. New histological observations. Am J Dermatopathol 1996;18:403–8.
272. Diaz-Cascajo C, Weyers W, Borghi S. Sclerosing dermatofibrosarcoma protuberans. J Cutan Pathol 1998;25:440–4.
273. Diaz-Cascajo C, Weyers W, Borrego L, Inarrea JB, Borghi S. Dermatofibrosarcoma protuberans with fibrosarcomatous areas: a clinico-pathologic and immunohistochemic study in four cases. Am J Dermatopathol 1997;19:562–7.
274. Ding JA, Hashimoto H, Sugimoto T, Tsuneyoshi M, Enjoji M. Bednar tumor (pigmented dermatofibrosarcoma protuberans). An analysis of six cases. Acta Pathol Jpn 1990;40:744–54.
275. Dupree WB, Langloss JM, Weiss SW. Pigmented dermatofibrosarcoma protuberans (Bednar tumor). A pathologic, ultrastructural, and immunohistochemical study. Am J Surg Pathol 1985;9:630–9.
276. Eckert F, Schaich B, Landthaler M. [Spinocellular cancers and myxoid atypical fibroxanthoma of an actinically damaged burn scar.] Hautarzt 1991;42:254–7. (German.)
277. Elgart GW, Hanly A, Busso M, Spencer JM. Bednar tumor (pigmented dermatofibrosarcoma protuberans) occurring in a site of prior immunization: immunochemical findings and therapy. J Am Acad Dermatol 1999;40(Pt 2):315–7.
278. England DM, Hochholzer L, McCarthy MJ. Localized benign and malignant fibrous tumors of the pleura. A clinicopathologic review of 223 cases. Am J Surg Pathol 1989;13:640–58.
279. Evans HL. Low-grade fibromyxoid sarcoma. A report of 12 cases. Am J Surg Pathol 1993;17:595–600.
280. Feldman PS, Barr RJ. Ultrastructure of spindle cell squamous carcinoma. J Cutan Pathol 1976;3:17–24.
281. Fetsch JF, Laskin WB, Tavassoli FA. Superficial angiomyxoma (cutaneous myxoma): a clinicopathologic study of 17 cases arising in the genital region. Int J Gynecol Pathol 1997;16:325–34.
282. Fetsch JF, Michal M, Miettinen M. Pigmented (melanotic) neurofibroma: a clinicopathologic and immunohistochemical analysis of 19 lesions from 17 patients. Am J Surg Pathol 2000;24:331–43.
283. Filipowicz EA, Ventura KC, Pou AM, Logrono R. FNAC in the diagnosis of recurrent dermatofibrosarcoma protuberans of the forehead. A case report. Acta Cytol 1999;43:1177–80.
284. Fletcher CD. Giant cell fibroblastoma of soft tissue: a clinicopathological and immunohistochemical study. Histopathology 1988;13:499–508.
285. Fletcher CD, Evans BJ, MacArtney JC, Smith N, Wilson Jones E, McKee PH. Dermatofibrosarcoma protuberans: a clinicopathological and immunohistochemical study with a review of the literature. Histopathology 1985;9:921–38.
286. Fletcher CD, Theaker JM, Flanagan A, Krausz T. Pigmented dermatofibrosarcoma protuberans (Bednar tumour): melanocytic colonization or neuroectodermal differentiation? A clinicopathological and immunohistochemical study. Histopathology 1988;13:631–43.
287. Fletcher CD, Tsang WY, Fisher C, Lee KC, Chan JK. Angiomyofibroblastoma of the vulva. A benign neoplasm distinct from aggressive angiomyxoma. Am J Surg Pathol 1992;16:373–82.

288. Folpe AL, Lane KL, Paull G, Weiss SW. Low-grade fibromyxoid sarcoma and hyalinizing spindle cell tumor with giant rosettes: a clinicopathologic study of 73 cases supporting their identity and assessing the impact of high-grade areas. Am J Surg Pathol 2000;24:1353–60.

289. Fretzin DF, Helwig EB. Atypical fibroxanthoma of the skin. A clinicopathologic study of 140 cases. Cancer 1973;31:1541–52.

290. Fukasawa Y, Takada A, Tateno M, et al. Solitary fibrous tumor of the pleura causing recurrent hypoglycemia by secretion of insulin-like growth factor II. Pathol Int 1998;48:47–52.

291. Fukunaga M, Nomura K, Matsumoto K, Doi K, Endo Y, Ushigome S. Vulval angiomyofibroblastoma. Clinicopathologic analysis of six cases. Am J Clin Pathol 1997;107:45–51.

292. Fukunaga M, Ushigome S, Fukunaga N. Low-grade fibromyxoid sarcoma. Virchows Arch 1996;429:301–3.

293. Garcia C, Clark RE, Buchanan M. Dermatofibrosarcoma protuberans. Int J Dermatol 1996;35:867–71.

294. Goldblum JR, Tuthill RJ. CD34 and factor-XIIIa immunoreactivity in dermatofibrosarcoma protuberans and dermatofibroma. Am J Dermatopathol 1997;19:147–53.

295. Goodlad JR, Mentzel T, Fletcher CD. Low grade fibromyxoid sarcoma: clinicopathological analysis of eleven new cases in support of a distinct entity. Histopathology 1995;26:229–37.

296. Granter SR, Nucci MR, Fletcher CD. Aggressive angiomyxoma: reappraisal of its relationship to angiomyofibroblastoma in a series of 16 cases. Histopathology 1997;30:3–10.

297. Hardisson D, Cuevas-Santos J, Contreras F. Solitary fibrous tumor of the skin. J Am Acad Dermatol 2002;46(2 Suppl Case Reports):S37–40.

298. Harvell JD, Kilpatrick SE, White WL. Histogenetic relations between giant cell fibroblastoma and dermatofibrosarcoma protuberans. CD34 staining showing the spectrum and a simulator. Am J Dermatopathol 1998;20:339–45.

299. Helwig EB. Tumor Seminar. Texas State J Med 1963;59:652–89.

300. Helwig EB, May D. Atypical fibroxanthoma of the skin with metastasis. Cancer 1986;57:368–76.

301. Hisaoka M, Kouho H, Aoki T, Daimaru Y, Hashimoto H. Angiomyofibroblastoma of the vulva: a clinicopathologic study of seven cases. Pathol Int 1995;45:487–92.

302. Hisaoka M, Okamoto S, Morimitsu Y, Tsuji S, Hashimoto H. Dermatofibrosarcoma protuberans with fibrosarcomatous areas. Molecular abnormalities of the p53 pathway in fibrosarcomatous transformation of dermatofibrosarcoma protuberans. Virchows Arch 1998;433: 323–9.

303. Hsi ED, Nickoloff BJ. Dermatofibroma and dermatofibrosarcoma protuberans: an immunohistochemical study reveals distinctive antigenic profiles. J Dermatol Sci 1996;11:1–9.

304. Iezzoni JC, Fechner RE, Wong LS, Rosai J. Aggressive angiomyxoma in males. A report of four cases. Am J Clin Pathol 1995;104:391–6.

305. Jacobs DS, Edwards WD, Ye RC. Metastatic atypical fibroxanthoma of skin. Cancer 1975;35:457–63.

306. Kaburagi Y, Hatta N, Kawara S, Takehara K. Pigmented dermatofibrosarcoma protuberans (Bednar tumor) occurring in a Japanese infant. Dermatology 1998;197:48–51.

307. Kagoura M, Toyoda M, Nagahori H, Makino T, Morohashi M. An ultrastructural and immunohistochemical study of pigmented dermatofibrosarcoma protuberans (Bednar tumor). Eur J Dermatol 1999;9:366–9.

308. Kahn LB, Saxe N, Gordon W. Dermatofibrosarcoma protuberans with lymph node and pulmonary metastases. Arch Dermatol 1978;114:599–601.

309. Kamino H, Jacobson M. Dermatofibroma extending into the subcutaneous tissue. Differential diagnosis from dermatofibrosarcoma protuberans. Am J Surg Pathol 1990;14:1156–64.

310. Karabela-Bouropoulou V, Liapi-Avgeri G, Mahera H, et al. Giant cell fibroblastoma: an entity or a reactive phenomenon? Pathol Res Pract 1999;195:413–9.

311. Kemp JD, Stenn KS, Arons M, Fischer J. Metastasizing atypical fibroxanthoma. Coexistence with chronic lymphocytic leukemia. Arch Dermatol 1978;114:1533–5.

312. Khan ZM, Cockerell CJ. Atypical fibroxanthoma with osteoclast-like multinucleated giant cells. Am J Dermatopathol 1997;19:174–9.

313. Klemperer P, Rabin, C.B. Primary neoplasm of the pleura: a report of five cases. Arch Pathol 1931;11:385–412.

314. Kobayashi T, Hasegawa Y, Konohana A, Nakamura N. A case of Bednar tumor. Immunohistochemical positivity for CD34. Dermatology 1997;195:57–9.

315. Kroe DJ, Pitcock JA. Atypical fibroxanthoma of the skin. Report of ten cases. Am J Clin Pathol 1969;51:487–92.

316. Lane KL, Shannon RJ, Weiss SW. Hyalinizing spindle cell tumor with giant rosettes: a distinctive tumor closely resembling low-grade fibromyxoid sarcoma. Am J Surg Pathol 1997;21:1481–8.

317. Laskin WB, Fetsch JF, Tavassoli FA. Angiomyofibroblastoma of the female genital tract: analysis of 17 cases including a lipomatous variant. Hum Pathol 1997;28:1046–55.

318. Lindberg GM, Maitra A, Gokaslan ST, Saboorian MH, Albores-Saavedra J. Low grade fibromyxoid sarcoma: fine-needle aspiration cytology with histologic, cytogenetic, immunohistochemical, and ultrastructural correlation. Cancer 1999;87:75–82.
319. Longacre TA, Smoller BR, Rouse RV. Atypical fibroxanthoma. Multiple immunohistologic profiles. Am J Surg Pathol 1993;17:1199–209.
320. Ma CK, Zarbo RJ, Gown AM. Immunohistochemical characterization of atypical fibroxanthoma and dermatofibrosarcoma protuberans. Am J Clin Pathol 1992;97:478–83.
321. Marcus JR, Few JW, Senger C, Reynolds M. Dermatofibrosarcoma protuberans and the Bednar tumor: treatment in the pediatric population. J Pediatr Surg 1998;33:1811–4.
322. McCluggage WG, Patterson A, Maxwell P. Aggressive angiomyxoma of pelvic parts exhibits oestrogen and progesterone receptor positivity. J Clin Pathol 2000;53:603–5.
323. Mezzelani A, Sozzi G, Nessling M, et al. Low grade fibromyxoid sarcoma. A further low-grade soft tissue malignancy characterized by a ring chromosome. Cancer Genet Cytogenet 2000; 122:144–8.
324. Michal M, Zamecnik M. Giant cell fibroblastoma with a dermatofibrosarcoma protuberans component. Am J Dermatopathol 1992; 14:549–52.
325. Michie BA, Reid RP, Fallowfield ME. Aneuploidy in atypical fibroxanthoma: DNA content quantification of 10 cases by image analysis. J Cutan Pathol 1994;21:404–7.
326. Mochizuki Y, Narisawa Y, Kohda H. A case of Bednar tumor recurring after 23 years. J Dermatol 1996;23:614–8.
327. Nakamura T, Ogata H, Katsuyama T. Pigmented dermatofibrosarcoma protuberans. Report of two cases as a variant of dermatofibrosarcoma protuberans with partial neural differentiation. Am J Dermatopathol 1987;9:18–25.
328. Nemoto T, Shinoda M, Komatsuzaki K, Hara T, Kojima M, Ogihara T. Myxoid leiomyoma of the vulva mimicking aggressive angiomyxoma. Pathol Int 1994;44:454–9.
329. Nichols GE, Cooper PH. Low-grade fibromyxoid sarcoma: case report and immunohistochemical study. J Cutan Pathol 1994;21:356–62.
330. Nielsen GP, Rosenberg AE, Young RH, Dickersin GR, Clement PB, Scully RE. Angiomyofibroblastoma of the vulva and vagina. Mod Pathol 1996;9:284–91.
331. O'Brien KP, Seroussi E, Dal Cin P, et al. Various regions within the alpha-helical domain of the COL1A1 gene are fused to the second exon of the PDGFB gene in dermatofibrosarcomas and giant-cell fibroblastomas. Genes Chromosomes Cancer 1998;23:187–93.
332. O'Connell JX, Trotter MJ. Fibrosarcomatous dermatofibrosarcoma protuberans with myofibroblastic differentiaion: a histologically distinctive variant [corrected]. Mod Pathol 1996;9:273–8.
333. O'Dowd J, Laidler P. Progression of dermatofibrosarcoma protuberans to malignant fibrous histiocytoma: report of a case with implications for tumor histogenesis. Hum Pathol 1988;19: 368–70.
334. Ockner DM, Sayadi H, Swanson PE, Ritter JH, Wick MR. Genital angiomyofibroblastoma. Comparison with aggressive angiomyxoma and other myxoid neoplasms of skin and soft tissue. Am J Clin Pathol 1997;107:36–44.
335. Ohtani N, Fukusato T, Tezuka F. Sarcomatous dermatofibrosarcoma protuberans metastasized to the lung: preservation of CD34 expression in tumor cells. Pathol Int 1998;48:989–93.
336. Okamura JM, Barr RJ, Battifora H. Solitary fibrous tumor of the skin. Am J Dermatopathol 1997;19:515–8.
337. Onoda N, Tsutsumi Y, Kakudo K, et al. Pigmented dermatofibrosarcoma protuberans (Bednar tumor). An autopsy case with systemic metastasis. Acta Pathol Jpn 1990;40:935–40.
338. Orlandi A, Bianchi L, Spagnoli LG. Myxoid dermatofibrosarcoma protuberans: morphological, ultrastructural and immunohistochemical features. J Cutan Pathol 1998;25:386–93.
339. Oshiro Y, Fukuda T, Tsuneyoshi M. Atypical fibroxanthoma versus benign and malignant fibrous histiocytoma. A comparative study of their proliferative activity using MIB-1, DNA flow cytometry, and p53 immunostaining. Cancer 1995;75:1128–34.
340. Parker TL, Zitelli JA. Surgical margins for excision of dermatofibrosarcoma protuberans. J Am Acad Dermatol 1995;32(Pt 1):233–6.
341. Parlette LE, Smith CK, Germain LM, Rolfe CA, Skelton H. Accelerated growth of dermatofibrosarcoma protuberans during pregnancy. J Am Acad Dermatol 1999;41(Pt 1):778–83.
342. Patterson JW, Jordan WP Jr. Atypical fibroxanthoma in a patient with xeroderma pigmentosum. Arch Dermatol 1987;123:1066–70.
343. Patterson JW, Konerding H, Kramer WM. "Clear cell" atypical fibroxanthoma. J Dermatol Surg Oncol 1987;13:1109–14.
344. Puig L, De Moragas JM, Matias-Guiu X, Moreno A. [Pigmented dermatofibrosarcoma protuberans (Bednar's tumor).] Med Cutan Ibero Lat Am 1988;16:314–8. (Spanish.)

345. Requena L, Sangueza OP, Sanchez Yus E, Furio V. Clear-cell atypical fibroxanthoma: an uncommon histopathologic variant of atypical fibroxanthoma. J Cutan Pathol 1997;24:176–82.
346. Sanz-Trelles A, Ayala-Carbonero A, Rodrigo-Fernandez I, Weil-Lara B. Leiomyomatous nodules and bundles of vascular origin in the fibrosarcomatous variant of dermatofibrosarcoma protuberans. J Cutan Pathol 1998;25:44–9.
347. Sasaki M, Ishida T, Horiuchi H, MacHinami R. Dermatofibrosarcoma protuberans: an analysis of proliferative activity, DNA flow cytometry and p53 overexpression with emphasis on its progression. Pathol Int 1999;49:799–806.
348. Sasano H, Date F, Yamamoto H, Nagura H. Angiomyofibroblastoma of the vulva: case report with immunohistochemical, ultrastructural and DNA ploidy studies and a review of the literature. Pathol Int 1997;47:647–50.
349. Sato N, Kimura K, Tomita Y. Recurrent dermatofibrosarcoma protuberans with myxoid and fibrosarcomatous changes paralleled by loss of CD34 expression. J Dermatol 1995;22:665–72.
350. Shidham VB, Ayala GE, Lahaniatis JE, Garcia FU. Low-grade fibromyxoid sarcoma: clinicopathologic case report with review of the literature. Am J Clin Oncol 1999;22:150–5.
351. Shmookler BM, Enzinger FM, Weiss SW. Giant cell fibroblastoma. A juvenile form of dermatofibrosarcoma protuberans. Cancer 1989;64:2154–61.
352. Siassi RM, Papadopoulos T, Matzel KE. Metastasizing aggressive angiomyxoma. N Engl J Med 1999;341:1772.
353. Sigel JE, Bergfeld WF, Goldblum JR. A morphologic study of dermatofibrosarcoma protuberans: expansion of a histologic profile. J Cutan Pathol 2000;27:159–63.
354. Sigel JE, Goldblum JR. Solitary fibrous tumor of the skin. Am J Dermatopathol 2001;23:275–8.
355. Silverman JS, Albukerk J, Tamsen A. Comparison of angiomyofibroblastoma and aggressive angiomyxoma in both sexes: four cases composed of bimodal CD34 and factor XIIIa positive dendritic cell subsets. Pathol Res Pract 1997;193:673–82.
356. Silverman JS, Tamsen A. A cutaneous case of giant cell angiofibroma occurring with dermatofibrosarcoma protuberans and showing bimodal CD34+ fibroblastic and FXIIIa+ histiocytic immunophenotype. J Cutan Pathol 1998;25:265–70.
357. Skalova A, Michal M, Husek K, Zamecnik M, Leivo I. Aggressive angiomyxoma of the pelvioperineal region. Immunohistological and ultrastructural study of seven cases. Am J Dermatopathol 1993;15:446–51.
358. Smith KJ, Skelton HG 3rd, Morgan AM, Barrett TL, Lupton GP. Spindle cell neoplasms coexpressing cytokeratin and vimentin (metaplastic squamous cell carcinoma). J Cutan Pathol 1992;19:286–93.
359. Steeper TA, Rosai J. Aggressive angiomyxoma of the female pelvis and perineum. Report of nine cases of a distinctive type of gynecologic soft-tissue neoplasm. Am J Surg Pathol 1983;7:463–75.
360. Taylor HB, Helwig EB. Dermatofibrosarcoma protuberans. A study of 115 cases. Cancer 1962;15:717–25.
361. Tomaszewski MM, Lupton GP. Atypical fibroxanthoma. An unusual variant with osteoclast-like giant cells. Am J Surg Pathol 1997;21:213–8.
362. Ugai K, Kizaki T, Morimoto K, Sashikata T. A case of low-grade fibromyxoid sarcoma of the thigh. Pathol Int 1994;44:793–9.
363. Val-Bernal JF, Corral J, Fernandez F, Gomez-Bellvert C. Atypical fibroxanthoma with osteoclast-like giant cells. Acta Derm Venereol 1994;74:467–70.
364. Vallat-Decouvelaere AV, Dry SM, Fletcher CD. Atypical and malignant solitary fibrous tumors in extrathoracic locations: evidence of their comparability to intra-thoracic tumors. Am J Surg Pathol 1998;22:1501–11.
365. Van der Griend MD, Burda P, Ferrier AJ. Angiomyofibroblastoma of the vulva. Gynecol Oncol 1994;54:389–92.
366. Vanni R, Faa G, Dettori T, Melis GB, Dumanski JP, O'Brien KP. A case of dermatofibrosarcoma protuberans of the vulva with a COL1A1/PDGFB fusion identical to a case of giant cell fibroblastoma. Virchows Arch 2000;437:95–100.
367. Velanovich V. Superficial angiomyxoma presenting as a groin hernia in a male toddler. Am Surg 1996;62:253–5.
368. Vella R, Calleri D. [Superficial angiomyxoma of the epidiymis. Presentation of a new case and clinical considerations.] Minerva Urol Nefrol 2000;52:77–9. (Italian.)
369. Weiss SW, Nickoloff BJ. CD-34 is expressed by a distinctive cell population in peripheral nerve, nerve sheath tumors, and related lesions. Am J Surg Pathol 1993;17:1039–45.
370. Westra WH, Grenko RT, Epstein J. Solitary fibrous tumor of the lower urogenital tract: a report of five cases involving the seminal vesicles, urinary bladder, and prostate. Hum Pathol 2000;31:63–8.

371. Wick MR, Ritter JH, Lind AC, Swanson PE. The pathological distinction between "deep penetrating" dermatofibroma and dermatofibrosarcoma protuberans. Semin Cutan Med Surg 1999;18:91–8.
372. Worrell JT, Ansari MQ, Ansari SJ, Cockerell CJ. Atypical fibroxanthoma: DNA ploidy analysis of 14 cases with possible histogenetic implications. J Cutan Pathol 1993;20:211–5.
373. Zamecnik M. Fibrosarcomatous dermatofibrosarcoma protuberans with giant rosettes. Am J Dermatopathol 2001;23:41–5.
374. Zamecnik M, Michal M. [Angiomyofibroblastoma of the lower genital tract in women.] Cesk Patol 1994;30:16–8. (Slovak.)
375. Zamecnik M, Michal M. Low-grade fibromyxoid sarcoma: a report of eight cases with histologic, immunohistochemical, and ultrastructural study. Ann Diagn Pathol 2000;4:207–17.
376. Zelger BW, Ofner D, Zelger BG. Atrophic variants of dermatofibroma and dermatofibrosarcoma protuberans. Histopathology 1995;26:519–27.

Malignant Fibrous Tissue Tumors

377. Alconchel MD, Olivares C, Alvarez R. Squamous cell carcinoma, malignant melanoma and malignant fibrous histiocytoma arising in burn scars. Br J Dermatol 1997;137:793–8.
378. Angervall L, Hagmar B, Kindblom LG, Merck C. Malignant giant cell tumor of soft tissues: a clinicopathologic, cytologic, ultrastructural, angiographic, and microangiographic study. Cancer 1981;47:736–47.
379. Beham A, Wirnsberger G, Schmid C. [Immunohistochemical studies in the differential diagnosis of malignant fibrous histiocytoma.] Wien Klin Wochenschr 1986;98:617–22. (German.)
380. Brecher ME, Franklin WA. Absence of mononuclear phagocyte antigens in malignant fibrous histiocytoma. Am J Clin Pathol 1986;86:344–8.
381. Corsi A, Perugia G, De Matteis A. Epithelioid sarcoma of the penis. Clinicopathologic study of a tumor with myogenic features and review of the literature concerning this unusual location. Pathol Res Pract 1999;195:441–8.
382. Dickersin GR. Synovial sarcoma: a review and update, with emphasis on the ultrastructural characterization of the nonglandular component. Ultrastruct Pathol 1991;15:379–402.
383. Enzinger FM. Angiomatoid malignant fibrous histiocytoma: a distinct fibrohistiocytic tumor of children and young adults simulating a vascular neoplasm. Cancer 1979;44:2147–57.
384. Feely MG, Fidler ME, Nelson M, Neff JR, Bridge JA. Cytogenetic findings in a case of epithelioid sarcoma and a review of the literature. Cancer Genet Cytogenet 2000;119:155–7.
385. Fisher C. Synovial sarcoma. Ann Diagn Pathol 1998;2:401–21.
386. Fletcher CD, McKee PH. Sarcomas—a clinicopathological guide with special reference to cutaneous manifestation. IV. Extraskeletal osteosarcoma, extraskeletal chondrosarcoma, alveolar soft part sarcoma, clear cell sarcoma and discussion. Clin Exp Dermatol 1985;10:523–39.
387. Flieder DB, Moran CA. Primary cutaneous synovial sarcoma: a case report. Am J Dermatopathol 1998;20:509–12.
388. Frable WJ, Kay S, Lawrence W, Schatzki PF. Epithelioid sarcoma. An electron microscopic study. Arch Pathol 1973;95:8–12.
389. Fu YS, Gabbiani G, Kaye GI, Lattes R. Malignant soft tissue tumors of probable histiocytic origin (malignant fibrous histiocytomas): general considerations and electron microscopic and tissue culture studies. Cancer 1975;35:176–98.
390. Fukunaka H, Etoh T, Nakagawa H, Tamaki K. A case of subcutaneous malignant fibrous histiocytoma circumscribed by fibrous tissue. J Dermatol 1996;23:836–9.
391. Gross E, Rao BN, Pappo A, et al. Epithelioid sarcoma in children. J Pediatr Surg 1996;31:1663–5.
392. Halling AC, Wollan PC, Pritchard DJ, Vlasak R, Nascimento AG. Epithelioid sarcoma: a clinicopathologic review of 55 cases. Mayo Clin Proc 1996;71:636–42.
393. Henderson SA, Davis R, Nixon JR. Synovial sarcoma: a clinicopathological review. Int Orthop 1991;15:251–5.
394. Iwasaki H, Ohjimi Y, Ishiguro M, et al. Epithelioid sarcoma with an 18q aberration. Cancer Genet Cytogenet 1996;91:46–52.
395. Kempson RL, Kyriakos M. Fibroxanthosarcoma of the soft tissues. A type of malignant fibrous histiocytoma. Cancer 1972;29:961–76.
396. Lazova R, Moynes R, May D, Scott G. LN-2 (CD74). A marker to distinguish atypical fibroxanthoma from malignant fibrous histiocytoma. Cancer 1997;79:2115–24.
397. Lopes JM, Hannisdal E, Bjerkehagen B, et al. Synovial sarcoma. Evaluation of prognosis with emphasis on the study of DNA ploidy and proliferation (PCNA and Ki-67) markers. Anal Cell Pathol 1998;16:45–62.
398. Lopez-Rios F, Rodriguez-Peralto JL, Castano E, Gil R. Epithelioid sarcoma masquerading as perforating granuloma annulare. Histopathology 1997;31:102–3.

399. Lushnikova T, Knuutila S, Miettinen M. DNA copy number changes in epithelioid sarcoma and its variants: a comparative genomic hybridization study. Mod Pathol 2000;13:1092–6.
400. Medenica M, Casas C, Lorincz AL, Van Dam DP. Epithelioid sarcoma: ultrastructural observation of lymphoid cell-induced lysis of tumor cells. Acta Derm Venereol 1979;59:333–9.
401. Miettinen M, Fanburg-Smith JC, Virolainen M, Shmookler BM, Fetsch JF. Epithelioid sarcoma: an immunohistochemical analysis of 112 classical and variant cases and a discussion of the differential diagnosis. Hum Pathol 1999;30:934–42.
402. Mills SE, Fechner RE, Bruns DE, Bruns ME, O'Hara MF. Intermediate filaments in eosinophilic cells of epithelioid sarcoma: a light-microscopic, ultrastructural, and electrophoretic study. Am J Surg Pathol 1981;5:195–202.
403. Moore SW, Wheeler JE, Hefter LG. Epitheloid sarcoma masquerading as Peyronie's disease. Cancer 1975;35:1706–10.
404. Padilla RS, Flynn K, Headington JT. Epithelioid sarcoma. Enzymatic histochemical and electron microscopic evidence of histiocytic differentiation. Arch Dermatol 1985;121:389–93.
405. Prat J, Woodruff JM, Marcove RC. Epithelioid sarcoma: an analysis of 22 cases indicating the prognostic significance of vascular invasion and regional lymph node metastasis. Cancer 1978;41:1472–87.
406. Ratnam AV, Naik KG. Epithelioid sarcoma—a case report. Br J Dermatol 1978;99:451–3.
407. Ross HM, Lewis JJ, Woodruff JM, Brennan MF. Epithelioid sarcoma: clinical behavior and prognostic factors of survival. Ann Surg Oncol 1997;4:491–5.
408. Rothman AE, Lowitt MH, Pfau RG. Pediatric cutaneous malignant fibrous histiocytoma. J Am Acad Dermatol 2000;42(Pt 2):371–3.
409. Saxe N, Botha JB. Epithelioid sarcoma. A distinctive clinical presentation. Arch Dermatol 1977;113:1106–8.
410. Scott SM, Reiman HM, Pritchard DJ, Ilstrup DM. Soft tissue fibrosarcoma. A clinicopathologic study of 132 cases. Cancer 1989;64:925–31.
411. Sonobe H, Ohtsuki Y, Sugimoto T, Shimizu K. Involvement of 8q, 22q, and monosomy 21 in an epithelioid sarcoma. Cancer Genet Cytogenet 1997;96:178–80.
412. Soule EH, Pritchard DJ. Fibrosarcoma in infants and children: a review of 110 cases. Cancer 1977;40:1711–21.
413. Spillane AJ, A'Hern R, Judson IR, Fisher C, Thomas JM. Synovial sarcoma: a clinicopathologic, staging, and prognostic assessment. J Clin Oncol 2000;18:3794–803.
414. Spillane AJ, Thomas JM, Fisher C. Epithelioid sarcoma: the clinicopathological complexities of this rare soft tissue sarcoma. Ann Surg Oncol 2000;7:218–25.
415. Stephen MR, Morton R. Myxoid malignant fibrous histiocytoma mimicking papular mucinosis. Am J Dermatopathol 1998;20:290–5.
416. Tjalma WA, Hauben EI, Deprez SM, Van Marck EA, van Dam PA. Epithelioid sarcoma of the vulva. Gynecol Oncol 1999;73:160–4.
417. Ugurlu K, Turgut G, Kabukcuoglu F, Ozcan H, Sanus Z, Bas L. Malignant fibrous histiocytoma developing in a burn scar. Burns 1999;25:764–7.
418. Weiss SW, Enzinger FM. Malignant fibrous histiocytoma: an analysis of 200 cases. Cancer 1978;41:2250–66.
419. Weiss SW, Enzinger FM. Myxoid variant of malignant fibrous histiocytoma. Cancer 1977;39:1672–85.
420. Wick MR, Manivel JC. Epithelioid sarcoma and isolated necrobiotic granuloma: a comparative immunocytochemical study. J Cutan Pathol 1986;13:253–60.
421. Wood GS, Beckstead JH, Turner RR, Hendrickson MR, Kempson RL, Warnke RA. Malignant fibrous histiocytoma tumor cells resemble fibroblasts. Am J Surg Pathol 1986;10:323–35.
422. Zagars GK, Mullen JR, Pollack A. Malignant fibrous histiocytoma: outcome and prognostic factors following conservation surgery and radiotherapy. Int J Radiat Oncol Biol Phys 1996;34:983–94.

SUPPLEMENTAL REFERENCES

Connective Tissue Nevi

Aroni K, Kyriazi E, Aivaliotis M, Davaris P. Familial localized connective tissue nevus of the scalp with alopecia (report of a very unusual case). J Eur Acad Dermatol Venereol 2004;18:340–1.

Yokogawa M, Kamakura T, Ishiguro H, Ikeda M, Kodama H. Mucinous nevus. J Dermatol 2005;32:30–3.

Fibrous Hamartoma of Infancy

Lakshminarayanan R, Konia T, Welborn J. Fibrous hamartoma of infancy: a case report with associated cytogenetic findings. Arch Pathol Lab Med 2005;129:520–2.

Dermatofibroma

Gonzalez-Vela MC, Val-Bernal JF, Martino M, Gonzalez-Lopez MA, Garcia-Alberdi E, Hermana S. Sclerotic fibroma-like dermatofibroma: an uncommon distinctive variant of dermatofibroma. Histol Histopathol 2005;20:801–6.

Li N, McNiff J, Hui P, Manfioletti G, Tallini G. Differential expression of HMGA1 and HMGA2 in dermatofibroma and dermatofibrosarcoma protuberans: potential diagnostic applications, and comparison with histologic findings, CD34, and factor XIIIa immunoreactivity. Am J Dermatopathol 2004;26:267–72.

Ohnishi T, Sasaki M, Nakai K, Watanabe S. Atrophic dermatofibroma. J Eur Acad Dermatol Venereol 2004;18:580–3.

Song Y, Sakamoto F, Ito M. Characterization of factor XIIIa+ dendritic cells in dermatofibroma: Immunohistochemical, electron and immuno-electron microscopical observations. J Dermatol Sci 2005;39:89–96.

Angiofibroma and Related Lesions

Bansal C, Stewart D, Li A, Cockerell CJ. Histologic variants of fibrous papule. J Cutan Pathol 2005;32:424–8.

Plexiform Fibrohistiocytic Tumor

Mori O, Hashimoto T. Plexiform fibrohistiocytic tumor. Eur J Dermatol 2004;14:118–20.

Superficial Acral Fibromyxoma

Andre J, Theunis A, Richert B, de Saint-Aubain N. Superficial acral fibromyxoma: clinical and pathological features. Am J Dermatopathol 2004;26:472–4.

Pleomorphic Fibroma

Mahmood MN, Salama ME, Chaffins M, et al. Solitary sclerotic fibroma of skin: a possible link with pleomorphic fibroma with immunophenotypic expression for O13 (CD99) and CD34. J Cutan Pathol 2003;30:631–6.

Sclerotic Fibroma

High WA, Stewart D, Essary LR, Kageyama NP, Hoang MP, Cockerell CJ. Sclerotic fibroma-like change in various neoplastic and inflammatory skin lesions: is sclerotic fibroma a distinct entity? J Cutan Pathol 2004;31:373–8.

Collagenous Fibroma

Bernal K, Nelson M, Neff JR, Nielsen SM, Bridge JA. Translocation (2;11)(q31;q12) is recurrent in collagenous fibroma (desmoplastic fibroblastoma). Cancer Genet Cytogenet 2004;149:161–3.

Dagli M, Eryilmaz A, Acar A, Kulacoglu S, Akmansu H. Collagenous fibroma (desmoplastic fibroblastoma). Yonsei Med J 2004;45:941–3.

Inflammatory Pseudotumor

El Shabrawi-Caelen L, Kerl K, Cerroni L, Soyer HP, Kerl H. Cutaneous inflammatory pseudotumor—a spectrum of various diseases? J Cutan Pathol 2004;31:605–11.

Keloid

Chevray PM, Manson PN. Keloid scars are formed by polyclonal fibroblasts. Ann Plast Surg 2004;52:605-8.

Jiang DY, Fu XB, Chen W, Sun TZ. [Relationship of overexpression of angiogenesis factors and their receptors with invasive growth of keloid.] Zhonghua Zheng Xing Wai Ke Za Zhi 2004;20:128-31. (Chinese.)

Lee JY, Yang CC, Chao SC, Wong TW. Histopathological differential diagnosis of keloid and hypertrophic scar. Am J Dermatopathol 2004;26:379–84.

Messadi DV, Doung HS, Zhang Q, et al. Activation of NFkappaB signal pathways in keloid fibroblasts. Arch Dermatol Res 2004;296:125–33.

Elastofibroma Dorsi

Guha AR, Raja RC, Devadoss VG. Elastofibroma dorsi—a case report and review of literature. Int J Clin Pract 2004;58:218-20.

Solivetti FM, Bacaro D, Di Luca Sidozzi A, Cecconi P. Elastofibroma dorsi: ultrasound pattern in three patients. J Exp Clin Cancer Res 2003;22:565–9.

Giant Cell Tumor of Tendon Sheath

Stefanato CM, Turner MS, Bhawan J. High-pressure paint-gun injury of the finger simulating giant cell tumor of tendon sheath. J Cutan Pathol 2005;32:179–83.

Giant Cell Epulis (Peripheral Giant Cell Granuloma)

Chaparro-Avendano AV, Berini-Aytes L, Gay-Escoda C. Peripheral giant cell granuloma. A report of five cases and review of the literature. Med Oral Patol Oral Cir Bucal 2005;10:53–7, 48–52.

Fibromatosis

Bhattacharya B, Dilworth HP, Iacobuzio-Donahue C, et al. Nuclear beta-catenin expression distinguishes deep fibromatosis from other benign and malignant fibroblastic and myofibroblastic lesions. Am J Surg Pathol 2005;29:653–9.

Dominguez-Malagon H. Intracellular collagen and fibronexus in fibromatosis and other fibroblastic tumors. Ultrastruct Pathol 2004;28:67–73.

Fen Li C, Kandel C, Baliko F, Nadesan P, Brunner N, Alman BA. Plasminogen activator inhibitor-1 (PAI-1) modifies the formation of aggressive fibromatosis (desmoid tumor). Oncogene 2005;24:1615–24.

Sawyer JR, Sammartino G, Gokden N, Nicholas RW. A clonal reciprocal t(2;7)(p13;p13) in plantar fibromatosis. Cancer Genet Cytogenet 2005;158:67–9.

Tipton DA, Woodard ES 3rd, Baber MA, Dabbous M. Role of the c-myc proto-oncogene in the proliferation of hereditary gingival fibromatosis fibroblasts. J Periodontol 2004;75:360–9.

Juvenile Hyaline Fibromatosis

Anadolu RY, Oskay T, Ozsoy N, Erdem C. Juvenile non-hyaline fibromatosis: juvenile hyaline fibromatosis without prominent hyaline changes. J Cutan Pathol 2005;32:235–9.

Thomas JE, Moossavi M, Mehregan DR, McFalda WL, Mahon MJ. Juvenile hyaline fibromatosis: a case report and review of the literature. Int J Dermatol 2004;43:785–9.

Nodular Fasciitis

Plaza JA, Mayerson J, Wakely PE Jr. Nodular fasciitis of the hand: a potential diagnostic pitfall in fine-needle aspiration cytopathology. Am J Clin Pathol 2005;123:388–93.

Solitary Fibrous Tumor

Chen HJ, Zhang HY, Li X, et al. [Solitary fibrous tumor: the clinicopathologic and immunohistochemical characteristics of 26 cases.] Sichuan Da Xue Xue Bao Yi Xue Ban 2004;35:675–9. (Chinese.)

Rakheja D, Wilson KS, Meehan JJ, Schultz RA, Maale GE, Timmons CF. Extrapleural benign solitary fibrous tumor in the shoulder of a 9-year-old girl: case report and review of the literature. Pediatr Dev Pathol 2004;7:653–60.

Dermatofibrosarcoma Protuberans

Domanski HA. FNA diagnosis of dermatofibrosarcoma protuberans. Diagn Cytopathol 2005;32:299–302.

McNiff JM, Subtil A, Cowper SE, Lazova R, Glusac EJ. Cellular digital fibromas: distinctive CD34-positive lesions that may mimic dermatofibrosarcoma protuberans. J Cutan Pathol 2005;32:413–8.

Saeki H, Tsunemi Y, Ohtsuki M, Kikuchi K, Tamaki K. Gene mutation analysis in five cases of dermatofibrosarcoma protuberans using formalin-fixed, paraffin-embedded tissues. Acta Derm Venereol 2005;85:221–4.

Szollosi Z, Nemes Z. Transformed dermatofibrosarcoma protuberans: a clinicopathological study of eight cases. J Clin Pathol 2005;58:751–6.

Takahira T, Oda Y, Tamiya S, et al. Microsatellite instability and p53 mutation associated with tumor progression in dermatofibrosarcoma protuberans. Hum Pathol 2004;35:240–5.

Weinrach DM, Wang KL, Wiley EL, Laskin WB. Immunohistochemical expression of matrix metalloproteinases 1, 2, 9, and 14 in dermatofibrosarcoma protuberans and common fibrous histiocytoma (dermatofibroma). Arch Pathol Lab Med 2004;128:1136–41.

Giant Cell Fibroblastoma

Soto L, Jie T, Saltzman DA. Giant cell fibroblastoma of the breast in a child—a case report and review of the literature. J Pediatr Surg 2004;39:229–30.

Aggressive Angiomyxoma, Superficial Angiomyxoma, Angiomyofibroblastoma

Amezcua CA, Begley SJ, Mata N, Felix JC, Ballard CA. Aggressive angiomyxoma of the female genital tract: a clinicopathologic and immunohistochemical study of 12 cases. Int J Gynecol Cancer 2005;15:140–5.

Cao D, Srodon M, Montgomery EA, Kurman RJ. Lipomatous variant of angiomyofibroblastoma: report of two cases and review of the literature. Int J Gynecol Pathol 2005;24:196–200.

Chatelain D, Lazure T, Manaouil D, et al. [Angiomyofibroblastoma of the male genital tract. Pathological and immunohistochemical study of three cases.] Ann Pathol 2005;25:58–62. (French.)

Perret AG, Perrot JL, Dutoit M, Fouilloux B, Peoc'h M, Cambazard F. [Superficial angiomyxoma: report of four cases, including two subungueal tumors.] Ann Pathol 2005;25:54–7. (French.)

van Roggen JF, van Unnik JA, Briaire-de Bruijn IH, Hogendoorn PC. Aggressive angiomyxoma: a clinicopathological and immunohistochemical study of 11 cases with long-term follow-up. Virchows Arch 2005;446:157–63.

Low-Grade Fibromyxoid Sarcoma

Antonescu CR, Baren A. Spectrum of low-grade fibrosarcomas: a comparative ultrastructural analysis of low-grade myxofibrosarcoma and fibromyxoid sarcoma. Ultrastruct Pathol 2004;28:321–32.

Billings SD, Giblen G, Fanburg-Smith JC. Superficial low-grade fibromyxoid sarcoma (Evans tumor): a clinicopathologic analysis of 19 cases with a unique observation in the pediatric population. Am J Surg Pathol 2005;29:204–10.

Franchi A, Massi D, Santucci M. Hyalinizing spindle cell tumor with giant rosettes and low-grade fibromyxoid sarcoma: an immunohistochemical and ultrastructural comparative investigation. Ultrastruct Pathol 2003;27:349–55.

Mertens F, Fletcher CD, Antonescu CR, et al. Clinicopathologic and molecular genetic characterization of low-grade fibromyxoid sarcoma, and cloning of a novel FUS/CREB3L1 fusion gene. Lab Invest 2005;85:408–15.

Panagopoulos I, Storlazzi CT, Fletcher CD, et al. The chimeric FUS/CREB3l2 gene is specific for low-grade fibromyxoid sarcoma. Genes Chromosomes Cancer 2004;40:218–28.

Atypical Fibroxanthoma

Cooper JZ, Newman SR, Scott GA, Brown MD. Metastasizing atypical fibroxanthoma (cutaneous malignant histiocytoma): report of five cases. Dermatol Surg 2005;31:221–5; discussion 225.

Ly H, Selva D, James CL, Huilgol SC. Superficial malignant fibrous histiocytoma presenting as recurrent atypical fibroxanthoma. Australas J Dermatol 2004;45:106–9.

Mihic-Probst D, Zhao J, Saremaslani P, et al. CGH analysis shows genetic similarities and differences in atypical fibroxanthoma and undifferentiated high grade pleomorphic sarcoma. Anticancer Res 2004;24:19–26.

Rudisaile SN, Hurt MA, Santa Cruz DJ. Granular cell atypical fibroxanthoma. J Cutan Pathol 2005;32:314–7.

Smith-Zagone MJ, Prieto VG, Hayes RA, Timperman WW Jr., Diwan AH. HMB-45 (gp103) and MART-1 expression within giant cells in an atypical fibroxanthoma: a case report. J Cutan Pathol 2004;31:284–6.

Malignant Fibrous Histiocytoma

Erlandson RA, Antonescu CR. The rise and fall of malignant fibrous histiocytoma. Ultrastruct Pathol 2004;28:283–9.

Fletcher CD. Pleomorphic malignant fibrous histiocytoma: fact or fiction? A critical reappraisal based on 159 tumors diagnosed as pleomorphic sarcoma. Am J Surg Pathol 1992;16:213–28.

Randall RL, Albritton KH, Ferney BJ, Layfield L. Malignant fibrous histiocytoma of soft tissue: an abandoned diagnosis. Am J Orthop 2004;33:602–8.

Szollosi Z, Nemeth T, Egervari K, Nemes Z. Histiocyte-like cells expressing factor XIIIa do not belong to the neoplastic cell population in malignant fibrous histiocytoma. Pathol Res Pract 2005;201:369–77.

Epithelioid Sarcoma

Lin L, Hicks D, Xu B, et al. Expression profile and molecular genetic regulation of cyclin D1 expression in epithelioid sarcoma. Mod Pathol 2005;18:705–9.

Lualdi E, Modena P, Debiec-Rychter M, et al. Molecular cytogenetic characterization of proximal-type epithelioid sarcoma. Genes Chromosomes Cancer 2004;41:283–90.

Nishio J, Iwasaki H, Nabeshima K, et al. Establishment of a new human epithelioid sarcoma cell line, FU-EPS-1: molecular cytogenetic characterization by use of spectral karyotyping and comparative genomic hybridization. Int J Oncol 2005;27:361–9.

Synovial Sarcoma

Nakasone J, Shimizu T, Gomyo H, et al. Assessment of microinvasion with reverse transcriptase polymerase chain reaction in a case of synovial sarcoma. J Orthop Sci 2004;9:162–5.

7 VASCULAR TUMORS AND PSEUDOTUMORS

There has been considerable interest in vascular neoplasms of the skin over the past two decades because of their potential association with the acquired immunodeficiency syndrome (AIDS). In addition, it has been recognized that such lesions are associated with several conditions that are hereditary. These include the Klippel-Trenaunay-Weber, "blue rubber bleb," Sturge-Weber, and Maffucci syndromes. This chapter considers the spectrum of benign, "borderline," and malignant vascular cutaneous neoplasms, and discusses the pseudotumoral proliferations that may be confused with them.

VASCULAR NEVUS

Clinical Features. The vascular connective tissue nevus, *nevus flammeus (port wine stain, stork bite)*, is common in the general population (fig. 7-1) (78), but is best known for its association with other pathologic elements of the Sturge-Weber, Klippel-Trenaunay-Weber, and Parkes-Weber syndromes (6,19,22,47,55,83). Clinically, nevus flammeus takes the form of a variably prominent red-violet patch or plaque that is usually confined to one side of the body. It may be relatively inconspicuous or involve a large portion of the skin surface; the latter eventuality is most often observed in syndromic rather than sporadic cases.

Cutaneous telangiectasias are part of the Osler-Weber-Rendu syndrome, in association with vascular abnormalities of the mucosae, ears, and nail beds. This autosomal dominant complex presents as a generalized profusion of tiny macular or papular red lesions in adolescents and young adults. Hemorrhage from the nose and gut is potentially life-threatening for patients with the Osler-Weber-Rendu syndrome. Similar lesions may appear sporadically during pregnancy in young women, as acquired dermatomal eruptions in middle adulthood, or in association with cirrhosis (*spider angioma, nevus araneus*). True hemangiomas may sometimes arise in nevus flammeus, particularly during gestation.

Pathologic Findings. The histologic appearance of nevus flammeus is that of dermal telangiectasia, rather than a true hemangioma. Dilated vascular spaces of varying sizes are dispersed throughout the corium, separated by relatively normal connective tissue and cutaneous appendages (78). With advancing age of the patient, the telangiectatic vessels may increase in caliber so that they resemble large veins (fig. 7-2). In children, this vascular malformation is often subtle, being composed by attenuated capillaries in the superficial dermis. The microscopic characteristics of cutaneous telangiectasias are analogous to those of early-stage nevus flammeus: numerous small caliber, thin-walled blood vessels that are randomly distributed throughout the corium or the submucosa of the oral cavity.

BENIGN VASCULAR NEOPLASMS

Benign vascular tumors of the skin are generally typified by the proliferation of both endothelial and pericytic neoplastic cells. Two such

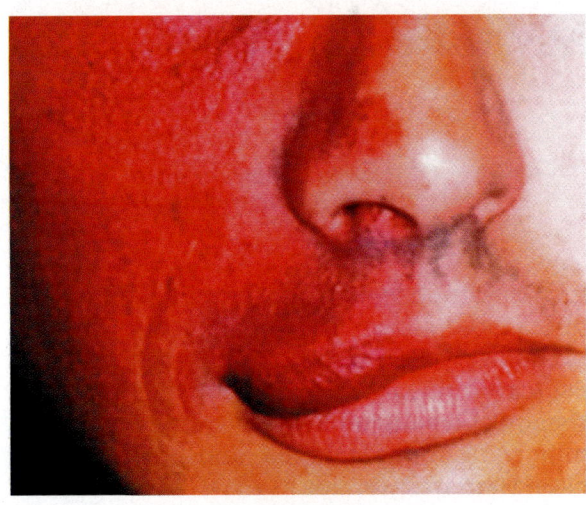

Figure 7-1

NEVUS FLAMMEUS

This lesion is on the face of an adult.

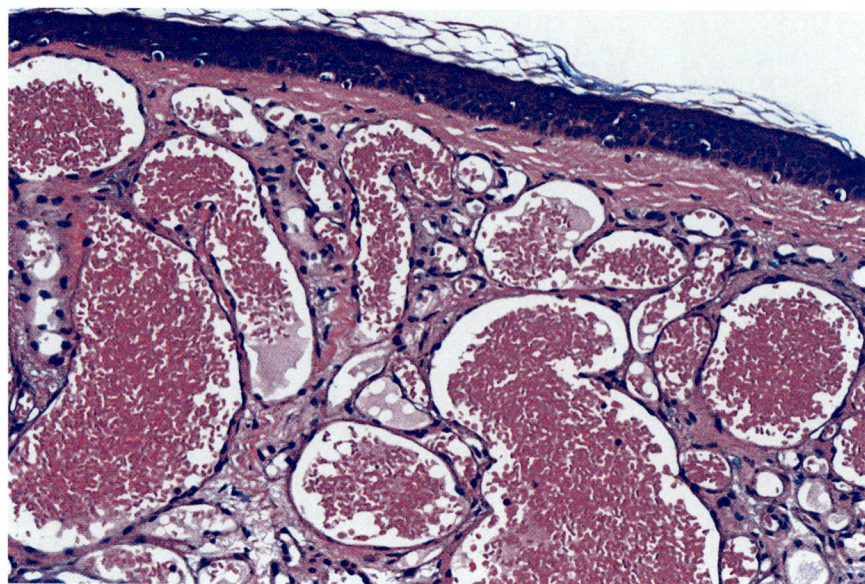

Figure 7-2

NEVUS FLAMMEUS

Dilated vein-like blood vessels are seen in the dermis.

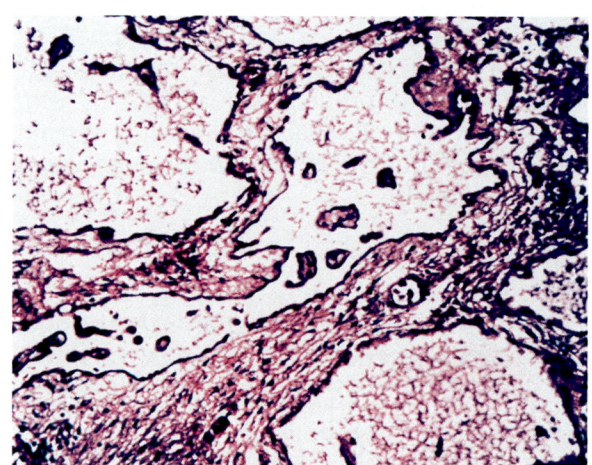
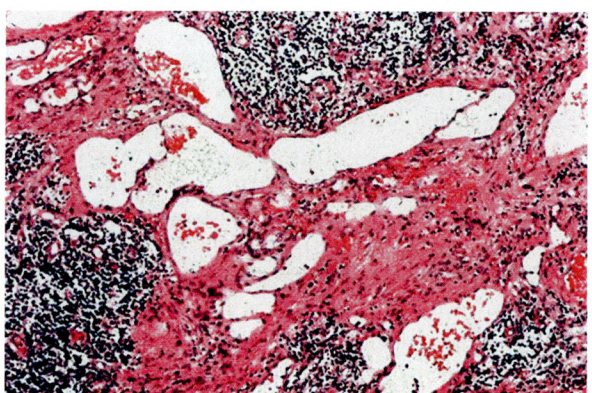

Figure 7-3

DEEP LYMPHANGIOMA OF THE SKIN

Left: Ectatic vascular spaces are filled with proteinaceous lymphatic fluid.
Right: Stromal lymphocytes are interspaced in the fluid.

tumors (lymphangioma and Kimura's tumor) feature a close morphologic relationship with immunologic cells (i.e., lymphocytes); the remainder (cavernous and capillary hemangiomas, epithelioid hemangioma, acral arteriovenous tumor, pyogenic granuloma, and other hemangioma variants) do not.

Lymphangioma

There are two types of cutaneous lymphangioma: *circumscribed-superficial (lymphangioma superficialis circumscriptum)* and *deep lymphangioma* (23,24,60,62,82). The latter tends to occur early in life, whereas the former may be seen at any age. Both favor the skin of the head, neck, and axillae, and present as fluctuant plaques (deep lymphangiomas) or multiple papular or verrucoid lesions (circumscribed lymphangiomas). Large areas of the skin surface may be involved by either form of this neoplasm.

Deep lymphangiomas display a profusion of thin-walled vessels at all levels of the dermis

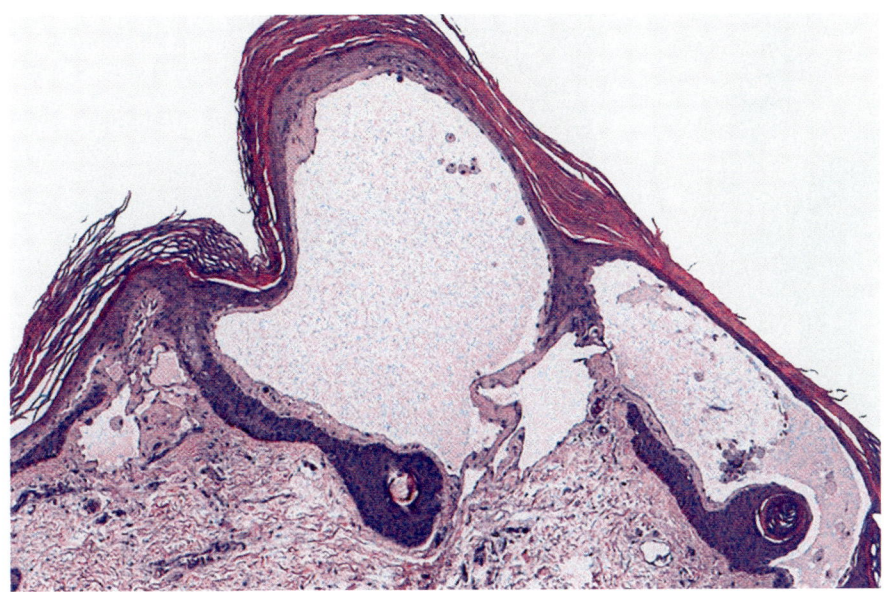

Figure 7-4

LYMPHANGIOMA SUPERFICIALIS CIRCUMSCRIPTUM

The lesion is a collection of lymphatic vessels in the upper dermis. The overlying epidermis has a tendency to engulf the lesion by forming collarettes.

and often involve the superficial subcutis as well. The endothelial lining cells are extremely attenuated, with flattened, inconspicuous nuclei, amphophilic cytoplasm, and no mitoses. The vascular channels comprising deep lymphangiomas are variable in diameter, but some attain large, cystic proportions. The intervening dermal connective tissue shows no alteration. Mature lymphocytes are often admixed throughout these tumors, and small collections of such cells may be observed within vascular lumens as well, along with serum (fig. 7-3) (24). Intravascular erythrocytes are typically scanty or absent.

In contrast, lymphangioma circumscriptum demonstrates numerous thin-walled lymphatic channels that are confined to the upper dermis (fig. 7-4). Indeed, most are so superficial that they are encompassed by surrounding rete pegs of the overlying epidermis (60,82). Acanthosis and hyperkeratosis of the epidermis may be observed. Accumulations of lymphocytes are much less prominent in lymphangioma circumscriptum in comparison with deep lymphangioma.

Despite the undoubted benign nature of all cutaneous lymphangiomas, postoperative recurrence is 15 to 20 percent (24,62). In all likelihood, this finding relates to the poor clinical definition of their margins.

Cavernous and Capillary Hemangiomas

Hemangiomas of the skin are often congenital lesions but may appear at any time throughout life (11,20,48–50,74). They assume a variety of clinical appearances, ranging from one simulating nevus flammeus to inconspicuous, pinpoint areas of redness (fig. 7-5). In cases featuring multiple cutaneous hemangiomas, associated lesions of other organs may be present. These include bony deformities and cartilaginous neoplasms (Maffucci's syndrome), meningeal hemangiomatosis and superficial cerebral gliosis (Sturge-Weber syndrome), gastrointestinal mucosal telangiectasia (Osler-Weber-Rendu syndrome), thrombocytopenia and congestive heart failure (Kasabach-Merritt syndrome), multiple lipomas and macrocephaly (Bannayan's syndrome), and cutaneous dysplasia (cutis marmorata telangiectasia congenita) (11,48–50). Because of the serious nature of many of these conditions, the dermatopathologist must be mindful of their relationship to benign vascular tumors of the skin in any case in which several specimens are received from the same patient.

Most cutaneous hemangiomas are divided into two categories based on the size of their constituent vascular channels. Those with blood-filled lumens that are larger than normal small veins are classified as *cavernous hemangiomas* (fig. 7-6), whereas those composed of more or less solid proliferations of bland endothelial cells with inconspicuous lumens are *capillary hemangiomas* (fig. 7-7). The latter may demonstrate marked mitotic activity in some cases, but division figures are never pathologic in shape.

Nonmelanocytic Tumors of the Skin

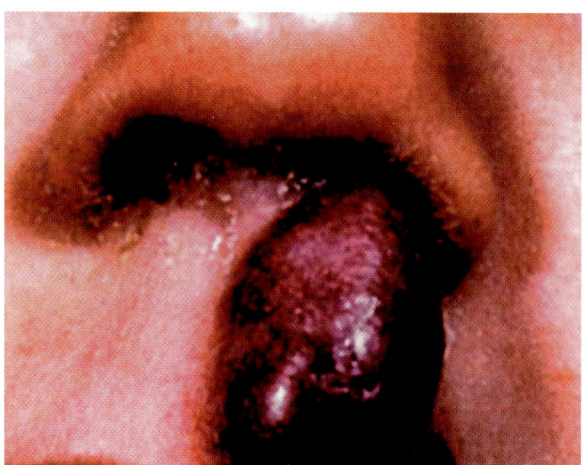 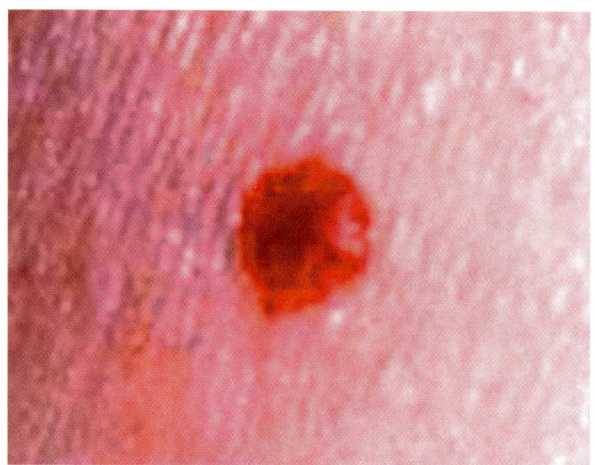

Figure 7-5

CAVERNOUS AND CAPILLARY HEMANGIOMAS

Left: A cavernous hemangioma of the lip in a child takes the form of a bulbous, reddish blue nodule.
Right: An ordinary capillary hemangioma.

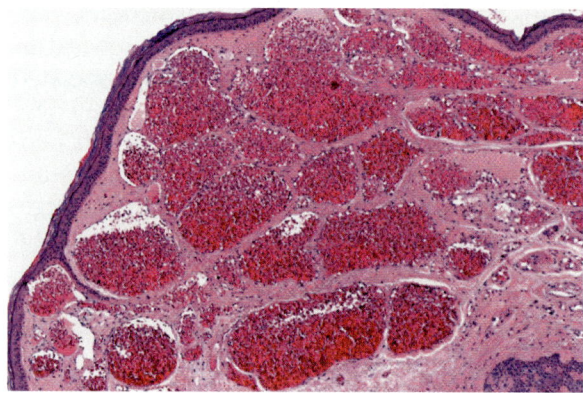 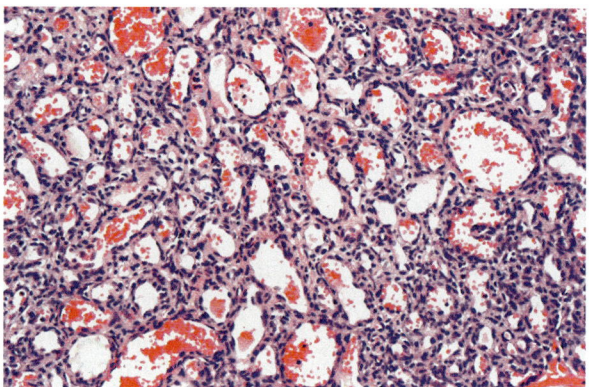

Figure 7-6

CAVERNOUS HEMANGIOMA

Histologically, cavernous hemangioma comprises a collection of closely apposed thin-walled vessels in the dermis.

Figure 7-7

CAPILLARY HEMANGIOMA

Lobular groups of tubular vessels are invested by pericytes.

Moreover, nuclei in both types of hemangioma of the skin are cytologically bland, attesting to their benign nature.

Most cutaneous hemangiomas are circumscribed but not encapsulated. Surrounding blood vessels of the dermis may be somewhat dilated, often leading to concern over the adequacy of surgical excision in such cases. Since dermal lesions rarely recur, even if subtotally resected, this point is of little significance.

Some authors have separated the lesion known as *infantile hemangioendothelioma* (61) from *cellular capillary hemangioma of infancy* (26). However, we believe the two tumors to be similar for practical purposes. Both are composed of lobulated masses of plump endothelial cells, as previously described (fig. 7-8); the only difference is their relative depths of cutaneous involvement. Infantile hemangioendothelioma is centered in the subcutis or deeper soft tissues,

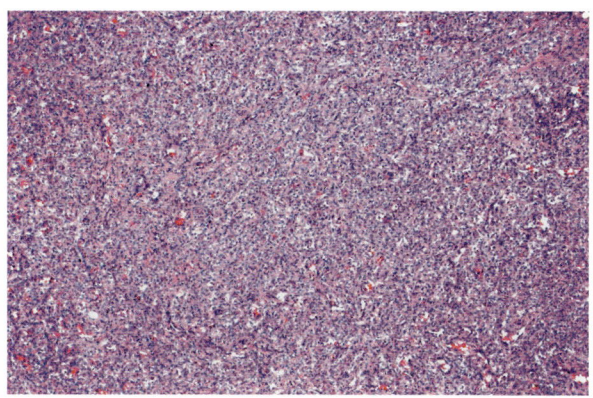 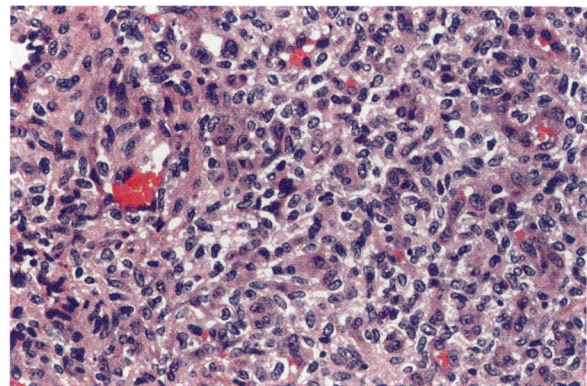

Figure 7-8

CELLULAR CAPILLARY HEMANGIOMA

Left: A relatively bloodless sheet of compact dermal vessels is seen on low magnification.
Right: Closer inspection shows that there are many small vascular lumens in the tumor.

and cellular capillary hemangioma is a more superficial lesion. This factor accounts for the observed difference in the efficacy of surgery for these neoplasms. Deep tumors of the soft tissue recur in roughly 10 percent of cases, whereas superficial capillary hemangiomas are virtually always cured by simple removal (48).

Lobular Capillary Hemangioma (Pyogenic Granuloma) and Related Lesions

Over 100 years after the description of the cutaneous vascular lesion known as *pyogenic granuloma* (30,63), this tumor continues to serve as the object of elucidative studies. Pyogenic granuloma was originally so named because of its clinical resemblance to polypoid granulation tissue and a presumed relationship to prior infections. Mills et al. (54) have shown convincingly that it is not merely a reaction to injury, but rather, a true neoplasm with reproducible microscopic features. Hence, the alternative designation of *lobular capillary hemangioma* has been embraced in recent years.

This lesion may occur at any age in any skin area, as a polypoid, strawberry-red excrescence (fig. 7-9). The mucosal surfaces are often involved as well, particularly in the oral cavity during pregnancy (fig. 7-10) (57).

Lobular capillary hemangioma features the proliferation of small vascular channels that are separated into lobules by fibrous connective tissue (38,54). The diameter of the constituent vessels is variable, even within the same lobule, but

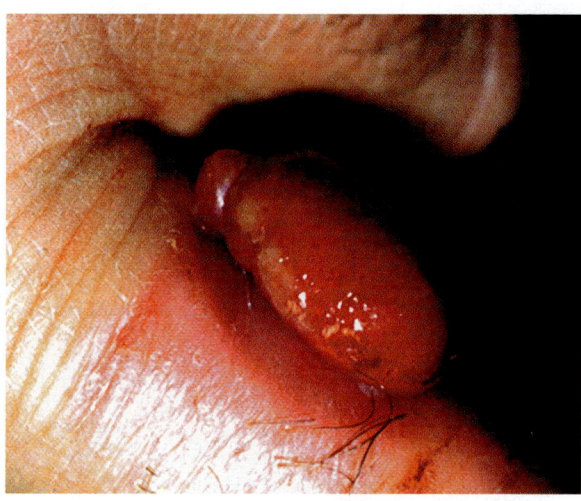

Figure 7-9

LOBULAR CAPILLARY HEMANGIOMA

A polypoid, red, friable lesion of the hand has an erythematous base.

all vessels are lined by plump, cytologically innocuous endothelial cells and supported by pericytic elements. Some nuclear atypia may be evident if the lesion has ulcerated or has been irritated, and mitoses are readily observed under such circumstances. Moreover, inflamed granulation tissue may be superimposed on lobular capillary hemangioma. This tumor virtually always retains its lobular profile on low-power microscopy, and polypoid examples often manifest an ingrowing collarette of epidermis at their bases (figs. 7-11, 7-12). These features serve to distinguish lobular capillary hemangioma from reactive fibrovascular proliferations.

Cooper et al. (15,16) have described two unusual variants of lobular capillary hemangioma that are located exclusively intravenously or subcutaneously. These occurrences lend credence to the premise that lobular capillary hemangioma is a true neoplasm. A closely related,

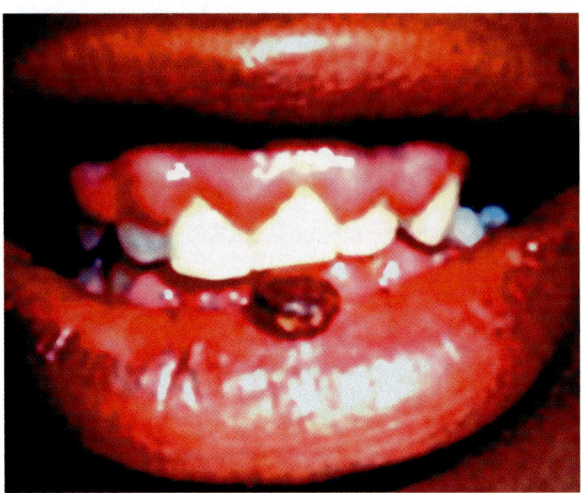

Figure 7-10

LOBULAR CAPILLARY HEMANGIOMA

The lesion may appear in the oral mucosa during pregnancy.

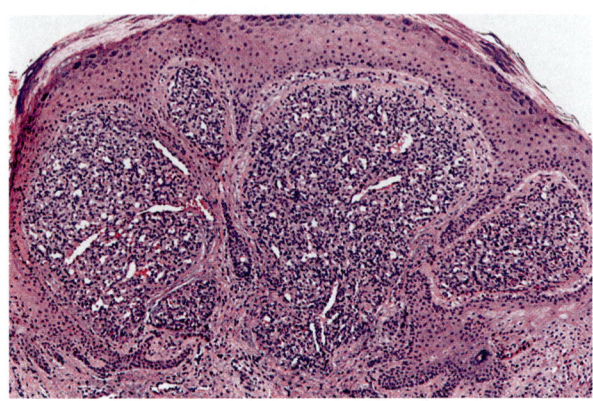

Figure 7-11

LOBULAR CAPILLARY HEMANGIOMA

Prototypically, the lesion is elevated and nodular, and bordered histologically by an adnexal collarette.

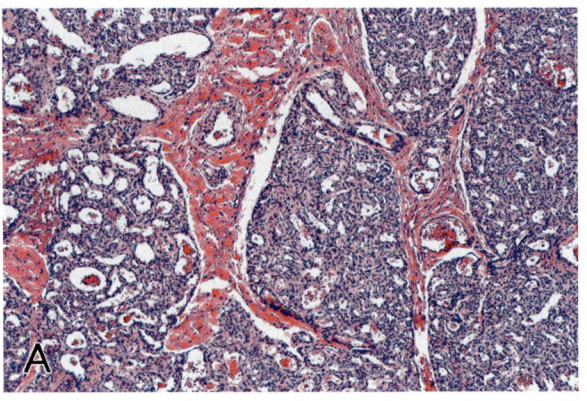

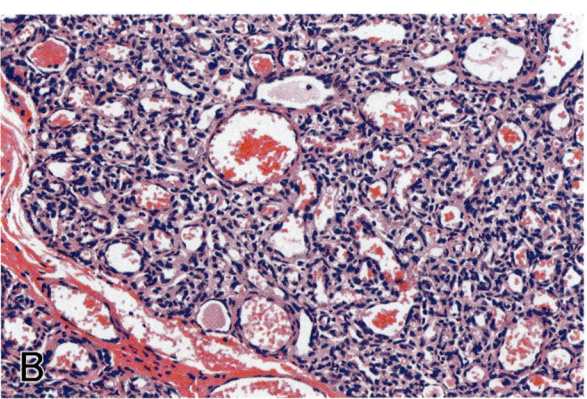

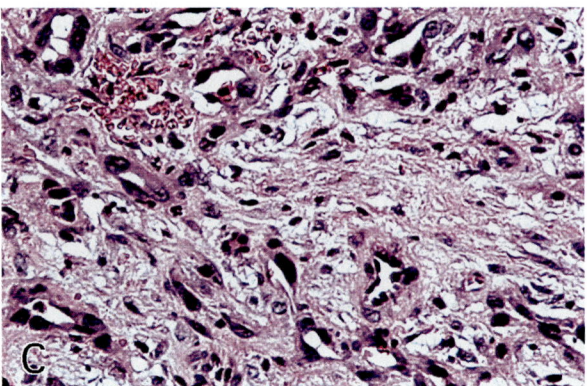

Figure 7-12

LOBULAR CAPILLARY HEMANGIOMA

A,B: Constituent vascular lobules have central "feeding" vessels that are larger than those at the periphery of the lobules.

C: Mechanical or inflammatory irritation of such lesions may cause mild nuclear atypia of the constituent endothelial cells, as shown here.

if not identical, lesion is known as *acquired tufted angioma* and has been documented by several other authors (1,40,59,71). This tumor is dermal and largely intravascular, and shows a somewhat more prominent pericytic component than the classic lobular capillary hemangioma (figs. 7-13, 7-14); however, these differences are minor. Padilla et al. (59) have offered the opinion (with which we agree) that *epulis gravidarum* and *angioblastoma of Nakagawa* represent additional variants of lobular capillary hemangioma.

Most examples of lobular capillary hemangioma are cured by simple excision. Nevertheless, there are reports of lesions that recur multiple times, have regional satellitosis, and have a disseminated distribution (fig. 7-15) (2,5,18, 56,75,80,84). The reasons underlying aberrant behaviors such as these are currently unknown, but the neoplasms in question have been histologically typical examples of benign lobular capillary hemangioma. Ultimately, the clinical outcome in such cases in excellent.

Kimura's Disease

In 1948, Kimura et al. (45) described an unusual neoplasm that affected the skin and subcutis. It was initially thought to represent a form of granuloma (33); however, subsequent study has shown that endothelial proliferation is the central feature of this lesion (69,77). *Kimura's disease,* or *Kimura's tumor,* favors the preauricular skin and has a strong predilection to occur in Asian patients. The average age at diagnosis is 40 years, but the lesion has often been present for several years before the patient seeks medical attention.

Clinically, Kimura's disease usually is represented by a single, deeply seated, red-violet nodule. Nonetheless, multiple, regionally clustered lesions are seen in as many as 45 percent of cases (fig. 7-16). Elevations of serum immunoglobulin (Ig)E levels and eosinophilia of the peripheral blood are evident in some cases (77).

Microscopically, the most striking finding in Kimura's disease is its lymphoid component. This accounts for the bulk of the proliferating cells, which are organized into follicular configurations, often with well-formed germinal centers (fig. 7-17) (69,77). In addition, reactive eosinophils and mast cells often are numerous. The vascular component of Kimura's disease is

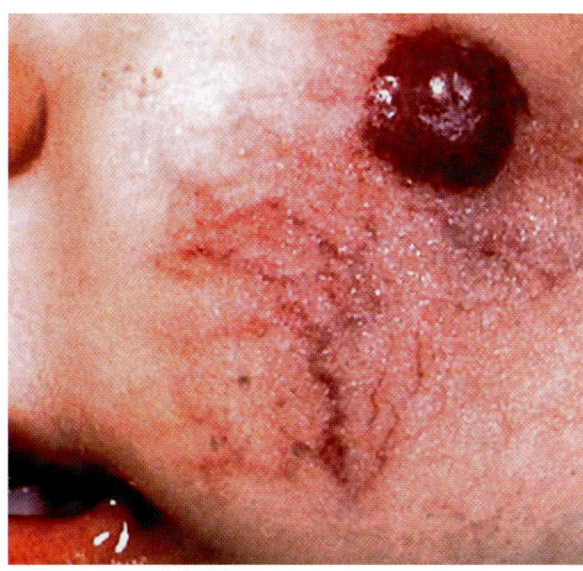

Figure 7-13

ACQUIRED TUFTED ANGIOMA

Central reddish nodule with peripheral serpentine profiles of dermal discoloration of facial skin in a child. This lesion is likely equivalent to intravascular lobular capillary hemangioma.

evident between and within such follicles, and is composed of elongated capillary-sized vessels containing plump, cytologically bland endothelial cells (fig. 7-18). Mitoses may be observed in the latter but are never conspicuous. Also, there usually is no relationship between proliferating vascular channels in Kimura's disease and preexisting blood vessels (77). The dermis demonstrates marked fibrosis immediately surrounding the bulk of the lesion and may become hyalinized.

Epithelioid (Histiocytoid) Hemangioma

A lesion that is closely related to Kimura's disease is *epithelioid hemangioma* (13,45,69,76, 77). Because the endothelial cells in the latter tumor are thought by some to resemble histiocytes, the lesion is also termed *histiocytoid hemangioma* (69). Epithelioid hemangiomas feature cords of proliferating endothelia, often with cytoplasmic vacuolization, in the dermis and subcutis. They are often organized around small luminal spaces and may merge with the walls of large, preexisting veins or arteries, with an interposed myxoid zone of connective tissue.

Nonmelanocytic Tumors of the Skin

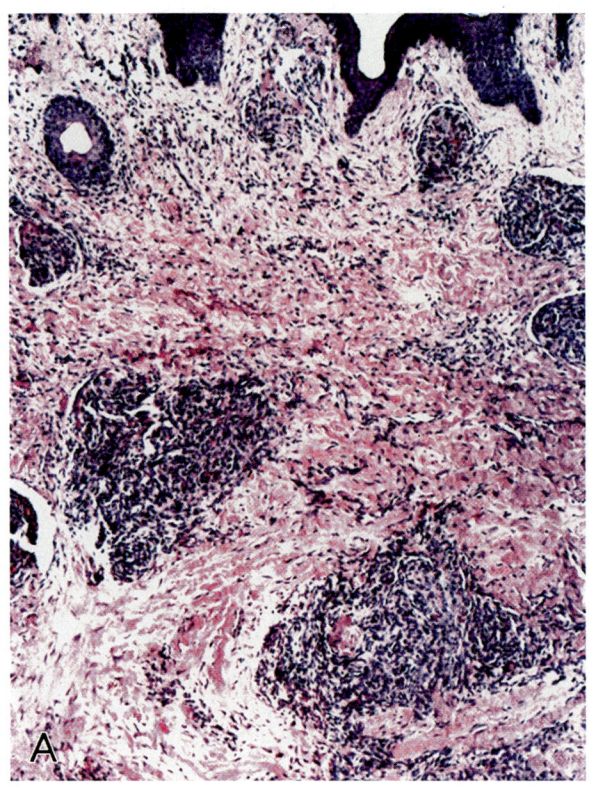
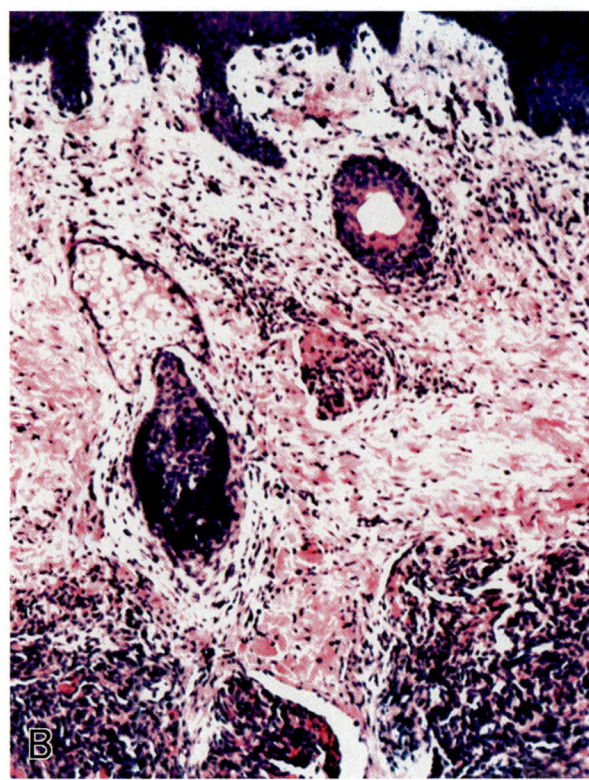
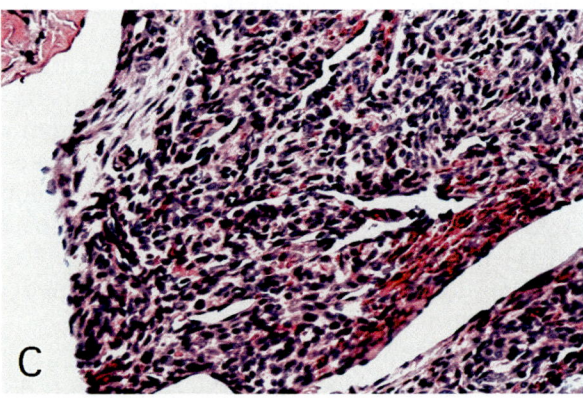

Figure 7-14

ACQUIRED TUFTED ANGIOMA

A,B: There is a multinodular profile in the dermis, which has been likened to collections of "cannon balls."

C: Lobules of endothelial and pericytic tumor cells protrude into preexisting vascular lumens.

An admixture of reactive eosinophils and lymphocytes is a variable finding in epithelioid hemangioma, leading to another alternative designation of *angiolymphoid hyperplasia with eosinophilia* (fig. 7-19) (7,13,39,51,53,58,79,81), but these cellular elements are not as prominent as they are in Kimura's disease. The formation of lymphoid follicles is uncommon.

As previously suggested, the nuclei of the endothelial cells of epithelioid hemangiomas show folded contours and pale, evenly dispersed chromatin (fig. 7-20); these features are like those of tissue histiocytes. Mitotic figures and nucleoli are rarely observed.

In contrast to Kimura's disease, only rare cases of epithelioid hemangioma are associated with peripheral eosinophilia and hyperglobulinemia of the IgE type (77). Moreover, the rate of recurrence of these lesions differs after surgical excision: approximately 10 percent of epithelioid hemangiomas reappear after surgery, contrasted with 75 percent of tumors in Kimura's disease. In addition, 50 to 60 percent of patients with Kimura's disease have regional lymphadenopathy,

Vascular Tumors and Pseudotumors

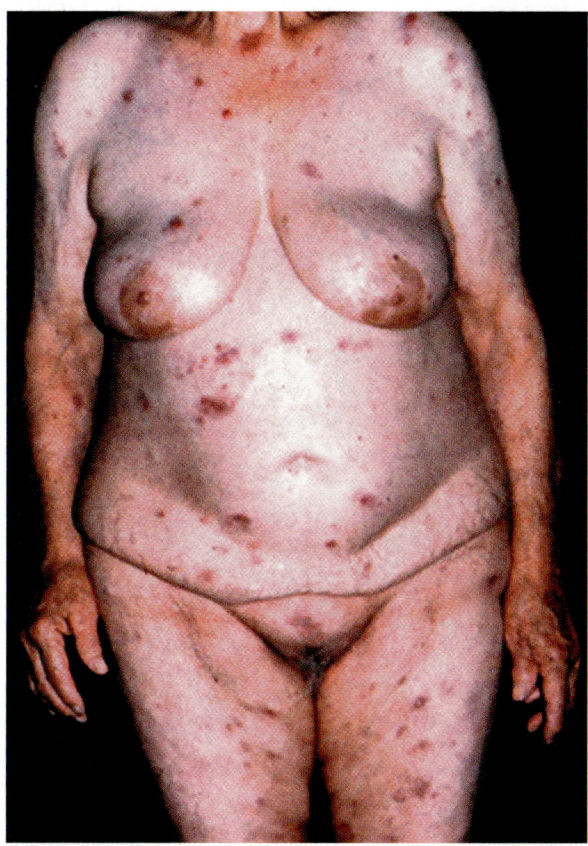

Figure 7-15

DISSEMINATED LOBULAR CAPILLARY HEMANGIOMA
Multiple reddish nodules and plaques are seen in the skin of the trunk and extremities of an elderly woman. It was observed that some of the lesions spontaneously regressed during a five-year period of observation.

whereas the lymph nodes are normal in individuals with epithelioid hemangioma.

Acral Arteriovenous Tumor/ (Arterio-)Venous Hemangioma

Through the work of Connelly and Winkelmann, Carapeto and colleagues, and Girard et al. (10,14,25), another distinctive group of benign vascular neoplasms has been characterized. These occur preferentially on the head and neck or extremities of adult patients (average age, 58 years) and variously have been termed *acral arteriovenous tumors, venous hemangiomas,* or *arteriovenous hemangiomas.* Most present as enlarging or bleeding nodular lesions, with or without tenderness, and average 4 mm in greatest dimension (14).

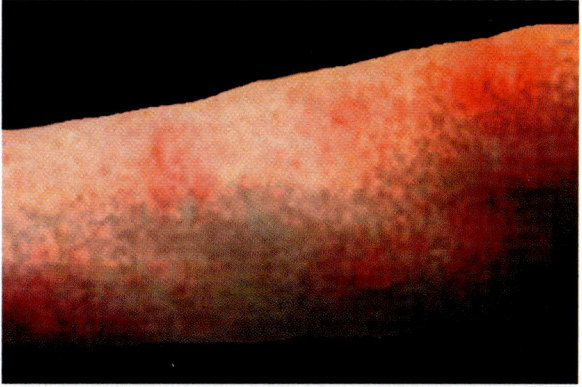

Figure 7-16

KIMURA'S DISEASE
Several reddish plaques and nodules are seen in the skin of the arm.

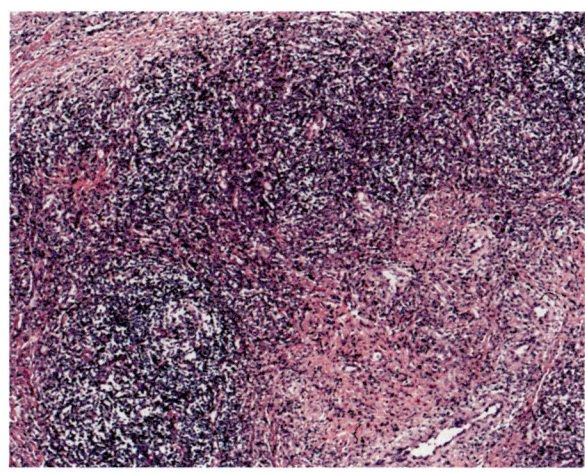

Figure 7-17

KIMURA'S DISEASE
Vascular proliferation is accompanied by a dense, chronic, inflammatory infiltrate with formation of lymphoid follicles.

The acral arteriovenous tumor is composed of large, closely apposed vascular channels with prominent fibromuscular coats, and is located in the superficial or middle dermis (figs. 7-21, 7-22). It is typically circumscribed but may be surrounded by ectatic blood vessels, particularly deep to the mass (25). This appearance may lead to confusion with true arteriovenous malformations. Dermal appendages, such as pilosebaceous units or sweat glands, and inflammatory cells may be entrapped within acral arteriovenous

Nonmelanocytic Tumors of the Skin

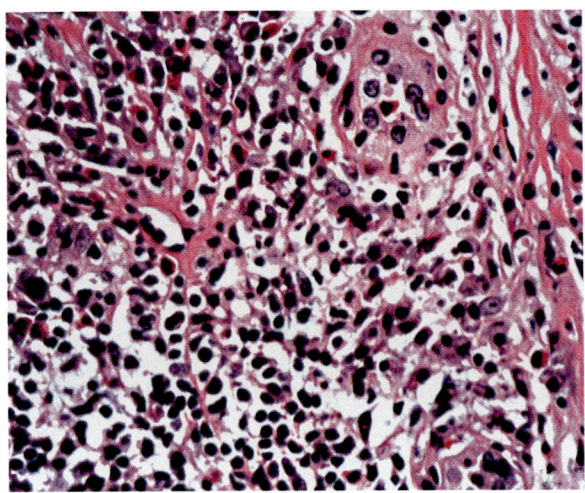

Figure 7-18
KIMURA'S DISEASE
Vascular profiles feature plump endothelial cells (top right), with numerous admixed lymphocytes and eosinophils.

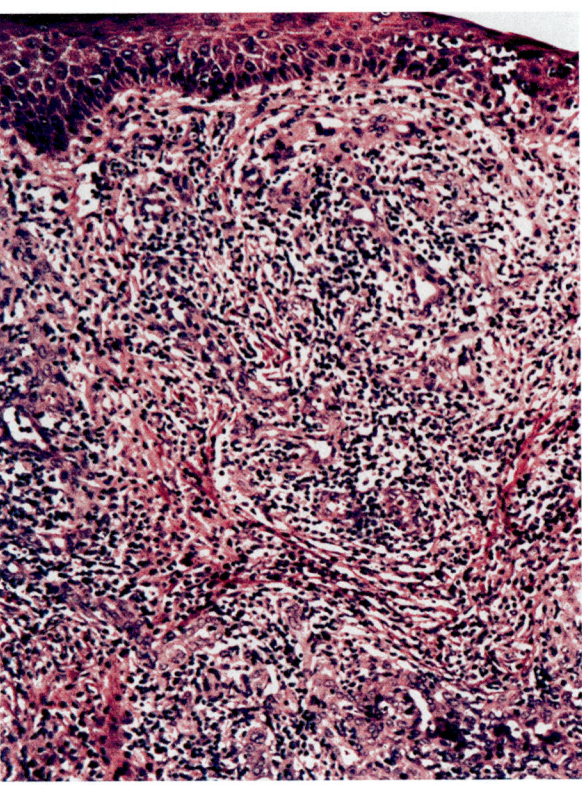

Figure 7-19
ANGIOLYMPHOID HYPERPLASIA WITH EOSINOPHILIA
This is a variant of epithelioid hemangioma in which lymphocytes and eosinophils permeate the tumor. These inflammatory elements are not as prominent as they are in Kimura's disease.

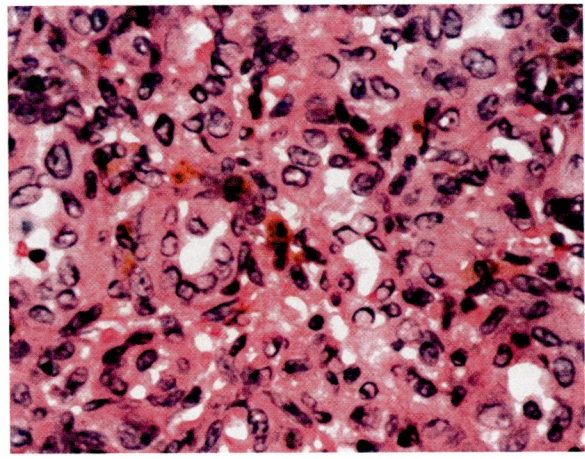

Figure 7-20
EPITHELIOID HEMANGIOMA
Tubular vessels are lined by plump endothelial cells with folded nuclear membranes.

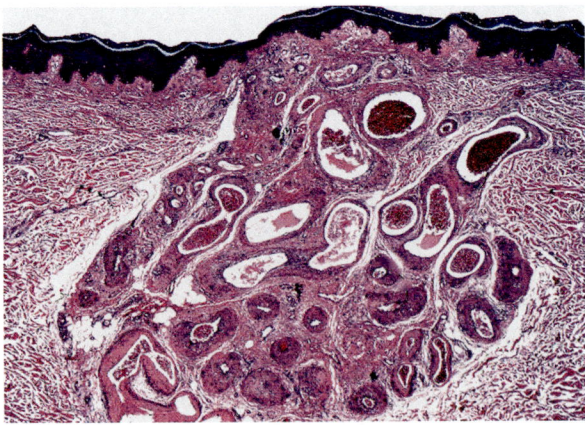

Figure 7-21
ACRAL ARTERIOVENOUS TUMOR
A closely grouped cluster of vein-like blood vessels in the reticular dermis contains smooth muscle cells in the vessel walls.

tumors. Attenuated, bland endothelial cells line the tumoral lumens. Surrounding fibromuscular tissue may contain elastic fibers, but these are not organized into lamellae as in normal blood vessels or arteriovenous malformations.

Cutaneous acral arteriovenous tumors are uniformly benign and are cured by simple ex-

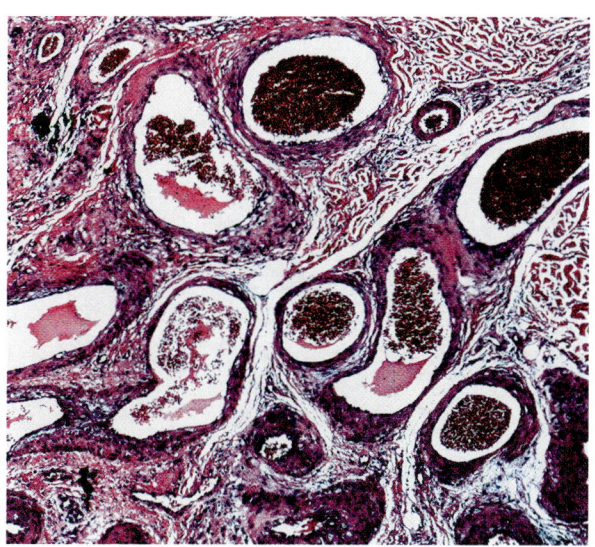

Figure 7-22

ACRAL ARTERIOVENOUS TUMOR

The blood vessels are distinct from one another, rather than merging imperceptibly as expected in vascular malformations of the skin.

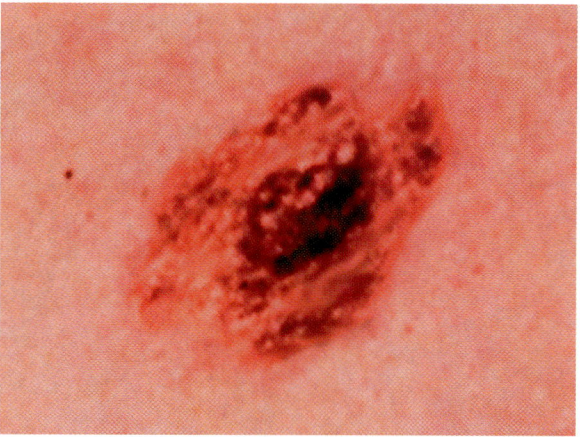

Figure 7-23

HOBNAIL (TARGETOID HEMOSIDEROTIC) HEMANGIOMA

The configuration resembles an archery target. (Courtesy of Dr. D. J. Santa Cruz, St. Louis, MO.)

cision. To date, there have been no accounts of consistent associations between these lesions and abnormalities of other organs.

Hobnail/Targetoid/"Atypical" Hemangioma

Santa Cruz and Aronberg (67,70) described five patients with a peculiar vascular tumor, originally termed *targetoid hemangioma* but recently renamed as *hobnail hemangioma* (27,52). The first designation derives from the clinical appearance of the lesion, which simulates that of an archery target, and is sharply circumscribed (fig. 7-23) (70).

The microscopic characteristics of this hemangioma are unexpectedly atypical for a benign endothelial proliferation. It demonstrates arrays of angulated vascular channels in the dermis, which dissect collagen bundles in a manner analogous to that of angiosarcoma (fig. 7-24). Papillary configurations of endothelial cells, many of which have a "hobnail" appearance (with luminally displaced nuclei), may be evident within these channels (fig. 7-25). Histologic findings that militate against a malignant diagnosis for this neoplasm include uniformly bland nuclear features, a lack of mitotic activity, and a common abundance of hemosiderin-laden macrophages in the tumoral stroma (27,52,67,70).

Mentzel et al. (52) have expanded the morphologic spectrum of hobnail hemangioma. In a study of 62 cases, they observed some lesions that shared microscopic features with lymphangioma, retiform hemangioendothelioma, and Dabska's tumor, as discussed later in this chapter.

Concern over the biological potential of an atypical hemangioma may largely be allayed by proper communication with the dermatologist. As mentioned previously, the clinical hallmarks of hobnail hemangioma do not overlap with those of angiosarcoma or Kaposi's sarcoma. In addition, analysis for human herpes virus 8 (HHV8), which is seen in most examples of Kaposi's sarcoma, are negative in hobnail hemangioma (29).

The differential diagnosis of hobnail hemangioma also includes other skin lesions with similar microscopic features, such as the so-called benign lymphangioendothelioma (also known as acquired progressive lymphangioma) (28,31, 41) and multinucleate cell angiohistiocytoma (3,4, 17,42,65,73). Benign lymphangioendothelioma is potentially seen throughout adulthood, and in most skin fields, as a flesh colored or pigmented papule or plaque. The tumor contains proteinaceous lymphatic fluid rather than intravascular erythrocytes; it also lacks stromal hemosiderin

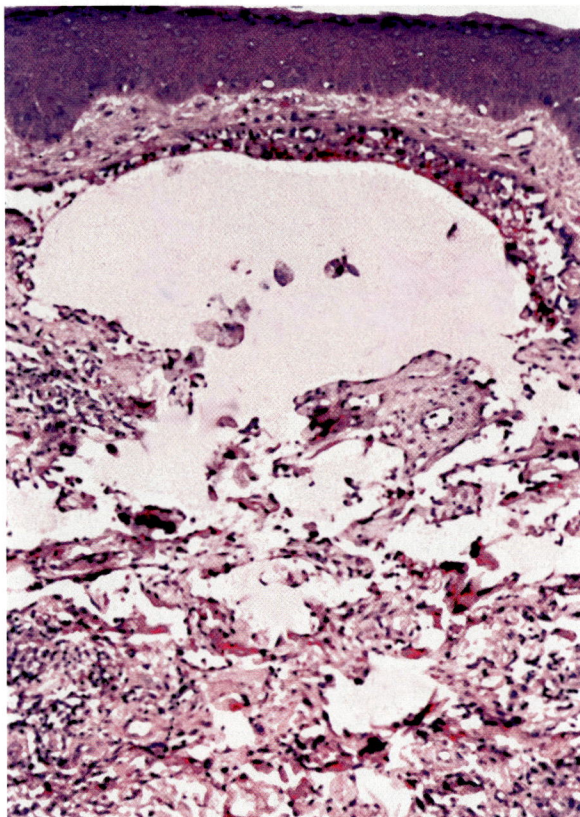

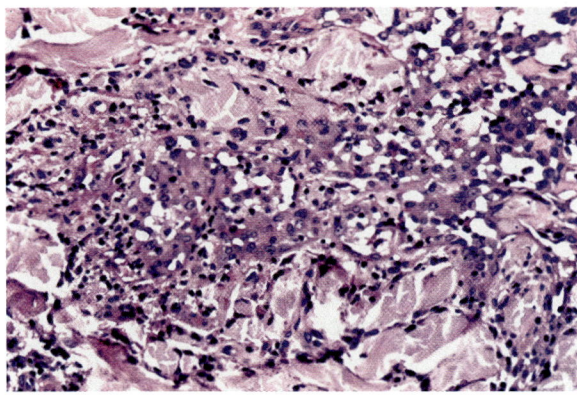

Figure 7-24

HOBNAIL (TARGETOID HEMOSIDEROTIC) HEMANGIOMA

Top: Haphazardly formed vascular spaces irregularly permeate the dermis.
Bottom: The racemose nature of the proliferation simulates that of a vascular malignancy.

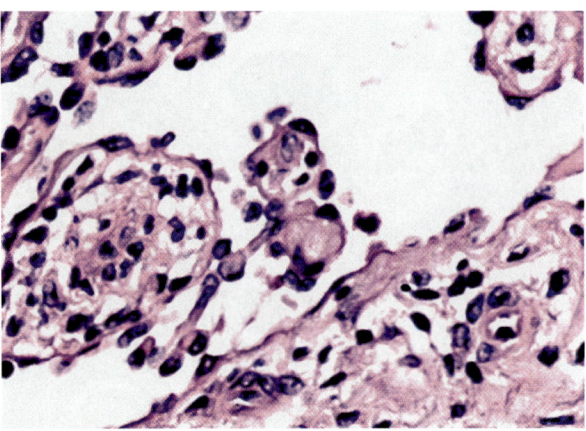

Figure 7-25

HOBNAIL (TARGETOID HEMOSIDEROTIC) HEMANGIOMA

Small micropapillae project into the vascular lumens of atypical cutaneous hemangiomas, and constituent nuclei have a "hobnail" configuration.

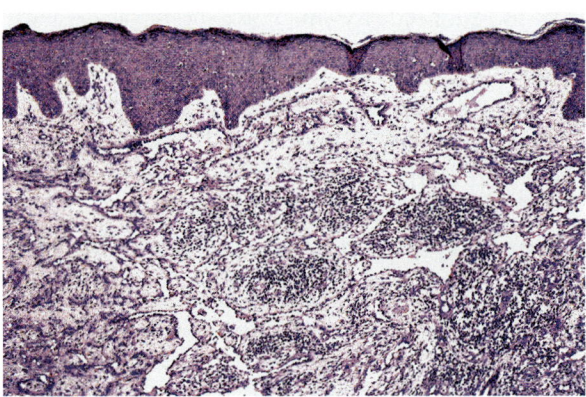

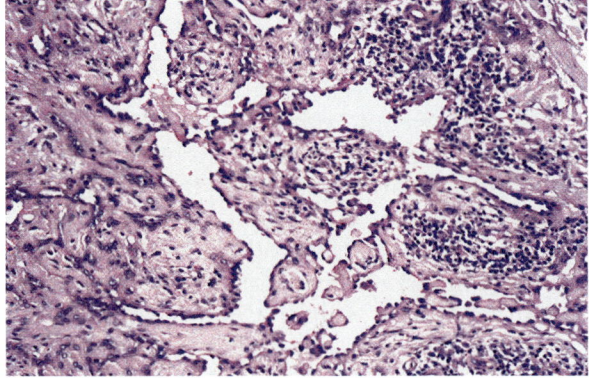

Figure 7-26

BENIGN LYMPHANGIOENDOTHELIOMA

Top: There is a relatively disorganized proliferation of dermal vascular channels, but endothelial cells are bland.
Bottom: Stromal lymphocytes are notable.

deposits, and is often invested by lymphoid infiltrates (fig. 7-26). Angiohistiocytoma is a multifocal papular lesion, usually located on the extremities. It contains multinucleated stromal

Vascular Tumors and Pseudotumors

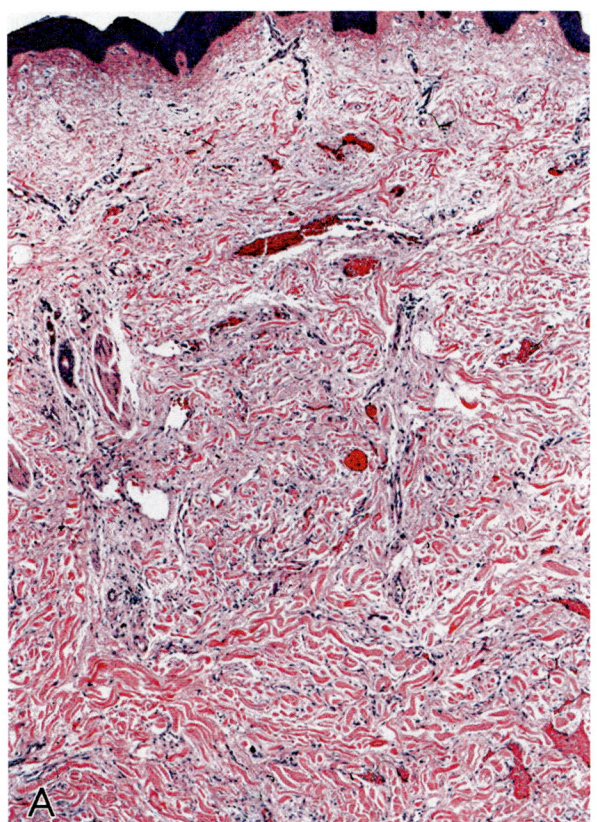
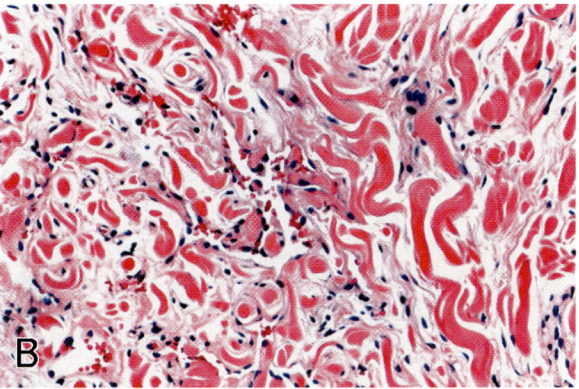
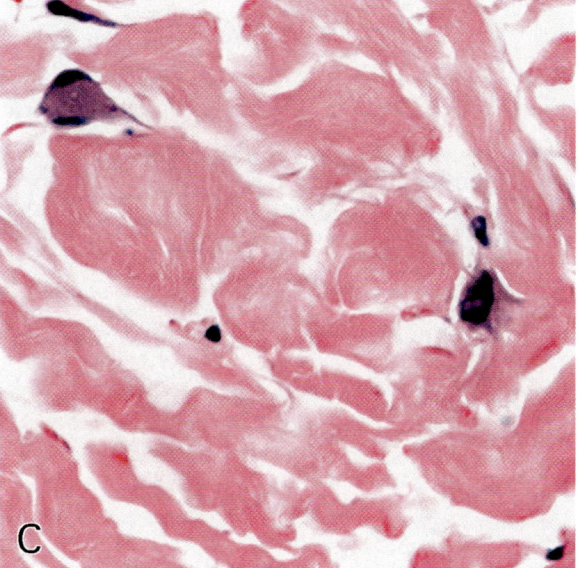

Figure 7-27

MULTINUCLEATE CELL ANGIOHISTIOCYTOMA

Irregularly disposed collections of thin-walled blood vessels in the dermis (A,B) are interspersed with multinucleated, "floret"-type stromal giant cells (C).

cells that are interspersed between randomly configured dermal vascular spaces (fig. 7-27). In some foci, the multinucleated cells may appear to line vascular (or pseudovascular) spaces, similar to the histologic profile of giant cell fibroblastoma.

Other Cutaneous Hemangioma Variants

Additional forms of cutaneous hemangioma exist, which together with hobnail hemangioma, can be considered generically as atypical hemangiomas. These are considered in the following section.

Acquired elastotic hemangioma (68) preferentially occurs in sun-exposed skin fields, particularly on the arms and neck, in middle-aged to elderly women. It usually is a reddish plaque but is not often interpreted clinically as a hemangioma. Histologically, this tumor exhibits a band-like proliferation of capillary-sized blood vessels in the papillary and upper reticular dermis (fig. 7-28). These vessels are often arranged parallel to the skin surface. In keeping with its diagnostic name, elastotic hemangioma also features marked solar elastosis in and around the lesional vessels.

Microvenular hemangioma also favors solar-damaged skin, especially on the arms, but arises in young or middle-aged persons with no sex preference (8,32,44). Its macroscopic image is like that of more ordinary hemangiomas. However, the microscopic configuration includes elongated tubular profiles of endothelial cells, resembling small veins in their luminal caliber, which are randomly disposed throughout the dermal collagen. They also may interconnect and demonstrate branching profiles (fig. 7-29).

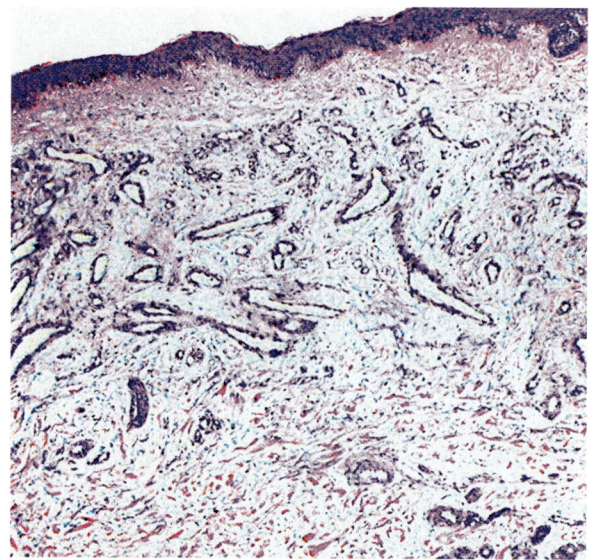

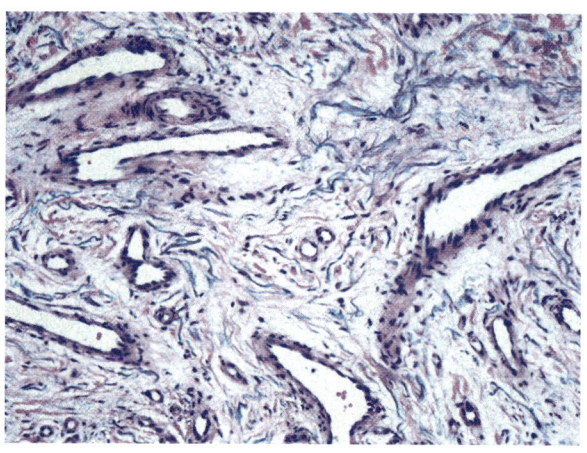

Figure 7-28

ACQUIRED ELASTOTIC CUTANEOUS HEMANGIOMA
Top: A plate-like proliferation of blood vessels is seen in the upper reticular dermis.
Bottom: The intervening dermal stroma shows marked solar elastosis.

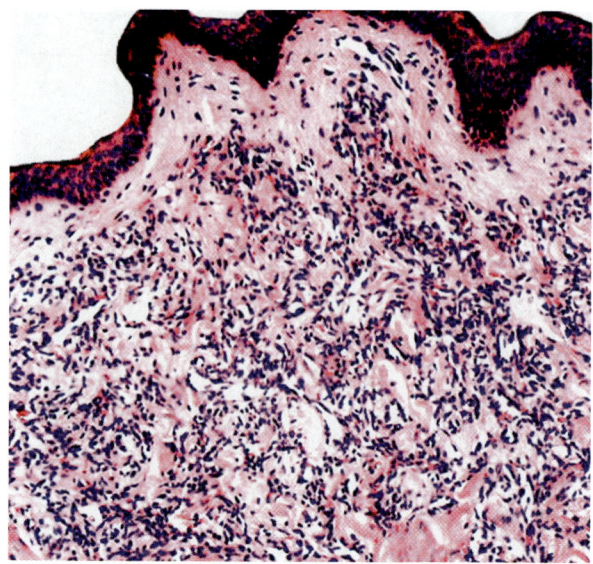

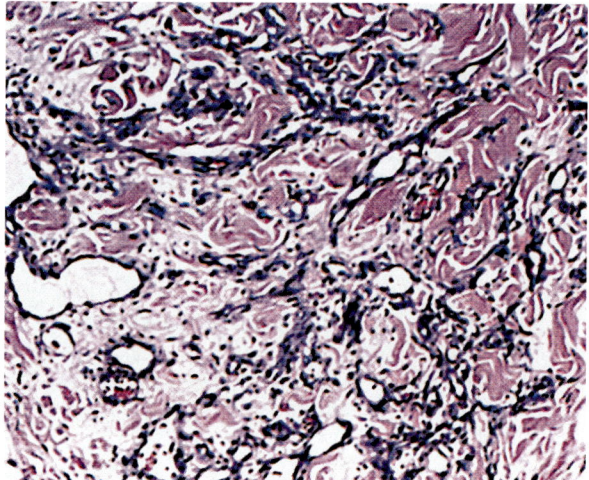

Figure 7-29

MICROVENULAR HEMANGIOMA
Top: Randomly arranged vascular profiles are seen in the dermis and subcutis.
Bottom: The vessels have compressed, narrow lumens and show a tendency to interconnect. They are, however, cytologically bland.

Nuclear atypia, mitotic activity, and intratumoral inflammation are absent, and microvenular hemangioma has a confined appearance on scanning microscopy. All of those attributes are unlike the characteristics of vascular malignancies in the skin.

Sinusoidal hemangioma is an unusual subtype of cavernous hemangioma (9,21). It is located in the deep dermis or subcutis, usually on the trunk and extremities, and shows a predilection for women. The histologic features include dilated, interanastomosing blood vessels with thin walls; focal pseudopapillary arrays of endothelial cells; modest nuclear pleomorphism and hyperchromasia; and limited areas of irregular growth into the subcutis. These characteristics often raise concern over a diagnosis of angiosarcoma, but the clinical setting of axial soft tissues rather than the head and neck, and a long evolution (9), favors a benign interpretation.

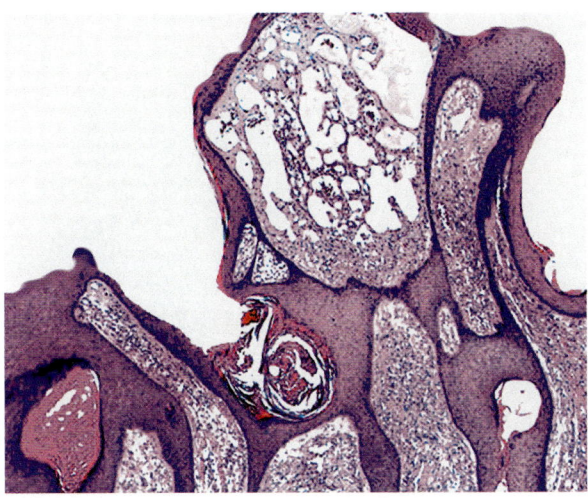

Figure 7-30

VERRUCOUS HEMANGIOMA

This cutaneous hemangioma has incited a markedly hyperplastic epidermal response, yielding the image of verrucous hemangioma.

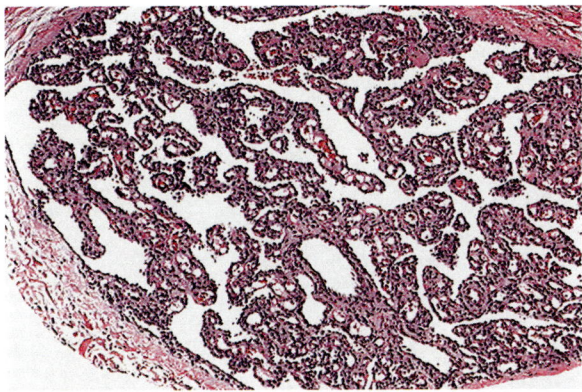

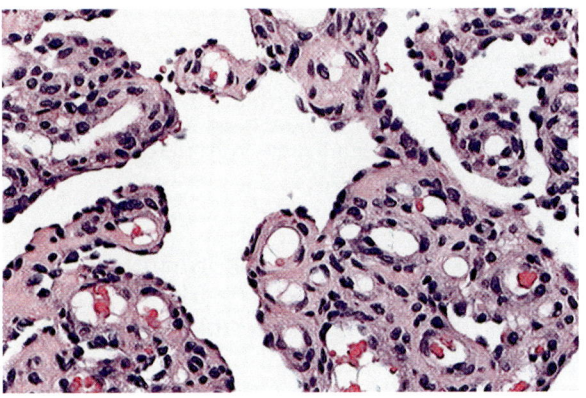

Figure 7-31

GLOMERULOID HEMANGIOMA

Constituent cells are aggregated into organoid structures resembling renal glomeruli.

Verrucous hemangioma is a variant of cavernous hemangioma that is typified by overlying epidermal papillomatosis, parakeratosis, and hyperkeratosis (fig. 7-30) (37). Epidermal rete ridges extend downward in this tumor to "embrace" or surround lesional blood vessels, much in the same manner as that observed in angiokeratoma (see below).

Glomeruloid hemangioma is a variant in which proliferating vascular channels are the size of dermal venules, and are grouped together in discrete clusters so that they passingly resemble glomeruli of the kidney on low-power microscopy (fig. 7-31) (12,46,75). Globules that stain with the periodic acid–Schiff (PAS) stain, and which may represent immunoglobulin deposits, are potentially seen in and between the tumor cells. The significance of these tumors resides in their association with the POEMS syndrome (polyneuropathy, organomegaly, endocrinopathies, monoclonal gammopathies, and skin lesions), which is usually linked to an underlying lymphoproliferative disease or plasma cell dyscrasia (5,12,65,75). Some publications have suggested that glomeruloid hemangioma is actually a form of reactive cutaneous endothelial hyperplasia, also given the name *angioendotheliomatosis*.

Infiltrating hemangioma is also composed of venule-sized channels, but this lesion differs from the others described thus far because it is not circumscribed. A disorganized proliferation of randomly arranged (but complete) luminal profiles is seen throughout the dermis and subcutis, and the lesion may involve underlying fascia and muscle as well (*intramuscular hemangioma*) (fig. 7-32). Viscera, bones, and multiple soft tissues are affected in some cases, justifying the diagnostic use of the term *angiomatosis* (66).

Angiokeratoma

Angiokeratomas are seen in two clinical settings: as isolated, sporadic, papulonodular, red-violet lesions or as multiple papules that tend to affect the genital skin and lower extremities in patients with Fabry's disease (angiokeratomatosis corporis diffusum universale, an X-linked recessive deficiency of trihexylceramide alpha-galactosidase that results in degeneration of the nervous system, and renal insufficiency) (fig.

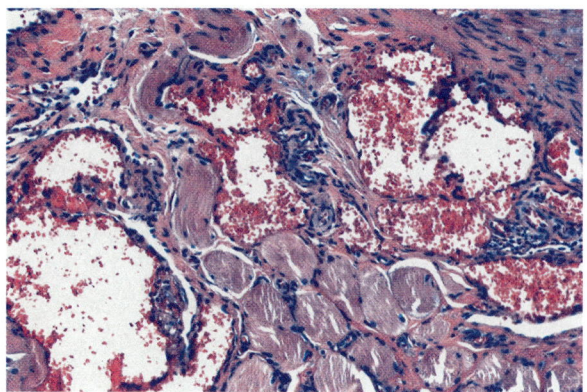

Figure 7-32

INFILTRATING HEMANGIOMA

Infiltrating hemangiomas may involve underlying striated muscle, as shown here. Despite their benign biological nature, this feature often leads to recurrence after attempts at surgical excision.

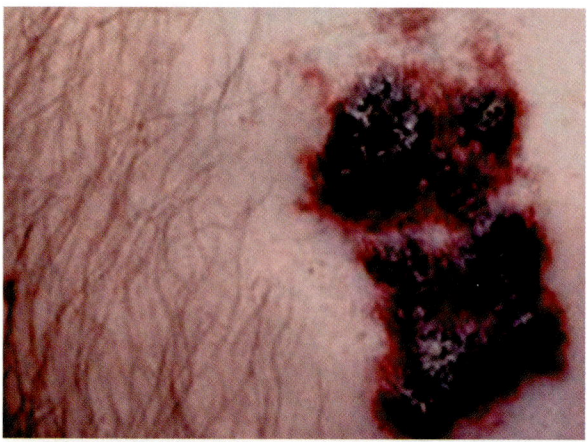
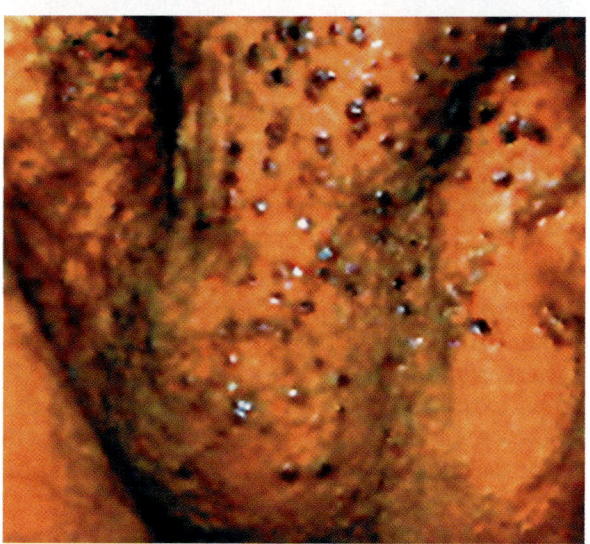

Figure 7-33

ANGIOKERATOMA

Top: An irregular, reddish brown plaque in the skin of the arm.

Bottom: In contrast, a patient with the multifocal syndromic form of this tumor, in association with Fabry's disease, has many shiny, flat-topped papular lesions in the skin of the scrotum.

7-33) (34–36). Syndromic abnormalities tend to present in adolescence or early adulthood, whereas isolated angiokeratoma is seen in individuals of all ages.

There is no difference in the light microscopic appearance of isolated and Fabry's disease–associated angiokeratomas. Blood lakes in the upper dermis are surrounded by complete collarettes of epidermis, with slight overlying hyperkeratosis and papillomatosis (fig. 7-34) (34). A resemblance to verrucous hemangioma therefore exists, but the latter proliferation affects the deep reticular dermis as well. Syndromic angiokeratomas may be distinguished from sporadic examples by electron microscopy. Ultrastructural analysis shows lamellated intralysosomal myelin figures in lesional endothelial cells, pericytes, and fibroblastic stromal cells of the dermis in patients with Fabry's disease (72), but not in those with sporadic angiokeratoma.

BORDERLINE VASCULAR TUMORS

Papillary Endovascular (Intralymphatic?) Angioendothelioma

Clinical Features. *Papillary endovascular angioendotheliomas* were first described by Dabska in 1969 (92), and have subsequently become known using her name as an eponym (i.e., *Dabska's tumor*). They are seen principally in children and adolescents as fluctuant, ill-defined, reddish plaques or nodules that range in size up to 5 cm. Rare cases have also been reported in noncutaneous sites and in adults (110,124,133). A zone of dermal edema may surround such neoplasms (92,93). "Metastases" to regional lymph nodes were reported in the seminal series of cases, but other authors have since suggested the alternative interpretation that the nodal implants actually represented tumor "satellites" as part of a field neoplasia phenomenon (109). Nevertheless, papillary endovascular angioendothelioma does have a propensity to recur locally after surgical excision, justifying its inclusion as a borderline proliferation (92,100,111,116,122).

Pathologic Findings. The microscopic features of are distinctive. As its name suggests, this tumor is confined to preexisting vascular spaces in the corium, most of which have the properties of dilated lymphatic channels (fig. 7-35). Indeed, based on a study of 12 cases, Fanburg-Smith et al. (97) have proposed that the tumor be renamed *papillary intralymphatic angioendothelioma*. Similar to deep lymphangiomas of the skin, papillary endovascular angioendothelioma features contiguous dermal fibrosis and intralesional aggregates of lymphocytes. The latter cells are also evident in intimate admixture with plump endothelial cell clusters inside of the affected vessels (92,93,97,100,109–111,116,122,124,131a,135).

The papillae are composed of polyhedral cells with round nuclei, dispersed chromatin, and small nucleoli. As mentioned, mature lymphocytes commonly mantle the peripheral aspects of the papillary formations, which contain internal, globular, intercellular eosinophilic deposits of basement membrane material (fig. 7-36). These inclusions may be labeled with the PAS stain or with immunostains for laminin and collagen type IV (97,131a).

Adjacent blood vessels that do not contain papillae are nonetheless lined by atypical endothelial cells that have hyperchromatic nuclei.

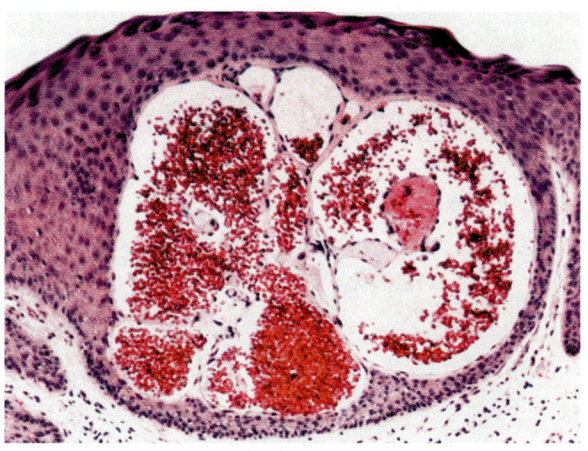

Figure 7-34

ANGIOKERATOMA

There is a proliferation of thin-walled blood vessels in the upper dermis, surrounded peripherally by epidermal collarettes.

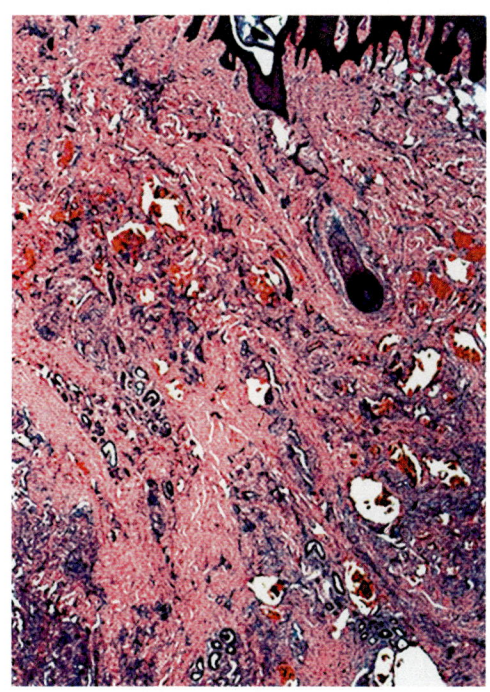

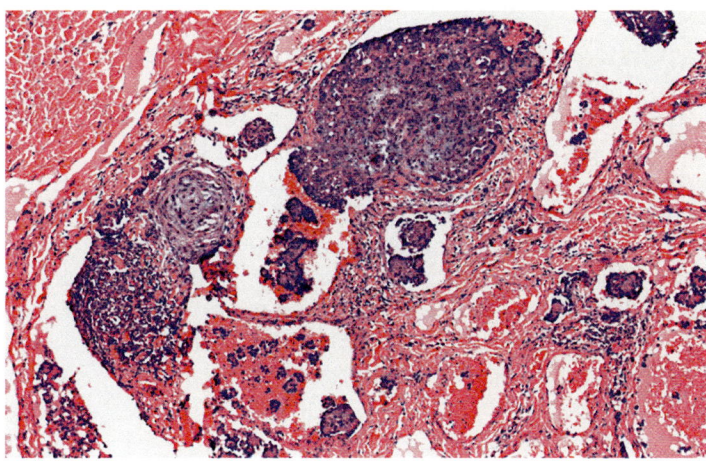

Figure 7-35

PAPILLARY ENDOVASCULAR ANGIOENDOTHELIOMA

Micropapillary arrays of plump endothelial cells are seen in dilated lymphatic-like dermal spaces.

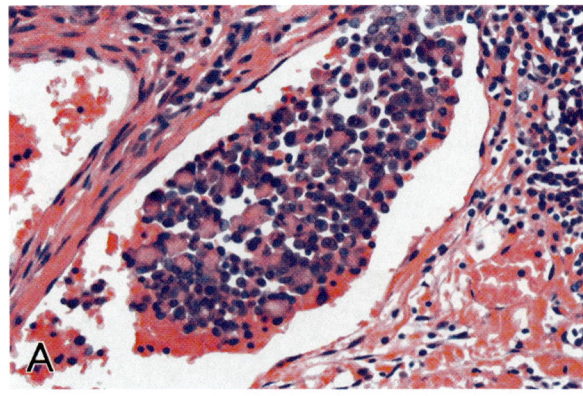
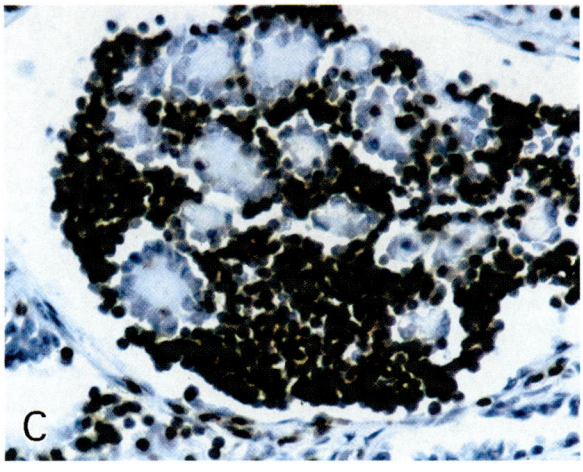
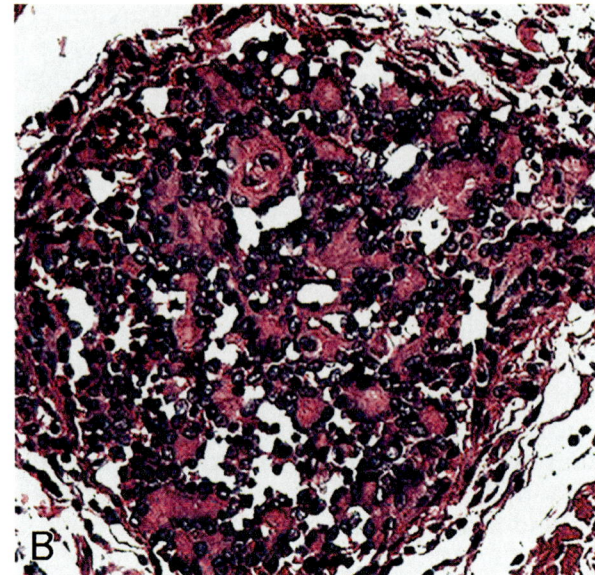

Figure 7-36

PAPILLARY ENDOVASCULAR ANGIOENDOTHELIOMA

A,B: Numerous lymphocytes are associated with the micropapillae of the tumor, and the endothelial cell aggregates synthesize globular deposits of eosinophilic basement membrane material.

C: An immunostain for CD45 demonstrates the intravascular lymphoid cells.

Small areas of racemose vascular proliferation also may be apparent in the dermis, as seen in well-differentiated angiosarcomas. Mitotic activity is present but limited.

Fukunaga (100) has raised the question of whether papillary endovascular angioendothelioma is simply a morphologic pattern, as opposed to a pathologic entity. That possibility was suggested by the observation that Dabska's tumor-like proliferations have been reported as secondary elements in hemangiomas and vascular malformations of the skin (85,119). In our experience, the histologic image is most often a "pure" one, justifying its continued recognition as a distinctive neoplasm.

Epithelioid Hemangioendothelioma

Clinical Features. *Epithelioid hemangioendotheliomas* are subcutaneous lesions that only uncommonly involve the dermis. They present as firm, tan-pink nodules and plaques measuring several centimeters in maximum diameter. Adults are primarily affected, with a slight predilection for women. The trunk and extremities are the usual sites of origin (fig. 7-37) (129, 131a). Some patients with epithelioid hemangioendothelioma of the skin concurrently have histologically identical tumors in the lung (where they were known in the past as intravascular bronchoalveolar tumors [IVBAT]), the liver, or both locations (89,131). Under such conditions, it is impossible to determine whether the visceral and cutaneous lesions are independent primary neoplasms, or whether they represent metastases of one another. The lesion recurs in up to 40 percent of patients, and in approximately 15 percent metastasize to distant extracutaneous locations (89,112,118,129).

Pathologic Findings. Epithelioid hemangioendothelioma is typified by disorganized sheets and cords of large polyhedral tumor cells with amphophilic cytoplasm, prominent cytoplasmic vacuoles, and round but eccentric nuclei (fig. 7-38). Chromatin is vesicular and small nucleoli are often seen (131). The neoplastic cells do not form complete intercellular vascular lumens, as is seen in epithelioid hemangioma (131a). However, like the latter tumor, epithelioid hemangioendothelioma has a proclivity for growth around preexisting large blood vessels. Mitotic activity and necrosis may be apparent, and Mentzel et al. (112) observed some tendency (albeit a statistically insignificant one) towards worsened behavior when such features were observed. The background stroma is variably fibrous or myxoid in character (131). Mentzel and colleagues have suggested that the tumor should be reclassified as a fully malignant endothelial neoplasm, rather than a borderline lesion, but the rationale for such a statement is not readily apparent to us. Indeed, Quante et al. (118) observed no examples of metastasis among eight patients with cutaneous lesions who were followed for up to 3 years after diagnosis.

Differential Diagnosis. Two particular diagnostic errors are possible in the evaluation of epithelioid hemangioendothelioma. First, focusing on the cord-like arrays of polygonal cells in some cases leads to a misinterpretation of metastatic carcinoma. Second, those lesions with extensive cytoplasmic vacuolization may erroneously be labeled as adipocytic in nature. The application of electron microscopy or immunohistochemical studies for epithelial and endothelial

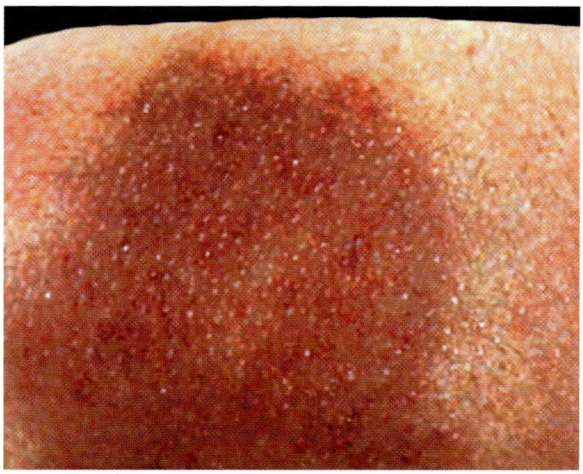

Figure 7-37

EPITHELIOID HEMANGIOENDOTHELIOMA

A large, ill-defined, reddish plaque on the arm.

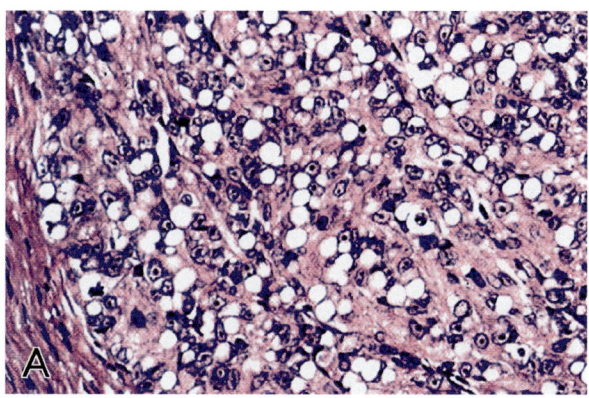

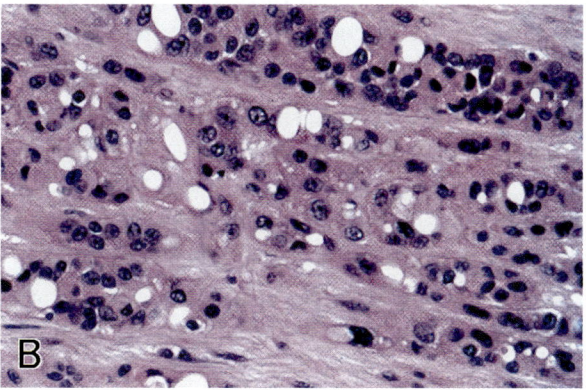

Figure 7-38

EPITHELIOID HEMANGIOENDOTHELIOMA

Sheet-like arrays (A) or clusters (B) of epithelioid endothelial cells permeate the soft tissue of the dermis and subcutis. Another example demonstrates the prominent intracytoplasmic vacuoles in this tumor (C).

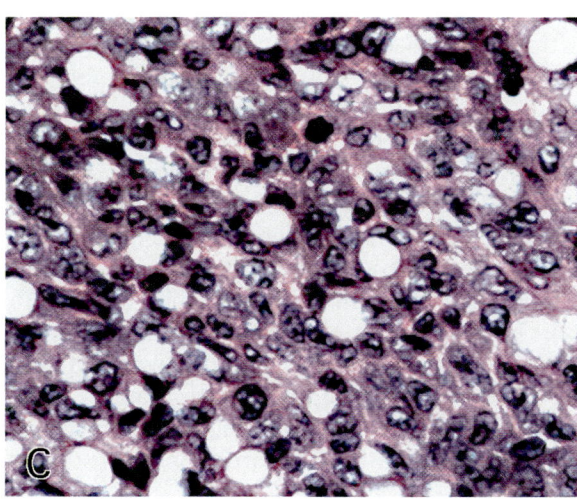

determinants is useful in resolving such uncertainties (131a). Weibel-Palade bodies are seen ultrastructurally (131), and there is consistent immunoreactive for von Willebrand factor, CD31, CD34, and thrombomodulin (118,131a).

Spindle Cell Hemangioendothelioma (Hemangioma)

Clinical Features. *Spindle cell hemangioendothelioma/hemangioma* is a tumor that is seemingly confined to the skin and subcutis (88,96, 98,105–107,117,123,125,130). It has a long period of evolution, up to 30 years, and usually presents in young adulthood (123,130). This neoplasm has a marked tendency for multifocality and a predilection for the skin of the extremities (fig. 7-39) (123). It also may arise in the setting of Maffucci's syndrome, in which multiple enchondromas of bone are also observed (117,123,130).

Spindle cell hemangioendothelioma is a multinodular, red-violet, fluctuant lesion that may attain a size of several centimeters. Its original borderline status stemmed from the fact that local recurrence after surgical excision was common, occurring in up to 70 percent of cases (130). Only one instance of distant metastasis has been reported to date, and that case was unusual in that the patient had received radiation therapy (130).

Two controversies that have surrounded this neoplasm center on whether it is, indeed, a neoplasm at all (98,105,106), and if so, whether it should more properly be classified as *spindle cell hemangioma* (126). The latter term is used increasingly at the present time. Spindle cell hemangioendothelioma is therefore somewhat arbitrarily and debatably included in this section on borderline vascular neoplasms, largely for historical reasons.

Pathologic Findings. The microscopic appearance is distinctive because it is an amalgamation of the attributes of cavernous hemangioma and Kaposi's sarcoma (98,123,130,131a). There is an intimate admixture of large, ectatic vascular spaces in the dermis, which often contain luminal thrombi and may harbor calcifications as well. Spindle cell foci show extravasation of erythrocytes and intracytoplasmic vacuoles (fig. 7-40). The latter finding is shared with epithelioid hemangioendothelioma, described

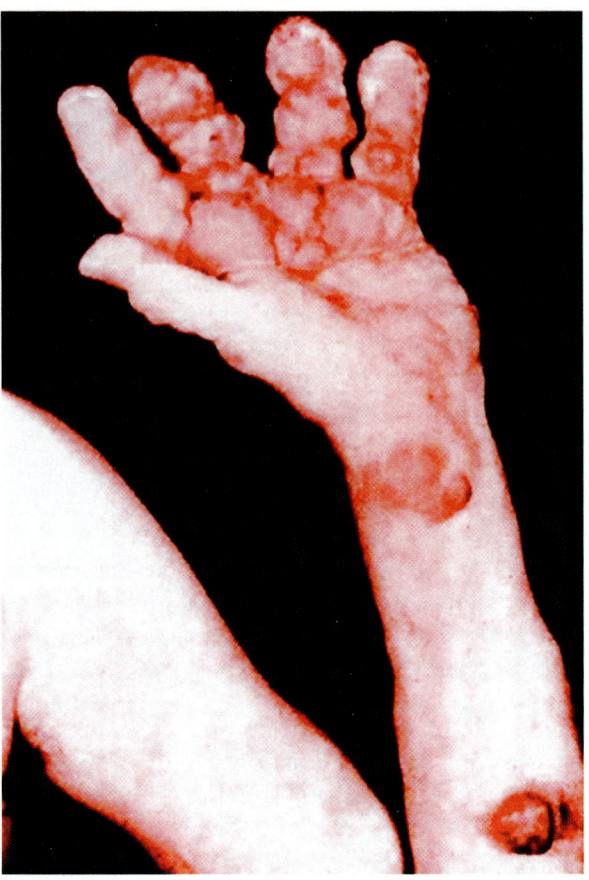

Figure 7-39

SPINDLE CELL HEMANGIOENDOTHELIOMA/HEMANGIOMA

Multiple exophytic reddish nodules in the skin of the arm of a patient with Maffucci's syndrome. (Courtesy of Dr. S. W. Weiss, Atlanta, GA.)

above. Immunohistologic markers of endothelial differentiation are typically lacking in the fusiform elements of spindle cell hemangioendothelioma, and they instead tend to demonstrate myofibroblastic features. The nuclei of the cells of both tumor components are relatively bland, and mitotic activity is limited. The peripheral borders of the proliferation are poorly defined, and small "satellite" lesions may be observed within several millimeters on either side of the main mass (123). Permeation into the subcutis or deeper soft tissues is common. Small areas featuring racemose, interanastomosing, dissecting vascular channels may be noted as well.

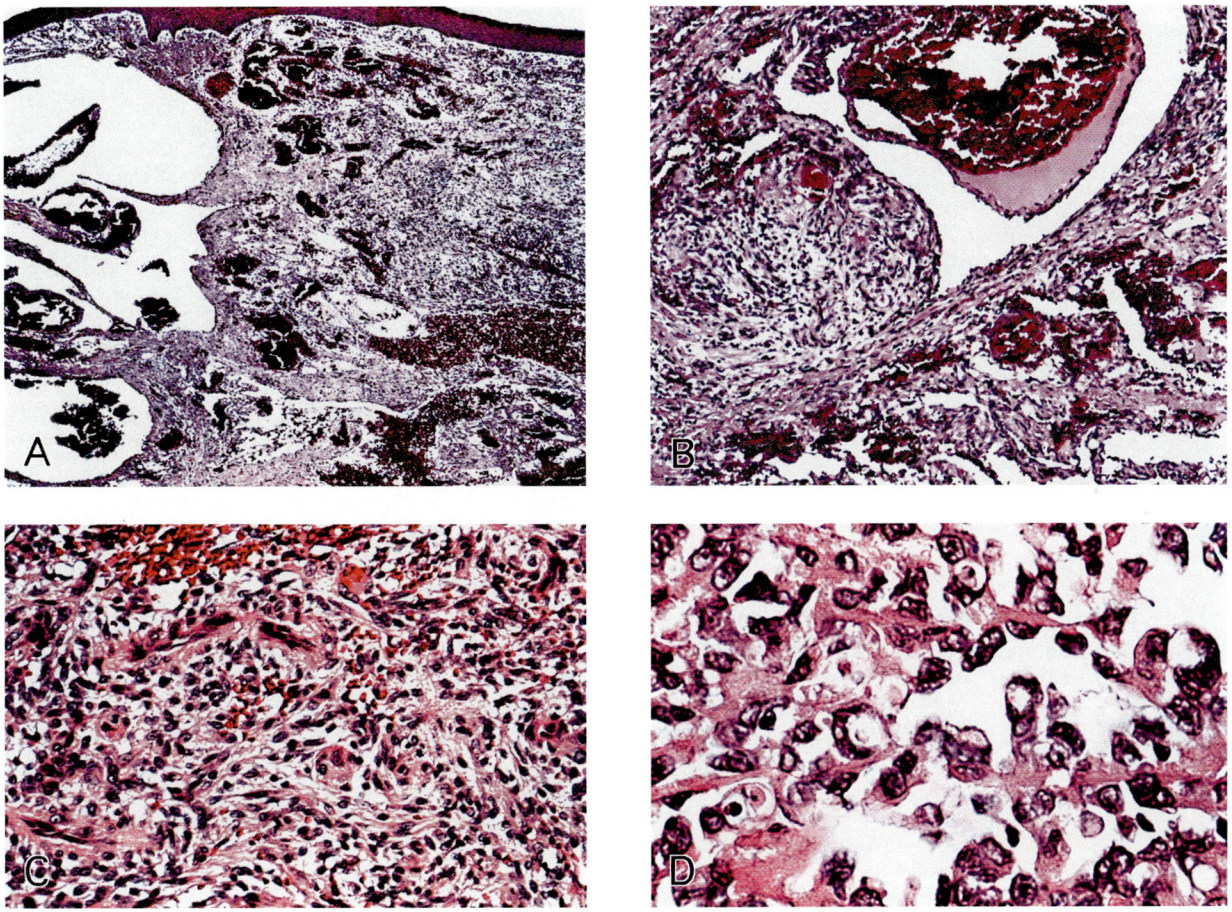

Figure 7-40

SPINDLE CELL HEMANGIOENDOTHELIOMA/HEMANGIOMA

A,B: A combination of dilated vein-like spaces and a spindle cell proliferation is seen in the dermis.
C: The spindle cell component has a disorganized growth pattern in the dermis.
D: Constituent cells focally demonstrate cytoplasmic vacuolization.

Kaposiform Hemangioendothelioma

Clinical Features. *Kaposiform hemangioendothelioma* is a neoplasm that is most commonly observed in children and adolescents, although examples also have been reported in adult patients as well (86,91,101,103,108,113,127,134,135). There is no apparent gender predilection. This cutaneous tumor may take the form of rapidly enlarging red-violet plaques, nodules, or grouped telangiectasias, and may reach a maximum size of several centimeters. Lesions in the skin may be accompanied by concomitant lesions in the deep soft tissues, and an association with lymphangiomatosis is common (127,132,135). Another peculiar clinical linkage is with the Kasabach-Merritt phenomenon (peripheral consumption of platelets and other formed blood elements), producing a potentially life-threatening coagulopathy (101,127,128,135).

The preferred therapy for this lesion is complete surgical excision, when possible; however, administration of interferon, steroids, and other agents may be necessary for unresectable tumors (86,94). Death may occur as a result of the cited complications of these neoplasms, and their aggressive local growth may produce considerable morbidity, but metastasis has not been documented.

Pathologic Findings. Kaposiform hemangioendothelioma is typified by the amalgamation of histologic findings that are seen in lymphangioma, hemangioma variants, other forms

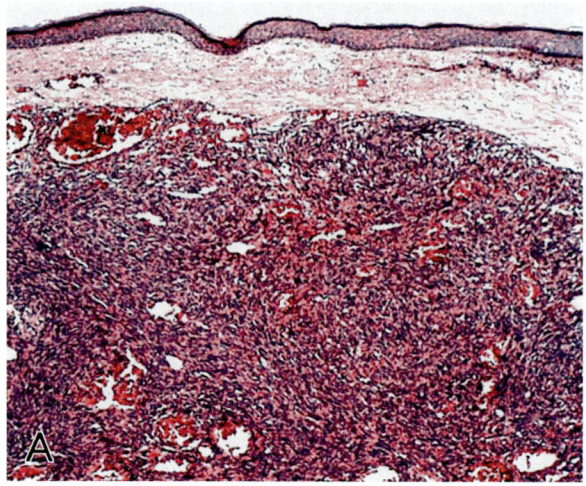

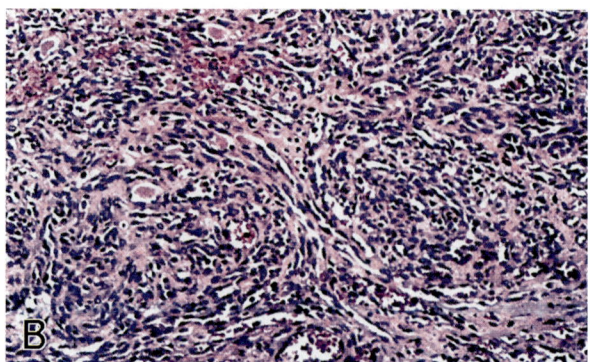

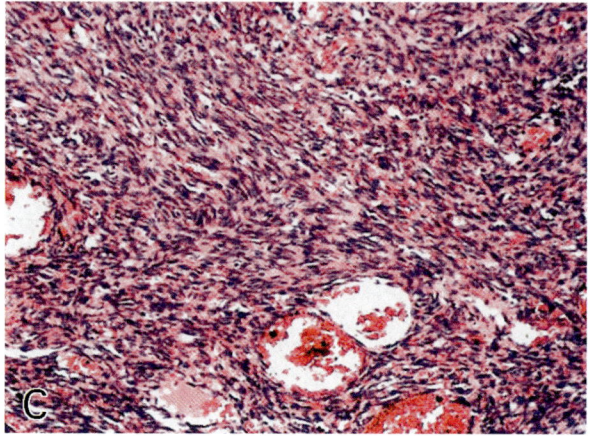

Figure 7-41

KAPOSIFORM HEMANGIOENDOTHELIOMA

There is an admixture of capillary hemangioma-like elements and a dermal spindle cell proliferation that simulates the appearance of Kaposi's sarcoma. The tumor cells are focally arranged in a micronodular fashion (A–C).

of hemangioendothelioma, and Kaposi's sarcoma. These findings include a proliferation of fusiform or compact polygonal endothelial cells, arranged in sheets or micronodular arrays in the dermis and subcutis (fig. 7-41). The endothelial cells also line interconnecting slit-like vascular channels or rounded capillary-type vessels, and some of the lumens in such structures contain microthrombi. Cytoplasmic hyaline droplets, extravasated erythrocytes, and stromal hemosiderin are seen in some tumors. Nuclear atypia is slight, and mitotic activity is variable but generally limited.

Differential Diagnosis. In contrast to true Kaposi's sarcoma, which is the principal differential diagnostic consideration, there is no molecular evidence of infection with HHV8 (104). Folpe et al. (99), however, have shown that kaposiform hemangioendothelioma does share potential immunoreactivity for vascular endothelial growth factor receptor-3 with Kaposi's sarcoma; Dabska's tumor and some angiosarcomas also may express that marker.

Retiform Hemangioendothelioma

Calonje et al. (90) described a cutaneous tumor that was named *retiform hemangioendothelioma*. It occurs in patients over a wide age range (from 9 to 78 years), with no gender predilection. The tumors are encountered in the skin of the trunk, extremities, scalp, and genital region. There is a potential association with chronic lymphedema and prior therapeutic irradiation. One of the neoplasms in the original series metastasized to regional lymph nodes, but none spread more distantly or resulted in death. Possible multicentric growth has subsequently been reported (95,120), as has a pathogenetic linkage with HHV8 (121).

The microscopic image is somewhat similar to that of Dabska's tumor, including a stromal lymphoid infiltrate and the formation of small intravascular papillae with hyaline collagenized cores. Retiform hemangioendothelioma has more elaborately arborizing vascular channels (fig. 7-42), however, which have been likened to the configuration of normal rete testis, and a

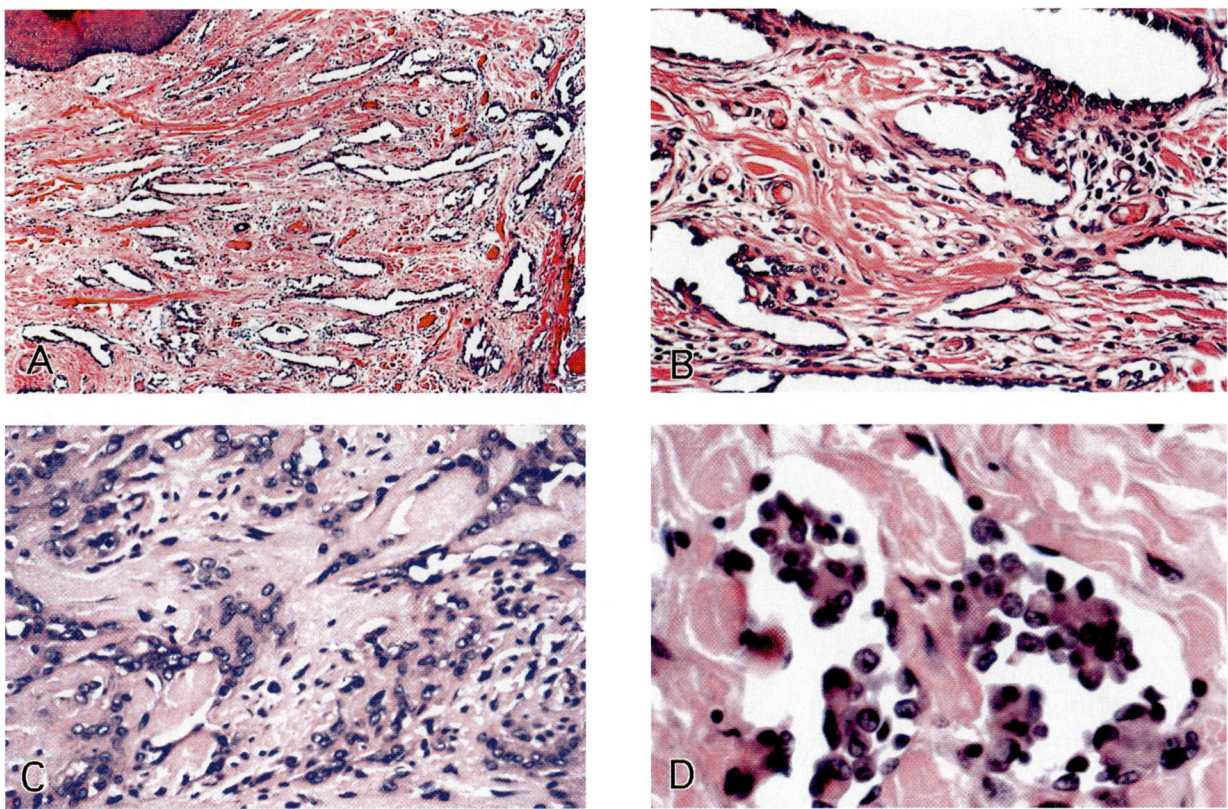

Figure 7-42

RETIFORM HEMANGIOENDOTHELIOMA

A: Elongated, slightly branching vascular spaces in the dermis resemble the normal rete testis.
B: The tumor cells lining the vascular channels are plump.
C: Relatively solid-looking cords are formed.
D: In other areas, the cells are aggregated focally into small micropapillations.

potential subpopulation of fusiform tumor cells. The nuclear features are relatively bland, and mitotic activity is limited. Necrosis is absent, and there is no "dissection" of dermal collagen by the lesion as would be expected in angiosarcoma. Benign lymphangioendothelioma also demonstrates a capacity for retiform vascular growth, but that neoplasm lacks intralesional erythrocytes and has a more prominent stromal lymphocytic infiltrate.

Other Hemangioendotheliomas

There are two other rare forms of hemangioendothelioma: *composite* and *epithelioid sarcoma-like cutaneous hemangioendothelioma*. The first of these lesions demonstrates a histologic admixture of elements resembling those seen in epithelioid, retiform, and spindle cell hemangioendotheliomas as well as angiosarcoma, but manifests no particularly distinctive clinical features (115). Epithelioid sarcoma-like hemangioendothelioma is composed of sheets of polygonal tumor cells with only vague vasogenesis (fig. 7-43) (87). It is reactive for keratin (as are approximately 30 to 40 percent of all epithelioid endothelial tumors), but also exhibits positivity for CD31, unlike true epithelioid sarcoma. Moreover, epithelioid sarcoma-like hemangioendothelioma has an indolent biological evolution, without metastasis in the majority of cases (87), differing from the behavior of true epithelioid sarcoma.

MALIGNANT VASCULAR NEOPLASMS

Those mesenchymal neoplasms that demonstrate a reproducible tendency for recurrence and distant metastasis are rightly considered

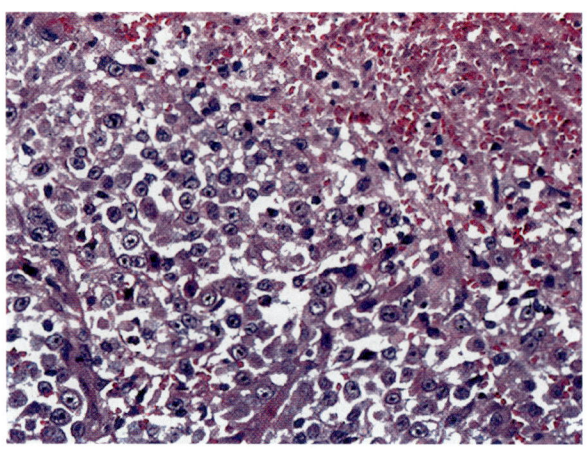

Figure 7-43

EPITHELIOID SARCOMA-LIKE HEMANGIOENDOTHELIOMA

Sheets of moderately atypical tumor cells have only vague vasogenesis. The neoplastic elements in this case were immunoreactive for both keratin and CD31.

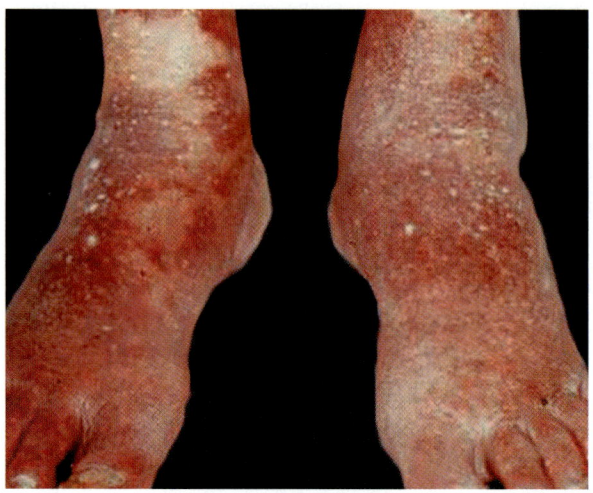

Figure 7-44

CLASSIC KAPOSI'S SARCOMA

Brown, indurated, confluent plaques in the skin of the lower legs in an elderly man of Italian descent.

to be overtly malignant. In specific regard to cutaneous vascular tumors, there are only two that truly fulfill those criteria: Kaposi's sarcoma and angiosarcoma. That statement reflects our bias that lymphangiosarcoma cannot be reliably separated from angiosarcoma, given current diagnostic tools.

Kaposi's Sarcoma

Clinical Features. The clinical characteristics of Kaposi's sarcoma are by now all too familiar to most physicians, because of the tremendous increase in the incidence of this tumor occasioned by the advent of the AIDS epidemic in the 1980s. Prior to that time, Kaposi's sarcoma was a lesion rarely encountered outside of the Mediterranean basin and Africa (147,193,196).

This neoplasm occurs in four well-defined clinical settings (193,196). *Classic Kaposi's sarcoma* is a disease that predominantly affects elderly men of Middle-Eastern or Italian heritage, and which manifests as multiple, coalescent, red-brown macules and plaques on the distal lower extremities (fig. 7-44). A subset of patients has lesions that resemble deep lymphangiomas (149), accompanied by lymphedema of the extremities. Nodular, sometimes ulcerated tumors of the skin and viscera eventually supervene in this variant, but only after a prolonged period of time. *African Kaposi's sarcoma* is seen in young black patients from restricted portions of the African continent. Women are almost as frequently afflicted as men, and their mean age is less than that of those with the classic form by two to three decades. The disorder is rapidly progressive, with the early appearance of nodular lesions (fig. 7-45) and involvement of lymph nodes and internal organs. *Kaposi's sarcoma associated with iatrogenic immunosuppression* shares clinical features with both the classic and African subtypes. It primarily affects recipients of allogeneic organ transplants (184). *AIDS-related Kaposi's sarcoma* is precipitated by infection with human immunodeficiency virus (HIV). In the AIDS pandemic, the sarcoma was noted in young homosexual men (157,158), with fewer cases in intravenous drug abusers and recipients of infected blood products.

Although the other manifestations of AIDS have become more evenly distributed among the infected patient populations, Kaposi's sarcoma has remained largely confined to gay males (189,193). Nevertheless, its incidence has already begun to decline, even though the number of HIV-infected individuals continues to rise on a worldwide scale. The reasons for these epidemiologic peculiarities are unknown at the present time (165,193).

AIDS-related Kaposi's sarcoma has a deceptively innocuous appearance at its onset, taking

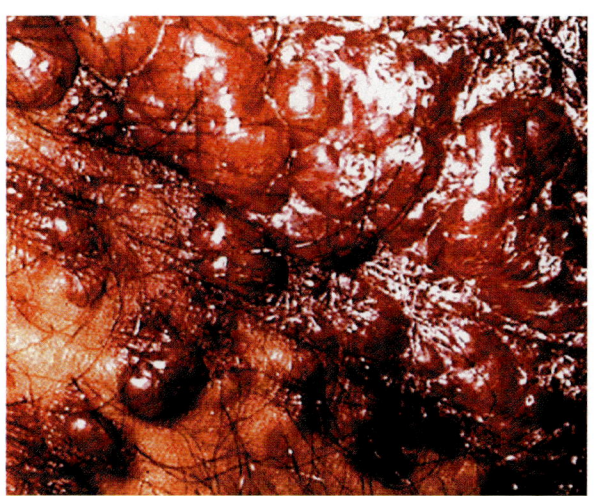

Figure 7-45
AFRICAN KAPOSI'S SARCOMA
Confluent nodules of tumor in the skin of the groin.

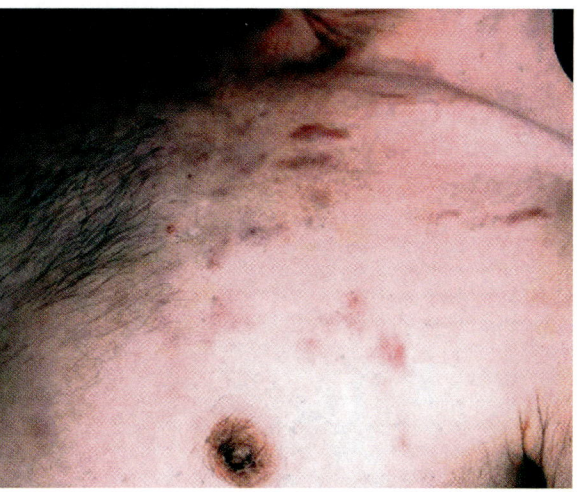

Figure 7-46
KAPOSI'S SARCOMA AND ACQUIRED IMMUNODEFICIENCY SYNDROME
The tumor is represented by several ecchymosis-like lesions in the skin of the thorax.

the form of ill-defined macular patches that often resemble ecchymoses (fig. 7-46) (136, 147, 157,196a). In contrast to the topographic confinement of the classic variant, in AIDS patients the tumor may affect virtually any skin field as well as the mucosa (158,166). Visceral involvement also appears rapidly, similar to that seen in the African form (164).

Several common threads have emerged that bind all of the variants of Kaposi's sarcoma together. One factor is the human leukocyte antigen (HLA)-DR5 allele, which is greatly over-represented in Kaposi's sarcoma patients when compared with the population at large (183). The second is seropositivity for cytomegalovirus (CMV) (144). In reference to that observation, some authors have advanced the hypothesis that Kaposi's sarcoma is not a neoplasm at all, but instead represents the direct result of a tissue reaction to an infectious agent (or agents) (150). We do not subscribe to the latter view. It has been shown that Kaposi's sarcoma cells express an activated oncogene, termed *K-FGF* (152). Moreover, the features of this proliferation in transfection studies are most consistent with those of a true neoplasm (152), and the pattern of visceral involvement seen in advanced cases (164,196) is unlike that of any known viral disease. Lastly, genomic sequences of HHV8 have been detected in Kaposi's sarcoma by molecular analyses, in common with several other irrefutable endothelial neoplasms of the skin (139,140,168,177–179). It would therefore appear tenable to conclude that Kaposi's sarcoma may result from the effects of HIV-CMV-HHV8 co-infection in susceptible (HLA-DR5-positive?) individuals, allowing viral agents to express a latent potential for cellular transformation and oncogenesis (154,177,166a,199a).

Classic Kaposi's sarcoma is an indolent process that only infrequently causes the death of the patient. African, transplant-associated, and HIV-related variants evolve more rapidly and are often fatal (147,151,196).

Pathologic Findings. Early Kaposi's sarcoma most often takes a macular or patch form (136, 147,157). Microscopically, this variant is extremely subtle. Often, only a limited proliferation of small, attenuated, interanastomosing but bland blood vessels are seen in the periappendageal reticular corium, together with an excess of nondescript spindle cells throughout the dermal connective tissue (fig. 7-47). In addition, small preexisting blood vessels are often invested by a lymphoplasmacytic infiltrate. The "promontory" sign, neovascular channels formed around native vessels yielding profiles that simulate the promontory of a cliff, is a helpful diagnostic finding (fig.7-48) (136,147,157,

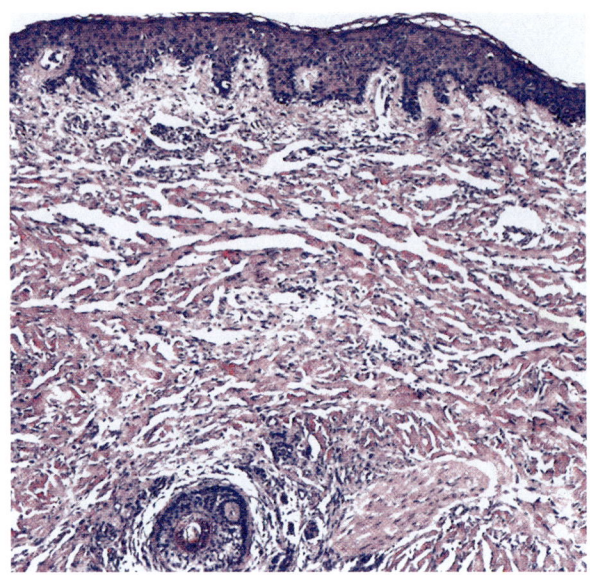
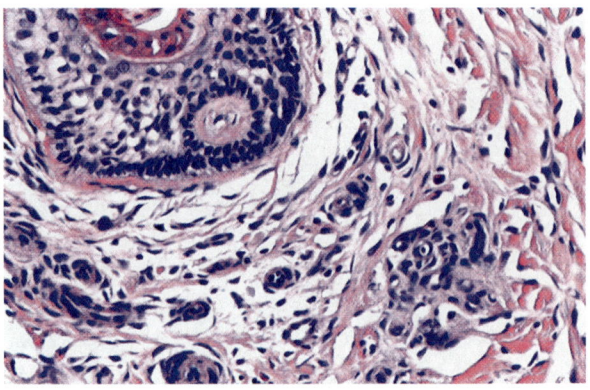

Figure 7-47

PATCH STAGE KAPOSI'S SARCOMA

The proliferation of thin-walled, disorganized, vascular channels between dermal collagen bundles (left) tends to surround and isolate dermal appendages (above).

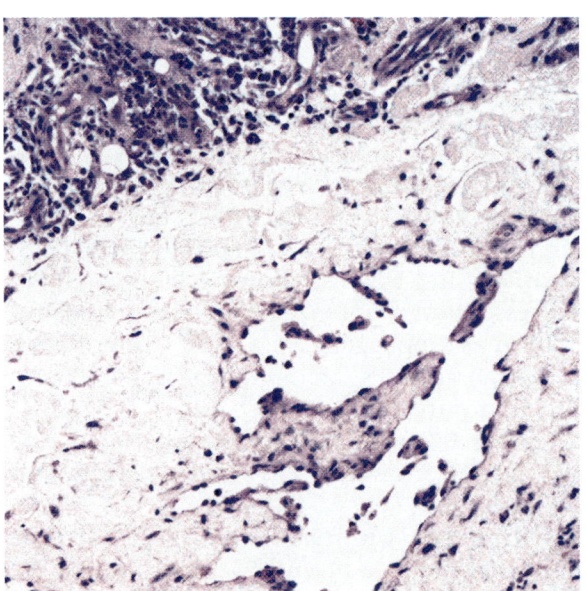
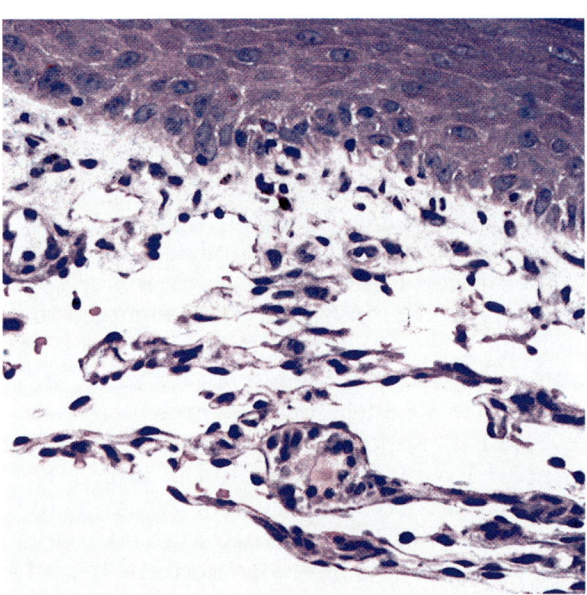

Figure 7-48

THE "PROMONTORY" SIGN OF KAPOSI'S SARCOMA

New tumoral vascular spaces form around preexisting dermal blood vessels.

196a). Small groupings of venule-like blood vessels are interspersed randomly throughout the dermis in some cases, and extravasated erythrocytes are inconspicuous, if they are present at all (147). McNutt et al. (171) have shown that endothelia within new (neoplastic) blood vessels are often apoptotic in the patch stage. This observation is unique, and would not be expected in benign vascular proliferations.

Plaque stage Kaposi's sarcoma features the appearance of more organized aggregates of spindle cells, which form small fascicles in admixture with capillary-sized neovascular channels, extravasated erythrocytes, hemosiderin,

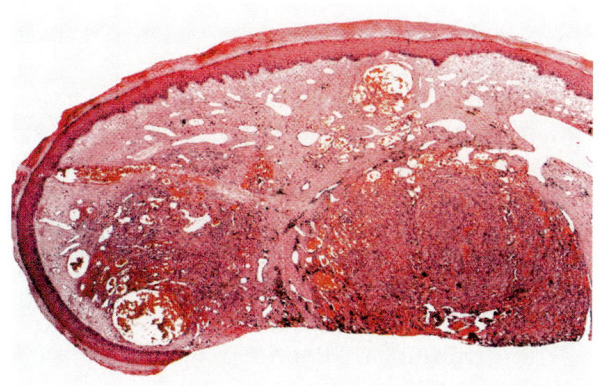
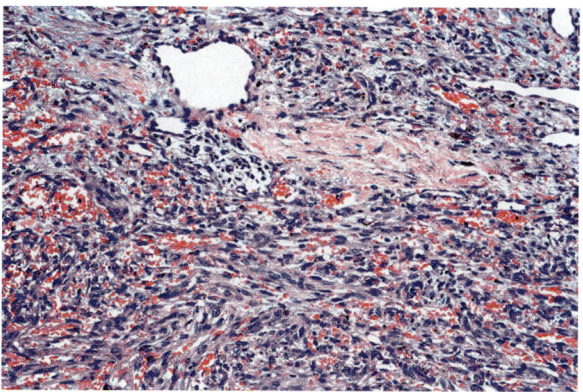

Figure 7-49

PLAQUE STAGE KAPOSI'S SARCOMA

An advanced lesion of Kaposi's sarcoma shows an internal spindle cell nodule.

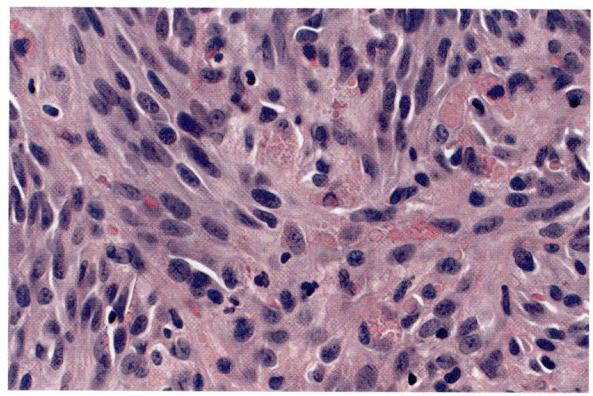
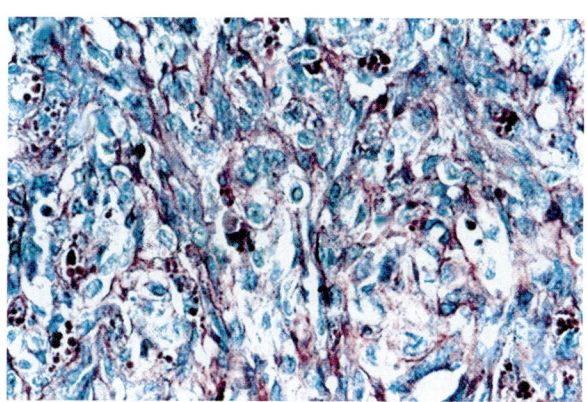

Figure 7-50

KAPOSI'S SARCOMA

Intracellular globules are often seen, as highlighted here with the periodic acid–Schiff (PAS) stain after diastase digestion.

and stromal hemosiderin granules (fig. 7-49) (143,147,196,196a). The groupings of neoplastic cells are often diffusely dispersed throughout the dermis, but sometimes assume a pseudolobular configuration (147). Another useful diagnostic clue that appears at this phase of tumor evolution is the presence of hyaline globules in the neoplastic endothelial cells (fig. 7-50). These represent phagocytosed erythrocytes, as documented by the peroxidase reaction; they also may be stained by the PAS-diastase method (147,157,196). The presence of hyaline globules alone is not sufficient for a diagnosis of Kaposi's sarcoma, because these globules can be seen in non-neoplastic vascular proliferations of the skin (143,147); however, their presence is helpful when interpreted in the proper context. Finally, small papillary projections of tumor cells may be observed within ectatic neovascular spaces in this stage of Kaposi's sarcoma, together with racemose, dissecting luminal profiles throughout the dermis (143).

The truly spindle cell stage of Kaposi's sarcoma is the nodular phase, where fusiform elements comprise the bulk of the proliferating cell population. The nuclei are only modestly hyperchromatic, with indistinct nucleoli, and cytoplasm is scant and amphophilic. A notable diagnostic feature is the presence of cytoplasmic vacuoles in the spindle cells (fig. 7-51),

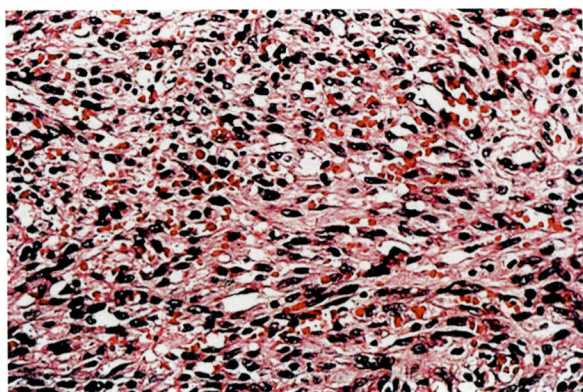

Figure 7-51

KAPOSI'S SARCOMA

Intracellular vacuolization is often evident in the spindle cells.

probably representing a primitive attempt at vascular lumen formation (157,190,196). The fusiform cells of Kaposi's sarcoma appear to spare dermal zones that surround preexisting vessels, leaving hypocellular cuffs around the latter structures, a helpful microscopic finding (194). Extravasated erythrocytes and stromal hemosiderin deposition are maximum in scope in the nodular stage, and hyaline globules often are numerous in the neoplastic cells.

A continuing controversy regarding Kaposi's sarcoma focuses on the nature of the proliferating elements of the spindle cell form. There is no question that patch stage and plaque stage disease features reproducible immunoreactivity for endothelial markers, but these determinants are only occasionally detected in the spindle cell variant. Some authors have contended that Kaposi's sarcoma is a modified lymphatic endothelial tumor (141), whereas others have concluded that it is not endothelial at all (160). We prefer the premise that Kaposi's sarcoma begins as a vascular endothelial neoplasm that undergoes reproducible clonal evolution to yield a cellular population resembling myofibroblasts, at which point it only partially retains a vascular immunophenotype.

Pantanowitz et al. (181) considered the morphologic features that represent biological regression in treated lesions. These include a diminution in the number of neoplastic spindle cells, increased perivascular infiltrates of lymphocytes, and a prominence of dermal hemosiderophages.

The overall image was felt to be somewhat similar to that of pigmented purpuras.

Differential Diagnosis. As mentioned earlier, atypical hemangiomas and benign lymphangioendothelioma can simulate the morphologic image of patch-stage Kaposi's sarcoma. The first two tumors do not demonstrate the promontory sign microscopically, and they both lack immunoreactivity for HHV8 latent nuclear antigen-1 (LNA1) (146a,159a,180a,181a).

The differential diagnosis of spindle cell Kaposi's sarcoma includes leiomyosarcoma, spindle cell melanoma, spindle cell squamous carcinoma, malignant peripheral nerve sheath tumor, fibrohistiocytic neoplasms (especially angiomatoid fibrous histiocytomas), and spindle cell angiosarcoma. All but the last are easily excluded by attention to histologic detail or application of special studies (Table 7-1) (143,147,190).

Spindle cell angiosarcoma is a rare lesion, with microscopic attributes nearly identical to those of nodular Kaposi's sarcoma (185,190, 196a). Nevertheless, the clinical features of the two conditions usually differ substantially. Spindle cell angiosarcoma also exhibits a much higher degree of nuclear atypia and mitotic activity. Moreover, studies for HHV8 are typically positive in Kaposi's sarcoma but not in spindle cell angiosarcoma (170).

Non-neoplastic simulants of Kaposi's sarcoma also exist. Those entities are considered separately at the end of this chapter.

Angiosarcoma

Clinical Features. *Angiosarcoma of the skin* is characteristically seen in one of several well-defined clinical contexts: idiopathic proliferations on the scalp or face of elderly patients; occurrence in a field of prior therapeutic irradiation after a lag period of 5 or more years; and development in an area of chronic cutaneous lymphedema (the so called Stewart-Treves syndrome) (fig. 7-52) (138,146,148,155,156,161–163,191,197,198). An exceedingly small number of tumors arise as lesions of the extremities or trunk in individuals with no apparent predisposing conditions.

Angiosarcomas likewise show a variety of macroscopic presentations. They may be large, multinodular, ill-defined, violaceous, bloody, and sometimes ulcerated masses (fig. 7-53); vague ecchymosis-like macular lesions; ligneous,

Table 7-1

DIFFERENTIAL DIAGNOSIS OF KAPOSI'S SARCOMA

Lesion	CHB[a]	CVS	EE	LSC	LGC	HHV8-LNA1	VBV	S-100	MSA	CHG
Kaposi's sarcoma	+	0	+	+	0	+	0	0	0	0
Lobular capillary hemangioma	0	0	0	0	0	0	0	0	0	0
MPNST[b]	0	0	0	+	0	0	0	+/–	0	0
Leiomyosarcoma	0	0	0	+	+/–	0	0	+/–	+	0
Desmoplastic malignant melanoma	0	0	0	+	+/–	0	0	+	0	0
Spindle cell angiosarcoma	0	0	+/–	+	+/–	0	0	0	0	0
Proliferative scar tissue	0	+/–	+/–	+	0	0	+	0	0	+/–
Acroangiodermatitis	0	+	+/–	0	0	0	0	0	0	+/–
Fibrohistiocytic tumors	0	0	0	+	+	0	0	0	0	+/–
Reactions to Monsel's solution	0	0	+/–	+/–	+/–	0	0	0	0	+

[a]CHB = cytoplasmic hyaline bodies; CVS = clinical venous stasis; EE = extravasated erythrocytes among proliferating cells; LSC = lesional spindle cells; LGC = lesional giant cells; HHV8-LNA1 = immunoreactivity for human herpesvirus-8 latent nuclear antigen-1; VBV = vertically oriented stromal blood vessels; S-100 = S-100 protein immunoreactivity; MSA = muscle-specific actin immunoreactivity; CHG = clumped intralesional hemosiderin granules.
[b]MPNST = malignant peripheral nerve sheath tumor.

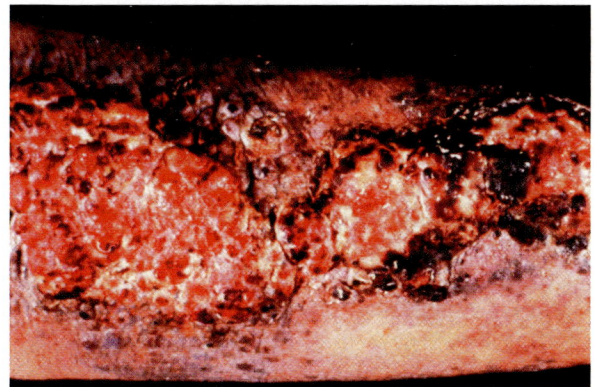 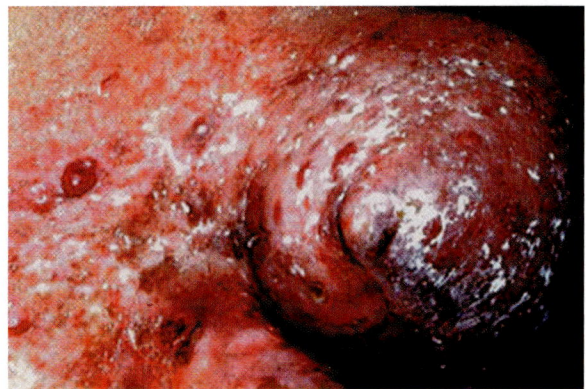

Figure 7-52

ANGIOSARCOMA

Left: Angiosarcoma of the right lower leg in the setting of chronic lymphedema (Stewart-Treves syndrome), several years after inguinal lymphadenectomy for the treatment of malignant melanoma.

Right: Another example of Stewart-Treves–type angiosarcoma has recurred locally following amputation of an arm, in a patient who had irradiation to the region for breast carcinoma.

"brawny" alterations in the skin that simulate erysipelas (fig. 7-54); and multifocal, seemingly discrete bluish red nodules that simulate cavernous hemangiomas (fig. 7-55) (196a).

The behavior of angiosarcoma is uniformly aggressive. Those patients whose neoplasms are less than 10 cm in maximum dimension may benefit from radical surgical excision and postoperative irradiation, but almost all affected individuals eventually die of unmanageable local tumor growth or distant metastases (162).

Pathologic Findings. In classic form, angiosarcoma is a disorganized proliferation of polyhedral, atypical endothelial cells with

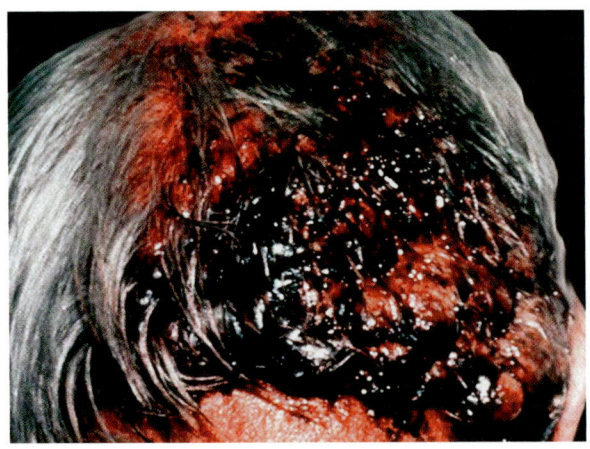

Figure 7-53

ANGIOSARCOMA

A multinodular, ulcerated, bloody mass in the scalp of an elderly woman represents idiopathic cutaneous angiosarcoma.

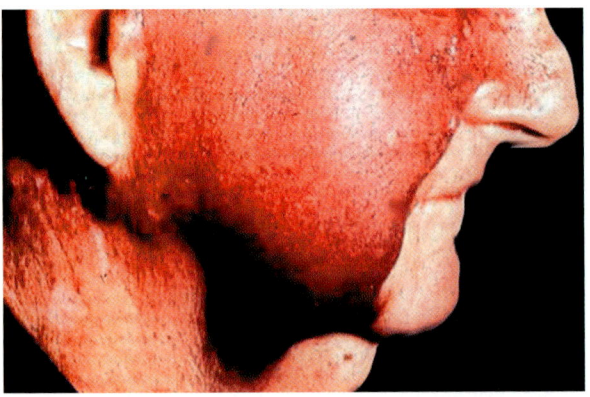

Figure 7-54

ANGIOSARCOMA

This angiosarcoma resembles the appearance of erysipelas, with "brawny" induration of the facial skin.

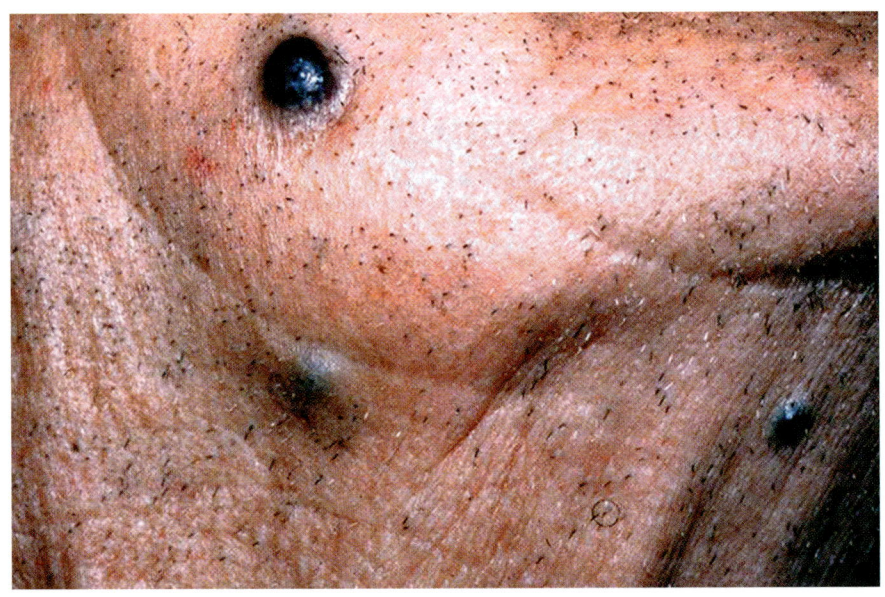

Figure 7-55

ANGIOSARCOMA

Deceptively hemangioma-like multicentric angiosarcomas are seen in the facial skin in this patient.

hyperchromatic nuclei and scant amphophilic cytoplasm. The tumor cells mantle racemose, interconnecting, "sieve"-like vascular channels in the skin that dissect through dermal collagen and deeper tissues, and contain luminal red blood cells (fig. 7-56) (148,155,161,162,169,197). Cutaneous appendages are variably entrapped or destroyed by the proliferation; hemosiderin and chronic inflammatory cells may be interspersed throughout the lesion. Large tumors may ulcerate the overlying epidermis multifocally.

Micropapillae of neoplastic cells are frequently seen projecting into the neovascular channels of angiosarcomas (fig. 7-57), and the supporting (stromal) blood vessels also may show nuclear atypia in endothelial cells. Mitotic activity is variable in scope but always present. Necrosis may or may not be observed (155,169).

Several microscopic variants of angiosarcoma are recognized. These include the spindle cell subtype, described above (fig. 7-58) (185,190, 196a), a solid epithelioid form (fig. 7-59) (112,174,

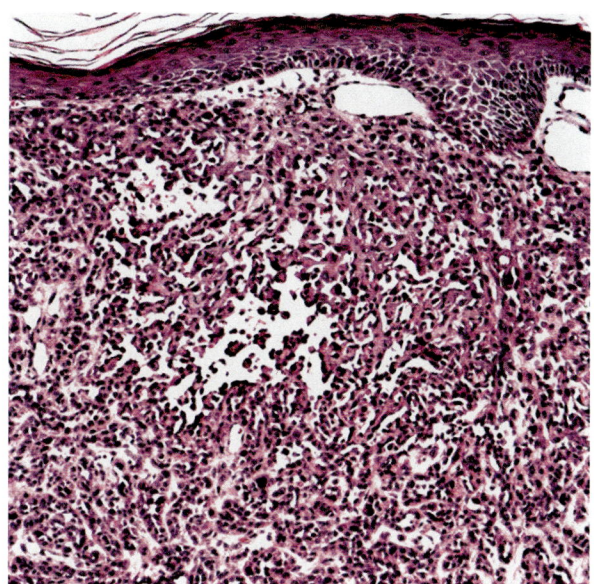
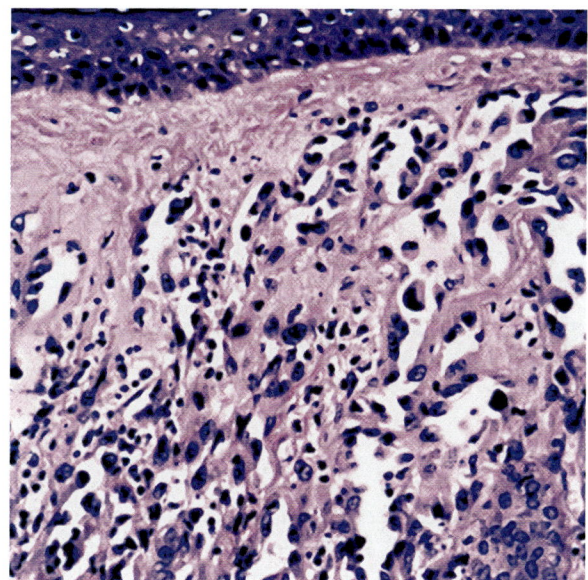

Figure 7-56

ANGIOSARCOMA

A "sieve"-like growth pattern, in which vascular channels permeate the dermis and deeper soft tissues.

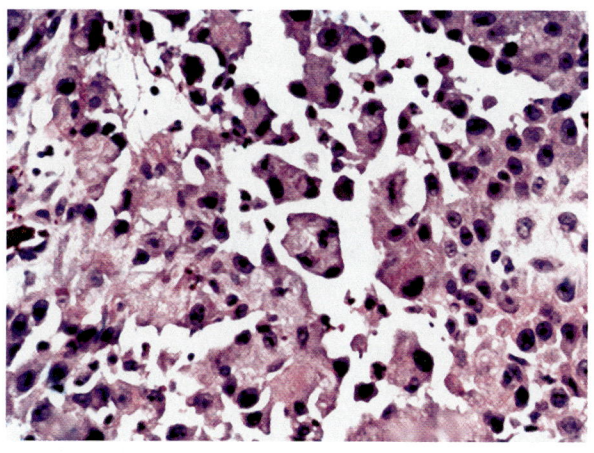
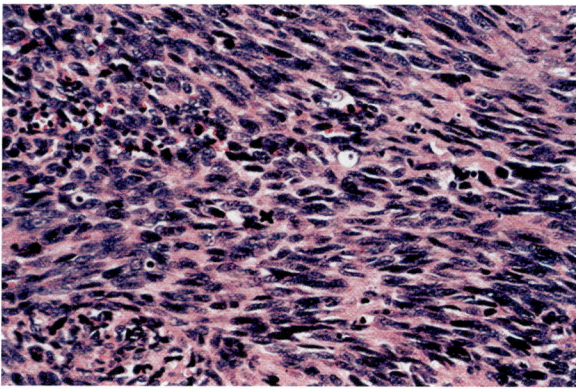

Figure 7-57

ANGIOSARCOMA

Micropapillary arrays of cytologically atypical endothelial cells are apparent.

Figure 7-58

SPINDLE CELL ANGIOSARCOMA

The neoplastic cells form only vague vascular channels and are characterized by a high degree of cytologic

182,186), minimal-deviation (hemangioma-like) angiosarcoma (fig. 7-60) (174,196a), a granular cell variant (fig. 7-61) (172), and a pleomorphic subtype with the potential to simulate atypical fibroxanthoma or malignant fibrous histiocytoma (fig. 7-62) (148). Akiyama et al. (137) also have reported two cases in which benign melanocytes and melanophages were intermixed with the neoplastic endothelial cells in the dermis.

Among these histologic forms, several merit further comment because they may be the source of diagnostic error. *Minimal deviation angiosarcoma* (MDAS) shows minimal cytologic atypia of the constituent endothelial cells, and forms more complete (tubular) vascular lumens

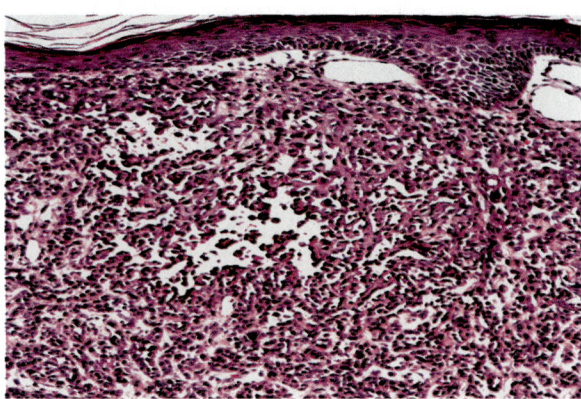
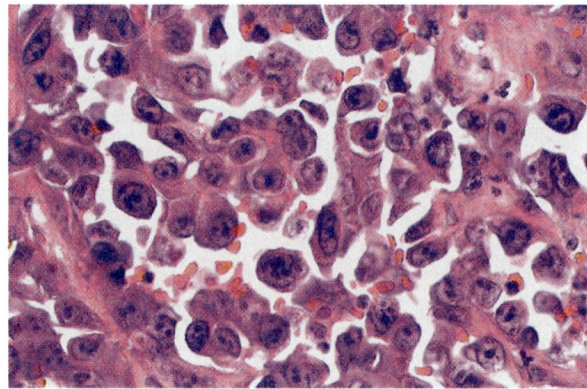

Figure 7-59

EPITHELIOID ANGIOSARCOMA

The epithelioid variant of angiosarcoma may be confused with metastatic carcinoma involving the skin because of its composition by large polygonal cells and few erythrocytes.

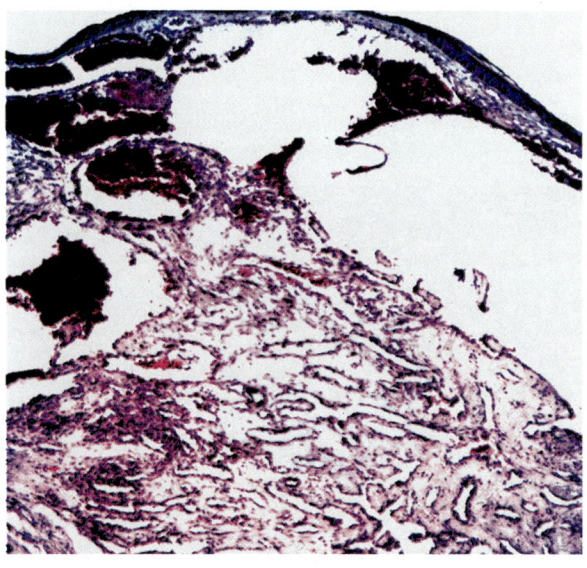

Figure 7-60

MINIMAL DEVIATION ANGIOSARCOMA

The minimal deviation variant of angiosarcoma demonstrates superficial cavernous vascular spaces, like those seen in banal hemangiomas. Deeper elements of the tumor, however, show a greater degree of cytologic and architectural anaplasia.

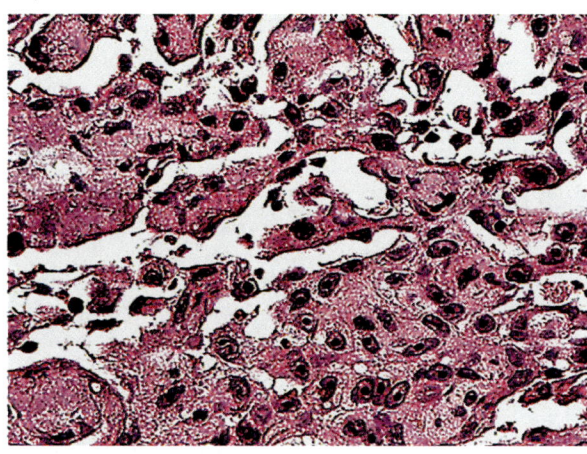

Figure 7-61

GRANULAR CELL ANGIOSARCOMA

Granular cell change is apparent in the tumor cells of this angiosarcoma, representing a potential trap with respect to the possible misdiagnosis of cutaneous granular cell tumor.

in the upper dermis than other variants (174, 196a). Nonetheless, biopsy specimens that include the deep dermis and subcutis inevitably reveal the racemose, dissecting, endothelial profiles that are characteristic. The danger here is in the interpretation of shallow punch biopsies or shave biopsies, such that MDAS may be mistaken for atypical hemangioma or benign lymphangioendothelioma. As described above, the latter two lesions have a permeative pattern of growth in the dermis which mimics the superficial aspect of MDAS. We believe that all tumors demonstrating an atypical, disorganized pattern of neovasogenesis should be excised totally.

Epithelioid angiosarcoma is composed entirely or predominantly of plump polyhedral cells that imitate true epithelia (145,148,182,186). These occupy much of the lumen in the vascular spaces formed by such lesions, and therefore

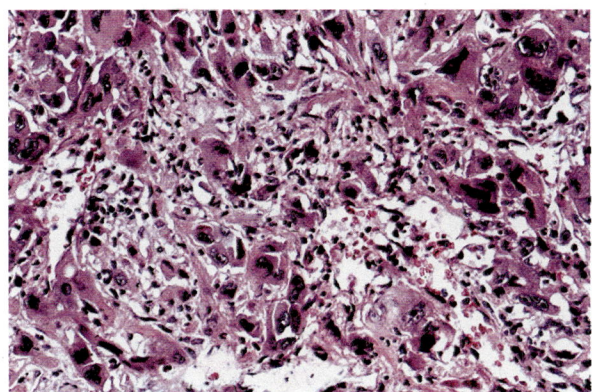

Figure 7-62

PLEOMORPHIC ANGIOSARCOMA

Pleomorphic angiosarcoma is basically indistinguishable at a morphologic level from other pleomorphic sarcomas of the skin. Ultrastructural or immunohistochemical proof of endothelial differentiation is often required for recognition of this tumor variant.

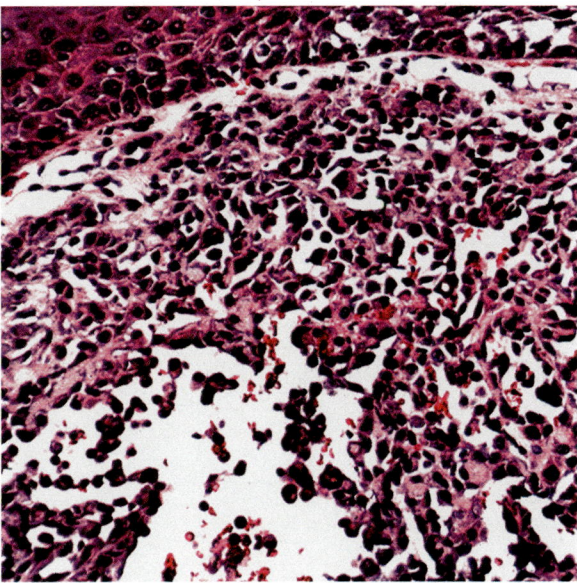

Figure 7-63

ANGIOSARCOMA-LIKE (PSEUDOVASCULAR) SUBTYPE OF CUTANEOUS SQUAMOUS CELL CARCINOMA

Acantholytic arrays of tumor cells closely simulate the racemose growth pattern of a vascular neoplasm. Special studies and clinical correlation are necessary for the effective diagnosis of this lesion.

the latter channels often contain few discernible erythrocytes and are not readily recognized as endothelial in nature.

Differential Diagnosis. Simulants of spindle cell angiosarcoma have been discussed above in connection with Kaposi's sarcoma. Epithelioid vascular tumors may mimic true epithelial neoplasms (particularly pseudovascular or angiomatoid squamous carcinomas [fig. 7-63] [176]), melanoma and clear-cell sarcoma, epithelioid sarcoma, epithelioid leiomyosarcoma, and large cell lymphoma (196a). Pleomorphic variants of angiosarcoma can be confused with atypical fibroxanthoma, primary or metastatic undifferentiated carcinomas, melanoma, and malignant fibrous histiocytoma (196a). Immunohistologic analysis is the most useful tool for diagnosing angiosarcoma. Endothelial tumors are reactive for vimentin, von Willebrand factor, CD31 and CD34 antigens, thrombomodulin, and Ulex europaeus I agglutinin receptors; they typically lack epithelial membrane antigen, p63 protein, desmin, muscle-specific actin, and S-100 protein (Table 7-2) (153,173,175,180,192,195,199). Interestingly, however, selected keratin proteins and epithelial tumor-associated glycoproteins, as recognized by the antibody designated as B72.3, may be seen in some epithelioid angiosarcomas (173,187). Miettinen and Fetsch (173) found that keratins 8 and 18 were most likely to be found in vascular neoplasms, and they recommended that those protein targets be avoided when choosing antikeratin antibodies to study endothelial tumors.

TUMEFACTIVE NON-NEOPLASTIC VASCULAR PROLIFERATIONS

Several proliferations of blood vessels in the skin have more than a passing histologic resemblance to true neoplasms, but are reparative or otherwise reactive in nature. These are considered in the following sections.

Lesions that Simulate Kaposi's Sarcoma

As a byproduct of the AIDS pandemic and the consequent increased interest in vascular lesions of the skin, several non-neoplastic proliferations have been identified that may simulate Kaposi's sarcoma. These include acroangiodermatitis, proliferating dermal scars, reactions to application of Monsel's solution, and certain infections.

Acroangiodermatitis. This is a proliferative reaction to dermal erythrocyte extravasation that occurs in the setting of severe venous stasis

Table 7-2

IMMUNOHISTOCHEMICAL DIFFERENTIAL DIAGNOSIS OF EPITHELIOID ANGIOSARCOMA

Tumor	CK[a]	p63	S-100	Mel-A	CAL-D	VIM	CD31	CD34	CD45
Epithelioid angiosarcoma	+/-	0	0	0	0	+	+	+	0
Angiosarcoma-like SCC	+	+	0	0	0	+/-	0	0	0
Angiomatoid melanoma	0	0	+	+	0	+	0	0	0
Melanoma of soft parts	0	0	+	+	0	+	0	0	0
Epithelioid sarcoma	+	0	+/-	0	+/-	+	0	+	0
Epithelioid leiomyosarcoma	0	0	+/-	0	+	+/-	0	0	0
Large cell ML	0	0	0	0	0	+/-	0	0	+
AFX/MFH	0	0	0	0	0	+	0	0	0

[a]CK = cytokeratin; p63 = p63 protein; Mel-A = Melan-A/MART-1; CAL-D = caldesmon; VIM = vimentin; SCC = squamous cell carcinoma; ML = malignant lymphoma; AFX = atypical fibroxanthoma; MFH = malignant fibrous histiocytoma.

in the lower extremities due to venous valvular insufficiency. It is therefore seen in patients with severe venous varicosities of the legs, who tend to be elderly (216,226,243,248). The lesions are typically slow-evolving, brawny, red-brown macules, papules, or plaques, but they also assume a more violaceous nodular character in some instances. Depending upon the symmetry or asymmetry of the venous insufficiency, one or both legs may be affected. The areas of skin surrounding the malleoli and dorsal surfaces of the feet are primarily involved by this process.

Patients with classic Kaposi's sarcoma do not tend to have venous stasis of the legs, except by coincidence. Physical examination and careful history taking regarding the course and pace of the eruption usually permit a diagnosis of acroangiodermatitis to be made solely on clinical grounds.

In those cases where these features are indeterminate, biopsy may be useful. The lesion shows a lobular pattern of capillary and venular proliferation in the dermis, particularly in its superficial aspect (fig. 7-64). There is no proclivity for new vessels to cluster around old ones (i.e., the promontory sign is lacking); there is no interstitial dermal hypercellularity; and the degree of lesional hemosiderin deposition greatly outstrips the extent of visible red blood cell extravasation (243,248). The latter microscopic features differ markedly from those seen in Kaposi's sarcoma.

Proliferating Scars. Not uncommonly, biopsies of proliferating scars (following episodes of injury that the patient may not remember) are performed under the impression that these lesions represent cutaneous neoplasms. The resulting histologic profile is essentially that of organizing granulation tissue, featuring a regimented proliferation of capillaries and venules that are typically oriented vertically within the dermis (143,248). Proliferation of intervening fibroblasts and myofibroblasts is frequent, with variable edema or dense collagen deposition in the surrounding dermal stroma. If the scar has been traumatized, red blood cell leakage and hemosiderin deposition may be observed. Nonetheless, the overall image of this lesion is only superficially like that of Kaposi's sarcoma and diagnostic separation of the two conditions is typically straightforward.

The characteristics of reactions to the application of Monsel's solution (a surgical styptic) are similar to those of proliferating scars. Because this pharmaceutical agent includes iron salts, large irregular or rhomboidal clusters of iron pigment are observed in tissue reactions to Monsel's preparation (fig. 7-65) (200).

Bacillary (Epithelioid) Angiomatosis. Caused by infection with *Bartonella henselae* (207,209,219,223,224,232,238), this condition is observed in patients who are infected with HIV, leading to particular concern that they have Kaposi's sarcoma. Red-violet cutaneous

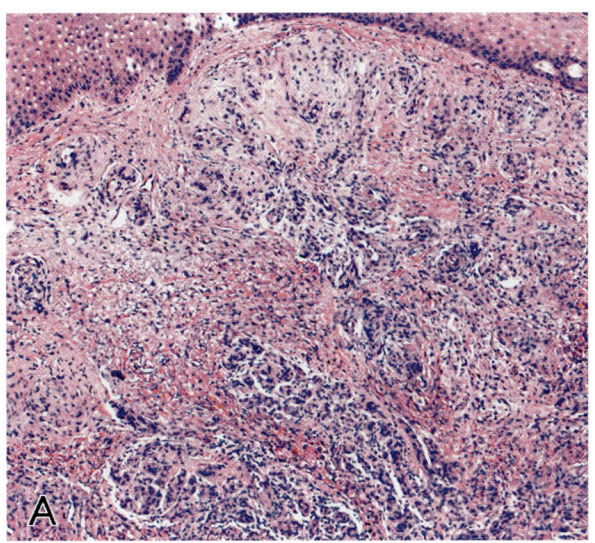
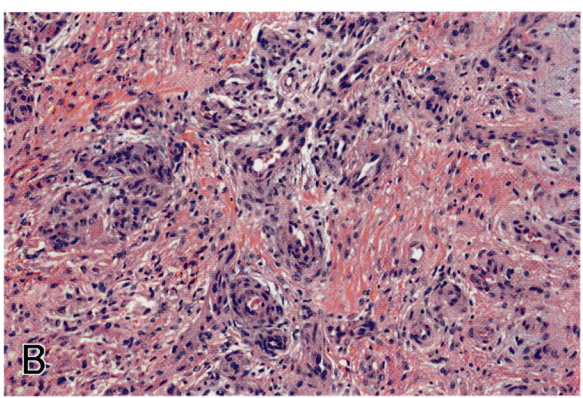
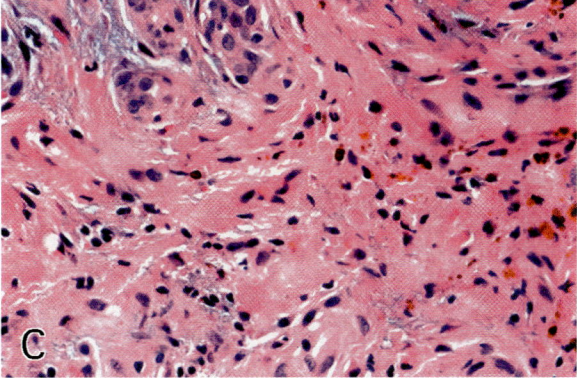

Figure 7-64

ACROANGIODERMATITIS

A: The low-power microscopic view of a proliferating dermal scar shows vertically oriented blood vessels.

B: Vascular proliferation in this condition occurs in "plates" in the dermis, and is represented by venules and capillaries.

C: Hemosiderin deposits and chronic inflammation are common.

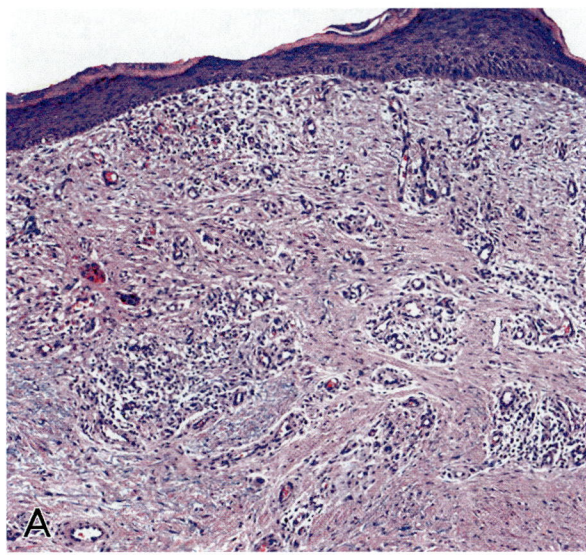
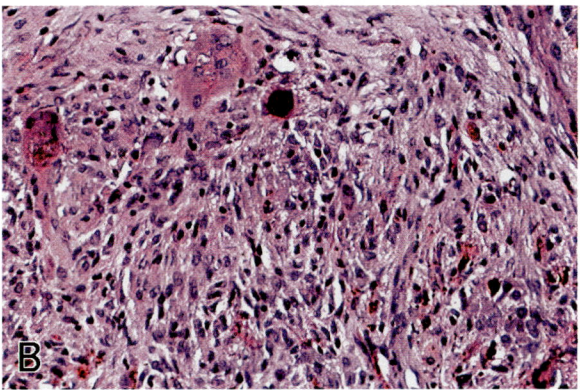
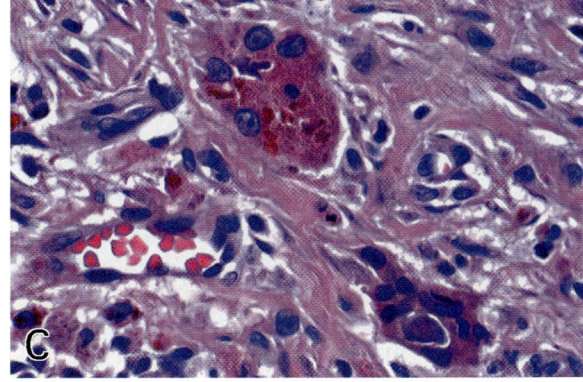

Figure 7-65

REACTION TO THE APPLICATION OF MONSEL'S SOLUTION

A,B: There is a spindle cell proliferation in the dermis.

C: Clumps of ferruginated material present among the spindle cells and in foreign body-type giant cells provide a helpful clue to the diagnosis.

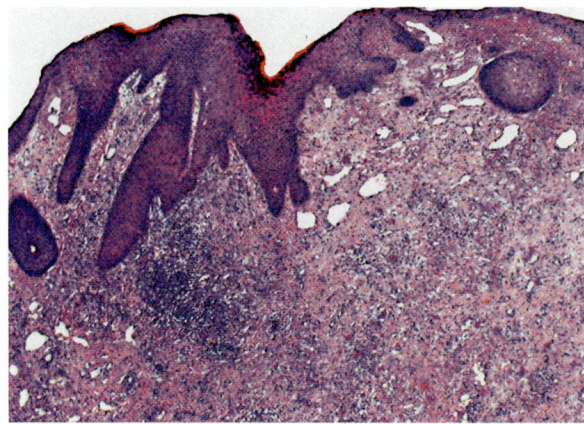

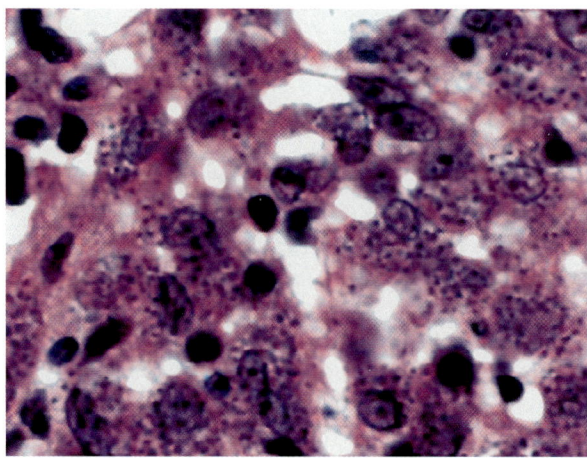

Figure 7-67

BACILLARY ANGIOMATOSIS

High-power microscopic inspection of the endothelial cells reveals cytoplasmic granularity due to the presence of numerous intracellular bacteria.

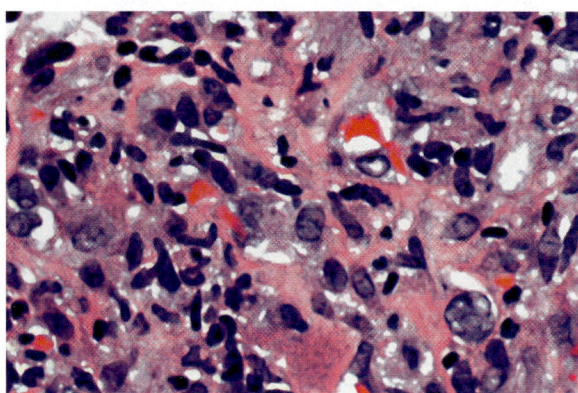

Figure 7-66

BACILLARY ANGIOMATOSIS

A proliferation of tubular dermal blood vessels (top) is admixed with numerous acute and chronic inflammatory cells (bottom).

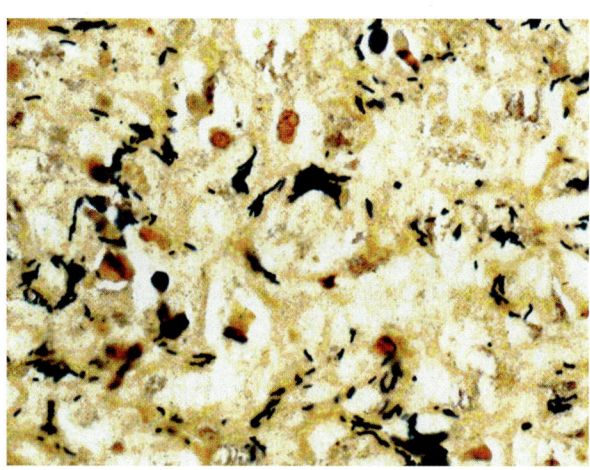

Figure 7-68

BACILLARY ANGIOMATOSIS

Innumerable intracellular bacilliform organisms are shown by the Warthin-Starry stain.

nodules and plaques of variable sizes are seen, without topographic predilections. The viscera also may be involved, heightening the mimicry of Kaposi's sarcoma (209,219,239).

The histologic features of bacillary angiomatosis differ substantially from those of Kaposi's sarcoma, and are instead more similar to those of epithelioid hemangioma. Organized sheets or clusters of completely formed vascular channels are observed in the dermis, with indistinctly lobular profiles (fig. 7-66); an epidermal collarette is frequently seen at the lateral borders of the proliferation. Constituent endothelial cells are plump, with abundant cytoplasm and bland nuclear features, although mitotic activity and limited foci of necrosis may be apparent (209, 223,248). Intralesional neutrophilia is a distinctive finding as well. Close examination of the cells shows granular cytoplasmic inclusions that represent clusters of bacilliform organisms (fig. 7-67) (223). These may be highlighted with the Warthin-Starry stain (fig. 7-68) (223,224,248). Virtually identical cutaneous lesions are also seen in association with infection by *Bartonella* sp in South American patients with Carrion's disease (verruga peruana) (202,203). Treatment of bacillary angiomatosis with appropriate antibiotics results in resolution of the

Vascular Tumors and Pseudotumors

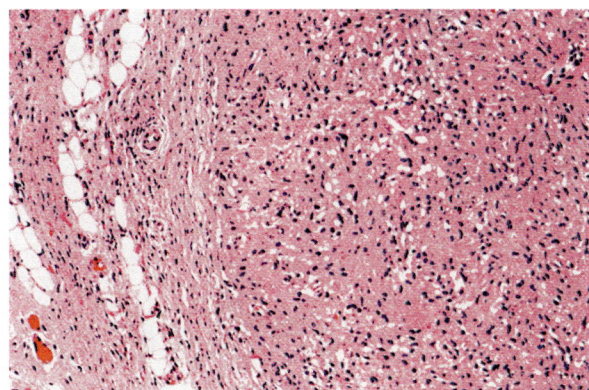
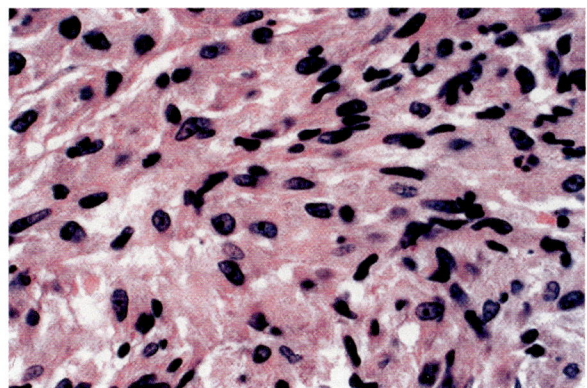

Figure 7-69

SPINDLE CELL REACTION TO MYCOBACTERIA

Mycobacterial pseudotumors of the dermis and subcutis may simulate spindle cell variants of Kaposi's sarcoma on low-power histologic examination (left), but the cytologic attributes of the latter tumor are lacking and no stromal erythrocyte extravasation is seen (right).

disease (223); thus, pathologic confusion of this process with Kaposi's sarcoma is a particularly serious error.

Spindle Cell Reactions to Mycobacteria. A related but histologically dissimilar cutaneous proliferation is seen in patients with AIDS who are infected with atypical mycobacteria. In this context, spindle cell lesions of the skin may be observed that emulate nodular Kaposi's sarcoma (206,248). They are composed of dermal fibroblast-like cells arranged in whorling fascicles, admixed with bands of sclerotic collagen, lymphocytes, and plasma cells (fig. 7-69). Careful scrutiny of the cytoplasm in the fusiform elements reveals granular inclusions that represent clumps of mycobacteria. These may be further delineated with the Ziehl-Nielsen or Fite stain (fig. 7-70) (206). Appropriate antibiotic treatment results in only variable resolution of the lesions, but they clearly should not be confused with Kaposi's sarcoma.

Potential Simulators of Angiosarcoma

There are two non-neoplastic cutaneous proliferations that may be mistaken for angiosarcoma by the unwary pathologist. These include *papillary intravascular endothelial hyperplasia (PIEH; Masson's vegetant intravascular hemangioendothelioma)* (201,204,208,213,221,229) and *rudimentary or true meningoceles* (203,206, 229). Both lesions occur in well-defined clinical settings that differ markedly from those at-

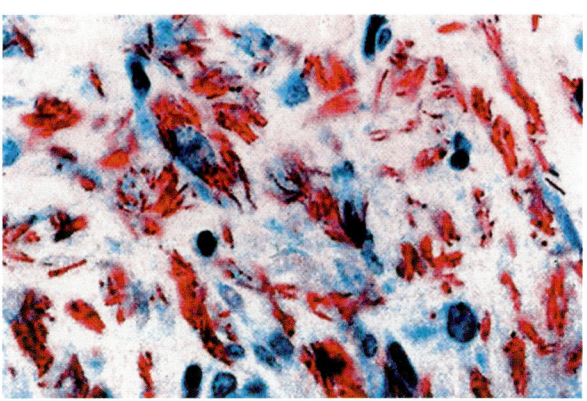

Figure 7-70

SPINDLE CELL REACTION TO MYCOBACTERIA

Histochemical stains for acid-fast bacteria show large groups of intracellular organisms in mycobacterial pseudotumors.

tending angiosarcomas. PIEH is seen as a consequence of trauma and thrombosis within preexisting hematomas, hemangiomas, varices, or otherwise-dilated blood vessels, usually on the distal extremities (213). Meningoceles are dysraphic dermal or subcuticular malformations of infants and children, and are situated near the midline of the body.

Microscopic examination of PIEH shows a racemose proliferation of bland endothelial cells that mantles hyalinized pseudopapillary cores of organized fibrinous thrombotic material (213, 221). Low-power histologic assessment clearly

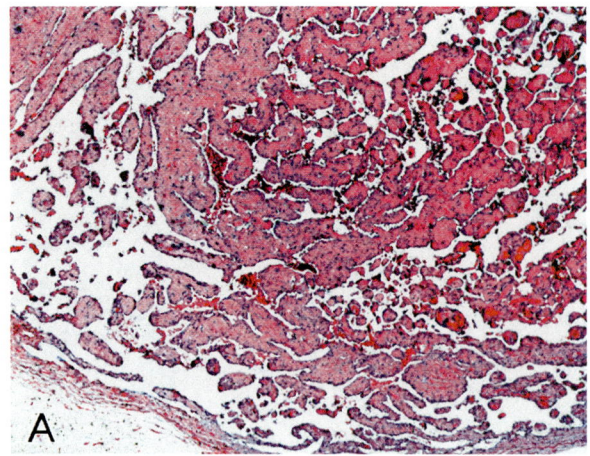
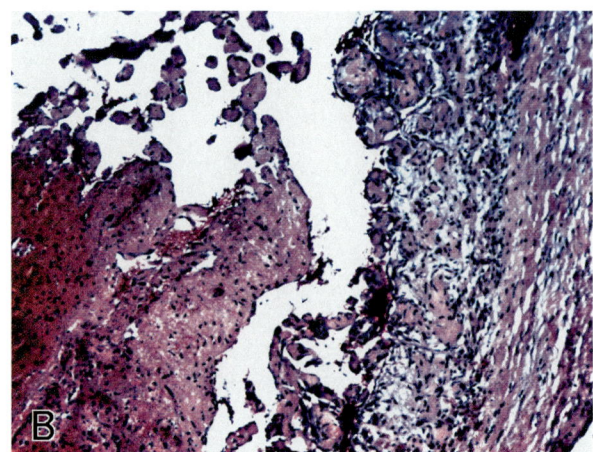
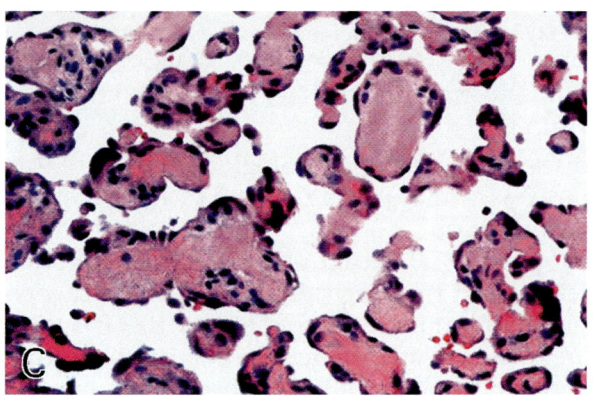

Figure 7-71

PAPILLARY INTRAVASCULAR ENDOTHELIAL HYPERPLASIA

The internal aspects of papillary intravascular endothelial hyperplasia in a dilated vein (A,B) demonstrate the mantling of organized fibrin by proliferating endothelial cells, superficially resembling an angiosarcoma (C).

demonstrates the sharp confinement of the lesion to the lumen of a thrombosed hematoma, a large vein, or an artery (fig. 7-71). The latter point is crucial to correct interpretation, because the internal aspects of PIEH may otherwise easily be mistaken for those of a low-grade angiosarcoma.

Meningoceles are composed of flattened or low-cuboidal polyhedral cells that permeate the dermis in a dissecting fashion, with formation of internal pseudovascular spaces (fig. 7-72) (see chapter 8). Focal aggregates of lesional cells may have a concentrically lamellated appearance, and microcalcifications of the psammomatous type may be identified (205,227,242,244). Rudimentary meningoceles arise almost exclusively in the skin of the scalp or posterior neck, whereas true meningoceles of the skin may be encountered anywhere along the neuraxis. The former of these malformations lacks histologic components other than those just described, but true meningoceles also may exhibit the presence of admixed glia, choroid plexus, fetal muscle, and embryonic vascular proliferations. Meningeal lesions are uniformly immunoreactive for epithelial membrane antigen, but they lack endothelial markers (227); the converse of this profile is expected in true vascular neoplasms.

Other Reactive Vascular Proliferations

Two other forms of non-neoplastic cutaneous endothelial proliferation may be mistaken for vascular tumors. These are reactive angioendotheliomatosis-angiomatosis and lymphangioma-like papules that are seen in previously irradiated skin fields.

Reactive Angioendotheliomatosis. Reactive angioendotheliomatosis (214,228,249) has been linked etiologically with a wide variety of coexisting disorders, including collagen vascular diseases, valvular heart disease (e.g., infectious and marantic endocarditis), cirrhosis, cryoglobulinemia, sarcoidosis, atherosclerotic peripheral vascular disease, antiphospholipid syndrome, dysproteinemias, cutaneous amyloid deposition, and Castleman's disease with POEMS syndrome (see foregoing section on

Vascular Tumors and Pseudotumors

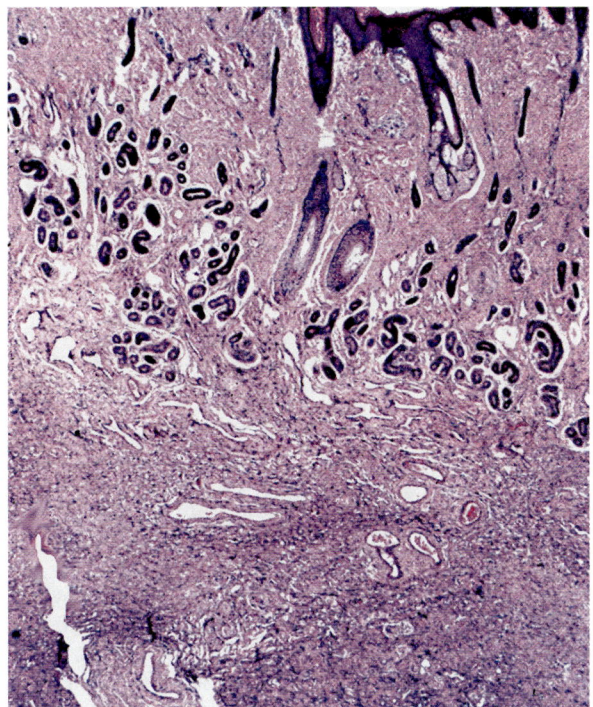

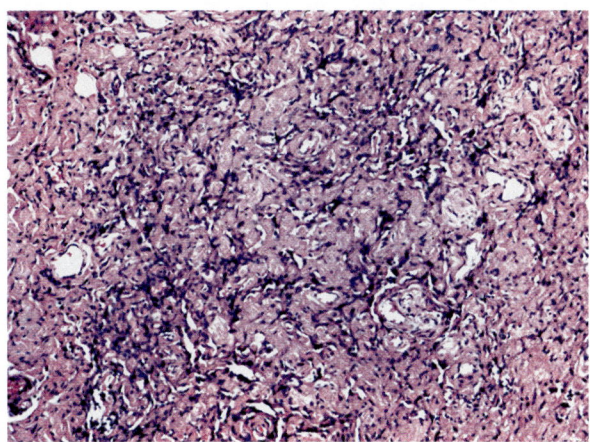

Figure 7-72

MENINGOCELE

Rudimentary meningocele of the scalp in a child shows a racemose configuration of pseudovascular spaces in the deep dermis. The lesion has an image like that of angiosarcoma, but is instead composed of meningothelial cells.

glomeruloid hemangioma) (210,215,217,218, 220,222,225,230,231,234,241,245,246). Some cases are apparently idiopathic in nature, however (231). Two other clinical conditions that may be associated with reactive angioendotheliomatosis are iatrogenic immunosuppression and arteriovenous fistulae (230,234).

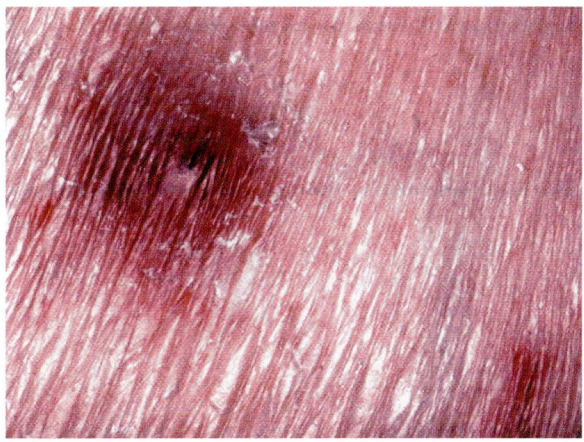

Figure 7-73

REACTIVE ANGIOENDOTHELIOMATOSIS

Reddish macules and plaques of variable sizes in the skin of the trunk in an adult.

Reactive angioendotheliomatosis has variable macroscopic manifestations, including multifocal formation of erythematous macules, papules, or plaques (fig. 7-73), as well as ulcers. It generally evolves over the span of months to years, and may spontaneously regress in some instances. Affected patients are of any age. Although the condition has a wide anatomic distribution, the extremities are favored.

Microscopically, the principal abnormality is a proliferation of dermal capillaries, which may assume either a lobular or diffuse configuration (fig. 7-74). Intravascular endothelial cells are variably epithelioid, and luminal microthrombi may be seen (fig. 7-75). The surrounding dermis may demonstrate a proliferation of pericytic cells (especially when the inciting cause is cryoprotein deposition) or fibroblasts. In one study by McMenamin and Fletcher (230), immunoreactivity for HHV8-LNA1 was present in 40 percent of cases. That finding represents yet another point of potential confusion with true neoplasms such as Kaposi's sarcoma.

Rongioletti and Rebora (237) have suggested that reactive angioendotheliomatosis is but one point in a spectrum of cutaneous disorders that includes acroangiodermatitis, dermal angiomatosis, intravascular histiocytosis (236), angiopericytomatosis, and glomeruloid angioendotheliomatosis. These lesions have been grouped together nosologically as cutaneous reactive

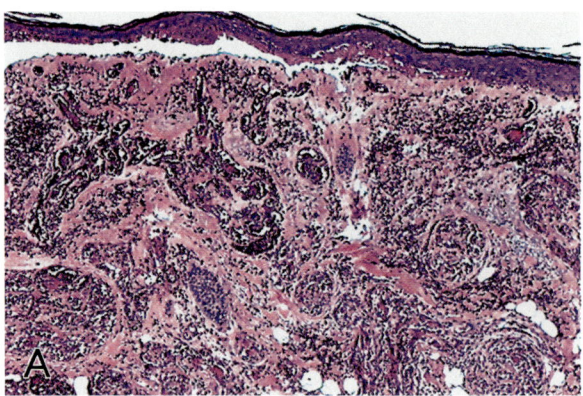
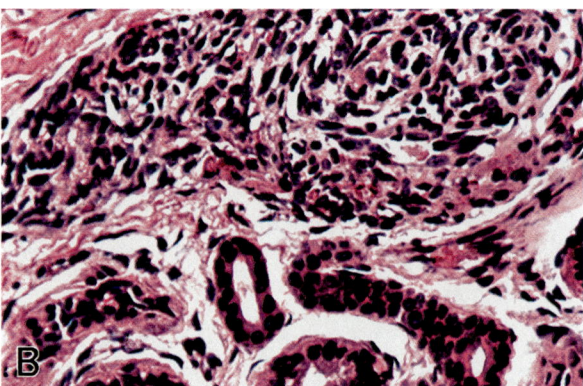
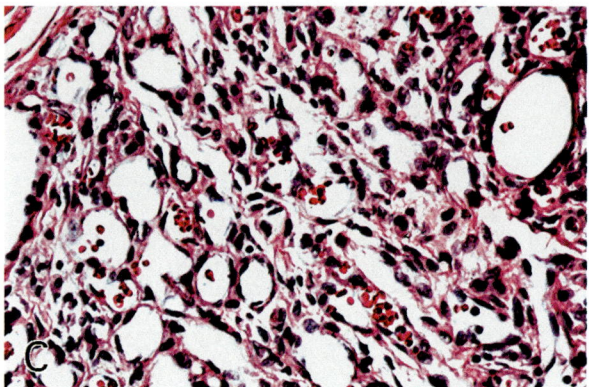

Figure 7-74

REACTIVE ANGIOENDOTHELIOMATOSIS

A: A proliferation of venule-like blood vessels is seen. Erythrocytes extravasate into the dermis.

B: This lesion has a lobular configuration, with pericytic and endothelial components.

C: Another example assumes a more diffuse profile in the corium, having the image of dermal angiomatosis.

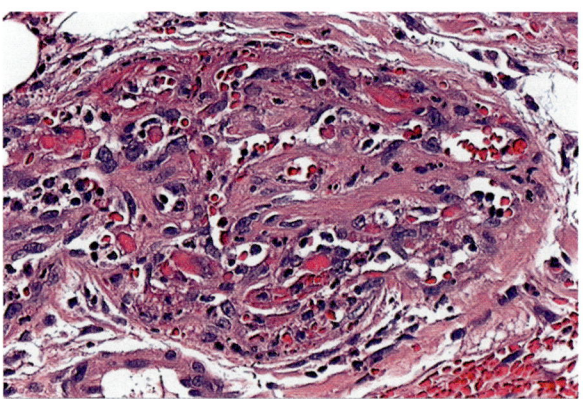

Figure 7-75

REACTIVE ANGIOENDOTHELIOMATOSIS

Deposition of platelet and fibrin microthrombi is apparent in this case of reactive angioendotheliomatosis caused by cryoglobulinemia.

angiomatoses, in recognition of the fact that they may imitate various forms of hemangioma in the skin (237).

Lymphangioma-like Papules Following Irradiation. Several reports have described the appearance of a peculiar pseudoneoplastic vascular proliferation in previously irradiated skin fields, which takes the form of solitary or multiple papules or vesicles (211,212,233,235,239, 240,247). Obviously, the principal concern in such circumstances is the appearance of an angiosarcoma (212).

Microscopically, the lesions exhibit variable degrees of atypia, with some showing a proliferation of lymphatic-like vessels that dissect the dermal collagen to a limited extent. The latter characteristic has prompted some authors to employ the diagnostic term of *atypical vascular lesion* (212,240). Little or no nuclear atypia is seen in constituent endothelial cells, however, and no micropapillary formations are present (fig. 7-76). The overall image is most like that of benign lymphangioendothelioma (progressive acquired lymphangioma) in miniature, and the biological evolution of the lesion has been uniformly benign. The diagnostic designation of *postirradiation lymphangioma-like papule* (248) appears to be best for this proliferation.

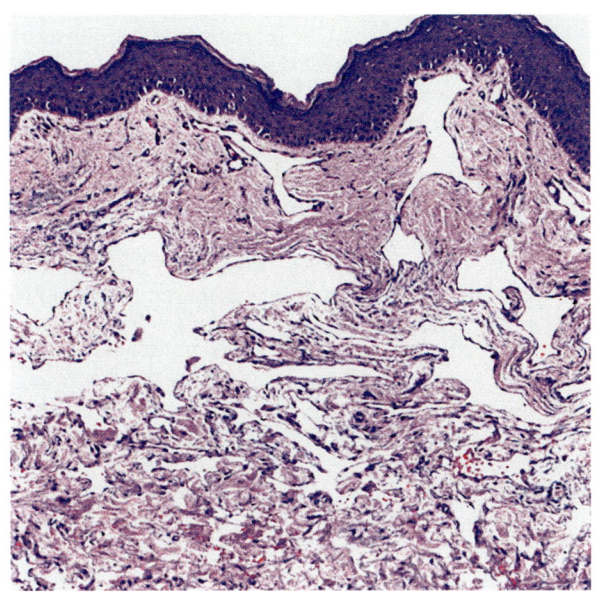
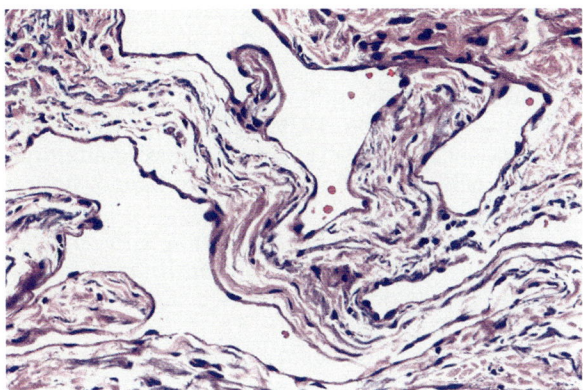

Figure 7-76

LYMPHANGIOMA-LIKE PAPULES FOLLOWING IRRADIATION

A proliferation of atypical lymphatic vascular profiles is seen in the dermis in a previously irradiated skin field. The patient had a history of breast carcinoma.

REFERENCES

Vascular Nevus and Benign Vascular Neoplasms

1. Alessi E, Berti E, Sala F. Acquired tufted angioma. Am J Dermatopathol 1986;8:426–9.
2. Allen RG, Rodman OG. Pyogenic granuloma recurrent with satellite lesions. J Dermatol Surg Oncol 1979;5:490–3.
3. Aloi F, Solaroli C, Tomasini C, Pippione M. Multinucleate cell angiohistiocytoma: a report of two cases. J Eur Acad Dermatol Venereol 1998;11:51–4.
4. Annessi G, Girolomoni G, Giannetti A. Multinucleate cell angiohistiocytoma. Am J Dermatopathol 1992;14:340–4.
5. Bardwick PA, Zvaifler NJ, Gill GN, Newman D, Greenway GD, Resnick DL. Plasma cell dyscrasia with polyneuropathy, organomegaly, endocrinopathy, M protein, and skin changes: the POEMS syndrome. Report of two cases. Medicine 1980;59:311–22.
6. Barsky SH, Rosen S, Geer DE, Noe JM. The nature and evolution of port wine stains: a computer-assisted study. J Invest Dermatol 1980;74:154–7.
7. Bendl BJ, Asano K, Lewis RJ. Nodular angioblastic hyperplasia with eosinophilia and lymphofolliculosis. Cutis 1977;19:327–9.
8. Black RJ, McCusker GM, Eedy DJ. Microvenular hemangioma. Clin Exp Dermatol 1995;20:260–62.
9. Calonje E, Fletcher CD. Sinusoidal hemangioma. A distinctive benign vascular neoplasm within the group of cavernous hemangiomas. Am J Surg Pathol 1991;15:1130–5.
10. Carapeto FJ, Garcia-Perez A, Winkelmann RK. Acral arteriovenous tumor. Acta Derm Venereol 1977;57:155–8.
11. Chabalko JJ, Fraumeni JF Jr. Blood vessel neoplasms in children: epidemiologic aspects. Med Pediatr Oncol 1975;1:135–40.
12. Chan JK, Fletcher CD, Hicklin GA, Rosai J. Glomeruloid hemangioma. A distinctive cutaneous lesion of multicentric Castleman's disease associated with POEMS syndrome. Am J Surg Pathol 1990;14:1036–46.

13. Chan JK, Hui PK, Ng CS, Yuen NW, Kung IT, Gwi E. Epithelioid hemangioma (angiolymphoid hyperplasia with eosinophilia) and Kimura's disease in Chinese. Histopathology 1989;15:557–74.
14. Connelly MG, Winkelmann RK. Acral arteriovenous tumor. A clinicopathologic review. Am J Surg Pathol 1985;9:15–21.
15. Cooper PH, McAllister HA, Helwig EB. Intravenous pyogenic granuloma. A study of 18 cases. Am J Surg Pathol 1979;3:221–8.
16. Cooper PH, Mills SE. Subcutaneous granuloma pyogenicum. Lobular capillary hemangioma. Arch Dermatol 1982;118:30–3.
17. Cribier B, Gambini C, Rainero M, Grosshans E. Multinucleate cell angiohistiocytoma. A review and report of four cases. Acta Derm Venereol 1995;75:337–9.
18. de Kaminsky AR, Otero AC, Kaminsky CA, Shaw M, Formentini E, Abulafia. Multiple disseminated pyogenic granulomas. Br J Dermatol 1978;98:461–4.
19. Dohil MA, Baugh WP, Eichenfield LF. Vascular and pigmented birthmarks. Pediatr Clin North Am 2000;47:783–812.
20. Donsky HJ. Vascular tumors of the skin. Can Med Assoc J 1968;99:993–1000.
21. Enjolras O, Wassef M, Brocheriou-Spelle I, Josset P, Tran Ba Huy P, Merland JJ. [Sinusoidal hemangioma.] Ann Dermatol Venereol 1998;125:575–80. (French.)
22. Finley JL, Noe JM, Arndt KA, Rosen S. Port-wine stains. Morphologic variations and developmental lesions. Arch Dermatol 1984;120:1453–5.
23. Fisher I, Orkin M. Acquired lymphangioma (lymphangiectasis). Report of a case. Arch Dermatol 1970;101:230–4.
24. Flanagan BP, Helwig EB. Cutaneous lymphangioma. Arch Dermatol 1977;113:24–30.
25. Girard C, Graham JH, Johnson WC. Arteriovenous hemangioma (arteriovenous shunt). A clinicopathological and histochemical study. J Cutan Pathol 1974;1:73–87.
26. Gonzalez-Crussi F, Reyes-Mugica M. Cellular hemangiomas ("hemangioendotheliomas") in infants. Light microscopic, immunohistochemical, and ultrastructural observations. Am J Surg Pathol 1991;15:769–78.
27. Guillou L, Calonje E, Speight P, Rosai J, Fletcher CD. Hobnail hemangioma: a pseudomalignant vascular lesion with a reappraisal of targetoid hemosiderotic hemangioma. Am J Surg Pathol 1999;23:97–105.
28. Guillou L, Fletcher CD. Benign lymphangioendothelioma (acquired progressive lymphangioma): a lesion not to be confused with well-differentiated angiosarcoma and patch-stage Kaposi's sarcoma. Clinicopathologic analysis of a series. Am J Surg Pathol 2000;24:1047–57.
29. Gutzmer R, Kaspari M, Herbst RA, Kapp A, Kiehl P. Absence of HHV8-DNA in hobnail hemangiomas. J Cutan Pathol 2002;29:154–8.
30. Hartzell MB. Granuloma pyogenicum (botryomycosis of French authors). J Cutan Dis 1904;22:520–3.
31. Herron GS, Rouse RV, Kosek JC, Smoller BR, Egbert BM. Benign lymphangioendothelioma. J Am Acad Dermatol 1994;31:362–8.
32. Hunt SJ, Santa Cruz DJ, Barr RJ. Microvenular hemangioma. J Cutan Pathol 1991;18:235–40.
33. Iizuka S. Eosinophilic lymphadenitis and granulomatosis: Kimura's disease. Nihon Univ Med J 1959;18:900–8.
34. Imperial R, Helwig EB. Angiokeratoma. A clinicopathological study. Arch Dermatol 1967;95:166–75.
35. Imperial R, Helwig EB. Angiokeratoma of the scrotum (Fordyce type). J Urol 1967;98:379–87.
36. Imperial R, Helwig EB. Angiokeratoma of the vulva. Obstet Gynecol 1967;29:307–12.
37. Imperial R, Helwig EB. Verrucous hemangioma. A clinicopathologic study of 21 cases. Arch Dermatol 1967;96:247–53.
38. Johnson WC. Pathology of cutaneous vascular tumors. Int J Dermatol 1976;15:239–70.
39. Jones EW, Bleehen SS. Inflammatory angiomatous nodules with abnormal blood vessels occurring about the ears and scalp (pseudo or atypical pyogenic granuloma). Br J Dermatol 1969;81:804–16.
40. Jones EW, Orkin M. Tufted angioma (angioblastoma). A benign progressive angioma, not to be confused with Kaposi's sarcoma or low-grade angiosarcoma. J Am Acad Dermatol 1989;20(Pt 1):214–25.
41. Jones EW, Winkelmann RK, Zachary CB, Reda AM. Benign lymphangioendothelioma. J Am Acad Dermatol 1990;23(Pt 1):229–38.
42. Jones WE, Cerio R, Smith NP. Multinucleate cell angiohistiocytoma: an acquired vascular anomaly to be distinguished from Kaposi's sarcoma. Br J Dermatol 1990;122:651–63.
43. Kanik AB, Oh CH, Bhawan J. Disseminated cutaneous epithelioid hemangioma. J Am Acad Dermatol 1996;35(Pt 2):851–3.
44. Kim YC, Park HJ, Cinn YW. Microvenular hemangioma. Dermatology 2003;206:161–4.
45. Kimura T, Yoshimura S, Ishikawa E. Abnormal granuloma with proliferation of lymphoid tissue. Trans Soc Pathol Jpn 1948;37:179–80.
46. Kishimoto S, Takenaka H, Shibagaki R, Noda Y, Yamamoto M, Yasuno H. Glomeruloid hemangioma in POEMS syndrome shows two different immunophenotypic endothelial cells. J Cutan Pathol 2000;27:87–92.

47. Lorenz S, Maier C, Segerer H, Landthaler M, Hohenleutner U. [Skin changes in newborn infants in the first 5 days of life.] Hautarzt 2000;51:396–400. (German.)
48. Margileth AM. Cutaneous vascular tumors. Mod Probl Pediatr 1975;17:101–10.
49. Margileth AM, Museles M. Current concepts in diagnosis and management of congenital cutaneous hemangiomas. Pediatrics 1965;36:410–26.
50. Margileth AM, Museles M. Cutaneous hemangiomas in children Diagnosis and conservative managment. JAMA 1965;194:523–6.
51. Mehregan AH, Shapiro L. Angiolymphoid hyperplasia with eosinophilia. Arch Dermatol 1971;103:50–7.
52. Mentzel T, Partanen TA, Kutzner H. Hobnail hemangioma ("targetoid hemosiderotic hemangioma"): clinicopathologic and immunohistochemical analysis of 62 cases. J Cutan Pathol 1999;26:279–86.
53. Merkel KH, Werhahn C. Epithelioid hemangioma—angiolymphoid hyperplasia with eosinophilia. Case report and review of the literature. Zentralbl Allg Pathol 1988;134:499–504.
54. Mills SE, Cooper PH, Fechner RE. Lobular capillary hemangioma: the underlying lesion of pyogenic granuloma. A study of 73 cases from the oral and nasal mucous membranes. Am J Surg Pathol 1980;4:470–9.
55. Mueller-Lessmann V, Behrendt A, Wetzel WE, Petersen K, Anders D. Orofacial findings in the Klippel-Trenaunay syndrome. Int J Paediatr Dent 2001;11:225–9.
56. Nappi O, Wick MR. Disseminated lobular capillary hemangioma (pyogenic granuloma). A clinicopathologic study of two cases. Am J Dermatopathol 1986; 8:379–85.
57. Nichols GE, Gaffey MJ, Mills SE, Weiss LM. Lobular capillary hemangioma. An immunohistochemical study including steroid hormone receptor status. Am J Clin Pathol 1992;97:770–5.
58. Olsen TG, Helwig EB. Angiolymphoid hyperplasia with eosinophilia: a clinicopathologic study of 116 patients. J Am Acad Dermatol 1985;12:781–96.
59. Padilla RS, Orkin M, Rosai J. Acquired "tufted" hemangioma (progressive capillary hemangioma). A distinctive clinicopathologic entity related to lobular capillary hemangioma. Am J Dermatopathol 1987;9:292–300.
60. Palmer LC, Strauch WG, Welton WA. Lymphangioma circumscriptum. Arch Dermatol 1978;114:394–7.
61. Park EA, Seo JW, Lee SW, Choi HY, Lee SJ. Infantile hemangioendothelioma treated with high dose methylprednisolone pulse therapy. J Korean Med Sci 2001;16:127–9.
62. Peachey RD, Lim CC, Whimster IW. Lymphangioma of skin. A review of 65 cases. Br J Dermatol 1970;83:519–26.
63. Poncet A, Dor L. Botryomycose humaine. Rev Chir 1897;18:996–1005.
64. Prieto VG, Shea CR. Selected cutaneous vascular neoplasms. A review. Dermatol Clin 1999;17:507–20.
65. Puig L, Fernandez-Figueras MT, Bielsa I, Lloveras B, Alomar A. Multinucleate cell angiohistiocytoma: a fibrohistiocytic proliferation with increased mast cell numbers and vascular hyperplasia. J Cutan Pathol 2002;29:232–7.
66. Rao VK, Weiss SW. Angiomatosis of soft tissue: an analysis of the histologic features and clinical outcome in 51 cases. Am J Surg Pathol 1992;16:764–71.
67. Rapini RP, Golitz LE. Targetoid hemosiderotic hemangioma. J Cutan Pathol 1990;17:233–5.
68. Requena L, Kutzner H, Mentzel T. Acquired elastotic hemangioma: a clinicopathologic variant of hemangioma. J Am Acad Dermatol 2002;47:371–6.
69. Rosai J, Gold J, Landy R. The histiocytoid hemangiomas. A unifying concept embracing several previously described entities of skin, soft tissue, large vessels, bone, and heart. Hum Pathol 1979;10:707–30.
70. Santa Cruz DJ, Aronberg J. Targetoid hemosiderotic hemangioma. J Am Acad Dermatol 1988;19:550–8.
71. Satomi I, Tanaka Y, Murata J, et al. A case of angioblastoma (Nakagawa). Rinsho Dermatol 1981;23:703–9.
72. Schatzki PF, Kipreos B, Payne J. Fabry's disease. Primary diagnosis by electron microscopy. Am J Surg Pathol 1979;3:211–19.
73. Shapiro PE, Nova MP, Rosmarin LA, Halperin AJ. Multinucleate cell angiohistiocytoma: a distinct entity diagnosable by clinical and histologic features. J Am Acad Dermatol 1994;30:417–22.
74. Simpson JR. Natural history of cavernous hemangiomata. Lancet 1959;2:1057–63.
75. Tsai CY, Lai CH, Chan HL, Kuo TT. Glomeruloid hemangiomaùa specific cutaneous marker of POEMS syndrome. Int J Dermatol 2001;40:403–6.
76. Tsang WY, Chan JK. The family of epithelioid vascular tumors. Histol Histopathol 1993;8:187–212.
77. Urabe A, Tsuneyoshi M, Enjoji M. Epithelioid hemangioma versus Kimura's disease. A comparative clinicopathologic study. Am J Surg Pathol 1987;11:758–66.
78. Van Aalst JA, Bhuller A, Sadove AM. Pediatric vascular lesions. J Craniofac Surg 2003;14:566–83.

79. Walker AN, Morton BD. Pathologic quiz case 1. Epithelioid hemangioma (histiocytoid hemangioma, angiolymphoid hyperplasia with eosinophilia). Arch Otolaryngol Head Neck Surg 1987;113:332–5.
80. Warner J, Jones EW. Pyogenic granuloma recurring with multiple satellites. A report of 11 cases. Br J Dermatol 1968;80:218–27.
81. Wells GC, Whimster IW. Subcutaneous angiolymphoid hyperplasia with eosinophilia. Br J Dermatol 1969;81:1–15.
82. Whimster IW. The pathology of lymphangioma circumscriptum. Br J Dermatol 1976;94:473–86.
83. Wick MR, Manivel JC. Vascular neoplasms of the skin: a current perspective. Adv Dermatol 1989;4:185–252; discussion 253.
84. Zaynoun ST, Juljulian HH, Kurban AK. Pyogenic granuloma with multiple satellites. Arch Dermatol 1974;109:689–91.

Borderline Endothelial Tumors

85. Argani P, Athanasian E. Malignant endovascular papillary angioendothelioma (Dabska tumor) arising within a deep intramuscular hemangioma. Arch Pathol Lab Med 1997;121:992–5.
86. Beaubien ER, Ball NJ, Storwick GS. Kaposiform hemangioendothelioma: a locally aggressive vascular tumor. J Am Acad Dermatol 1998;38:799–802.
87. Billings SD, Folpe AL, Weiss SW. Epithelioid sarcoma-like hemangioendothelioma. Am J Surg Pathol 2003;27:48–57.
88. Bodemer C, Fraitag S, Amoric JC, Benaceur S, Brunelle F, De Prost Y. [Spindle cell hemangioendothelioma with monomelia and multifocal form in a child.] Ann Dermatol Venereol 1997;124:857–60. (French.)
89. Bollinger BK, Laskin WB, Knight CB. Epithelioid hemangioendothelioma with multiple site involvement. Literature review and observations. Cancer 1994;73:610–5.
90. Calonje E, Fletcher CD, Wilson-Jones E, Rosai J. Retiform hemangioendothelioma. A distinctive form of low-grade angiosarcoma delineated in a series of 15 cases. Am J Surg Pathol 1994;18:115–25.
91. Cooper JG, Edwards SL, Holmes JD. Kaposiform hemangioendothelioma: case report and review of the literature. Br J Plast Surg 2002;55:163–5.
92. Dabska M. Malignant endovascular papillary angioendothelioma of the skin in childhood. Clinicopathologic study of 6 cases. Cancer 1969;24:503–10.
93. De Dulanto F, Armijo-Moreno M. Malignant endovascular papillary hemangioendothelioma of the skin. The nosological situation. Acta Derm Venereol 1973;53:403–8.
94. Deb G, Jenkner A, De Sio L, et al. Spindle cell (kaposiform) hemangioendothelioma with Kasabach-Merritt syndrome in an infant: successful treatment with alpha-2A interferon. Med Pediatr Oncol 1997;28:358–61.
95. Duke D, Dvorak A, Harris TJ, Cohen LM. Multiple retiform hemangioendotheliomas. A low-grade angiosarcoma. Am J Dermatopathol 1996;18:606–10.
96. Eltorky M, McChesney T, Sebes J, Hall JC. Spindle cell hemangioendothelioma. Report of three cases and review of the literature. J Dermatol Surg Oncol 1994;20:196–202.
97. Fanburg-Smith JC, Michal M, Partanen TA, Alitalo K, Miettinen M. Papillary intralymphatic angioendothelioma (PILA): a report of twelve cases of a distinctive vascular tumor with phenotypic features of lymphatic vessels. Am J Surg Pathol 1999;23:1004–10.
98. Fletcher CD, Beham A, Schmid C. Spindle-cell hemangioendothelioma: a clinicopathological and immunohistochemical study indicative of a non-neoplastic lesion. Histopathology 1991;18:291–301.
99. Folpe AL, Veikkola T, Valtola R, Weiss SW. Vascular endothelial growth factor receptor-3 (VEGFR-3): a marker of vascular tumors with presumed lymphatic differentiation, including Kaposi's sarcoma, kaposiform and Dabska-type hemangioendotheliomas, and a subset of angiosarcomas. Mod Pathol 2000;13:180–5.
100. Fukunaga M. Endovascular papillary angioendothelioma (Dabska tumor). Pathol Int 1998;48:840–1.
101. Fukunaga M, Ushigome S, Ishikawa E. Kaposiform hemangioendothelioma associated with Kasabach-Merritt syndrome. Histopathology 1996;28:281–4.
102. Gianotti R, Gelmetti C, Alessi E. Congenital cutaneous multifocal kaposiform hemangioendothelioima. Am J Dermatopathol 1999;21:557–61.
103. Hardisson D, Prim MP, De Diego JI, Patron M, Escribano A, Rabanal I. Kaposiform hemangioendothelioma of the external auditory canal in an adult. Head Neck 2002;24:614–7.
104. Hisaoka M, Hashimoto H, Iwamasa T. Diagnostic implication of Kaposi's sarcoma-associated herpesvirus with special reference to the distinction between spindle-cell hemangioendothelioma and Kaposi's sarcoma. Arch Pathol Lab Med 1998;122:72–6.
105. Imayama S, Murakamai Y, Hashimoto H, Hori Y. Spindle-cell hemangioendothelioma exhibits the ultrastructural features of reactive vascular proliferation rather than of angiosarcoma. Am J Clin Pathol 1992;97:279–87.

106. Kumarasinghe MP, Bian NS, Hai LB. Spindle cell hemangioendothelioma—an acquired vascular lesion of uncertain nature. Ceylon Med J 1999; 44:89–91.
107. Lessard M, Barnhill RL. Spindle cell hemangioendothelioma of the skin. J Am Acad Dermatol 1988;18:393–5.
108. Mac-Moune Lai F, To KF, Choi PC, et al. Kaposiform hemangioendothelioma: five patients with cutaneous lesions and long follow-up. Mod Pathol 2001;14:1087–92.
109. Manivel JC, Wick MR, Swanson PE, Patterson K, Dehner LP. Endovascular papillary angioendothelioma of childhood: a vascular tumor possibly characterized by "high" endothelial differentiation. Hum Pathol 1986;17:1240–4.
110. McCarthy EF, Lietman S, Argani P, Frassica FJ. Endovascular papillary angioendothelioma (Dabska tumor) of bone. Skeletal Radiol 1999;28:100–3.
111. Mentzel T. [Hemangioendotheliomas—evolution of a concept of a heterogeneous group of vascular neoplasms.] Verh Dtsch Ges Pathol 1998;82:99–111. (German.)
112. Mentzel T, Beham A, Calonje E, Katenkamp D, Fletcher CD. Epithelioid hemangioendothelioma of skin and soft tissues: clinicopathologic and immunohistochemical study of 30 cases. Am J Surg Pathol 1997;21:363–74.
113. Mentzel T, Mazzoleni G, Dei Tos AP, Fletcher CD. Kaposiform hemangioendothelioma in adults. Clinicopathologic and immunohistochemical analysis of three cases. Am J Clin Pathol 1997;108:450–5.
114. Morgan J, Robinson MJ, Rosen LB, Unger H, Niven J. Malignant endovascular papillary angioendothelioma (Dabska tumor). A case report and review of the literature. Am J Dermatopathol 1989;11:64–8.
115. Nayler SJ, Rubin BP, Calonje E, Chan JK, Fletcher CD. Composite hemangioendothelioma: a complex, low-grade vascular lesion mimicking angiosarcoma. Am J Surg Pathol 1000;24:352–61.
116. Patterson K, Chandra RS. Malignant endovascular papillary angioendothelioma. Cutaneous borderline tumor. Arch Pathol Lab Med 1985;109:671–3.
117. Pellegrini AE, Drake RD, Qualman SJ. Spindle cell hemangioendothelioma: a neoplasm associated with Maffucci's syndrome. J Cutan Pathol 1995;22:173–6.
118. Quante M, Patel NK, Hill S, et al. Epithelioid hemangioendothelioma presenting in the skin: a clinicopathologic study of eight cases. Am J Dermatopathol 1998;20:541–6.
119. Quecedo E, Martinez-Escribano JA, Febrer I, Oliver V, Velasco M, Aliaga A. Dabska tumor developing within a preexisting vascular malformation. Am J Dermatopathol 1996;18:302–7.
120. Requena L, Sangueza OP. Cutaneous vascular proliferations. Part III. Malignant neoplasms, other cutaneous neoplasms with significant vascular component, and disorders erroneously considered as vascular neoplasms. J Am Acad Dermatol 1998;38:143–75.
121. Schommer M, Herbst RA, Brodersen JP, et al. Retiform hemangioendothelioma: another tumor associated with human herpesvirus type 8? J Am Acad Dermatol 2000;42(Pt 1):290–2.
122. Schwartz RA, Dabski C, Dabska M. The Dabska tumor: a thirty-year retrospect. Dermatology 2000;201:1–5.
123. Scott GA, Rosai J. Spindle-cell hemangioendothelioma. Report of seven additional cases of a recently described vascular neoplasm. Am J Dermatopathol 1988;10:281–8.
124. Takaoka K, Sakurai K, Noguchi K, Hashitani S, Urade M. Endovascular papillary angioendothelioma (Dabska tumor) of the tongue: report of a case. J Oral Pathol Med 2003;32:492–5.
125. Terashi H, Itami S, Kurata S, Sonoda T, Takayasu S, Yokoyma S. Spindle cell hemangioendothelioma: report of three cases. J Dermatol 1991; 18:104–11.
126. Tomasini C, Aloi F, Soro E, Elia V. Spindle cell hemangioma. Dermatology 1999;199:274–6.
127. Vin-Christian K, McCalmont TH, Frieden IJ. Kaposiform hemangioendothelioma. An aggressive, locally invasive vascular tumor that can mimic hemangioma of infancy. Arch Dermatol 1997;133:1573–8.
128. Walker GM, Abu-Rajab R, MacLennan A, Haji Vassiliou CA, Howatson AG, Carachi R. Kasabach-Merritt syndrome in a neonate caused by a kaposiform hemangioendothelioma. Med Pediatr Oncol 2002;38:424–7.
129. Weiss SW, Enzinger FM. Epithelioid hemangioendothelioma: a vascular tumor often mistaken for a carcinoma. Cancer 1982;50:970–81.
130. Weiss SW, Enzinger FM. Spindle-cell hemangioendothelioma. A low-grade angiosarcoma resembling a cavernous hemangioma and Kaposi's sarcoma. Am J Surg Pathol 1986;10: 521–30.
131. Weiss SW, Ishak KG, Dail DH, Sweet DE, Enzinger FM. Epithelioid hemangioendothelioma and related lesions. Semin Diagn Pathol 1986;3:259–87.
131a. Wick MR, Manivel JC. Vascular neoplasms of the skin: a current perspective. Adv Dermatol 1989;4:185–252; discussion 253.
132. Wilken JJ, Meier FA, Kornstein MJ. Kaposiform hemangioendothelioma of the thymus. Arch Pathol Lab Med 1000;124:1542–4.

133. Yamada A, Uematsu K, Yashoshima H, et al. Endovascular papillary angioendothelioma (Dabska tumor) in an elderly woman. Pathol Int 1998;48:164–7.
134. Zamecnik M, Koys F, Mikleova Z, Michal M. Additional case of kaposiform hemangioendothelioma in an adult. Cesk Patol 2001;37:128–9.
135. Zukerberg LR, Nickoloff BJ, Weiss SW. Kaposiform hemangioendothelioma of infancy and childhood. An aggressive neoplasm associated with Kasabach-Merritt syndrome and lymphangiomatosis. Am J Surg Pathol 1993; 17:321–8.

Malignant Endothelial Neoplasms

136. Ackerman AB. Subtle clues to diagnosis by conventional microscopy. The patch stage of Kaposi's sarcoma. Am J Dermatopathol 1979;1:165–72.
137. Akiyama M, Naka W, Harada T, Nishikawa T. Angiosarcoma with dermal melanocytosis. J Cutan Pathol 1989;16:149–53.
138. Alessi E, Sala F, Berti E. Angiosarcomas in lymphedematous limbs. Am J Dermatopathol 1986;8:371–8.
139. Alkan S, Eltoum IA, Tabbara S, Day E, Karcher DS. Usefulness of molecular detection of human herpes-virus-8 in the diagnosis of Kaposi sarcoma by fine-needle aspiration. Am J Clin Pathol 1999;111:91–6.
140. Alkan S, Karcher DS, Ortiz A, Khalil S, Akhtar M, Ali MA. Human herpesvirus 8/Kaposi's sarcoma-associated herpesvirus in organ transplant patients with immunosuppression. Br J Hematol 1997;96:412–4.
141. Beckstead JH, Wood GS, Fletcher V. Evidence for the origin of Kaposi's sarcoma from lymphatic endothelium. Am J Pathol 1985;119:294–300.
142. Bennett RG, Keller JW, Ditty JF Jr. Hemangiosarcoma subsequent to radiotherapy for a hemangioma in infancy. J Dermatol Surg Oncol 1978;4:881–3.
143. Blumenfeld W, Egbert BM, Sagebiel RW. Differential diagnosis of Kaposi's sarcoma. Arch Pathol Lab Med 1985;109:123–7.
144. Boldogh I, Beth E, Huang ES, Kyalwazi SK, Giraldo G. Kaposi's sarcoma: IV. Detection of CMV-DNA, CMV-RNA, and CMNA in tumor biopsies. Int J Cancer 1981;28:469–74.
145. Boucher LD, Swanson PE, Stanley MW, Silverman JF, Raab SS, Geisinger KR. Cytology of angiosarcoma: findings in fourteen fine-needle aspiration biopsy specimens and one pleural fluid specimen. Am J Clin Pathol 2000;114:210–9.
146. Chen KT, Gilbert EF. Angiosarcoma complicating generalized lymphangiectasia. Arch Pathol Lab Med 1979;103:86–8.
146a. Cheuk W, Wong KO, Wong CS, Dinkel JE, Ben-Dor D, Chan JK. Immunostaining for human herpesvirus 8 latent nuclear antigen-1 helps distinguish Kaposi sarcoma from its mimickers. Am J Clin Pathol 2004;121:335–42.
147. Chor PJ, Santa Cruz DJ. Kaposi's sarcoma. A clinicopathologic review and differential diagnosis. J Cutan Pathol 1992;19:6–20.
148. Cooper PH. Angiosarcomas of the skin. Semin Diagn Pathol 1987;4:2-17.
149. Cossu S, Satta R, Cottoni F, Massarelli G. Lymphangioma-like variant of Kaposi's sarcoma: clinicopathologic study of seven cases with review of the literature. Am J Dermatopathol 1997;19:16–22.
150. Costa J, Rabson AS. Generalized Kaposi's sarcoma is not a neoplasm. Lancet 1983;1:58.
151. Dantzig PE. Chemotherapy for Kaposi's sarcoma [Letter]. Arch Dermatol 1976;112:1179.
152. Delli-Bovi P, Basilico C. Isolation of a rearranged human transforming gene following transfection of Kaposi's sarcoma DNA. Proc Natl Acad Sci USA 1987;84:5660–4.
153. DeYoung BR, Swanson PE, Argenyi ZB, et al. CD31 immunoreactivity in mesenchymal neoplasms of the skin and subcutis: report of 145 cases and review of putative immunohistologic markers of endothelial differentiation. J Cutan Pathol 1995;22:215–22.
154. Fenoglio CM, Oster M, Lo Gerfo P, et al. Kaposi's sarcoma following chemotherapy for testicular cancer in a homosexual man: demonstration of cytomegalovirus RNA in sarcoma cells. Hum Pathol 1982;13:955–9.
155. Girard C, Johnson WC, Graham JH. Cutaneous angiosarcoma. Cancer 1970;26:868–83.
156. Goette DK, Detlefs RL. Postirradiation angiosarcoma. J Am Acad Dermatol 1985;12(Pt 2):922–6.
157. Gottlieb GJ, Ackerman AB. Kaposi's sarcoma: an extensively disseminated form in young homosexual men. Hum Pathol 1982;13:882–92.
158. Gottlieb GJ, Ackerman AB, eds. Kaposi's sarcoma: a text and atlas. Philadelphia: Lea & Febiger; 1988:73–112.
159. Hamels J, Blondiau B, Mirgaux M. Cutaneous angiosarcoma arising in a mastectomy scar after therapeutic irradiation. Bull Cancer 1981;68:353–6.
159a. Hammock L, Reisenauer A, Wang W, Cohen C, Birdsong G, Folpe AL. Latency-associated nuclear antigen expression and human herpesvirus-8 polymerase chain reaction in the evaluation of Kaposi sarcoma and other vascular tumors in HIV-positive patients. Mod Pathol 2005;18:463–8.

160. Harrison AC, Kahn LB. Myogenic cells in Kaposi's sarcoma: an ultrastructural study. J Pathol 1978;124:157–60.
161. Hodgkinson DJ, Soule EH, Woods JE. Cutaneous angiosarcoma of the head and neck. Cancer 1979;44:1106–113.
162. Holden CA, Spittle MF, Jones EW. Angiosarcoma of the face and scalp, prognosis and treatment. Cancer 1987;59:1046–57.
163. Hultberg BM. Angiosarcomas in chronically lymphedematous extremities. Two cases of Stewart-Treves syndrome. Am J Dermatopathol 1987;9:406–12.
164. Ioachim HL, Adsay V, Giancotti FR, Dorsett B, Melamed J. Kaposi's sarcoma of internal organs. A multiparameter study of 86 cases. Cancer 1995;75:1376–85.
165. Jaffe HW. AIDS: epidemiologic features. J Am Acad Dermatol 1990;22(Pt 2):1167–71.
166. Jordan RC, Regezi JA. Oral spindle cell neoplasms: a review of 307 cases. Oral Surg Oral Med Oral Pathol Oral Radiol Endod 2003;95:717–24.
166a. Lan K, Kuppers DA, Robertson ES. Kaposi's sarcoma-associated herpesvirus reactivation is regulated by interaction of latency-associated nuclear antigen with recombination signal sequence-binding protein Jkappa, the major downstream effector of the Notch signaling pathway. J Virol 2005;79;3468–78.
167. Lo TC, Silverman ML, Edelstein A. Postirradiation hemangiosarcoma of the chest wall. Report of a case. Acta Radiol Oncol 1985;24:237–40.
168. Luppi M, Torelli G. The new lymphotropic herpesviruses (HHV-6, HHV-7, HHV-8) and hepatitis C virus (HCV) in human lymphoproliferative diseases: an overview. Haematologica 1996;81:265–81.
169. Maddox JC, Evans HL. Angiosarcoma of skin and soft tissue: a study of forty-four cases. Cancer 1981;48:1907–21.
170. Martinez-Escribano JA, del Pino Gil-Mateo M, Miquel J. Ledesma F, Aliga A. Human herpesvirus 8 is not detectable by polymerase chain reaction in angiosarcoma. Br J Dermatol 1998;138:546–7.
171. McNutt NS, Fletcher V, Conant MA. Early lesions of Kaposi's sarcoma in homosexual men. An ultrastructural comparison with other vascular proliferations in skin. Am J Dermatopathol 1983;3:62–77.
172. McWilliam LJ, Harris M. Granular cell angiosarcoma of the skin: histology, electron microscopy, and immunohistochemistry of a newly recognized tumor. Histopathology 1985;9:1205–16.
173. Miettinen M, Fetsch JF. Distribution of keratins in normal endothelial cells and a spectrum of vascular tumors: implications in tumor diagnosis. Hum Pathol 2000;31:1062–7.
174. Miyachi Y, Imamura S. Very low-grade angiosarcoma. Dermatologica 1981;162:206–8.
175. Mukai K, Rosai J. Factor VIII-related antigen: an endothelial marker, In: DeLellis RA, ed. Diagnostic immunohistochemistry. New York: Masson; 1984:253–61.
176. Nappi O, Wick MR, Pettinato G, Ghiselli RW, Swanson PE. Pseudovascular adenoid squamous cell carcinoma of the skin. A neoplasm that may be mistaken for angiosarcoma. Am J Surg Pathol 1992;16:429–38.
177. Nickoloff BJ, Foreman KE. Etiology and pathogenesis of Kaposi's sarcoma. Recent Results Cancer Res 2002;160:332–42.
178. Noel JC, Hermans P, Andre J, et al. Herpesvirus-like DNA sequences and Kaposi's sarcoma: relationship with epidemiology, clinical spectrum, and histologic features. Cancer 1996;77:2132–6.
179. Nuovo M, Nuovo G. Utility of HHV8 RNA detection for differentiating Kaposi's sarcoma from its mimics. J Cutan Pathol 2001;28:248–55.
180. Ordonez NG, Batsakis JG. Comparison of Ulex europaeus I lectin and factor VIII-related antigen in vascular lesions. Arch Pathol Lab Med 1984;108:129–32.
180a. Pak F, Pyakural P, Kokhaei P, et al. HHV-8/KSHV during the development of Kaposi's sarcoma: evaluation by polymerase chain reaction and immunohistochemistry. J Cutan Pathol 2005;32:21–7.
181. Pantanowitz L, Dezube BJ, Pinkus GS, Tahan SR. Histological characterization of regression in acquired immunodeficiency syndrome-related Kaposi's sarcoma. J Cutan Pathol 2004;31:26–34.
181a. Patel RM, Goldblum JR, Hsi ED. Immunohistochemical detection of human herpesvirus-8 latent nuclear antigen-1 is useful in the diagnosis of Kaposi sarcoma. Mod Pathol 2004;17;456–60.
182. Perez-Atayde AR, Achenbach H, Lack EE. High-grade epithelioid angiosarcoma of the scalp. An immunohistochemical and ultrastructural study. Am J Dermatopathol 1986;8:411–8.
183. Pollack MS, Safai B, Myskowski PL, Gold JW, Pandey J, DuPont B. Frequencies of HLA and Gm immunogenetic markers in Kaposi's sarcoma. Tissue Antigens 1983;21:1–8.
184. Roszkiewicz A, Roszkiewicz J, Lange M, Tukaj C. Kaposi's sarcoma following long-term immunosuppressive therapy: clinical, histologic, and ultrastructural study. Cutis 1998;61:137–41.
185. Schwartz RA, Kardashian JF, McNutt NS, Crain WR, Welch KL, Choy SH. Cutaneous angiosarcoma resembling anaplastic Kaposi's sarcoma in a homosexual man. Cancer 1983;51:721–6.

186. Sidbury R, Heintz PW, Beckstead JH, White CR Jr. Cutaneous malignant epithelioid neoplasms. Adv Dermatol 1999;14:285–306.
187. Sirgi KE, Wick MR, Swanson PE. B72.3 and CD34 immunoreactivity in malignant epithelioid soft tissue tumors. Adjuncts in the recognition of endothelial neoplasms. Am J Surg Pathol 1993;17:179–85.
188. Smith KJ, Lupton GP, Skelton HG. Cutaneous angiosarcomas with a starry-sky pattern. Arch Pathol Lab Med 1997;121(Pt 1):980–4.
189. Smith KJ, Nelson A, Angritt P, Morz A, Skelton HG. Kaposi's sarcoma in women: a clinicopathologic study. J Cutan Med Surg 1999;3:132–9.
190. Snover DC, Rosai J. Vascular sarcomas of the skin. In: Wick MR, ed. Pathology of unusual malignant cutaneous tumors. New York: Marcel Dekker; 1985:181–209.
191. Stewart FW, Treves N. Lymphangiosarcoma in postmastectomy lymphedema. A report of six cases in elephantiasis chirurgica. Cancer 1948;1:64–81.
192. Swanson PE, Wick MR. Immunohistochemical evaluation of vascular neoplasms. Clin Dermatol 1991;9:243–53.
193. Tappero JW, Conant MA, Wolfe SF, Berger TG. Kaposi's sarcoma. Epidemiology, pathogenesis, histology, clinical spectrum, staging criteria, and therapy. J Am Acad Dermatol 1993;28:371–95.
194. Templeton AC. Kaposi's sarcoma. Pathol Annu 1981;17(Pt 2):315–36.
195. Traweek ST, Kandalaft PL, Mehta P, Battifora H. The human hematopoietic progenitor cell antigen (CD34) in vascular neoplasia. Am J Clin Pathol 1991;96:25–31.
196. Wick MR. Kaposi's sarcoma unrelated to the acquired immunodeficiency syndrome. Curr Opin Oncol 1991;3:377–83.
196a. Wick MR, Manivel JC. Vascular neoplasms of the skin: a current perspective. Adv Dermatol 1989;4:185–252; discussion 253.
197. Wilson-Jones E. Malignant angioendothelioma of the skin. Br J Dermatol 1964;76:21–39.
198. Woodward AH, Ivins JC, Soule EH. Lymphangiosarcoma arising in chronic lymphedematous extremities. Cancer 1972;30:562–72.
199. Yonezawa S, Maruyama I, Sakae K, Igata A, Majerus PW, Sato E.. Thrombomodulin as a marker for vascular tumors. Comparative study with factor VIII and Ulex europaeus I lectin. Am J Clin Pathol 1987;88:405–11.
199a. Zhang J, Wang J, Wood C, Zhang L. Kaposi's sarcoma-associated herpesvirus/human herpesvirus-8 replication and transcription activator regulates viral and cellular genes via interferon-stimulated response elements. J Virol 2005;79:5640–52.

Tumefactive Non-Neoplastic Vascular Proliferations

200. Amazon K, Robinson MD, Rywlin AM. Ferrugination caused by Monsel's solution. Clinical observations and experimentations. Am J Dermatopathol 1980;2:197–205.
201. Amerigo J, Berry CL. Intravascular papillary endothelial hyperplasia in the skin and subcutaneous tissue. Virchows Arch Pathol Anat 1980;387:81–91.
202. Arias-Stella J, Lieberman PH, Erlandson RA, Arias-Stella J Jr. Histology, immunochemistry, and ultrastructure of the verruga in Carrion's disease. Am J Surg Pathol 1986;10:595–610.
203. Arias-Stella J, Lieberman PH, Garcia-Caceres U, Erlandson RA, Kruger H, Arias-Stella J Jr. Verruga peruana mimicking malignant neoplasms. Am J Dermatopathol 1987;9:279–91.
204. Barr RJ, Graham JH, Sherwin LA. Intravascular papillary endothelial hyperplasia. A benign lesion mimicking angiosarcoma. Arch Dermatol 1978;114:723–6.
205. Berry AD 3rd, Patterson JW. Meningoceles, meningomyeloceles, and encephaloceles: a neuro-dermatopathologic study of 132 cases. J Cutan Pathol 1991;18:164–77.
206. Brandwein M, Choi HS, Strauchen J, Stoler M, Jagirdar J. Spindle-cell reaction to nontuberculous mycobacteriosis in AIDS mimicking a spindle-cell neoplasm. Evidence for dual histiocytic and fibroblast-like characteristics of spindle cells. Virchows Arch A Pathol Anat Histopathol 1990;416:281–6.
207. Chian CA, Arrese JE, Pierard GE. Skin manifestations of Bartonella infections. Int J Dermatol 2002;41:461–6.
208. Clearkin KP, Enzinger FM. Intravascular papillary endothelial hyperplasia. Arch Pathol Lab Med 1976;100:441–4.
209. Cockerell CJ, Whitlow MA, Webster GF, Friedman-Kien AE. Epithelioid angiomatosis: a distinct vascular disorder in patients with the acquired immunodeficiency syndrome or AIDS-related complex. Lancet 1987;2:654–6.
210. Creamer D, Black MM, Calonje E. Reactive angioendotheliomatosis in association with the antiphospholipid syndrome. J Am Acad Dermatol 2000;42(Pt 2):903–6.
211. Diaz-Cascajo C, Borghi S, Weyers W, Retzlaff H, Requena L, Metze D. Benign lymphangiomatous papules of the skin following radiotherapy: a report of five new cases and review of the literature. Histopathology 1999;35:319–27.

212. Fineberg S, Rosen PP. Cutaneous angiosarcoma and atypical vascular lesions of the skin and breast after radiation therapy for breast carcinoma. Am J Clin Pathol 1994;102:757–63.
213. Hashimoto H, Daimaru Y, Enjoji M. Intravascular papillary endothelial hyperplasia. A clinicopathologic study of 91 cases. Am J Dermatopathol 1983;5:539–46.
214. Heid E, Ball C, Grosshans E. [Reactive cutaneous angioendotheliomatosis.] Ann Dermatol Venereol 1990;117:35–6. (French.)
215. Judge MR, McGibbon DH, Thompson RP. Angioendotheliomatosis associated with Castleman's lymphoma and POEMS syndrome. Clin Exp Dermatol 1993;18:360–2.
216. Kapdagli H, Gunduz K, Ozturk G, Kandiloglu G. Pseudo-Kaposi's sarcoma (Mali type). Int J Dermatol 1998;37:223–5.
217. Kim S, Elenitsas R, James WD. Diffuse dermal angiomatosis: a variant of reactive angioendotheliomatosis associated with peripheral vascular atherosclerosis. Arch Dermatol 2002;138:456–8.
218. Kimyai-Asadi A, Nousari HC, Ketabchi N, Henneberry JM, Costarangos C. Diffuse dermal angiomatosis: a variant of reactive angioendotheliomatosis associated with atherosclerosis. J Am Acad Dermatol 1999;40(Pt 1):257–9.
219. Koehler JE. Bartonella-associated infections in HIV-infected patients. AIDS Clin Care 1995;7:97–102.
220. Krell JM, Sanchez RL, Solomon AR. Diffuse dermal angiomatosis: a variant of reactive cutaneous angioendotheliomatosis. J Cutan Pathol 1994;21:363–70.
221. Kuo T, Sayers CP, Rosai J. Masson's "vegetant intravascular hemangioendothelioma:" a lesion often mistaken for angiosarcoma: study of seventeen cases located in the skin and soft tissues. Cancer 1976;38:1227–36.
222. Lazova R, Slater C, Scott G. Reactive angioendotheliomatosis. Case report and review of the literature. Am J Dermatopathol 1996;18:63–9.
223. LeBoit PE, Berger TG, Egbert BM, Beckstead JH, Yen TS, Stoler MH. Bacillary angiomatosis. The histopathology and differential diagnosis of a pseudoneoplastic infection in patients with immunodeficiency virus disease. Am J Surg Pathol 1989;13:909–20.
224. LeBoit PE, Berger TG, Egbert BM, et al. Epithelioid hemangioma-like vascular proliferation in AIDS: manifestation of cat-scratch bacillus infection? Lancet 1988;1:960–3.
225. LeBoit PE, Solomon AR, Santa Cruz DJ, Wick MR. Angiomatosis with luminal cryoprotein deposition. J Am Acad Dermatol 1992;27(Pt 1):969–73.
226. Mali JW, Kuiper JP, Hamers AA. Acro-angiodermatitis of the foot. Arch Dermatol 1965;92:515–8.
227. Marrogi AJ, Swanson PE, Kyriakos M, Wick MR. Rudimentary meningocele of the skin. Clinicopathologic features and differential diagnosis. J Cutan Pathol 1991;18:178–88.
228. Martin S, Pitcher D, Tschen J, Wolfe JE Jr. Reactive angioendotheliomatosis. J Am Acad Dermatol 1980;2:117–23.
229. Masson P. Hemangioendotheliome vegetant intravasculaire. Bull Soc Anat 1923;93:517–27.
230. McMenamin ME, Fletcher CD. Reactive angioendotheliomatosis: a study of 15 cases demonstrating a wide clinicopathologic spectrum. Am J Surg Pathol 2002;26:685–97.
231. Ortonne N, Vignon-Pennamen MD, Majdalani G, Pinquier L, Janin A. Reactive angioendotheliomatosis secondary to dermal amyloid angiopathy. Am J Dermatopathol 2001;23:315–9.
232. Plettenberg A, Lorenzen T, Burtsche BT, et al. Bacillary angiomatosis in HIV-infected patients—an epidemiological and clinical study. Dermatology 2000;201:326–31.
233. Prioleau PG, Santa Cruz DJ. [Lymphangioma circumscriptum following radical mastectomy and radiation therapy.] Cancer 1978;42:1989–91. (German.)
234. Requena L, Farina MC, Renedo G, Alvarez A, Yus ES, Sangueza OP. Intravascular and diffuse dermal reactive angioendotheliomatosis secondary to iatrogenic arteriovenous fistulas. J Cutan Pathol 1999;26:159–64.
235. Requena L, Kutzner H, Mentzel T, Duran R, Rodriguez-Peralto JL. Benign vascular proliferations in irradiated skin. Am J Surg Pathol 2002;26:328–37.
236. Rieger E, Soyer HP, Leboit PE, Metze D, Slovak R, Kerl H. Reactive angioendotheliomatosis or intravascular histiocytosis? An immunohistochemical and ultrastructural study in two cases of intravascular histiocytic cell proliferation. Br J Dermatol 1999;140:497–504.
237. Rongioletti F, Rebora A. Cutaneous reactive angiomatoses: patterns and classification of reactive vascular proliferation. J Am Acad Dermatol 2003;49:887–96.
238. Rosales CM, McLaughlin MD, Sata T, et al. AIDS presenting with cutaneous Kaposi's sarcoma and bacillary angiomatosis in the bone marrow mimicking Kaposi's sarcoma. AIDS Patient Care STDS 2002;16:573–7.
239. Rosso R, Gianelli U, Carnevali L. Acquired progressive lymphangioma of the skin following radiotherapy for breast carcinoma. J Cutan Pathol 1995;22:164–7.

240. Sener SF, Milos S, Feldman JL, et al. The spectrum of vascular lesions in the mammary skin, including angiosarcoma, after breast conservation treatment for breast cancer. J Am Coll Surg 2001;193:22–8.
241. Shyong EQ, Gorevic P, Lebwohl M, Phelps RG. Reactive angioendotheliomatosis and sarcoidosis. Int J Dermatol 2002;41:894–7.
242. Sibley DA, Cooper PH. Rudimentary meningocele: a variant of "primary cutaneous meningioma." J Cutan Pathol 1989;16:72–80.
243. Strutton G, Weedon D. Acro-angiodermatitis. A simulant of Kaposi's sarcoma. Am J Dermatopathol 1987;9:85–9.
244. Suster S, Rosai J. Hamartoma of the scalp with ectopic meningothelial elements. A distinctive benign soft tissue lesion that may simulate angiosarcoma. Am J Surg Pathol 1990;14:1–11.
245. Thai KE, Barrett W, Kossard S. Reactive angioendotheliomatosis in the setting of antiphospholipid syndrome. Australas J Dermatol 2003;44:151–5.
246. Tomasini C, Soro E, Pippione M. Angioendotheliomatosis in a woman with rheumatoid arthritis. Am J Dermatopathol 2000;22:334–8.
247. Weyers W, Nilles M, Konig M. Lymphangioma circumscriptum cysticum following surgical and radiologic therapy. Hautarzt 1990;41:102–4.
248. Wick MR, Ritter JH, Humphrey PA. Pseudoneoplastic lesions of the skin and superficial soft tissues. In: Wick MR, Humphrey PA, Ritter JH, eds. Pathology of pseudoneoplastic lesions. Philadelphia: Lippincott-Raven; 1997:545–86.
249. Wick MR, Rocamora A. Reactive and malignant "angioendotheliomatosis": a discriminant clinicopathological study. J Cutan Pathol 1988;15: 260–71.

SUPPLEMENTAL REFERENCES

Vascular Malformations

Chiller KG, Frieden IJ, Arbiser JL. Molecular pathogenesis of vascular anomalies: classification into three categories based upon clinical and biochemical characteristics. Lymphat Res Biol 2003;1:267–81.

Devriendt K, Swillen A, Stalmans I, Casteels I. Pulmonary atresia/ventricular septal defect associated with facial port-wine stain and retinal vascular abnormality: a new constellation or deletion in chromosome 22q11.2? Am J Med Genet 2005;132:340–1.

Feller L, Lemmer J. Encephalotrigeminal angiomatosis. SADJ 2003;58:370–3.

Hoeger PH, Martinez A, Maerker J, Harper JI. Vascular anomalies in Proteus syndrome. Clin Exp Dermatol 2004;29:222–30.

Leech SN, Taylor AE, Ramesh V, Birchall D, Ann Lynch S. Widespread capillary malformation associated with global developmental delay and megalencephaly. Clin Dysmorphol 2004;13:169–72.

Sanchez-Carpintero I, Mihm MC, Mizeracki A, Waner M, North PE. Epithelial and mesenchymal hamartomatous changes in a mature port-wine stain: morphologic evidence for a multiple germ layer field defect. J Am Acad Dermatol 2004;50:608–12.

Lymphangioma

Fukunaga M. Expression of D2-40 in lymphatic endothelium of normal tissues and in vascular tumors. Histopathology 2005;46:396–402.

Hwang LY, Guill CK, Page RN, Hsu S. Acquired progressive lymphangioma. J Am Acad Dermatol 2003;49(Suppl 5):S250–1.

North PE, Kahn T, Cordisco MR, Dadras SS, Detmar M, Frieden IJ. Multifocal lymphangioendotheliomatosis with thrombocytopenia: a newly-recognized clinicopathological entity. Arch Dermatol 2004;140:599–606.

Hemangioma Variants

Adegboyega PA, Qiu S. Hemangioma versus vascular malformation: presence of nerve bundle is a diagnostic clue for vascular malformation. Arch Pathol Lab Med 2005;129:772–5.

Bhattacharjee P, Hui P, McNiff J. Human herpesvirus-8 is not associated with angiolymphoid hyperplasia with eosinophilia. J Cutan Pathol 2004;31:612–5.

Brenn T, Fletcher CD. Cutaneous epithelioid angiomatous nodule: a distinct lesion in the morphologic spectrum of epithelioid vascular tumors. Am J Dermatopathol 2004;26:14–21.

Buckmiller LM. Update on hemangiomas and vascular malformations. Curr Opin Otolaryngol Head Neck Surg 2004;12:476–87.

Franke FE, Steger K, Marks A, Kutzner H, Mentzel T. Hobnail hemangiomas (targetoid hemosiderotic haemangiomas) are true lymphangiomas. J Cutan Pathol 2004;31:362–7.

Hunt SJ, Santa Cruz DJ. Vascular tumors of the skin: a selective review. Semin Diagn Pathol 2004;21:166–218.

Leon-Villapalos J, Wolfe K, Kangesu L. GLUT-1: an extra diagnostic tool to differentiate between hemangiomas and vascular malformations. Br J Plast Surg 2005;58;348–52.

Ramchandani PL, Sabesan T, Hussein K. Angiolymphoid hyperplasia with eosinophilia masquerading as Kimura disease. Br J Oral Maxillofac Surg 2005;43:249–52.

Rossi S, Orvieto E, Furlanetto A, Laurino L, Ninfo V, Dei Tos AP. Utility of the immunohistochemical detection of FLI-1 expression in round cell and vascular neoplasm using a monoclonal antibody. Mod Pathol 2004;17:547–52.

Wang G, Li C, Gao T. Verrucous hemangioma. Int J Dermatol 2004;43:745–6.

Kimura's Disease

Chen H, Thompson LD, Aguilera NS, Abbondanzo SL. Kimura disease: a clinicopathologic study of 21 cases. Am J Surg Pathol 2004;28:505–13.

Chim CS, Fung A, Shek TW, Liang R, Ho WK, Kwong YL. Analysis of clonality in Kimura's disease. Am J Surg Pathol 2002;26:1083–6.

Yuen HW, Goh YH, Low WK, Lim-Tan SK. Kimura's disease: a diagnostic and therapeutic challenge. Singapore Med J 2005;46:179–83.

Angiokeratoma

Lee MW, Choi JH, Sung KJ, Moon KC, Koh JK. Acral pseudolymphomatous angiokeratoma of children (APACHE). Pediatr Dermatol 2003;20:457–8.

Lucke T, Hoppner W, Schmidt E, Illsinger S, Das AM. Fabry disease: reduced activities of respiratory chain enzymes with decreased levels of energy-rich phosphates in fibroblasts. Mol Genet Metab 2004;82:93–7.

Ozdemir R, Karaaslan O, Tiftikcioglu YO, Kocer U. Angiokeratoma circumscriptum. Dermatol Surg 2004;30:1364–6.

Hemangioendothelioma Variants

Al-Shraim M, Mahboub B, Neligan PC, Chamberlain D, Ghazarian D. Primary pleural epithelioid hemangioendothelioma with metastases to the skin. A case report and literature review. J Clin Pathol 2005;58:107–9.

Gruman A, Liang MG, Mulliken JB, et al. Kaposiform hemangioendothelioma without Kasabach-Merritt phenomenon. J Am Acad Dermatol 2005;52:616–22.

Lyons LL, North PE, Mac-Moune Lai F, Stoler MH, Folpe AL, Weiss SW. Kaposiform hemangioendothelioma: a study of 33 cases emphasizing its pathologic, immunophenotypic, and biologic uniqueness from juvenile hemangioma. Am J Surg Pathol 2004;28:559–68.

Martinez AE, Robinson MJ, Alexis JB. Kaposiform hemangioendothelioma associated with nonimmune fetal hydrops. Arch Pathol Lab Med 2004;128:678–81.

Kaposi's Sarcoma

Aoki Y, Tosato G. Neoplastic conditions in the context of HIV-1 infection. Curr HIV Res 2004;2:343–9.

Berber I, Altaca G, Aydin C, et al. Kaposi's sarcoma in renal transplant patients: predisposing factors and prognosis. Transplant Proc 2005;37;967–8.

Cheung L, Rockson SG. The lymphatic biology of Kaposi's sarcoma. Lymphat Res Biol 2005;3:25–35.

Cohen A, Wolf DG, Guttman-Yassky E, Sarid R. Kaposi's sarcoma-associated herpesvirus: clinical, diagnostic, and epidemiological aspects. Crit Rev Clin Lab Sci 2005;42:101–53.

Huang JY, Chiang YJ, Lai PC, et al. Posttransplant Kaposi's sarcoma: report from a single center. Transplant Proc 2004;36:2145–7.

Kempf W, Cathomas G, Burg G, Trueb RM. Micronodular Kaposi's sarcoma—a new variant of classic-sporadic Kaposi's sarcoma. Dermatology 2004;208:255–8.

Pantanowitz L, Schwartz EJ, Dezube BJ, Kohler S, Dorfman RF, Tahan SR. C-Kit (CD117) expression in AIDS-related, classic, and African endemic Kaposi sarcoma. Appl Immunohistochem Mol Morphol 2005;13:162–6.

Ramirez JA, Laskin WB, Guitart J. Lymphangioma-like Kaposi sarcoma. J Cutan Pathol 2005;32:286–92.

Rigopoulos D, Paparizos V, Katsambas A. Cutaneous markers of HIV infection. Clin Dermatol 2004;22:487–98.

Schwartz RA. Kaposi's sarcoma: an update. J Surg Oncol 2004;87:146–51.

Seo T, Park J, Choe J. Kaposi's sarcoma-associated herpesvirus viral IFN regulatory factor 1 inhibits transforming growth factor-beta signaling. Cancer Res 2005;65:1738–47.

Angiosarcoma

Billings SD, McKenney KJ, Folpe AL, Hardacre MC, Weiss SW. Cutaneous angiosarcoma following breast-conserving surgery and radiation: an analysis of 27 cases. Am J Surg Pathol 2004;28:781–8.

Gherardi G, Rossi S, Perrone S, Scanni A. Angiosarcoma after breast-conserving therapy: fine needle aspiration biopsy, immunocytochemistry, and clinicopathologic correlates. Cancer 2005;105:145–51.

Manning T, Smoller BR, Horn TD, et al. Evaluation of anti-thrombomodulin antibody as a tumor marker for vascular neoplasms. J Cutan Pathol 2004;31:652–6.

Morgan MB, Swann M, Somach S, Eng W, Smoller BR. Cutaneous angiosarcoma: a case series with prognostic correlation. J Am Acad Dermatol 2004;50:867–74.

Puizina-Ivic N, Bezic J, Marasovic D, Gotovac V, Carija A, Bozic M. Angiosarcoma arising in sclerodermatous skin. Acta Dermatovenereol Alp Panonica Adriat 2005;14:20–5.

Simonart T, Heenen M. Radiation-induced angiosarcomas. Dermatology 2004;209:175–6.

Pseudoneoplastic Lesions Simulating Vascular Tumors

Boyd AS, Robbins J. Cutaneous Mycobacterium avium intracellulare infection in an HIV+ patient mimicking histoid leprosy. Am J Dermatopathol 2005;27:39–41.

Singhi MK, Kachhawa D, Ghiya BC. A retrospective study of clinico-histopathological correlation in leprosy. Indian J Pathol Microbiol 2003;46:47–8.

8 TUMORS AND TUMOR-LIKE CONDITIONS SHOWING NEURAL, NERVE SHEATH, AND ADIPOCYTIC DIFFERENTIATION

This chapter, on neural and lipocytic neoplasms, is an abbreviated treatment of such lesions, with particular reference to those that affect the skin. Readers are reminded that separate tumor Atlases are devoted to soft tissue tumors and neoplasms of the peripheral nerves, and they are referred to those resources for more detailed information.

NEURAL LESIONS

Neuroma and Ganglioneuroma

Clinical Features. Two types of cutaneous neuroma are generally recognized: *post-traumatic neuroma* (99,108) and *palisading/encapsulated (Reed's) neuroma* (8,28,34,35,37,41,69,81,100). Both variants present as small, nodular, tan-pink lesions; post-traumatic neuromas, which are often painful, tend to affect the extremities (where mechanical injuries are most common), whereas palisading neuromas are painless and occur almost exclusively on the face. Both favor adult patients, with no predilection for gender.

Ganglioneuromas rarely arise in the skin (51,57,75,98), but rather are typically found in mucosal surfaces such as the lips, mouth, and conjunctiva, or in modified mucosa (e.g., genital skin). They are largely restricted to patients with the multiple endocrine neoplasia syndrome, type 2b (23), in which medullary thyroid carcinoma, pheochromocytoma, parathyroid hyperplasia, and a marfanoid habitus are also seen. Mucosal ganglioneuromas are typically multiple, and take the form of irregular nodules of variable size; however, rare cases of solitary ganglioneuroma of the skin have been reported, sometimes under the rubric of *ganglion cell choristoma* (101). The appearance of such lesions is as nondescript, tan, firm nodules; some may be congenital.

Pathologic Findings and Differential Diagnosis. Post-traumatic neuromas are actually misnamed, in that they are not truly neoplastic proliferations of peripheral nerves. They are the result of aberrant attempts at reinnervation after traumatic disruption of neural axons and consequent intraneural scarring (99). Accordingly, relatively banal nerve bundles are distorted by fibrous bands within them and surrounding them. Regenerating axonal fibers may be "blocked" from establishing continuity with distal portions of the axon by such zones of fibrosis, yielding micronodular proliferations of axons and accompanying Schwann cells. Adjacent blood vessels may contain organizing microthrombi.

Palisading neuromas, on the other hand, are actual neoplasms. They are centered in the middermis, and often have a peripheral attenuated fibrous capsule. Fascicles of bland, amitotic spindle cells are separated by artifactual clefts and are internally intertwined around one another. No fibrous sheaths surround them, as would be seen in post-traumatic neuromas. Tumor cell nuclei in palisading neuromas manifest a tendency to align in parallel within each fascicle (figs. 8-1, 8-2). Nuclear contours are sometimes serpiginous, as the profiles of individual cells themselves may be. The cytoplasm is amphophilic. Palisading neuroma lacks the intracellular fibrillation, cytoplasmic eosinophilia, and blunt-ended nuclear profile that would be expected in benign smooth muscle tumors, which represent the most likely pathologic diagnostic alternative. Similarly, tumor cell fascicles that are cut in cross section do not exhibit the zones of perinuclear cytoplasmic clarity that are seen in leiomyomas.

Ganglioneuromas differ from the description just given in that they are not encapsulated, and, more importantly, contain well-formed ganglion cells interspersed throughout the lesion (fig. 8-3). The ganglion cells are variable in number, and are easily recognized by their polyhedral shape, vesicular nuclei, and prominent

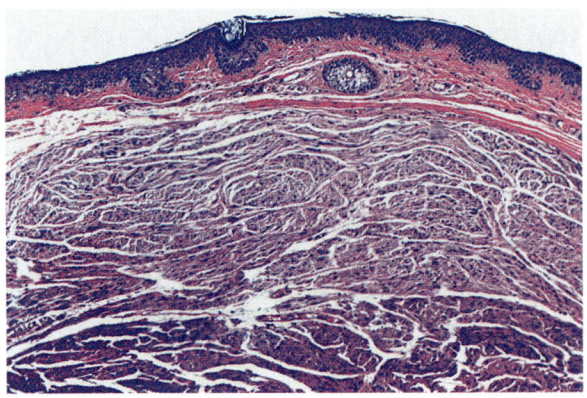

Figure 8-1

PALISADING NEUROMA

An attenuated fibrous capsule surrounds a fascicular proliferation of bland spindle cells that demonstrate nuclear palisading.

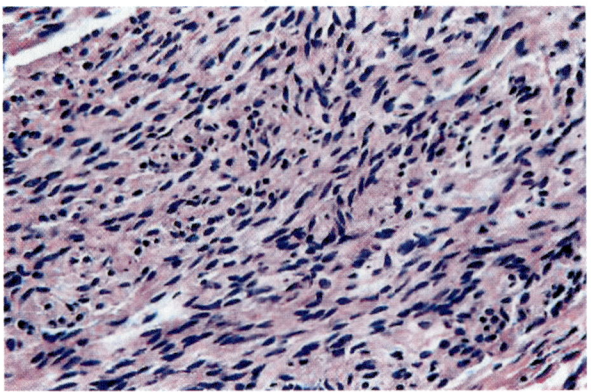

Figure 8-2

PALISADING NEUROMA

There are serpiginous nuclear contours in the lesional cells and a lack of mitotic activity.

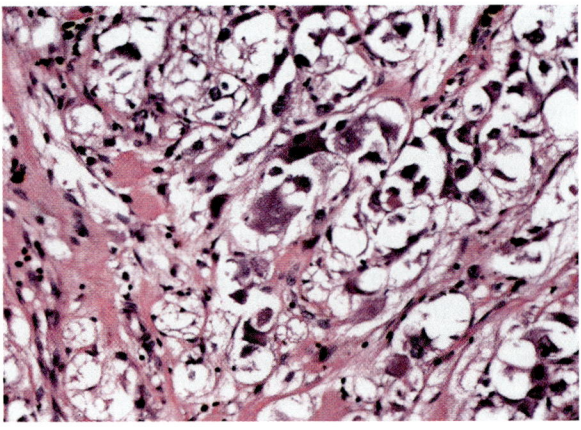

Figure 8-3

GANGLIONEUROMA

Large cells with irregular nuclear contours and abundant cytoplasm are admixed with compact spindle cells. The former are ganglion cells and can be labeled with antibodies to synaptophysin or microtubule-associated protein-2.

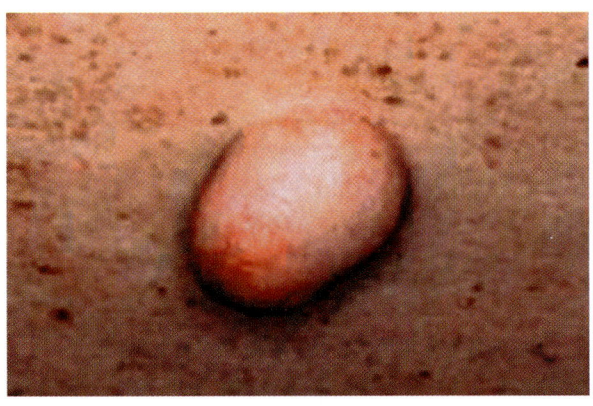

Figure 8-4

SOLITARY NEUROFIBROMA

A nondescript, soft, raised, nodular lesion in the skin of the trunk.

nucleoli. Franchi and colleagues (46) studied a case showing notable stromal desmoplasia. Drut et al. (36) documented a case of giant congenital nevus that contained an extensive zone of ganglioneuromatous differentiation. The differential diagnosis principally centers on the possibility of ganglioneuromatous "maturation" of metastatic neuroblastoma in the skin (49), but the clinical setting typically makes the interpretation straightforward.

Neurofibroma

Clinical Features. *Neurofibroma of the skin* is common as a sporadic neoplasm, in which case it is a nondescript, soft papule or nodule measuring up to 3 cm in greatest dimension (fig. 8-4). Any skin field may be affected by solitary neurofibroma (including modified mucosa), as well as any age group (13,93,118).

Multiple neurofibromas (fig. 8-5), particularly if they are accompanied by "cafe au lait" lesions and are seen in patients under 10 years of age, strongly suggest a diagnosis of *von Recklinghausen's disease* (70,77,103). The plexiform variant

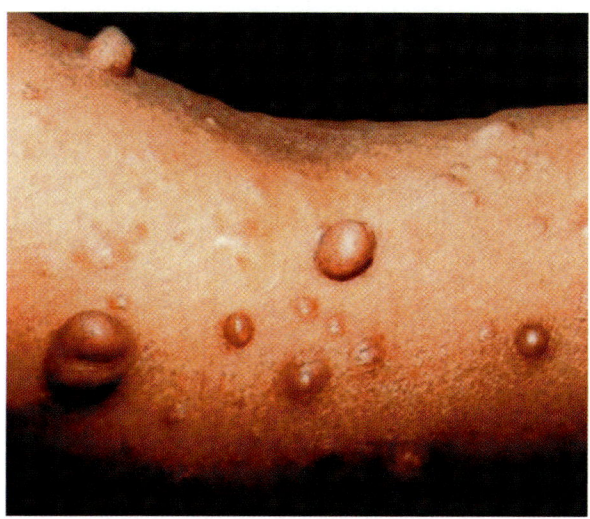

Figure 8-5

VON RECKLINGHAUSEN'S DISEASE (NEUROFIBROMATOSIS)

Multiple raised nodules are present in the skin of the arm.

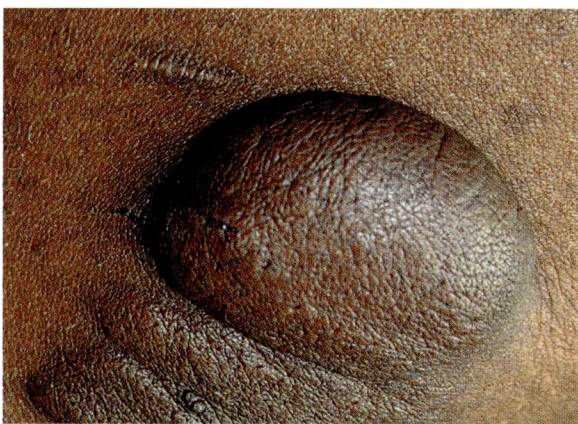

Figure 8-6

VON RECKLINGHAUSEN'S DISEASE

This plexiform neurofibroma has a multicompartmental appearance, like that of "waves against the shore."

of neurofibroma, which is regarded as presumptive evidence of von Recklinghausen's disease even if solitary (fig. 8-6) (127,129), may attain a size of more than 20 cm. The lesion can greatly distort the superficial soft tissue, so that the affected skin acquires a pendulous appearance (elephantiasis neuromatosa). The cut surface of plexiform neurofibroma resembles a "bag of worms."

Pathologic Findings. Neurofibromas are spindle cell tumors with a bland cytologic appearance and serpiginous nucleocytoplasmic contour. Solitary nodular forms are usually circumscribed but not encapsulated, but a diffuse variant exists that shows a tendency to blend with the surrounding dermis or soft tissue. Microscopically, these lesions are usually internally uniform (fig. 8-7), and may be restricted to the corium or extend deeply into the subcutis. Myxoid stromal change is relatively common, but a tendency toward nuclear palisading is generally not appreciated. The tumor cells are arranged haphazardly, in thin fascicles, or in a vaguely storiform pattern in sporadic neurofibromas, with entrapment of dermal collagen and appendages (fig. 8-8). Intralesional mast cells are often numerous, and some lesions also contain entrapped adipocytes (2,124). Variants include tumors with partial melaninization of the tumor cells (39,62),

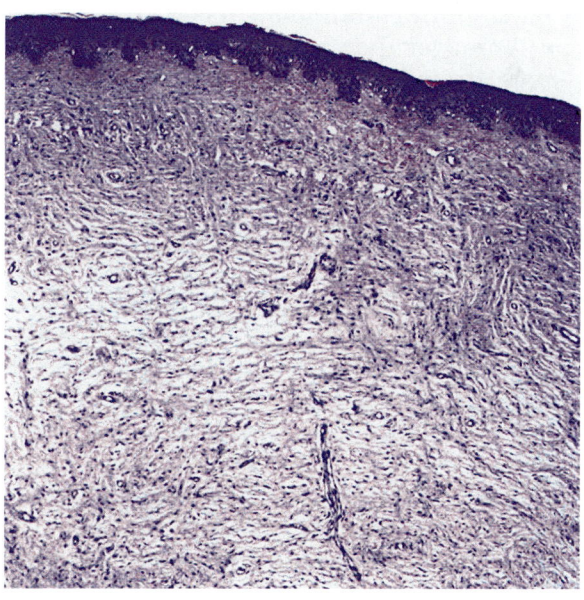

Figure 8-7

NEUROFIBROMA

An ill-defined proliferation of cytologically bland spindle cells is present in the dermis. The background stroma is vaguely myxoid.

and a peculiar, recently described subtype called *dendritic cell neurofibroma with pseudorosettes*, a dermal spindle cell neoplasm that also contains many circular aggregates of small round cells which encompass stromal material (85).

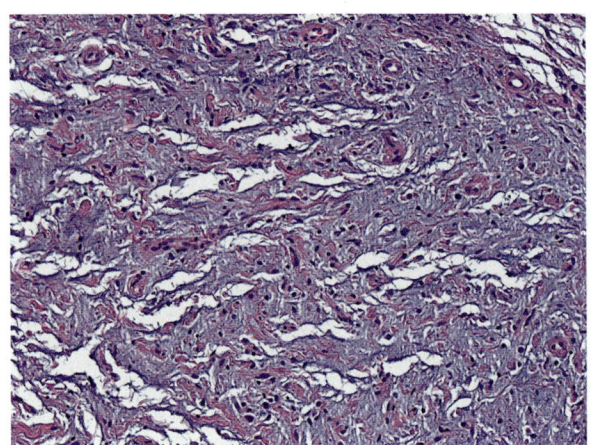

Figure 8-8

NEUROFIBROMA

A formless proliferation of bland spindle cells is set in a fibromyxoid stroma.

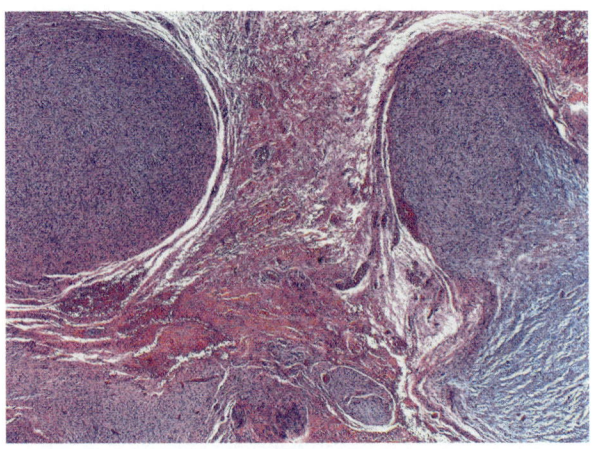

Figure 8-9

PLEXIFORM NEUROFIBROMA

Several micronodules are composed of fibromyxoid and neural tissue. The overall image is like that of distorted miniature nerve trunk.

Plexiform neurofibroma has a distinctive configuration that recalls a distorted neural plexus. Irregular fascicles of proliferating but banal Schwann cells are separated from one another by a myxofibrous stroma or adipose tissue, such that each grouping of spindle cells resembles a miniature nerve trunk (fig. 8-9) (119). Occasionally, structures resembling Meissner or pacinian corpuscles may punctuate these proliferations (106). The histologic interpretation of plexiform neurofibroma strongly suggests a diagnosis of von Recklinghausen's disease; therefore, the above-cited microscopic features should all be present before making that diagnosis.

Differential Diagnosis. Mitotic activity, local hypercellularity, necrosis, and nuclear atypia are worrisome features in lesions thought to be neurofibromas. It is well known that great difficulty may be encountered in distinguishing such neoplasms from selected malignant peripheral nerve sheath tumors (MPNSTs) of low histologic grade, particularly if they are several centimeters in size (26,119). Special note should be made of lesions with the alarming features just cited, and the preferred diagnostic terminology in such instances is "peripheral nerve sheath tumor of indeterminate biologic potential." Recent studies have suggested that positive immunostains for mutant p53 protein and Ki-67 may be helpful in separating MPNSTs from other nerve sheath tumors, which are negative for those markers (56,67,78).

The dendritic neurofibroma with pseudorosettes may be confused with another malignant neoplasm, namely, primitive neuroectodermal tumor/extraskeletal Ewing's sarcoma (58). The former lacks CD99 immunoreactivity and contains zones of spindle cell growth, both of which are features not expected in primitive neuroectodermal tumors.

An additional problem is distinguishing neurofibroma from ordinary but extensively neurotized melanocytic intradermal nevi, as well as amelanotic and neuroid variants of blue nevus or Spitz's nevus (16,117). Serial sections are often required to search for small foci of obvious melanocytes in the latter, and it is admittedly impossible to make the distinction in some cases. Our pragmatic approach to this problem is to rely on the "rule of association." If a single polypoid lesion is present with a neural histologic image, the diagnosis is that of neurofibroma; on the other hand, if the patient in question also has several melanocytic nevi, the best interpretation is that of a neurotized nevus. Most neurofibromas and neurotized nevi share immunoreactivity for S-100 protein (fig. 8-10) but they lack specialized melanocytic determinants; hence, immunohistology is usually not discriminatory in that context. Gray et al. (53a), however, have suggested that immunoreactivity for

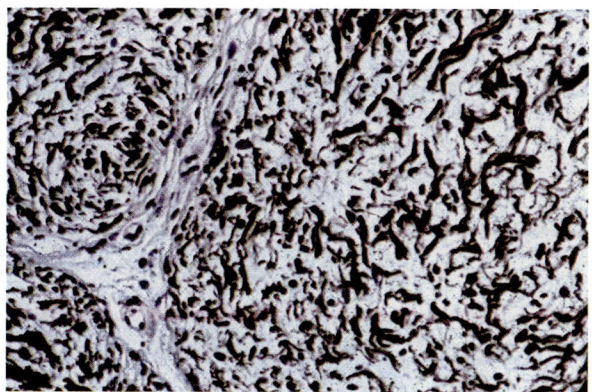

Figure 8-10

NEUROFIBROMA

There is diffuse immunoreactivity for S-100 protein.

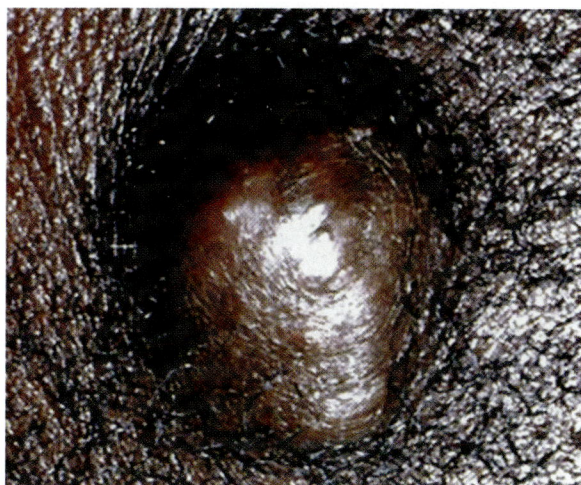

Figure 8-11

NEURILEMMOMA

A fleshy nodular lesion protrudes above the skin surface.

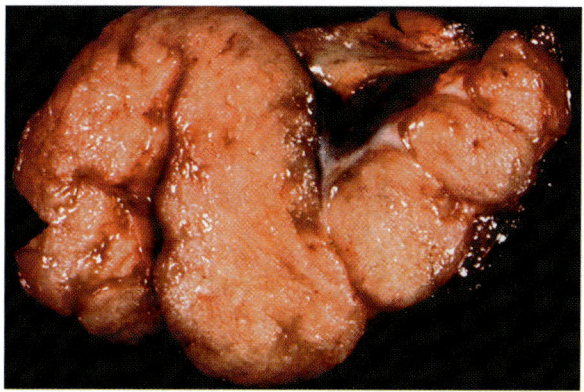

Figure 8-12

NEURILEMMOMA

An unusual finding is the presence of macroscopic plexiform change in the lesion. This finding does not imply the presence of von Recklinghausen's disease, as would be true with plexiform neurofibroma.

factor XIIIa is restricted to neurofibromas in this particular differential diagnostic setting.

Another possible differential diagnostic consideration is perineurioma, a form of peripheral nerve sheath tumor that is characterized by concentric, "onion-bulb" configurations of spindle cells (132,133). Like neurofibroma, this neoplasm also may assume a plexiform configuration. Perineurioma is recognizable by its immunoreactivity for epithelial membrane antigen, as well as its typical morphologic image (112).

There are other cutaneous tumors that may assume a plexiform appearance. These include Spitz's nevus, plexiform fibrohistiocytic tumor, and plexiform dermatofibroma. None of these tumors occurs in patients with von Recklinghausen's disease, and their immunohistologic profiles, as presented elsewhere in this book, are dissimilar from those of neurofibroma.

Neurilemmoma

Clinical Features. Neurilemmomas (schwannomas) are essentially clinically identical to sporadic neurofibromas (fig. 8-11). There is a potential association between cutaneous variants and von Recklinghausen's disease if the lesions are multifocal and grossly plexiform (fig. 8-12); however, this is a rare occurrence (9,82,119).

Pathologic Findings. Neurilemmomas differ from neurofibromas in two major respects. First, they demonstrate a biphasic cellular growth pattern; second, they are often encapsulated and contain internal, thick-walled, stromal blood vessels (118).

The two major microscopic patterns in neurilemmoma are the Antoni A and Antoni B configurations. These feature the presence of dense spindle cell foci with potential nuclear palisading (the Verocay bodies), and myxoid or edematous paucicellular areas composed of bland myxoid or stellate tumor cells, respectively (figs. 8-13, 8-14) (107,119). Intratumoral mast cells are numerous. The nuclear characteristics are usually bland, although traumatized, long-standing superficial ("ancient") neurilemmomas may

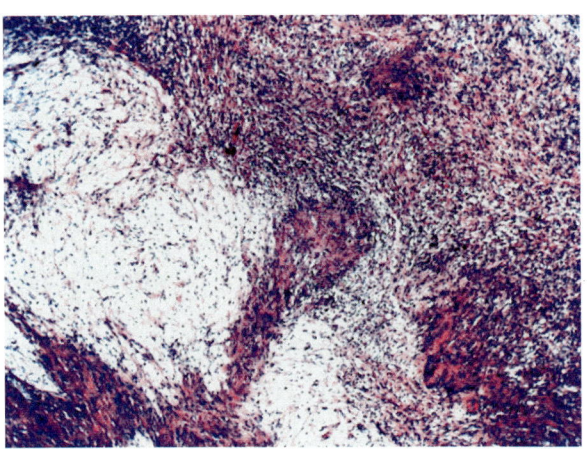
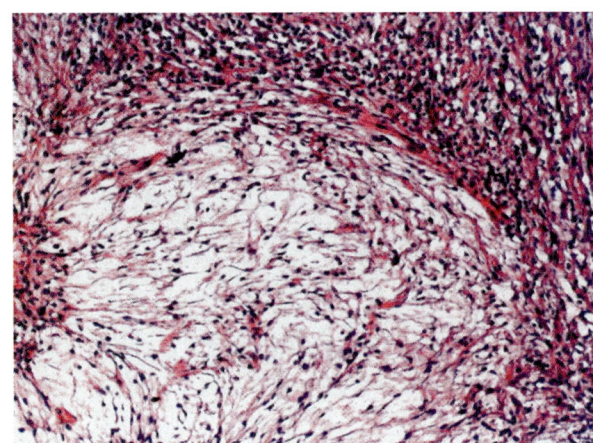

Figure 8-13

NEURILEMMOMA

Left: Compact cellular (Antoni A) areas and zones of loose fibromyxoid (Antoni B) tissue are juxtaposed.
Right: The interface between Antoni A and Antoni B foci is clearer here.

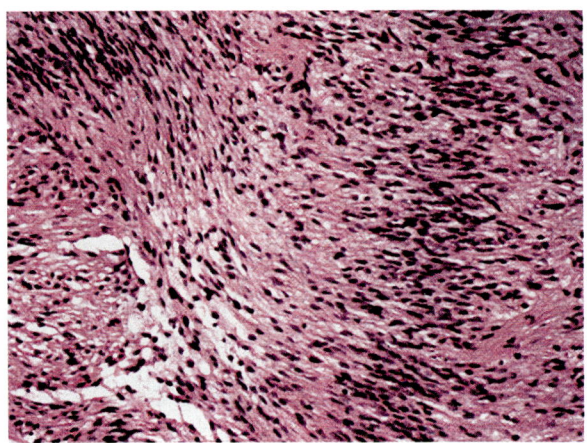
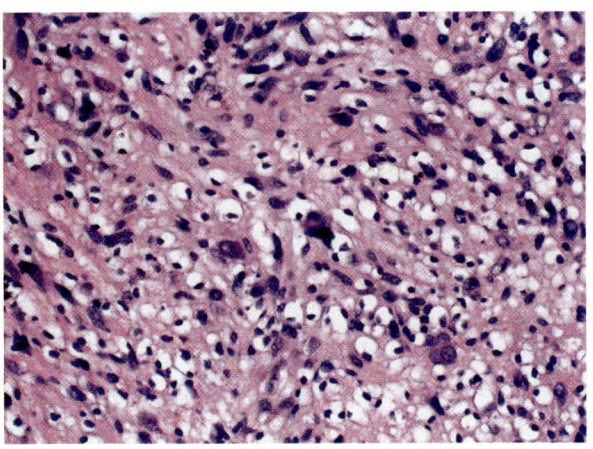

Figure 8-14

NEURILEMMOMA

Nuclei in Antoni A foci demonstrate prominent palisading. This arrangement is known as a Verocay body.

Figure 8-15

"ANCIENT" NEURILEMMOMA

Notable nuclear pleomorphism and hyperchromasia, in the absence of mitotic activity or alterations in the nucleocytoplasmic ratio, are seen. These changes are degenerative and have no prognostic significance.

show nuclear enlargement and hyperchromasia as secondary changes (fig. 8-15). Mitotic activity is scanty, but unlike neurofibroma, some division figures may be tolerated without alarm regarding possible malignancy. Indeed, malignant change in neurilemmoma is rare (79), and is, for practical purposes, restricted to large and deep-seated tumors.

Neurilemmoma is much more versatile than other peripheral nerve sheath tumors with respect to its modes of microscopic differentiation. Variants of this neoplasm include one containing small groups of epithelium, with or without mucin production *(glandular neurilemmoma)* (fig. 8-16) (130); another showing an admixture of melaninized cells *(melanotic neurilemmoma)* (fig. 8-17) (45,83); a *plexiform neurilemmoma* in which the macroscopic appearance of the tumor simulates that of plexiform neurofibroma (see above) (43,63,66); a variant dominated by plump epithelioid tumor cells

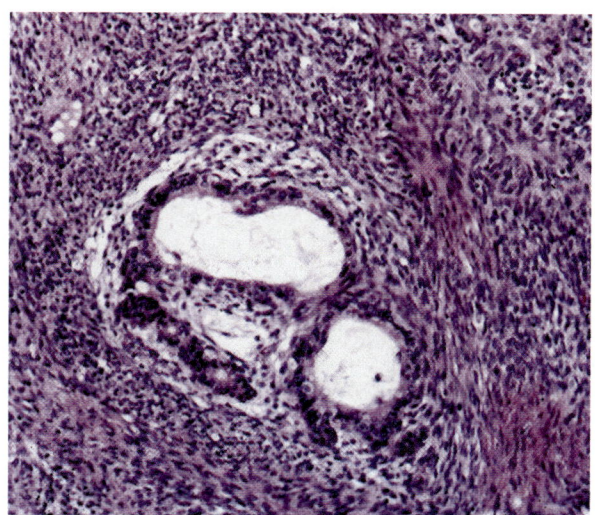

Figure 8-16

NEURILEMMOMA

True glandular tissue is apparent with an Antoni A focus. Gland formation is likely metaplastic.

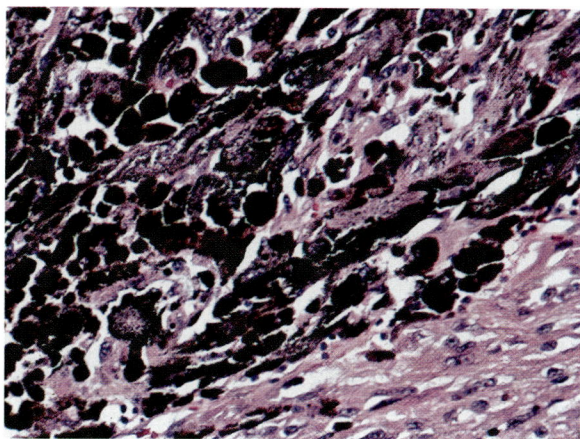

Figure 8-17

MELANOTIC NEURILEMMOMA

Densely pigmented cytoplasm is evident. Lesions such as this may be black or brown grossly.

(*epithelioid neurilemmoma*) (92,110,120); and a form in which both melaninization and psammomatous calcification are apparent (*psammomatous-melanotic neurilemmoma*) (22). Some observers use the term *cellular schwannoma* in describing some cutaneous tumors with extremely dense Antoni A areas. The latter designation is most properly applied to a restricted subset of neurilemmoma that occurs in the deep soft tissues of the midline (44); we do not use this term in the context of skin pathology.

Differential Diagnosis. Cutaneous smooth muscle tumors occasionally show variation in cellular density and a tendency towards nuclear palisading, mirroring the attributes of neurilemmoma. Leiomyomas are consistently immunoreactive for desmin, actin, caldesmon, and calponin, however, and only sporadically for S-100 protein; neurilemmomas exhibit the converse of that profile. Examples of neuroid basal cell carcinoma with prominent nuclear palisading have been reported by San Juan et al. (105). Those lesions are immunoreactive for keratin and lack neural determinants.

Neurothekeoma

Like virtually any pathologic entity, the tumor now known as *neurothekeoma* has undergone substantial conceptual metamorphosis since its original description by Gallagher and Helwig in 1980 (48). Relatively shortly thereafter, an alternate term for a putatively related superficial soft tissue tumor, *dermal nerve sheath myxoma*, was introduced (97). Diagnostic complexity in this group of lesions was further amplified by publications on a lesion dubbed *cellular neurothekeoma*, originally described by Rosati et al. in 1986 (15,21,102). We consider each of these tumor types to represent distinct and mutually exclusive neoplasms, as substantiated by the results of immunohistologic and electron microscopic studies; however, that is not necessarily the nosologic synthesis of this neoplastic family that other observers may embrace.

Clinical Features. Lesions currently grouped under the rubrics of neurothekeoma and dermal nerve sheath myxoma primarily affect young individuals with a mean age of 22 years at diagnosis. Females predominate by a ratio of 2 to 1, and the tumors are most often located on the face, shoulders, and arms. They are uncommonly ulcerated, nonpigmented, variably firm, dome-shaped papules or nodules, sometimes with a translucent quality (fig. 8-18) (6,15,21,42,48,53,97,102).

Pathologic Findings. In our opinion, the term neurothekeoma should be used in reference to a tumor that is composed of bland to moderately atypical plump spindle cells and epithelioid elements in the dermis, and which

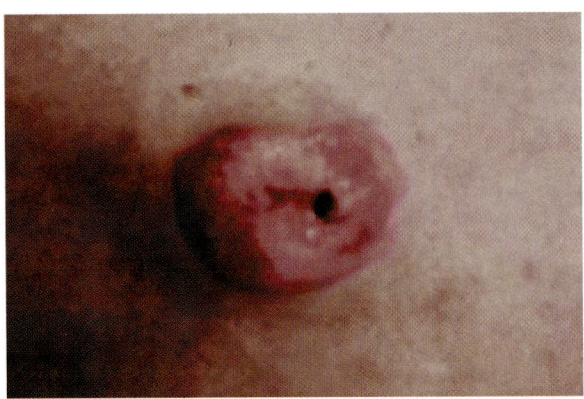

Figure 8-18

NEUROTHEKEOMA

Seen in the upper back of an adolescent boy.

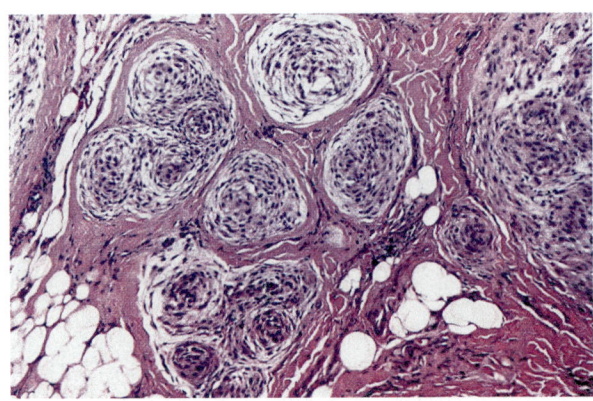

Figure 8-19

CLASSIC NEUROTHEKEOMA

Concentric profiles of bluntly fusiform and cytologically bland tumor cells typify the microscopic appearance of classic cutaneous neurothekeoma.

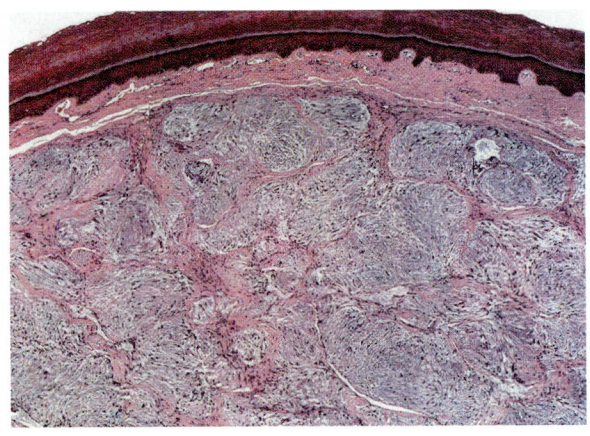

Figure 8-20

DERMAL NERVE SHEATH MYXOMA

Nested arrays of bland spindle cells contain abundant fibromyxoid stroma.

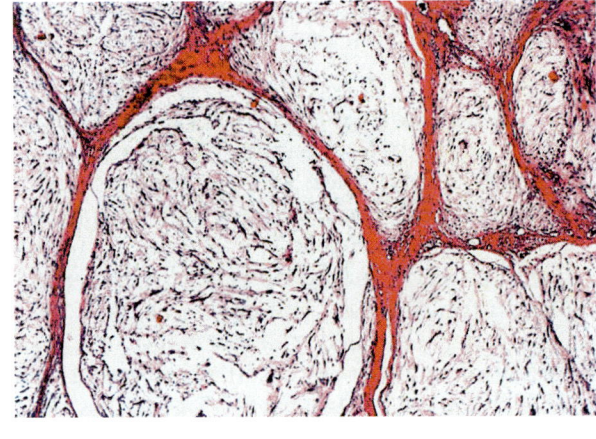

Figure 8-21

DERMAL NERVE SHEATH MYXOMA

Rounded configurations of fusiform tumor cells are in a fibromyxoid matrix.

simulates the appearance of melanocytic theques (fig. 8-19). Mitoses may be numerous in these lesions, but they are never pathologic in shape. In contrast, dermal nerve sheath myxomas are extremely mucomyxoid tumors that show broadly separated and concentric proliferations of spindle cells, which are separated by their matrix (figs. 8-20, 8-21). Nuclear atypia and mitotic figures are variably seen but usually inconspicuous. Cellular neurothekeoma consists of solid aggregates of epithelioid, vaguely nevoid cells in the dermis, without concentration into nests (fig. 8-22). These neoplasms may demonstrate moderate nuclear hyperchromasia, and mitotic figures are usually easily found.

Immunohistologically, there is evidence that dermal nerve sheath myxoma shows schwannian or perineurial cell differentiation, because it is only variably reactive for S-100 protein, CD57 antigen, and epithelial membrane antigen (10, 122). In contrast, all of these markers are absent in classic neurothekeoma and cellular neurothekeoma. The last of these lesions is further distinguished by its positivity for myogenous

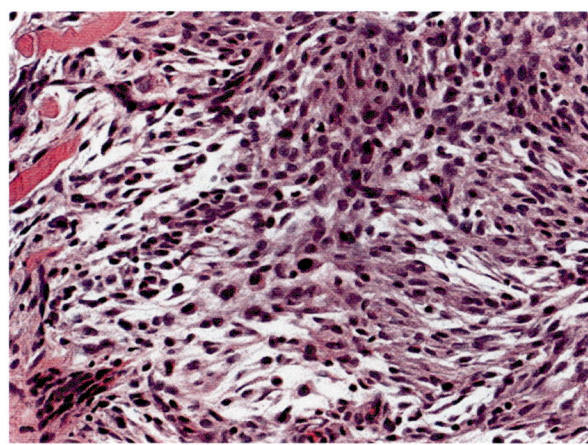 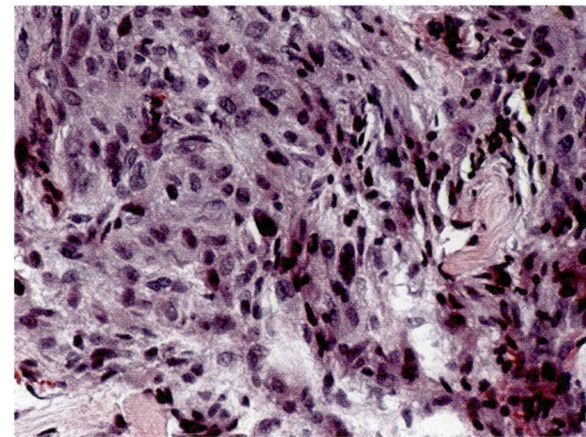

Figure 8-22

CELLULAR NEUROTHEKEOMA

Left: The growth pattern is less organoid than that of classic neurothekeoma or dermal nerve sheath myxoma.
Right: Moderate nuclear pleomorphism, relative dense cellularity, and at least focal sheet-like growth characterize cellular neurothekeoma.

determinants such as actin, as demonstrated by Calonje et al. (21); hence, cellular neurothekeoma may, in fact, be a form of epithelioid cutaneous leiomyoma.

Ultrastructural studies of dermal nerve sheath myxoma have shown evidence of nerve sheath differentiation, as manifested by the production of pericellular basal laminar material and the presence of elongated and partially overlapping cellular processes (14). These characteristics are not present in either classic neurothekeoma or cellular neurothekeoma, which demonstrate more primitive and fibroblast-like morphologic attributes.

Differential Diagnosis. The differential diagnosis of neurothekeoma principally centers on epithelioid neurofibroma, epithelioid neurilemmoma, and low-grade epithelioid MPNST of the skin and subcutis (particularly the plexiform variety), as well as dermal epithelioid (Spitz's) nevus and nevoid melanoma. These entities can be distinguished from one another by immunohistologic studies (10,14,15,61): nerve sheath tumors and melanocytic nevi are both reactive for S-100 protein, and a sizable proportion of melanocytic proliferations, both benign and malignant, express the HMB45 antigen, MART-1/Melan-A, and tyrosinase, whereas neurothekeomas lack all of these determinants. Neurothekeoma is "allowed" to manifest a fair degree of nuclear hyperchromasia as well as mitotic activity, without any connotation of malignancy; however, the presence of spontaneous necrosis, striking cellular pleomorphism, or pathologically shaped division figures seriously questions an interpretation of neurothekeoma and suggests an alternative diagnosis of melanoma or epithelioid MPNST.

Treatment and Prognosis. The treatment for neurothekeoma is simple excision. To date, there have been no recurrences, providing that the lesions in question have been completely removed. Busam et al. (19) studied 10 neurothekeomas that were larger than 6 cm, grew deep into the subcutis or skeletal muscle, had infiltrative borders, and showed vascular invasion, brisk mitotic activity, and notable cytologic atypia. Despite such features, none of those lesions behaved adversely.

Benign Granular Cell Tumor

Clinical Features. *Granular cell tumors* are tan, dome-shaped nodules with a smooth surface, measuring up to 3 cm in greatest dimension (fig. 8-23). They occur at all ages and all topographic locations, with no preference for either gender (18,71). They may be multifocal (5,11,54).

Pathologic Findings. The hallmark of a granular cell tumor is its exclusive composition by polyhedral cells with eccentric oval nuclei,

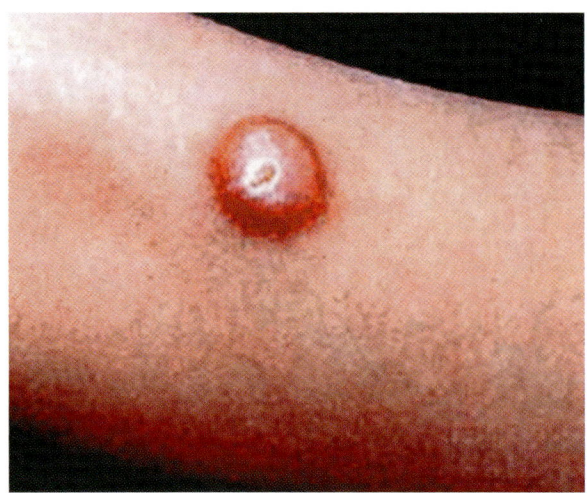
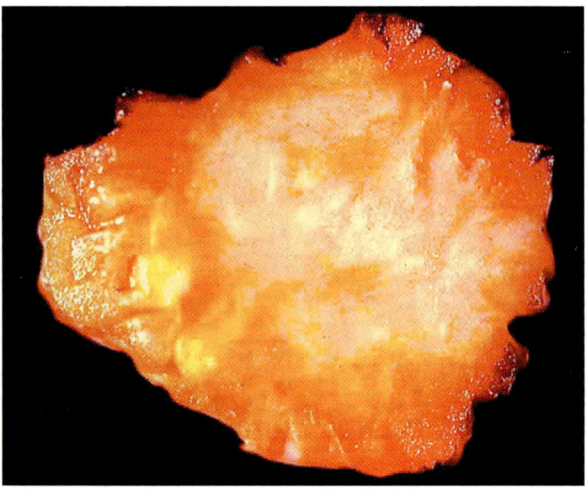

Figure 8-23

GRANULAR CELL TUMOR

Left: The lesion is an umbilicated erythematous nodule in the skin of the arm.
Right: The cut surface of the excised lesion demonstrates internal irregularity and involvement of the subcutis.

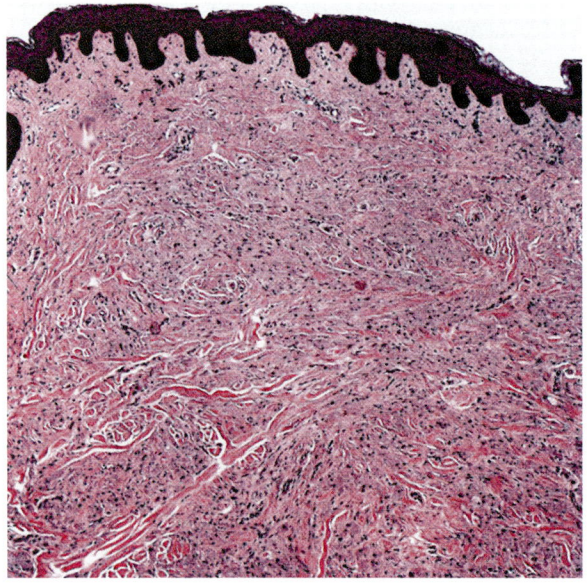

Figure 8-24

GRANULAR CELL TUMOR

Cutaneous granular cell tumor occupies the entirety of the corium and shows a disorganized growth pattern that dissects through the dermal collagen.

dispersed nuclear chromatin, and overtly granular eosinophilic cytoplasm (114). The overlying epidermis is typically induced to proliferate, sometimes producing such striking pseudoepitheliomatous hyperplasia that a diagnosis of squamous carcinoma may be entertained in small superficial biopsies. The neoplastic cells permeate the dermis irregularly, entrapping collagen bundles and cutaneous adnexa, and may extend into the superficial subcutis (fig. 8-24). The low-power microscopic appearance of this lesion is circumscribed but not encapsulated (7,115). Rare mitotic figures may be seen.

The cells of benign granular cell tumors are monotonous, with bland nuclear features and abundant eosinophilic or amphophilic cytoplasm (fig. 8-25). Atypical division figures, necrosis, vascular permeation, and overlying ulceration should prompt consideration of malignancy (87).

The justification for including granular cell tumor in this section on nerve sheath tumors is obtained from data on its ultrastructural and immunohistologic features (1). Most neoplasms of this type (approximately 85 percent) show electron microscopic evidence of Schwann cell differentiation (1,116); likewise, immunoreactivity for S-100 protein, calretinin, CD56, and CD57 links such lesions to other neural lesions (1,40).

Differential Diagnosis. In a minority of cases, granular cell change may simply be a nonspecific degenerative alteration (reflecting an abundance of secondary cytoplasmic phagolysosomes [fig. 8-26]) in neoplasms that are not

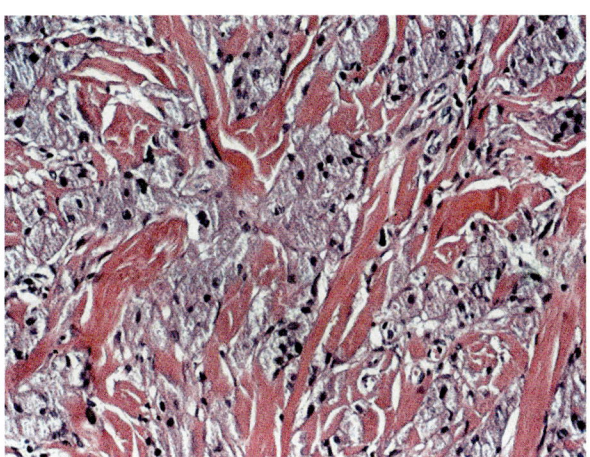 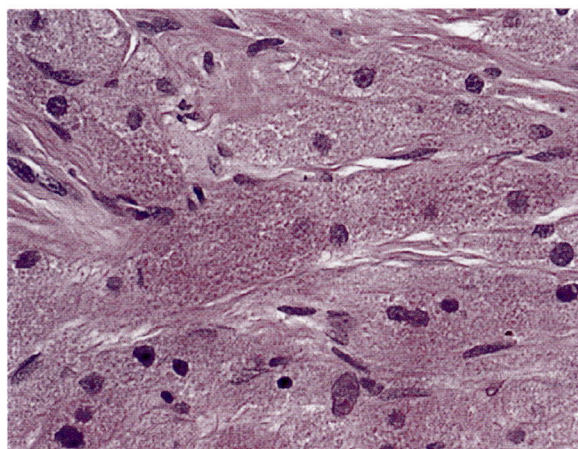

Figure 8-25

GRANULAR CELL TUMOR

Left: Disruption of the dermal collagen bundles by groups of tumor cells is apparent.
Right: The neoplastic cells are cytologically bland, with prominent cytoplasmic stippling and slightly eccentric compact nuclei.

neural in nature, such as dermatofibroma, atypical fibroxanthoma, leiomyoma, leiomyosarcoma, angiosarcoma, and basal cell carcinoma (1,60,72, 73,84,91,111,123). Granular cell variants of the latter lesions do not show any differences in behavior when compared with their conventional forms; their specialized pathologic features are covered elsewhere in this monograph.

Peripheral Neuroepithelioma/ Primitive Neuroectodermal Tumor

Clinical Features. *Peripheral neuroepithelioma* (59) (formerly called *extraskeletal Ewing's sarcoma* and now known as *primitive neuroectodermal tumor* [PNET] [12,29,30,64,65,86,94,95,104,113, 121]) is rarely encountered in the superficial subcutis and dermis (fig. 8-27), where it presents as a nodular, red-violet, ill-defined mass. Patients with cutaneous PNET are usually children, adolescents, or young adults, but older individuals are occasionally affected as well. The neoplasms may attain a maximum dimension of 10 cm and grow rapidly. The trunk and extremities are favored locations (58,94,95,104).

The clinical behavior of this tumor is aggressive. Even with prompt diagnosis and therapy, PNET is associated with a 5-year disease-free survival rate of approximately 60 percent; distant metastases to lungs, liver, bones, and brain are common (55).

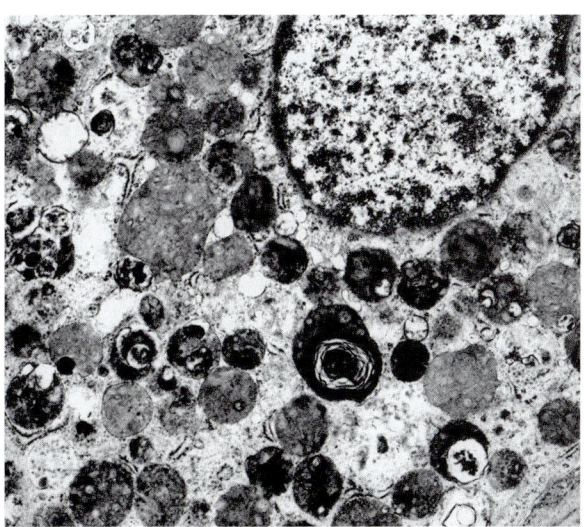

Figure 8-26

GRANULAR CELL TUMOR

Numerous secondary and tertiary cytoplasmic phagolysosomes are seen in this electron photomicrograph.

Pathologic Findings. PNET represents one of the prototypical small round cell tumors. There are sheets, vague nests, and occasional cords of closely apposed, monomorphic neoplastic cells that are approximately two to three times the size of mature lymphocytes (figs. 8-28, 8-29). These aggregates are separated from one another

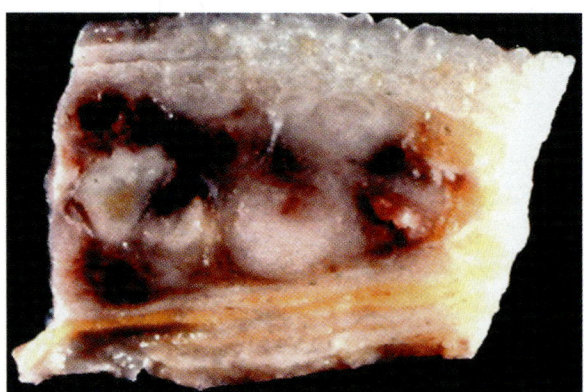

Figure 8-27

SUBCUTANEOUS PRIMITIVE NEUROECTODERMAL TUMOR

This multinodular and hemorrhagic lesion has ill-defined borders.

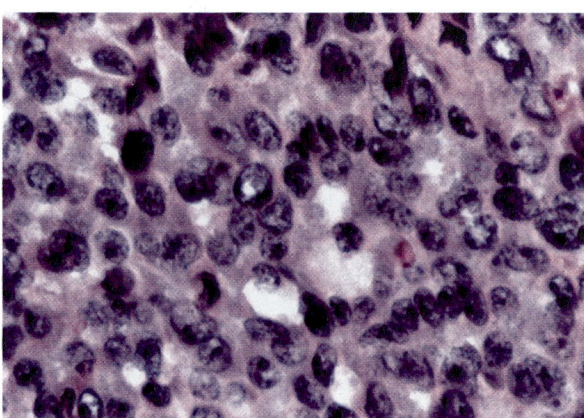

Figure 8-29

SUBCUTANEOUS PRIMITIVE NEUROECTODERMAL TUMOR

The neoplastic cells are relatively uniform, with dispersed chromatin and relatively sparse mitotic activity.

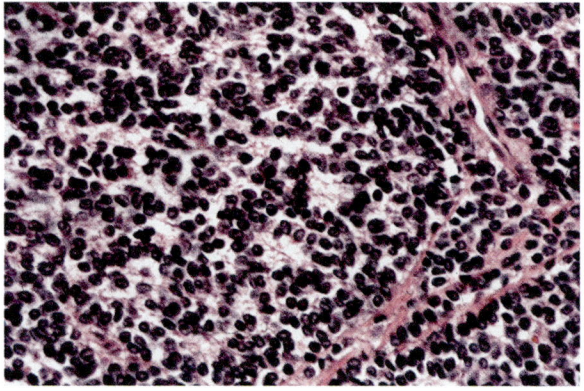

Figure 8-28

SUBCUTANEOUS PRIMITIVE NEUROECTODERMAL TUMOR

Monotonous small round cells focally form vague rosettes.

by a delicate but complex fibrovascular stromal network. Mitotic activity is variable but may be surprisingly sparse; similarly, cellular apoptosis and regional necrosis may or may not be present.

The nuclear detail of PNET is one of the most helpful clues to its recognition. Chromatin is typically evenly distributed, and nucleoli, if present, are small. The cytoplasm is modest in amount, and is amphophilic.

Differential Diagnosis. A minority of PNETs exhibit the presence of intercellular rosettes, betraying the primitive neural nature of this neoplasm (59). The fibrillary intercellular meshwork seen in many examples of metastatic neuroblastoma, an important differential diagnostic alternative, is lacking in PNET. Similarly, focal nuclear pleomorphism and multinucleation are absent, in contrast to the characteristics of small round cell (embryonal or alveolar) rhabdomyosarcoma. Merkel cell carcinoma is a diagnostic consideration because this tumor may arise deep in the skin without any intervening dermal component. Because it is somewhat related to PNET in terms of cellular differentiation, electron microscopy or immunohistology are often necessary to obtain a final distinction between these lesions. PNET is typified by immunoreactivity for CD99 (fig. 8-30) and, in most cases, negativity or only focal labeling for pankeratin, and an absence of actin, desmin, microtubule-associated protein-2 (MAP2), and cytokeratin (CK) 20 (58,90). Merkel cell carcinoma is diffusely reactive for pankeratin and CK20; neuroblastoma is uniformly CD99 negative and reacts for MAP2; and rhabdomyosarcoma is consistently positive for actin and desmin.

Cytogenetic analysis in this group of lesions shows a t(11;22) chromosomal translocation in PNET; abnormalities of chromosomes 1 and 6 in Merkel cell tumors; aberrations of chromosomes 1, 11, and 17 in neuroblastomas; and allelic losses at 11p, or t(1;13) or t(2;13) translocations in rhabdomyosarcomas (50,74,125,131).

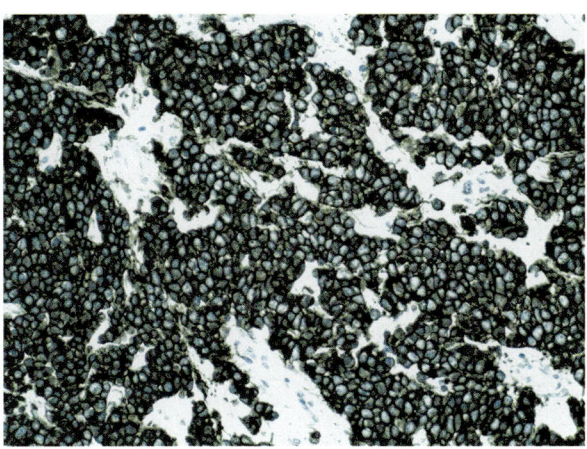

Figure 8-30

SUBCUTANEOUS PRIMITIVE NEUROECTODERMAL TUMOR

Diffuse and intense immunoreactivity for CD99 (MIC2 protein).

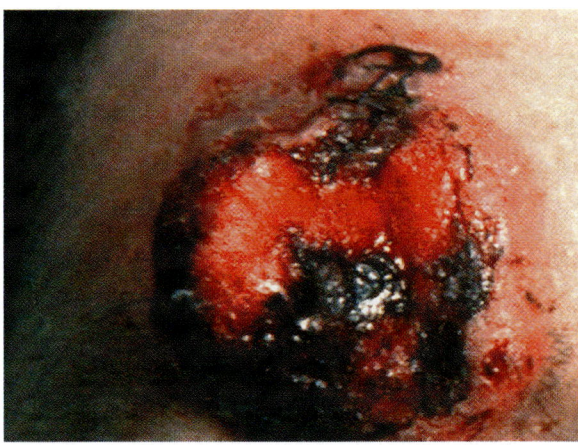

Figure 8-31

MALIGNANT PERIPHERAL NERVE SHEATH TUMOR

The lesion presents as an ulcerated nodule in the skin of the forehead.

Malignant lymphoma of the subcutis also may simulate any of the other small cell neoplasms, including PNET. The nuclei of the lymphoid cells differ from those in other diagnostic alternatives because they are more irregular in contour and have a greater tendency to overlap. The most certain indicator of hematopoietic differentiation is the CD45 antigen, which is only seen in lymphoproliferative lesions.

Nonepithelioid Malignant Peripheral Nerve Sheath Tumor

Clinical Features. Outside the setting of von Recklinghausen's disease, the existence of *cutaneous malignant peripheral nerve sheath tumor* (MPNST) has been questioned in the past. It is well recognized that approximately 1 to 3 percent of patients with von Recklinghausen's disease, both children and adults, develop malignant transformation of superficial neurofibromas, which rapidly expand in size and often become painful (25,89,96).

Sporadic cutaneous MPNST has been accepted as a bona fide entity over the last few years. These are nodules or plaques with variable growth rates, that have a propensity to arise on the trunk or extremities of adults (24,52). Ulceration may supervene (fig. 8-31), and local paresthesias or dysesthesias are sometimes observed if the masses are associated with major nerves.

The behavior of MPNST is generally predicated upon its size, location, and surgical resectability. Tumors arising in the skin more often demonstrate local recurrence (in approximately 80 percent of cases) than distant metastasis (15 to 20 percent) (24,38).

Pathologic Findings. The microscopic features of MPNST are variable; indeed, this neoplasm is one of the great "chameleons" of pathology. In most cases, a modestly pleomorphic proliferation of spindle cells is seen in the dermis and subcutis; the degree of cellularity varies from region to region (fig. 8-32). The tumors cells are randomly arranged or configured in fascicles that may intersect at acute angles (the "herringbone" growth pattern), and many contain "wavy" or serpiginous nuclei (fig. 8-33). Myxoid stromal change is evident in approximately one third of cases, and a focally storiform arrangement of tumor cells is often observed as well (24).

These lesions entrap cutaneous appendages rather than destroy them, but the peripheral margins of growth are indistinct. Permeation into the subcutis and underlying soft tissue is common. Nuclear atypia is modest to moderate, and mitotic activity is present but not striking.

Occasional examples of cutaneous MPNST, particularly those occurring in patients with von Recklinghausen's disease, exhibit divergent mesenchymal differentiation. Tumors showing

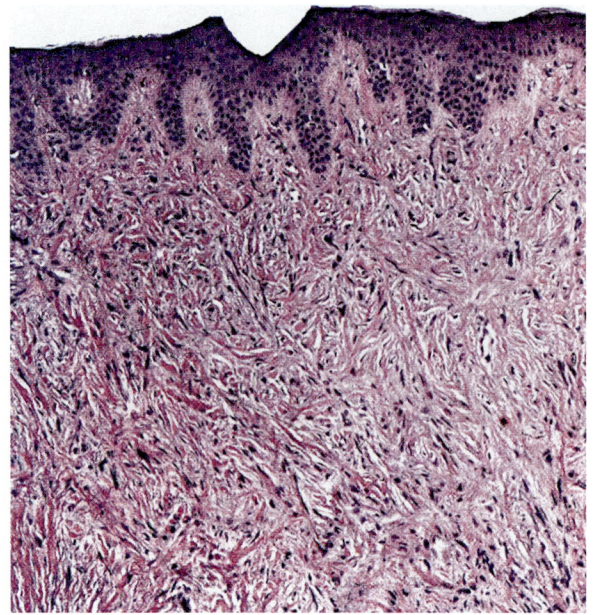

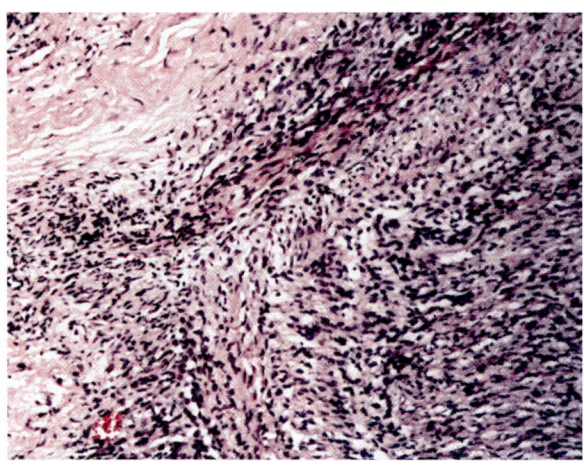

Figure 8-32

MALIGNANT PERIPHERAL NERVE SHEATH TUMOR

Top: A haphazard growth of atypical spindle cells is present in the dermis.

Bottom: On closer inspection, nuclear atypia and variation in cellular density are apparent within the mass.

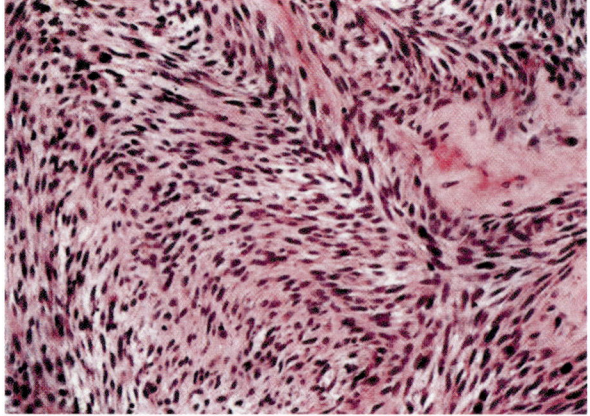

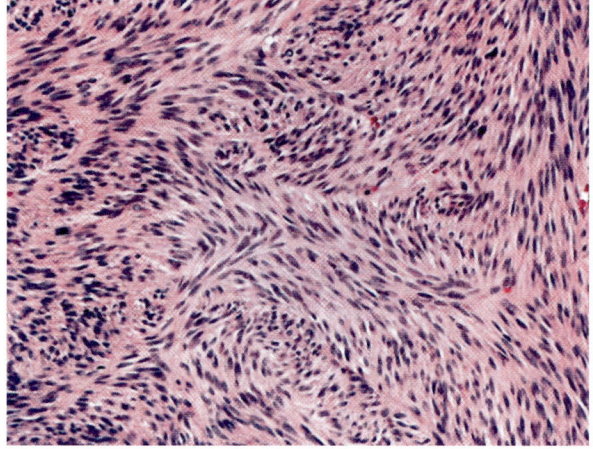

Figure 8-33

MALIGNANT PERIPHERAL NERVE SHEATH TUMOR

Top: A "herringbone" growth pattern of fusiform tumor cells is evident.

Bottom: Another example shows vague nuclear palisading, analogous to the image of selected benign nerve sheath tumors.

an admixture of rhabdomyosarcomatous elements with the spindle cell population are known as *malignant triton tumors* (fig. 8-34) (27,68,129). Although de novo rhabdomyosarcoma is a highly aggressive neoplasm, triton tumors are paradoxically no different biologically than conventional MPNST. Other divergent elements that have been reported in such lesions include those resembling osteosarcoma, pigmented malignant melanoma (*melanotic MPNST*), chondrosarcoma, adenocarcinoma (*glandular MPNST*), and angiosarcoma (24,38).

Electron microscopic evaluation demonstrates elongated, overlapping cytoplasmic processes in the spindle cells of MPNST (fig. 8-35). Focal formation of pericellular basal lamina is also common, as are primitive appositional plaques between adjacent tumor cells.

Immunohistologic studies show reactivity for CD56 in 60 percent of cases, S-100 protein in approximately 50 percent, and CD57 in 33 percent (figs. 8-36, 8-37) (80,119,128). When used as a panel, one or more of these markers is

Tumors and Tumor-Like Conditions Showing Neural and Adipocytic Differentiation

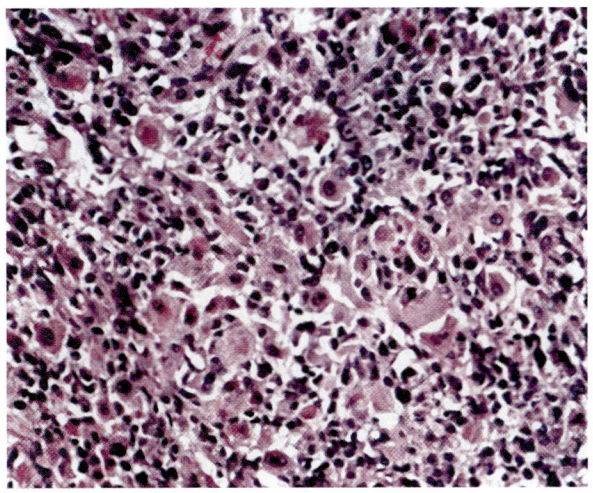

Figure 8-34

MALIGNANT PERIPHERAL NERVE SHEATH TUMOR

Divergent rhabdomyoblastic differentiation, represented by round cells with notably eosinophilic cytoplasm, is seen. The presence of this element confers the designation of malignant triton tumor.

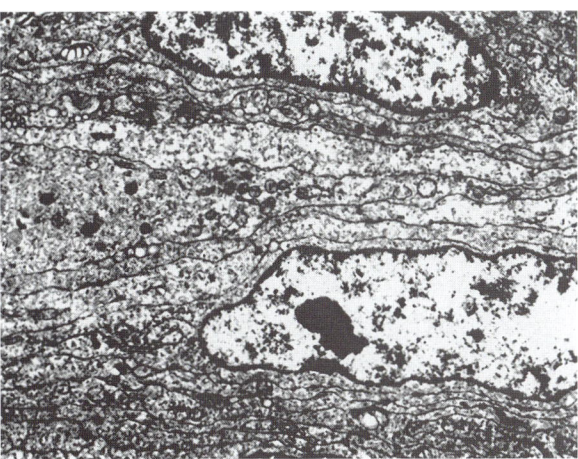

Figure 8-35

MALIGNANT PERIPHERAL NERVE SHEATH TUMOR

Elaborately overlapping and attenuated cytoplasmic processes are invested by basal lamina. Premelanosomes are absent in this electron photomicrograph.

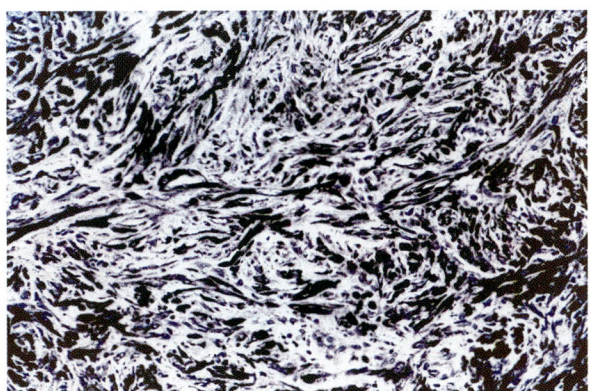

Figure 8-36

MALIGNANT PERIPHERAL NERVE SHEATH TUMOR
Multifocal immunoreactivity for S-100 protein.

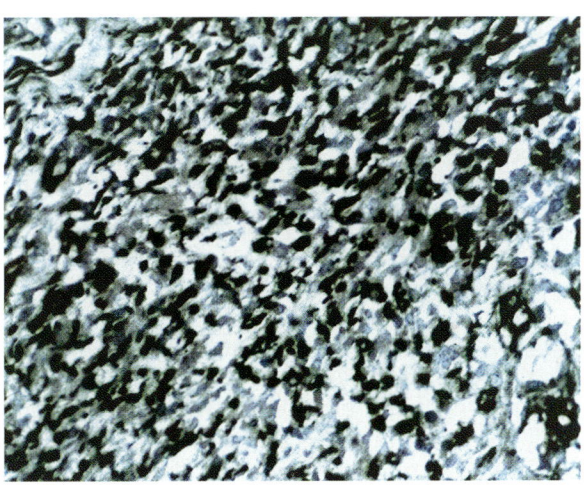

Figure 8-37

MALIGNANT PERIPHERAL NERVE SHEATH TUMOR
Positivity for CD57.

present in 70 percent of lesions. Divergent tumors also express desmin or muscle-specific actin, keratin, or the CD31 or CD34 antigen. In light of this heterogeneity in the immunophenotype of MPNST, ultrastructural assessments are usually more definitive in resolving diagnostic difficulties.

Differential Diagnosis. The differential diagnosis includes leiomyosarcoma, spindle cell squamous carcinoma, dermatofibrosarcoma protuberans, atypical fibroxanthoma, and desmoplastic or neurotropic melanoma. All but the last of these possibilities are adequately distinguished from MPNST by electron microscopy and immunohistology (119).

Neuroid spindle cell melanomas and true nerve sheath tumors share many similarities (31,127). Ultrastructural features of the two groups are virtually identical, since spindle cell melanomas fail to demonstrate cytoplasmic

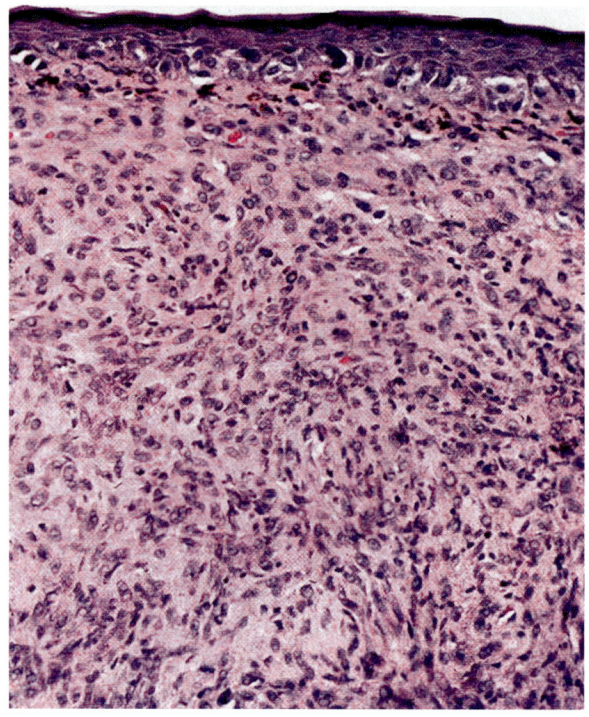

Figure 8-38

NEUROID SPINDLE CELL MELANOMA

Neuroid spindle cell melanoma is similar morphologically to malignant peripheral nerve sheath tumor of the skin, but the former neoplasm, shown here, may demonstrate the presence of atypical melanocytic proliferation at the dermoepidermal junction.

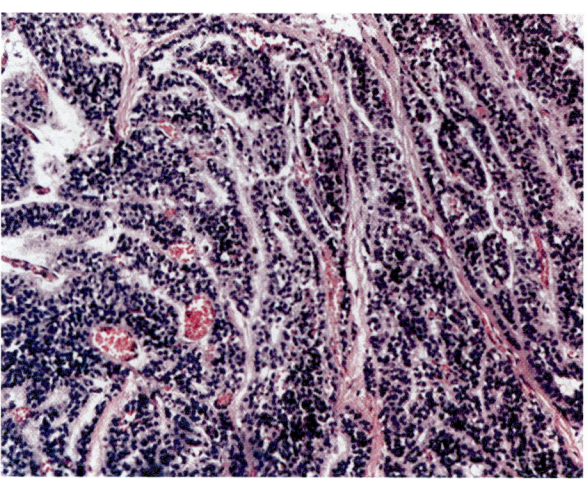

Figure 8-39

EPITHELIOID MALIGNANT PERIPHERAL NERVE SHEATH TUMOR

Cords and clusters of atypical polygonal tumor cells are in a fibromyxoid stroma.

premelanosomes (33). HMB45, MART-1, and tyrosinase, which are specific determinants of melanocytic cells, are absent in almost all neuroid melanomas and are also not seen in MPNST (126). Thus, the distinction between neuroid melanoma and cutaneous MPNST may be difficult, in the absence of a concurrent or previous intraepidermal melanocytic proliferation (fig. 8-38). Whether separation of the two tumors is necessary is a contentious point because of the similarity in their biologic potential and behavior (127).

Pending resolution of this issue, we require that a diagnosis of sporadic cutaneous MPNST be made only under the following circumstances: an epidermal melanocytic lesion must be absent; electron microscopy and immunohistology must be performed; and the results should not support the presence of melanocytic differentiation.

Epithelioid Malignant Peripheral Nerve Sheath Tumor

Clinical Features. The clinical features of *epithelioid MPNST* are identical to those of the spindle cell form of this tumor, as described above.

Pathologic Findings. Epithelioid MPNST differs substantially from spindle cell nerve sheath sarcomas microscopically. The former neoplasm is composed solely of polyhedral cells that are arranged in cords, clusters, and sheets, often separated by myxoid or mucinous stromal material. Nuclei are vesicular with prominent nucleoli, mitotic activity is brisk, and the cytoplasm is amphophilic or eosinophilic and modest in quantity (figs. 8-39, 8-40) (32,88,110). Interpretation of this relatively nondescript image (compared with that of other epithelioid cell sarcomas) is aided in some cases by an obvious association between the tumor and a large cutaneous or subcutaneous nerve. Nevertheless, it is complicated in other instances by the fact that the neoplastic cells of epithelioid MPNST may show obvious melanin production, similar to melanotic neurilemmoma.

Differential Diagnosis. The pigment production in epithelioid MPNST brings metastatic melanoma (particularly the myxoid variant [17]) and clear cell sarcoma into the differential diagnosis. Electron microscopy shows the

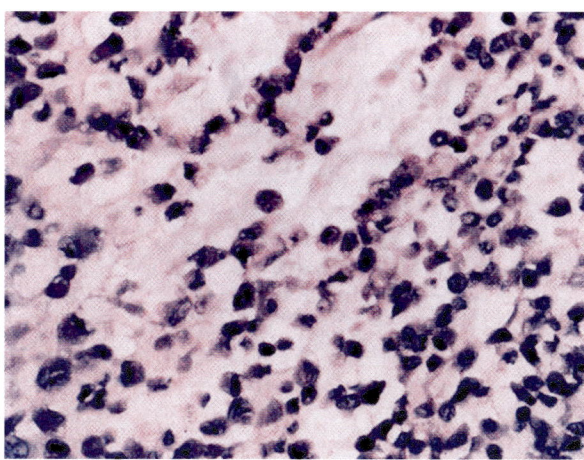

Figure 8-40

MALIGNANT PERIPHERAL NERVE SHEATH TUMOR

The tumor cells demonstrate open nuclear chromatin, discernible nucleoli, and amphophilic cytoplasm. They are set in a fibromyxoid stroma.

generic ultrastructural features of MPNST, but may demonstrate premelanosomes in the pigmented elements. Immunohistologic melanocytic markers are generally not observed in epithelioid MPNST.

Malignant Granular Cell Tumor

Clinical Features. *Malignant cutaneous granular cell tumors* (MGCT) are uncommon: less than 50 examples have been documented (3,4,20,76,87,109). They have an average size of 4 cm and are seemingly restricted to adult patients, with a predominance in women. Although no anatomic location is unknown as a site of origin for MGCT of the skin, most occur on the proximal extremities or trunk as subcutaneous nodules or ill-defined plaques.

Recurrence after adequate surgical excision is the usual indicator of aggressive biologic potential. Metastases of MGCT have been seen in over 50 percent of reported cases, and involve the regional lymph nodes, lung, liver, bone, and brain. Mortality approximates 80 percent (87).

Pathologic Findings. The microscopic features of MGCT are similar to those of its benign counterpart, as described above. Presumptive histologic signs of malignancy include broad zones of spontaneous necrosis, obvious invasion of stromal blood vessels, and numerous mitotic figures with atypical forms. It is also likely that the gross size of the tumor plays a role in determining its biology: tumors that are larger than 3 cm are at principal risk for recurrence or metastasis, provided that they also demonstrate the above-cited atypical microscopic features (109). Althausen et al. (4) have further suggested that a microscopically irregular (infiltrative) advancing tumor margin correlates with a risk of recurrence.

Although most MGCTs, like their benign counterpart, demonstrate a Schwannian phenotype by electron microscopy and immunohistologic analysis, a subset of granular cell tumors exists that is microscopically atypical and which has an "uncommitted" immunophenotype (73). These lesions are usually polypoid, with a maximum size of 2 cm or less. They may recur, but metastasis has not been reported.

Differential Diagnosis. The differential diagnosis of MGCT of the skin includes other primary cutaneous neoplasms as well as metastatic tumors with a granular cell appearance. Leiomyosarcoma of the skin may have a predominantly granular cell phenotype, as may basal cell carcinoma or angiosarcoma (60,72,73,84,91,111,123). Likewise, selected examples of metastatic adenocarcinoma with granular cell change may simulate the appearance of primary MGCT of the skin (47).

PSEUDOTUMORS OF THE SKIN RELATED TO THE NERVOUS SYSTEM

Rudimentary Meningocele (Primary Cutaneous Meningioma, Meningotheliomatous Hamartoma)

In 1974, Lopez et al. (144) reviewed the clinicopathologic attributes of several apparently meningothelial cutaneous lesions and adopted the term "acoelic meningeal hamartoma" to describe them. This term implies that the masses in question had no connection to the central nervous system or its coverings, and it also indicates that they were thought to be non-neoplastic. Sibley and Cooper (149), in 1989, had a similar interpretation: that a subset of cutaneous meningothelial lesions probably represented developmental malformations. These were called *rudimentary meningoceles,* signifying that they were formed by non-neoplastic rests of the meninges that had become entrapped within

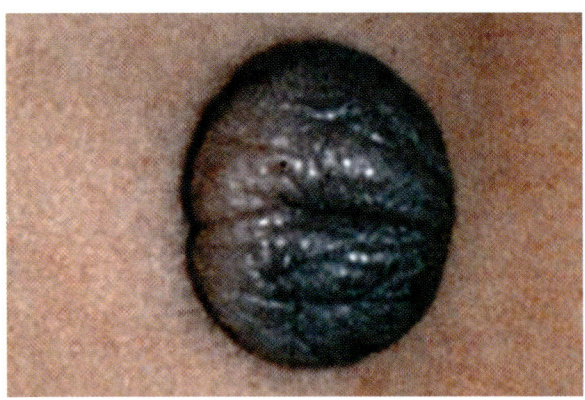

Figure 8-41

RUDIMENTARY MENINGOCELE

The lesion, in the skin of the lower neck in a child, is exophytic and fluctuant.

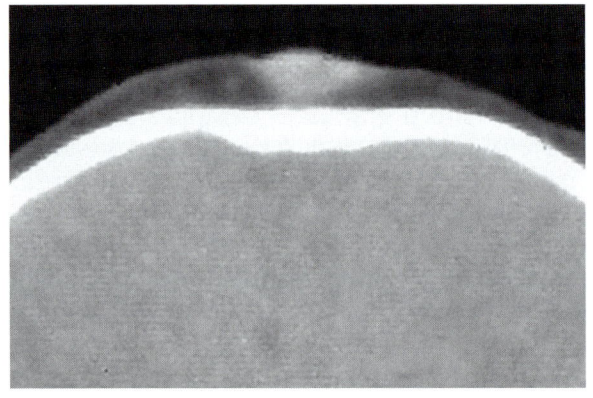

Figure 8-42

RUDIMENTARY MENINGOCELE

Computerized tomogram of the head shows a rudimentary meningocele in the occipital soft tissue. No underlying abnormalities in the cranial bones are apparent.

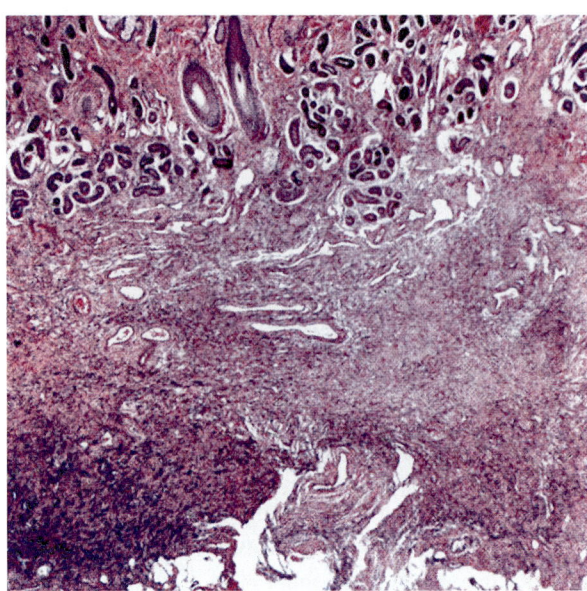

Figure 8-43

RUDIMENTARY MENINGOCELE

A racemose proliferation of spindle cells mantles pseudovascular spaces in the deep dermis and subcutis.

the integument early in life. This same interpretation was espoused by Suster and Rosai (151), except that the alternative term, *meningotheliomatous hamartoma*, was chosen for the lesion under discussion.

Clinical Findings. Whichever of these designations is preferred to describe them, rudimentary meningoceles have reproducible clinical features. Unlike true meningoceles, which are typically noted in the neonatal period and show radiographic evidence of continuity with the cerebral investments, rudimentary meningoceles manifest later in childhood as nodular, dermal-based lesions, usually in the skin of the posterior scalp or neck (fig. 8-41), sometimes in association with annular alopecia or an abnormal tuft of hair (134,139,143,146,150). There may be subjacent defects in cranial suture lines (fig. 8-42), but no underlying nervous system abnormalities are evident (145,149,151). These same features distinguish the rudimentary meningocele from secondary cutaneous meningiomas. The latter are seen typically in the frontal or superior scalp in middle-aged or elderly patients, and the lesions derive from direct cutaneous extension by true neoplasms of the meninges (144).

Pathologic Findings. The microscopic appearance is potentially deceptive. It features the deep dermal and subcutaneous proliferation of polygonal cells with oval nuclei, dispersed chromatin, and a moderate amount of amphophilic cytoplasm, arranged in a dyshesive, dissecting, permeative pattern in the supporting connective tissue (figs. 8-43, 8-44). Like meningothelial cells in general, the proliferating elements of rudimentary meningoceles are immunoreactive for epithelial membrane antigen and vimentin (145,149,151).

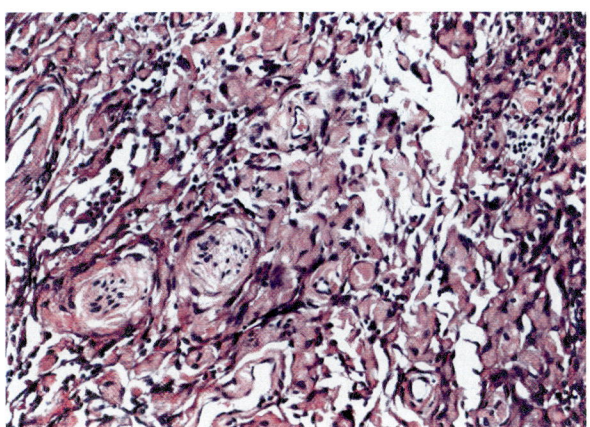

Figure 8-44

RUDIMENTARY MENINGOCELE

Cytologically bland spindle cells dissect through the dermal collagen and surround neurovascular structures.

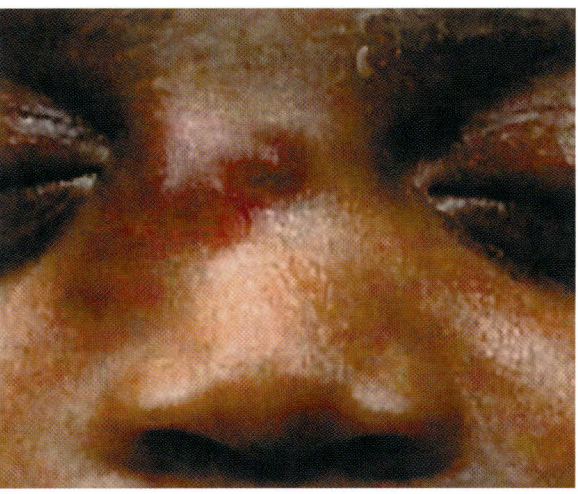

Figure 8-45

CUTANEOUS GLIAL HETEROTOPIA

Heterotopic glial tissue in the skin over the bridge of the nose (nasal glioma) in an infant is represented by multinodular cutaneous growth.

Differential Diagnosis. The intercellular spaces that are formed in rudimentary meningoceles and the overall image that is produced are reminiscent of the features of angiosarcomas or atypical hemangiomas (151). There are no erythrocytes in meningoceles, and serial sections may demonstrate the presence of small psammomatoid calcifications. The latter findings are not expected in vascular tumors, which are epithelial membrane antigen negative. Another differential diagnostic consideration is the neoplasm known as giant cell fibroblastoma (138), which similarly features the presence of intratumoral angiectoid channels. That lesion is found preferentially on the extremities of adolescents, it has a second constituent growth pattern that is composed of a more solid fibroblastic proliferation, and it is epithelial membrane antigen negative (145).

Cutaneous Glial Heterotopia (Nasal Glioma)

Clinical Features. Another malformation that is pathogenetically similar to rudimentary meningocele is *cutaneous glial heterotopia* (CGH), also known inaccurately as *nasal glioma* (136, 137,140–142,147,148,152). This lesion is seen in children; in pure form, it represents the growth of cerebral matter which has become detached completely from the subjacent brain during development. Other clinically similar masses are, instead, accompanied by patent subjacent meningeal tracts through the skull that are definable radiographically; these should be regarded technically as encephaloceles rather than heterotopias (152). Because gross examination is incapable of distinguishing CGH from an encephalocele, and casual excision of the latter lesion carries a major risk of iatrogenic meningitis, all patients with these abnormalities should be given a thorough neuroradiologic evaluation (135).

Both CGH and encephalocele characteristically present in the skin of the nasal bridge as single, asymptomatic, firm, and pink, tan, or violaceous nodules (fig. 8-45). Extension of the masses into the nasal cavity is seen in a minority of cases. There are typically no associated neural defects in these patients (140,148).

Pathologic Findings and Differential Diagnosis. The microscopic features of CGH are responsible for its having been assigned the erroneous designation of "glioma." A proliferation of astrocytes, with or without a minor population of oligodendroglia or the formation of plump eosinophilic Rosenthal fibers, is observed histologically, with compartmentalization by delicate fibrovascular stroma (figs. 8-46, 8-47). There is a fibrillary background neuropil, and scattered ganglion cells are apparent in a minority of cases. No secondary features of true glioma, such as perivascular hypercellu-

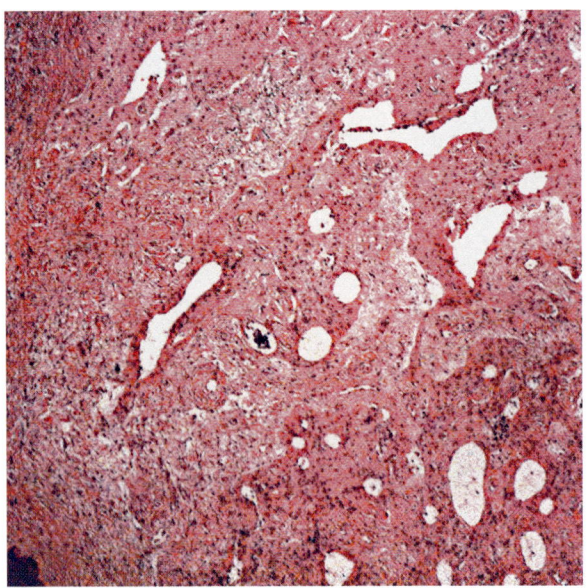

Figure 8-46

CUTANEOUS GLIAL HETEROTOPIA

Vague fascicles of bland stellate cells are punctuated by prominent stromal blood vessels in the dermis.

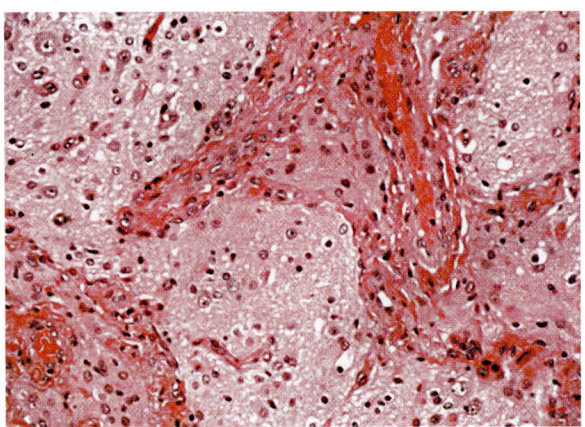

Figure 8-47

CUTANEOUS GLIAL HETEROTOPIA

The mixture of glial and neuronal elements is seen clearly.

larity or submeningeal astrocytic proliferation, are evident in CGH. Mitoses and necrosis are similarly absent (140,142,147,148,151).

If a demonstration of the non-neoplastic nature of CGH is desired, the proliferating glial cells can be labeled for glial fibrillary acidic protein immunohistologically; the matrical neuropil is reactive for neurofilament protein. Gan-

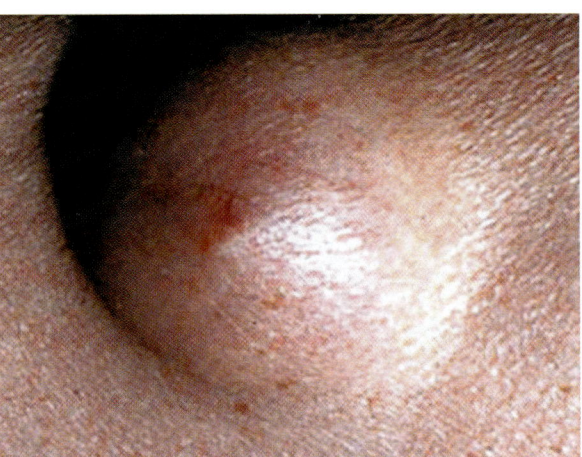

Figure 8-48

LIPOMA

Ordinary superficial lipoma of the upper arm is represented clinically by a compressible soft nodule in the subcutis.

glion cells are recognizable by stains for synaptophysin and MAP2. These conjoint observations are incompatible with the diagnosis of a true glioma (137).

TUMORS WITH ADIPOCYTIC DIFFERENTIATION

Primary cutaneous tumors with lipocytic features are, in our opinion, benign. These are considered individually in the following section. Liposarcoma does not arise in the skin, although it may secondarily involve the integument by extension from a contiguous but deeper anatomic origin, or via metastasis. Thus, readers are referred to texts on primary soft tissue tumors for a discussion of malignant adipocytic neoplasms.

Lipoma Variants

Clinical Features. Lipomas are almost ubiquitous in the adult population. When they arise in cosmetically unacceptable locations or in patients who are naturally anxious about "growths," they are excised.

Lipomas are easily compressible, mobile, irregularly nodular lesions that may be located in the deep soft tissues or the subcutis (fig. 8-48); they can attain an impressive size. The fatty nature of such tumors on cut section is usually obvious.

Particular clinical variants of lipoma with which the dermatologist must be familiar include

Tumors and Tumor-Like Conditions Showing Neural and Adipocytic Differentiation

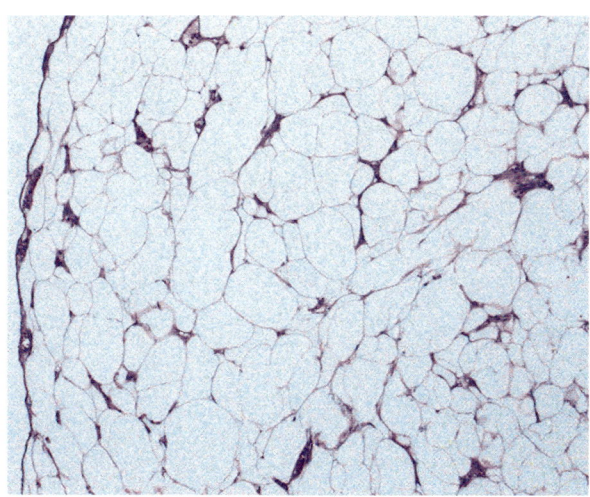

Figure 8-49

LIPOMA

Lipomas are composed of mature adipocytes bound by an attenuated fibrous capsule.

the *spindle cell* (153,160,161,163–165,167,181), *pleomorphic/atypical* (153,155,165,181), *sclerotic* (192), *fibrohistiocytic* (177), *glandular* (169), *chondroid* (175,180,182), and *vascular (angiolipomatous)* (159,170) subtypes. The first of these is most often seen on the upper trunk of elderly patients, with males predominating. The base of the neck and the interscapular region are particularly common sites of origin for spindle cell lipomas, and they occasionally may be multiple and familial (162,163). These lesions are firmer and more fixed to surrounding tissue than the usual lipoma, and therefore may engender some concern. Pleomorphic/atypical lipomas likewise have a firm consistency, and are observed on the extremities or the head and neck (187). Angiolipomas have a broader anatomic distribution, but are distinguished from other lipoma variants by their tendency to be painful when traumatized or palpated (170). Sclerotic, glandular, chondroid, and fibrohistiocytic lipomas are purely histologically defined subtypes, and their clinical features do not differ from those of ordinary benign adipocytic neoplasms.

Rare patients manifest the syndrome of familial lipomatosis, in which hundreds of fatty lesions appear throughout adult life in all topographic sites (174,183). Lipomas also may be components of Gardner's syndrome along with familial adenomatous polyposis of the colon (183).

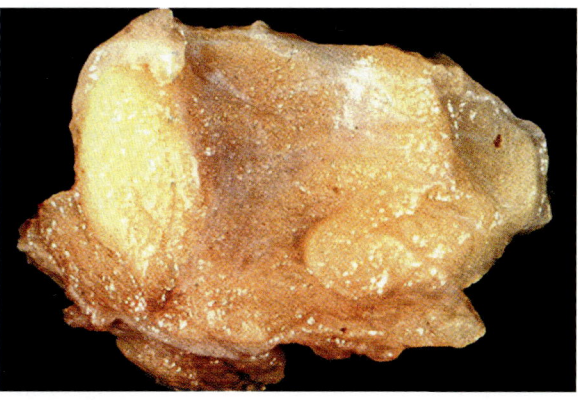

Figure 8-50

SPINDLE CELL LIPOMA

A variegated cut surface in which dense white-gray tissue punctuates obvious adipocytic areas.

Pathologic Findings and Differential Diagnosis. In their usual banal form, lipomas represent localized overgrowths of mature adipocytes that are bound by a thin fibrous capsule (fig. 8-49). The internal stroma is delicate and inconspicuous, and there is no tendency for matrical sclerosis with increasing size (183,186). Simple entrapment of adnexal epithelial structures (especially eccrine glands) in superficial lipomas yields the image of "adenolipoma" (glandular lipoma) (169); accordingly, we are unconvinced that the latter designation refers to a distinct pathologic entity.

Spindle cell lipoma is a triphasic neoplasm in which lobules of mature fat cells are interposed with dense zones of bland spindle cell growth and other areas of prominent myxoid stromal change (figs. 8-50, 8-51) (159,164). In some cases, the latter two components are dominant, leading to diagnostic consideration of a neural or fibroblastic proliferation; in rare examples, metaplastic osteoid or cartilage is seen in such tumors, or a prominent vascular stroma leads to diagnostic consideration of an endothelial lesion (pseudoangiomatous spindle cell lipoma) (168). French et al. (165) have described a purely dermal variant of spindle cell lipoma, which differs from subcutaneous lesions in showing a wider anatomic distribution and lack of histologic circumscription.

The differential diagnosis of spindle cell lipoma also includes mammary-type myofibroblastoma (179). This superficial soft tissue tumor

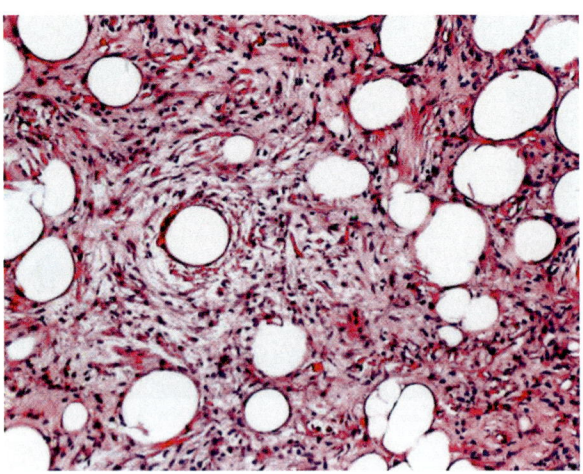
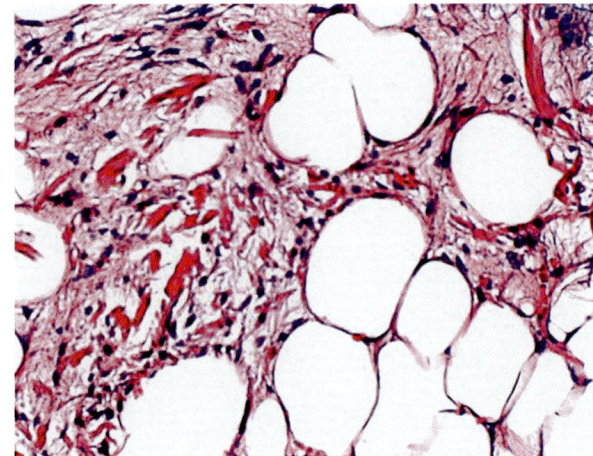

Figure 8-51

SPINDLE CELL LIPOMA

Left: There is an admixture of nondescript bland spindle cells, myxoid stroma, and mature lipocytes.
Right: The fusiform tumor cells are shown clearly in this figure.

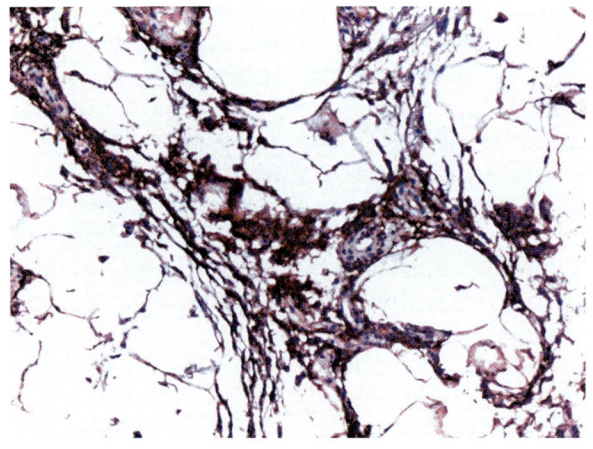

Figure 8-52

SPINDLE CELL LIPOMA

Immunoreactivity for CD34 is apparent.

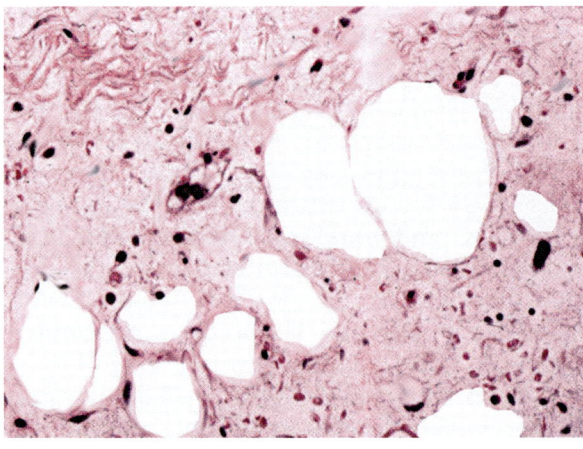

Figure 8-53

PLEOMORPHIC (ATYPICAL) LIPOMA

Scattered multinucleated ("floret") tumor cells with hyperchromatic nuclei are present.

is histologically indistinguishable from spindle cell lipoma; however, it is immunoreactive for myogenous markers such as desmin and muscle-specific actin, as well as CD34, whereas spindle cell lipoma labels only for the last of those determinants (fig. 8-52) (188). Another lesion that resembles spindle cell lipoma is the fibrous hamartoma of infancy. These proliferations occur in mutually exclusive patient populations and the CD34 positivity of spindle cell lipoma distinguishes it from fibrous hamartoma.

Pleomorphic, or atypical, lipoma differs from the usual type by its content of "floret" cells (fig. 8-53) (155,165,181,187). These are multinucleated and atypical but cytologically bland elements that are interspersed throughout the background population of mature adipocytes. A modest increase in stromal fibrous tissue also may be apparent within such masses, recalling the image of well-differentiated sclerosing liposarcoma of deep soft tissue. The overall configuration of the mass, including sharp circumscription, a

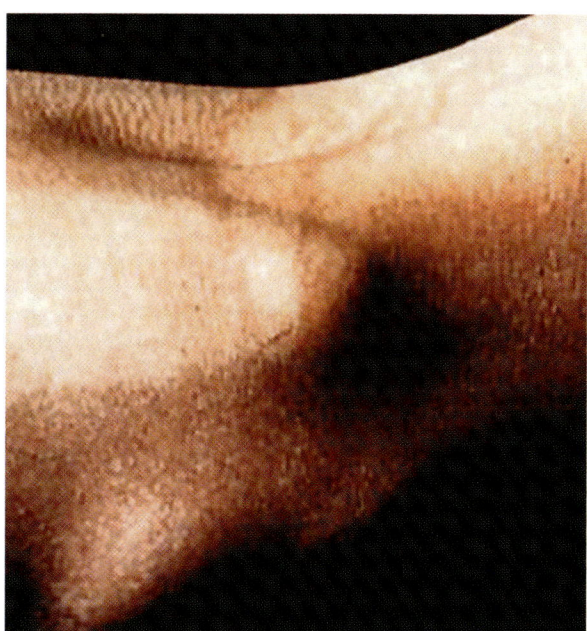

Figure 8-54

SUBCUTANEOUS ANGIOLIPOMA

The lesion is in the antecubital fossa. The overall appearance is superimposable with that of ordinary lipoma (see figure 8-48), but angiolipomas may be tender on palpation whereas simple lipomas are not.

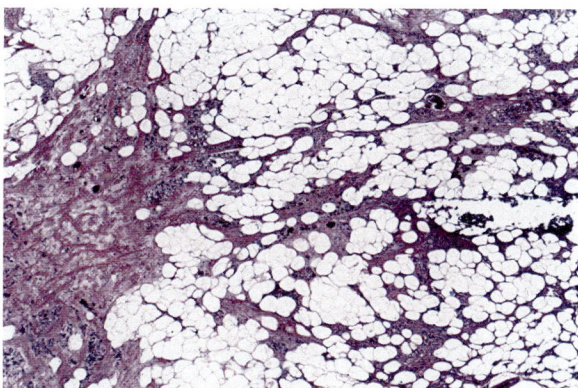

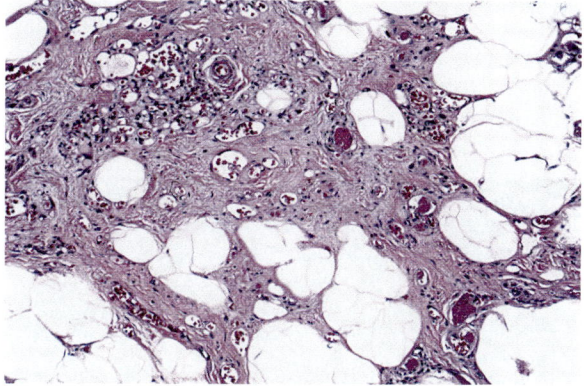

Figure 8-55

SUBCUTANEOUS ANGIOLIPOMA

Top: Small caliber blood vessels concentrate at the periphery of lesional fat lobules.

Bottom: Congeries of blood vessels in angiolipoma are often associated with intraluminal fibrin microthrombi, as shown here.

superficial location, and a lack of mitotic activity and lipoblasts, serves to allay concern over a diagnosis of malignancy (187). As stated previously, liposarcoma virtually never begins its growth in the subcutis.

Angiolipoma is typified by the proliferation of small groups of capillary- or venule-sized blood vessels in the setting of otherwise typical lipoma (159,170). The vascular clusters tend to be disposed toward the periphery of the adipocytic lobules, and may be associated with small collections of nondescript spindle cells (figs. 8-54, 8-55). One form of angiolipoma features the prominent overgrowth of vascular elements containing fibrin microthrombi, such that they actually dominate the mass. Such tumors, known as *cellular angiolipomas* (171,172), can be confused with angioleiomyomas, angiomyolipomas (also known as angiolipoleiomyomas) (154), and other lesions that are basically spindle cell proliferations. The consistent presence of lobulated aggregates of fat cells, microthrombi in stromal blood vessels, and foci of myxoid stromal change separate angiolipomas from these other possibilities. Moreover, angiomyolipomas show a greater integration of constituent blood vessels and smooth muscle cells throughout the lesions, as well as immunoreactivity with HMB45 (figs. 8-56, 8-57), unlike angiolipomas (154). Finally, a particular cytogenetic abnormality, deletion of chromosome 13q, is unique to spindle cell lipoma in this specific context (161). Based on its aggregated pathologic characteristics, it is very likely that yet another lipoma subtype, known as *dendritic fibromyxolipoma* (189), is simply a myxoid variant of spindle cell lipoma.

Sclerotic lipoma is a subcutaneous variant that is dominated by dense fibrosclerotic matrix, in which adipocytes are scattered (192). The collagenized zones often show a storiform pattern, like that of storiform collagenoma (sclerotic fibroma).

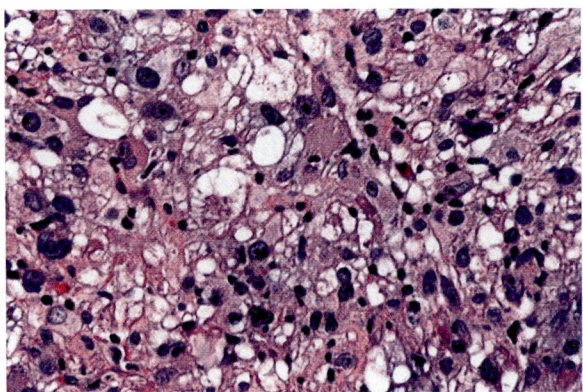

Figure 8-56

CELLULAR ANGIOMYOLIPOMA OF THE SUBCUTIS

Moderately pleomorphic polygonal and stellate cells are admixed with scant adipocytes.

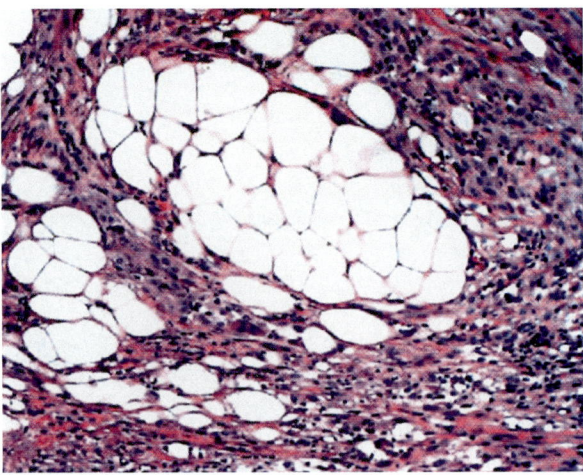

Figure 8-58

FIBROHISTIOCYTIC LIPOMA

Lesional fat lobules are partially effaced by a spindle cell proliferation like that seen in dermatofibroma or dermatofibrosarcoma.

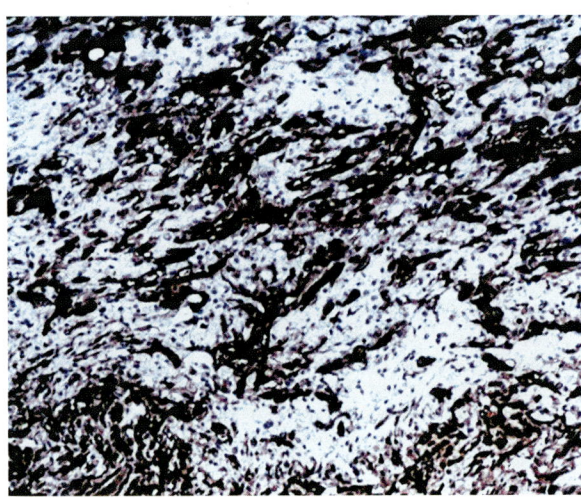

Figure 8-57

CELLULAR ANGIOMYOLIPOMA OF THE SUBCUTIS

Immunoreactivity with HMB45 and other melanocytic markers distinguishes angiomyolipoma of the subcutis from other skin tumors containing adipocytes.

Chondroid lipoma is a microscopically distinctive lesion that has the hybrid features of a lipoblastic proliferation and a chordoid/myxoid neoplasm and resembles extraskeletal chondrosarcoma (175,180,182). Lipocytic elements having eccentric nuclei and univacuolated cytoplasm are admixed with tumor cells that are more nondescript and polygonal, in a myxochondroid stroma. A diagnosis of malignancy is suggested by microscopy at high magnification, but this can be avoided by noting that the lesion is superficial (subcutaneous) and well-demarcated or even encapsulated. These features are not consonant with interpretations of either liposarcoma or chondrosarcoma.

Other ordinary lipomas may contain simple islands of mature cartilage. These should not be labeled as chondroid lipoma, and can instead be called *metaplastic lipoma*.

Fibrohistiocytic lipoma is similarly an amalgamated neoplasm that has conjoint microscopic features of simple lipoma with engrafted spindle cell zones that resemble dermatofibroma or dermatofibrosarcoma protuberans (DFSP) (fig. 8-58) (177). Despite the fact that both DFSP and fibrohistiocytic lipoma are CD34 positive, misdiagnosis can be avoided by attention to the circumscription of the tumor; moreover, the t(17;22) chromosomal translocation of DFSP (190) has not been reported in fibrohistiocytic lipoma. The fusiform elements in this lipoma variant are also immunoreactive for calponin (a myogenous marker), which has not been observed in DFSP. In our opinion, another tumor type, called *hemosiderotic fibrohistiocytic lipomatous lesion* (178), is simply a fibrohistiocytic lipoma that arises in the distal extremities. Because of that localization, the neoplasm is likely to be traumatized and accrue hemosiderin pigment in its stroma.

Lipoblastoma

Clinical Features. *Lipoblastoma* is confined to patients under the age of 5 years, and may occur singly or as part of a disseminated process (*lipoblastomatosis*) (157,173,176). Most lesions occur in the subcutis of the arms and legs as firm but compressible nodules of variable sizes (191). On cut section, they are well demarcated, and have a variably white-yellow appearance.

Pathologic Findings. Lipoblastoma demonstrates a range of embryonic-type adipocytic differentiation: a mixture of mature fat cells, bland stellate cells in a myxoid stroma, and lipoblasts with eccentric nuclei and univacuolated cytoplasm (157). The overall growth pattern is lobular, with aggregates of tumor cells separated from one another by delicate fibrovascular septa. Myxoid zones are often most prominent at the periphery of the cellular lobules; areas of prominent stromal vascularity may be apparent within myxoid areas, similar to those seen in angiolipomas. Mitotic activity may be observed in some lipoblastomas, but typically it is absent.

Differential Diagnosis. Because of the presence of lipoblasts and myxoid foci, lipoblastoma has been confused in the past with myxoid liposarcoma. Liposarcoma is rare in early childhood (173), and it virtually never arises in superficial soft tissue. Furthermore, myxoid liposarcoma shows a t(12;16) chromosomal translocation, whereas abnormalities in chromosome 8q typify lipoblastoma (185).

Hibernoma

Clinical Features. *Hibernomas* are rare tumors that demonstrate differentiation towards brown (fetal) fat (158,184). They are observed in patients of all ages; the subcuticular soft tissues of the head and neck, upper trunk, and axillae are the favored cutaneous sites of origin. The clinical appearance of such tumors is identical to that of conventional lipoma, but hibernomas are tan-brown rather than yellow on cut section (fig. 8-59) (156,184). They may be regarded simply as fetal lipomas because of these features.

Pathologic Findings. Hibernomas closely recapitulate the appearance of banal lipomas microscopically, except for the detailed features of the tumor cells. In contrast to a composition of mature adipocytes with uniformly lu-

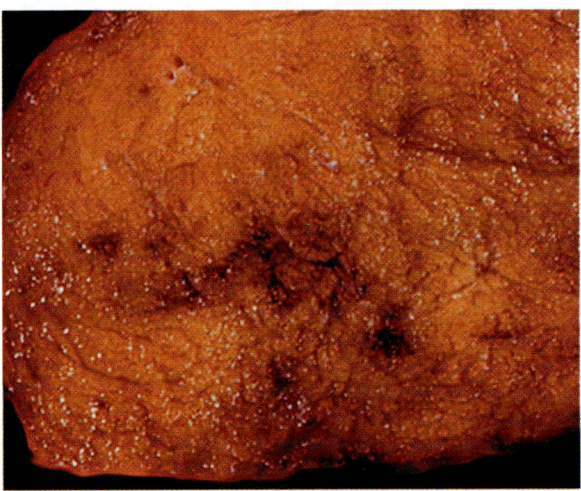

Figure 8-59

SUBCUTANEOUS HIBERNOMA

The cut surface of the lesion has a darker color than that of ordinary lipoma, owing to differentiation towards brown (fetal) fat.

cent single vacuoles, the cells of typical hibernomas are multivacuolated, with eosinophilic cytoplasm (figs. 8-60, 8-61) and internal lipofuscin granules. These lesions are usually well circumscribed or encapsulated, lobulated, and devoid of mitoses (158). Furlong et al. (166) have described three additional microscopic variants of hibernoma: myxoid, spindle cell, and lipoma-like. These correspondingly demonstrate a striking mucomyxoid stroma; zones that resemble the image of spindle cell lipoma (see above); and a scarcity of brown fat-type lipocytes.

Differential Diagnosis. As implied by the foregoing comments, hibernoma may resemble ordinary lipoma or lipoblastoma. The distinctive qualities of brown fat are usually sufficient to assure easy recognition of this lesion.

ADIPOCYTIC PSEUDOTUMORS

Nevus Lipomatosus

Clinical Features. *Nevus lipomatosus* is a cutaneous mesenchymal malformation that is commonly congenital in nature, rather than a true neoplasm (193,195,197,200,203). This lesion most often presents as multiple, sometimes agminated, soft, yellow-tan papules or nodules in the skin of the buttock, trunk, or extremities

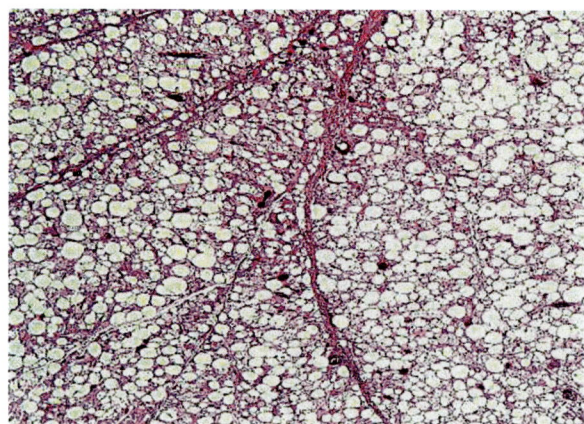

Figure 8-60

SUBCUTANEOUS HIBERNOMA

Lobules of adipocytes with notably amphophilic or eosinophilic cytoplasmic globules are apparent.

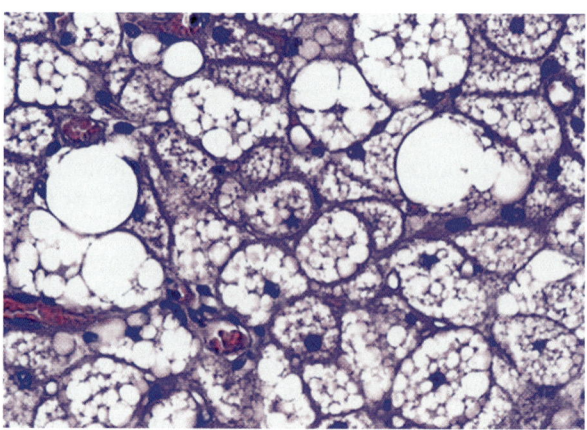

Figure 8-61

SUBCUTANEOUS HIBERNOMA

The tumor cells of hibernoma are identical to those seen in fetal fat.

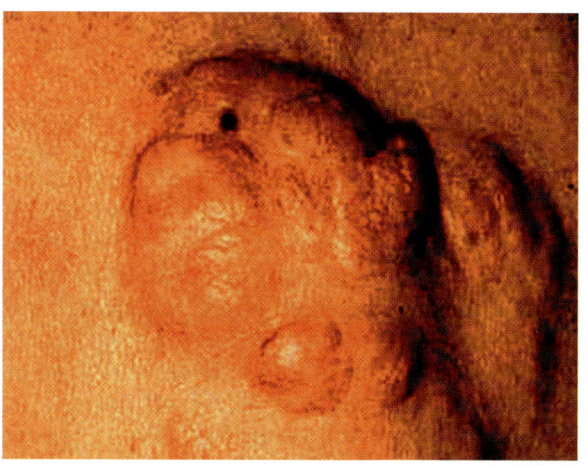

Figure 8-62

NEVUS LIPOMATOSUS

The lesion is on the truncal skin.

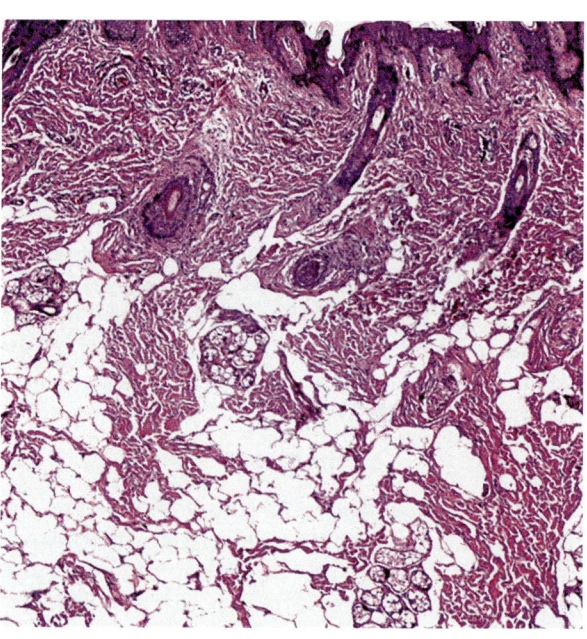

Figure 8-63

NEVUS LIPOMATOSUS

Groups of mature lipocytes are scattered irregularly throughout the dermis.

(fig. 8-62). The lesions may coalesce to form irregular plaques. Rarely, infants have disseminated nevus lipomatosus and extensively folded skin (the "Michelin tire baby" syndrome) (199, 204). Isolated lesions may be observed in children and adults, and these are nearly impossible to separate clinically from acrochordons.

Pathologic Findings. The primary microscopic feature of nevus lipomatosus is the presence of small groups of mature adipocytes at all levels of the dermis, particularly centered around adnexa and blood vessels (fig. 8-63). Accordingly, the junction between the corium and subcutis is often blurred (200). Lesions that clinically simulate acrochordons are polypoid, and their connective tissue cores show a mixed constitution of mature fat cells, collagen fibers, and small caliber stromal blood vessels. Some

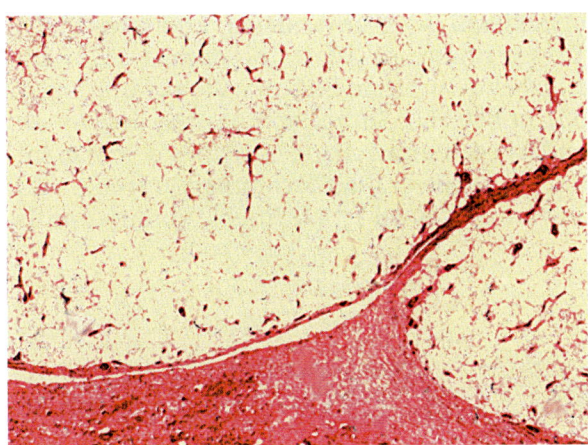

Figure 8-64

TUMEFACTIVE LIPEDEMA

Lobules of subcutaneous fat demonstrate the presence of intercellular and intracellular edema fluid.

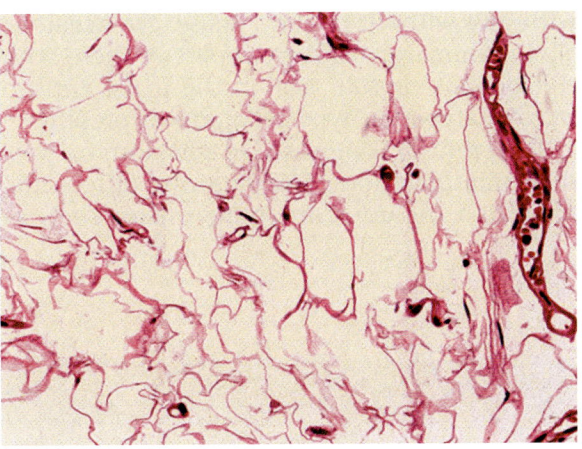

Figure 8-65

TUMEFACTIVE LIPEDEMA

Intercellular and intracellular adipocytic edema.

examples of the latter variant of nevus lipomatosus may, in actuality, represent resolving intradermal melanocytic nevi, as evidenced by the fact that small collections of nevocytes are sometimes present. The nevus cells may be highlighted with immunostains for S-100 protein. A morphologic overlap between nevus lipomatosus and connective tissue nevus has also been noted (203).

Differential Diagnosis. The differential diagnosis principally concerns the separation of nevus lipomatosus from true lipoma. If there is no intercalation of adipocytes into the interstices of the dermis, and especially if the lesion in question has an apparent fibrous capsule, we prefer a diagnosis of simple lipoma.

Tumefactive Localized Lipedema

Clinical Features. Lipedema is a condition that is less familiar to pathologists than it is to surgeons and physicians in cardiovascular medicine (194,205,206). The classic form affects women almost exclusively and is seen in middle life. Typical clinical findings include enlargement of both buttocks, bilaterally enlarged legs with an appearance like that of "Egyptian columns," sparing of the soft tissue of the feet, persistence of swelling even after prolonged elevation of the extremities, and a lack of pitting edema. Angiologic studies fail to show evidence of lymphatic or venous insufficiency in lymphedema, and the precise mechanism for the progressive accumulation of interstitial fluid is unknown. Treatment is either expectant or surgical, if the lesion interferes with limb function or is unsatisfactory cosmetically.

There is also a solitary form of the disease known as the *tumefactive localized lipedema* (TLL). *Lipedematous alopecia* represents that variant; it was initially described over 65 years ago by Cornbleet (196), who saw a female patient with hair loss whose scalp was said to feel like cotton batting. Several other examples of this disease have been recorded (198,201); all of the affected patients have been women, and none had lipedema of the legs or any other significant health problems. It is felt that alopecia evolves in this setting because of disturbances in the local oncotic environment of the scalp, and the effects of these disturbances on the viability of hair bulbs or papillae (198). We have encountered one example of TLL in the skin of the leg as well, and the clinical similarity to lipoma was striking in that case.

Pathologic Findings. Spaces are evident between and within the adipocytes in lipedema; the material they contain lacks tinctorial affinity, and yet the overall image is not that of an artifactual separation of the tissue elements (figs. 8-64, 8-65). No dilatation of lymphatic or vascular lumens is seen, nor is there an increase in the density of fibrous matrix. Colloidal iron stains, with and without hyaluronidase, are negative. No inflammatory cells are apparent, there is no collagenous capsule around the mass, and no nuclear atypia or hypercellularity is present.

Differential Diagnosis. In addition to a possible interpretation of lipoma, the differential diagnosis includes myxomucinoses such as myxedema, scleromyxedema, and scleredema. These conditions affect the dermis (202) and all label with Alcian blue or colloidal iron methods, unlike TLL. Simple lipomas may acquire secondary edematous change, but they do not manifest the scope of fluid accumulation seen in TLL and are contained by a definable fibrous capsule.

REFERENCES

Neural Lesions

1. Abenoza P, Sibley RK. Granular cell myoblastoma and schwannoma: fine structural and immunohistochemical study. Ultrastruct Pathol 1987;11:19–28.
2. Ahn SK, Ahn HJ, Kim TH, Hwang SM, Choi EH, Lee SH. Intratumoral fat in neurofibroma. Am J Dermatopathol 2002;24:326–9.
3. al-Sarraf M, Loud A, Vaitkevicius V. Malignant granular cell tumor. Histochemical and electron microscopic study. Arch Pathol 1971;91:550–8.
4. Althausen AM, Kowalski DP, Ludwig ME, Curry SL, Greene JF. Granular cell tumors: a new clinically important histologic finding. Gynecol Oncol 2000;77:310–3.
5. Altman CE, Hamill R, Pujals J. Multiple cutaneous granular cell tumors of the scrotum. Cutis 1999;63:77–80.
9. Angervall L, Kindblom LG, Haglid K. Dermal nerve sheath myxoma. A light and electron microscopic, histochemical an immunohistochemical study. Cancer 1984;53:1752–9.
10. Apisarnthanarax P. Granular cell tumor. An analysis of 16 cases and review of the literature. J Am Acad Dermatol 1981;5:171–83.
6. Argenyi ZB. Immunohistochemical characterization of palisaded encapsulated neuroma. J Cutan Pathol 1990;17:329–35.
7. Argenyi ZB. Newly recognized neural neoplasms relevant to the dermatopathologist. Dermatol Clin 1992;10:219–34.
8. Argenyi ZB, LeBoit PE, Santa Cruz D, Swanson PE, Kutzner H. Nerve sheath myxoma (neurothekeoma) of the skin: light microscopic and immunohistochemical reappraisal of the cellular variant. J Cutan Pathol 1993;20:294–303.
11. Bakos L. Multiple cutaneous granular cell tumors with systemic defects: a distinct entity? Int J Dermatol 1993;32:432–5.
12. Banerjee SS, Agbamu DA, Eyden BP, Harris M. Clinicopathological characteristics of peripheral primitive neuroectodermal tumor of skin and subcutaneous tissue. Histopathology 1997;31:355–66.
13. Barbagallo JS, Kolodzieh MS, Silverberg NB, Weinberg JM. Neurocutaneous disorders. Dermatol Clin 2002;20:547–60.
14. Barnhill RL, Dickersin GR, Nickeleit V, et al. Studies on the cellular origin of neurothekeoma: clinical, light microscopic, immunohistochemical, and ultrastructural observations. J Am Acad Dermatol 1991;25:80–8.
15. Barnhill RL, Mihm MC Jr. Cellular neurothekeoma. A distinctive variant of neurothekeoma mimicking nevomelanocytic tumors. Am J Surg Pathol 1990;14:113–20.
16. Bhawan J, Cao SL. Amelanotic blue nevus: a variant of blue nevus. Am J Dermatopathol 1999;21:225–8.
17. Bhuta S, Mirra JM, Cochran AJ. Myxoid malignant melanoma. A previously undescribed histologic pattern noted in metastatic lesions. Am J Surg Pathol 1986;10:203–11.
18. Billeret-Lebranchu V. [Granular cell tumor. Epidemiology of 263 cases.] Arch Anat Cytol Pathol 1999;47:26–30. (French.)
19. Busam KJ, Mentzel T, Colpaert C, Barnhill RL, Fletcher CD. Atypical or worrisome features in cellular neurothekeoma: a study of 10 cases. Am J Surg Pathol 1998;22:1067–72.
20. Cadotte M. Malignant granular-cell myoblastoma. Cancer 1974;33:1417–22.
21. Calonje E, Wilson-Jones E, Smith NP, Fletcher CD. Cellular neurothekeoma: an epithelioid variant of pilar leiomyoma? Morphological and immunohistochemical analysis of a series. Histopathology 1992;20:397–404.
22. Carney JA. Psammomatous melanotic schwannoma. A distinctive, heritable tumor with special associations, including cardiac myxoma and the Cushing syndrome. Am J Surg Pathol 1990;14:206–22.

23. Carney JA, Sizemore GW, Lovestedt SA. Mucosal ganglioneuromatosis, medullary thyroid carcinoma, and pheochromocytoma: multiple endocrine neoplasia, type 2b. Oral Surg 1976; 41:739–52.
24. Dabski C, Reiman HM Jr, Muller SA. Neurofibrosarcoma of skin and subcutaneous tissues. Mayo Clin Proc 1990;65:164–72.
25. D'Agostino AN, Soule EH, Miller RH. Sarcomas of the peripheral nerves and somatic soft tissues associated with multiple neurofibromatosis (von Recklinghausen's disease). Cancer 1963;16:1015–27.
26. Daimaru Y, Hashimoto H, Enjoji M. Malignant peripheral nerve-sheath tumors (malignant schwannomas). An immunohistochemical study of 29 cases. Am J Surg Pathol 1985;9:434–44.
27. Daimaru Y, Hashimoto H, Enjoji M. Malignant "triton" tumors: a clinicopathologic and immunohistochemical study of nine cases. Hum Pathol 1984;15:768–78.
28. Dakin MC, Leppard B, Theaker JM. The palisaded encapsulated neuroma (solitary circumscribed neuroma). Histopathology 1992;20:405–10.
29. Dehner LP. Peripheral and central neuroectodermal tumors. A nosologic concept seeking a consensus. Arch Pathol Lab Med 1986;110:997–1005.
30. Dehner LP. Primitive neuroectodermal tumor and Ewing's sarcoma. Am J Surg Pathol 1993; 17:1–13.
31. Diaz-Cascajo C, Hoos A. Histopathologic features of malignant peripheral nerve sheath tumor are not restricted to metastatic malignant melanoma and can be found in primary malignant melanoma also. Am J Surg Pathol 2000; 24:1438–9.
32. DiCarlo EF, Woodruff JM, Bansal M, Erlandson RA. The purely epithelioid malignant peripheral nerve sheath tumor. Am J Surg Pathol 1986;10:478–90.
33. DiMaio SM, Mackay B, Smith JL Jr, Dickersin GR. Neurosarcomatous transformation in malignant melanoma: an ultrastructural study. Cancer 1982;50:2345–54.
34. Dover JS, From L, Lewis A. Clinicopathologic findings in palisaded encapsulated neuromas. J Cutan Pathol 1986;13:77–82.
35. Dover JS, From L, Lewis A. Palisaded encapsulated neuromas. A clinicopathologic study. Arch Dermatol 1989;125:386–9.
36. Drut R, Drut RM, Cohen M. Adnexal-centered giant congenital melanocytic nevus with extensive ganglioneuromatous component and trisomy 7. Pediatr Dev Pathol 1999;2:473–7.
37. Dubovy SR, Clark BJ. Palisaded encapsulated neuroma (solitary circumscribed neuroma of skin) of the eyelid: report of two cases and review of the literature. Br J Ophthalmol 2001; 85:949–51.
38. Ducatman BS, Scheithauer BW, Piepgras DG, Reiman HM, Ilstrup DM. Malignant peripheral nerve sheath tumors. A clinicopathologic study of 120 cases. Cancer 1986;57:2006–21.
39. Fetsch JF, Michal M, Miettinen M. Pigmented (melanotic) neurofibroma: a clinicopathologic and immunohistochemical analysis of 19 lesions from 17 patients. Am J Surg Pathol 2000; 24:331–43.
40. Fine SW, Li M. Expression of calretinin and the alpha-subunit of inhibin in granular cell tumors. Am J Clin Pathol 2003;119:259–64.
41. Fletcher CD. Solitary circumscribed neuroma of the skin (so-called palisaded encapsulated neuroma). A clinicopathologic and immunohistochemical study. Am J Surg Pathol 1989; 13:574–80.
42. Fletcher CD, Chan JK, McKee PH. Dermal nerve sheath myxoma: a study of three cases. Histopathology 1986;10:135–45.
43. Fletcher CD, Davies SE. Benign plexiform (multinodular) schwannoma: a rare tumor unassociated with neurofibromatosis. Histopathology 1986;10:971–80.
44. Fletcher CD, Davies SE, McKee PH. Cellular schwannoma: a distinct pseudosarcomatous entity. Histopathology 1987;11:21–35.
45. Font RL, Truong LD. Melanotic schwannoma of soft tissues. Electron-microscope observations and review of the literature. Am J Surg Pathol 1984;8:129–38.
46. Franchi A, Massi D, Santucci M. Desmoplastic cutaneous ganglioneuroma. Histopathology 1999;34:82–4.
47. Franzblau MJ, Manwaring J, Plumhof C, Listrom MB, Burgdorf WH. Metastatic breast carcinoma mimicking granular cell tumor. J Cutan Pathol 1989;16:218–22.
48. Gallager RL, Helwig EB. Neurothekeoma—a benign cutaneous tumor of neural origin. Am J Clin Pathol 1980;74:759–64.
48. Gambini C, Rongioletti F. Primary congenital cutaneous ganglioneuroma. J Am Acad Dermatol 1996;35:353–4.
50. Gancberg D, Feoli F, Hamels J, et al. Trisomy 6 in Merkel cell carcinoma: a recurrent chromosomal aberration. Histopathology 2000;37:445–51.
51. Geffner RE, Hassell CM. Ganglioneuroma of the skin. Arch Dermatol 1986;122:377–8.
52. George E, Swanson PE, Wick MR. Malignant peripheral nerve sheath tumors of the skin. Am J Dermatopathol 1989;11:213–21.

53. Goldstein J, Lifshitz T. Myxoma of the nerve sheath. Report of three cases, observations by light and electron microscopy and histochemical analysis. Am J Dermatopathol 1985;7:423–9.

53a. Gray MH, Smoller BR, McNutt NS, Hsu A. Immunohistochemical demonstration of factor XIIIa expression in neurofibromas. A practical means of differentiating these tumors from neurotized melanocytic nevi and schwannomas. Arch Dermatol 1990;126:472–6.

54. Gross VL, Lynfield Y. Multiple cutaneous granular cell tumors: a case report and review of the literature. Cutis 2000;69:343–6.

55. Gururangan S, Marina NM, Luo X, et al. Treatment of children with peripheral primitive neuroectodermal tumor or extraosseous Ewing's tumor with Ewing's-directed therapy. J Pediatr Hematol Oncol 1998;20:55–61.

56. Halling KC, Scheithauer BW, Halling AC, et al. p53 expression in neurofibroma and malignant peripheral nerve sheath tumor. An immunohistochemical study of sporadic and NF1-associated tumors. Am J Clin Pathol 1996;106:282–8.

57. Hammond RR, Walton JC. Cutaneous ganglioneuromas: a case report and review of the literature. Hum Pathol 1996;27:735–8.

58. Hasegawa SL, Davison JM, Rutten A, Fletcher JA, Fletcher CD. Primary cutaneous Ewing's sarcoma: immunophenotypic and molecular cytogenetic evaluation of five cases. Am J Surg Pathol 1998;22:310–8.

59. Hashimoto H, Enjoji M, Nakajima T, Kiryu H, Daimaru Y. Malignant neuroepithelioma (peripheral neuroblastoma). A clinicopathologic study of 15 cases. Am J Surg Pathol 1983;7:309–18.

60. Hayden AA, Shamma HN. Ber-EP4 and MNF-16 in a previously undescribed morphologic pattern of granular basal cell carcinoma. Am J Dermatopathol 2001;23:530–2.

61. Husain S, Silvers DN, Halperin AJ, McNutt NS. Histologic spectrum of neurothekeoma and the value of immunoperoxidase staining for S-100 protein in distinguishing it from melanoma. Am J Dermatopathol 1994;16:496–503.

62. Inaba M, Yamamoto T, Minami R, Ohbayashi C, Hanioka K. Pigmented neurofibroma: report of two cases and literature review. Pathol Int 2001;51:565–9.

63. Iwashita T, Enjoji M. Plexiform neurilemmoma: a clinicopathological and immunohistochemical analysis of 23 tumours from 20 patients. Virchows Arch A Pathol Anat Histopathol 1987;411:305–9.

64. Jacinto CM, Grant-Kels JM, Knibbs DR, Daman LA, Piorkowski RJ. Malignant peripheral neuroectodermal tumor presenting as a scalp nodule. Am J Dermatopathol 1991;13:63–70.

65. Jurgens H, Bier V, Harms D, et al. Malignant peripheral neuroectodermal tumors. A retrospective analysis of 42 patients. Cancer 1988;61:349–57.

66. Kao GF, Laskin WB, Olsen TG. Solitary cutaneous plexiform neurilemmoma (schwannoma): a clinicopathologic, immunohistochemical, and ultrastructural study of 11 cases. Mod Pathol 1989;2:20–6.

67. Kindblom LG, Ahlden M, Meis-Kindblom JM, Stenman G. Immunohistochemical and molecular analysis of p53, MDM2, proliferating cell nuclear antigen, and Ki-67 in benign and malignant peripheral nerve sheath tumors. Virchows Arch 1995;427:19–26.

68. Kiryu H, Urabe H. Malignant Triton tumor. A case with protein histopathological patterns. Am J Dermatopathol 1992;14:255–62.

69. Kossard S, Kumar A, Wilkinson B. Neural spectrum: palisaded encapsulated neuroma and verocay body poor dermal schwannoma. J Cutan Pathol 1999;26:31–6.

70. Kuo LA, Kuo RS. Plexiform neurofibromatosis: a difficult surgical problem. Aust NZ J Surg 1990;60:732–5.

71. Lack EE, Worsham GF, Callihan MD, et al. Granular cell tumor: a clinicopathologic study of 110 patients. J Surg Oncol 1980;13:301–16.

72. Lacroix-Triki M, Rochaix P, Marques B, Coindre JM, Voigt JJ. [Granular cell tumors of the skin of non-neural origin: report of 8 cases.] Ann Pathol 1999;19:94–8. (French.)

73. LeBoit PE, Barr RJ, Burall S, Metcalf JS, Yen TS, Wick MR. Primitive polypoid granular-cell tumor and other cutaneous granular cell neoplasms of apparent nonneural origin. Am J Surg Pathol 1991;15:48–58.

74. Lee CS, Southey MC, Slater H, Auldist AW, Chow CW, Venter DJ. Primary cutaneous Ewing's sarcoma/peripheral primitive neuroectodermal tumors in childhood. A molecular, cytogenetic, and immunohistochemical study. Diagn Molec Pathol 1995;4:174–81.

75. Lee JY, Martinez AJ, Abell E. Ganglioneuromatous tumor of the skin: a combined heterotopia of ganglion cells and hamartomatous neuroma: report of a case. J Cutan Pathol 1988;15:58–61.

76. MacKenzie DH. Malignant granular cell myoblastoma. J Clin Pathol 1967;20:739–42.

77. McCarroll HR. Clinical manifestations of congenital neurofibromatosis. J Bone Joint Surg 1950;32A:601–17.

78. McCarron KF, Goldblum JR. Plexiform neurofibroma with and without associated malignant peripheral nerve sheath tumor: a clinicopathologic and immunohistochemical analysis of 54 cases. Mod Pathol 1998;11:612–7.
79. McMenamin ME, Fletcher CD. Expanding the spectrum of malignant change in schwannomas: epithelioid malignant change, epithelioid malignant peripheral nerve sheath tumor, and epithelioid angiosarcoma: a study of 17 cases. Am J Surg Pathol 2001;25:13–25.
80. Mechtersheimer G, Staudter M, Moller P. Expression of the natural killer cell-associated antigens CD56 and CD57 in human neural and striated muscle cells and in their tumors. Cancer Res 1991;51:1300–7.
81. Megahed M. Palisaded encapsulated neuroma (solitary circumscribed neuroma). A clinicopathologic and immunohistochemical study. Am J Dermatopathol 1994;16:120–5.
82. Megahed M. Plexiform schwannoma. Am J Dermatopathol 1994;16:288–93.
83. Mennemeyer RP, Hallman KO, Hammar SP, Raisis JE, Tytus JS, Bockus D. Melanotic schwannoma. Clinical and ultrastructural studies of three cases with evidence of intracellular melanin synthesis. Am J Surg Pathol 1979;3:3–10.
84. Mentzel T, Wadden C, Fletcher CD. Granular cell change in smooth muscle tumors of skin and soft tissue. Histopathology 1994;24:223–31.
85. Michal M, Fanburg-Smith JC, Mentzel T, et al. Dendritic neurofibroma with pseudorosettes: a report of 18 cases of a distinct and hitherto unrecognized neurofibroma variant. Am J Surg Pathol 2001;25:587–94.
86. Mierau GW. Extraskeletal Ewing's sarcoma (peripheral neuroepithelioma). Ultrastruct Pathol 1985;9:91–8.
87. Miracco C, Andreassi A, Laurini L, De Santi MM, Taddeucci P, Tosi P. Granular cell tumor with histological signs of malignancy: report of a case and comparison with 10 benign and 4 atypical cases. Br J Dermatol 1999;141:573–5.
88. Morgan KG, Gray C. Malignant epithelioid schwannoma of superficial soft tissue? A case report with immunohistology and electron microscopy. Histopathology 1985;9:765–75.
89. Murakami T, Kiyosawa T, Murata S, Usui K, Ohtsuki M, Nakagawa H. Malignant schwannoma with melanocytic differentiation arising in a patient with neurofibromatosis. Br J Dermatol 2000;143:1078–82.
90. Nicholson SA, McDermott MB, Swanson PE, Wick MR. CD99 and cytokeratin-20 in small-cell and basaloid tumors of the skin. Appl Immunohistochem Molec Morphol 2000;8:37–41.
91. Orosz Z. Atypical fibroxanthoma with granular cells. Histopathology 1998;33:88–9.
92. Orosz Z. Cutaneous epithelioid schwannoma: an unusual benign neurogenic tumor. J Cutan Pathol 1999;26:213–4.
93. Oshman RG, Phelps RG, Kantor I. A solitary neurofibroma on the finger. Arch Dermatol 1988;122:1185–6.
94. Patterson JW, Maygarden SJ. Extraskeletal Ewing's sarcoma with cutaneous involvement. J Cutan Pathol 1986;13:46–58.
95. Peters MS, Reiman HM, Muller SA. Cutaneous extraskeletal Ewing's sarcoma. J Cutan Pathol 1985;12:476–85.
96. Preston FW, Walsh WS, Clarke TH. Cutaneous neurofibromatosis (von Recklinghausen's disease): clinical manifestations and incidence of sarcoma in 61 male patients. Arch Surg 1952;64:813–27.
97. Pulitzer DR, Reed RJ. Nerve-sheath myxoma (perineurial myxoma). Am J Dermatopathol 1985;7:409–18.
98. Radice F, Gianotti R. Cutaneous ganglion cell tumor of the skin. Case report and review of the literature. Am J Dermatopathol 1993;15:488–91.
99. Reed RJ, Bliss BO. Morton's neuroma. Regressive and productive intermetatarsal elastofibrositis. Arch Pathol 1973;95:123–9.
100. Reed RJ, Fine RM, Meltzer HD. Palisaded encapsulated neuromas of the skin. Arch Dermatol 1972;106:865–70.
101. Rios JJ, Diaz-Cano SJ, Rivera-Hueto F, Villar JL. Cutaneous ganglion cell choristoma. Report of a case. J Cutan Pathol 1991;18:469–73.
102. Rosati LA, Fratamico CM, Eusebi V. Cellular neurothekeoma. Appl Pathol 1986;4:186–91.
103. Ross DE. Skin manifestations of von Recklinghausen's disease and associated tumors (neurofibromatosis). Am Surg 1965;31:729–40.
104. Sangueza OP, Sangueza P, Valda LR, Meshul CK, Requena L. Multiple primitive neuroectodermal tumors. J Am Acad Dermatol 1994;31:356–61.
105. San Juan J, Monteagudo C, Navarro P, Terradez JJ. Basal cell carcinoma with prominent central palisading of epithelial cells mimicking schwannoma. J Cutan Pathol 1999;26:528–32.
106. Saxen E. Tumours of tactile end-organs. Acta Pathol Microbiol Scand 1948;25:66–79.
107. Saxen E. Tumors of the sheaths of the peripheral nerves (studies on their structure). Acta Pathol Microbiol Scand 1948;79(Suppl):1–135.
108. Scotti TM. The lesion of Morton's metatarsalgia (Morton's toe). AMA Arch Pathol 1957;63:91–102.

109. Shimamura K, Osamura RY, Ueyama Y, et al. Malignant granular cell tumor of the right sciatic nerve. Report of an autopsy case with electron microscopic, immunohistochemical, and enzyme histochemical studies. Cancer 1984; 53:524–9.
110. Sidbury R, Heintz PW, Beckstead JH, White CR Jr. Cutaneous malignant epithelioid neoplasms. Adv Dermatol 1999;14:285–306.
111. Sironi M, Assi A, Pasquinelli G, Cenacchi G. Not all granular cell tumors show schwann cell differentiation: a granular cell leiomyosarcoma of the thumb, a case report. Am J Dermatopathol 1999;21:307–9.
112. Skelton HG, Williams J, Smith KJ. The clinical and histologic spectrum of cutaneous fibrous perineuriomas. Am J Dermatopathol 2001; 23:190–6.
113. Smith LM, Adams RH, Brothman AR, Vanderhooft SL, Coffin CM. Peripheral primitive neuroectodermal tumor presenting with diffuse cutaneous involvement and 7;22 translocation. Med Pediatr Oncol 1998;30:357–63.
114. Sobel HJ, Churg J. Granular cells and granular cell lesions. Arch Pathol 1964;77:132–41.
115. Sobel HJ, Marquet E. Granular cells and granular cell lesions. Pathol Annu 1974;9:43–79.
116. Sobel HJ, Schwartz R, Marquet E. Light- and electron-microscopic study of the origin of granular-cell myoblastoma. J Pathol 1973; 109:101–11.
117. Spatz A, Peterse S, Fletcher CD, Barnhill RL. Plexiform spitz nevus: an intradermal spitz nevus with plexiform growth pattern. Am J Dermatopathol 1999;21:542–6.
118. Stout AP. Neurofibroma and neurilemoma. Clin Proc 1946;5:1–12.
119. Swanson PE, Scheithauer BW, Wick MR. Peripheral nerve sheath neoplasms. Clinicopathologic and immunohistochemical observations. Pathol Annu 1995;30(Pt 2):1–82.
120. Taxy JB, Battifora H. Epithelioid schwannoma: diagnosis by electron microscopy. Ultrastruct Pathol 1981;2:19–24.
121. Taylor GB, Chan YF. Subcutaneous primitive neuroectodermal tumor in the abdominal wall of a child: long-term survival after local excision. Pathology 2000;32:294–8.
122. Theaker JM, Fletcher CD. Epithelial membrane antigen expression by the perineurial cell: further studies of peripheral nerve lesions. Histopathology 1989;14:581–92.
123. Val-Bernal JF. Dermatofibroma with granular cells. Histopathology 1997;31:481–2.
124. Val-Bernal JF, de sa Dehesa J, Garijo MF, Val D. Cutaneous lipomatous neurofibroma. Am J Dermatopathol 2002;24:246–50.
125. Westermann F, Schwab M. Genetic parameters of neuroblastomas. Cancer Lett 2002;184:127–47.
126. Wick MR. Immunohistology of melanocytic neoplasms. In: Dabbs DJ, ed. Diagnostic immunohistochemistry. Philadelphia: WB Saunders; 2002.
127. Wick MR. Malignant peripheral nerve sheath tumors of the skin. Mayo Clin Proc 1990;65: 279–82.
128. Wick MR, Swanson PE, Scheithauer BW, Manivel JC. Malignant peripheral nerve sheath tumor. An immunohistochemical study of 62 cases. Am J Clin Pathol 1987;87:425–33.
129. Wong TY, Suster S. Primary cutaneous sarcomas showing rhabdomyoblastic differentiation. Histopathology 1995;26:25–32.
130. Woodruff JM. Peripheral nerve tumors showing glandular differentiation (glandular schwannomas). Cancer 1976;37:2399–413.
131. Xia SJ, Pressey JG, Barr FG. Molecular pathogenesis of rhabdomyosarcoma. Cancer Biol Ther 2002;1:97–104.
132. Zamecnik M, Michal M. Perineurial cell differentiation in neurofibromas. Report of eight cases including a case with composite perineurioma-neurofibroma features. Pathol Res Pract 2001;197:537–44.
133. Zelger B, Weinlich G, Zelger B. Perineurioma. A frequently unrecognized entity with emphasis on a plexiform variant. Adv Clin Pathol 2000;4:25–33.

Pseudotumors of the Skin Related to the Nervous System

134. Argenyi ZB. Cutaneous neural heterotopias and related tumors relevant for the dermatopathologist. Semin Diagn Pathol 1996;13:60–71.
135. Barkovich AJ, Vandermarck P, Edwards MS, Cogen PH. Congenital nasal masses: CT and MR imaging features in 16 cases. Am J Neuroradiol 1991;12:105–16.
136. Brunsting HA. Nasal glioma. Cutis 1981;27:43–6.
137. Cerda-Nicolas M, Sanchez-Fernandez de Sevilla C, Lopez-Gines C, Peydro-Olaya A, Llombart-Bosch A. Nasal glioma or nasal glial heterotopia? Morphological, immunohistochemical, and ultrastructural study of two cases. Clin Neuropathol 2002;21:66–71.
138. Dymock RB, Allen PW, Stirling JW, Gilbert EF, Thombery JM. Giant cell fibroblastoma. A distinctive recurrent tumor of childhood. Am J Surg Pathol 1987;11:263–71.
139. El Shabrawi-Caelen L, White WL, Soyer HP, Kim BS, Frieden IJ, McCalmont TH. Rudimentary meningocele: remnant of a neural tube defect? Arch Dermatol 2001;137:45–50.

140. Fletcher CD, Carpenter G, McKee PH. Nasal glioma. A rarity. Am J Dermatopathol 1986;8:341–6.
141. Gambini C, Rongioletti F, Rebora A. Proliferation of eccrine sweat ducts associated with heterotopic neural tissue (nasal glioma). Am J Dermatopathol 2000;22:179–82.
142. Gebhart W, Hohlbrugger H, Lassmann H, Ramadan W. Nasal glioma. Int J Dermatol 1982;21:212–5.
143. Kishimoto H, Nagata S, Yamada A, Nishioka K. Rudimentary meningocele presenting with an annular alopecia. Eur J Dermatol 2000;10:215–6.
144. Lopez DA, Silvers DN, Helwig EB. Cutaneous meningioma—a clinicopathologic study. Cancer 1974;34:728–44.
145. Marrogi AJ, Swanson PE, Kyriakos M, Wick MR. Rudimentary meningocele of the skin. Clinicopathologic features and differential diagnosis. J Cutan Pathol 1991;18:178–88.
146. Mihara Y, Miyamoto T, Hagari Y, Mihara M. Rudimentary meningocele of the scalp. J Dermatol 1997;24:606–10.
147. Mirra SS, Pearl GS, Hoffman JC, Campbell WG Jr. Nasal 'glioma' with prominent neuronal component: report of a case. Arch Pathol Lab Med 1981;105:540–1.
148. Patterson K, Kapur S, Chandra RS. "Nasal glioma" and related brain heterotopias: a pathologist's perspective. Ped Pathol 1986;5:353–62.
149. Sibley DA, Cooper PH. Rudimentary meningocele: a variant of "primary cutaneous meningioma." J Cutan Pathol 1989;16:72–80.
150. Stone MS, Walker PS, Kennard CD. Rudimentary meningocele presenting with a scalp hair tuft. Report of two cases. Arch Dermatol 1994;130:775–7.
151. Suster S, Rosai J. Hamartoma of the scalp with ectopic meningothelial elements. A distinctive benign soft tissue lesion that may simulate angiosarcoma. Am J Surg Pathol 1990;14:1–11.
152. Younus M, Coode PE. Nasal glioma and encephalocele: two separate entities. Report of two cases. J Neurosurg 1986;64:516–9.

Tumors with Adipocytic Differentiation

153. Allen PW, Strungs I, MacCormac LB. Atypical subcutaneous fatty tumors: a review of 37 referred cases. Pathology 1998;30:123–35.
154. Buyukbabani N, Tetikkurt S, Ozturk AS. Cutaneous angiomyolipoma: report of two cases with emphasis on HMB-45 utility. J Eur Acad Dermatol Venereol 1998;11:151–4.
155. Challis D. Atypical subcutaneous fatty tumors. Adv Anat Pathol 2000;7:94–9.
156. Chen DY, Wang CM, Chan HL. Hibernoma. Case report and literature review. Dermatol Surg 1998;24:393–5.
157. Chung EB, Enzinger FM. Benign lipoblastomatosis. An analysis of 35 cases. Cancer 1973;32:482–92.
158. Dardick I. Hibernoma: a possible model of brown fat histogenesis. Hum Pathol 1978;9:321–9.
159. Dixon AY, McGregor DH, Lee SH. Angiolipomas: an ultrastructural and clinicopathologic study. Hum Pathol 1981;12:739–47.
160. Domanski HA, Carlen B, Jonsson K, Mertens F, Akerman M. Distinct cytologic features of spindle cell lipoma. A cytologic-histologic study with clinical, radiologic, electron microscopic, and cytogenetic correlations. Cancer 2001;93:381–9.
161. Dumollard JM, Ranchere-Vince D, Burel F, et al. [Spindle cell lipoma and 13q deletion: diagnostic utility of cytogenetic analysis.] Ann Pathol 2001;21:303–10. (French.)
162. Enzinger FM, Harvey DA. Spindle-cell lipoma. Cancer 1975;36:1852–9.
163. Fanburg-Smith JC, Devaney KO, Miettinen M, Weiss SW. Multiple spindle cell lipomas: a report of 7 familial and 11 nonfamilial cases. Am J Surg Pathol 1998;22:40–8.
164. Fletcher CD, Martin-Bates E. Spindle-cell lipoma: a clinicopathological study with some original observations. Histopathology 1987;11:803–17.
165. French CA, Mentzel T, Kutzner H, Fletcher CD. Intradermal spindle cell/pleomorphic lipoma: a distinct subset. Am J Dermatopathol 2000;22:496–502.
166. Furlong MA, Fanburg-Smith JC, Miettinen M. The morphologic spectrum of hibernoma: a clinicopathologic study of 170 cases. Am J Surg Pathol 2001;25:809–14.
167. Haas AF, Fromer ES, Bricca GM. Spindle cell lipoma of the scalp: a case report and review. Dermatol Surg 1999;25:68–71.
168. Hawley IC, Krausz T, Evans DJ, Fletcher CD. Spindle cell lipoma—a pseudoangiomatous variant. Histopathology 1994;24:565–9.
169. Hitchcock MG, Hurt MA, Santa Cruz DJ. Adenolipoma of the skin: a report of nine cases. J Am Acad Dermatol 1993;29:82–5.
170. Howard WR, Helwig EB. Angiolipoma. Arch Dermatol 1960;82:924–31.
171. Hunt SJ, Santa Cruz DJ, Barr RJ. Cellular angiolipoma. Am J Surg Pathol 1990;14:75–81.
172. Kanik AB, Oh CH, Bhawan J. Cellular angiolipoma. Am J Dermatopathol 1995;17:312–5.
173. Kauffman SL, Stout AP. Lipoblastic tumors of children. Cancer 1959;12:912–25.

174. Kurzweg FT, Spencer R. Familial multiple lipomatosis. Am J Surg 1951;82:762–5.
175. Lakshmiah SR, Scott KW, Whear NM, Monoghan A. Chondroid lipoma: a rare but diagnostically important lesion. Int J Oral Maxillofac Surg 2000;29:445–6.
176. Mahour GH, Bryan BJ, Isaacs H Jr. Lipoblastoma and lipoblastomatosis—a report of six cases. Surgery 1988;104:577–9.
177. Marshall-Taylor C, Fanburg-Smith JC. Fibrohistiocytic lipoma: twelve cases of a previously undescribed benign fatty tumor. Ann Diagn Pathol 2000;4:354–60.
178. Marshall-Taylor C, Fanburg-Smith JC. Hemosiderotic fibrohistiocytic lipomatous lesion: ten cases of a previously undescribed fatty lesion of the foot/ankle. Mod Pathol 2000;13:1192–9.
179. McMenamin ME, Fletcher CD. Mammary-type myofibroblastoma of soft tissue: a tumor closely related to spindle cell lipoma. Am J Surg Pathol 2001;25:1022–9.
180. Meis JM, Enzinger FM. Chondroid lipoma. A unique tumor simulating liposarcoma and myxoid chondrosarcoma. Am J Surg Pathol 1993;17:1103–12.
181. Mentzel T. Cutaneous lipomatous neoplasms. Semin Diagn Pathol 2001;18:250–7.
182. Mentzel T, Remmler K, Katenkamp D. [Chondroid lipoma. Clinicopathological, immunohistochemical, and ultrastructural analysis of six cases of a distinct entity in the spectrum of lipomas.] Pathologe 1999;20:330–4. (German.)
183. Osment LS. Cutaneous lipomas and lipomatosis. Surg Gynecol Obstet 1968;127:129–32.
184. Rigor VU, Goldstone SE, Jones J, Bernstein R, Gold MS, Weiner S. Hibernoma. A case report and discussion of a rare tumor. Cancer 1986;57:2207–11.
185. Rubin BP, Dal Cin P. The genetics of lipomatous tumors. Semin Diagn Pathol 2001;18:286–93.
186. Sahl WJ Jr. Mobile encapsulated lipomas. Formerly called encapsulated angiolipomas. Arch Dermatol 1978;114:1684–6.
187. Shmookler BM, Enzinger FM. Pleomorphic lipoma: a benign tumor simulating liposarcoma. A clinicopathologic analysis of 48 cases. Cancer 1981;47:126–33.
188. Suster S, Fisher C. Immunoreactivity for the human hematopoietic progenitor cell antigen (CD34) in lipomatous tumors. Am J Surg Pathol 1997;21:195–200.
189. Suster S, Fisher C, Moran CA. Dendritic fibromyxolipoma: clinicopathologic study of a distinctive benign soft tissue lesion that may be mistaken for a sarcoma. Ann Diagn Pathol 1998;2:111–20.
190. Terrier-Lacombe MJ, Guillou L, Maire G, et al. Dermatofibrosarcoma protuberans, giant cell fibroblastoma, and hybrid lesions in children: clinicopathologic comparative analysis of 28 cases with molecular data—a study from the French Federation of Cancer Centers Sarcoma Group. Am J Surg Pathol 2003;27:27–39.
191. Young RJ 3rd, Warschaw KE, Elston DM, Perry VE. Acral lipoblastoma. Cutis 2000;65:243–5.
192. Zelger BG, Zelger B, Steiner H, Rutten A. Sclerotic lipoma: lipomas simulating sclerotic fibroma. Histopathology 1997;31:174–81.

Adipocytic Pseudotumors

193. Armstrong DK, Walsh MY, Bingham A, McMillan C. Nevus lipomatosus cutaneus superficialis. Australas J Dermatol 1997;38:88–90.
194. Bilancini S, Lucchi M, Tucci S. [Lipedema: clinical and diagnostic criteria.] Angiologia 1990;42:133–7. (Spanish.)
195. Chanoki M, Sugamoto I, Suzuki S, Hamada T. Nevus lipomatosus cutaneus superficialis of the scalp. Cutis 1989;43:143–4.
196. Cornbleet T. Cutis verticis gyrata? Lipoma? Arch Dermatol Syphilol 1935;32:688–98.
197. Dotz W, Prioleau PG. Nevus lipomatosus cutaneus superficialis. A light and electron microscopic study. Arch Dermatol 1984;120:376–9.
198. Fair KP, Knoell KA, Patterson JW, Rudd RJ, Greer KE. Lipedematous alopecia: a clinicopathologic, histologic, and ultrastructural study. J Cutan Pathol 2000;27:49–53.
199. Gardner EW, Miller HM, Lowney ED. Folded skin associated with underlying nevus lipomatosus. Arch Dermatol 1979;115:978–9.
200. Jones EW, Marks R, Pongsehirun D. Nevus superficialis lipomatosus. A clinicopathological report of twenty cases. Br J Dermatol 1975;93:121–3.
201. Lee JH, Sung YH, Yoon JS, Park JK. Lipedematous scalp. Arch Dermatol 1994;130:802–3.
202. Matsuoka LY, Wortsman J, Carlisle KS, Kupchella CK, Dietrich JG. The acquired cutaneous mucinoses. Arch Intern Med 1984;144:1974–80.
203. Orteu CH, Hughes JR, Rustin MH. Nevus lipomatosus cutaneus superficialis: overlap with connective tissue nevi. Acta Derm Venereol 1996;76:243–5.
204. Ross CM. Generalized folded skin with an underlying lipomatous nevus. "The Michelin tire baby." Arch Dermatol 1969;100:320–3.
205. Schmitz R. [Lipedema from the differential diagnostic and therapeutic viewpoint.] Z Hautkr 1987;62:146–57. (German.)
206. Wienert V, Leeman S. [Lipedema.] Hautarzt 1991;42:484–6. (German.)

SUPPLEMENTAL REFERENCES

Neuroma

Baltalarli B, Demirkan N, Yagci B. Traumatic neuroma: unusual benign lesion occurring in the mastectomy scar. Clin Oncol (R Coll Radiol) 2004;16:503–4.

Dubovy SR, Clark BJ. Palisaded encapsulated neuroma (solitary circumscribed neuroma of skin) of the eyelid: report of two cases and review of the literature. Br J Ophthalmol 2001;85:949–51.

Golod O, Soriano T, Craft N. Palisaded encapsulated neuroma—a classic presentation of a commonly misdiagnosed neural tumor. J Drugs Dermatol 2005;4:92–4.

Neurofibroma and Neurilemmoma (Schwannoma)

Claessens N, Heymans O, Arrese JE, Garcia R, Oelbrandt B, Pierard GE. Cutaneous psammomatous melanotic schwannoma: non-recurrence with surgical excision. Am J Clin Dermatol 2003;4:799–802.

Endo H, Oikawa A, Utani A, Shinkai H. Plexiform neurofibromas express the transcription factor Gli1. Dermatology 2004;209:284–7.

Gray MH, Smoller BR, McNutt NS, Hsu A. Immunohistochemical demonstration of factor XIIIa expression in neurofibromas. A practical means of differentiating these tumors from neurotized melanocytic nevi and schwannomas. Arch Dermatol 1990;126:472–6.

Kazakov DV, Pitha J, Sima R, et al. Hybrid peripheral nerve sheath tumors: Schwannoma-perineurioma and neurofibroma-perineurioma. A report of three cases in extradigital locations. Ann Diagn Pathol 2005;9:16–23.

Kovarik CL, Hsu MY, Cockerell CJ. Neurofibromatous changes in dermatofibrosarcoma protuberans: a potential pitfall in the diagnosis of a serious cutaneous soft tissue neoplasm. J Cutan Pathol 2004;31:492–6.

Kurtkaya-Yapicier O, Scheithauer B, Woodruff JM. The pathobiologic spectrum of Schwannomas. Histol Histopathol 2003;18:925–34.

Saad AG, Mutema GK, Mutasim DF. Benign cutaneous epithelioid schwannoma: case report and review of the literature. Am J Dermatopathol 2005;27;45–7.

Terasaki K, Mera Y, Uchimiya H, Katahira Y, Kanzaki T. Plexiform schwannoma. Clin Exp Dermatol 2003;28:372–4.

Val-Bernal JF, Gonzalez-Vela MC. Cutaneous lipomatous neurofibroma: characterization and frequency. J Cutan Pathol 2005;32:274–9.

Neurothekeoma

Bhatia S, Chu P, Weinberg JM. Atypical cellular neurothekeoma. Dermatol Surg 2003;29:1154–7.

Laskin WB, Fetsch JF, Miettinen M. The "neurothekeoma": immunohistochemical analysis distinguishes the true nerve sheath myxoma from its mimics. Hum Pathol 2000;31:1230–41.

Misago N, Satoh T, Narisawa Y. Cellular neurothekeoma with histiocytic differentiation. J Cutan Pathol 2004;31:568–72.

Page RN, King R, Mihm MC Jr, Googe PB. Microophthalmia transcription factor and NKI/C3 expression in cellular neurothekeoma. Mod Pathol 2004;17:230–4.

Ward JL, Prieto VG, Joseph A, Chevray P, Kronowitz S, Sturgis EM. Neurothekeoma. Otolaryngol Head Neck Surg 2005;132:86–9.

Watanabe K, Kusakabe T, Hoshi N, Suzuki T. Subcutaneous cellular neurothekeoma: a pseudosarcomatous tumor. Br J Dermatol 2001;144:1273-4.

Granular Cell Tumors

El-Gamal HM, Robinson-Bostom L, Saddler KD, Pan T, Mihm MC Jr. Compound melanocytic nevi with granular cell changes. J Am Acad Dermatol 2004;50:765–6.

Le BH, Boyer PJ, Lewis JE, Kapadia SB. Granular cell tumor: immunohistochemical assessment of inhibin-alpha, protein gene product 9.5, S100 protein, CD68, and Ki-67 proliferative index with clinical correlation. Arch Pathol Lab Med 2004;128:771–5.

Rudisaile SN, Hurt MA, Santa Cruz DJ. Granular cell atypical fibroxanthoma. J Cutan Pathol 2005;32:314–7.

Primitive Neuroectodermal Tumor

Grayson W, Mare LR. Ganglioneuroblastic differentiation in a primary cutaneous malignant melanoma. Am J Dermatopathol 2003;25:40–4.

Peydro-Olaya A, Llombart-Bosch A, Carda-Batalla C, Lopez-Guerrero JA. Electron microscopy and other ancillary techniques in the diagnosis of small round cell tumors. Semin Diagn Pathol 2003;20;25–45.

Somers GR, Shago M, Zielenska M, Chan HS, Ngan BY. Primary subcutaneous primitive neuroectodermal tumor with aggressive behavior and an unusual karyotype: case report. Pediatr Dev Pathol 2004;7:538–45.

Adipocytic Tumors

Val-Bernal JF, Gonzalez-Vela MC, Cuevas J. Primary purely intradermal pleomorphic liposarcoma. J Cutan Pathol 2003;30:516–20.

9 TUMORS OF MUSCLE, CARTILAGE, AND BONE

There are relatively few primary cutaneous tumors of muscular, cartilaginous, or osseous differentiation. Cartilage in skin is unusual except in the form of heterotopia, e.g., accessory tragi, or "wattles" (5,14). Osteosarcoma, a true primary osseous neoplasia, only rarely arises in skin; other "osseous" tumors that are considered in this chapter are more accurately categorized as fibrous tissue tumors that ossify. Bone can also form in the skin as a congenital anomaly: as miliary osteomas of the face, as a manifestation of the X-linked dominant disorder Albright's hereditary osteodystrophy, in fibrodysplasia ossificans progressiva, or as a secondary phenomenon in a variety of inflammatory disorders or tumors of the skin. Bone formation also occurs in pilomatricoma, and bone can form through enchondral ossification in the mixed tumor of skin, or chondroid syringoma. Of primary significance is the role that some of these tumors play in differential diagnosis; for example, leiomyosarcoma is frequently included in the differential diagnosis of malignant spindle cell tumors of the skin.

SMOOTH MUSCLE TUMORS

Smooth Muscle Hamartoma

Clinical Features. *Smooth muscle hamartoma* is an uncommon lesion that may present at birth, during childhood, or occasionally in adult life. The congenital type is reported to have a prevalence of 1 in 2,600 live births, with a slight male predominance (66). It typically presents as a patch or slightly elevated plaque on the trunk (particularly the lumbosacral region [66]) or proximal extremities. Cases have also involved the dartos muscle of the scrotum (49) or the orbital region (31), including the conjunctival fornix (52). Generalized cutaneous involvement in infants has on rare occasion produced large folds of skin, resembling the "Michelin tire baby" syndrome (17,22,54). These cases have also been associated with hypertrichosis (22,54).

Smooth muscle hamartomas have been reported to demonstrate a pseudo-Darier's sign. A true Darier's sign consists of urtication (occurrence of a wheal and flare) upon stroking a lesion of cutaneous mastocytosis; the urtication is the result of the release of histamine from the increased numbers of dermal mast cells in that disorder. In smooth muscle hamartoma, stroked lesions develop transient erythema, edema, induration, or piloerection that can mimic Darier's sign (21,31); however, in one case in which this sign was demonstrated, the mast cells were not increased in number (21).

Some lesions are composed of follicular or perifollicular papules; hypertrichosis and hyperpigmentation are present in a variable proportion of cases (6,7,15). *Becker's nevus (Becker's melanosis)*, a skin lesion characterized by hyperpigmentation and hypertrichosis, is associated with hyperplasia of smooth muscle. Most authors now consider Becker's nevus and smooth muscle hamartoma to be related conditions, perhaps ends of a spectrum of lesions consisting of follicular, melanocytic, and smooth muscle elements (15,17,31,62). One patient with Michelin tire baby syndrome had other mesodermal anomalies, seizures, and developmental delay, and showed a paracentric inversion of the long arm of chromosome 7 (54). Lesions may become less prominent over time. Malignant transformation has not been reported (21,66).

Pathologic Findings. Within the dermis are numbers of well-differentiated smooth muscle bundles, oriented in apparently random arrangements (fig. 9-1). Some of these muscle bundles are associated with the follicular units that accompany smooth muscle hamartoma (7,17). As would be expected, these smooth muscle bundles stain red with the trichrome method and are positive for muscle-associated immunostains. Nerve fibers are also a component of these lesions (23), as are CD34-positive dendritic cells (32). Exaggerated budding of rete ridges and basilar hypermelanosis may be present, particularly

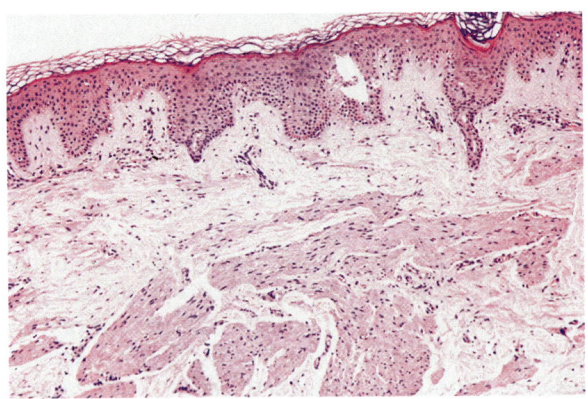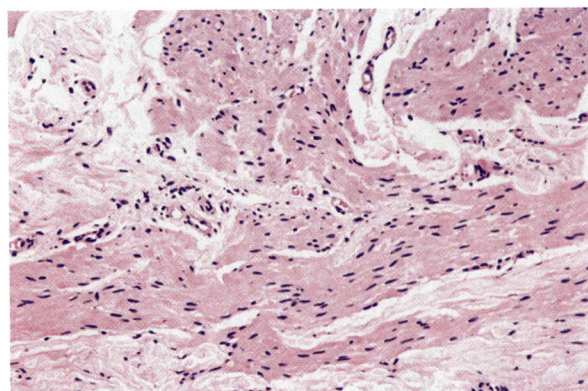

Figure 9-1

SMOOTH MUSCLE HAMARTOMA

Left: Well-differentiated smooth muscle bundles are in random arrangements. The overlying epidermis is somewhat acanthotic, but microscopic changes suggesting an associated Becker's nevus are not observed.

Right: Detail of randomly oriented smooth muscle bundles.

in those cases associated with Becker's nevus. Hypertrichosis can be difficult to demonstrate in random, vertically oriented sections, but may be more effectively evaluated in horizontal sections, particularly when compared to a similarly prepared biopsy of normal skin from the same region. Ultrastructural studies show smooth muscle cells, including pale cells, dark cells, and intermediate types, as well as varying proportions of myelinated and unmyelinated nerve (23).

Differential Diagnosis. Lesions associated with significant rete ridge proliferation, basilar hypermelanosis, and hypertrichosis may actually represent Becker's nevus with an associated smooth muscle hamartoma. The scattered, random orientation of smooth muscle bundles separated by abundant dermal collagen, seen in smooth muscle hamartoma, differs from the usual picture in piloleiomyoma, in which intersecting smooth muscle bundles are arranged in larger, tumor-like aggregates.

Leiomyoma

Clinical Features. Leiomyomas as a group are relatively common cutaneous tumors. They are often divided into three types: *piloleiomyoma,* derived from or differentiating toward arrector pili muscle; *leiomyoma of the nipple, areola, or genital region;* and *angioleiomyoma (angiomyoma),* derived from vessel walls.

Piloleiomyomas may be solitary or multiple, grouped or linear. The sexes are affected equally. There is some evidence that truncal tumors are more common in patients who have multiple lesions (50). Multiple piloleiomyomas may be familial (42), and an association with uterine leiomyoma has been reported in some familial cases (18,39). There has been a report of a piloleiomyoma arising in an organoid nevus of the scalp (8). Piloleiomyomas are firm, red-brown papules or nodules that tend to be painful, either spontaneously or to touch (41). Individually, piloleiomyoma can resemble dermatofibroma, but with the interesting property of contracting with application of an ice cube.

Solitary leiomyoma arises in the nipple or areolar region of both men and women, and presents as an ill-defined or infiltrative mass (1,61,64). It may also be painful, but there has been at least one case in which an incidental tumor was identified in a mastectomy specimen (43).

Scrotal leiomyoma arises from the tunica dartos (12) or between the tunica dartos and tunica vaginalis testis (40). This tumor presents as a firm mass (40) that may be pedunculated (12) or have a verrucous surface (53). Vulvar leiomyoma has also been reported (2,28,44,45), and in this location the tumor can clinically mimic a variety of inflammatory and neoplastic processes.

Angioleiomyomas are typically solitary lesions that usually arise in the subcutis but can

Tumors of Muscle, Cartilage, and Bone

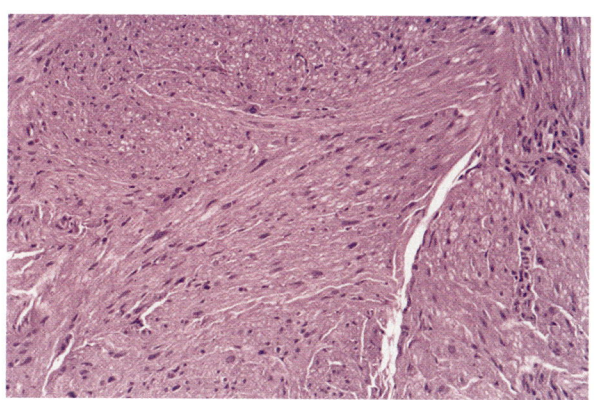

Figure 9-2

PILOLEIOMYOMA

There are interconnecting bundles of smooth muscle cells, "cigar-shaped" nuclei in longitudinally sectioned cells, and a vacuolated appearance of the cytoplasm of those cells oriented in cross section.

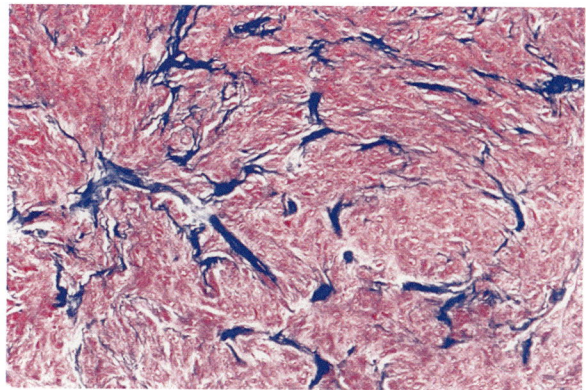

Figure 9-3

PILOLEIOMYOMA

The smooth muscle appears red with the trichrome stain.

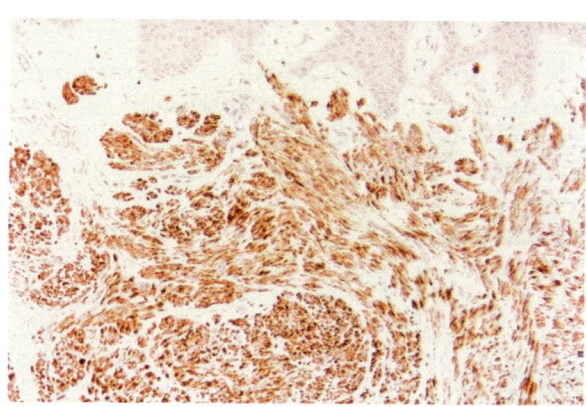

Figure 9-4

PILOLEIOMYOMA

The cells of leiomyoma are desmin positive.

also be dermal (24,46). They occur with particular frequency on the lower extremities (48), but they also arise on the upper extremities, head, and (uncommonly) trunk (24). These lesions are somewhat more common in women than men (24). As is true for other types of cutaneous leiomyoma, angioleiomyoma is usually painful (34,41).

Pathologic Findings. Piloleiomyoma and nipple/areola or genital type of leiomyoma have similar microscopic features, consisting of interconnecting bundles of smooth muscle cells in straight or whorled arrangements (fig. 9-2). The fibrillar quality of the cytoplasm in longitudinally sectioned cells can sometimes be discerned on hematoxylin and eosin (H&E)- stained sections, and can be better demonstrated with the phosphotungstic acid-hematoxylin (PTAH) stain (19). In cross section, the cytoplasm of these cells appears vacuolated. Their nuclei are slightly elongated but blunt-ended ("cigar shaped") (fig. 9-2). Proliferating cells largely replace the dermal connective tissue, but admixed collagen fibers are present. Interlacing nerve fibers have been identified with a variety of staining methods (50,60). Unusual features include myxoid and epithelioid changes (both reported in vulvar leiomyomas) (2,28,44), granular cells (38), and Verocay bodies (33). Mitotic figures are frequently absent but an occasional one may be seen. Raj et al. (50) indicate that up to 1 mitosis per 10 high-power fields can be encountered in these lesions without conveying an adverse prognosis. The overlying epidermis may appear normal or the rete ridge pattern may be effaced, but epidermal hyperplasia (acanthosis) is present in over half of cases (50). The smooth muscle bundles stain red with the trichrome method (fig. 9-3), and are positive with immunohistochemical stains such as smooth muscle actin, muscle-specific actin, and desmin (fig. 9-4).

Angioleiomyomas are sharply circumscribed nodules composed of smooth muscle. Vessels are identified within these nodules, and possess lumens with varying degrees of patency.

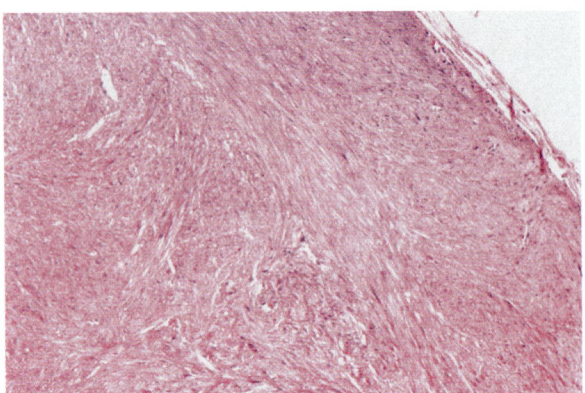 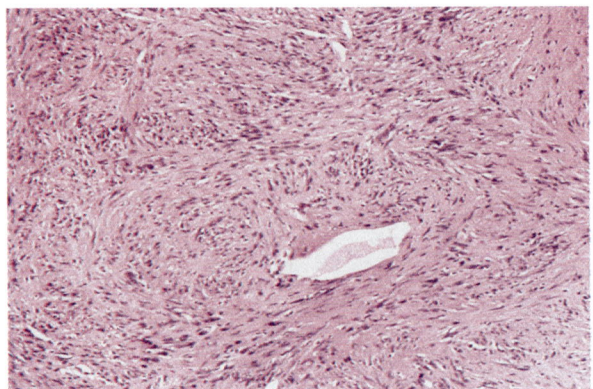

Figure 9-5

ANGIOLEIOMYOMA

Left: These tumors are sharply circumscribed.
Right: Smooth muscle surrounding constituent vessels merges to form the tumor mass.

Closer inspection shows that the smooth muscle surrounding these vessels merges with adjacent smooth muscle to form the tumor mass (fig. 9-5). In their study of 562 cases, Hachisuga et al. (24) identified three histologic types of angioleiomyoma, based upon features of the constituent vessels: a capillary type, with numerous small vascular channels; a cavernous type, with dilated vascular channels and relatively small amounts of smooth muscle; and a venous type, composed of veins with thick muscular walls (24). An *epithelioid angioleiomyoma* has been reported (27), and atypical nuclei with degenerative changes have been observed, a feature of so-called *symplastic leiomyoma* (11). Mucinous changes also occur (34). Small clusters of mature lipocytes can be found in a minority of cases (24). Lesions with a substantial component of lipocytes may be termed *angiomyolipoma* (see below). An ultrastructural study of one lesion by Siefert (55) showed vessels with prominent endothelial cells that contained numerous Weibel-Palade bodies and were enveloped by typical smooth muscle cells.

Differential Diagnosis. Generally, leiomyomas are sufficiently distinctive that there are no major problems in the differential diagnosis. Piloleiomyomas sometimes resemble other benign spindle cell tumors of skin, including dermatofibroma or neurofibroma. The morphologic characteristics of the cells and their nuclei often permit distinction of these lesions. In contrast to leiomyomas, dermatofibromas may have a significant inflammatory component, show xanthomatization, and possess Touton-like multinucleated giant cells. The "buckled," or "S-shaped" nuclei of neurofibromas are distinctly different from the blunt-ended, cigar-shaped nuclei of leiomyoma. Immunohistochemistry can be useful in difficult cases, because of the positivity for smooth muscle markers in leiomyomas, the factor XIIIa predominance in dermatofibromas, and the expression of S-100 protein and other neural markers in neurofibromas. Dermatomyofibromas and dermatofibromas with a myofibroblastic component are positive for smooth muscle actin, but unlike leiomyomas they are usually desmin negative.

Rarely, piloleiomyomas with palisading or Verocay body formation resemble neurilemmoma, but a lack of encapsulation, as well as the cytologic features and negativity for neural markers, should permit recognition of the former. A greater degree of difficulty could be encountered in angioleiomyomas with palisading, since these tumors appear to be encapsulated, but again, cytologic details (angiocentricity, cytoplasmic myofibrils, nuclear features) and special stains (positivity for PTAH, actin, and desmin) should permit correct identification of angioleiomyoma.

Myxoid leiomyoma of the vulva has been confused with aggressive angiomyxoma, and it should be noted that cells of the latter tumor

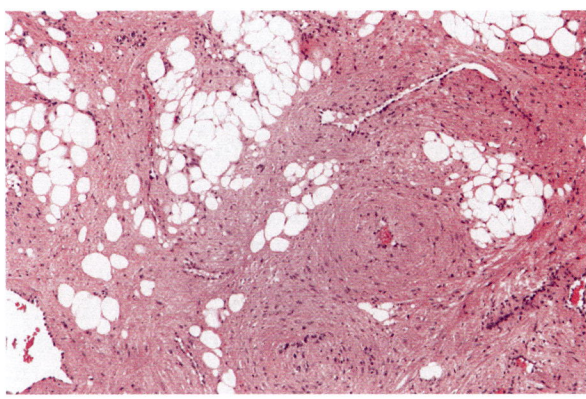 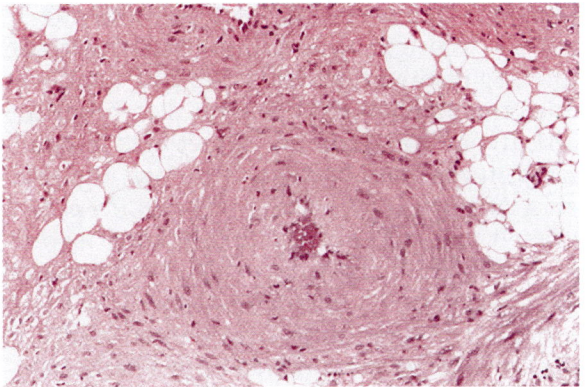

Figure 9-6

ANGIOMYOLIPOMA OF SUBCUTANEOUS TISSUE

Left: Adipose tissue and blood vessels are surrounded by smooth muscle that extends into connective tissue septa.
Right: High-power view.

can express both actin and desmin. The presence of interlacing cells with characteristics of smooth muscle cells is a distinctive feature of myxoid leiomyoma (44).

The cellular variant of neurothekeoma features intradermal nests and fascicles of epithelioid to spindle-shaped cells that are smooth muscle actin positive. These cells have also been reported to be NK1/C3 positive, weakly neuron-specific enolase positive, and desmin negative. Nevertheless, it has been suggested that these tumors may actually represent variants of piloleiomyoma (10).

Superficial leiomyosarcomas can be distinguished from leiomyomas by their increased cellularity and pleomorphism. In addition, leiomyosarcomas display a greater degree of mitotic activity (usually more than 2 mitoses per 10 high-power fields, in contrast to the less than 1 mitosis per 10 high-power fields expected in leiomyomas), and often show atypical mitotic forms.

Cutaneous Angiomyolipoma (Angiolipoleiomyoma)

Clinical Features. Only a few examples of *cutaneous angiomyolipoma* have been reported. It was first described in an abstract by Argenyi et al. (4), and these authors provided greater detail in a subsequent publication (3). Fitzpatrick et al. (20) reported eight additional cases under the term *angiolipoleiomyoma*, a designation they preferred in order to avoid confusion with the renal angiomyolipoma encountered in tuberous sclerosis. There have been a number of subsequent case reports. Cutaneous (or, more accurately, subcutaneous) angiomyolipomas are benign tumors that typically occur in acral locations; two cases have been reported that arose in the nasal cavity (65). There is no known association with tuberous sclerosis.

Pathologic Findings. These are sharply circumscribed tumors that are composed of smooth muscle bundles, blood vessels, and adipose tissue. The smooth muscle both surrounds vascular spaces and extends into septa within adipose tissue (fig. 9-6) (37). Since several studies have described small clusters of mature lipocytes in angioleiomyomas (24,35), a strong case could be made that cutaneous angiomyolipomas are simply variants of that better known tumor. It has been recommended, however, that a separate designation be maintained, both because of sex incidence (thus far, cutaneous angiomyolipomas are more common in men, in contrast to angioleiomyoma) and histopathologic differences.

Differential Diagnosis. Elastic laminae are commonly seen among blood vessels of angiomyolipoma but are usually not demonstrable in angioleiomyoma (4,20). The prominent lipomatous component of angiomyolipoma incorporates a differential diagnosis that differs from that of angioleiomyoma, and includes angiolipoma and arteriovenous hemangioma

(20). In renal angiomyolipomas, smooth muscle may be arranged in a diffuse pattern without forming distinct fascicles, as seen in cutaneous angiomyolipomas (20). Nuclear pleomorphism and hyperchromasia are sometimes encountered in the renal tumors. Although the presence of nuclear pleomorphism had been considered to be a possible differentiating feature, pleomorphic changes have since been reported in cutaneous angiomyolipoma as well (51). One other microscopic difference between renal and cutaneous angiomyolipomas is the HMB45 positivity of the large interstitial cells of renal angiomyolipomas (56). Thus far, cutaneous and mucocutaneous angiomyolipomas have been HMB45 negative (9,63,65).

Leiomyosarcoma

Clinical Features. *Leiomyosarcomas of skin* are generally divided into two types, *dermal* and *subcutaneous*, based upon clinical, histopathologic, and prognostic differences. In addition, leiomyosarcomas can metastasize to skin from other sites, including uterus (36) and deep extracutaneous tissues (59). Leiomyosarcomas arise most often on the extremities, particularly the hip, thigh, and knee (16,19,25,30), but truncal lesions also occur (13). The unusual *epithelioid variant of leiomyosarcoma* may have a somewhat different distribution, as these lesions have been reported in the head and neck regions (57). Adults of widely ranging ages have developed the tumor, with a predominance among middle-aged to older individuals (16,19). While initial studies suggested a male predominance (16), more recent studies have shown a greater frequency in women (25,47).

Leiomyosarcomas present as one or a few dermal or subcutaneous nodules that may be painful. In our experience, both dermal and subcutaneous varieties are often clinically suspected to be epidermal cysts. Multiple studies have shown that the intradermal tumors have a relatively low recurrence rate and rarely result in metastasis and death, while the reverse is true for subcutaneous lesions (16,19,29,30,59). The lung is a common metastatic site (16,30). Hashimoto et al. (25) found that the depth of the initial tumor was a critical factor in prognosis, since among their cases, patients with tumors confined to the subcutis did well, while seven of nine patients with muscle involvement died within 5 years of excision. Nevertheless, local recurrence, distant metastasis, and death have been associated with a dermal lesion (59). Wide local excision is the treatment of choice for leiomyosarcoma.

Pathologic Findings. Intradermal leiomyosarcomas are usually poorly demarcated, consisting of interwoven fascicles of spindled cells merging with a collagenous stroma. Involvement of the subcutis is sometimes observed. Better-differentiated foci resemble piloleiomyoma, since the tumor cells in these areas feature cytoplastic myofibrils and cigar-shaped nuclei; poorly differentiated areas are densely cellular, with scattered atypical nuclei and mitotic figures (fig. 9-7). Subcutaneous leiomyosarcomas tend to be more sharply circumscribed and usually display prominent blood vessels, consistent with the presumed vascular origin of these tumors (16,19). In epithelioid leiomyosarcoma, tumor cells have round to oval contours and generous amounts of eosinophilic cytoplasm (57). A case of *granular cell leiomyosarcoma* has also been reported; the granules were periodic acid–Schiff (PAS) positive, diastase resistant (58).

The number of mitoses that is required for a diagnosis is a question that has not been completely resolved. In an earlier study, Headington et al. (26) suggested that a high mitotic count is not an appropriate criterion for primary dermal leiomyosarcomas, as it is for noncutaneous tumors. Chow et al. (13) required 1 or more mitoses per 5 high-power fields in cellular areas in order to make the diagnosis. Tumor size appears to be an independent prognostic variable by multivariate analysis, and tumors greater than 5 cm in diameter are associated with poor survival (30). In fact, tumor size and depth of involvement are more important prognostic indicators than are the usual microscopic criteria for grading tumors: cellularity, anaplasia, and mitotic activity. Thus, intradermal leiomyosarcomas tend to behave in a benign fashion regardless of tumor grade (30).

Immunohistochemical staining generally shows that tumor cells are positive for vimentin and smooth muscle actin (fig. 9-8) (59). Desmin staining has been somewhat more variable, with some studies showing positivity in all cases (59), while in others less than half of the cases

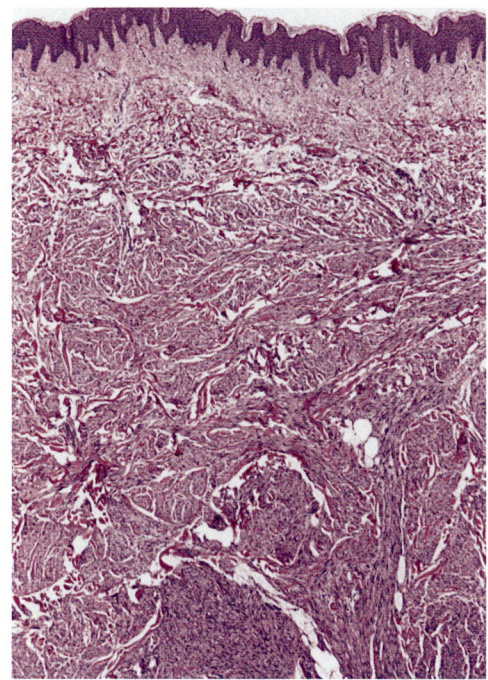

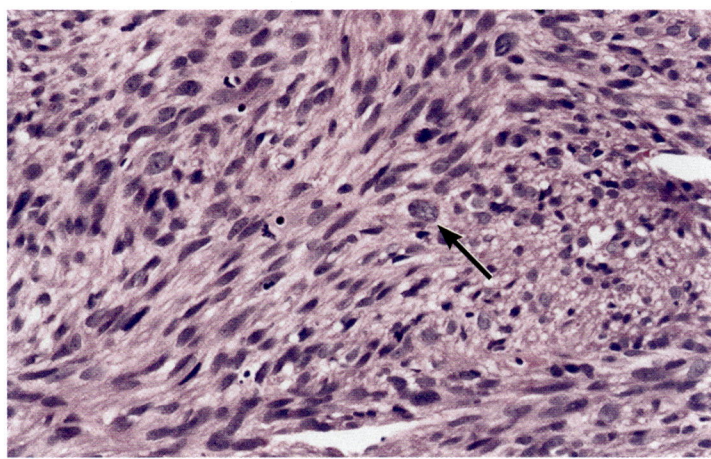

Figure 9-7

CUTANEOUS LEIOMYOSARCOMA

Left: This tumor is present within the dermis but also extends into the subcutis.

Above: High-power view. Nuclear pleomorphism, karyorrhexis, and a mitotic figure are seen (arrow).

are desmin positive (25,47). Oliver et al. (47) have suggested that desmin staining may be less frequent in higher-grade tumors. Tumor cells may sometimes express cathepsin B, myelin basic protein, epithelial membrane antigen, S-100 protein, and leu-7. Swanson et al. (59) provided evidence that dermal tumors were more likely than extracutaneous tumors to express S-100 protein, while the reverse appeared to be true for leu-7. In the study of epithelioid leiomyosarcoma, Suster (57) found that tumor cells were actin and vimentin positive but desmin, S-100 protein, cytokeratin, epithelial membrane antigen, HMB45, factor VIII, and alpha-1-antichymotrypsin negative.

Ultrastructurally, the tumor cells have the characteristics of smooth muscle cells, with varying degrees of differentiation (25,26,55,57). Edematous cells with scant myofilaments (55) and histiocyte-like tumor cells (25) have been reported. Seifert (55) found multiple accumulated centrioles in tumor cells. In one study of DNA pattern in cutaneous and subcutaneous leiomyosarcomas, all five aneuploid or nonclassifiable tumors metastasized, while there were no metastases among eight diploid cases (47).

Differential Diagnosis. Tumor size, cellularity, cytologic atypia, and mitotic activity should permit differentiation from leiomyoma. Cuta-

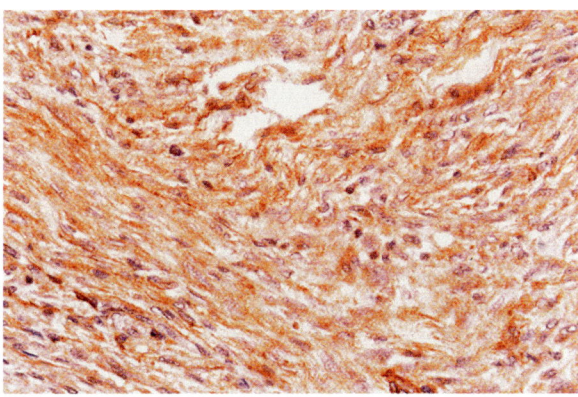

Figure 9-8

CUTANEOUS LEIOMYOSARCOMA

This tumor is smooth muscle actin positive.

neous leiomyosarcoma must often be differentiated from other malignant spindle cell tumors that arise in skin, including dermatofibrosarcoma protuberans and malignant fibrous histiocytoma (25). Subcutaneous varieties with vascular prominence may resemble hemangiopericytoma. Epithelioid leiomyosarcomas must be differentiated from malignant melanoma, epithelioid sarcoma, and primary or metastatic carcinomas. In most leiomyosarcomas, better differentiated areas can be found that show recognizable

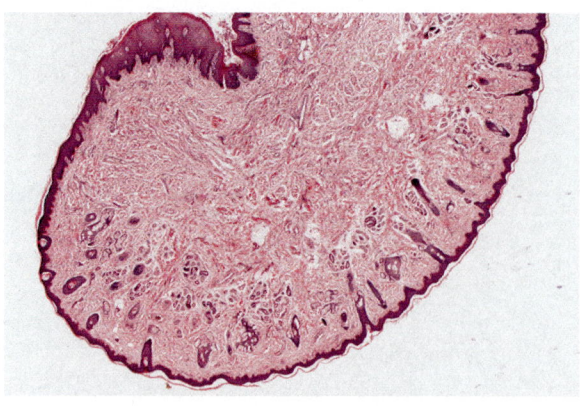 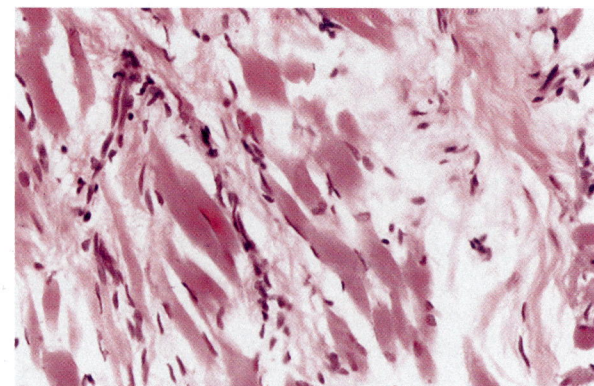

Figure 9-9

RHABDOMYOMATOUS MESENCHYMAL HAMARTOMA

Left: Low-power view shows a polypoid lesion containing numerous vellus follicles and eccrine sweat coils.
Right: Skeletal muscle bundles occupy the subcutaneous core of the polyp.

smooth muscle differentiation, and these morphologic clues can be supplemented by immunohistochemistry or electron microscopy. Although some dermal leiomyosarcomas express S-100 protein (59), in contrast to melanoma, these cells should be actin positive and negative for other melanocytic markers. Fortunately, the epithelioid leiomyosarcomas reported by Suster (57) were S-100 protein and HMB45 negative. Although both leiomyosarcomas and epithelioid sarcomas are vimentin positive, leiomyosarcomas are cytokeratin negative and show either weak or negative staining for epithelial membrane antigen (57,59).

STRIATED MUSCLE TUMORS AND RHABDOID TUMOR

Rhabdomyomatous Mesenchymal Hamartoma

Clinical Features. Also known as *congenital midline hamartoma* and *striated muscle hamartoma, rhabdomyomatous mesenchymal hamartoma* (RMH) is a lesion that consists of single or multiple congenital polypoid lesions. Affected infants usually present with central facial polyps, with the chin (67,75,84,96) and nostrils (76,86) favored sites. Other locations on the head and neck, including periorbital and preauricular regions, have also been described (83,95), and unusual locations have included the chest (96) and perianal region (98). The lesions have the interesting property of showing spontaneous movement, e.g., during feeding (95). RMH is mainly of cosmetic importance, but an association with other congenital anomalies has been reported (80). These anomalies include cleft lip, thyroglossal duct sinus (96), preauricular sinus, low-set ears and bilateral sclerocorneas (96), amniotic band syndrome and lipoma of brain (86), and limbal dermoid and coloboma in a patient with RMH of the eyelid (93). It has been proposed that at least some of the polypoid skin lesions that occur in the oculocerebrocutaneous syndrome (Delleman's syndrome) are examples of RMH (73,96).

Pathologic Findings. The polyps of RMH are lined by stratified squamous epithelium and contain vellus follicles (with associated arrectores pilorum muscles) and varying numbers of eccrine sweat glands (fig. 9-9, left). Skeletal muscle, arranged in bundles or as single fibers, is present in the subcutaneous fat and may extend into the dermis (fig. 9-9, right) (75,80,95). Cross-striations are readily identifiable. Both type 1 and type 2 muscle fibers have been identified in frozen sections using reduced nicotinamide adenine dinucleotide (NADH) and adenosine triphosphatase (ATPase) stains, and the typical ultrastructural characteristics of skeletal muscle are seen (95).

Differential Diagnosis. The microscopic characteristics of RMH are unique. This tumor somewhat resembles fibroepithelial polyp, nevus lipomatosus, and particularly accessory tragus (75), but the finding of a skeletal muscle

Tumors of Muscle, Cartilage, and Bone

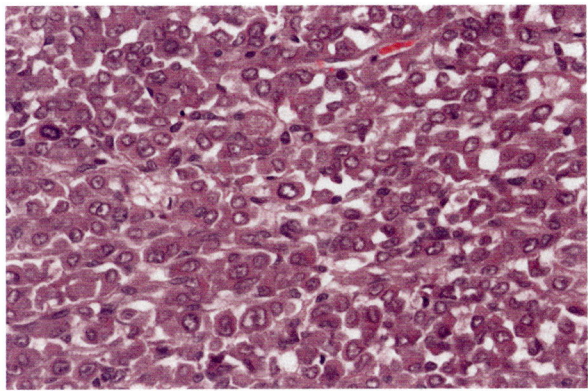

Figure 9-10

RHABDOMYOSARCOMA

The alveolar rhabdomyosarcoma, shown here, is the type most frequently reported in the skin.

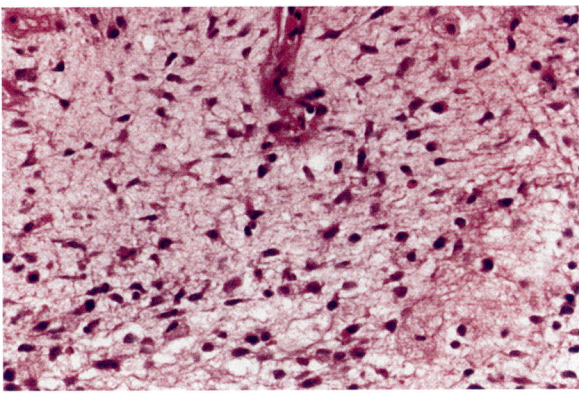

Figure 9-11

RHABDOMYOSARCOMA

The embryonal type is also described in skin.

component is decisive. These superficial cutaneous lesions are unlikely to be confused with deeper or more primitive tumors such as fetal rhabdomyoma, fibrous hamartoma of infancy, or Triton tumor (95).

Rhabdomyosarcoma

Clinical Features. The presentation of rhabdomyosarcoma as a cutaneous tumor is a rare event, but examples have been reported (70,74, 79,82,87,91,100,103). These tumors arise most commonly in children and young adults, with an apparent predilection for the head and neck, particularly the nose and cheeks (69,74,79,91, 103); however, these tumors can also arise in older adults (99,100) and in other locations, such as the trunk (70,87). In contrast to the improved prognosis associated with the superficial variants of some malignant mesenchymal tumors, cutaneous rhabdomyosarcomas are prone to metastasize. Sites of metastasis include skin (79, 87,99), lymph nodes (69,87), brain (82), and other tissues in a disseminated fashion (69).

Pathologic Findings. The histologic types of rhabdomyosarcoma are *alveolar*, *embryonal* (including *botryoid* and *spindle cell* subtypes), and *pleomorphic* (figs. 9-10, 9-11). All three major types are represented among the cases of cutaneous rhabdomyosarcoma, with the alveolar type being the most frequently reported to date (fig. 9-10) (69,74,79,82). One elderly adult presented with the pleomorphic type of rhabdomyosarcoma, a form of the tumor that typically presents in adults (72,100). Rhabdomyosarcoma may also be the mesenchymal element in carcinosarcoma of the skin (89,94).

Cytologically, tumor cells range from undifferentiated, small, rounded to spindled cells to larger, polygonal or strap-shaped cells that may possess eosinophilic cytoplasm and show cross-striations. Irregular cytoplasmic vacuoles and intracellular glycogen can be demonstrated. Immunohistochemistry is of immense help in the diagnosis. Tumor cells stain for vimentin, desmin, muscle-specific actin, and myoglobin, although the staining may not be as intense (and myoglobin may be negative) in more primitive tumors (68,70,72,79). Ultrastructural examination may delineate features of rhabdomyoblasts, including the presence of thick and thin filaments (70).

Differential Diagnosis. In a tumor with this degree of microscopic variability, the differential diagnosis would be expected to be broad, although perhaps somewhat more limited for cutaneous tumors than for those of deeper soft tissues. Small cell tumors can resemble metastatic neuroblastoma (79), lymphoma, malignant melanoma, primitive neuroectodermal tumor (PNET), or small cell carcinoma. Pleomorphic varieties can mimic melanoma as well as pleomorphic liposarcoma, leiomyosarcoma, or malignant fibrous histiocytoma (68,102). Immunohistochemistry and electron microscopy are helpful in the differential diagnosis of these tumors. In fact, in a retrospective immunohistochemical study of pleomorphic sarcomas,

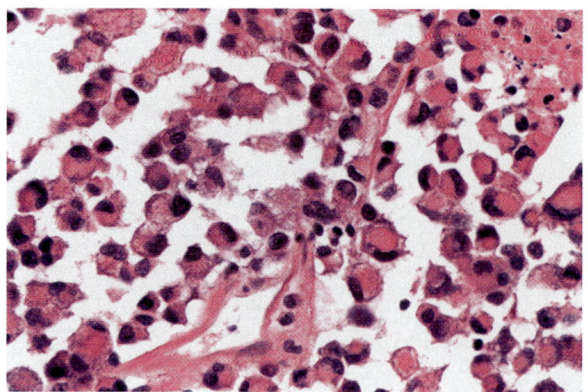
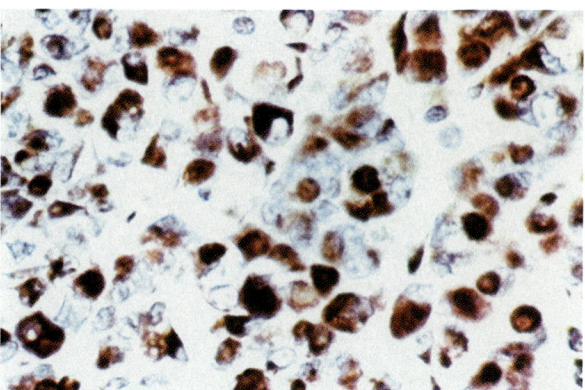

Figure 9-12

MALIGNANT RHABDOID TUMOR

Left: There are polygonal to rounded cells with eosinophilic cytoplasmic inclusions.
Right: Tumor cells are vimentin positive.

deJong et al. (72) found that the majority of tumors originally diagnosed as rhabdomyosarcoma were reclassified as malignant fibrous histiocytoma or leiomyosarcoma, while one pleomorphic sarcoma was reclassified as a rhabdomyosarcoma.

(Extrarenal) Malignant Rhabdoid Tumor

Clinical Features. *Malignant rhabdoid tumor* was originally identified in the kidney as a possible subset of Wilms' tumor with features resembling rhabdomyosarcoma (71). It has since been reported in a number of deep soft tissue sites and in several internal organs (77,81). Tumors with the microscopic features ascribed to malignant rhabdoid tumor have also been identified in the skin. These have occurred as primary lesions (71,97), as second neoplasms arising from other cutaneous tumors such as a neurovascular hamartoma (90) or benign mesenchymal tumor (78), or as presumed metastases from primary tumors of the kidney or deep soft tissues (81). Patients with classic malignant rhabdoid tumors are infants or young children, but similar appearing tumors also arise in middle-aged or older adults (85,97). This tumor is generally aggressive, with the rapid occurrence of metastasis and death (77,92,101).

Pathologic Findings. Malignant rhabdoid tumor is composed of polygonal or rounded cells with generous amounts of cytoplasm and hyaline, eosinophilic, PAS-positive (diastase resistant) inclusions (fig. 9-12, left). Large, rounded, vesicular nuclei with prominent, centrally located nucleoli are seen.

Ultrastructurally, the inclusions consist of whorled aggregates of 10-nm intermediate filaments (71,101). The cytoplasmic material of classic examples stains for vimentin (fig. 9-12, right), epithelial membrane antigen, and cytokeratin but not for S-100 protein, muscle-related protein, and neural protein (101). Other tumors with morphologic features consistent with malignant rhabdoid tumor have expressed desmin (97), muscle-specific actin (78), S-100 protein and synaptophysin (85), or vimentin only (71). This variability in immunohistochemical phenotype has suggested to some that extrarenal malignant rhabdoid tumor is not a single entity but a heterogeneous group of undifferentiated tumors, all of which share rhabdoid microscopic features (88). DNA analysis has revealed a diploid profile (78).

Differential Diagnosis. In view of the immunohistochemical heterogeneity of lesions reported as malignant rhabdoid tumors, it is apparent that a number of different tumors can present with similar features. Poorly differentiated squamous cell carcinoma and malignant melanoma are two that are of particular importance in dermatopathology. There is also a close resemblance between epithelioid sarcoma and malignant rhabdoid tumor, both in terms of cytomorphology and immunohistochemical profile. A distinction between the two may depend upon the patient's age, and the clinical location

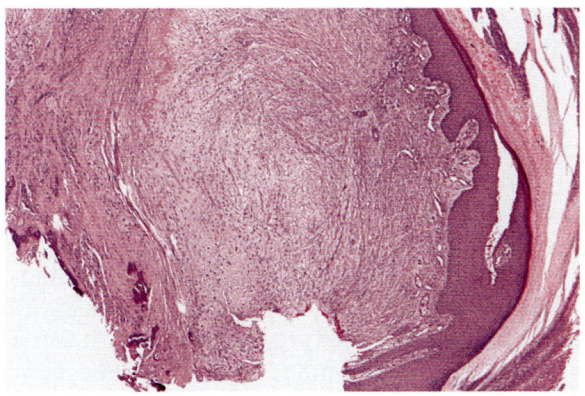 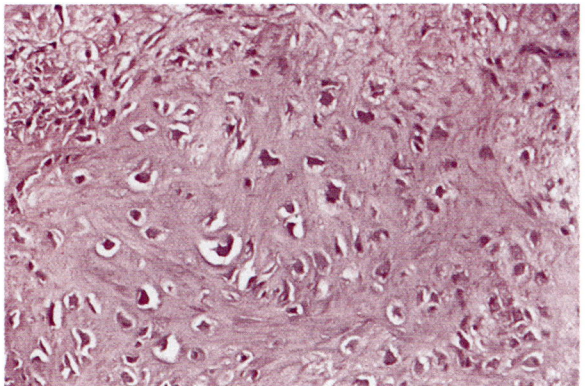

Figure 9-13

EXTRASKELETAL CHONDROMA

Left: This is a lobulated, well-circumscribed tumor.
Right: High-power view shows mature-appearing hyaline cartilage.

of the tumor and its overall microscopic configuration. Occurrence on the forearm or hand of a young adult favors epithelioid sarcoma, as do the histopathologic features of multinodularity and central necrosis mimicking a palisaded necrobiotic granuloma (92).

CARTILAGINOUS TUMORS AND PARACHORDOMA

Extraskeletal Chondroma

Clinical Features. *Extraskeletal chondromas* are uncommon tumors that usually arise in the soft tissues of the hands and feet of adults. Although true skin involvement by these tumors is rare (107,123), the subcutaneous mass created by an enlarging soft tissue lesion in these locations may result in a tissue sample that finds its way to a dermatopathologist. Related lesions include *enchondroma,* a tumor arising within cartilage or bone; *ecchondroma,* which develops at the surface of cartilage; and *periosteal chondroma.* If sufficiently large, these lesions produce cutaneous symptoms, including swelling, which mimics paronychia and is associated with nail dystrophy (139,143). Radiographic studies are therefore important, both to accurately categorize these tumors and to provide guidance for appropriate surgical management. On radiologic examination, extraskeletal chondromas show ring-like or curvilinear calcifications (144), and despite their extraosseous location, may be associated with erosions of adjacent bone. These are not aggressive tumors and they respond well to local excision, although recurrences are possible. Cutaneous cartilaginous rests, also known as wattles, are sometimes encountered in the lateral neck in infancy and early childhood. These lesions may be of branchial cleft origin (108,111,126).

Pathologic Findings. Extraskeletal chondromas are lobulated, well-circumscribed lesions composed of hyaline cartilage, with varying degrees of fibrosis and mucin deposition (fig. 9-13). Calcification can be a prominent feature (114), particularly in the central portion of the lesion (fig. 9-14), and ossification has been reported (113). Granuloma formation may be present at the periphery of the tumor (141). Pleomorphic cells or chondroblasts are sometimes seen, but these tend to be concentrated centrally, with more mature-appearing cells at the periphery of the tumor (141,144). An unusual related lesion has been reported as *extraskeletal chondroma with lipoblast-like cells* (110). As would be expected of chondrocytes, the cells comprising extraskeletal chondroma are positive for S-100 protein and vimentin.

Differential Diagnosis. The microscopic features of extraskeletal chondromas are relatively distinctive. The presence of prominent granulomas with giant cells could lead to confusion with giant cell tumor of tendon sheath, while lesions with extensive calcification might resemble forms of calcinosis cutis. The most important entity to exclude is chondrosarcoma,

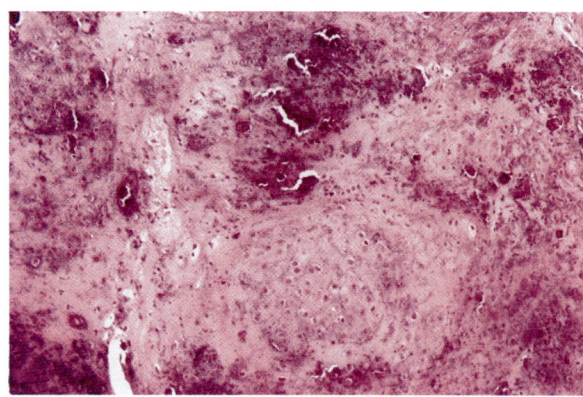

Figure 9-14
EXTRASKELETAL CHONDROMA
There is extensive calcification in the central portion of the lesion.

but the anatomic distribution, small size, and tendency toward peripheral maturation associated with extraskeletal chondroma normally permits its accurate recognition.

Subungual Osteochondroma and Exostosis

Clinical Features. *Subungual osteochondroma* has been described as a rare manifestation of an otherwise common tumor of bone (104,122,127). Its "rarity," however, may depend upon the rigor with which it is distinguished from subungual exostosis (Dupuytren's exostosis), which has similar microscopic characteristics. Subungual osteochondromas occur on the fingers and toes, and are commonly encountered in children and young adults (127,131,136). The presentation is that of an expanding, tender mass involving the digit, with deformity of the overlying nail plate. The clinical differential diagnosis includes cyst, fibroma, subungual verruca, amelanotic melanoma, glomus tumor, and subungual hematoma (104,120,127,142); however, the radiographic findings are typical (104,115, 122,136). Excision is curative, although lesions do recur (129,131).

Pathologic Findings. The microscopic changes of subungual osteochondroma include a cap of hyaline cartilage and underlying trabecular bone that forms through enchondral ossification (127). Despite proliferative activity of cells comprising the cartilaginous cap, the typical organization of these tumors, as demonstrated radiographically and histopathologically, should permit distinction from sarcomas, including chondrosarcoma (129).

Differential Diagnosis. Although subungual exostosis and osteochondroma may represent variants of the same lesion, there are some clinical and microscopic differences between the two, leading some authors to conclude that they are distinctive. In contrast to subungual osteochondromas, exostoses occur in females more often than males, are often preceded by trauma or infection (and may therefore represent pseudotumors), arise in the distal tuft of the phalanx rather than the epiphyseal line, and possess a cap of fibrocartilage rather than hyaline cartilage (115,120,136).

Parachordoma

Clinical Features. *Parachordoma* is a tumor of uncertain histogenesis that resembles both chordoma and extraskeletal myxoid chondrosarcoma. It is discussed here because of its histologic similarities to chondroid tumors, although it is not regarded as a tumor of true cartilaginous differentiation.

Parachordoma usually arises in deep soft tissues of the extremities or trunk, near tendons, synovium, or bone (112,119). Cutaneous or superficial subcutaneous examples are rare, but have been reported on the finger (135), thigh, and forearm (124). These lesions present most often in young to middle-aged adults, although examples in children and teenagers have been reported (118,119,138). Thus far, reported tumors have demonstrated slow growth and only local invasion (112). They respond well to complete excision, although recurrence is possible (112,132). Convincing evidence for metastasis of a parachordoma has not been presented to date (117,124).

Pathologic Findings. Histologically, parachordomas are lobulated tumors. They are composed of nodules containing aggregates of cells within a myxoid or hyaline matrix. These nodules may be separated by bands of fibrous connective tissue (124). The constituent cells are polygonal, with eosinophilic cytoplasm, and these may merge with smaller, rounded to spindled cells. Some of the cells have vacuolated cytoplasm, resembling the physaliphorous cells of chordoma (119,124). Pseudoglandular arrangements of these cells are sometimes observed (118).

The myxoid matrix is Alcian blue positive and hyaluronidase sensitive (119). The cells of parachordoma are regularly vimentin and S-100 protein positive (118,119,121,124,132,135). Epithelial membrane antigen staining is variably positive (119,124). Certain cytokeratins have also been reported to be positive, including pancytokeratin (124,135), CAM5.2 (118), and cytokeratin (CK) 8/18 (119), but negative results have been obtained for AE1 and CK1/10, CK7, CK19, and CK20 (118,119). Type IV collagen is present in a linear distribution around nests of cells (119).

Electron microscopy shows cells with cytoplasmic vacuoles, intermediate filaments, pinocytotic vesicles, junctional complexes, and microvillous processes (118,124). Flow cytometry of one case showed a diploid histogram (132), but cytogenetic analyses have shown a variety of chromosomal anomalies (119,132,138), including trisomy 15 and monosomies of 1, 16, and 17 (119).

Differential Diagnosis. The chief considerations in the differential diagnosis of parachordoma are two biologically more aggressive tumors, myxoid chondrosarcoma and chordoma. Parachordomas are more likely than the other two tumors to show positivity for type IV collagen deposition around nests of cells (119). In contrast to parachordomas, extraskeletal myxoid chondrosarcomas are cytokeratin negative and have a different cytogenetic profile, including the t(9:22)(q22;q12) rearrangement (119,133).

Chordomas are more often cytokeratin and epithelial membrane antigen positive than are parachordomas (124), although there is overlap in this regard. Chordomas tend to have a different cytokeratin profile, since they are positive for AE1, CK8/18, CK1/10, and CK19, and negative for CK7 and CK20, while parachordomas are CK8/18 positive but negative for AE1, CK1/10, CK19, CK7, and CK20 (118,119). Chordomas also have the distinguishing ultrastructural feature of numerous rough endoplasmic reticulum-mitochondrial complexes (124). Cytogenetic abnormalities also differ from those of parachordoma, since chordomas have shown monosomies of 3, 4, 10, and 13 (119).

The lack of myoepithelial markers in parachordoma would argue against soft tissue myoepithelioma, a tumor that may be related to the eccrine mixed tumor of skin (117–119).

Chondrosarcoma

Clinical Features. Chondrosarcoma involves the skin in several ways. It can present as a cutaneous metastasis from a primary lesion of bone (106,125,128,130,137), rarely as a metastasis from a primary soft tissue tumor (105), or as a lesion centered in the subcutis. In a rare case, a patient first presented with cutaneous metastases of a dedifferentiated chondrosarcoma that was later found to have derived from a tumor arising in the right humerus (106).

Pathologic Findings. Two varieties are encountered in skin: *myxoid chondrosarcoma* and *mesenchymal chondrosarcoma*. Myxoid chondrosarcoma consists of aggregates of cells with hyperchromatic nuclei within a (sulfated) mucinous matrix (fig. 9-15) (116); mesenchymal chondrosarcoma features sheets of undifferentiated cells and islands of well-differentiated cartilaginous tissue (109). The diagnosis depends upon the recognition of cartilaginous differentiation, together with immunohistochemical and ultrastructural features (134,140). Chondrosarcomas are vimentin, S-100 protein, and leu-7 positive and are usually negative for epithelial markers (140).

Differential Diagnosis. The above findings usually permit distinction from tumors such as myxoid liposarcoma (which features lipoblasts, numerous proliferative blood vessels, and nonsulfated mucin), and chondroid syringoma and malignant chondroid syringoma (which display epithelial cells that are cytokeratin positive).

CALCIFYING AND OSSIFYING TUMORS

Ossifying Fibromyxoid Tumor

Clinical Features. *Ossifying fibromyxoid tumor* is a soft tissue tumor first reported by Enzinger, Weiss, and Liang in 1989 (152). It commonly arises in the subcutis (146,152,154–156,162, 168), and typically presents as a painless mass that develops in adults, with a slight male predominance. The extremities are usually involved, but lesions also arise in the head and neck region and in the trunk. Recurrence following removal is common (146,152). Metastasis has been reported, both to subcutaneous tissue (of an opposite extremity) and lung, although this is rare (152,156). For these reasons,

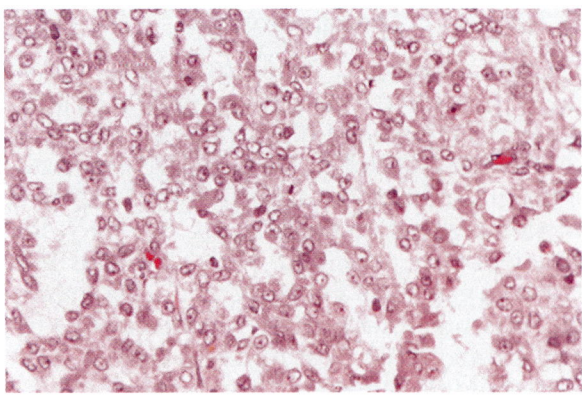

Figure 9-15

MYXOID CHONDROSARCOMA

Tumor cells are present within a matrix composed of sulfated mucin.

complete excision with assurance of free margins is indicated (146).

Pathologic Findings. Microscopically, ossifying fibromyxoid tumor has lobulated contours and is composed of small, rounded to spindled cells grouped in cords and nests (152), storiform or whorled configurations (154), or pseudoalveolar arrangements (fig. 9-16A) (162). These groups of cells are present within a myxoid to hyaline matrix, with foci of osteoid formation (152,156). Bone formation is present, most characteristically as a discontinuous shell within the fibrous capsule of the tumor (fig. 9-16B) (152,162,168). Cytologic atypia is minimal and mitoses are infrequent (fig. 9-16C), although they numbered as high as 2 per 10 high-power fields in the atypical variants of the tumor reported by Kilpatrick et al. (156).

Results of immunohistochemical staining have been variable. Vimentin and S-100 protein are usually positive (152,155,156), although the latter may stain focally and in one case appeared to stain only associated dendritic cells (146). In some studies, cells have also stained for neuron-specific enolase (154,168), glial fibrillary acidic protein (149,160), leu-7 (154,160), and desmin (154,156), although in other reports each of these was negative (146,162). There can be weak stromal staining for type IV collagen and laminin (146), but a type II collagen stain has been negative, which argues against a cartilaginous derivation of the tumor (149). Consistently negative results have been obtained with antibodies to cytokeratins, epithelial membrane antigen, and actin (146,160,162,168). Ultrastructural studies have shown cells with complex cell processes and reduplicated basal lamina (160,162). The staining pattern and electron microscopic findings are suggestive of a Schwann cell origin for this tumor (146, 149,160,162), although some authors have proposed a fibroblastic or myofibroblastic derivation (154,155). One investigated tumor had an aneuploid DNA content (154).

Differential Diagnosis. When all the elements are present, the diagnosis of ossifying fibromyxoid tumor is relatively straightforward. However, examples with sparse or absent bone formation may be confused with other tumors of fibrohistiocytic, myofibroblastic, or neural origin (163,164).

Fibro-osseous Pseudotumor of the Digits

Clinical Features. *Fibro-osseous pseudotumor of the digits* occurs in the soft tissues of the fingers and toes of young adults, predominantly women. It presents as a fusiform swelling or polypoid nodule that may be associated with rapid growth, pain, or ulceration of the overlying skin (147,150,167). A history of trauma can sometimes be elicited (150). Despite a sometimes alarming clinical and microscopic appearance, this tumor is cured by complete excision. It is considered by many to be closely related to *myositis ossificans*.

Pathologic Findings. The microscopic features include a nodular fasciitis-like proliferation of fibroblasts in a myxoid stroma, immature osteoid formation lined by osteoblasts, and formation of mature lamellar bone. These elements may be combined without the zonal arrangement characteristic of myositis ossificans (i.e., fibroblastic proliferation merging with immature osteoid, with a peripheral zone of lamellar bone) (150). Sleater et al. (167) were able to discern some degree of zonation in their cases. Mitotic activity is noted within zones of fibroblast proliferation. In the study by Sleater et al., the fibroblastic cells stained for vimentin and smooth muscle actin but not for S-100 protein, cytokeratins, CD34, and factor VIII; these results favor myofibroblastic differentiation. In a case presented by Chan et al. (147), however, actin staining was negative,

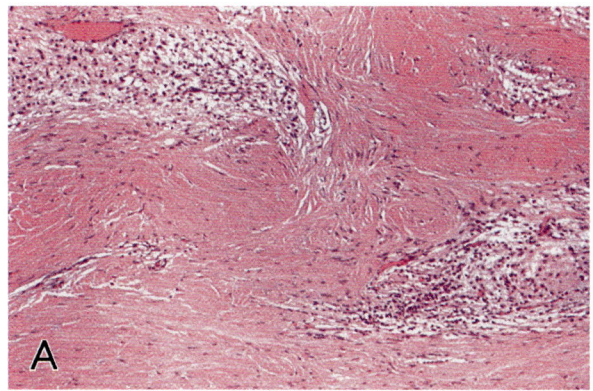
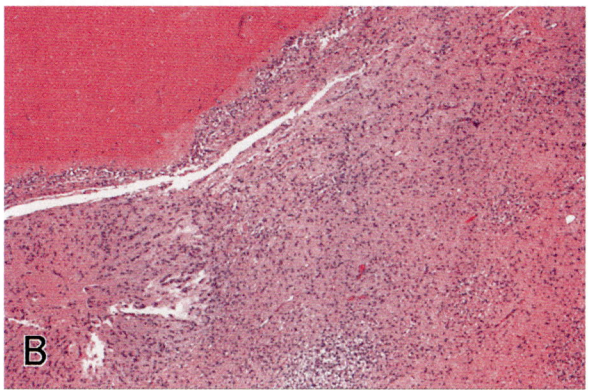
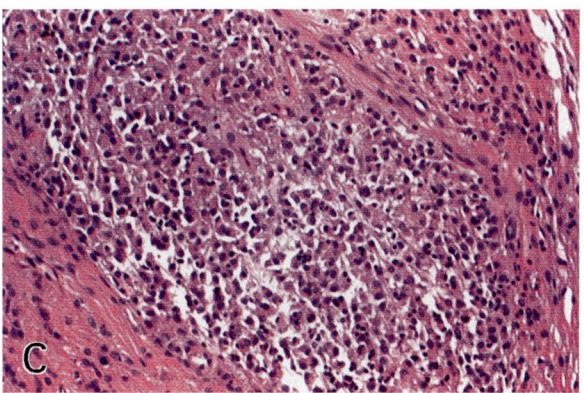

Figure 9-16

OSSIFYING FIBROMYXOID TUMOR

A: Cords and nests of tumor cells are present within a sclerotic, somewhat hyaline matrix.
B: Bone formation is evident in this low-power view.
C: Tumor cells are rounded to spindled, and display minimal cytologic atypia.

and dense bodies were not observed ultrastructurally. The proliferation marker Ki-67 is moderately positive in fibroblast areas (167).

Differential Diagnosis. The evidence suggests that fibro-osseous pseudotumor of the digits is closely related to myositis ossificans. The major differences include anatomic location (myositis ossificans occurs in large muscles) and sex incidence (myositis ossificans is more common in men). Microscopically and immunohistochemically, these lesions are similar, and while the zonal arrangement is generally better developed in myositis ossificans, some zoning can be identified in fibro-osseous pseudotumor (167).

The rapid growth and mitotic activity of fibro-osseous pseudotumor can raise concerns about extraskeletal osteosarcoma. The latter tumor, however, occurs in an older age group, rarely involves the digits, and features significant pleomorphism and atypical mitotic figures. In osteosarcoma, zonation is either absent or reversed, in which case immature spindle cell areas tend to be present at the periphery rather than in central portions of the tumor (165,167).

In one reported case of a polypoid nodule, initial incomplete excision led to an erroneous diagnosis of pyogenic granuloma (147), emphasizing the importance of complete excision for accurate histopathologic evaluation.

Calcifying Aponeurotic Fibroma

Clinical Features. *Calcifying aponeurotic fibroma* mainly affects children and young adults. It most often involves the palm or fingers, plantar portion of the foot, or the ankle, but unusual locations have also been reported, such as the back, knee, and thigh (153,161). It presents as a slow-growing, painless mass, associated with the fascia, tendons, or aponeuroses. It is poorly circumscribed and prone to recurrence. Although rare, metastasis has been reported, in the form of a fibrosarcoma that metastasized to lung and bone (159).

Pathologic Findings. Proliferations of plump, spindled to epithelioid fibroblasts form fascicular arrangements and extend irregularly into adjacent connective tissues. There are centrally located foci of chondroid metaplasia and

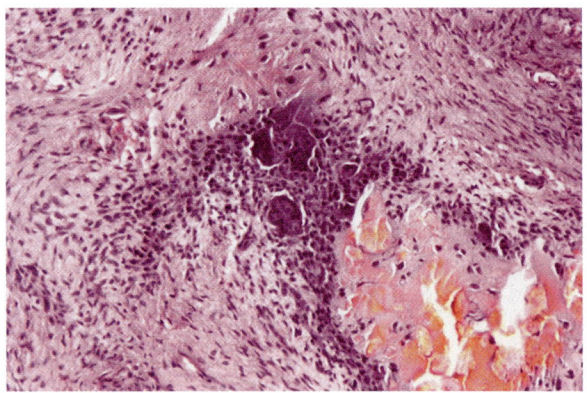

Figure 9-17

CALCIFYING APONEUROTIC FIBROMA

The central portion of this lesion shows chondroid metaplasia and calcification. Note the surrounding spindled fibroblasts.

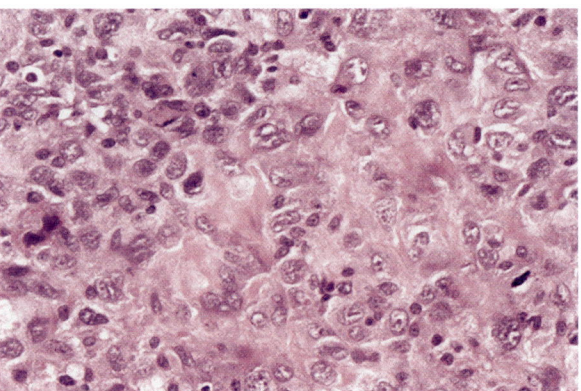

Figure 9-18

OSTEOSARCOMA

The cellular component of this tumor mimics other soft tissue sarcomas.

calcification (fig. 9-17), which are more pronounced in tumors from older individuals, and may become more pronounced with progressive recurrences (161). Osteoclast-like giant cells may be identified at the periphery of the foci of chondroid metaplasia; however, ossification is rare (151). Pleomorphism is mild, mitoses are infrequent, and atypical mitoses are generally not observed (161). As expected, sulfated mucin is identified in the chondroid foci. In one study, fibroblasts were vimentin, CD68, CD99, and S-100 protein positive; in three of six tumors, cells were smooth muscle actin and muscle-specific actin positive (153).

Differential Diagnosis. Examples of calcifying aponeurotic fibroma with minimal chondroid or calcium deposition may be confused with forms of fibromatosis or spindle cell sarcoma (161). On the other hand, lesions with more prominent chondroid material and calcification resemble extraskeletal chondroma. The latter tumor occurs in an older age group, is lobulated and sharply demarcated from the adjacent connective tissue, possesses better developed cartilage, and shows more diffuse calcification (151,161).

Osteosarcoma

Extraskeletal osteosarcoma rarely occurs in the skin, but it can arise in the subcutis or dermis (145,148,157,158), extend to the skin from a deep soft tissue focus, or metastasize to skin from another primary site (166). Extraskeletal osteosarcoma can also develop in an area that has received radiation therapy, in which case there may be overlying changes of chronic radiodermatitis. Patients with extraskeletal osteosarcoma have a poor prognosis (145).

The microscopic findings are consistent with those found in traditional forms of osteosarcoma: foci of neoplastic bone, osteoid, or cartilage and a cellular component that can mimic other soft tissue sarcomas (fig. 9-18) (145,148). The atypical microscopic characteristics usually permit distinction from benign cartilaginous and osseous tumors, but it may be difficult to distinguish osteosarcoma from other malignant tumors that occasionally show metaplastic ossification, such as malignant fibrous histiocytoma (145,148).

REFERENCES

Smooth Muscle Tumors

1. Allison JG, Dodds HM. Leiomyoma of the male nipple. A case report and literature review. Am Surg 1989;55:501–2.
2. Aneiros J, Beltran E, Garcia del Moral R, Nogales FF Jr. Epithelioid leiomyoma of the vulva. Diagn Gynecol Obstet 1982;4:351–6.
3. Argenyi ZB, Piette WW, Goeken JA. Cutaneous angiomyolipoma. A light-microscopic, immunohistochemical, and electron-microscopic study. Am J Dermatopathol 1991;13:497–502.
4. Argenyi ZB, Piette, WW, Goeken J. Cutaneous angiomyolipoma: a light microscopic, immunohistochemical, and electron microscopic study [Abstract]. J Cutan Pathol 1986;13:434.
5. Bendet E. A wattle (cervical accessory tragus). Otolaryngol Head Neck Surg 1999;121:508–9.
6. Berberian BJ, Burnett JW. Congenital smooth muscle hamartoma: a case report. Br J Dermatol 1986;115:711–4.
7. Bronson DM, Fretzin DF, Farrell LN. Congenital pilar and smooth muscle nevus. J Am Acad Dermatol 1983;8:111–4.
8. Burden PA, Gentry RH, Fitzpatrick JE. Piloleiomyoma arising in an organoid nevus: a case report and review of the literature. J Dermatol Surg Oncol 1987;13:1213–8.
9. Buyukbabani N, Tetikkurt S, Ozturk AS. Cutaneous angiomyolipoma: report of two cases with emphasis on HMB-45 utility. J Eur Acad Dermatol Venereol 1998;11:151–4.
10. Calonje E, Wilson-Jones E, Smith NP, Fletcher CD. Cellular 'neurothekeoma': an epithelioid variant of pilar leiomyoma? Morphological and immunohistochemical analysis of a series. Histopathology 1992;20:397–404.
11. Carla TG, Filotico R, Filotico M. Bizarre angiomyomas of superficial soft tissues. Pathologica 1991;83:237–42.
12. Chang SG, Lee SC, Park YK, Chai SE. Pedunculated leiomyoma of scrotum. J Korean Med Sci 1991;6:284–6.
13. Chow J, Sabet LM, Clark BL, Coire CI. Cutaneous leiomyosarcoma: case reports and review of the literature. Ann Plast Surg 1987;18:319–22.
14. Christensen P, Barr RJ. Wattle: an unusual congenital anomaly. Arch Dermatol 1985;121:22–3.
15. Civatte J, Marinho E, Oliver Santos R. [Smooth muscle hamartoma or nevus of Becker? Apropos of 4 cases.] Med Cutan Ibero Lat Am 1988;16:145–8. (Spanish.)
16. Dahl I, Angervall L. Cutaneous and subcutaneous leiomyosarcoma. A clinicopathologic study of 47 patients. Pathol Eur 1974;9:307–15.
17. de la Espriella J, Grossin M, Marinho E, Belaich S. [Smooth muscle hamartoma: anatomoclinical characteristics and nosological limits.] Ann Dermatol Venereol 1993;120:879–83. (French.)
18. Fearfield LA, Smith JR, Bunker CB, Staughton RC. Association of multiple familial cutaneous leiomyoma with a uterine symplastic leiomyoma. Clin Exp Dermatol 2000;25:44–7.
19. Fields JP, Helwig EB. Leiomyosarcoma of the skin and subcutaneous tissue. Cancer 1981;47:156–69.
20. Fitzpatrick JE, Mellette JR Jr, Hwang RJ, Golitz LE, Zaim MT, Clemons D. Cutaneous angiolipoleiomyoma. J Am Acad Dermatol 1990;23(Pt 1):1093–8.
21. Gagne EJ, Su WP. Congenital smooth muscle hamartoma of the skin. Pediatr Dermatol 1993;10:142–5.
22. Glover MT, Malone M, Atherton DJ. Michelin-tire baby syndrome resulting from diffuse smooth muscle hamartoma. Pediatr Dermatol 1989;6:329–31.
23. Goldman MP, Kaplan RP, Heng MC. Congenital smooth-muscle hamartoma. Int J Dermatol 1987;26:448–52.
24. Hachisuga T, Hashimoto H, Enjoji M. Angioleiomyoma. A clinicopathologic reappraisal of 562 cases. Cancer 1984;54:126–30.
25. Hashimoto H, Daimaru Y, Tsuneyoshi M, Enjoji M. Leiomyosarcoma of the external soft tissues. A clinicopathologic, immunohistochemical, and electron microscopic study. Cancer 1986;57:2077–88.
26. Headington JT, Beals TF, Niederhuber JE. Primary leiomyosarcoma of skin: a report and critical appraisal. J Cutan Pathol 1977;4:308–17.
27. Heffernan MP, Smoller BR, Kohler S. Cutaneous epithelioid angioleiomyoma. Am J Dermatopathol 1998;20:213–7.
28. Hopkins-Luna AM, Chambers DC, Goodman MD. Epithelioid leiomyoma of the vulva. J Natl Med Assoc 1999;91:171–3.
29. Jegasothy BV, Gilgor RS, Hull M. Leiomyosarcoma of the skin and subcutaneous tissue. Arch Dermatol 1981;117:478–81.
30. Jensen ML, Jensen OM, Michalski W, Nielsen OS, Keller J. Intradermal and subcutaneous leiomyosarcoma: a clinicopathological and immunohistochemical study of 41 cases. J Cutan Pathol 1996;23:458–63.

31. Johnson MD, Jacobs AH. Congenital smooth muscle hamartoma. A report of six cases and a review of the literature. Arch Dermatol 1989;125:820–2.
32. Koizumi H, Kodama K, Tsuji Y, Matsumura T, Nabeshima M, Ohkawara A. CD34-positive dendritic cells are an intrinsic part of smooth muscle hamartoma. Br J Dermatol 1999;140:172–4.
33. Lespi PJ, Smit R. Verocay body-prominent cutaneous leiomyoma. Am J Dermatopathol 1999;21:110–1.
34. MacDonald DM, Sanderson KV. Angioleiomyoma of the skin. Br J Dermatol 1974;91:161–8.
35. Magner D, Hill DP. Encapsulated angiomyoma of the skin and cutaneous tissues. Am J Clin Pathol 1961;35:137–41.
36. McIntosh GS, Li AK, Hobbs KE. Late cutaneous and muscular metastases of a uterine leiomyosarcoma after an initial simultaneous presentation with an adenocarcinoma. Ann Chir Gynaecol 1983;72:229–31.
37. Mehregan DA, Mehregan DR, Mehregan AH. Angiomyolipoma. J Am Acad Dermatol 1992;27(Pt 2):331–3.
38. Mentzel T, Wadden C, Fletcher CD. Granular cell change in smooth muscle tumours of skin and soft tissue. Histopathology 1994;24:223–31.
39. Mezzadra G. [Multiple hereditary cutaneous leiomyoma. Study of a systemic case in a male subject related to a family with cutaneous leiomyomatosis and uterine fibromyomatosis.] Minerva Dermatol 1965;40:388–93. (Italian.)
40. Minami M, Inoue W, Uchida M. [Leiomyoma of the scrotum: a case report.] Hinyokika Kiyo 1999;45:207–9. (Japanese.)
41. Montgomery H. Smooth-muscle tumors of the skin. Arch Dermatol 1959;79:32–41.
42. Nair BK. Familial cutaneous leiomyoma. Indian J Pathol Bacteriol 1973;16:75–7.
43. Nascimento AG, Karas M, Rosen PP, Caron AG. Leiomyoma of the nipple. Am J Surg Pathol 1979;3:151–4.
44. Nemoto T, Shinoda M, Komatsuzaki K, Hara T, Kojima M, Ogihara T. Myxoid leiomyoma of the vulva mimicking aggressive angiomyxoma. Pathol Int 1994;44:454–9.
45. Neri A, Peled Y, Braslavski D. Vulvar leiomyoma. Acta Obstet Gynecol Scand 1993;72(3):221–2.
46. Neviaser RJ, Newman W. Dermal angiomyoma of the upper extremity. J Hand Surg [Am] 1977;2:271–4.
47. Oliver GF, Reiman HM, Gonchoroff NJ, Muller SA, Umbert IJ. Cutaneous and subcutaneous leiomyosarcoma: a clinicopathological review of 14 cases with reference to antidesmin staining and nuclear DNA patterns studied by flow cytometry. Br J Dermatol 1991;124:252–7.
48. Pastore RL, Ianiro G. Cutaneous angioleiomyoma. J Am Podiatr Med Assoc 1999;89:145–7.
49. Quinn TR, Young RH. Smooth-muscle hamartoma of the tunica dartos of the scrotum: report of a case. J Cutan Pathol 1997;24:322–6.
50. Raj S, Calonje E, Kraus M, Kavanagh G, Newman PL, Fletcher CD. Cutaneous pilar leiomyoma: clinicopathologic analysis of 53 lesions in 45 patients. Am J Dermatopathol 1997;19:2–9.
51. Rodriguez-Fernandez A, Caro-Mancilla A. Cutaneous angiomyolipoma with pleomorphic changes. J Am Acad Dermatol 1993;29:115–6.
52. Roper GJ, Smith MS, Lueder GT. Congenital smooth muscle hamartoma of the conjunctival fornix. Am J Ophthalmol 1999;128:643–4.
53. Runne U, Antz H, Pullmann H. [Verrucous leiomyoma of the scrotum presenting as condyloma acuminatum.] Z Hautkr 1980;55:652–60. (German.)
54. Schnur RE, Herzberg AJ, Spinner N, et al. Variability in the Michelin tire syndrome. A child with multiple anomalies, smooth muscle hamartoma, and familial paracentric inversion of chromosome 7q. J Am Acad Dermatol 1993;28(Pt 2):364–70.
55. Seifert HW. [Electron microscopic investigation on cutaneous leiomyosarcoma (author's transl).] Arch Dermatol Res 1978;263:159–69. (German.)
56. Sturtz CL, Dabbs DJ. Angiomyolipomas: the nature and expression of the HMB45 antigen. Mod Pathol 1994;7:842–5.
57. Suster S. Epithelioid leiomyosarcoma of the skin and subcutaneous tissue. Clinicopathologic, immunohistochemical, and ultrastructural study of five cases. Am J Surg Pathol 1994;18:232–40.
58. Suster S, Rosen LB, Sanchez JL. Granular cell leiomyosarcoma of the skin. Am J Dermatopathol 1988;10:234–9.
59. Swanson PE, Stanley MW, Scheithauer BW, Wick MR. Primary cutaneous leiomyosarcoma. A histological and immunohistochemical study of 9 cases, with ultrastructural correlation. J Cutan Pathol 1988;15:129–41.
60. Thyresson HN, Su WP. Familial cutaneous leiomyomatosis. J Am Acad Dermatol 1981;4:430–4.
61. Tsujioka K, Kashihara M, Imamura S. Cutaneous leiomyoma of the male nipple. Dermatologica 1985;170:98–100.
62. Urbanek RW, Johnson WC. Smooth muscle hamartoma associated with Becker's nevus. Arch Dermatol 1978;114:104–6.
63. Val-Bernal JF, Mira C. Cutaneous angiomyolipoma. J Cutan Pathol 1996;23:364–8.

64. Velasco M, Ubeda B, Autonell F, Serra C. Leiomyoma of the male areola infiltrating the breast tissue. AJR Am J Roentgenol 1995;164:511–2.
65. Watanabe K, Suzuki T. Mucocutaneous angiomyolipoma. A report of 2 cases arising in the nasal cavity. Arch Pathol Lab Med 1999;123:789–92.
66. Zvulunov A, Rotem A, Merlob P, Metzker A. Congenital smooth muscle hamartoma. Prevalence, clinical findings, and follow-up in 15 patients. Am J Dis Child 1990;144:782–4.

Striated Muscle Tumors and Rhabdoid Tumor

67. Ashfaq R, Timmons CF. Rhabdomyomatous mesenchymal hamartoma of skin. Pediatr Pathol 1992;12:731–5.
68. Beham A, Wirnsberger G, Schmid C. [Immunohistochemical studies in the differential diagnosis of malignant fibrous histiocytoma.] Wien Klin Wochenschr 1986;98:617–22. (German.)
69. Brocker EB, Hamm H, Ritter J, Happle R, Schmidt D. [Rhabdomyosarcoma: differential diagnosis of cutaneous tumors in childhood.] Hautarzt 1992;43:590–3. (German.)
70. Chang Y, Dehner LP, Egbert B. Primary cutaneous rhabdomyosarcoma. Am J Surg Pathol 1990;14:977–82.
71. Dabbs DJ, Park HK. Malignant rhabdoid skin tumor: an uncommon primary skin neoplasm. Ultrastructural and immunohistochemical analysis. J Cutan Pathol 1988;15:109–15.
72. de Jong AS, van Kessel-van Vark M, Albus-Lutter CE. Pleomorphic rhabdomyosarcoma in adults: immunohistochemistry as a tool for its diagnosis. Hum Pathol 1987;18:298–303.
73. Delleman JW, Oorthuys JW. Orbital cyst in addition to congenital cerebral and focal dermal malformations: a new entity? Clin Genet 1981;19:191–8.
74. Deneo H, Carlevaro A, Espasandin J, Carzoglio JC, Cendan ME, Vignale RA. [Alveolar rhabdomyosarcoma of the skin.] Med Cutan Ibero Lat Am 1983;11:437–41. (Spanish.)
75. Elgart GW, Patterson JW. Congenital midline hamartoma: case report with histochemical and immunohistochemical findings. Pediatr Dermatol 1990;7:199–201.
76. Farris PE, Manning S, Vuitch F. Rhabdomyomatous mesenchymal hamartoma. Am J Dermatopathol 1994;16:73–5.
77. Frierson HF Jr, Mills SE, Innes DJ Jr. Malignant rhabdoid tumor of the pelvis. Cancer 1985;55:1963–7.
78. Garcia-Bustinduy M, Alvarez-Arguelles H, Guimera F, et al. Malignant rhabdoid tumor beside benign skin mesenchymal neoplasm with myofibromatous features. J Cutan Pathol 1999;26:509–15.
79. Hayashi K, Ohtsuki Y, Takahashi K, et al. Congenital alveolar rhabdomyosarcoma with multiple skin metastases. Report of a case. Acta Pathol Jpn 1988;38:241–8.
80. Hendrick SJ, Sanchez RL, Blackwell SJ, Raimer SS. Striated muscle hamartoma: description of two cases. Pediatr Dermatol 1986;3:153–7.
81. Hsueh C, Kuo TT. Congenital malignant rhabdoid tumor presenting as a cutaneous nodule: report of 2 cases with review of the literature. Arch Pathol Lab Med 1998;122:1099–102.
82. Ito F, Watanabe Y, Harada T, Horibe K. Cerebral metastases of alveolar rhabdomyosarcoma in an infant with multiple skin nodules. J Pediatr Hematol Oncol 1997;19:466–9.
83. Katsumata M, Keong CH, Satoh T. Rhabdomyomatous mesenchymal hamartoma of skin. J Dermatol 1990;17:384–7.
84. Mills AE. Rhabdomyomatous mesenchymal hamartoma of skin. Am J Dermatopathol 1989;11:58–63.
85. Morgan MB, Stevens L, Patterson J, Tannenbaum M. Cutaneous epithelioid malignant nerve sheath tumor with rhabdoid features: a histologic, immunohistochemical, and ultrastructural study of three cases. J Cutan Pathol 2000;27:529–34.
86. Nakanishi H, Hashimoto I, Takiwaki H, Urano Y, Arase S. Striated muscle hamartoma of the nostril. J Dermatol 1995;22:504–7.
87. Ndiaye B, Grosshans E, Dieng MT, et al. [Cutaneous rhabdomyosarcoma.] Ann Dermatol Venereol 1994;121:814–6. (French.)
88. Parham DM, Weeks DA, Beckwith JB. The clinicopathologic spectrum of putative extrarenal rhabdoid tumors. An analysis of 42 cases studied with immunohistochemistry or electron microscopy. Am J Surg Pathol 1994;18:1010–29.
89. Patel NK, McKee PH, Smith NP, Fletcher CD. Primary metaplastic carcinoma (carcinosarcoma) of the skin. A clinicopathologic study of four cases and review of the literature. Am J Dermatopathol 1997;19:363–72.
90. Perez-Atayde AR, Newbury R, Fletcher JA, Barnhill R, Gellis S. Congenital "neurovascular hamartoma" of the skin. A possible marker of malignant rhabdoid tumor. Am J Surg Pathol 1994;18:1030–8.
91. Perez-Guillermo M, Bonmati-Limorte C, Garcia-Rojo B, Hernandez-Gil A. Infantile cutaneous rhabdomyosarcoma (Li-Fraumeni syndrome): cytological presentation of fine-needle aspirate biopsy, report of a case. Diagn Cytopathol 1992;8:621–6.

92. Perrone T, Swanson PE, Twiggs L, Ulbright TM, Dehner LP. Malignant rhabdoid tumor of the vulva: is distinction from epithelioid sarcoma possible? A pathologic and immunohistochemical study. Am J Surg Pathol 1989;13:848–58.
93. Read RW, Burnstine M, Rowland JM, Zamir E, Rao NA. Rhabdomyomatous mesenchymal hamartoma of the eyelid: report of a case and literature review. Ophthalmology 2001;108:798–804.
94. Saboorian MH, Kenny M, Ashfaq R, Albores-Saavedra J. Carcinosarcoma arising in eccrine spiradenoma of the breast. Report of a case and review of the literature. Arch Pathol Lab Med 1996;120:501–4.
95. Sahn EE, Garen PD, Pai GS, Levkoff AH, Hagerty RC, Maize JC. Multiple rhabdomyomatous mesenchymal hamartomas of skin. Am J Dermatopathol 1990;12:485–91.
96. Sanchez RL, Raimer SS. Clinical and histologic features of striated muscle hamartoma: possible relationship to Delleman's syndrome. J Cutan Pathol 1994;21:40–6.
97. Sangueza OP, Meshul CK, Sangueza P, Mendoza R. Rhabdoid tumor of the skin. Int J Dermatol 1992;31:484–7.
98. Scrivener Y, Petiau P, Rodier-Bruant C, Cribier B, Heid E, Grosshans E. Perianal striated muscle hamartoma associated with hemangioma. Pediatr Dermatol 1998;15:274–6.
99. Simsir A, Ioffe OB, Henry M. Adult rhabdomyosarcoma with skin metastases: diagnosis by fine needle aspiration biopsy. Acta Cytol 2001;45:106–8.
100. Staindl O, Zelger J. [Rhabdomyosarcoma of the skin.] Hautarzt 1977;28:574–7. (German.)
101. Tsuneyoshi M, Daimaru Y, Hashimoto H, Enjoji M. Malignant soft tissue neoplasms with the histologic features of renal rhabdoid tumors: an ultrastructural and immunohistochemical study. Hum Pathol 1985;16:1235–42.
102. Weiss SW, Enzinger FM. Malignant fibrous histiocytoma: an analysis of 200 cases. Cancer 1978;41:2250–66.
103. Wiss K, Solomon AR, Raimer SS, Lobe TE, Gourley W, Headington JT. Rhabdomyosarcoma presenting as a cutaneous nodule. Arch Dermatol 1988;124:1687–90.

Cartilaginous Tumors and Parachordoma

104. Apfelberg DB, Druker D, Maser MR, Lash H. Subungual osteochondroma. Differential diagnosis and treatment. Arch Dermatol 1979;115:472–3.
105. Aramburu-Gonzalez JA, Rodriguez-Justo M, Jimenez-Reyes J, Santonja C. A case of soft tissue mesenchymal chondrosarcoma metastatic to skin, clinically mimicking keratoacanthoma. Am J Dermatopathol 1999;21:392–4.
106. Arce FP, Pinto J, Portero I, Echevarria S, Val-Bernal JF. Cutaneous metastases as initial manifestation of dedifferentiated chondrosarcoma of bone. An autopsy case with review of the literature. J Cutan Pathol 2000;27:262–7.
107. Ayala F, Lembo G, Montesano M. A rare tumor: subungual chondroma. Report of a case. Dermatologica 1983;167:339–40.
108. Bendet E. A wattle (cervical accessory tragus). Otolaryngol Head Neck Surg 1999;121:508–9.
109. Bertoni F, Picci P, Bacchini P, et al. Mesenchymal chondrosarcoma of bone and soft tissues. Cancer 1983;52:533–41.
110. Chan JK, Lee KC, Saw D. Extraskeletal chondroma with lipoblast-like cells. Hum Pathol 1986;17:1285–7.
111. Christensen P, Barr RJ. Wattle: an unusual congenital anomaly. Arch Dermatol 1985;121:22–3.
112. Dabska M. Parachordoma: a new clinicopathologic entity. Cancer 1977;40:1586–92.
113. Dahlin DC, Salvador AH. Cartilaginous tumors of the soft tissues of the hands and feet. Mayo Clin Proc 1974;49:721–6.
114. DelSignore JL, Torre BA, Miller RJ. Extraskeletal chondroma of the hand. Case report and review of the literature. Clin Orthop 1990;(254):147–52.
115. Eliezri YD, Taylor SC. Subungual osteochondroma. Diagnosis and management. J Dermatol Surg Oncol 1992;18:753–8.
116. Enzinger FM, Shiraki M. Extraskeletal myxoid chondrosarcoma. An analysis of 34 cases. Hum Pathol 1972;3:421–35.
117. Fisher C. Parachordoma exists—but what is it? Adv Anat Pathol 2000;7:141–8.
118. Fisher C, Miettinen M. Parachordoma: a clinicopathologic and immunohistochemical study of four cases of an unusual soft tissue neoplasm. Ann Diagn Pathol 1997;1:3–10.
119. Folpe AL, Agoff SN, Willis J, Weiss SW. Parachordoma is immunohistochemically and cytogenetically distinct from axial chordoma and extraskeletal myxoid chondrosarcoma. Am J Surg Pathol 1999;23:1059–67.
120. Grisafi PJ, Lombardi CM, Sciarrino AL, Rainer GF, Buffone WF. Three select subungual pathologies: subungual exostosis, subungual osteochondroma, and subungual hematoma. Clin Podiatr Med Surg 1989;6:355–64.
121. Hirokawa M, Manabe T, Sugihara K. Parachordoma of the buttock: an immunohistochemical case study and review. Jpn J Clin Oncol 1994;24:336–9.
122. Hodgkinson DJ. Subungual osteochondroma. Plast Reconstr Surg 1984;74:833–4.

123. Holmes HS, Bovenmeyer DA. Cutaneous cartilaginous tumor. Arch Dermatol 1976;112:839–40.
124. Imlay SP, Argenyi ZB, Stone MS, McCollough ML, Henghold WB. Cutaneous parachordoma. A light microscopic and immunohistochemical report of two cases and review of the literature. J Cutan Pathol 1998;25:279–84.
125. Karabela-Bouropoulou V, Patra-Malli F, Agnantis N. Chondrosarcoma of the thumb: an unusual case with lung and cutaneous metastases and death of the patient 6 years after treatment. J Cancer Res Clin Oncol 1986;112:71–4.
126. Karlin CA, De Smet AA, Neff J, Lin F, Horton W, Wertzberger JJ. The variable manifestations of extraarticular synovial chondromatosis. AJR Am J Roentgenol 1981;137:731–5.
127. Kim SW, Moon SE, Kim JA. A case of subungual osteochondroma. J Dermatol 1998;25:60–2.
128. King DT, Gurevitch AW, Hirose FM. Multiple cutaneous metastases of a scapular chondrosarcoma. Arch Dermatol 1978;114:584–6.
129. Landon GC, Johnson KA, Dahlin DC. Subungual exostoses. J Bone Joint Surg Am 1979;61:256–9.
130. Leal-Khouri SM, Barnhill RL, Baden HP. An unusual cutaneous metastasis of a chondrosarcoma. J Cutan Pathol 1990;17:274–7.
131. Miller-Breslow A, Dorfman HD. Dupuytren's (subungual) exostosis. Am J Surg Pathol 1988;12:368–78.
132. Niezabitowski A, Limon J, Wasilewska A, Rys J, Lackowska B, Nedoszytko B. Parachordoma—a clinicopathologic, immunohistochemical, electron microscopic, flow cytometric, and cytogenetic study. Gen Diagn Pathol 1995;141:49–55.
133. Orndal C, Carlen B, Akerman M, et al. Chromosomal abnormality t(9;22)(q22;q12) in an extraskeletal myxoid chondrosarcoma characterized by fine needle aspiration cytology, electron microscopy, immunohistochemistry and DNA flow cytometry. Cytopathology 1991;2:261–70.
134. Povysil C, Matejovsky Z. A comparative ultrastructural study of chondrosarcoma, chordoid sarcoma, chordoma and chordoma periphericum. Pathol Res Pract 1985;179:546–59.
135. Sangueza OP, White CR Jr. Parachordoma. Am J Dermatopathol 1994;16:185–8.
136. Schulze KE, Hebert AA. Diagnostic features, differential diagnosis, and treatment of subungual osteochondroma. Pediatr Dermatol 1994;11:39–41.
137. Sherr DL, Fountain KS, Kalb RE. Cutaneous metastases from chondrosarcoma. J Dermatol Surg Oncol 1986;12:146–9.
138. Tihy F, Scott P, Russo P, Champagne M, Tabet JC, Lemieux N. Cytogenetic analysis of a parachordoma. Cancer Genet Cytogenet 1998;105:14–9.
139. Wawrosch W, Rassner G. [Monstrous enchondroma of the ungual phalanx of the forefinger with nail deformity.] Hautarzt 1985;36:168–9. (German.)
140. Wick MR, Burgess JH, Manivel JC. A reassessment of "chordoid sarcoma." Ultrastructural and immunohistochemical comparison with chordoma and skeletal myxoid chondrosarcoma. Mod Pathol 1988;1:433–43.
141. Williams DS, Zichichi S. Extraskeletal chondroma of the foot. J Am Podiatr Med Assoc 1998;88:506–9.
142. Woo TY, Rasmussen JE. Subungual osteocartilaginous exostosis. J Dermatol Surg Oncol 1985;11:534–6.
143. Yaffee HS. Peculiar nail dystrophy caused by an enchondroma. Arch Dermatol 1965;91:361.
144. Zlatkin MB, Lander PH, Begin LR, Hadjipavlou A. Soft-tissue chondromas. AJR Am J Roentgenol 1985;144:1263–7.

Calcifying and Ossifying Tumors

145. Bane BL, Evans HL, Ro JY, et al. Extraskeletal osteosarcoma. A clinicopathologic review of 26 cases. Cancer 1990;65:2762–70.
146. Barrett TL, Skelton HG, Smith KJ, O'Grady TC, Proctor-Shipman L. Ossifying fibromyxoid tumor of soft parts: a case report and review. J Cutan Pathol 1996;23:378–80.
147. Chan KW, Khoo US, Ho CM. Fibro-osseous pseudotumor of the digits: report of a case with immunohistochemical and ultrastructural studies. Pathology 1993;25:193–6.
148. Chung EB, Enzinger FM. Extraskeletal osteosarcoma. Cancer 1987;60:1132–42.
149. Donner LR. Ossifying fibromyxoid tumor of soft parts: evidence supporting Schwann cell origin. Hum Pathol 1992;23:200–2.
150. Dupree WB, Enzinger FM. Fibro-osseous pseudotumor of the digits. Cancer 1986;58:2103–9.
151. Enzinger FM, Weiss SW. Fibrous tumors of infancy and childhood soft tissue tumors, 3rd ed. St. Louis: Mosby-Year Book, Inc; 1995:256–61.
152. Enzinger FM, Weiss SW, Liang CY. Ossifying fibromyxoid tumor of soft parts. A clinicopathological analysis of 59 cases. Am J Surg Pathol 1989;13:817–27.
153. Fetsch JF, Miettinen M. Calcifying aponeurotic fibroma: a clinicopathologic study of 22 cases arising in uncommon sites. Hum Pathol 1998;29:1504–10.

154. Fukunaga M, Ushigome S, Ishikawa E. Ossifying subcutaneous tumor with myofibroblastic differentiation: a variant of ossifying fibromyxoid tumor of soft parts? Pathol Int 1994;44:727–34.
155. Hanski W, Lewicki Z. New observations on three cases of ossifying fibromyxoid tumor of soft parts. Pol J Pathol 1994;45:231–8.
156. Kilpatrick SE, Ward WG, Mozes M, Miettinen M, Fukunaga M, Fletcher CD. Atypical and malignant variants of ossifying fibromyxoid tumor. Clinicopathologic analysis of six cases. Am J Surg Pathol 1995;19:1039–46.
157. Kobos JW, Yu GH, Varadarajan S, Brooks JS. Primary cutaneous osteosarcoma. Am J Dermatopathol 1995;17:53–7.
158. Kuo TT. Primary osteosarcoma of the skin. J Cutan Pathol 1992;19:151–5.
159. Lafferty KA, Nelson EL, Demuth RJ, Miller SH, Harrison MW. Juvenile aponeurotic fibroma with disseminated fibrosarcoma. J Hand Surg [Am] 1986;11:737–40.
160. Miettinen M. Ossifying fibromyxoid tumor of soft parts. Additional observations of a distinctive soft tissue tumor. Am J Clin Pathol 1991;95:142–9.
161. Murphy BA, Kilpatrick SE, Panella MJ, White WL. Extra-acral calcifying aponeurotic fibroma: a distinctive case with 23-year follow-up. J Cutan Pathol 1996;23:369–72.
162. Nakayama F, Kuwahara T. Ossifying fibromyxoid tumor of soft parts of the back. J Cutan Pathol 1996;23:385–8.
163. Orosz Z, Sapi Z, Szentirmay Z. Unusual benign neurogenic soft tissue tumour. Epithelioid schwannoma or an ossifying fibromyxoid tumour? Pathol Res Pract 1993;189:601–5; discussion 605–7.
164. Rooney MT, Nascimento AG, Tung RL. Ossifying plexiform tumor. Report of a cutaneous ossifying lesion with histologic features of neurothekeoma. Am J Dermatopathol 1994;16:189–92.
165. Schutte HE, van der Heul RO. Pseudomalignant, nonneoplastic osseous soft-tissue tumors of the hand and foot. Radiology 1990;176:149–53.
166. Setoyama M, Kanda A, Kanzaki T. Cutaneous metastasis of an osteosarcoma. A case report. Am J Dermatopathol 1996;18:629–32.
167. Sleater J, Mullins D, Chun K, Hendricks J. Fibro-osseous pseudotumor of the digit: a comparison to myositis ossificans by light microscopy and immunohistochemical methods. J Cutan Pathol 1996;23:373–7.
168. Velasco-Pastor AM, Martinez-Escribano J, del Pino Gil-Mateo M, Quecedo-Estebanez E, Fortea-Baixauli JM, Aliaga-Boniche A. Ossifying fibromyxoid tumor of soft parts. J Cutan Pathol 1996;23:381–4.

SUPPLEMENTAL REFERENCES

Smooth Muscle Hamartoma

Oiso N, Fukai K, Ishii M, Hayashi T, Uda H, Imanishi M. A case of acquired smooth muscle hamartoma of the scrotum. Clin Exp Dermatol 2005;30:523–4.

Sbano P, Sbano E, Alessandrini C, Criscuolo M, Fimiani M. Igloo-like prepuce: a peculiar aspect of smooth-muscle hamartoma of the genitalia? J Cutan Pathol 2005;32:184–7.

van Kooten EO, Hage JJ, Meinhardt W, Horenblas S, Mooi WJ. Acquired smooth-muscle hamartoma of the scrotum: a histological simulator? J Cutan Pathol 2004;31:388–92.

Leiomyoma

Cairey-Remonnay S, Salard D, Algros MP, Laurent R. [Multiple familial cutaneous leiomyoma.] Ann Dermatol Venereol 2003;130:1017–20. (French.)

Marrazzo A, Taormina P, Noto A, Cardinale G, Casa L, Lo Gerfo D. Nipple leiomyoma in man: a case report. G Chir 2004;25:132–3.

Matthews JH, Pichardo RO, Hitchcock MG, Leshin B. Cutaneous leiomyoma with cytologic atypia, akin to uterine symplastic leiomyoma. Dermatol Surg 2004;30:1249–51.

Ramesh P, Annapureddy SR, Khan F, Sutaria PD. Angioleiomyoma: a clinical, pathological and radiological review. Int J Clin Pract 2004;58:587–91.

Sevilla Chica F, Meseguer Garcia P, Roca Estelles MJ, Gomez Castro A, Mola Arizo MJ, Sala Aznar A. [Atypical or bizarre leiomyoma of the scrotum. Report of one case and bibliographic review.] Arch Esp Urol 2004;57:428–31. (Spanish.)

Cutaneous Angiomyolipoma

Tsuruta D, Maekawa N, Ishii M. Cutaneous angiomyolipoma. Dermatology 2004;208:231–2.

Leiomyosarcoma

Bellezza G, Sidoni A, Cavaliere A, Scheibel M, Bucciarelli E. Primary cutaneous leiomyosarcoma: a clinicopathological and immunohistochemical study of 7 cases. Int J Surg Pathol 2004;12:39–44.

Cho YH, Park SG, Kim SH, Park JS, Lee MG. Cutaneous metastatic malignant mixed mullerian tumour mimicking cutaneous leiomyosarcoma: a case report. Br J Dermatol 2004;151:947–9.

Sabah M, Cummins R, Leader M, Kay E. Leiomyosarcoma and malignant fibrous histiocytoma share similar allelic imbalance pattern at 9p. Virchows Arch 2005;446:251–8.

Seemann N, Lehmann P. [Varying characteristics of subcutaneous and dermal leiomyosarcomas. Two case reports and literature review.] Hautarzt 2005 April 22. [Epub ahead of print.]

Tsuruta D, Maekawa N, Ishii M. Cutaneous angiomyolipoma. Dermatology 2004;208:231–2.

Rhabdomyomatous Mesenchymal Hamartoma

Chang CP, Chen GS. Rhabdomyomatous mesenchymal hamartoma: a plaque-type variant in an adult. Kaohsiung J Med Sci 2005;21:185–8.

Takeyama J, Hayashi T, Sanada T, Shimanuki Y, Saito M, Shirane R. Rhabdomyomatous mesenchymal hamartoma associated with nasofrontal meningocele and dermoid cyst. J Cutan Pathol 2005;32:310–3.

Rhabdomyosarcoma

Ilyas EN, Goldsmith K, Lintner R, Manders SM. Rhabdomyosarcoma arising in a giant congenital melanocytic nevus. Cutis 2004;73:39–43.

Tanzarella S, Lionello I, Valentinis B, Russo V, Lollini PL, Traversari C. Rhabdomyosarcomas are potential target of MAGE-specific immunotherapies. Cancer Immunol Immunother 2004;53:519–24.

Extrarenal Rhabdoid Tumor

Gambini C, Sementa A, Rongioletti F. "Proximal-type" epithelioid sarcoma in a young girl. Pediatr Dermatol 2004;21:117–20.

Subungual Osteochondroma and Exostosis

Vazquez-Flores H, Dominguez-Cherit J, Vega-Memije ME, Saez-De-Ocariz M. Subungual osteochondroma: clinical and radiologic features and treatment. Dermatol Surg 2004;30:1031–4.

Ossifying Fibromyxoid Tumor

Saadat P, Pullarkat S, Kelly L, Vadmal M. Ossifying fibromyxoid tumor of the skin: a report of 2 cases with light microscopic, immunohistochemical, and electron microscopic characterization. J Am Acad Dermatol 2005;52:644–7.

10 HISTIOCYTIC PROLIFERATIONS

This chapter describes a group of disorders characterized by the cutaneous infiltration of "histiocytes" and other cells considered to be derived from blood monocytes, including Langerhans cells, indeterminate cells, interdigitating cells, and other dendritic cells (125). The term histiocyte is outmoded, and largely of historical interest (58); it is understood that these cells have the characteristics attributed to macrophages (58,125). Nevertheless, the term histiocyte has become ingrained in the literature, and in fact, at least nine of the entities covered in this section bear the histiocyte label. For that reason, and to promote ease of reference, we have retained the term, although wherever possible we use the expression "histiocyte (macrophage)" or some other means to emphasize the monocyte-macrophage lineage of these cells.

NON-LANGERHANS CELL HISTIOCYTIC INFILTRATES

Many of the non-Langerhans cell histiocytoses could be termed "orphan diseases," as they are rarely encountered in routine practice. There has been an attempt to unify these histiocytoses (at least conceptually), since despite some clinical and histopathologic differences, all appear to be derived from the monocyte/macrophage. Their differing microscopic features may result, at least in part, from the effects of cytokines (134). Included in this group are juvenile xanthogranuloma, benign cephalic histiocytosis, generalized eruptive histiocytoma, xanthoma disseminatum, progressive nodular histiocytosis, and reticulohistiocytoma. Of the more common histiocytic proliferative disorders, juvenile xanthogranuloma can mimic, or be mimicked by, such diverse entities as Langerhans cell histiocytosis and epithelioid melanocytic tumors. Reticulohistiocytomas are most often encountered in the solitary form. Langerhans cell histiocytosis continues to be an important diagnostic consideration and challenge; some examples of the latter that manifest as eruptive cutaneous lesions in childhood appear to have a benign clinical course. Finally, cutaneous involvement with Rosai-Dorfman disease is increasingly diagnosed, and there are instances of this disorder that either first present in or are limited to the skin.

(Juvenile) Xanthogranuloma

Clinical Features. *(Juvenile) xanthogranuloma* consists of one or more cutaneous or subcutaneous nodules that contain proliferations of histiocytes (macrophages) in a characteristic configuration. As the name implies, these lesions are most common in infancy or childhood (59), but they also arise during adult life (97), and occurrence in a 77-year-old man has been reported (84). Males are predominantly affected.

The lesions most often occur in the head and neck region, but also appear on the trunk and extremities (109). Patients with multiple lesions are not unusual (109). Juvenile xanthogranuloma typically presents as red to yellow-orange papules or nodules ranging between 0.5 and 1.0 cm in diameter, but plaque-like (21) and macronodular (94) examples have also been reported, as have lesions of the deep soft tissues (65). Many other organs may be involved, including the eye (75), testis (59), pericardium (121), lung (55), kidney (47), and retroperitoneum and spleen (42). Eye involvement is probably the best known extracutaneous manifestation, and usually accompanies papular skin lesions (137); the chorioretinal region, ciliary body, corneoscleral limbus, and iris are involved (31,75). Anterior chamber hemorrhage and glaucoma can be associated with iris lesions.

A link between juvenile xanthogranuloma, neurofibromatosis, and juvenile chronic myelogenous leukemia has been repeatedly described, and is considered to be a true disease association (138). A patient with neurofibromatosis type 2, juvenile xanthogranuloma, and multiple neurilemmomas has also been reported (63). Lesions tend to involute spontaneously in

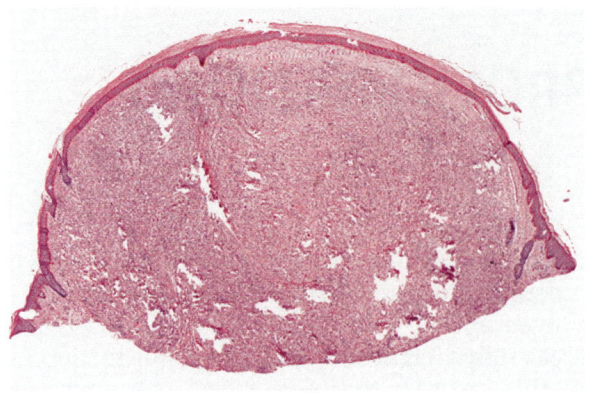 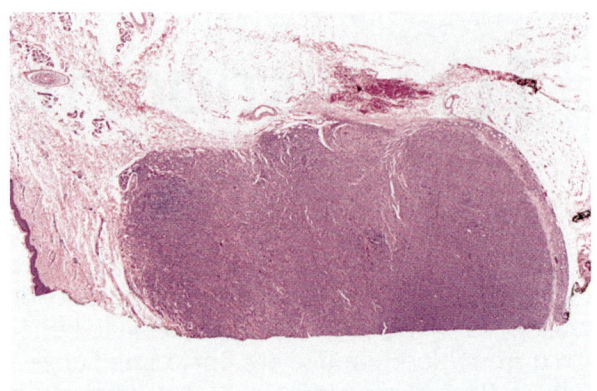

Figure 10-1

JUVENILE XANTHOGRANULOMA

Left: This is the typical configuration, consisting of a protuberant papule or small nodule.
Right: An example of deep xanthogranuloma, with extension into the subcutis.

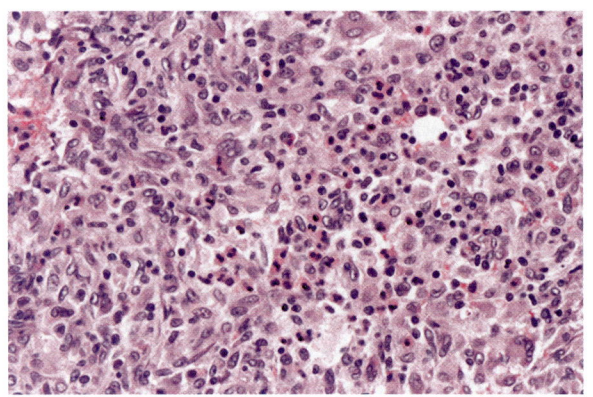 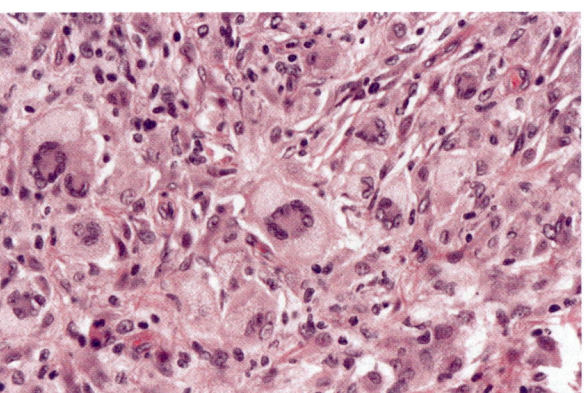

Figure 10-2

JUVENILE XANTHOGRANULOMA

Left: Eosinophils are numerous in this lesion.
Right: Foam-laden macrophages are present, and Touton giant cells are readily identified.

one to several years (97). The issue of whether juvenile xanthogranuloma is a reactive or neoplastic process is still unsettled, but it is generally grouped among the non-Langerhans cell histiocytoses (125).

Pathologic Findings. Lesions often have the configuration of papules or small nodules (fig. 10-1, left). There are deep variants that may spare the superficial dermis and extend into the subcutis (fig. 10-1, right). The microscopic appearance varies, depending partly upon the stage of the process. Initially, there is an influx of histiocytes (macrophages), with small amounts of lipid that can be identified with fat stains (34), although the use of such stains in a particular clinical situation requires a degree of diagnostic prescience. In a fully developed lesion, several cell types can be identified, including vacuolated or foamy, spindled, or oncocytic cells (131), and eosinophils (fig. 10-2, left). Giant cells are common and may be of "ground-glass," foreign body, or Touton type (131). Touton giant cells are a histopathologic hallmark of juvenile xanthogranuloma and may be numerous. These cells consist of cores of eosinophilic cytoplasm, a surrounding wreath of nuclei, and an outer lipid

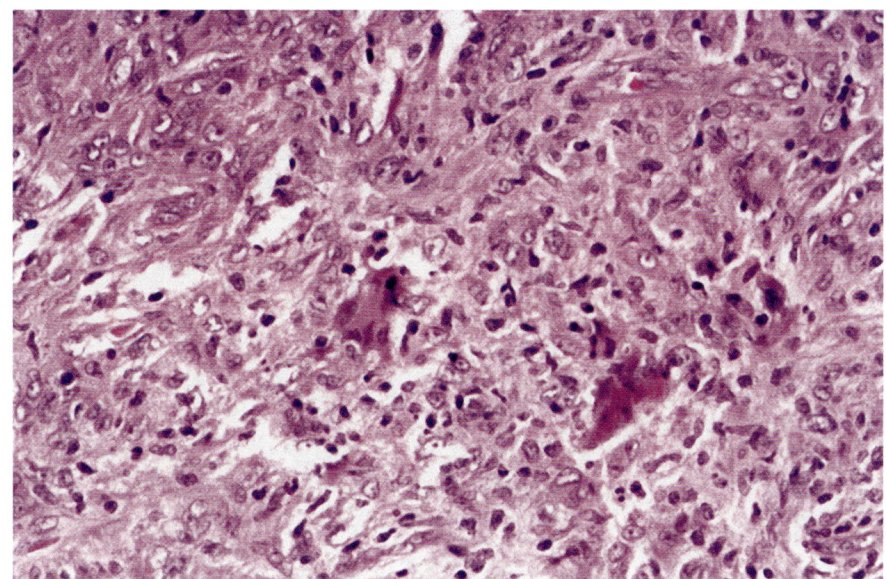

Figure 10-3

JUVENILE XANTHOGRANULOMA, LATE-STAGE LESION

Involutional changes are seen; however, distorted multinucleated cells can still be identified.

layer (fig. 10-2, right). Touton giant cells may be absent (109), however, particularly in early- or late-stage lesions. They are rare in deep forms of juvenile xanthogranuloma (65) and more prominent in adult than in juvenile lesions (131). Shapiro et al. (105) described 17 cases in which lipidized and giant cells were inconspicuous or absent. Newman et al. (81) reported five lesions composed mainly of nonlipidized cells; four of these occurred in infants. In late-stage lesions, fibroblasts and accompanying fibrosis replace these cellular elements. Even in later stages, remnants of eosinophils or giant cells that have been distorted by the fibrosing process may be identified (fig. 10-3). Bang et al. (8) identified Sézary cell-like atypical lymphocytes in involuting lesions of juvenile xanthogranuloma.

Immunohistochemical studies have been extensive. The histiocytic cells are regularly vimentin positive. They are usually positive for the macrophage markers HAM56, lysozyme, and CD68, but results have been variable or negative when stained for alpha-1-antitrypsin or -antichymotrypsin, or MAC387 (65,78,103). In most instances, the constituent cells are factor XIIIa positive (65,69,78,81,103,113). Although staining for S-100 protein has usually been negative except for dendritic cells (103, 110,136), two studies have reported staining of xanthoma cells, larger histiocytes, and Touton giant cells in 25 to 30 percent of cases (69,113). CD1a was negative in both studies. Kraus et al. (69) concluded that there is morphologic and phenotypic overlap between the lesional cells of juvenile xanthogranuloma and plasmacytoid monocytes, which they suggest may explain the occasional extracutaneous involvement observed with these lesions. Vasconcelos et al. (118) found cytomegaloviral antigens in some of the histiocytes in an oral lesion, suggesting a possible association with this infectious agent (7).

Ultrastructural studies have confirmed the presence of histiocytes in varying stages of development; some have been reported to have desmosome-like junctional complexes (104). Myofibroblasts have also been identified (65). Features of Langerhans cells are not observed (34).

Differential Diagnosis. Difficulties arise in distinguishing between juvenile xanthogranuloma and Langerhans cell histiocytosis. The latter is more apt to show histiocytes with reniform nuclei and epidermal infiltration, while well-formed Touton giant cells are uncommon. In most instances, the cells of juvenile xanthogranuloma are S-100 protein negative; the occasional S-100–positive examples are CD1a negative (113), in contrast to Langerhans cell histiocytosis.

Lipidized dermatofibromas also have some features in common with juvenile xanthogranuloma, but these lesions tend to feature overlying epidermal acanthosis and a characteristic "curlicue" arrangement of cells. The Touton-like giant cells in dermatofibromas tend to be angulated, have some clumping of nuclei without

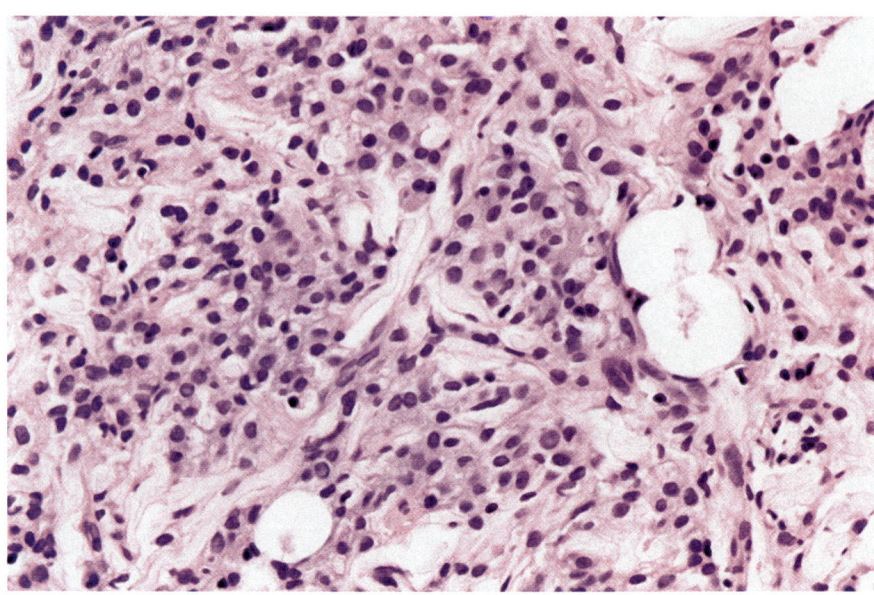

Figure 10-4

JUVENILE XANTHOGRANULOMA

The oncocytic cells in this lesion resemble mast cells.

the classic wreath-like arrangement, and have a lipid layer that often contains hemosiderin. The cells of both lesions can be factor XIIIa positive, although this stain is more likely to be strong and evenly distributed among the cells of dermatofibroma. In contrast to juvenile xanthogranuloma, dermatofibroma cells tend to be positive for LN3, and negative for CD68 and peanut agglutinin (131).

Morphologically, the prevalence of lipidized cells and Touton giant cells usually allows distinction from reticulohistiocytoma, whose cells have a characteristic ground-glass cytoplasm and nuclei with sharply defined nuclear membranes and prominent nucleoli. This differentiation is fortunate, for there can be considerable immunohistochemical overlap of the two lesions.

S-100 protein–positive examples of juvenile xanthogranuloma can be confused with intradermal variants of epithelioid cell (Spitz's) nevus. Staining for CD68 may not help in their differentiation, since melanocytic tumors sometimes express this antigen. The presence of junctional nests, or staining for HMB45, MART-1, or tyrosinase indicates a melanocytic lesion. Of additional help would be a stain for factor XIIIa, since most examples of juvenile xanthogranuloma are at least focally positive, while melanocytic nevi and malignant melanomas are factor XIIIa negative (3,80).

We have encountered rare cases of juvenile xanthogranuloma with a predominance of oncocytic or nonlipidized cells, resembling mastocytoma (fig. 10-4). Depending upon the quality of the tissue sections, simple distinction on morphologic grounds alone may not be possible. In such instances, negative results with stains for mast cells, such as Giemsa, Leder (chloroacetate esterase), or CD117, may be diagnostically helpful.

Benign Cephalic Histiocytosis

Clinical Features. This benign condition was first reported by Gianotti, Caputo, and Ermacora in 1971 (44). Since that time there have been sporadic reports of the disorder, usually appearing as single case reports or small series. Classically, *benign cephalic histiocytosis* appears during the first 3 years of life (45) as yellow to red-brown papules that eventually become flat and pigmented (45). There is a male to female ratio of approximately 2 to 1 (85). As the name implies, lesions predominate on the head and neck region, but involvement of the trunk and extremities has been reported (33,85). Eventual resolution of these lesions by late childhood is the rule (45,67). In one reported case, there was an association with diabetes insipidus, a condition usually linked to forms of Langerhans cell histiocytosis or xanthoma disseminatum (124). There was one report of xanthomatized, eruptive cephalic histiocytomas in an adult patient with T-cell lymphoma (4). A close relationship between benign cephalic histiocytosis and other members of the non-Langerhans cell histiocytosis group of disorders has been repeatedly proposed (46,98,133).

Pathologic Findings. Typically, there is a well-circumscribed, upper to mid-dermal infiltrate of histiocytes (macrophages), although the deep dermis may also be involved. Gianotti, Alessi, and Caputo (46) have described three patterns of histiocytic proliferation: papillary dermal, lichenoid, and diffuse. The histiocytes tend to be small and rounded, with irregular nuclei and little if any xanthomatization. Gianotti et al. found larger, pleomorphic histiocytes with generous amounts of eosinophilic cytoplasm, indented nuclei, and prominent nucleoli in their cases with the papillary dermal pattern. There may be an associated perivascular and interstitial lymphocytic and eosinophilic infiltrate (33,46).

Immunohistochemically, the histiocytic cells are S-100 protein and CD1a negative, which distinguishes them from Langerhans cells (30,98). They are variably positive for HAM56, factor XIIIa, CD68, and peanut agglutinin, with the expression of these antigens being partly dependent upon the stage of development of the lesions investigated (98,133).

Electron microscopy plays a key role in the diagnosis of benign cephalic histiocytosis. The most distinctive feature consists of "comma-shaped" or "worm-like" bodies in the cytoplasm of the histiocytes. These bodies are composed of two parallel electron-dense structures, each 60-nm wide, separated by an 80-nm space of lesser density (9,30,33,45,85). They are present in 5 to 30 percent of the cells in a given lesion (45). They are not entirely diagnostic for this disorder, since they are also sometimes observed in lesions of generalized eruptive histiocytoma (46). Other relatively characteristic findings include desmosome-like junctions (30,46,85) and coated vesicles (45,85). Gianotti et al. (46) have only observed desmosome-like junctions between histiocytes in cases of benign cephalic histiocytosis. Laminated bodies are also present (133), but they are not sufficiently distinctive to be diagnostically useful (46). Birbeck granules are absent from the proliferating cells (30,85).

Differential Diagnosis. The diagnosis of benign cephalic histiocytosis is not difficult in an ideal setting: multiple lesions on the face of a young child, a dermal infiltrate of nonxanthomatized histiocytes lacking the features of Langerhans cells, and the presence of comma-shaped bodies on ultrastructural examination. The close relationship between this disorder and other forms of non-Langerhans cell histiocytosis has been alluded to; for example, one reported case of eruptive histiocytoma in an adult closely resembled benign cephalic histiocytosis (115). A comparison of two cases of giant solitary xanthogranuloma and benign cephalic histiocytosis showed similar histopathologic features and evolutionary characteristics over time (133), and a case of benign cephalic histiocytosis evolving into juvenile xanthogranuloma has been reported (98). In a careful study of this issue by Gianotti et al. (46), blinded histopathologic evaluations of specimens representing benign cephalic histiocytosis, generalized eruptive histiocytoma, papular xanthoma, and juvenile xanthogranuloma were performed. With few exceptions, there was a close relationship among the findings in benign cephalic histiocytosis, generalized eruptive histiocytoma, and early, nonxanthomatized juvenile xanthogranuloma, suggesting that these three disorders may well be part of a spectrum of a single disease process.

Progressive Nodular Histiocytosis

Clinical Features. *Progressive nodular histiocytosis* was first described in 1974 by Rodriguez et al. (96) and named by Gianotti and Caputo in 1985 (43). Since that time only a few cases have been reported (16,51,111,114,135). This rare condition is characterized by the progressive, widespread development of cutaneous lesions of two types: papules ranging from 2 to 10 mm in diameter, and nodules measuring 1 to 3 cm in diameter. It is neither a familial nor a congenital dermatosis, and cases have been reported in both children and adults. Lesions occur on the face, trunk, and extremities (14, 114); the facial lesions can produce the marked deformation of a leonine appearance. Lesions also occur in the conjunctiva, oral mucosa, and central nervous system (14). One case was associated with a variety of systemic disorders, including chronic myelogenous leukemia (51). The combination of clinical and microscopic features has led some to conclude that this condition is a variant form of juvenile xanthogranuloma (14,51,134). Although, as the name implies, this is a progressive disorder, regression of individual lesions can occur (114). The case described by Winkelmann et al. (126), which probably constitutes an example of progressive nodular histiocytosis, responded to vinblastine therapy.

Pathologic Findings. Lesions are composed of spindled cells that may form storiform arrangements (135). Aggregates of histiocytes (macrophages) with eosinophilic, vacuolated, or xanthomatized cytoplasm are also identified (16,114,135). Multinucleated cells, including Touton giant cells, may be observed, but are not invariably present (114,126,135). Lymphocytes are often present and may be numerous, and eosinophils and plasma cells are sometimes seen as well (114,126).

Immunohistochemically, the predominating cells have features of macrophages and dermal dendrocytes: positive for lysozyme, alpha-1-antitrypsin, CD68, HAM56, and factor XIIIa (114,135). They also express muscle-specific and smooth muscle actins (135). The negative reaction for S-100 protein argues against a Langerhans cell origin (114). This latter finding is supported by ultrastructural findings that have demonstrated an absence of Birbeck granules (114,126,135). Other electron microscopic features are cytoplasmic inclusions with laminated or highly complex structures (22,126,135), and lipid phagocytosis (16). Torres et al. (114) identified dense granules, some comma-shaped and some with electron-lucent centers, in their case of progressive nodular histiocytosis.

Differential Diagnosis. There is such a close microscopic resemblance to juvenile xanthogranuloma (particularly to those with a spindle cell component) that this lesion and progressive nodular histiocytosis are now widely considered variants of the same disorder (14, 134,135). The microscopic findings also closely resemble those of dermatofibroma, however, the clinical presentation of a progressive eruption of papules and nodules is distinct from that of dermatofibroma. Zelger et al. (135) have described a solitary variant of progressive nodular histiocytosis (*spindle cell xanthogranuloma*) that is diagnostically more problematic. In contrast to dermatofibroma, these solitary tumors include a lack of overlying epidermal hyperplasia or sclerotic collagen, a prominent xanthogranulomatous reaction and peripheral lymphocytic infiltrate, and regular reactivity for macrophage markers (135). Dermatofibromas can be virtually identical to the lesions of progressive nodular histiocytosis, however, and it remains to be seen whether the concept of a solitary version of progressive nodular histiocytosis will (or should) be accepted by the dermatopathology community.

The complex inclusion bodies seen on ultrastructural examination of lesions of progressive nodular histiocytosis are similar to those of reticulohistiocytoma, but in other respects the clinical and microscopic features differ significantly from both reticulohistiocytoma and multicentric reticulohistiocytosis (see below).

Generalized Eruptive Histiocytoma

Clinical Features. *Generalized eruptive histiocytoma* is an uncommon dermatosis, first reported by Winkelmann and Muller in 1963 (127). Numerous red-brown papules and nodules develop, sometimes in crops, over the face, trunk, and arms (122). Lesions tend to be symmetrical, with flexural sparing (48). Generalized eruptive histiocytoma is known to occur in adults of all ages, but numerous cases have also been reported in children (23,64,122). Childhood lesions tend to have an asymmetrical distribution and do not involve mucous membranes, in contrast to adult lesions (23). Although lesions may involute spontaneously, new ones develop more or less continuously, so that the condition may last for years (5,127). Lesions associated with high fever and drug eruption (106), and with rheumatic fever (77), suggest that at least in some instances the proliferation of histiocytes may be reactive. Another case that progressed to xanthoma disseminatum, complete with the development of diabetes insipidus, provides a possible link to other non-Langerhans cell histiocytoses (93).

Pathologic Findings. There is usually a monomorphous dermal infiltrate comprised of cells with pale to amphophilic cytoplasm and oval nuclei (106,127); in one case, both small and large cells were present (48). Foam cells and multinucleated cells are usually absent (48,64,127) but may be observed, especially in lesions of long duration (5,127). There may be an accompanying infiltrate of lymphocytes (64,127) or eosinophils (102). Support for the monocyte/macrophage origin of these cells is provided by staining for vimentin, alpha-1-antichymotrypsin, CD68, MAC387, and MS-1 (a marker of sinusoidal endothelial cells and dendritic cells) (48,64,77). Lysozyme expression has varied in the two studies in which it was investigated (64,77), and in one report, staining for alpha-1-antitrypsin was negative (102). The cells are typically S-100 protein and CD1a negative. In the case of Saijo et al. (102), some S-100 protein- and OKT6-positive cells were identified, but Birbeck granules were not observed, suggesting the presence of indeterminate cells. Ultrastructural studies have demonstrated a variety of dense, laminated or myeloid and annular bodies within the cytoplasm of histiocyte-like cells, the specificity of which is unclear (19,106).

Differential Diagnosis. The microscopic features are similar to those of early lesions of juvenile xanthogranuloma. Rare reports of transition to xanthoma disseminatum also suggest a close relationship to that condition (93,122). In contrast to these disorders, foam cell and giant cell formation are not usually features of generalized eruptive histiocytoma. Lesions of reticulohistiocytosis differ from those of generalized eruptive histiocytoma by possessing cells with ground-glass cytoplasm and more frequent multinucleated cells; the latter are particularly prominent in older lesions.

Xanthoma Disseminatum

Clinical Features. *Xanthoma disseminatum* is a rare dermatosis that affects both children and adults. Numerous orange to red-brown papules and nodules develop in a widespread distribution, with a tendency to coalesce and involve flexural surfaces such as the axilla, antecubital fossa, and groin. Enlargement and fibrosis of cutaneous lesions can produce significant cosmetic and functional defects (15). Skin lesions are persistent, although individual lesions may regress. Mucous membrane involvement is common, with several reports of laryngeal and pharyngeal lesions (112). In one case, bronchial involvement was associated with death due to acute respiratory failure (28). Other organs affected by the disease have included the eyes (68), brain (56,68), and bone, the latter showing osteolytic lesions (13,17). Diabetes insipidus is frequently described, and there is sometimes an associated monoclonal gammopathy;

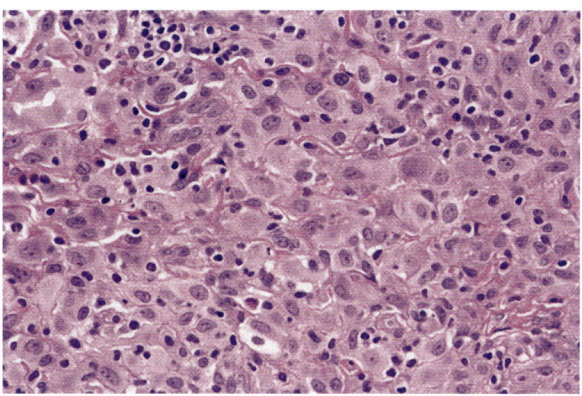

Figure 10-5

XANTHOMA DISSEMINATUM

Although many of the cells have rounded contours, a few possess scalloped borders. The nuclei are ovoid.

both multiple myeloma and Waldenström's macroglobulinemia have been reported (52,73, 76). Blood lipid levels are normal (11). A few cases of generalized eruptive histiocytoma have evolved into a picture of xanthoma disseminatum, suggesting a link between these two disorders (35,93), and with other non-Langerhans cell histiocytoses, as previously discussed.

Pathologic Findings. The dermis contains a proliferation of histiocytes (macrophages) within a fibrillary connective tissue stroma. These histiocytes possess scalloped borders and ovoid, vesicular nuclei (fig. 10-5) (134). Elastophagocytosis by these cells has been demonstrated (70). In older lesions, xanthoma cells and admixtures of other inflammatory cells are present, and multinucleated giant cells of both foreign body and Touton varieties can be found (fig. 10-6) (1,70,123). The lipid within the histiocytes is doubly refractile, indicating the presence of cholesterol esters (79). In a variant of the disorder, known as *xanthosiderohistiocytosis*, extensive hemosiderin deposition is observed (10,73).

Immunohistochemical staining shows that the histiocytes in xanthoma disseminatum are factor XIIIa and CD68 positive. They also express CD14, CD11b, and CD11c (117). They are negative for CD1a, S-100 protein, CD1b, CD15, and CD34 (130). They are weakly positive for peanut agglutinin (130), and staining for MAC387 has been variable (35,130). Ultrastructurally,

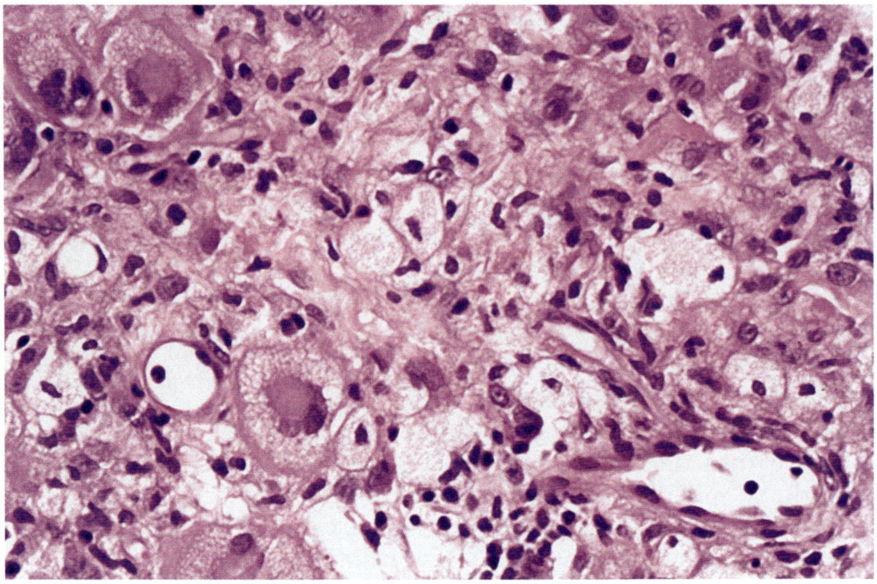

Figure 10-6

XANTHOMA DISSEMINATUM

An older lesion shows xanthoma cells and Touton giant cells.

phagosomes, vacuoles, lamellar bodies, and even worm-like bodies have been found within histiocytes (35,70), but to date no specific or diagnostic inclusions have been described.

Differential Diagnosis. In a fully developed case, the clinical features are characteristic, but early xanthoma disseminatum can resemble other non-Langerhans cell histiocytoses. Examples with numerous Touton giant cells can be confused with juvenile xanthogranuloma. Immunohistochemistry is usually of little help in distinguishing these two conditions, except perhaps in cases of xanthogranuloma in which the cells express S-100 protein.

Zelger et al. (130) have considered in detail the morphologic and immunohistochemical differences between xanthoma disseminatum and Langerhans cell histiocytosis. The latter has a more diffuse, band-like infiltrate with epidermal infiltration. Langerhans cells have a higher nuclear to cytoplasmic ratio than do the cells of xanthoma disseminatum, and possess reniform nuclei (130). In addition, the cells of Langerhans cell histiocytosis are S-100 protein and CD1a positive and stain strongly with peanut agglutinin (35,117,130).

Reticulohistiocytosis

Clinical Features. Reticulohistiocytosis presents in two ways. In *multicentric reticulohistiocytosis* (MRH), papular or nodular skin lesions are associated with mutilating arthritis, involvement of mucous membranes and other organ systems, and constitutional symptoms. *Reticulohistiocytoma* (RH) manifests as single or occasionally multiple cutaneous lesions in the absence of arthritis or other signs and symptoms. It is important to distinguish these disorders from two quite different conditions with similar-sounding names: congenital self-healing reticulohistiocytosis, best regarded as a Langerhans cell histiocytosis, and reticulohistiocytoma of the dorsum, which is more accurately classified as a primary cutaneous follicular center cell (B-cell) lymphoma.

MRH is most common among middle-aged women (100), but it is not confined to this group, and has been reported in children (18,20). This condition primarily involves skin and joints. Polyarthritis is the initial manifestation in about two thirds of patients; of the remainder, half develop skin lesions first and half develop changes in both sites simultaneously (74,95). Skin lesions are reddish brown to flesh-colored papules or nodules that are particularly common on the face and upper half of the body, including the hands. The bilaterally symmetrical arthritis particularly involves the distal interphalangeal joints of the hands, but other affected joints include the shoulders, knees, ankles, feet, and spine. The arthritis is often rapidly progressive, and in about half of patients, severe joint destruction produces arthritis mutilans, although with disproportionately

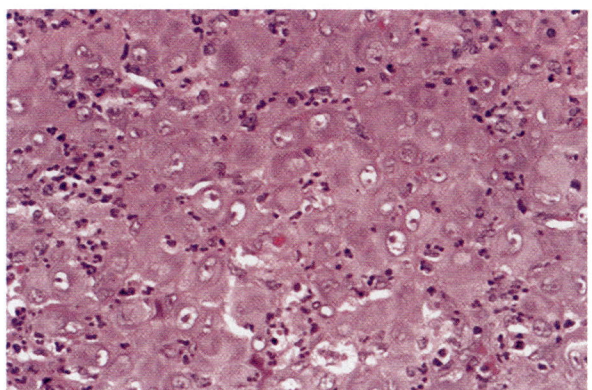 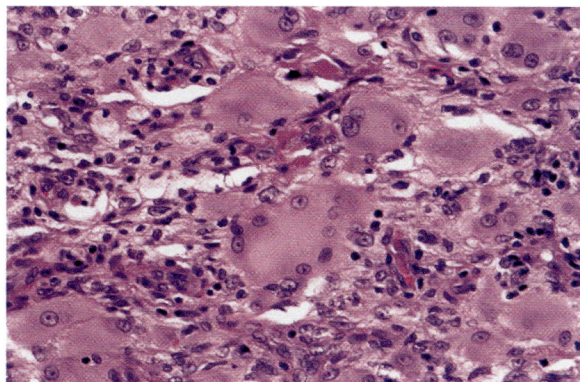

Figure 10-7

RETICULOHISTIOCYTOMA

Left: Mononucleated oncocytic cells have ground-glass cytoplasm. The nuclei possess sharply delineated membranes and prominent nucleoli. Note the infiltrate of neutrophils; these cells tend to be encountered in early lesions of reticulohistiocytoma, and are said to be more common in these lesions than in multicentric reticulohistiocytosis.

Right: This example has multinucleated giant cells, which tend to be larger and more numerous in older lesions.

mild symptoms (50). Radiographic changes of the bones and articular surfaces are sufficiently distinctive to suggest the diagnosis even in the absence of known cutaneous disease (37). There may be involvement of mucous membranes and other organs, including salivary glands, thyroid gland, and pericardium (36,41). Symptoms include fever, weight loss, and weakness. An association with internal malignancy is reported in about 24 percent of cases, representing a broad spectrum of solid tumors and lymphomas (24,82,108). The diagnosis of MRH most often precedes that of the malignancy (82). The disease may remit despite persistent malignancy, while on the other hand, removal of the malignancy may have no effect on MRH (24). The course of the disease is highly variable. Skin lesions and (less commonly) arthropathy may improve over a period of several years, but persistence or progression of disease is common (57).

RH consists of single or, less commonly, multiple red-brown papules or nodules that develop on the head and neck, trunk, or legs (89). Both spontaneous regression and recurrences of lesions are reported. Patients do not develop arthritis, mucous membrane involvement, or constitutional symptoms. In an unusual case reported by Goette et al. (49), diffuse cutaneous lesions spontaneously involuted, followed by the development of subacute myelogenous leukemia.

Pathologic Findings. Both MRH and RH show dermal infiltrates of large, oncocytic cells with a characteristic ground-glass appearance of the cytoplasm. The cells may be both mononucleated (fig. 10-7, left) and multinucleated (fig. 10-7, right), the latter showing irregular nuclear arrangements. The nuclei feature sharply delineated membranes and prominent nucleoli; occasional mitoses can be identified. Giant cells of the Touton type have been described, but they are not common and do not represent a characteristic feature. The number and size of the giant cells tend to increase in older lesions (27). These same cell types are identified in synovium and other affected organs (41,83). Varying numbers of spindled cells are present in the surrounding stroma (fig. 10-8). Early lesions, in particular, tend to have associated inflammatory infiltrates that include lymphocytes, neutrophils, and eosinophils in varying proportions (fig. 10-7, left), while later-stage lesions are accompanied by fibrosis. The cytoplasm of the oncocytic cells is periodic acid–Schiff (PAS) positive, diastase resistant. Stains for lipid performed on frozen sections are usually negative, but positive results have occasionally been reported (29,83). Phagocytosis of collagen by these cells has been observed (20,41), and in one case associated with paraproteinemia, gamma heavy chains were detected in giant cells (92). An abundant reticulin network surrounds individual cells.

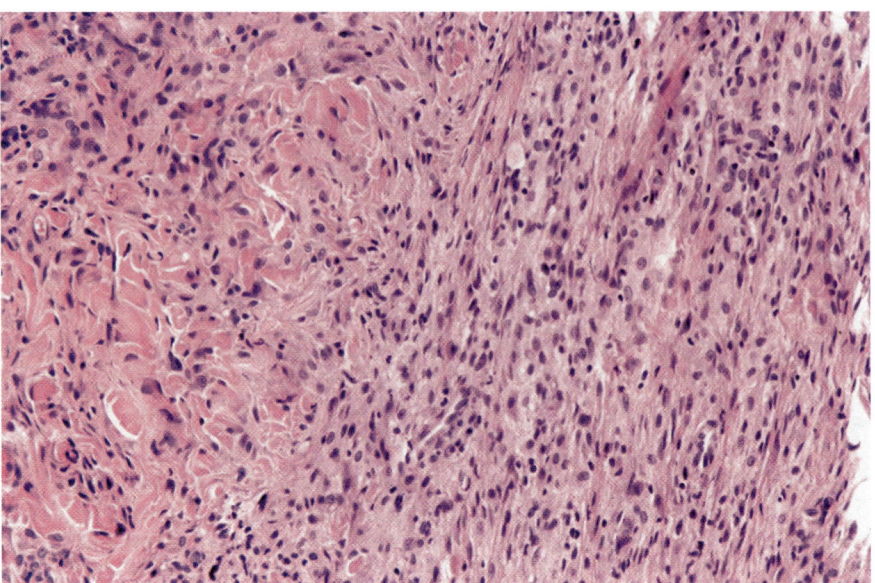

Figure 10-8
RETICULOHISTIOCYTOMA
Spindled cells are featured.

Immunohistochemically, the cells of MRH and RH stain for CD68, HAM56, lysozyme, alpha-1-antitrypsin, and vimentin; they are negative for MAC387, CD15, CD34, desmin, and muscle-specific actin (132). S-100 protein is typically negative, but positive cases have been reported (61,87). Factor XIIIa staining has been identified, particularly in cases of RH (61,132) but also in one case of MRH (87). Regarding traditional lymphocyte markers, the cells of MRH show membranous staining for CD45 and CD3 but are negative for CD45RO, CD20, and CD30 (108). On ultrastructural study, there are complex interdigitations between cells, which may represent a distinguishing feature of reticulohistiocytosis (27,71). Other findings include dense bodies, numerous mitochondria, and cytoplasmic vacuoles (27,49,71,74). One study showed intracytoplasmic inclusions of long-spacing collagen (type VI) in MRH (38). These morphologic and immunohistochemical findings all point to a monocyte/macrophage lineage for the constituent cells of reticulohistiocytosis (41,108).

Despite significant histologic similarities between MRH and RH, there are major clinical differences between the two conditions. This has led to a search for any possible distinguishing pathologic features. It has been suggested that RH lesions have a more prominent neutrophilic infiltrate and spindle cell stroma (100). The multinucleated cells of RH tend to be larger and more bizarre in appearance than those of MRH (fig. 10-9). Zelger et al. (132) found that vacuolated, spindle-shaped, and xanthomatized mononuclear histiocytes and Touton multinucleated cells were present only in lesions of RH. Although there were generally minor differences in antigenic expression between the two conditions, the cells of RH expressed factor XIIIa and HHF35 (a marker for smooth muscle cells and myofibroblasts), while those of MRH were negative for those markers (132). Further studies are needed to determine the diagnostic value of these findings.

Differential Diagnosis. The cytologic characteristics of the cells of both types of RH, with their characteristic ground-glass cytoplasm, ordinarily permit ready distinction from juvenile xanthogranuloma, in which lipidized cells and Touton giant cells predominate (109). Similarly, distinction from other conditions characterized by lipidized cells, including xanthomas, dermatofibroma, and lepromatous leprosy, is usually not difficult. Confusion with Langerhans cell histiocytosis is possible, particularly in those cases of RH that are S-100 protein positive; however, the nuclei of RH cells lack the reniform features of Langerhans cell histiocytosis. In one S-100 protein–positive case of RH, no Birbeck granules were found (61), and staining for OKT6 (CD1) was negative (54).

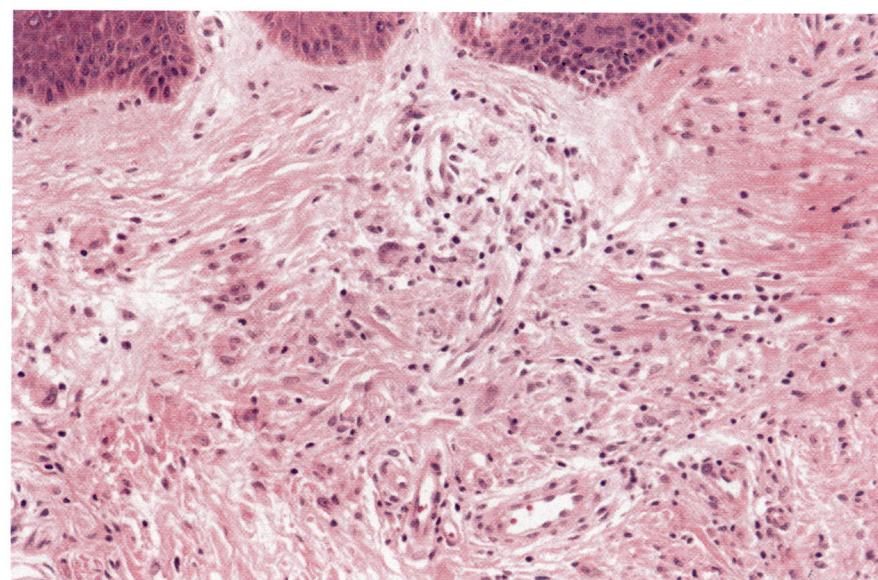

Figure 10-9

MULTICENTRIC RETICULOHISTIOCYTOSIS

The constituent cells are smaller than those encountered in reticulohistiocytoma.

Familial Histiocytic Dermatoarthritis

Clinical Features. *Familial histiocytic dermatoarthritis* is a particularly rare condition, first described by Zayid and Farraj in 1973 (129). Few reports have appeared since that time (116,128). The cutaneous lesions consist of widespread papules and nodules that develop during childhood. Other features include a symmetrical, steroid-resistant polyarthritis and eye involvement that can manifest as glaucoma, uveitis, or cataracts.

Pathologic Findings. Microscopically, there is a dermal infiltrate of nonlipidized histiocytes (macrophages) with varying numbers of lymphocytes, plasma cells, and eosinophils. Multinucleated giant cells have been observed. The cytoplasm of these cells was initially reported to be PAS negative, but a more recent case showed PAS-positive, diastase-sensitive intracellular material, representing glycogen (116). Fibrosis occurs in older lesions. Ultrastructural examination has shown pleomorphic cytoplasmic inclusions consisting of dense, irregularly shaped bodies.

Differential Diagnosis. Familial histiocytic dermatoarthritis and multicentric reticulohistiocytosis (MRH) are both dermatoarthritides that can include giant cells, PAS-positive intracytoplasmic material, and the ultrastructural finding of pleomorphic inclusions. A family history, early onset of disease, and ocular abnormalities are features not associated with MRH. In contrast to familial histiocytic dermatoarthritis, the PAS-positive cytoplasmic material in MRH is diastase resistant. Multinucleated giant cells are not invariably present in MRH (this is particularly the case in early lesions), and the classic ground glass cytoplasm and nuclear features of the cells of MRH have not been reported in cases of familial histiocytic dermatoarthritis.

Rosai-Dorfman Disease (Sinus Histiocytosis with Massive Lymphadenopathy)

Clinical Features. *Rosai-Dorfman disease* was first described by Rosai and Dorfman in 1969 (101). It classically consists of bilateral, painless but sometimes massive adenopathy (cervical, inguinal), fever, polyclonal hyperglobulinemia (60), an elevated erythrocyte sedimentation rate (62), and immune dysfunction (40). Reaction to an infectious agent has been proposed as one possible cause (53), and there are reports of an association with mycetoma (99), herpes zoster (32), and herpes simplex and bacterial urinary tract infections (86). More than 40 percent of patients have extranodal involvement (26), including the orbit, upper respiratory track, and bone (72). The skin is the most common site of extranodal disease, appearing in about 27 percent of patients with lymph node involvement (25).

Cutaneous Rosai-Dorfman disease in the absence of lymph node infiltration has been reported but is rare. In our experience, patients with Rosai-Dorfman disease who first present

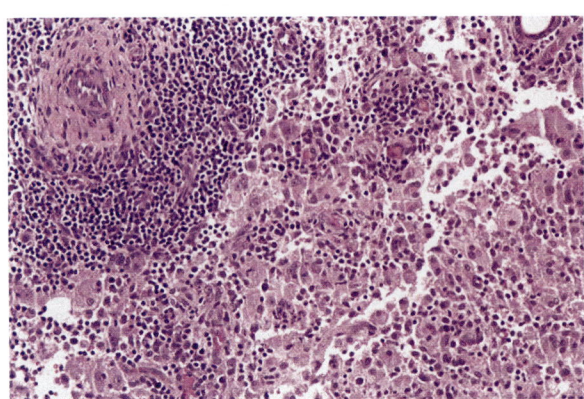 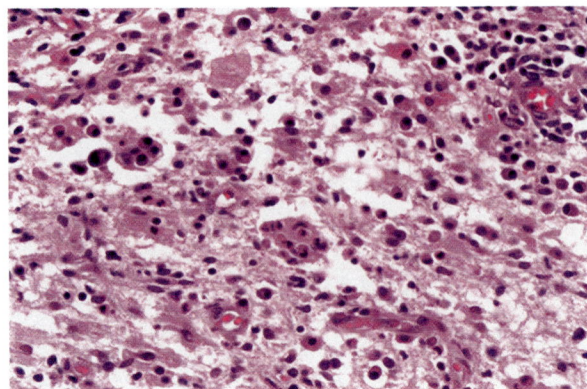

Figure 10-10

ROSAI-DORFMAN DISEASE

Left: There are aggregates of histiocytes (macrophages) with abundant granular cytoplasm. A lymphoplasmacellular infiltrate surrounds a thick-walled vessel at the upper left.

Right: The histiocytes (macrophages) demonstrate emperipolesis.

with skin lesions may have subtle lymphadenopathy that is missed on initial examination. Skin lesions are typically nodules or plaques (25), but a papular eruption (62) and pustular/acneiform lesions (2) have also been reported. Lesions may involve spontaneously (2,107), but the condition may persist for many years (12). Death can occur, usually from complications related to immunologic dysfunction or infection, although rarely is death directly attributable to Rosai-Dorfman disease itself (39).

Pathologic Findings. The principal microscopic finding consists of nodular or diffuse aggregates of large histiocytes (macrophages) with abundant, granular to vacuolated cytoplasm and rounded to reniform nuclei (6). These cells resemble the sinus histiocytes of lymph nodes (26). Their cytoplasm often contains lymphocytes and other cells (fig. 10-10). This is believed to occur through a process termed emperipolesis, defined as an ability of one cell to penetrate the cytoplasm of another cell, where it may remain for a time, wander freely within its cytoplasm, and eventually pass through it (91,119). Cells are not damaged in the process, thereby differing from the more familiar process of phagocytosis (119). Xanthomatous changes occur, particularly in older lesions (90), and Touton giant cells have been reported (12). An infiltrate of neutrophils and plasma cells may accompany the aggregates of histiocytes (macrophages), and lymphoid aggregates and plasma cells surrounding thick-walled vessels may be found at the periphery of a lesion (26).

The immunohistochemical hallmark of these lesions is the cytoplasmic expression of S-100 protein in the large histiocytes (macrophages), in the face of CD1a negativity (88,90). These cells have also been reported to express factor XIIIa, CD4 (88), the macrophage markers CD68 and MAC387 (66,107), and a variety of adhesion molecules that are known to be employed by tissue macrophages (62,90). Ultrastructurally, the large histiocytes (macrophages) lack Birbeck granules (120).

Differential Diagnosis. Lesions with foamy histiocytes (macrophages) and Touton giant cells could be confused with xanthoma or juvenile xanthogranuloma (90). Finding evidence for emperipolesis involving the large macrophages, however, points to a diagnosis of Rosai-Dorfman disease. This is further supported by the cytoplasmic S-100 protein positivity of these cells. In contrast to the S-100 protein–positive cells of Langerhans cell histiocytosis, those of Rosai-Dorfman disease are CD1a negative and lack Birbeck granules. Other microscopic features more characteristic of Rosai-Dorfman disease include prominent lymphocytic and plasmacellular infiltrates and thick-walled vessels.

MALIGNANT HISTIOCYTOSIS

Clinical Features. Two related, uncommon malignant conditions characterized by proliferations of histiocytes are *histiocytic lymphoma* and *malignant histiocytosis*, the latter previously termed *histiocytic medullary reticulosis*. In the current World Health Organization Classification of Tumors (148), these are grouped under the term *histiocytic sarcoma*. Histiocytic lymphoma is said to derive from the fixed tissue histiocyte (macrophage), and malignant histiocytosis from the circulating monocyte or tissue macrophage (144).

In recent years, sophisticated immunohistochemical and genetic studies have shown that many cases formerly considered examples of malignant histiocytosis were in fact B-cell lymphomas, T-cell lymphomas, anaplastic CD30-positive large cell lymphomas, or infection-related hemophagocytic syndromes (139). Thus, in a reassessment of cases reported as malignant histiocytosis in 1975, Wilson et al. (149) showed that most would now be recognized as anaplastic large cell lymphoma. Similarly, Arai et al. (140) found that only one of seven cases previously diagnosed as histiocytic lymphoma, and two of four cases diagnosed as malignant histiocytosis, were truly histiocytic in origin. Egeler et al. (144) classified only one of nine cases previously diagnosed as malignant histiocytosis as a histiocytic malignancy. It is evident that forms of malignant histiocytosis are even rarer than formerly believed; moreover, much of the historical information regarding the clinical and histopathologic features of malignant histiocytosis is inaccurate and therefore in need of revision.

Malignant histiocytosis is mainly a disease of adults, and shows a slight male predominance (148). An association with mediastinal germ cell tumor has been reported in some patients (143). Sites of involvement include lymph nodes, skin, and a variety of other extranodal sites, including the gastrointestinal tract, kidney, and breast (140,146,148). Systemic symptoms and signs include fatigue, fever, weight loss, hepatosplenomegaly, lytic bone lesions, intestinal obstruction, and pancytopenia. Skin lesions consist of solitary or multiple nodules involving the face, trunk, and extremities. Ulceration of nodules occurs (140). Malignant histiocytosis usually follows an aggressive clinical course, and most patients succumb to complications of the disease.

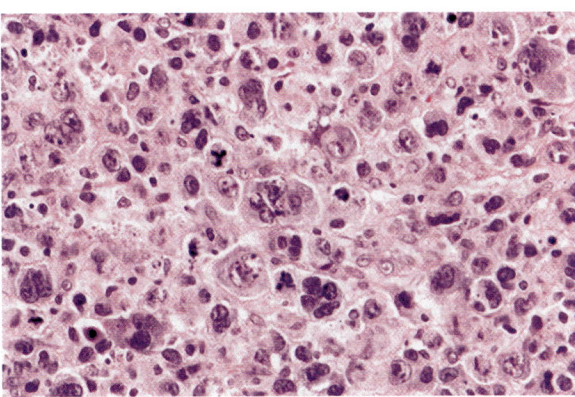

Figure 10-11

MALIGNANT HISTIOCYTOSIS

The tumor cells feature pink-staining cytoplasm and large, irregularly shaped nuclei.

Pathologic Findings. There is typically a diffuse, noncohesive dermal infiltrate (140,142), involving particularly the mid to deep dermis. Neither epidermotropism nor formation of a distinct grenz zone is observed. The constituent cells have varying amounts of pink-staining, sometimes foamy cytoplasm and eccentrically placed nuclei with a high nuclear to cytoplasmic ratio. These nuclei have vesicular chromatin, are rounded to reniform, and sometimes show substantial folding of their nuclear membranes (fig. 10-11) (140,142). Multinucleated cells are sometimes observed. Mitotic figures are present and may be numerous (147). Other cell types include lymphocytes, ordinary histiocytes (macrophages), plasma cells, and eosinophils (148).

Immunohistochemical studies show that the tumor cells express the histiocyte (macrophage)-related antigens CD68, lysozyme, CD11c, and CD14, but lack myeloid markers such as myeloperoxidase (148). These cells also stain for CD45, CD45RO, HLA-DR, and for CD4 (142,145,146). The latter antigen is characteristic of helper T cells, but is also known to be expressed in monocytes/histiocytes (145). Tumor cells do not otherwise express typical B- or T-cell antigens and are negative for CD30 (140). Weak, focal S-100 protein positivity is sometimes found, but the cells are negative for CD1a and other dendritic cell markers (142,146,148). The ultrastructural features of the tumor cells are nonspecific (141), but Birbeck granules or cell junctions are not found (148).

Differential Diagnosis. There is considerable resemblance to some B- and T-cell lymphomas and to anaplastic large cell, CD30-positive lymphoma, and, in fact, many tumors formerly classified as malignant histiocytosis or histiocytic lymphoma have proven on reevaluation to actually represent one of these other types of lymphoma. Marker studies are obviously keys to assuring an accurate diagnosis of malignant histiocytosis. A resemblance to Langerhans cell histiocytosis is also possible, but the latter condition tends to show epidermotropism, may be granulomatous, or may have a significant component of eosinophils. In addition, the cells of Langerhans cell histiocytosis are CD1a as well as S-100 protein positive and possess Birbeck granules that can be visualized ultrastructurally.

LANGERHANS CELL HISTIOCYTOSIS AND INDETERMINATE CELL HISTIOCYTOSIS

Langerhans Cell Histiocytosis

Clinical Features. *Langerhans cell histiocytosis,* formerly termed *histiocytosis X,* is characterized by a proliferation of cells, in the skin and other organ systems, with the immunophenotypic and ultrastructural characteristics of Langerhans cells. A related disorder, termed *congenital self-healing reticulohistiocytosis,* is discussed in the next section.

Langerhans cell histiocytosis is primarily a disease of children, although it also occurs in adults, including the elderly (152,169,192). It is more common in boys than girls. Classically it is divided into three types: 1) the *Letterer-Siwe* type is prone to occur during the first year of life, and is characterized by multifocal, multisystem involvement that includes the skin, bone, lung, liver, spleen, and lymph nodes. Patients may present with fever, anemia, thrombocytopenia, and hepatosplenomegaly. Most patients have skin lesions, which may be the first sign of the disease. These consist of crusted papules that are especially prominent on the scalp, face, and trunk in a "seborrheic dermatitis-like" distribution. The lesions can closely resemble severe seborrheic dermatitis clinically, except that purpura is a frequent accompaniment to the lesions; 2) the *Hand-Schuller-Christian* type involves several sites within one organ system, particularly bone. The classic findings are diabetes insipidus, exophthalmos, and bony defects involving cranial and long bones. Otitis media and pathologic fractures occur. Lymphadenopathy, hepatosplenomegaly, or both are also reported. About one third of patients develop skin lesions, which may resemble those of the Letterer-Siwe type or present as ulcerated plaques or xanthomatous papules and nodules (150,173); and 3) *unifocal disease,* or *eosinophilic granuloma,* which usually occurs in older children and adults. This mainly involves bone, particularly the skull, ribs, pelvis, and femur, but lesions of skin, lung, and lymph nodes have been described. Skin lesions consist of crusted papules or ulcerated plaques (155). As might be imagined, there are cases that show overlap of these three types of disease. Reported disease associations with Langerhans cell histiocytosis include acute lymphoblastic leukemia, neonatal infection, lymphoma, and a viral-associated hemophagocytic syndrome (170,179).

Several variant forms of Langerhans cell histiocytosis have been described. A generalized cutaneous eruption of the Letterer-Siwe type is seen in infants or (more rarely) in adults in the absence of systemic involvement. This eruption has a favorable prognosis (152,195). A pulmonary form occurs in young adults and appears to be related to cigarette smoking (154,187). Disease localized to the genitalia of elderly adults has been reported. The prognosis for these patients is generally excellent, although there have been reports of progression to multiorgan involvement (177). A rare multifocal form of the disease with markedly atypical cytologic features has been reported. This disorder has been designated *Langerhans cell sarcoma* in the World Health Organization Classification of Tumors (188). It occurs in both children and adults; median patient age is 41 years (152).

The prognosis of patients with Langerhans cell histiocytosis depends heavily upon the number of organs involved (161). The poorest survival rates are associated with multisystem disease types such as classic Letterer-Siwe disease and Langerhans cell sarcoma.

Pathologic Findings. The constituent cells are found in the dermis, in a dispersed or clustered fashion, and show a particular propensity for infiltrating the epidermis (fig. 10-12). These cells range from 10 to 15 µm in diameter;

have eosinophilic cytoplasm; and have nuclei with grooves or folds (sometimes producing a reniform appearance), finely dispersed chromatin, and relatively inconspicuous nucleoli (fig. 10-13). In Langerhans cell sarcoma, cells are larger, possess nuclei with abnormal chromatin and prominent nucleoli, and show frequent mitotic figures (151,169,192). Even in examples of the latter disorder, nuclear indentations or grooves can be identified among some of the tumor cells (169). Generally, the degree of morphologic atypia is not an accurate predictor of the clinical course of the disease (151). The accompanying inflammatory infiltrate often includes eosinophils, but also neutrophils, lymphocytes, and plasma cells. Extravasated erythrocytes are common, as would be expected in purpuric lesions. Foam-laden macrophages and multinucleated cells can be observed, particularly in older, fibrotic lesions (189).

Immunohistochemically, the cells express S-100 protein, CD1a (162,172), vimentin, and human leukocyte antigen (HLA)-DR. Positive staining with peanut agglutinin is also a characteristic of these cells, and the yield of positive results with this marker can be increased by prior trypsinization and a three-step staining procedure (181). The immunophenotype of the cells is similar to that of normal, intraepidermal Langerhans cells except that the tumor cells express CD4 and placental alkaline phosphatase and show a different pattern of adhesion molecule expression (156,163). Other B- and T-cell markers, and markers for follicular dendritic cells, are negative. On ultrastructural evaluation, Birbeck granules can be identified in 2 to 79 percent of tumor cells, with an average of 50 percent (158,160,190). Other less specific findings include myelin figures, worm-like bodies, and dense bodies (165).

One flow cytometric study of cases of Langerhans cell histiocytosis that lacked significant cytologic atypia failed to detect aneuploid subpopulations of cells (182). On the other hand, significant expression of proliferation markers

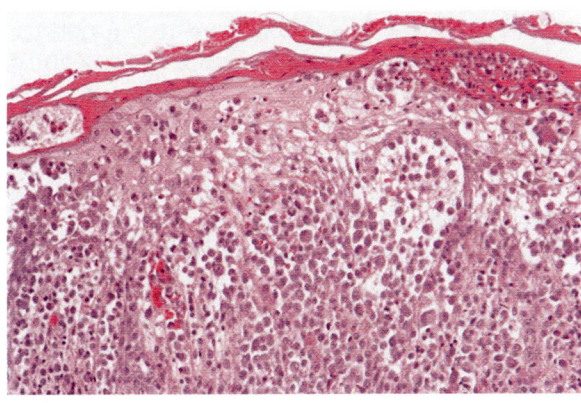

Figure 10-12

LANGERHANS CELL HISTIOCYTOSIS

There is extensive infiltration of the epidermis by the proliferating cells.

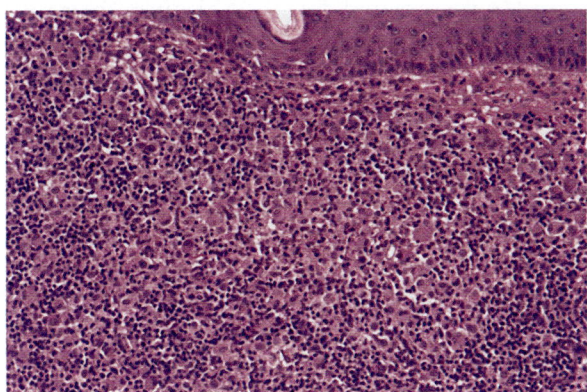 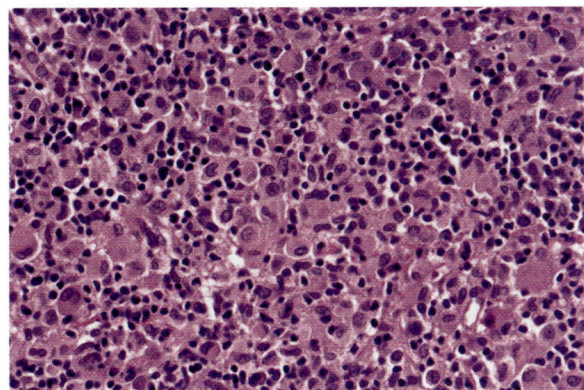

Figure 10-13

LANGERHANS CELL HISTIOCYTOSIS

Left: Low-power view shows the characteristic cells and an accompanying inflammatory infiltrate.
Right: The cells have eosinophilic cytoplasm and nuclei that are grooved or reniform. Among the inflammatory cells, eosinophils can be identified.

such as proliferating cell nuclear antigen (PCNA), Ki-S1, and Ki-67 has been reported (162). In addition, several studies employing assays for human androgen receptor gene (HUMARA) have demonstrated nonrandom X inactivation patterns, indicating that this tumor represents a clonal proliferation of cells bearing the Langerhans cell phenotype (169,190,194).

Differential Diagnosis. The lesions of juvenile xanthogranuloma may resemble Langerhans cell histiocytosis, particularly later-stage lesions in which the foamy histiocytes and multinucleated cells may be present. The cells of juvenile xanthogranuloma lack the characteristic reniform nuclei of Langerhans cell histiocytosis and usually do not show epidermotropism. Numerous, well-formed Touton giant cells are often seen in the former but not the latter. Examples of S-100 protein–positive juvenile xanthogranuloma have been reported (186), but these lesions are reliably CD1a negative, while at the same time they express factor XIIIa and CD68.

Xanthoma disseminatum also shares certain clinical and pathologic features with Langerhans cell histiocytosis, but the former condition lacks epidermotropism, its cells possess scalloped borders and ovoid nuclei, and they express factor XIIIa and CD68 rather than S-100 protein and CD1a (197).

The extensive epidermotropism seen in some cases of Langerhans cell histiocytosis can mimic that of cutaneous T-cell lymphoma, and in addition, the expression of CD4 among cells of the former could contribute to further confusion. The cell morphology of Langerhans cell histiocytosis (large cells with eosinophilic cytoplasm and reniform nuclei) is quite different from that in cutaneous T-cell lymphoma, however, and other T-cell markers are absent. Expression of S-100 protein and CD1a are not seen in the cells of cutaneous T-cell lymphoma.

Congenital Self-Healing Reticulohistiocytosis

Clinical Features. Hashimoto and Pritzker first described this variant of Langerhans cell histiocytosis in 1973 (166). Papules and nodules or, rarely, papulovesicular lesions (168) develop at birth or up to several weeks later. Patients usually present with multiple lesions, but solitary lesions have been reported in about 25 percent of cases (153). Locations include the scalp, face, trunk, and extremities, and a patient with eye involvement has recently been described (196). Lesions develop rapidly, tend to ulcerate, and then involute over a period of several months to a year (168). Systemic involvement does not occur.

Pathologic Findings. Within the dermis are aggregates of cells with abundant eosinophilic cytoplasm, some of which have a ground-glass appearance (fig. 10-14) (166). They may also infiltrate the epidermis (176). The cytoplasm of these cells is PAS positive, diastase resistant (166). Eosinophils, neutrophils, lymphocytes, and foamy histiocytes (macrophages) may accompany the process (180). With immunohistochemical methods, the cells express S-100 protein, CD1a, and HLA-DR (164,184). Up to 25 percent have Birbeck granules on electron microscopic examination. Laminated dense bodies are also present within these cells (167,168), and there is some evidence that the Birbeck granules may be transformed to dense bodies, possibly as part of a degenerative process (164,184).

Differential Diagnosis. The ground-glass appearance of the cytoplasm of some of the cells is reminiscent of true reticulohistiocytosis. The clinical setting of congenital self-healing lesions is distinctive, however, and in contrast to reticulohistiocytosis, the cells are regularly S-100 protein and CD1a positive.

Indeterminate Cell Histiocytosis

Clinical Features. Indeterminate cells are found in the normal dermis. Although their role is still being investigated, they are widely regarded as members of the antigen-presenting cell system. They may be either precursors of or incompletely developed Langerhans cells (171,178). A proliferation of these cells, known as *indeterminate cell histiocytosis*, was first described by Wood et al. in 1985 (193), although this designation also applies to cases reported by Winkelmann et al. in 1982 (191), and Fowler et al. in 1985 (159).

Indeterminate cell histiocytosis is recognized by its immunohistochemical and ultrastructural characteristics. Clinically, there is an eruption of reddish to yellow-brown papules on the face, trunk, or extremities (174). The lesions may remain discrete or coalesce to form plaques (159,185). Children and adults of both sexes are affected. The condition tends to be persistent,

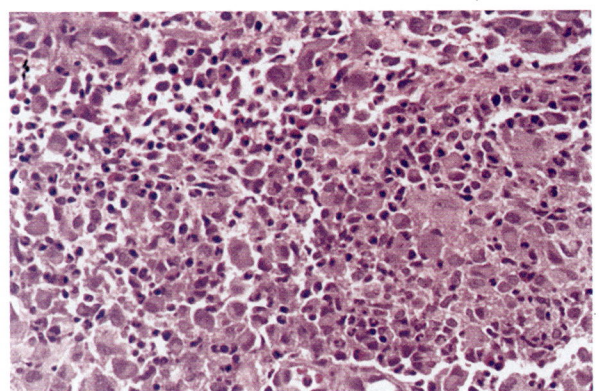 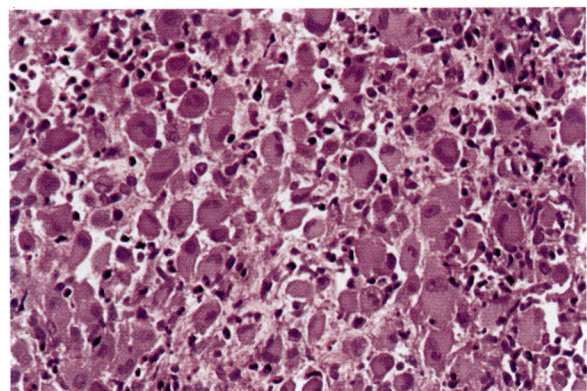

Figure 10-14

CONGENITAL SELF-HEALING RETICULOHISTIOCYTOSIS

Left: Cells with abundant eosinophilic cytoplasm are accompanied by inflammatory cells.
Right: High-power view shows cytologic detail. Ground-glass features are not apparent in this example.

although individual lesions may regress while new ones develop. Systemic involvement may be absent, but individual cases have been associated with hypercalcemia or hypergammaglobulinemia (157), bone involvement (175), and mast cell leukemia (171). A malignant clinical course resulting in death has been reported in an infant (175).

Pathologic Findings. There is a diffuse dermal infiltrate composed of cells with the characteristics of histiocytes (macrophages). These cells are variably vacuolated (185) or foamy (159,171), and multinucleated cells may be present (185). A lack of epidermotropism has been pointed out by several authors (174,185). Occasional cells have reniform nuclei (174). Lymphocytes are present, and may be either intermingled with the histiocytic infiltrate or arranged in clusters (174,183). Eosinophils have also been reported (183).

Immunohistochemical studies show expression of macrophage markers such as CD68, HAM56, MAC387, lysozyme, and alpha-1-antitrypsin (174,185), but a proportion of the cells also expresses factor XIIIa, S-100 protein, and CD1a (174,183,185). Examples that are S-100 protein negative but CD1a positive have been reported (157). The absence of Birbeck granules on electron microscopic examination, along with S-100 protein and/or CD1a positivity, defines this entity as an indeterminate cell disorder (159,174,183,185).

Differential Diagnosis. The microscopic features closely resemble those of other non-Langerhans cell histiocytoses. In particular, cases initially regarded as generalized eruptive histiocytoma (183) or juvenile xanthogranuloma (157) have been shown to have indeterminate cell components, suggesting a link among these disorders. Similarities to Langerhans cell histiocytosis may include the finding of some cells with reniform nuclei in the dermal infiltrate as well as the immunohistochemical features of S-100 protein and/or CD1a positivity. A lack of epidermotropism in the face of a substantial dermal infiltrate provides a clue to the diagnosis of indeterminate cell histiocytosis, but definitive diagnosis hinges upon the ultrastructural absence of Birbeck granules among proliferating cells.

REFERENCES

Non-Langerhans Cell Histiocytic Infiltrates

1. Altman J, Winkelmann RK. Xanthoma disseminatum. Arch Dermatol 1962;86:582–96.
2. Ang P, Tan SH, Ong BH. Cutaneous Rosai-Dorfman disease presenting as pustular and acneiform lesions. J Am Acad Dermatol 1999;41(Pt 2):335–7.
3. Anstey A, Cerio R, Ramnarain N, Orchard G, Smith N, Jones EW. Desmoplastic malignant melanoma. An immunocytochemical study of 25 cases. Am J Dermatopathol 1994;16:14–22.
4. Arnold ML, Anton-Lamprecht I. Multiple eruptive cephalic histiocytomas in a case of T-cell lymphoma. A xanthomatous stage of benign cephalic histiocytosis in an adult patient? Am J Dermatopathol 1993;15:581–6.
5. Arnold ML, Wirth H, Anton-Lamprecht I, Petzoldt D. [Generalized eruptive histiocytoma.] Hautarzt 1982;33:428–37. (German.)
6. Balestrieri GP, Salvi A, Spandrio S, Guerini A. [Skin involvement in Rosai-Dorfman disease. Description of a case.] G Ital Dermatol Venereol 1989;124:159–62. (Italian.)
7. Balfour HH Jr, Speicher CE, McReynolds DG, Nesbit ME. Juvenile xanthogranuloma associated with cytomegalovirus infection. Am J Med 1971;50:380–4.
8. Bang D, Cho NJ, Lee IJ, Ahn SK. Appearance of Sezary-like atypical lymphocytes in the regressing lesions of juvenile xanthogranuloma. Its role in the spontaneous regression. Acta Derm Venereol 1996;76:37–9.
9. Barsky BL, Lao I, Barsky S, Rhee HL. Benign cephalic histiocytosis. Arch Dermatol 1984;120: 650–5.
10. Battaglini J, Olsen TG. Disseminated xanthosiderohistiocytosis, a variant of xanthoma disseminatum, in a patient with a plasma cell dyscrasia. J Am Acad Dermatol 1984;11(Pt 2):750–5.
11. Beurey J, Lamaze B, Weber M, Delrous JL, Kremer B, Chaulieu Y. [Xanthoma disseminatum (Montgomery's syndrome) (author's transl).] Ann Dermatol Venereol 1979;106:353–9. (French.)
12. Biess B, Gartmann H. [Skin manifestations in sinus histiocytosis with massive lymphadenopathy (Rosai-Dorfman syndrome).] Z Hautkr 1985;60:219–28. (German.)
13. Blobstein SH, Caldwell D, Carter M. Bone lesions in xanthoma disseminatum. Arch Dermatol 1985;121:1313–7.
14. Botella-Estrada R, Sanmartin O, Grau M, Alegre V, Mas C, Aliaga A. Juvenile xanthogranuloma with central nervous system involvement. Pediatr Dermatol 1993;10:64–8.
15. Bromley GS, Goulian D Jr. Xanthoma disseminatum: an unusual cause of facial and limb deformity. Plast Reconstr Surg 1983;72:552–6.
16. Burgdorf WH, Kusch SL, Nix TE Jr, Pitha J. Progressive nodular histiocytoma. Arch Dermatol 1981;117:644–9.
17. Calverly DC, Wismer J, Rosenthal D, deSa D, Barr RD. Xanthoma disseminatum in an infant with skeletal and marrow involvement. J Pediatr Hematol Oncol 1995;17:61–5.
18. Candell Chalom E, Elenitsas R, Rosenstein ED, Kramer N. A case of multicentric reticulohistiocytosis in a 6-year-old child. J Rheumatol 1998;25:794–7.
19. Caputo R, Alessi E, Allegra F. Generalized eruptive histiocytoma. A clinical, histologic, and ultrastructural study. Arch Dermatol 1981;117: 216–21.
20. Caputo R, Alessi E, Berti E. Collagen phagocytosis in multicentric reticulohistiocytosis. J Invest Dermatol 1981;76:342–6.
21. Caputo R, Cambiaghi S, Brusasco A, Gelmetti C. Uncommon clinical presentations of juvenile xanthogranuloma. Dermatology 1998;197:45–7.
22. Caputo R, Crosti C, Cainelli T. A unique cytoplasmic structure in papular histiocytoma. J Invest Dermatol 1977;68:98–104.
23. Caputo R, Ermacora E, Gelmetti C, Berti E, Gianni E, Nigro A. Generalized eruptive histiocytoma in children. J Am Acad Dermatol 1987;17:449–54.
24. Catterall MD. Multicentric reticulohistiocytosis: a review of eight cases. Clin Exp Dermatol 1980;5:267–79.
25. Child FJ, Fuller LC, Salisbury J, Higgins EM. Cutaneous Rosai-Dorfman disease. Clin Exp Dermatol 1998;23:40–2.
26. Chu P, LeBoit PE. Histologic features of cutaneous sinus histiocytosis (Rosai-Dorfman disease): study of cases both with and without systemic involvement. J Cutan Pathol 1992;19:201–6.
27. Coode PE, Ridgway H, Jones DB. Multicentric reticulohistiocytosis: report of two cases with ultrastructure, tissue culture and immunology studies. Clin Exp Dermatol 1980;5:281–93.
28. Davies CW, Marren P, Juniper MC, Gray W, Wojnorowska F, Benson MK. Xanthoma disseminatum with respiratory tract involvement and fatal outcome. Thorax 2000;55:170–2.

29. Davies NE, Roenigk HH Jr, Hawk WA, O'Duffy JD. Multicentric reticulohistiocytosis. Report of a case with histochemical studies. Arch Dermatol 1968;97:543–7.
30. de Luna ML, Glikin I, Golberg J, Stringa S, Schroh R, Casas J. Benign cephalic histiocytosis: report of four cases. Pediatr Dermatol 1989;6:198–201.
31. DeBarge LR, Chan CC, Greenberg SC, McLean IW, Yannuzzi LA, Nussenblatt RB. Chorioretinal, iris, and ciliary body infiltration by juvenile xanthogranuloma masquerading as uveitis. Surv Ophthalmol 1994;39:65–71.
32. Delisle B, Gilbert M. [Sinus histiocytosis with cutaneous lesions and thoracic herpes zoster.] Ann Dermatol Venereol 1988;115:1205–7. (French.)
33. Eisenberg EL, Bronson DM, Barsky S. Benign cephalic histiocytosis. A case report and ultrastructural study. J Am Acad Dermatol 1985;12(Pt 1):328–31.
34. Esterly NB, Sahihi T, Medenica M. Juvenile xanthogranuloma. An atypical case with study of ultrastructure. Arch Dermatol 1972;105:99–102.
35. Ferrando J, Campo-Voegeli A, Soler-Carrillo J, et al. Systemic xanthohistiocytoma: a variant of xanthoma disseminatum? Br J Dermatol 1998;138:155–60.
36. Finelli LG, Tenner LK, Ratz JL, Long BD. A case of multicentric reticulohistiocytosis with thyroid involvement. J Am Acad Dermatol 1986;15(Pt 2):1097–100.
37. Fiumicelli A, Bruni L. [Multicentric reticulohistiocytosis (lipoid dermato-arthritis). A radiologic study of 3 cases.] Radiol Med (Torino) 1990;80:277–85. (Italian.)
38. Fortier-Beaulieu M, Thomine E, Boullie MC, Le Loet X, Lauret P, Hemet J. New electron microscopic findings in a case of multicentric reticulohistiocytosis. Long spacing collagen inclusions. Am J Dermatopathol 1993;15:587–9.
39. Foucar E, Rosai J, Dorfman RF. Sinus histiocytosis with massive lymphadenopathy. An analysis of 14 deaths occurring in a patient registry. Cancer 1984;54:1834–40.
40. Foucar E, Rosai J, Dorfman RF, Eyman JM. Immunologic abnormalities and their significance in sinus histiocytosis with massive lymphadenopathy. Am J Clin Pathol 1984;82:515–25.
41. Furey N, Di Mauro J, Eng A, Shaw J. Multicentric reticulohistiocytosis with salivary gland involvement and pericardial effusion. J Am Acad Dermatol 1983;8:679–85.
42. Garcia-Pena P, Mariscal A, Abellan C, Zuasnabar A, Lucaya J. Juvenile xanthogranuloma with extracutaneous lesions. Pediatr Radiol 1992;22:377–8.
43. Gianotti F, Caputo R. Histiocytic syndromes: a review. J Am Acad Dermatol 1985;13:383–404.
44. Gianotti F, Caputo R, Ermacora E. [Singular "infantile histiocytosis with cells with intracytoplasmic vermiform particles."] Bull Soc Fr Dermatol Syphiligr 1971;78:232–3. (French.)
45. Gianotti F, Caputo R, Ermacora E, Gianni E. Benign cephalic histiocytosis. Arch Dermatol 1986;122:1038–43.
46. Gianotti R, Alessi E, Caputo R. Benign cephalic histiocytosis: a distinct entity or a part of a wide spectrum of histiocytic proliferative disorders of children? A histopathological study. Am J Dermatopathol 1993;15:315–9.
47. Gilbert TJ, Parker BR. Juvenile xanthogranuloma of the kidney. Pediatr Radiol 1988;18:169–71.
48. Goerdt S, Bonsmann G, Sunderkotter C, Grabbe S, Luger T, Kolde G. A unique non-Langerhans cell histiocytosis with some features of generalized eruptive histiocytoma. J Am Acad Dermatol 1994;31(Pt 2):322–6.
49. Goette DK, Odom RB, Fitzwater JE, Jr. Diffuse cutaneous reticulohistiocytosis. Arch Dermatol 1982;118:173–6.
50. Gold RH, Metzger AL, Mirra JM, Weinberger HJ, Killebrew K. Multicentric reticulohistiocytosis (lipoid dermato-arthritis). An erosive polyarthritis with distinctive clinical, roentgenographic and pathologic features. Am J Roentgenol Radium Ther Nucl Med 1975;124:610–24.
51. Gonzalez Ruiz A, Bernal Ruiz AI, Aragoneses Fraile H, Peral Martinez I, Garcia Munoz M. Progressive nodular histiocytosis accompanied by systemic disorders. Br J Dermatol 2000;143:628–31.
52. Goodenberger ME, Piette WW, Macfarlane DE, Argenyi ZB. Xanthoma disseminatum and Waldenstrom's macroglobulinemia. J Am Acad Dermatol 1990;23(Pt 2):1015–8.
53. Grabczynska SA, Toh CT, Francis N, Costello C, Bunker CB. Rosai-Dorfman disease complicated by autoimmune haemolytic anaemia: case report and review of a multisystem disease with cutaneous infiltrates. Br J Dermatol 2001;145:323–6.
54. Green CA, Walker DJ, Malcolm AJ. A case of multicentric reticulohistiocytosis: uncommon clinical signs and a report of T-cell marker characteristics. Br J Dermatol 1986;115:623–8.
55. Gupta AK, Bhargava S. Juvenile xanthogranuloma with pulmonary lesions. Pediatr Radiol 1988;18:70.
56. Hammond RR, Mackenzie IR. Xanthoma disseminatum with massive intracranial involvement. Clin Neuropathol 1995;14:314–21.
57. Hansen E, Nilsen R, Milde EJ. Multicentric reticulohistiocytosis: a case report. Acta Derm Venereol 1983;63:175–6.

58. Headington JT. The histiocyte. In memoriam. Arch Dermatol 1986;122:532–3.
59. Helwig EB, Hackney VC. Juvenile xanthogranuloma (nevoxanthoendothelioma). Am J Pathol 1954;30:625–6.
60. Huang HY, Yang CL, Chen WJ. Rosai-Dorfman disease with primary cutaneous manifestations—a case report. Ann Acad Med Singapore 1998;27:589–93.
61. Hunt SJ, Shin SS. Solitary reticulohistiocytoma in pregnancy: immunohistochemical and ultrastructural study of a case with unusual immunophenotype. J Cutan Pathol 1995;22:177–81.
62. Innocenzi D, Silipo V, Giombini S, Ruco L, Bosman C, Calvieri S. Sinus histiocytosis with massive lymphadenopathy (Rosai-Dorfman disease): case report with nodal and diffuse mucocutaneous involvement. J Cutan Pathol 1998;25:563–7.
63. Iyengar V, Golomb CA, Schachner L. Neurilemmomatosis, NF2, and juvenile xanthogranuloma. J Am Acad Dermatol 1998;39(Pt 2):831–4.
64. Izaki S, Kitamura K, Arai E. Generalized eruptive histiocytoma: report of a pediatric case. J Dermatol 1993;20:105–8.
65. Janney CG, Hurt MA, Santa Cruz DJ. Deep juvenile xanthogranuloma. Subcutaneous and intramuscular forms. Am J Surg Pathol 1991;15:150–9.
66. Kang JM, Yang WI, Kim SM, Lee MG. Sinus histiocytosis (Rosai-Dorfman disease) clinically limited to the skin. Acta Derm Venereol 1999;79:363–5.
67. Khoo BP, Tay YK. Benign cephalic histiocytosis in Singapore—a review of 8 cases. Singapore Med J 1999;40:697–9.
68. Knobler RM, Neumann RA, Gebhart W, Radaskiewicz T, Ferenci P, Widhalm K. Xanthoma disseminatum with progressive involvement of the central nervous and hepatobiliary systems. J Am Acad Dermatol 1990;23(Pt 2):341–6.
69. Kraus MD, Haley JC, Ruiz R, Essary L, Moran CA, Fletcher CD. "Juvenile" xanthogranuloma: an immunophenotypic study with a reappraisal of histogenesis. Am J Dermatopathol 2001;23:104–11.
70. Kumakiri M, Sudoh M, Miura Y. Xanthoma disseminatum. Report of a case, with histological and ultrastructural studies of skin lesions. J Am Acad Dermatol 1981;4:291–9.
71. Kuwabara H, Uda H, Tanaka S. Multicentric reticulohistiocytosis. Report of a case with electron microscopic studies. Acta Pathol Jpn 1992;42:130–5.
72. Lazar AP, Esterly NB, Gonzalez-Crussi F. Sinus histiocytosis clinically limited to the skin. Pediatr Dermatol 1987;4:247–53.
73. Lazrak K, Machet MC, Forest JL, Machet L, Lorette G, Pasquiou C. [Disseminated xanthosidero-histiocytosis with cardiac involvement and monoclonal gammapathy.] Ann Dermatol Venereol 1993;120:904–6. (French.)
74. Lesher JL Jr, Allen BS. Multicentric reticulohistiocytosis. J Am Acad Dermatol 1984;11(Pt 2):713–23.
75. Lewis JR, Drummond GT, Mielke BW, Hassard DT, Astle WF. Juvenile xanthogranuloma of the corneoscleral limbus. Can J Ophthalmol 1990;25:351–4.
76. Maize JC, Ahmed AR, Provost TT. Xanthoma disseminatum and multiple myeloma. Arch Dermatol 1974;110:758–61.
77. Matsushima Y, Ohnishi K, Ishikawa O. Generalized eruptive histiocytoma of childhood associated with rheumatic fever. Eur J Dermatol 1999;9:548–50.
78. Misery L, Boucheron S, Claudy AL. Factor XIIIa expression in juvenile xanthogranuloma. Acta Derm Venereol 1994;74:43–4.
79. Mishkel MA, Cockshott WP, Nazir DJ, Rosenthal D, Spaulding WP, Wynn-Williams A. Xanthoma disseminatum. Clinical, metabolic, pathologic, and radiologic aspects. Arch Dermatol 1977;113:1094–100.
80. Nemeth AJ, Penneys NS, Bernstein HB. Fibrous papule: a tumor of fibrohistiocytic cells that contain factor XIIIa. J Am Acad Dermatol 1988;19:1102–6.
81. Newman CC, Raimer SS, Sanchez RL. Nonlipidized juvenile xanthogranuloma: a histologic and immunohistochemical study. Pediatr Dermatol 1997;14:98–102.
82. Nunnink JC, Krusinski PA, Yates JW. Multicentric reticulohistiocytosis and cancer: a case report and review of the literature. Med Pediatr Oncol 1985;13:273–9.
83. Orkin M, Goltz RW, Good RA, et al. A study of multicentric reticulohistiocytosis. Arch Dermatol 1964;89:640–54.
84. Pehr K, Elie J, Watters AK. "Juvenile" xanthogranuloma in a 77-year-old man. Int J Dermatol 1994;33:438–41.
85. Pena-Penabad C, Unamuno P, Garcia-Silva J, Ludena MD, Armijo M. Benign cephalic histiocytosis: case report and literature review. Pediatr Dermatol 1994;11:164–7.
86. Perez A, Rodriguez M, Febrer I, Aliaga A. Sinus histiocytosis confined to the skin. Case report and review of the literature. Am J Dermatopathol 1995;17:384–8.

87. Perrin C, Lacour JP, Michiels JF, Flory P, Ziegler G, Ortonne JP. Multicentric reticulohistiocytosis. Immunohistological and ultrastructural study: a pathology of dendritic cell lineage. Am J Dermatopathol 1992;14:418–25.
88. Perrin C, Michiels JF, Lacour JP, Chagnon A, Fuzibet JG. Sinus histiocytosis (Rosai-Dorfman disease) clinically limited to the skin. An immunohistochemical and ultrastructural study. J Cutan Pathol 1993;20:368–74.
89. Purvis WE, Helwig EB. Reticulohistiocytic granuloma ("reticulohistiocytoma") of the skin. Am J Clin Pathol 1954;24:1005–15.
90. Quaglino P, Tomasini C, Novelli M, Colonna S, Bernengo MG. Immunohistologic findings and adhesion molecule pattern in primary pure cutaneous Rosai-Dorfman disease with xanthomatous features. Am J Dermatopathol 1998;20:393–8.
91. Reid FM, Sandilands GP, Gray KG, Anderson JR. Lymphocyte emperipolesis revisited. II. Further characterization of the lymphocyte subpopulation involved. Immunology 1979;36:367–72.
92. Rendall JR, Vanhegan RI, Robb-Smith AH, Bowers RE, Ryan TJ, Vickers HR. Atypical multicentric reticulohistiocytosis with paraproteinemia. Arch Dermatol 1977;113:1576–82.
93. Repiso T, Roca-Miralles M, Kanitakis J, Castells-Rodellas A. Generalized eruptive histiocytoma evolving into xanthoma disseminatum in a 4-year-old boy. Br J Dermatol 1995;132:978–82.
94. Resnick SD, Woosley J, Azizkhan RG. Giant juvenile xanthogranuloma: exophytic and endophytic variants. Pediatr Dermatol 1990;7:185–8.
95. Ringel E, Moschella S. Primary histiocytic dermatoses. Arch Dermatol 1985;121:1531–41.
96. Rodriguez HA, Saul A, Galloso de Bello L, Tay J, Peyro E. Nodular cutaneous reactive histiocytosis caused by an unidentified microorganism: report of a case. Int J Dermatol 1974;13:248–60.
97. Rodriguez J, Ackerman AB. Xanthogranuloma in adults. Arch Dermatol 1976;112:43–4.
98. Rodriguez-Jurado R, Duran-McKinster C, Ruiz-Maldonado R. Benign cephalic histiocytosis progressing into juvenile xanthogranuloma: a non-Langerhans cell histiocytosis transforming under the influence of a virus? Am J Dermatopathol 2000;22:70–4.
99. Rongioletti F, Heid E, Grosshans E. [Sinus histiocytosis with massive lymphadenopathy (Destombes-Rosai-Dorfman) of cutaneous localization associated with a mycetoma.] G Ital Dermatol Venereol 1985;120:419–23. (Italian.)
100. Roper SS, Spraker MK. Cutaneous histiocytosis syndromes. Pediatr Dermatol 1985;3:19–30.
101. Rosai J, Dorfman RF. Sinus histiocytosis with massive lymphadenopathy. A newly recognized benign clinicopathological entity. Arch Pathol 1969;87:63–70.
102. Saijo S, Hara M, Kuramoto Y, Tagami H. Generalized eruptive histiocytoma: a report of a variant case showing the presence of dermal indeterminate cells. J Cutan Pathol 1991;18:134–6.
103. Sangueza OP, Salmon JK, White CR Jr, Beckstead JH. Juvenile xanthogranuloma: a clinical, histopathologic and immunohistochemical study. J Cutan Pathol 1995;22:327–35.
104. Seo IS, Min KW, Mirkin LD. Juvenile xanthogranuloma. Ultrastructural and immunocytochemical studies. Arch Pathol Lab Med 1986;110:911–5.
105. Shapiro PE, Silvers DN, Treiber RK, Cooper PH, True LD, Lattes R. Juvenile xanthogranulomas with inconspicuous or absent foam cells and giant cells. J Am Acad Dermatol. 1991;24(Pt 1):1005–9.
106. Shimizu N, Ito M, Sato Y. Generalized eruptive histiocytoma: an ultrastructural study. J Cutan Pathol 1987;14:100–5.
107. Skiljo M, Garcia-Lora E, Tercedor J, Massare E, Esquivias J, Garcia-Mellado V. Purely cutaneous Rosai-Dorfman disease. Dermatology 1995;191:49–51.
108. Snow JL, Muller SA. Malignancy-associated multicentric reticulohistiocytosis: a clinical, histological and immunophenotypic study. Br J Dermatol 1995;133:71–6.
109. Sonoda T, Hashimoto H, Enjoji M. Juvenile xanthogranuloma. Clinicopathologic analysis and immunohistochemical study of 57 patients. Cancer 1985;56:2280–6.
110. Tahan SR, Pastel-Levy C, Bhan AK, Mihm MC Jr. Juvenile xanthogranuloma. Clinical and pathologic characterization. Arch Pathol Lab Med 1989;113:1057–61.
111. Taunton OD, Yeshurun D, Jarratt M. Progressive nodular histiocytoma. Arch Dermatol 1978;114:1505–8.
112. Tietge UJ, Maschek H, Schneider A, et al. [Xanthoma disseminatum with marked mucocutaneous involvement.] Dtsch Med Wochenschr 1998;123:1337–42. (German.)
113. Tomaszewski MM, Lupton GP. Unusual expression of S-100 protein in histiocytic neoplasms. J Cutan Pathol 1998;25:129–35.
114. Torres L, Sanchez JL, Rivera A, Gonzalez A. Progressive nodular histiocytosis. J Am Acad Dermatol 1993;29(2 Pt 1):278–80.
115. Umbert IJ, Winkelmann RK. Eruptive histiocytoma. J Am Acad Dermatol 1989;20(Pt 2):958–64.

116. Valente M, Parenti A, Cipriani R, Peserico A. Familial histiocytic dermatoarthritis. Histologic and ultrastructural findings in two cases. Am J Dermatopathol 1987;9:491–6.
117. Varotti C, Bettoli V, Berti E, Cavicchini S, Caputo R. Xanthoma disseminatum: a case with extensive mucous membrane involvement. J Am Acad Dermatol 1991;25(Pt 2):433–6.
118. Vasconcelos FO, Oliveira LA, Naves MD, Castro WH, Gomez RS. Juvenile xanthogranuloma: case report with immunohistochemical identification of early and late cytomegalovirus antigens. J Oral Sci 2001;43:21–5.
119. Vlasov PA. [Emperipolesis and interrelations of megakaryocytes and neutrophilic granulocytes in the bone marrow of healthy dogs]. Arkh Anat Gistol Embriol 1989;96:60–3.
120. Wang JS, Hsieh SP, Shih DF, Tseng HH. Cutaneous Rosai-Dorfman disease manifesting as recurrent breast tumor: a case report. Chung Hua I Hsueh Tsa Chih (Taipei) 1997;59:269–73.
121. Webster SB, Reister HC, Harman LE Jr. Juvenile xanthogranuloma with extracutaneous lesions. A case report and review of the literature. Arch Dermatol 1966;93:71–6.
122. Wee SH, Kim HS, Chang SN, Kim DK, Park WH. Generalized eruptive histiocytoma: a pediatric case. Pediatr Dermatol 2000;17:453–5.
123. Weiss N, Keller C. Xanthoma disseminatum: a rare normolipemic xanthomatosis. Clin Investig 1993;71:233–8.
124. Weston WL, Travers SH, Mierau GW, Heasley D, Fitzpatrick J. Benign cephalic histiocytosis with diabetes insipidus. Pediatr Dermatol 2000;17:296–8.
125. Winkelmann RK. Cutaneous syndromes of non-X histiocytosis. A review of the macrophage-histiocyte diseases of the skin. Arch Dermatol 1981;117:667–72.
126. Winkelmann RK, Hu CH, Kossard S. Response of nodular non-X histiocytosis to vinblastine. Arch Dermatol 1982;118:913–7.
127. Winkelmann RK, Muller SA. Generalized eruptive histiocytoma. A benign papular histiocytic reticulosis. Arch Dermatol 1963;88:586–96.
128. Yokoyama Y. [Dermatoarthritis, familial histiocytic.] Ryoikibetsu Shokogun Shirizu 2001;33:548. (Japanese.)
129. Zayid I, Farraj S. Familial histiocytic dermatoarthritis. A new syndrome. Am J Med 1973;54:793–800.
130. Zelger B, Cerio R, Orchard G, Fritsch P, Wilson-Jones E. Histologic and immunohistochemical study comparing xanthoma disseminatum and histiocytosis X. Arch Dermatol 1992;128:1207–12.
131. Zelger B, Cerio R, Orchard G, Wilson-Jones E. Juvenile and adult xanthogranuloma. A histological and immunohistochemical comparison. Am J Surg Pathol 1994;18:126–35.
132. Zelger B, Cerio R, Soyer HP, Misch K, Orchard G, Wilson-Jones E. Reticulohistiocytoma and multicentric reticulohistiocytosis. Histopathologic and immunophenotypic distinct entities. Am J Dermatopathol 1994;16:577–84.
133. Zelger BG, Zelger B, Steiner H, Mikuz G. Solitary giant xanthogranuloma and benign cephalic histiocytosis—variants of juvenile xanthogranuloma. Br J Dermatol 1995;133:598–604.
134. Zelger BW, Sidoroff A, Orchard G, Cerio R. Non-Langerhans cell histiocytoses. A new unifying concept. Am J Dermatopathol 1996;18:490–504.
135. Zelger BW, Staudacher C, Orchard G, Wilson-Jones E, Burgdorf WH. Solitary and generalized variants of spindle cell xanthogranuloma (progressive nodular histiocytosis). Histopathology 1995;27:11–9.
136. Zelger BW, Steiner H, Kutzner H. Clear cell dermatofibroma. Case report of an unusual fibrohistiocytic lesion. Am J Surg Pathol 1996;20:483–91.
137. Zimmerman LE. Ocular lesions of juvenile xanthogranuloma. Nevoxanthoedothelioma. Am J Ophthalmol 1965;60:1011–35.
138. Zvulunov A, Barak Y, Metzker A. Juvenile xanthogranuloma, neurofibromatosis, and juvenile chronic myelogenous leukemia. World statistical analysis. Arch Dermatol 1995;131:904–8.

Malignant Histiocytosis

139. Akiyama M, Inamoto N, Nakamura K, Kakamura K. Malignant histiocytosis presenting as multiple erythematous plaques and cutaneous depigmentation. Am J Dermatopathol 1997;19:299–302.
140. Arai E, Su WP, Roche PC, Li CY. Cutaneous histiocytic malignancy. Immunohistochemical re-examination of cases previously diagnosed as cutaneous "histiocytic lymphoma" and "malignant histiocytosis." J Cutan Pathol 1993;20:115–20.
141. Cattoretti G, Villa A, Vezzoni P, Giardini R, Lombardi L, Rilke F. Malignant histiocytosis. A phenotypic and genotypic investigation. Am J Pathol 1990;136:1009–19.
142. Copie-Bergman C, Wotherspoon AC, Norton AJ, Diss TC, Isaacson PG. True histiocytic lymphoma: a morphologic, immunohistochemical, and molecular genetic study of 13 cases. Am J Surg Pathol 1998;22:1386–92.
143. deMent SH. Association between mediastinal germ cell tumors and hematologic malignancies: an update. Hum Pathol 1990;21:699–703.

144. Egeler RM, Schmitz L, Sonneveld P, Mannival C, Nesbit ME. Malignant histiocytosis: a reassessment of cases formerly classified as histiocytic neoplasms and review of the literature. Med Pediatr Oncol 1995;25:1–7.
145. Hanson CA, Jaszcz W, Kersey JH, et al. True histiocytic lymphoma: histopathologic, immunophenotypic and genotypic analysis. Br J Haematol 1989;73:187–98.
146. Kamel OW, Gocke CD, Kell DL, Cleary ML, Warnke RA. True histiocytic lymphoma: a study of 12 cases based on current definition. Leuk Lymphoma 1995;18:81–6.
147. Soria C, Orradre JL, Garcia-Almagro D, Martinez B, Algara P, Piris MA. True histiocytic lymphoma (monocytic sarcoma). Am J Dermatopathol 1992;14:511–7.
148. Weiss LM, Grogan TM, Muller-Hermelink HK, et al. Histiocytic sarcoma. In: Jaffe ES, Harris NL, Stein H, Vardiman JW, eds. Pathology and genetics of tumours of haematopoietic and lymphoid tissues. Lyon: IARC Press; 2001:278–9.
149. Wilson MS, Weiss LM, Gatter KC, Mason DY, Dorfman RF, Warnke RA. Malignant histiocytosis. A reassessment of cases previously reported in 1975 based on paraffin section immunophenotyping studies. Cancer 1990;66:530–6.

Langerhans Cell Histiocytoses and Indeterminate Cell Histiocytosis

150. Altman J, Winkelmann RK. Xanthomatous cutaneous lesions of histiocytosis X. Arch Dermatol 1963;87:164–70.
151. Ben-Ezra J, Bailey A, Azumi N, et al. Malignant histiocytosis X. A distinct clinicopathologic entity. Cancer 1991;68:1050–60.
152. Benisch B, Peison B, Carter H. Histiocytosis X of the skin in an elderly man. Am J Clin Pathol 1977;67:36–40.
153. Bernstein EF, Resnik KS, Loose JH, Halcin C, Kauh YC. Solitary congenital self-healing reticulohistiocytosis. Br J Dermatol 1993;129:449–54.
154. Colby TV, Lombard C. Histiocytosis X in the lung. Hum Pathol 1983;14:847–56.
155. Curtis AC, Cawley EP. Eosinophilic granuloma of bone with cutaneous manifestations. Arch Dermatol 1947;55:810–8.
156. de Graaf JH, Tamminga RY, Dam-Meiring A, Kamps WA, Timens W. The presence of cytokines in Langerhans' cell histiocytosis. J Pathol 1996;180:400–6.
157. de Graaf JH, Timens W, Tamminga RY, Molenaar WM. Deep juvenile xanthogranuloma: a lesion related to dermal indeterminate cells. Hum Pathol 1992;23:905–10.
158. Favara BE, McCarthy RC, Mierau GW. Histiocytosis X. Hum Pathol 1983;14:663–76.
159. Fowler JF, Callen JP, Hodge SJ, Verdi G. Cutaneous non-X histiocytosis: clinical and histologic features and response to dermabrasion. J Am Acad Dermatol 1985;13:645–9.
160. Gianotti F, Caputo R. Skin ultrastructure in Hand-Schuller-Christian disease. Report on abnormal Langerhans' cells. Arch Dermatol 1969;100:342–9.
161. Greenberger JS, Crocker AC, Vawter G, Jaffe N, Cassady JR. Results of treatment of 127 patients with systemic histiocytosis. Medicine (Baltimore) 1981;60:311–38.
162. Hage C, Willman CL, Favara BE, Isaacson PG. Langerhans' cell histiocytosis (histiocytosis X): immunophenotype and growth fraction. Hum Pathol 1993;24:840–5.
163. Harrist TJ, Bhan AK, Murphy GF, et al. Histiocytosis-X: in situ characterization of cutaneous infiltrates with monoclonal antibodies. Am J Clin Pathol 1983;79:294–300.
164. Hashimoto K, Bale GF, Hawkins HK, Langston C, Pritzker MS. Congenital self-healing reticulohistiocytosis (Hashimoto-Pritzker type). Int J Dermatol 1986;25:516–23.
165. Hashimoto K, Kagetsu N, Taniguchi Y, Weintraub R, Chapman-Winokur RL, Kasiborski A. Immunohistochemistry and electron microscopy in Langerhans cell histiocytosis confined to the skin. J Am Acad Dermatol 1991;25(Pt 1):1044–53.
166. Hashimoto K, Pritzker MS. Electron microscopic study of reticulohistiocytoma. An unusual case of congenital, self-healing reticulohistiocytosis. Arch Dermatol 1973;107:263–70.
167. Hashimoto K, Takahashi S, Lee RG, Krull EA. Congenital self-healing reticulohistiocytosis. Report of the seventh case with histochemical and ultrastructural studies. J Am Acad Dermatol 1984;11:447–54.
168. Herman LE, Rothman KF, Harawi S, Gonzalez-Serva A. Congenital self-healing reticulohistiocytosis. A new entity in the differential diagnosis of neonatal papulovesicular eruptions. Arch Dermatol 1990;126:210–2.
169. Itoh H, Miyaguni H, Kataoka H, et al. Primary cutaneous Langerhans cell histiocytosis showing malignant phenotype in an elderly woman: report of a fatal case. J Cutan Pathol 2001;28:371–8.
170. Klein A, Corazza F, Demulder A, Van Beers D, Ferster A. Recurrent viral associated hemophagocytic syndrome in a child with Langerhans cell histiocytosis. J Pediatr Hematol Oncol 1999;21:554–6.

171. Kolde G, Brocker EB. Multiple skin tumors of indeterminate cells in an adult. J Am Acad Dermatol 1986;15(Pt 1):591–7.
172. Krenacs L, Tiszalvicz L, Krenacs T, Boumsell L. Immunohistochemical detection of CD1A antigen in formalin-fixed and paraffin-embedded tissue sections with monoclonal antibody 010. J Pathol 1993;171:99–104.
173. Mahzoon S, Wood MG. Multifocal eosinophilic granuloma with skin ulceration. Histiocytosis X of the Hand-Schuller-Christian type. Arch Dermatol 1980;116:218–20.
174. Manente L, Cotellessa C, Schmitt I, et al. Indeterminate cell histiocytosis: a rare histiocytic disorder. Am J Dermatopathol 1997;19:276–83.
175. Martin Flores-Stadler E, Gonzalez-Crussi F, Greene M, Thangavelu M, Kletzel M, Chou PM. Indeterminate-cell histiocytosis: immunophenotypic and cytogenetic findings in an infant. Med Pediatr Oncol 1999;32:250–4.
176. Mascaro JM, Aliaga A, Mascaro-Galy C. [Autoinvolutive congenital reticulosis (Hashimoto-Pritzker type).] Ann Dermatol Venereol 1978;105:223–7. (French.)
177. Meehan SA, Smoller BR. Cutaneous Langerhans cell histiocytosis of the genitalia in the elderly: a report of three cases. J Cutan Pathol 1998;25:370–4.
178. Murphy GF, Bhan AK, Harrist TJ, Mihm MC Jr. In situ identification of T6-positive cells in normal human dermis by immunoelectron microscopy. Br J Dermatol 1983;108:423–31.
179. Neumann MP, Frizzera G. The coexistence of Langerhans' cell granulomatosis and malignant lymphoma may take different forms: report of seven cases with a review of the literature. Hum Pathol 1986;17:1060–5.
180. Ofuji S, Tachibana S, Kanato M, Horiguchi Y. Congenital self-healing reticulohistiocytosis (Hashimoto-Pritzker): a case report with a solitary lesion. J Dermatol 1987;14:182–4.
181. Rabkin MS, Kjeldsberg CR, Wittwer CT, Marty J. A comparison study of two methods of peanut agglutinin staining with S100 immunostaining in 29 cases of histiocytosis X (Langerhans' cell histiocytosis). Arch Pathol Lab Med 1990;114:511–5.
182. Rabkin MS, Wittwer CT, Kjeldsberg CR, Piepkorn MW. Flow-cytometric DNA content of histiocytosis X (Langerhans cell histiocytosis). Am J Pathol 1988;131:283–9.
183. Saijo S, Hara M, Kuramoto Y, Tagami H. Generalized eruptive histiocytoma: a report of a variant case showing the presence of dermal indeterminate cells. J Cutan Pathol 1991;18:134–6.
184. Schaumburg-Lever G, Rechowicz E, Fehrenbacher B, Moller H, Nau P. Congenital self-healing reticulohistiocytosis—a benign Langerhans cell disease. J Cutan Pathol 1994;21:59–66.
185. Sidoroff A, Zelger B, Steiner H, Smith N. Indeterminate cell histiocytosis—a clinicopathological entity with features of both X- and non-X histiocytosis. Br J Dermatol 1996;134:525–32.
186. Tomaszewski MM, Lupton GP. Unusual expression of S-100 protein in histiocytic neoplasms. J Cutan Pathol 1998;25:129–35.
187. Vassallo R, Ryu JH, Colby TV, Hartman T, Limper AH. Pulmonary Langerhans'-cell histiocytosis. N Engl J Med 2000;342:1969–78.
188. Weiss LM, Grogan TM, Pileri SA, et al. Langerhans cell sarcoma. In: Jaffe ES, Harris NL, Stein H, Vardiman JW, eds. Pathology and genetics of tumours of haematopoietic and lymphoid tissues. Lyon: IARC Press; 2001.
189. Wells GC. The pathology of adult type Letterer-Siwe disease. Clin Exp Dermatol 1979;4:407–12.
190. Willman CL, Busque L, Griffith BB, et al. Langerhans'-cell histiocytosis (histiocytosis X)—a clonal proliferative disease. N Engl J Med 1994;331:154–60.
191. Winkelmann RK, Hu CH, Kossard S. Response of nodular non-X histiocytosis to vinblastine. Arch Dermatol 1982;118:913–7.
192. Wood C, Wood GS, Deneau DG, Oseroff A, Beckstead JH, Malin J. Malignant histiocytosis X. Report of a rapidly fatal case in an elderly man. Cancer 1984;54:347–52.
193. Wood GS, Hu CH, Beckstead JH, Turner RR, Winkelmann RK. The indeterminate cell proliferative disorder: report of a case manifesting as an unusual cutaneous histiocytosis. J Dermatol Surg Oncol 1985;11:1111–9.
194. Yu RC, Chu C, Buluwela L, Chu AC. Clonal proliferation of Langerhans cells in Langerhans cell histiocytosis. Lancet 1994;343:767–8.
195. Zachariae H. Histiocytosis X in two infants—treated with topical nitrogen mustard. Br J Dermatol 1979;100:433–8.
196. Zaenglein AL, Steele MA, Kamino H, Chang MW. Congenital self-healing reticulohistiocytosis with eye involvement. Pediatr Dermatol 2001;18:135–7.
197. Zelger B, Cerio R, Orchard G, Fritsch P, Wilson-Jones E. Histologic and immunohistochemical study comparing xanthoma disseminatum and histiocytosis X. Arch Dermatol 1992;128:1207–12.

SUPPLEMENTAL REFERENCES

(Juvenile) Xanthogranuloma

Chantranuwat C. Systemic form of juvenile xanthogranuloma: report of a case with liver and bone marrow involvement. Pediatr Dev Pathol 2004;7: 646–8.

Gamo R, Ortiz-Romero P, Sopena J, Guerra A, Rodriguez-Peralto JL, Iglesias L. Anetoderma developing in juvenile xanthogranuloma. Int J Dermatol 2005;44:503–6.

Janssen D, Harms D. Juvenile xanthogranuloma in childhood and adolescence: a clinicopathologic study of 129 patients from the Kiel pediatric tumor registry. Am J Surg Pathol 2005;29:21–8.

Benign Cephalic Histiocytosis

Sidwell RU, Francis N, Slater DN, Mayou SC. Is disseminated juvenile xanthogranulomatosis benign cephalic histiocytosis? Pediatr Dermatol 2005;22:40–3.

Xanthoma Disseminatum

Alexander AS, Turner R, Uniate L, Pearcy RG. Xanthoma disseminatum: a case report and literature review. Br J Radiol 2005;78:153–7.

Reticulohistiocytosis

Ho SG, Yu RC. A case of multicentric reticulohistiocytosis with multiple lytic skull lesions. Clin Exp Dermatol 2005;30:515–8.

Luz FB, Gaspar AP, Ramos-e-Silva M, et al. Immunohistochemical profile of multicentric reticulohistiocytosis. Skinmed 2005;4:71–7.

Rosai-Dorfman Disease

Lu CI, Kuo TT, Wong WR, Hong HS. Clinical and histopathologic spectrum of cutaneous Rosai-Dorfman disease in Taiwan. J Am Acad Dermatol 2004;51:931–9.

Rodriguez-Galindo C, Helton KJ, Sanchez ND, Rieman M, Jeng M, Wang W. Extranodal Rosai-Dorfman disease in children. J Pediatr Hematol Oncol 2004;26:19–24.

Van Zander J. Cutaneous Rosai-Dorfman disease. Dermatol Online J 2004;10:12.

Malignant Histiocytosis

Lu CL, Li GD, Liu WP, et al. [Detection of TCR-gamma chain gene rearrangement in malignant histiocytosis.] Zhonghua Xue Ye Xue Za Zhi 2004;25:220–2. (Chinese.)

Langerhans Cell Histiocytosis

Anlauf M, Schafer MK, Depboylu C, et al. The vesicular monoamine transporter 2 (VMAT2) is expressed by normal and tumor cutaneous mast cells and Langerhans cells of the skin but is absent from Langerhans cell histiocytosis. J Histochem Cytochem 2004;52:779–88.

Braier J, Latella A, Balancini B, et al. Outcome in children with pulmonary Langerhans cell histiocytosis. Pediatr Blood Cancer 2004;43:765–9.

Kini U, Bhat PI, Jayaseelan E. FNA diagnosis of primary adult onset lymphocutaneous Langerhans' cell histiocytosis masquerading as deep fungal mycosis. Diagn Cytopathol 2005;32:292–5.

Patrizi A, Neri I, Bianchi F, et al. Langerhans cell histiocytosis and juvenile xanthogranuloma. Two case reports. Dermatology 2004;209:57–61.

Rolland A, Guyon L, Gill M, et al. Increased blood myeloid dendritic cells and dendritic cell-poietins in Langerhans cell histiocytosis. J Immunol 2005; 174:3067–71.

Congenital Self-Healing Reticulohistiocytosis

Ricart J, Jimenez A, Marquina A, Villanueva A. Congenital self-healing reticulohistiocytosis: report of a case and review of the literature. Acta Paediatr 2004;93:426–9.

Indeterminate Cell Histiocytosis

Wang CH, Chen GS. Indeterminate cell histiocytosis: a case report. Kaohsiung J Med Sci 2004;20:24–30.

11 PLASMACELLULAR INFILTRATIVE DISORDERS

Although plasma cells are commonly observed in the skin in a wide variety of inflammatory processes or as a response to tumors, primary plasmacellular disorders that directly involve the skin are rare. This chapter reviews the few plasmacellular infiltrative disorders that are encountered in dermatopathology practice: plasmacytoma, multiple myeloma, macroglobulinemia of Waldenström, and Castleman's disease.

MULTIPLE MYELOMA

Clinical Features. *Multiple myeloma* is a bone marrow–derived plasma cell neoplasm associated with serum monoclonal protein. The clinical characteristics typically include osteolytic lesions, bone pain, pathologic fractures, hypercalcemia, and anemia (22,34). Although autopsy study indicates that extraosseous involvement with multiple myeloma is common (26), the detection of extraosseous mass lesions during life is less frequent (19). Most patients have a monoclonal (M) component in the serum, identified by protein or immunoelectrophoresis. This is most commonly immunoglobin (Ig)G, but sometimes (in descending order) IgA, light chain (Bence-Jones) protein, or IgD. Bence-Jones protein is usually found in the urine of myeloma patients (51). Disease variants include *nonsecretory myeloma*, in which no M component is detectable (7), *plasma cell leukemia*, and *myeloma with plasmablastic morphology*. The latter two variants are associated with aggressive disease and a particularly poor prognosis (18,21).

The survival rates of patients with multiple myeloma who are treated with conventional chemotherapy appear to correlate with age: a median of 31 months for those over the age of 66 years, 44 months for those 66 years or less, and 57 months for those under 55 (49). The primary causes of death are infection and renal insufficiency (34).

Cutaneous involvement in multiple myeloma often reflects a secondary manifestation of the disease, such as amyloidosis, cryoglobulinemic purpura, xanthoma disseminatum (38), or deposition of crystalline proteinaceous material within follicular epithelium or in the dermis (28,48). Specific skin lesions are rare, and have been estimated to occur in 2 percent of patients (16,68); nevertheless, numerous case reports exist. Skin lesions usually occur late in the course of multiple myeloma (1), but they occasionally precede other manifestations of the disease (52). Cutaneous involvement most often represents direct extension from an underlying bony focus of disease (27,46), but skin lesions without underlying bone involvement do occur. These most often present as erythematous to violaceous nodules located on the scalp, neck, trunk, or extremities (19,27,31). The nodules may be solitary, localized to one particular region, or widespread. In one reported case, pathologic fracture of the humerus resulted in multiple regional cutaneous metastases (29). Specific cutaneous lesions typically portend an adverse prognosis and rapid demise, but long survival periods have been reported following the onset of cutaneous disease (46).

Kato et al. (31) reviewed the immunoglobulin types in reported cases of multiple myeloma with cutaneous involvement: 52 percent expressed IgG; 23 percent, IgA; 16 percent, IgD; and 6 percent, Bence-Jones protein. The incidence of cutaneous or soft tissue involvement in IgD myeloma appears to be disproportionately high, since only 2 percent of myeloma cases overall express IgD (19,31,45).

Pathologic Findings. There is infiltration of the dermis and subcutis by plasma cells. These may be arranged in large, densely populated masses or as individual cells that line up in cords between collagen bundles (46). Morphologically, the cells may vary in degree of maturity. Some are indistinguishable from normal plasma cells, while others display nuclei that are large, irregular in shape, or hyperchromatic (fig. 11-1)

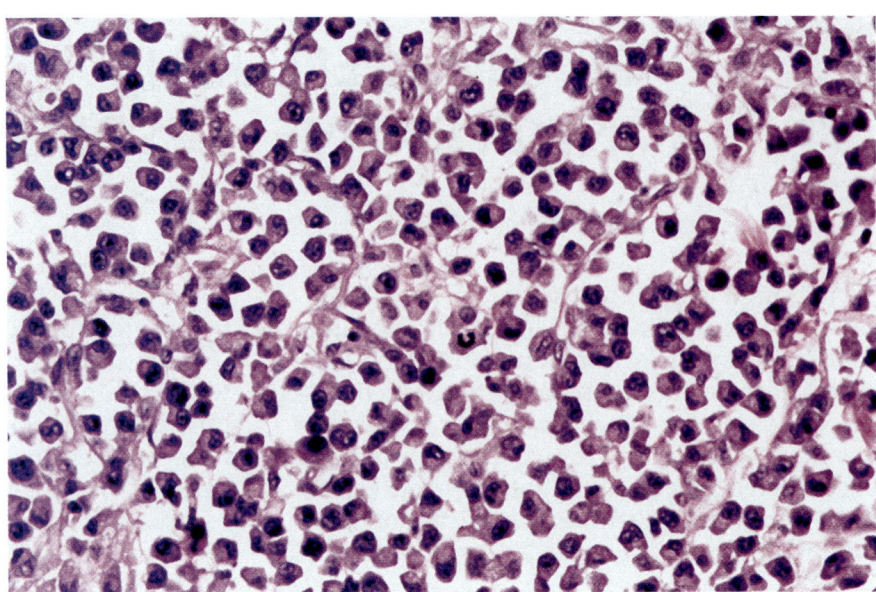

Figure 11-1

MULTIPLE MYELOMA INVOLVING THE SKIN

The cells resemble normal plasma cells, but many possess large, irregularly shaped or hyperchromatic nuclei. Nucleoli can be identified in some of the cells.

(19,30,46). Multinucleated cells are sometimes present (65). Some immature cells resemble lymphocytes (50,68); occasionally there are cells with a high nuclear to cytoplasmic ratio and prominent nucleoli, characteristic of plasmablasts (22). A plasmablastic morphology generally portends an adverse prognosis (22). The cytoplasm of these plasma cells stains red with methyl green-pyronin, reflecting their RNA content.

Demonstration of the immunoglobulin and light chain content of these cells by immunofluorescent or immunoperoxidase methods is only variably successful (29,62,68), but positive results have confirmed the electrophoretic findings (27,46). In situ hybridization is a more reliable method (64). Ultrastructurally, the neoplastic cells possess prominent rough endoplasmic reticulum containing immunoglobulin, sometimes in crystalline form (32,58).

Differential Diagnosis. The histopathologic distinction between multiple myeloma with cutaneous involvement and extraosseous plasmacytoma of skin cannot be made based upon the maturity of the plasma cell infiltration (61). A significant diagnostic dilemma is the differentiation between myeloma or plasmacytoma in skin and a reactive plasmacellular infiltrate. The latter can be seen in a variety of infectious processes (e.g., secondary syphilis) or as a response to malignancy of another type (e.g., basal or squamous cell carcinoma). The presence of immature plasma cells is a strong indicator of plasma cell neoplasia, since these atypical forms are rarely encountered in reactive infiltrates (22). In cases with a high percentage of mature-appearing plasma cells, in situ hybridization, or immunohistochemical staining for immunoglobulin and light chains may be useful in assessing clonality.

EXTRAOSSEOUS PLASMACYTOMA

Clinical Features. *Extraosseous plasmacytoma* is a neoplastic aggregation of plasma cells that arises outside of bone and bone marrow. Most patients are adults, with a male to female ratio of 2 to 1 (22). Most lesions arise in the upper respiratory passages (1), but they can appear in a variety of other organs, including bladder, gastrointestinal tract, and central nervous system. Skin involvement rarely has been reported, but can present in the form of a solitary lesion (63,67) or as multiple metastases. The metastatic lesions originate from several extramedullary sites (1,58), including the skin itself (9). Lesions consist of nodules or plaques, and arise in the skin of the trunk or extremities (36,63,67). Circulating monoclonal immunoglobulins or Bence-Jones protein can be detected in large or metastatic tumors, but not in smaller solitary lesions (44,47).

Solitary lesions tend to respond to conservative therapy (surgery or radiation) and are generally associated with a favorable prognosis (43,63,67), but some patients with solitary tumors, as well as those with multiple cutaneous plasmacytomas, have a high mortality rate

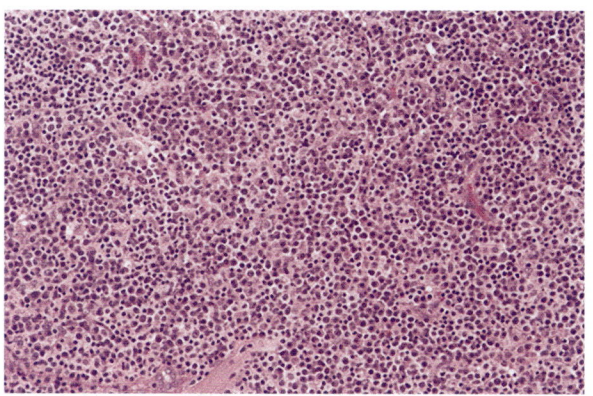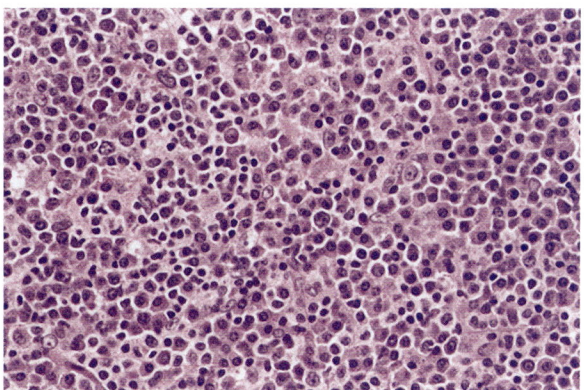

Figure 11-2

EXTRAOSSEOUS PLASMACYTOMA INVOLVING THE SKIN

Left: Low-power view shows a dense dermal infiltrate.

Right: In a higher-power view, some cells are recognizable as plasma cells, but others have an immature, anaplastic appearance.

(47,63). In their review of the literature, Wong et al. (67) documented disease-related deaths in 40 percent of patients with primary cutaneous plasmacytomas, suggesting that these tumors may be more aggressive than their noncutaneous extramedullary counterpart.

Pathologic Findings. There is usually a dense dermal infiltrate of plasma cells that may be morphologically bland in appearance but may also appear immature and anaplastic, with multinucleated cells and frequent mitoses (fig. 11-2) (32,41). In some cases, the microscopic appearance more closely resembles that of a B-cell lymphoma with marked plasma cell differentiation (22,58). As expected, the plasma cells are pyroninophilic (22,46,58), and monoclonal immunoglobulin, light chain restriction, or both can be detected with immunohistochemical techniques or by in situ hybridization (36,64,70). Kato et al. (31) reviewed 18 cases of primary cutaneous plasmacytoma and found that 56 percent expressed IgG; 11 percent, IgA; 17 percent, Bence-Jones protein; and none expressed IgD.

Other reported findings have included an association with histiocytes (macrophages) (32,46), and needle-shaped crystals in histiocytes that probably represent phagocytosis of proteinaceous material produced by the plasma cells (32). Interleukin-6, a cytokine that induces B-cell differentiation, may be expressed by tumor cells, and is present in elevated levels in plasma and in peripheral blood mononuclear cells of patients with cutaneous plasmacytomas (69).

Differential Diagnosis. The comments regarding multiple myeloma with cutaneous involvement also pertain to extraosseous plasmacytoma of the skin. Well-differentiated variants are difficult to distinguish morphologically from reactive plasmacellular infiltrates, but can be recognized by demonstrating monoclonality. The presence of immature forms argues against a reactive infiltrate. In some cases, a distinction from B-cell lymphoma with plasmacytic differentiation (immunocytoma, extranodal marginal zone lymphoma of mucosa-associated lymphoid tissue [MALT] type) can be difficult if not impossible. A distinction between multiple myeloma and extraosseous plasmacytoma of the skin cannot be reliably made on microscopic grounds alone. Both tend to show dense aggregates of plasma cells, although in a study of five cases that included examples of both lesions, only the myeloma cases showed the configuration of plasma cells dispersed singly or in small cords between dermal collagen bundles (46).

MACROGLOBULINEMIA OF WALDENSTRÖM

Clinical Features. *Macroglobulinemia of Waldenström* is a monoclonal, IgM gammopathy associated with a B-cell lymphoproliferative disorder. It usually accompanies lymphoplasmacytic lymphoma, a neoplasm that involves bone

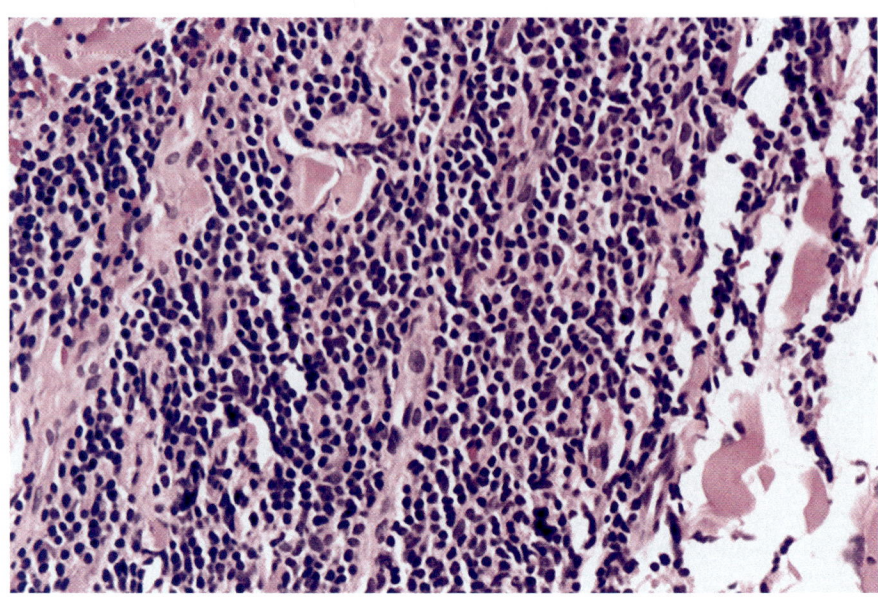

Figure 11-3

MACROGLOBULINEMIA OF WALDENSTRÖM

This skin lesion consists of a dermal infiltrate of lymphocytes and plasmacytoid cells.

marrow, lymph nodes, and spleen. IgM paraproteins, however, are also produced in association with other disorders, including B-cell chronic lymphocytic leukemia and extranodal marginal zone B-cell lymphoma of MALT type (5). The underlying lymphoplasmacytic lymphoma most commonly arises in elderly adults, more often in men than women. The disease is slowly progressive and patients have a median survival period of 5 years (15). The IgM paraprotein is responsible for a number of complications, including cerebrovascular accidents, neuropathy, and cryoglobulinemia.

Nonspecific cutaneous manifestations of macroglobulinemia result from the hyperviscosity state or from the cryoglobulinemia, and include urticaria, purpura, and ulcers (3). An immunobullous disease has also been reported, associated with deposition of linear IgM along the epidermal-dermal basement membrane zone (66).

There are two specific skin lesions of macroglobulinemia. The first consists of red-brown to violaceous papules, nodules, and plaques associated with lymphoplasmacellular infiltrates; these lesions have also been termed *immunocytoma, lymphoplasmacytic type* (6,39). The second specific skin lesion is a pink to flesh-colored papule composed of monoclonal immunoglobulin, the so-called *storage papules* (3,37,39).

Pathologic Findings. Of the two specific skin lesions of macroglobulinemia, the violaceous papules, nodules, and plaques show perivascular and diffuse, dermal and subcutaneous infiltrates of lymphocytes, plasmacytoid cells (resembling plasma cells but without the characteristic nuclear features), and more mature-appearing plasma cells (fig. 11-3). Some of the plasma cells may have periodic acid–Schiff (PAS)-positive intranuclear inclusions known as Dutcher bodies (8). Transformation to high-grade lymphoma rarely has been reported (3).

The pink to flesh-colored papules known as storage papules are composed of intradermal deposits of homogeneous, PAS–positive eosinophilic material that may demonstrate fissuring in the manner of amyloid or colloid (fig. 11-4) (24,37,39). Lesions characterized by lymphoplasmacellular infiltrates have demonstrated monoclonality for IgM and kappa light chains by immunofluorescent or immunoperoxidase methods (6,42). The amorphous material in storage papules contains IgM (24,39). Reported ultrastructural findings in the storage papules have varied. In one study, the papules contained thick (56-nm wide), nonbranching linear material with cross striations at 12-nm intervals (37), while in another report the material was granular and fibrillar with no periodicity (35).

Differential Diagnosis. The lymphoplasmacellular lesions may resemble reactive inflammatory infiltrates, but differ due to the presence of plasmacytoid or other atypical forms of lymphocytes and the demonstrability of IgM monoclonality by immunohistochemical methods.

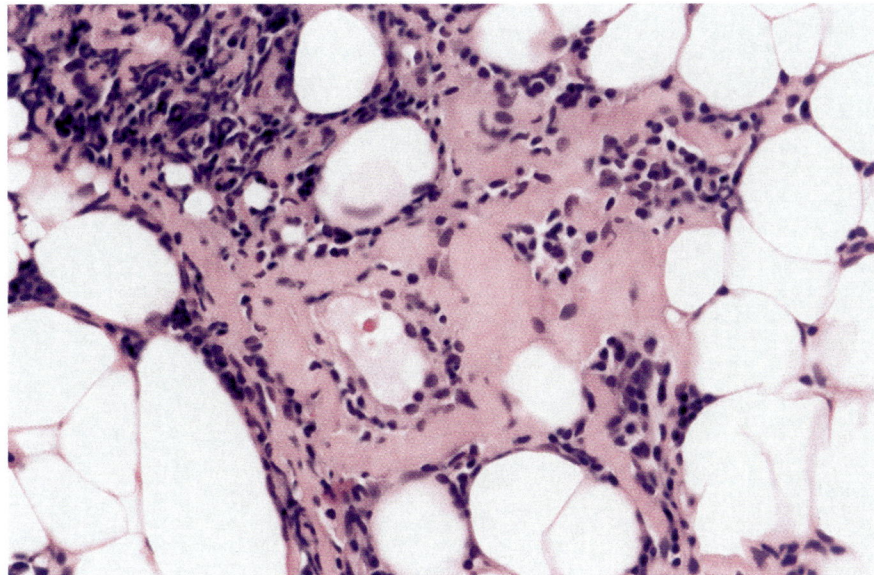

Figure 11-4

MACROGLOBULINEMIA OF WALDENSTRÖM

Intradermal deposits of homogeneous, eosinophilic material contain IgM.

These lesions may also be difficult to distinguish from other B-cell lymphomas with plasma cell or plasmacytoid components that are not associated with IgM paraprotein production and its complications. Electrophoretic or immunoelectrophoretic evidence of monoclonal IgM is indicated to confirm the presence of macroglobulinemia of Waldenström. This could be supplemented by immunohistochemical staining of tissue sections to demonstrate IgM monoclonality.

The storage papules can be confused with amyloidosis or colloid milium. The amorphous material fails to stain as amyloid or colloid (37), however, while at the same time it contains IgM. Although there has been some variation in the reported ultrastructural appearance of storage papules, they clearly differ from amyloid, which is characterized by straight, nonbranching filaments 6 to 7 nm in diameter and from juvenile colloid milium, which is composed of wavy filaments 8 to 10 nm in diameter. The ultrastructural resemblance may be similar to adult colloid milium, but in the latter case, there is usually evidence of derivation from the elastic fibers of solar elastosis (25).

CASTLEMAN'S DISEASE

Clinical Features. *Castleman's disease,* also known as *giant lymph node hyperplasia* or *angiofollicular lymph node hyperplasia,* was first reported in 1954 (53). This lymphoid hyperplasia most often occurs in the mediastinum or neck of young to middle-aged adults (56). There are two major histopathologic variants, and these closely correlate with the clinical presentation. The *hyaline-vascular type* is present in about 90 percent of cases, and usually occurs as localized disease without systemic complications. The *plasma cell type* is often associated with fever, anemia, thrombocytopenia, and polyclonal hypergammaglobulinemia. There is also an *intermediate type* with mixed histopathologic features. Like the hyaline-vascular variant, it usually presents as localized, asymptomatic disease. Both the hyaline-vascular and intermediate types can present with anemia or hypergammaglobulinemia (17). Multicentric Castleman's disease tends to occur among older individuals and to have a more severe clinical course (14). Treatment for localized Castleman's disease usually involves surgical excision, while radiation therapy or chemotherapy is sometimes used for multicentric or other forms of the disease (17,56).

The cause of Castleman's disease is not entirely clear. It is usually considered to be a B-cell proliferation caused by dysregulation of the immune system. Interleukin-6 may be involved in the pathogenesis of these lesions because of its role in the maturation of B cells to plasma cells and in the development of endothelial hyperplasia (53). A number of links have been described between this disorder and malignancy. Examples of Castleman's disease have

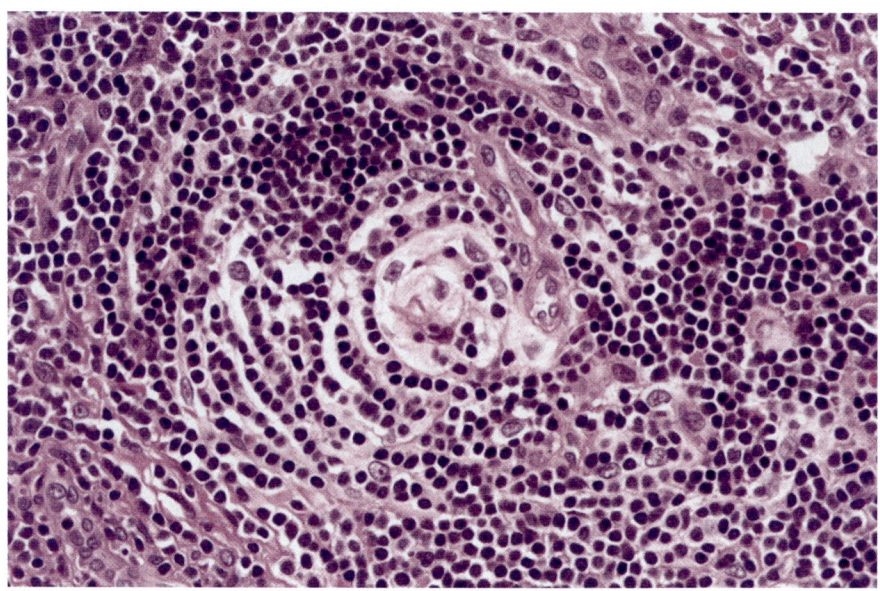

Figure 11-5

CASTLEMAN'S DISEASE

There is a lymphoid follicle with a small, atrophic germinal center, surrounded by an "onion-skin" layering of lymphocytes. The follicle is permeated by hyalinized capillaries.

accompanied POEMS syndrome (polyneuropathy, organomegaly, endocrinopathy, monoclonal gammopathy, and skin changes) (4,11), herpesvirus 8 infection with Kaposi's sarcoma and primary effusion lymphoma (4,10,20,60), follicular dendritic cell sarcoma (12), and cutaneous T-cell lymphoma (59).

Nonspecific cutaneous manifestations of Castleman's disease include skin changes of POEMS syndrome, such as glomeruloid hemangioma (11), paraneoplastic pemphigus (13), plane xanthomas, and vasculitis (54). Specific cutaneous or subcutaneous involvement is rarely reported. Cases have presented as single or (in one report) multicentric cutaneous or subcutaneous nodules (23,33,55,56), and locations have included the upper extremities (23,56), face, and trunk (33). The affected patients have otherwise been asymptomatic.

Pathologic Findings. The characteristic microscopic changes are described in lymph nodes. The common, hyaline-vascular type of Castleman's disease shows hyperplastic lymphoid follicles with small, atrophic germinal centers and an "onion-skin" layering of lymphocytes in the mantle zone; this is permeated by hyalinized capillaries in radial array (fig. 11-5). The interfollicular zones show hyalinized vessels within sclerotic collagen (fig. 11-6) (55,56). In the plasma cell type, hyperplastic lymphoid follicles are accompanied by prominent plasmacellular infiltration in the interfollicular zones, in the absence of hyalinized vessels (2). The intermediate type shows varying combinations of features of the hyaline-vascular and plasmacellular types (56). To some extent, these same patterns are also observed in cutaneous and subcutaneous lesions, although at present it is questionable whether accurate subtyping of the disease is possible on the basis of skin biopsy alone. Immunohistochemical staining usually reveals a polyclonal population of plasma cells (23), but occasionally, clonality (with lambda restriction) can be detected. Immunoglobulin and (rarely) T-cell receptor gene rearrangements have been detected in a minority of cases of Castleman's disease (40,57).

Differential Diagnosis. The differential diagnosis of cutaneous lesions of Castleman's disease includes lymphocytoma cutis, which could also show lymphoid follicles and small vessel proliferation. That lesion lacks atrophic germinal centers, the onion-skin layering of mantle lymphocytes, and the hyalinized appearance of the vessels. Angiolymphoid hyperplasia with eosinophilia most commonly (but not exclusively) involves the ear or periauricular tissues, usually lacks well-formed lymphoid follicles, contains numerous eosinophils, and possesses vessels that are not hyalinized but feature protuberant, histiocytoid endothelial cells (23,56). Kimura's disease shows hyperplastic lymphoid

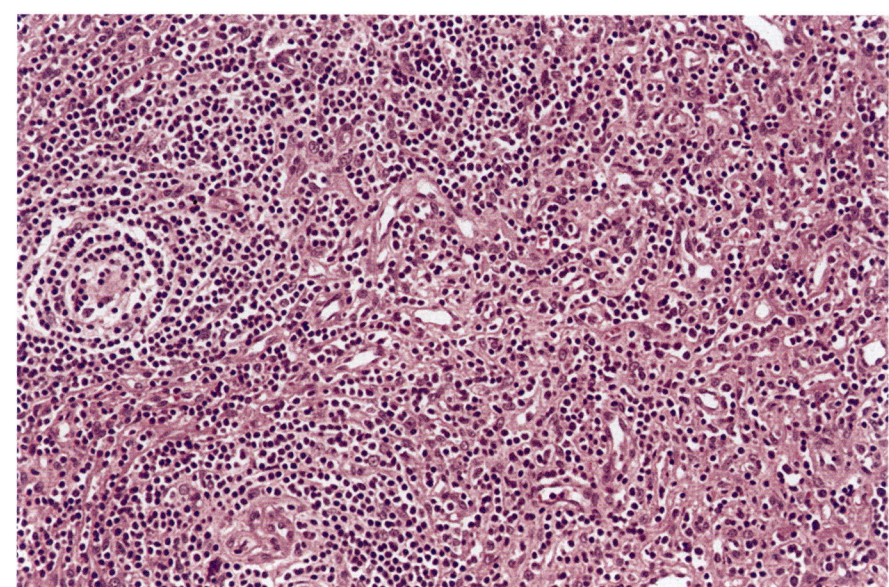

Figure 11-6

CASTLEMAN'S DISEASE

Hyalinized vessels are present in the interfollicular zones.

follicles but lacks the hyalinized vessels. Castleman's disease lacks the atypical forms or monotony seen in lymphomas or angioimmunoblastic lymphadenopathy. Despite the prominence of plasma cells in many cases of Castleman's disease, their usual polyclonality, combined with the presence of lymphoid follicles, distinguishes this condition from cutaneous involvement with multiple myeloma or plasmacytoma.

REFERENCES

1. Alberts DS, Lynch P. Cutaneous plasmacytomas in myeloma. Relationship to tumor cell burden. Arch Dermatol 1978;114:1784–7.
2. Anagnostou D, Harrison CV. Angiofollicular lymph node hyperplasia (Castleman). J Clin Pathol 1972;25:306–11.
3. Appenzeller P, Leith CP, Foucar K, Scott AA, Bigler CF, Thompson CT. Cutaneous Waldenstrom macroglobulinemia in transformation. Am J Dermatopathol 1999;21:151–5.
4. Belec L, Salmon-Ceron D, Blanche P, Dreyfus F, Zuber M, Sicard D. [POEMS syndrome (polyneuropathy, organomegaly, endocrinopathy, monoclonal gammopathy, skin changes), multicentric Castleman disease, renal chromophobe carcinoma and herpes virus type 8 infection.] Ann Pathol 1999;19:373–4. (French.)
5. Berger F, Isaacson PG, Piris MA, et al. Lymphoplasmacytic lymphoma/Waldenstrom macroglobulinemia. In: Jaffe ES, Harris NL, Stein H, Vardiman JW, eds. Pathology and genetics of tumours of haematopoietic and lymphoid tissues. Lyon: IARC Press; 2001:132–4.
6. Bergroth V, Reitamo S, Konttinen YT, Wegelius O. Skin lesions in Waldenstrom's macroglobulinaemia. Characterization of the cellular infiltrate. Acta Med Scand 1981;209:129–31.
7. Bosman C, Fusilli S, Bisceglia M, Musto P, Corsi A. Oncocytic nonsecretory multiple myeloma. A clinicopathologic study of a case and review of the literature. Acta Haematol 1996;96:50–6.
8. Bureau Y, Barriere H, Bureau B, Litoux P, de Galassus G. [Cutaneous localization of Waldenstrom's macroglobulinemia.] Ann Dermatol Syphiligr (Paris) 1968;95:125–37. (French.)
9. Canlas MS, Dillon ML, Loughrin JJ. Primary cutaneous plasmacytoma. Report of a case and review of the literature. Arch Dermatol 1979;115:722–4.

10. Cesarman E, Chang Y, Moore PS, Said JW, Knowles DM. Kaposi's sarcoma-associated herpesvirus-like DNA sequences in AIDS-related body-cavity-based lymphomas. N Engl J Med 1995;332:1186–91.
11. Chan JK, Fletcher CD, Hicklin GA, Rosai J. Glomeruloid hemangioma. A distinctive cutaneous lesion of multicentric Castleman's disease associated with POEMS syndrome. Am J Surg Pathol 1990;14:1036–46.
12. Chan JK, Tsang WY, Ng CS. Follicular dendritic cell tumor and vascular neoplasm complicating hyaline-vascular Castleman's disease. Am J Surg Pathol 1994;18:517–25.
13. Chorzelski T, Hashimoto T, Maciejewska B, Amagai M, Anhalt GJ, Jablonska S. Paraneoplastic pemphigus associated with Castleman tumor, myasthenia gravis and bronchiolitis obliterans. J Am Acad Dermatol 1999;41(Pt 1):393–400.
14. Couch WD. Giant lymph node hyperplasia associated with thrombotic thrombocytopenic purpura. Am J Clin Pathol 1980;74:340–4.
15. Dimopoulos MA, Panayiotidis P, Moulopoulos LA, Sfikakis P, Dalakas M. Waldenstrom's macroglobulinemia: clinical features, complications, and management. J Clin Oncol 2000;18:214–26.
16. Edwards GA, Zawadzki ZA. Extraosseous lesions in plasma cell myeloma. A report of six cases. Am J Med 1967;43:194–205.
17. Frizzera G. Castleman's disease and related disorders. Semin Diagn Pathol 1988;5:346–64.
18. Garcia-Sanz R, Orfao A, Gonzalez M, et al. Primary plasma cell leukemia: clinical, immunophenotypic, DNA ploidy, and cytogenetic characteristics. Blood 1999;93:1032–7.
19. Gomez EC, Margulies M, Rywlin A, Cabello B, Dominguez C. Cutaneous involvement by IgD myeloma. Arch Dermatol 1978;114:1700–3.
20. Granel B, Serratrice J, Zandotti C, et al. Conjugal HHV-8 infection with cutaneous Kaposi's sarcomas and Castleman's disease: fortuitous association or not? Dermatology 2000;200:153–4.
21. Greipp PR, Leong T, Bennett JM, et al. Plasmablastic morphology—an independent prognostic factor with clinical and laboratory correlates: Eastern Cooperative Oncology Group (ECOG) myeloma trial E9486 report by the ECOG Myeloma Laboratory Group. Blood 1998;91:2501–7.
22. Grogan TM, Van Camp B, Kyle RA, Muller-Hermelink HK, Harris NL. Plasma cell neoplasms [myeloma]. In: Jaffe ES, Harris NL, Stein H, Vardiman JW, eds. Pathology and genetics of tumours of haematopoietic and lymphoid tissues. Lyon: IARC Press; 2001:142–56.
23. Grossin M, Crickx B, Aitken G, Belaich S, Bocquet L. [Subcutaneous localizations of Castleman's pseudolymphoma. Review of the literature apropos of a case.] Ann Dermatol Venereol 1985;112:497–506. (French.)
24. Hanke CW, Steck WD, Bergfeld WF, et al. Cutaneous macroglobulinosis. Arch Dermatol 1980;116:575–7.
25. Hashimoto K, Black M. Colloid milium: a final degeneration product of actinic elastoid. J Cutan Pathol 1985;12:147–56.
26. Hayes DW, Bennett WA, Heck FJ. Extramedullary lesions in multiple myeloma. Arch Pathol 1952;53:262–72.
27. Jegou J, Derancourt C, Coindre JM, Leleu T, Perceau G, Bernard P. [Skin location of multiple myeloma mimicking a vascular tumor]. Ann Dermatol Venereol 2001;128:753–5.
28. Jenkins RE, Calonje E, Fawcett H, Greaves MW, Wilson-Jones E. Cutaneous crystalline deposits in myeloma. Arch Dermatol 1994;130:484–8.
29. Jorizzo JL, Gammon WR, Briggaman RA. Cutaneous plasmacytomas. A review and presentation of an unusual case. J Am Acad Dermatol 1979;1:59–66.
30. Kanno M, Nakamura S, Danno D, et al. [Gross spreading multiple extramedullary plasmacytomas to the skin in the terminal stage of multiple myeloma.] Rinsho Ketsueki 2001;42:554–8. (Japanese.)
31. Kato N, Kimura K, Yasukawa K, Aikawa K. Metastatic cutaneous plasmacytoma: a case report associated with IgA lambda multiple myeloma and a review of the literature of metastatic cutaneous plasmacytomas associated with multiple myeloma and primary cutaneous plasmacytomas. J Dermatol 1999;26:587–94.
32. Klein M, Grishman E. Single cutaneous plasmacytoma with crystalloid inclusions. Arch Dermatol 1977;113:64–8.
33. Kubota Y, Noto S, Takakuwa T, Tadokoro M, Mizoguchi M. Skin involvement in giant lymph node hyperplasia (Castleman's disease). J Am Acad Dermatol 1993;29(Pt 1):778–80.
34. Kyle RA. Multiple myeloma: review of 869 cases. Mayo Clin Proc 1975;50:29–40.
35. Lipsker D, Cribier B, Spehner D, Boehm N, Heid E, Grosshans E. Examination of cutaneous macroglobulinosis by immunoelectron microscopy. Br J Dermatol 1996;135:287–91.
36. Llamas-Martin R, Postigo-Llorente C, Vanaclocha-Sebastian F, Gil-Martin R, Iglesias-Diez L. Primary cutaneous extramedullary plasmacytoma secreting lambda IgG. Clin Exp Dermatol 1993;18:351–5.

37. Lowe L, Fitzpatrick JE, Huff JC, Shanley PF, Golitz LE. Cutaneous macroglobulinosis. A case report with unique ultrastructural findings. Arch Dermatol 1992;128:377–80.
38. Maize JC, Ahmed AR, Provost TT. Xanthoma disseminatum and multiple myeloma. Arch Dermatol 1974;110:758-61.
39. Mascaro JM, Montserrat E, Estrach T, et al. Specific cutaneous manifestations of Waldenstrom's macroglobulinaemia. A report of two cases. Br J Dermatol 1982;106:217–22.
40. Menke DM, DeWald GW. Lack of cytogenetic abnormalities in Castleman's disease. South Med J 2001;94:472–4.
41. Mikhail GR, Spindler AC, Kelly AP. Malignant plasmacytoma cutis. Arch Dermatol 1970;101:59–62.
42. Mozzanica N, Finzi AF, Facchetti G, Villa ML. Macular skin lesion and monoclonal lymphoplasmacytoid infiltrates. Occurrence in primary Waldenstrom's macroglobulinemia. Arch Dermatol 1984;120:778–81.
43. Muscardin LM, Pulsoni A, Cerroni L. Primary cutaneous plasmacytoma: report of a case with review of the literature. J Am Acad Dermatol 2000;43(Pt 2):962–5.
44. Parra CA, Rivero I, Martinez Moncunill AL. Mucocutaneous gamma G polyclonal plasmacytoma with two Bence Jones proteins (BJK and BJL). Arch Dermatol Forsch 1972;242:353–60.
45. Patel K, Carrington PA, Bhatnagar S, Houghton JB, Routledge RC. IgD myeloma with multiple cutaneous plasmacytomas. Clin Lab Haematol 1998;20:53–5.
46. Patterson JW, Parsons JM, White RM, Fitzpatrick JE, Kohout-Dutz E. Cutaneous involvement of multiple myeloma and extramedullary plasmacytoma. J Am Acad Dermatol 1988;19(Pt 1):879–90.
47. Prost C, Reyes F, Wechsler J, Gaston A, Richard I, Poirier J. High-grade malignant cutaneous plasmacytoma metastatic to the central nervous system. A case report with electron microscopy, immunohistological, and neuropathological studies. Am J Dermatopathol 1987;9:30–6.
48. Requena L, Sarasa JL, Ortiz Masllorens F, et al. Follicular spicules of the nose: a peculiar cutaneous manifestation of multiple myeloma with cryoglobulinemia. J Am Acad Dermatol 1995;32(Pt 2):834–9.
49. Riccardi A, Mora O, Brugnatelli S, et al. Relevance of age on survival of 341 patients with multiple myeloma treated with conventional chemotherapy: updated results of the MM87 prospective randomized protocol. Cooperative Group of Study and Treatment of Multiple Myeloma. Br J Cancer 1998;77:485–91.
50. River GL, Schorr WF. Malignant skin tumors in multiple myeloma. Arch Dermatol 1966;93:432–8.
51. Salmon SE, Cassady JR. Plasma cell neoplasms. In: DeVita VT, Hellman S, Rosenberg S, eds. Cancer, principles and practice of oncology. Philadelphia: JB Lippincott; 1988:1854.
52. Shah A, Klimo P, Worth A. Multiple myeloma first observed as multiple cutaneous plasmacytomas. Arch Dermatol 1982;118:922–4.
53. Shahidi H, Myers JL, Kvale PA. Castleman's disease. Mayo Clin Proc 1995;70:969–77.
54. Sherman D, Ramsay B, Theodorou NA, et al. Reversible plane xanthoma, vasculitis, and peliosis hepatis in giant lymph node hyperplasia (Castleman's disease): a case report and review of the cutaneous manifestations of giant lymph node hyperplasia. J Am Acad Dermatol 1992;26:105–9.
55. Skelton HG, Smith KJ. Extranodal multicentric Castleman's disease with cutaneous involvement. Mod Pathol 1998;11:93–8.
56. Sleater J, Mullins D. Subcutaneous Castleman's disease of the wrist. Am J Dermatopathol 1995;17:174–8.
57. Soulier J, Grollet L, Oksenhendler E, et al. Molecular analysis of clonality in Castleman's disease. Blood 1995;86:1131–8.
58. Swanson NA, Keren DF, Headington JT. Extramedullary IgM plasmacytoma presenting in skin. Am J Dermatopathol 1981;3:79–83.
59. Takubo T, Ohkura H, Kumura T, et al. Lymphoma in Castleman's disease, acute lymphocytic leukemia, adult T-cell leukemia and cutaneous T-cell lymphoma accompanied with high serum soluble Fas ligand levels. Haematologia 2000;30:23–6.
60. Teruya-Feldstein J, Zauber P, Setsuda JE, et al. Expression of human herpesvirus-8 oncogene and cytokine homologues in an HIV-seronegative patient with multicentric Castleman's disease and primary effusion lymphoma. Lab Invest 1998;78:1637–42.
61. Torne R, Su WP, Winkelmann RK, Smolle J, Kerl H. Clinicopathologic study of cutaneous plasmacytoma. Int J Dermatol 1990;29:562–6.
62. Tschen JA, Migliore PJ, McGavran MH. Multiple myeloma with cutaneous involvement. Arch Dermatol 1980;116:1394.
63. Tuting T, Bork K. Primary plasmacytoma of the skin. J Am Acad Dermatol 1996;34(Pt 2):386-90.
64. Walker E, Robertson AG, Boorman JG, McNicol AM. Primary cutaneous plasmacytoma: the use of in situ hybridization to detect monoclonal immunoglobulin light-chain mRNA. Histopathology 1992;20:135–8.

65. Walzer RA, Shapiro L. Multiple myeloma with cutaneous involvement. Dermatologica 1967;134:449–54.
66. Whittaker SJ, Bhogal BS, Black MM. Acquired immunobullous disease: a cutaneous manifestation of IgM macroglobulinaemia. Br J Dermatol 1996;135:283–6.
67. Wong KF, Chan JK, Li LP, Yau TK, Lee AW. Primary cutaneous plasmacytoma—report of two cases and review of the literature. Am J Dermatopathol 1994;16:392–7.
68. Wuepper KD, MacKenzie MR. Cutaneous extramedullary plasmacytomas. Arch Dermatol 1969;100:155–64.
69. Yamamoto T, Katayama I, Nishioka K. Increased plasma interleukin-6 in cutaneous plasmacytoma: the effect of intralesional steroid therapy. Br J Dermatol 1997;137:631–6.
70. Yamazaki T, Matsuura S, Watanabe K, et al. [Amylase-producing extramedullary plasmacytoma with multiple cutaneous metastasis following a solitary plasmacytoma of bone.] Rinsho Ketsueki 1990;31:391–5. (Japanese.)

SUPPLEMENTAL REFERENCES

Multiple Myeloma

Alexandrescu DT, Koulova L, Wiernik PH. Unusual cutaneous involvement during plasma cell leukaemia phase in a multiple myeloma patient after treatment with thalidomide: a case report and review of the literature. Clin Exp Dermatol 2005;30:391–4.

Damaj G, Mohty M, Vey N, et al. Features of extramedullary and extraosseous multiple myeloma: a report of 19 patients from a single center. Eur J Haematol 2004;73:402–6.

Paredes-Suarez C, Fernandez-Redondo V, Blanco MV, Sanchez-Aguilar D, Toribio J. Multiple myeloma with scleroderma-like changes. J Eur Acad Dermatol Venereol 2005;19:500–2.

Sanchez NB, Canedo IF, Garcia-Patos PE, de Unamuno Perez P, Benito AV, Pascual AM. Paraneoplastic vasculitis associated with multiple myeloma. J Eur Acad Dermatol Venereol 2004;18:731–5.

Extraosseous Plassmacytoma

Donner LR. Epstein-Barr virus-induced transformation of cutaneous plasmacytoma into CD30+ diffuse large B-cell lymphoma. Am J Dermatopathol 2004;26:63–6.

Fabbian F, Tessari G, Colato C, et al. Cutaneous plasmacytoma in a hemodialysis patient. Int J Artif Organs 2004;27:907–9.

Tessari G, Fabbian F, Colato C, et al. Primary cutaneous plasmacytoma after rejection of a transplanted kidney: case report and review of the literature. Int J Hematol 2004;80:361–4.

Macroglobulinemia of Waldenström

Ghobrial IM, Uslan DZ, Call TG, Witzig TE, Gertz MA. Initial increase in the cryoglobulin level after rituximab therapy for type II cryoglobulinemia secondary to Waldenstrom macroglobulinemia does not indicate failure of response. Am J Hematol 2004;77:329–30.

Castleman's Disease

Klein WM, Rencic A, Munshi NC, Nousari CH. Multicentric plasma cell variant of Castleman's disease with cutaneous involvement. J Cutan Pathol 2004;31:448–52.

Kojima M, Nakamura S, Nishikawa M, Itoh H, Miyawaki S, Masawa N. Idiopathic multicentric Castleman's disease. A clinicopathologic and immunohistochemical study of five cases. Pathol Res Pract 2005;201:325–32.

12 CUTANEOUS MASTOCYTOSIS

SYSTEMIC MASTOCYTOSIS

Mastocytosis is the term for a group of conditions characterized by accumulations of mast cells in a variety of tissues, with the skin being the most common single target organ. Cutaneous mastocytosis is usually an indolent disease; on the other hand, mast cell proliferations in other sites can be associated with an aggressive clinical course and death. Although the subject of this chapter is cutaneous mastocytosis, a few words should be said about systemic mastocytosis, in order to place the cutaneous form of the disease into proper perspective. The current World Health Organization classification of mastocytosis (26) is seen in Table 12-1.

Clinical involvement is limited to the skin in about 80 percent of cases. Among patients with systemic mastocytosis, about half develop skin lesions. Most of these patients have disease that follows an indolent clinical course (9), although at least one study was unable to detect a uniform correlation between the presence/absence of cutaneous involvement and prognosis among patients with systemic mast cell disease (25).

Mast cells are considered to be derivatives of hematopoietic progenitor cells (26), and the association of systemic mast cell disease with anemia and other hematologic malignancies suggests that mastocytosis may be a component of a broader, myeloid stem cell disorder (25). It is therefore not surprising that systemic mastocytosis regularly involves bone marrow, and is typically diagnosed by bone marrow biopsy (25). Other organs that are commonly infiltrated in this disease include the liver, spleen, lymph nodes, and gastrointestinal tract. Symptoms include flushing, diarrhea, fever, pruritus, urticaria, dermatographism, and bone pain. Many of these changes are related to the expected release of histamine. Other mediators also play a role, including heparin, platelet activating factor and its endogenous inhibitor (whose interactions may be responsible in part for flushing, pallor, and fluctuations in blood pressure (12), prostaglandin metabolites, and proteinases such as chymase and tryptase (8).

The diagnosis is confirmed by identifying aggregates of mast cells in tissue sections. These cells often have the morphologic characteristics of conventional mast cells, but there may also be less mature forms that have multilobated nuclei, lack cytoplasmic granules, or mimic the cells of leukemias or lymphomas (9). Histochemical and immunohistochemical methods that are helpful in confirming the mast cell nature of an infiltrate include the traditional stains of Giemsa, toluidine blue, and chloroacetate esterase (Leder), and stains for CD117 (c-kit). Staining for tryptase is the most sensitive and specific marker for mast cells, including those that occur in the various types of mast cell disease (6).

The prognosis of patients with systemic mastocytosis is variable. Some cases are indolent and have little or no effect on survival, while other forms of the disease are particularly aggressive; these include mast cell leukemia and mast cell sarcoma (9,25). Among those patients with systemic disease, findings that portend a poor prognosis are hepatosplenomegaly, hypercellular

Table 12-1

WORLD HEALTH ORGANIZATION CLASSIFICATION OF MASTOCYTOSIS

Cutaneous mastocytosis

Indolent systemic mastocytosis

Systemic mastocytosis with associated clonal, hematologic, non-mast cell lineage disease (AHNMD)

Aggressive systemic mastocytosis

Mast cell leukemia

Mast cell sarcoma

Extracutaneous mastocytoma

bone marrow, and a lack of cutaneous involvement (25). Histopathologic predictors of poor prognosis include cytologic atypia and constituent tumor cells that are Giemsa negative, tryptase positive or chloroacetate esterase negative, tryptase positive (6,25).

CUTANEOUS MASTOCYTOSIS (URTICARIA PIGMENTOSA)

Clinical Features. Cutaneous mastocytosis most commonly occurs in infants and small children, but it can also develop in adults, usually during the third and fourth decades of life (21). Although a family history is often not demonstrable, there have been several reports of familial mastocytosis that suggest an autosomal dominant inheritance pattern (2,14,19).

The skin lesions can present in several ways: as widespread maculopapules, nodules, or plaques; as a solitary nodule; as diffuse erythroderma with thickened skin described as having a "pseudolichenoid" appearance (14); or as telangiectatic lesions termed *telangiectasia macularis eruptiva perstans* (often shortened for convenience to TMEP). Although lesions with these clinical features can occur at any age, the erythrodermic form is most common in early infancy, while TMEP characteristically presents in adults (5,22). Lesions of mastocytosis often have the property of forming wheals (urticating) after stroking, a phenomenon called Darier's sign; however, Darier's sign is usually not demonstrable in TMEP lesions. Bullae can also develop, most often in childhood and particularly in association with the nodular or erythrodermic variants (15). Lesions are often hyperpigmented. These properties account for the name *urticaria pigmentosa*, which is sometimes used as a general term for all forms of cutaneous mastocytosis. The hyperpigmentation is believed to result from the effects of mast cell growth factor (the ligand for the product of the *c-kit* proto-oncogene), which stimulates both mast cell proliferation and melanin production by melanocytes (10). In rare cases, skin lesions can be virtually invisible, and then the diagnosis depends upon either recognition of increased numbers of mast cells in biopsy specimens or elevated basal serum tryptase levels (11). Pruritus, flushing, dermatographism, or rarely, diarrhea may accompany the condition.

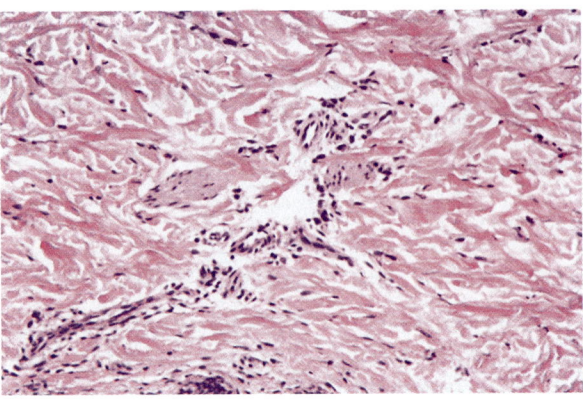

Figure 12-1

TELANGIECTASIA MACULARIS ERUPTIVA PERSTANS

A sparse perivascular infiltrate, composed mainly of mast cells, is observed in this variant of cutaneous mastocytosis.

Most children with cutaneous mastocytosis have no detectable systemic disease, and their skin lesions usually regress about the time of puberty. Bone marrow involvement, hepatosplenomegaly, diarrhea, and malnutrition have occurred in the diffuse erythrodermic type (27), and histamine shock and hemorrhagic episodes have been reported in some cases (17,20). Among adults with cutaneous disease, systemic involvement is common, as are such symptoms as generalized pruritus, flushing episodes, or gastrointestinal symptoms (22). In addition, skin lesions in adults do not regress spontaneously (18). For those with mastocytosis, the presence of cutaneous disease is considered a favorable prognostic factor, since the clinical course of the systemic disease tends to be indolent in these individuals (25).

Pathologic Findings. The diagnosis depends upon the identification of increased numbers of mast cells in skin biopsy specimens. In maculopapular lesions and in TMEP, mast cells are arranged in a perivascular distribution. The cells are often spindled but may also have round to oval contours; they possess granular cytoplasm and round to oval nuclei with homogeneous chromatin. Mast cells may be particularly sparse in TMEP (fig. 12-1). An unusual *fibrous mastocytoma*, composed of spindled mast cells, has been reported in a patient with generalized cutaneous disease (29). Mast cell infiltrates are

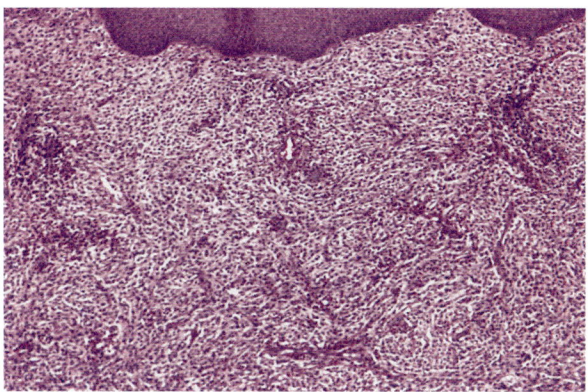 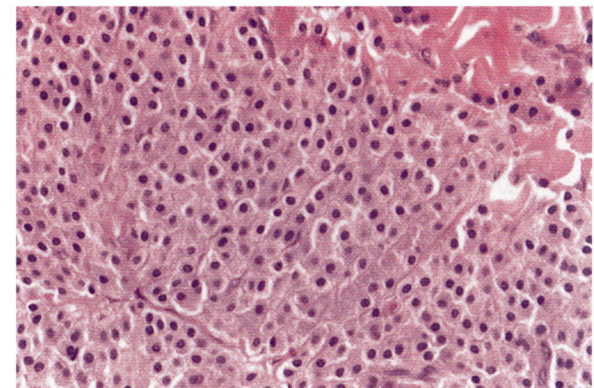

Figure 12-2

NODULAR MASTOCYTOSIS

Left: Dense aggregates of mast cells spare the epidermis.
Right: High-power view of another case of nodular mastocytosis. The cells are round to cuboidal, with centrally placed nuclei.

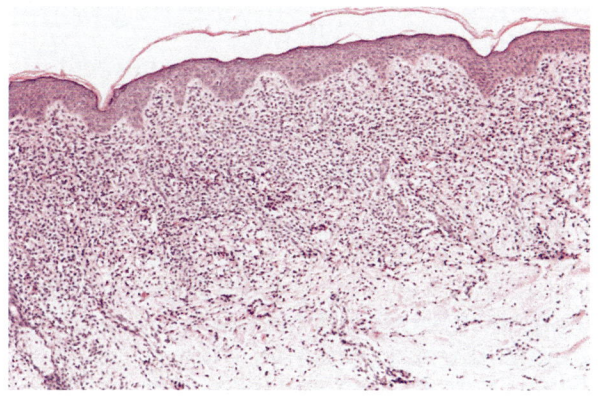 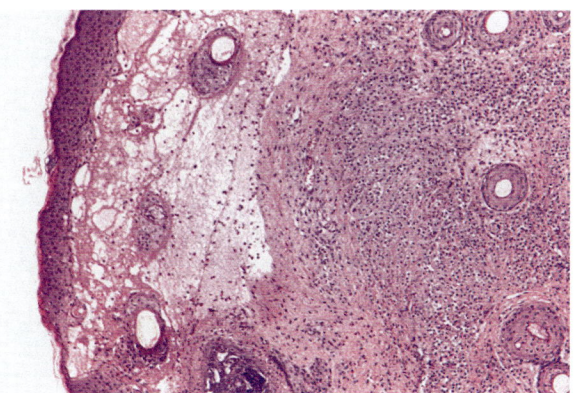

Figure 12-3

ERYTHRODERMIC MASTOCYTOSIS

A band-like arrangement of mast cells is seen in the superficial dermis.

Figure 12-4

BULLOUS MASTOCYTOSIS

The bullae arise subepidermally.

dense in the nodular and erythrodermic types (fig. 12-2), and in the case of erythroderma they tend to form band-like arrangements in the superficial dermis (fig. 12-3). Characteristically, these cells do not encroach upon the epidermis. In these densely cellular variants, the cells are usually round to cuboidal. If biopsies are obtained following lesional trauma, degranulation of mast cells may have occurred. Eosinophils often accompany the mast cell infiltrates due to the effect of eosinophil chemotactic factor. Bullae can arise subepidermally (fig. 12-4).

Mast cell granules stain metachromatically purple with the Giemsa or toluidine blue method (fig. 12-5). They also stain red with the chloroacetate esterase (Leder) stain (fig. 12-6). The authors have found the latter stain particularly useful and often easier to interpret than the metachromatic stains, although mature cells of the myelocytic series can also be positive using the Leder stain. Immunohistochemical staining for the c-kit proto-oncogene product (CD117) is also characteristic for mast cells (fig. 12-7) (3,4). Although this method is also not

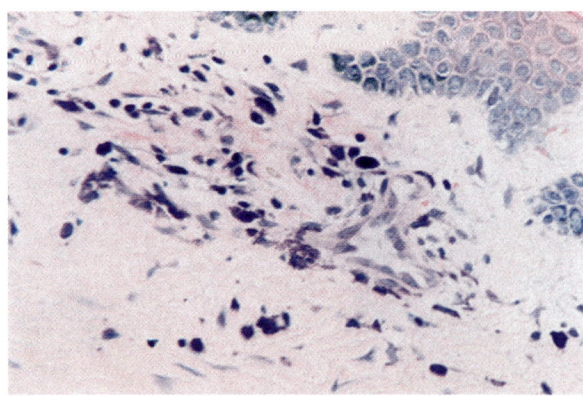

Figure 12-5

TELANGIECTASIA MACULARIS ERUPTIVA PERSTANS

The mast cells appear metachromatically purple with the Giemsa stain.

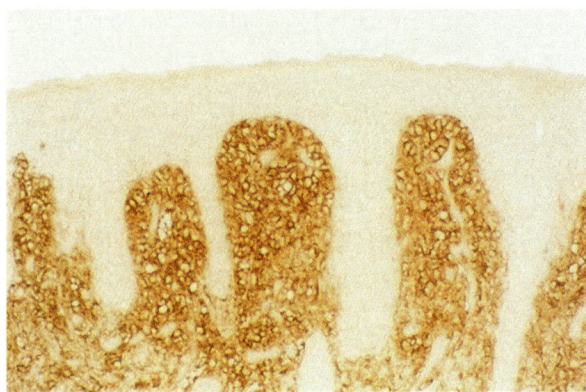

Figure 12-7

MASTOCYTOSIS

Positive immunohistochemical staining for the c-kit proto-oncogene product (CD117) is characteristic for mast cells.

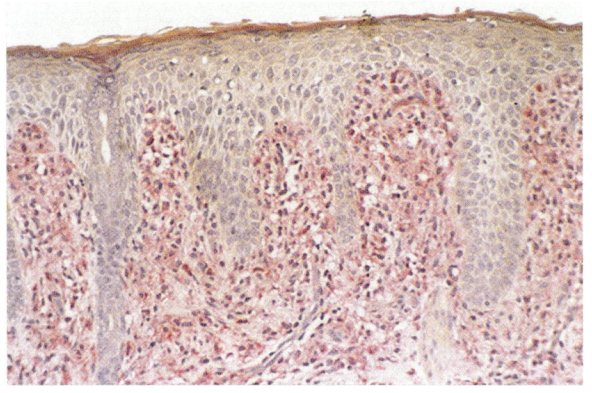

Figure 12-6

MASTOCYTOSIS

Mast cells stain red with the chloroacetate esterase (Leder) method.

entirely specific, it can be extremely useful in the context of cutaneous infiltration, and offers the advantage that mature granulocytes do not express c-kit. As mentioned before, immunohistochemical staining for tryptase is the most specific and sensitive marker for mast cells (6). As is the case in normal skin mast cells, the cells of cutaneous mastocytosis are both chymase and tryptase positive (7). Mast cells also commonly express monocyte/macrophage markers, such as alpha-1-antitrypsin and alpha-1-antichymotrypsin (13). They may also be positive for vimentin, CD20, leukocyte common antigen, and factor VIII (1).

Ultrastructurally, the cells of mastocytosis have many of the characteristics of normal cutaneous mast cells, although there may be variations in the appearance of the granules (13), nuclei may be indented or bilobed, and there may be prominent digitate cytoplasmic projections (14,23). Mast cells from lesional skin of adults with systemic disease appear to have more cytoplasm, larger nuclear size, and greater granule diameter, than do those of adults or infants with nonsystemic mastocytosis (24).

Differential Diagnosis. There are three major issues in the differential diagnosis of cutaneous mastocytosis. First is recognition of a lesion as true mastocytosis when infiltration is sparse. This problem arises particularly in connection with TMEP, in which only a few perivascular spindle cells may be observed, differing only slightly from the appearance of normal skin. The diagnosis then hinges on the recognition that virtually all of the infiltrating cells are mast cells, a determination aided by special stains such as chloroacetate esterase.

A second issue is the distinction of a primary mast cell disorder from an inflammatory dermatosis in which mast cells are fairly numerous. Examples of such conditions include spongiotic (eczematous) dermatoses, lichen planus, and erythema multiforme (16). Recognition of the defining features of these other disorders (spongiosis in eczematous dermatoses, interface changes in lichen planus, keratinocyte apoptosis and vacuolar degeneration of the epidermal basal layer in erythema multiforme), together with an appreciation of the polymorphous nature of the dermal infiltrate, should ordinarily permit recognition of those disorders. In addition, computerized image analysis of chloroacetate esterase–stained sections has shown more numerous and larger mast cells in skin lesions of adults with mastocytosis than in either inflammatory dermatoses or normal skin (28).

A final issue is the separation of mastocytosis from other nevi or neoplasms whose constituent cells resemble mast cells. Langerhans cell histiocytosis occurs in infants and adults, and may present as lesions containing numerous round to cuboidal cells and eosinophils. These cells, however, lack the characteristic cytoplasmic granules of mast cells; feature folded, indented, or reniform nuclei; and often permeate the epidermis. They fail to stain as mast cells and instead express S-100 protein, CD1a, and peanut agglutinin. The cells of melanocytic nevi can sometimes closely resemble mast cells; however, these cells may show nests along the junctional zone of the epidermis and dermis, and tend to be aggregated in nests and cords within the dermis. They lack the characteristic cytoplasmic granules or staining characteristics of mast cells, and are characteristically S-100 positive. A rare example of juvenile xanthogranuloma without the distinguishing morphologic features of lipidized cells or Touton giant cells can resemble mastocytosis microscopically. In such a case, a panel of special stains should provide the answer, since a positive metachromatic stain, or positive stains for chloroacetate esterase, c-kit, or tryptase, clearly favor a diagnosis of mastocytosis.

REFERENCES

1. Akiyama M, Watanabe Y, Nishikawa T. Immunohistochemical characterization of human cutaneous mast cells in urticaria pigmentosa (cutaneous mastocytosis). Acta Pathol Jpn 1991;41:344–9.
2. Chang A, Tung RC, Schlesinger T, Bergfeld WF, Dijkstra J, Kahn TA. Familial cutaneous mastocytosis. Pediatr Dermatol 2001;18:271–6.
3. Haas N, Hamann K, Grabbe J, Algermissen B, Czarnetzki BM. Phenotypic characterization of skin lesions in urticaria pigmentosa and mastocytomas. Arch Dermatol Res 1995;287:242–8.
4. Hamann K, Haas N, Grabbe J, Czarnetzki BM. Expression of stem cell factor in cutaneous mastocytosis. Br J Dermatol 1995;133:203–8.
5. Hannaford R, Rogers M. Presentation of cutaneous mastocytosis in 173 children. Australas J Dermatol 2001;42:15–21.
6. Horny HP, Sillaber C, Menke D, et al. Diagnostic value of immunostaining for tryptase in patients with mastocytosis. Am J Surg Pathol 1998;22:1132–40.
7. Irani AA, Garriga MM, Metcalfe DD, Schwartz LB. Mast cells in cutaneous mastocytosis: accumulation of the MCTC type. Clin Exp Allergy 1990;20:53–8.
8. Lazarus GS. Mastocytosis: new understandings in cutaneous pathophysiology. J Dermatol 1996;23:769–72.
9. Lennert K, Parwaresch MR. Mast cells and mast cell neoplasia: a review. Histopathology 1979;3:349–65.
10. Longley BJ Jr, Morganroth GS, Tyrrell L, et al. Altered metabolism of mast-cell growth factor (c-kit ligand) in cutaneous mastocytosis. N Engl J Med 1993;328:1302–7.
11. Ludolph-Hauser D, Schopf P, Rueff F, Przybilla B. [Occult cutaneous mastocytosis.] Hautarzt 2001;52:390–3. (German.)
12. Macpherson JL, Kemp A, Rogers M, et al. Occurrence of platelet-activating factor (PAF) and an endogenous inhibitor of platelet aggregation in diffuse cutaneous mastocytosis. Clin Exp Immunol 1989;77:391–6.
13. Mirowski G, Austen KF, Chiang L, et al. Characterization of cellular dermal infiltrates in human cutaneous mastocytosis. Lab Invest 1990;63:52–62.
14. Oku T, Hashizume H, Yokote R, Sano T, Yamada M. The familial occurrence of bullous mastocytosis (diffuse cutaneous mastocytosis). Arch Dermatol 1990;126:1478–84.

15. Orkin M, Good RA, Clawson CC, Fisher I, Windhorst DB. Bullous mastocytosis. Arch Dermatol 1970;101:547–64.
16. Patterson JW, Parsons JM, Blaylock WK, Mills AS. Eosinophils in skin lesions of erythema multiforme. Arch Pathol Lab Med 1989;113:36–9.
17. Poterack CD, Sheth KJ, Henry DP, Eisenberg C. Shock in an infant with bullous mastocytosis. Pediatr Dermatol 1989;6:122–5.
18. Roberts PL, McDonald HB, Wells RF. Systemic mast cell disease in a patient with unusual gastrointestinal and pulmonary abnormalities. Am J Med 1968;45:638–42.
19. Shaw JM. Genetic aspects of urticaria pigmentosa. Arch Dermatol 1968;97:137–8.
20. Smith TF, Welch TR, Allen JB, Sondheimer JM. Cutaneous mastocytosis with bleeding: probable heparin effect. Cutis 1987;39:241–4.
21. Soter NA. Mastocytosis and the skin. Hematol Oncol Clin North Am 2000;14:537–55, vi.
22. Tebbe B, Stavropoulos PG, Krasagakis K, Orfanos CE. Cutaneous mastocytosis in adults. Evaluation of 14 patients with respect to systemic disease manifestations. Dermatology 1998;197:101–8.
23. Tharp MD, Chaker B, Glass MJ, Burton R, Seelig LL Jr. In vitro functional reactivities of cutaneous mast cells from patients with mastocytosis. J Invest Dermatol 1987;89:264–8.
24. Tharp MD, Glass MJ, Seelig LL Jr. Ultrastructural morphometric analysis of lesional skin: mast cells from patients with systemic and nonsystemic mastocytosis. J Am Acad Dermatol 1988;18(Pt 1):298–306.
25. Travis WD, Li CY, Bergstralh EJ, Yam LT, Swee RG. Systemic mast cell disease. Analysis of 58 cases and literature review. Medicine (Baltimore) 1988;67:345–68.
26. Valent P, Horny HP, Li CY, et al. Mastocytosis. In: Jaffe ES, Harris NL, Stein H, Vardiman JW, eds. Pathology and genetics of tumours of haematopoietic and lymphoid tissues. Lyon: IARC Press; 2001:293–302.
27. Waxtein LM, Vega-Memije ME, Cortes-Franco R, Dominguez-Soto L. Diffuse cutaneous mastocytosis with bone marrow infiltration in a child: a case report. Pediatr Dermatol 2000;17:198–201.
28. Wilkinson B, Jones A, Kossard S. Mast cell quantitation by image analysis in adult mastocytosis and inflammatory skin disorders. J Cutan Pathol 1992;19:366–70.
29. Wood C, Sina B, Webster CG, Kurgansky D, Drachenberg CB, Reedy EA. Fibrous mastocytoma in a patient with generalized cutaneous mastocytosis. J Cutan Pathol 1992;19:128–33.

SUPPLEMENTAL REFERENCES

Cutaneous Mastocytosis (Urticaria Pigmentosa)

Arock M. [Mastocytosis, classification, biological diagnosis and therapy.] Ann Biol Clin (Paris) 2004;62:657–69. (French.)

Ben-Amitai D, Metzker A, Cohen HA. Pediatric cutaneous mastocytosis: a review of 180 patients. Isr Med Assoc J 2005;7:320–2.

Brockow K, Akin C, Huber M, Metcalfe DD. IL-6 levels predict disease variant and extent of organ involvement in patients with mastocytosis. Clin Immunol 2005;115:216–23.

Castells MC. Mastocytosis: classification, diagnosis, and clinical presentation. Allergy Asthma Proc 2004;25:33–6.

Kiszewski AE, Duran-Mckinster C, Orozco-Covarrubias L, Gutierrez-Castrellon P, Ruiz-Maldonado R. Cutaneous mastocytosis in children: a clinical analysis of 71 cases. J Eur Acad Dermatol Venereol 2004;18:285–90.

Lappe U, Aumann V, Mittler U, Gollnick H. Familial urticaria pigmentosa associated with thrombocytosis as the initial symptom of systemic mastocytosis and Down's syndrome. J Eur Acad Dermatol Venereol 2003;17:718–22.

Nguyen NQ. Telangiectasia macularis eruptiva perstans. Dermatol Online J 2004;10:1.

Noack F, Sotlar K, Notter M, Thiel E, Valent P, Horny HP. Aleukemic mast cell leukemia with abnormal immunophenotype and c-kit mutation D816V. Leuk Lymphoma 2004;45:2295–302.

13 LYMPHOID INFILTRATES, LYMPHOMA, AND HEMATOPOIETIC PROLIFERATIONS

The subject of lymphoid and hematopoietic neoplasia is extremely complex, and new knowledge is being acquired at a rapid pace. A full understanding of lymphomas, for example, requires an understanding of epidemiology, lymph node anatomy and physiology, lymphocyte differentiation pathways and corresponding morphologic changes, antigen expression, and genetics. Similar demands are required when studying the leukemias. Numerous volumes are devoted to these subjects, including several in the Atlas of Tumor Pathology series. Our purpose here is to emphasize those aspects of lymphomas and leukemias that are pertinent to cutaneous pathology.

LYMPHOID INFILTRATES AND LYMPHOMAS

Two major problems present themselves to pathologists when assessing cutaneous lymphoid infiltrates: 1) deciding whether a particular infiltrate is reactive or neoplastic and 2) assigning a malignant infiltrate to an appropriate diagnostic category within an established lymphoma classification scheme. The first problem typically arises in the setting of a dense, diffuse dermal infiltrate with only focal cytologic atypia and an intermingling of other cell types (e.g., eosinophils, mature plasma cells, and macrophages). Morphologic findings and histologic pattern alone are known to be inaccurate tools for diagnosing such cases (21), and immunophenotyping is not without its hazards. This issue is further addressed below.

The second problem is the selection of a proper classification scheme. New knowledge of immunophenotyping and genetics has certainly been beneficial to our understanding of the lymphomas. As a result, however, much of the older information regarding the diagnosis of lymphomas, based as it was upon purely morphologic criteria, has become outmoded, and several different classification systems have been devised, each of which has gained adherents but has later been replaced by newer, more accurate systems. Examples of these classifications include the Kiel system, the Working Formulation, and more recently, the Revised European-American Classification of Lymphoid Neoplasms (the REAL classification) (25). Because these systems were primarily designed for use by hematopathologists, some experts felt that they did not sufficiently address specific issues related to primary cutaneous lymphomas, which often display biological behaviors that are different from their nodal counterparts. For this reason, the Cutaneous Lymphoma Study Group of the European Organization for Research and Treatment of Cancer (EORTC) developed a classification system specifically for primary cutaneous lymphomas (31). Meanwhile, a newer World Health Organization (WHO) classification scheme (13) has recently been devised, based to a large extent upon the REAL classification, but with additional attention to clinical aspects of the lymphomas.

In choosing a classification scheme, we realize that it is not possible to satisfy every reader, but we use the WHO system in this text. This is because we have been persuaded by arguments that such a unified system enhances communication among pathologists and clinicians, while at the same time allows recognition of the unique features of some primary cutaneous lymphomas.

The WHO classification of lymphomas is shown in Table 13-1 (13). Note the overwhelming predominance of T-cell disorders among lymphomas that frequently involve the skin. This is the case not only in terms of the variety of conditions but also in frequency of occurrence: T-cell lymphomas account for more than 70 percent of all primary cutaneous lymphomas (31).

This discussion concentrates on those B-, T-, and NK (natural killer)-cell lymphomas that have frequent cutaneous involvement. Lymphomas that arise primarily in the skin are so designated. After each section, there is a brief consideration of those remaining lymphomas that

Table 13-1
WORLD HEALTH ORGANIZATION CLASSIFICATION OF LYMPHOMAS

B-Cell Neoplasms	T-Cell and NK (Natural Killer)-Cell Neoplasms
Precursor B-Cell Lymphoblastic Leukemia/Lymphoma	Precursor T-Cell Neoplasms
Mature B-Cell Neoplasms	**Precursor T-cell lymphoblastic leukemia/lymphoma**
Chronic lymphocytic leukemia/small cell lymphocytic lymphoma	Blastic NK-cell lymphoma
	Mature T-Cell and NK-Cell Neoplasms
B-cell prolymphocytic leukemia	T-cell prolymphocytic leukemia
Lymphoplasmacytic lymphoma/Waldenström's macroglobulinemia[a]	T-cell large granular lymphocytic leukemia
Splenic marginal zone lymphoma	**Aggressive NK-cell leukemia**
Hairy cell leukemia	**Adult T-cell leukemia/lymphoma**
Plasma cell myeloma[a]	**Extranodal NK/T-cell lymphoma, nasal type**
Solitary plasmacytoma of bone	Enteropathy-type T-cell lymphoma
Extraosseous plasmacytoma[a]	Hepatosplenic T-cell lymphoma
Extranodal marginal zone B-cell lymphoma of mucosa-associated lymphoid tissue (MALT lymphoma)[b]	**Subcutaneous panniculitis-like T-cell lymphoma**
	Mycosis fungoides
	Pagetoid reticulosis
	Granulomatous slack skin
Nodal marginal zone B-cell lymphoma	*Mycosis fungoides-associated follicular mucinosis*
Follicular lymphoma	**Sézary's syndrome**
Reticulohistiocytoma of the dorsum	**Primary cutaneous anaplastic large cell lymphoma**
Mantle cell lymphoma	**Peripheral T-cell lymphoma, unspecified**
Diffuse large B-cell lymphoma	*Lennert's lymphoma*
B-cell lymphoma of the leg	**Angioimmunoblastic T-cell lymphoma**
Mediastinal (thymic) large B-cell lymphoma	**Anaplastic large cell lymphoma**
Intravascular large B-cell lymphoma	T-cell Proliferation of Uncertain Malignant Potential
Primary effusion lymphoma	**Lymphomatoid papulosis**
Burkitt's lymphoma/leukemia	Hodgkin's Disease
B-Cell Proliferations of Uncertain Malignant Potential	Nodular lymphocyte-predominant Hodgkin's disease
Lymphomatoid granulomatosis	Classic Hodgkin's disease
Post-transplant lymphoproliferative disorder, polymorphic	Nodular sclerosis classic Hodgkin's disease
	Lymphocyte-rich classic Hodgkin's disease
	Mixed cellularity classic Hodgkin's disease
	Lymphocyte-depleted classic Hodgkin's disease

[a]These entities have been discussed in the chapter on plasmacellular tumors.
[b]Entities of particular importance to dermatologists and dermatopathologists are written in bold face; individual entities included in the European Organization for Research and Treatment of Cancer (EORTC) system but not specifically listed in the World Health Organization (WHO) classification are indicated in italics.

uncommonly involve the skin. Hodgkin's disease is considered separately.

LYMPHOCYTOMA CUTIS (REACTIVE LYMPHOID INFILTRATE, CUTANEOUS LYMPHOID HYPERPLASIA, PSEUDOLYMPHOMA, LYMPHADENOSIS BENIGNA CUTIS)

Clinical Features. These designations generally refer to localized or disseminated proliferations of lymphocytes in the skin that are considered to be benign or reactive in nature. For purposes of this discussion, the term *lymphocytoma cutis* is used unless otherwise specified.

Lymphocytoma cutis was first described in 1894 by Spiegler, and early on it was noted that, despite a clinical appearance resembling sarcoma, these lesions tended to follow a benign clinical course. It is seen in all age groups, although the disseminated variety predominates among older adults. Women are affected somewhat more frequently than men.

There are two patterns of distribution: localized and disseminated. Localized lesions present as solitary tumors ranging up to 4 cm in diameter or as groupings of small papular lesions. Tumors tend to be reddish brown, while papular lesions are firm, pink to violet, and translucent. Anetoderma (macular atrophy) can develop in these lesions (14). The most common locations are the head and neck regions, particularly the forehead, cheeks, nose, and earlobes. Other locations include the trunk, proximal arms, and genitalia. Disseminated lesions are much less common, and are widespread over the trunk, face, and extremities. Similar lesions involve the salivary and thyroid glands; oral, vulvar, or rectal mucosae; and the orbit (3).

Several specific causes of lymphocytoma cutis have been identified. Occasional lesions had been known to regress following penicillin therapy, and it has since been established that lymphocytoma cutis (often reported as *lymphadenosis benigna cutis* in the relevant literature) is one of the clinical manifestations of *Borrelia* infection, and can coexist with other cutaneous changes of Lyme disease (1,12). Arthropod bites in the absence of documented *Borrelia* infection have also been associated with the lesion. Lymphocytoma cutis as a postherpes zoster phenomenon has been reported on several occasions (24). These lesions also occur in patients with human immunodeficiency virus (HIV) infection, and one study has found oligoclonal expansion of HIV-specific CD8-positive lymphocytes in the skin of these individuals (2). Other antigenic stimuli have been associated with the condition, including tattoos, heavy metals such as gold and nickel, vaccinations (16), and drugs such as phenytoin (5), antihistamines (18), and antidepressants (8). In many and perhaps a majority of cases, however, a likely etiologic factor is not identified.

Typically, the general health of the patient is good, and lymphadenopathy or hepatosplenomegaly are not observed. Localized lesions reach maximum size in 3 weeks to 2 years and then tend to spontaneously involute, while disseminated lesions are more persistent. Cases induced by drug therapy, particularly phenytoin, may undergo dramatic resolution once the medication is discontinued (5,9). Other examples considered histologically benign have progressed over a period of years into a lymphoma.

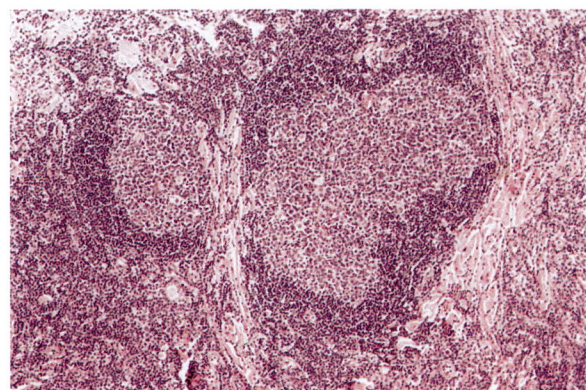

Figure 13-1

LYMPHOCYTOMA CUTIS

There are well-formed secondary lymphoid follicles with germinal centers.

Pathologic Findings. The following is a review of the morphologic and other laboratory findings that have been used in the past to identify cases as lymphocytoma cutis (22), although none of these criteria is absolutely diagnostic for a reactive lymphoid process. Findings may include varying degrees of acanthosis or even pseudoepitheliomatous hyperplasia, especially in cases associated with arthropod bites. There is typically a patchy, nodular or diffuse infiltrate composed largely of lymphocytes. The infiltrate tends to be "top-heavy," concentrated in the superficial to mid-dermis. A predominance of mature-appearing lymphocytes with sparse mitoses is usual; well-formed secondary lymphoid follicles are sometimes present (fig. 13-1). There are often admixtures of plasma cells, eosinophils, and macrophages, including epithelioid cells, and occasionally, multinucleated giant cells (fig. 13-2). Tingible body macrophages are frequently present (fig. 13-3) (7,10). These features are often accompanied by prominent vasculature, consisting of thick-walled vessels with plump endothelial cells (fig. 13-4). The separation of the infiltrate from the epidermis or adnexal epithelia by a grenz zone of uninvolved connective tissue is not regarded as a useful feature in differentiating benign from neoplastic lymphoid infiltrates (17).

Lymphocytoma cutis does not show a loss of B lineage antigens, a loss of pan-T-cell antigens, or abnormal coexpression of antigens among lymphocytes; polytypic light chain

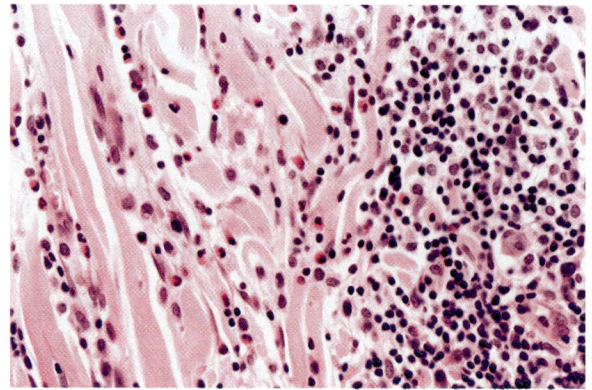

Figure 13-2

LYMPHOCYTOMA CUTIS

In addition to lymphocytes, other types of inflammatory cells are present, including eosinophils.

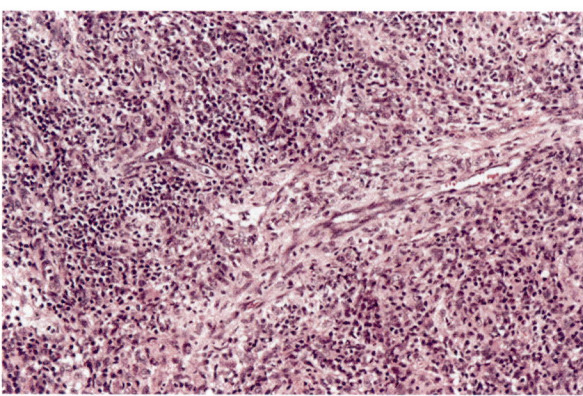

Figure 13-4

LYMPHOCYTOMA CUTIS

Thick-walled vessels are prominent.

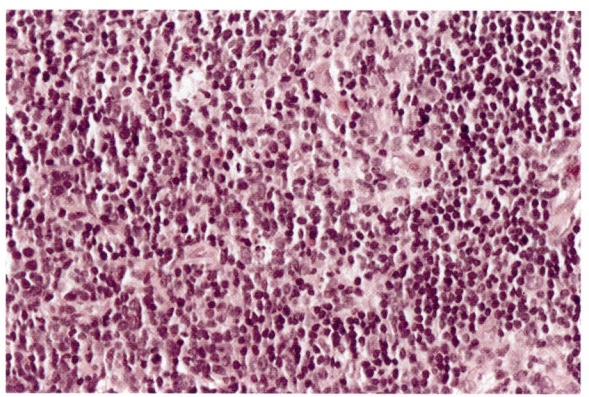

Figure 13-3

LYMPHOCYTOMA CUTIS

Tingible body macrophages are seen.

expression is the rule (19). Ploidy analysis shows a predominantly diploid cell population (11); clonal rearrangements of either immunoglobin (Ig) heavy chain or T-cell receptor genes is not detected (5,11). Identification of specific triggering factors, such as tick mouth parts, tattoo pigments, spirochetes, or ingested medications such as phenytoin, may provide crucial supporting evidence that a particular infiltrate is reactive rather than neoplastic.

Differential Diagnosis. Unfortunately, many of the morphologic features listed above have also been described in cutaneous lymphomas. These include vascular proliferation (19), formation of lymphoid follicles with germinal centers (6,21), and presence of eosinophils (17). At the same time, pleomorphic infiltrates can occur in lesions associated with a benign clinical course (10), or in lymphomas with a favorable prognosis (28). It has been stated that no single feature reliably differentiates lymphocytoma cutis from lymphoma in all cases (23), and that there is often a poor correlation between the microscopic features and clinical course of extranodal lymphoid lesions (27). Sometimes, even the more sophisticated diagnostic studies produce surprising results in cutaneous infiltrates that are morphologically bland; for example, markers of activation or proliferation such as CD25, CD38, CD71, and Ki-67 can be expressed in benign infiltrates (19). Monotypic plasma cells have been found in benign forms of cutaneous lymphoid hyperplasia (26), and lesions classified as "cutaneous lymphoid hyperplasia" by morphology and immunophenotyping rarely demonstrate B-cell monoclonality (29).

It is apparent that the differential diagnosis of cutaneous lymphoproliferative lesions can be one of the most challenging problems in dermatopathology. Still, combinations of morphologic, immunohistochemical, and genetic features are most often used successfully in distinguishing lymphocytoma cutis from lymphoma. A full complement of the characteristic histopathologic findings listed above, together with clinical data, provides reasonable assurance that a given infiltrate is benign or reactive. In addition, despite some limitations, investigations for abnormal antigen expression (30) or clonal gene rearrangements (5) are mainstays in the diagnostic workup of problematic cutaneous lymphoid infiltrates.

Many of the studies touching upon the differential diagnosis of lymphocytoma cutis have focused on the distinction from follicular lymphoma. A top-heavy infiltrate that features a mixture of inflammatory cells, lymphoid follicles, and nuclear debris favors the former over lymphoma (23). Miracco et al. (20) found that a lower apoptotic index (an expression of the relative numbers of apoptotic forms among all lymphoid cells) is typical of lymphocytoma cutis. Infiltrates containing a higher percentage of small lymphocytes, macrophages, and epithelioid and giant cells are typical of lymphocytoma cutis, while a predominance of medium and large lymphoid cells are seen in follicular lymphoma (20). An assessment of the nuclear characteristics by computerized image analysis can also be useful; the mean nuclear profile area of lymphoid cells appears to be the feature that permits the best discrimination between lymphocytoma cutis and follicular lymphoma (29). Regarding immunohistochemistry, a diagnosis of follicular lymphoma would be favored over lymphocytoma cutis when there are immunoglobulin-negative B cells, loss of B lineage antigens, CD5-positive B cells, or monotypic light chains (19). True follicular lymphoma in the skin shows expression of CD10 (common acute lymphocytic leukemia antigen) and bcl-2 protein in germinal centers (21).

Marginal zone lymphoma of the skin can closely mimic lymphocytoma cutis, in that it may feature a top-heavy infiltrate, frequently contains reactive follicles, and has a component of eosinophils (4,21). These lymphomas, however, show diffuse proliferations of marginal zone cells and sometimes sheets of plasma cells that demonstrate monotypic light chains. Dutcher bodies (eosinophilic intranuclear inclusions) are characteristic of the plasma cells in marginal zone lymphoma (4). A predominance of B cells, in some cases with a B to T cell ratio of 3 to 1, is characteristic of this lymphoma, in contrast to lymphocytoma cutis, which usually shows a T-cell predominance (4).

Primary cutaneous immunocytoma (see chapter 11, Macroglobulinemia of Waldenström) can also closely resemble lymphocytoma cutis. It may feature a top-heavy infiltrate, lymphoid follicles, eosinophils, macrophages, and bland-appearing lymphocytes (17). Distinctive features include T cells at the center of cutaneous nodules, monotypic light chain expression, and a lack of CD20 expression among the cells comprising the lymphoma (17).

In contrast to lymphocytoma cutis, T-cell lymphomas show a loss of pan-T-cell antigens, abnormal co-expression among T cells (CD4, CD8 positive or CD4, CD8 negative), or CD7 "dropout" to less than 20 percent of the total cell population (19). Even more problematic is the cutaneous T-cell–rich B-cell lymphoma in which relatively sparse neoplastic B cells are surrounded by small T cells (21). Detecting rearrangements of T-cell receptor or immunoglobulin heavy chain genes helps establish the diagnosis, respectively, of T-cell (5) or B-cell (30) lymphoma.

Lymphocytoma cutis may be difficult to distinguish from other benign dermatoses with heavy lymphocytic infiltrates, such as lymphocytic infiltration of Jessner, lupus erythematosus, or polymorphic light eruption. In addition to the traditional morphologic clues to these other diagnoses, lymphocytoma cutis is characterized by a greater proportion of CD20-positive B cells (15).

Situations inevitably arise in which a definitive diagnosis of a cutaneous lymphoid infiltrate cannot be rendered. In such cases, there should be a full description of the microscopic and immunohistochemical findings as well as a discussion of the possible interpretations of the results. These patients should undergo close clinical surveillance and rebiopsy of any new or recurrent lesions for further histopathologic study. Gene rearrangement or other cytogenetic studies should be considered in problematic cases.

B-CELL NEOPLASMS

Cutaneous Marginal Zone B-Cell Lymphoma (Mucosa-Associated Lymphoid Tissue [MALT] Lymphoma)

Clinical Features. *Marginal zone B-cell lymphoma* (MZL) is composed of cells with the characteristics of the B cells of the marginal zone of lymph nodes (centrocytes). This lymphoma most often arises in extranodal sites, particularly

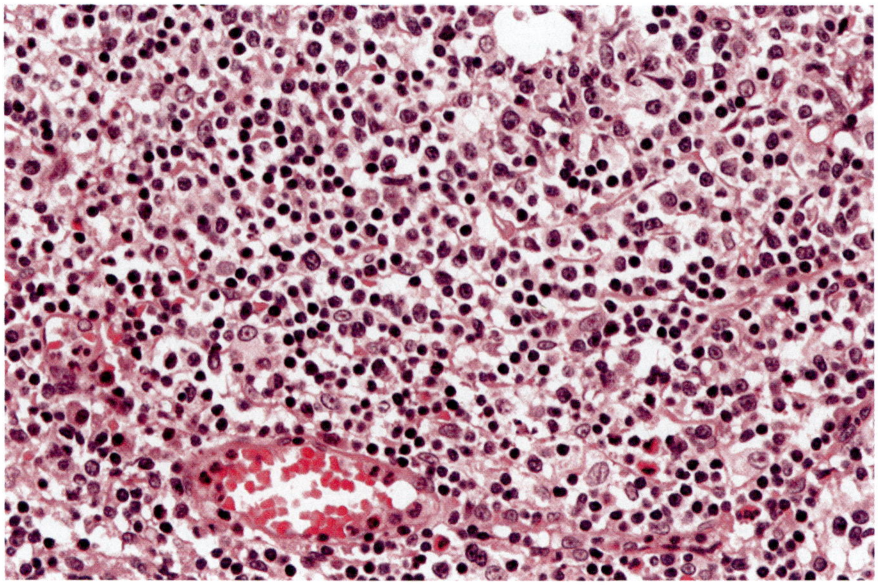

Figure 13-5

MARGINAL ZONE LYMPHOMA

There is a dense, diffuse infiltrate of small lymphocytes.

the gastrointestinal tract, although other sites include the lung, head and neck, periocular tissues, thyroid gland, breast, and skin. Primary nodal MZL does occur but is rare. Cutaneous involvement may be primary, or may represent secondary spread from another site. At least one group of authors regards MZL as possibly the most common subtype of primary cutaneous B-cell lymphoma (56).

MZL is considered to be a tumor of mucosa-associated (or skin-associated) lymphoid tissue, and has been referred to as such in previous classifications. It sometimes arises in the setting of chronic inflammation due to infectious agents (e.g., *Helicobacter pylori* gastritis) or autoimmune diseases (e.g., Sjögren's syndrome, Hashimoto's thyroiditis), suggesting a pathogenic role for chronic antigenic stimulation or persistent inflammation. In the skin, an association with *Borrelia burgdorferi* infection has been demonstrated on several occasions using polymerase chain reaction (PCR) methods (52,71,109).

The median age of patients with cutaneous MZL is within the sixth decade of life, and there is a slight female predominance (39,51,121). Patients present with red-brown papules, nodules, or plaques; an erythematous halo has been reported to surround some lesions (51). The upper half of the body is most commonly affected, with roughly equal distribution among head and neck, trunk, and upper extremity sites (40, 57,121). Although many patients have disease confined to the skin and subcutis, some present with concurrent involvement of other organ systems, and others develop secondary skin lesions following primary tumors in other sites (39). Symptoms directly referable to cutaneous MZL are not reported. There have been rare examples of a hyperviscosity syndrome in patients with Waldenström's macroglobulinemia that is related to extranodal MZL; skin was reported as one of the sites of lymphoma involvement (122).

Extranodal MZL in general, and primary cutaneous MZL in particular, are considered to be low-grade lymphomas with a good to excellent prognosis, although recurrences are common. Death attributed to the disease is rare, but has been reported in a patient who presented with concurrent cutaneous and extracutaneous disease (39). Involvement of multiple extranodal sites does not appear to adversely affect prognosis (120). Treatment usually includes radiation therapy and/or surgical excision; chemotherapy is sometimes employed. Antibiotics can be effective, particularly in cases of MZL associated with *Borrelia* infection (51,109).

Pathologic Findings. Epidermal changes are typically absent. There is a dense, diffuse dermal and subcutaneous infiltrate composed of small lymphocytes (fig. 13-5). Some of these have the features of centrocytes, or marginal zone cells: slightly irregular or indented nuclei and generous amounts of pale-staining cytoplasm. Other cells have monocytoid or plasmacytoid

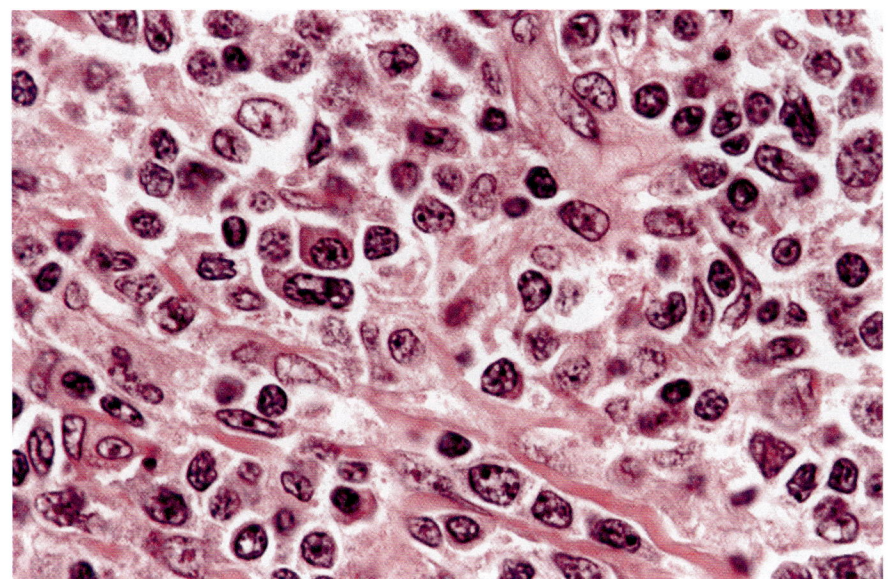

Figure 13-6

MARGINAL ZONE LYMPHOMA

Many cells possess pale-staining cytoplasm and indented nuclei. Plasma cells and plasmacytoid forms are also seen.

characteristics (fig. 13-6) (40,51). Scattered blasts may be present but generally represent a minor feature. Plasma cells are often present, arranged in zones or sheets. Dutcher bodies may be identified. Reactive germinal centers are frequently present, and these may be permeated by small, atypical lymphocytes (121). In addition, neoplastic lymphocytes may permeate adnexal epithelia, producing lymphoepithelial lesions.

The neoplastic cells of MZL have the following immunohistochemical profile: positive for CD20, CD79a, CD21, and bcl-2; negative for bcl-6, CD5, CD10, CD23, and CD35 (51,56,57, 76,122). These cells have also been reported to express the monocytoid B antibody, Ki-M1p (51). They are variably positive for CD43 and CD11c (76,122) and are negative for cyclin D1 (122). These cells express IgM, G, or A (51,76) and regularly show light chain restriction (40, 51,121,122). Rearrangements of immunoglobulin heavy and light chain genes have been reported (51,63), but in one study, no rearrangement of the *bcl-2* oncogene was detected among 12 patients tested (51). Trisomy 3 and the t(11;18)(q21;q21) translocation have been detected in some cases (103,132). In a few reported cases of cutaneous MZL, *Borrelia burgdorferi* genes have been detected with PCR methods (71,109).

Differential Diagnosis. The chief diagnostic consideration is the distinction of cutaneous MZL from a reactive lymphoid infiltrate. Morphologic clues to the identification of MZL have been discussed above in the section on lymphocytoma cutis. Confirmation of an initial morphologic impression of MZL can be obtained by identifying light chain restriction in tissues (40,121) or, if necessary, by gene rearrangement studies. A combination of morphologic and immunohistochemical findings usually permits distinction from other lymphomas involving the skin. Cutaneous infiltrates of immunocytoma are typically more monomorphous, with a predominance of lymphoplasmacytoid cells (51). The CD5 negativity of MZL may allow its distinction from most mantle cell lymphomas (an uncommon lymphoma in skin) and small cell lymphocytic lymphoma, although a CD5-negative mantle cell lymphoma in skin has been reported (100). Similarly, cyclin D1 expression is seen in mantle cell lymphoma but not in MZL (100). A more difficult problem is the differentiation of MZL from follicular lymphoma, another relatively common cutaneous B-cell lymphoma that may have a follicular configuration. The immunophenotypes of these two tumors are different: follicular lymphomas are bcl-6 and usually CD10 and bcl-2 positive, while MZL cells are bcl-6 and CD10 negative, and bcl-2 positive. Distinctive staining of the follicular structures of these two tumors can be demonstrated by identifying these antigens together with CD21, a marker for follicular mantle and dendritic cells (57).

Nonmelanocytic Tumors of the Skin

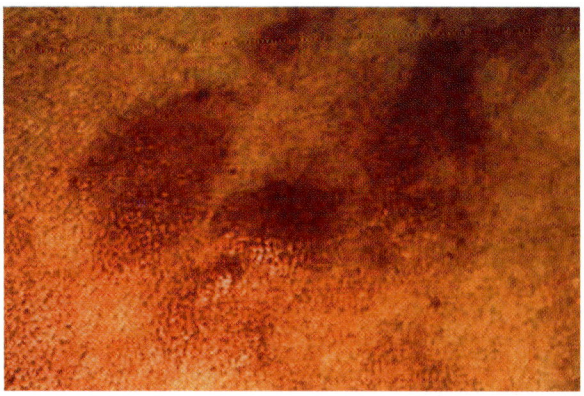

Figure 13-7

FOLLICULAR LYMPHOMA

Confluent reddish nodules and plaques are in the skin of the upper trunk.

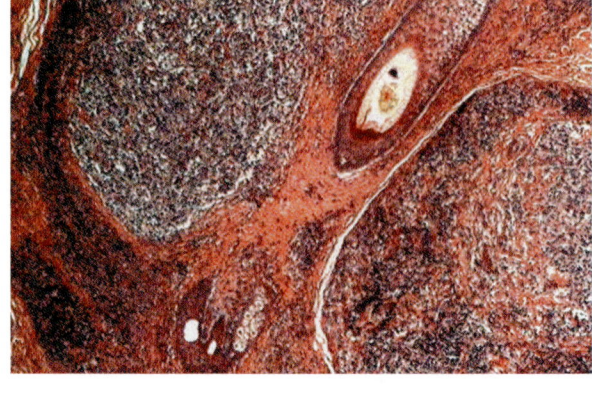

Figure 13-9

FOLLICULAR LYMPHOMA

Neoplastic follicles are apparent.

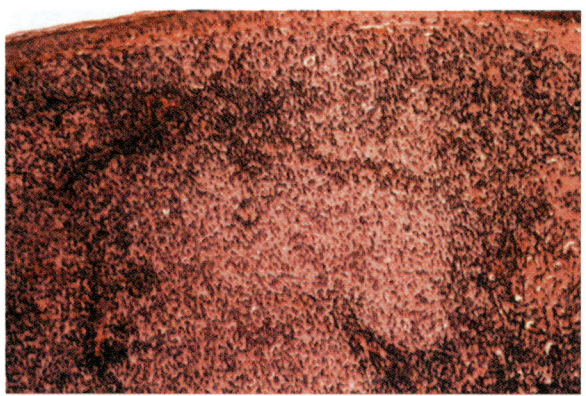

Figure 13-8

FOLLICULAR LYMPHOMA

This tumor occupies virtually the entire dermis. Obvious follicular lymphoid structures are present.

Follicular Lymphoma

Clinical Features. *Follicular lymphoma* (formerly known as *follicular center cell lymphoma* or *nodular small cleaved cell lymphoma*) may either arise in the skin or involve it secondarily. These eventualities account for roughly 40 percent of all cutaneous B-cell lymphomas, regardless of patient age and lesion site (33,43,50,65,72,99). In our experience, approximately 60 percent of cutaneous follicular lymphomas (CFLs) are primary lesions, and these have a predilection for the head and neck of middle-aged or elderly individuals.

As is true of B-cell lymphomas of the skin in general, CFLs present as red to violaceous plaques and nodules that gradually but persistently enlarge (fig. 13-7). Those lesions that arise in the corium typically remain confined to the skin for a prolonged period of time, and, although recurrences in the skin are common after local therapies for such lesions, involvement of extracutaneous tissues, including lymph nodes, is distinctly atypical. Chemotherapy is not usually administered in such cases and the clinical course is protracted (33,43,72).

Pathologic Findings. CFL usually occupies nearly the entire dermis in incisional or punch biopsies, often extending into the superficial subcutis as well (fig. 13-8). It is separated from the epidermis by a grenz zone in nearly all instances. Neoplastic follicles, which are composed of a variable mixture of centrocytic, centroblastic, and intermediate lymphoid cells, as well as dendritic cells, are easily seen on scanning microscopy of these lesions (fig. 13-9). The intervening tissue is occupied by small cells with irregular, often cleaved, nuclear contours. No mantles of mature small lymphocytes are seen around them, as would be expected in hyperplastic processes. The internal aspects of the neoplastic follicles in CFL do not contain tingible body macrophages or organized germinal centers, and the follicular aggregates have a relatively uniform size and shape (fig. 13-10). No polarity of cell density is observed within them; mitoses and apoptotic activity are infrequent.

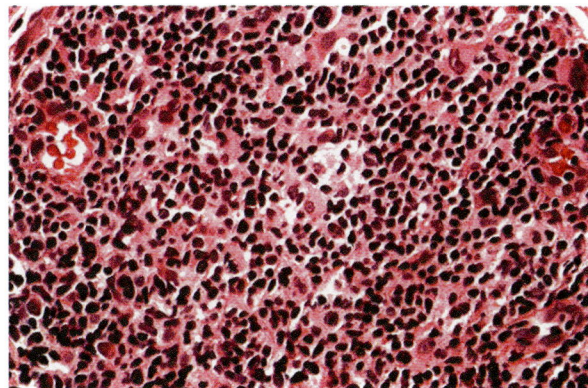 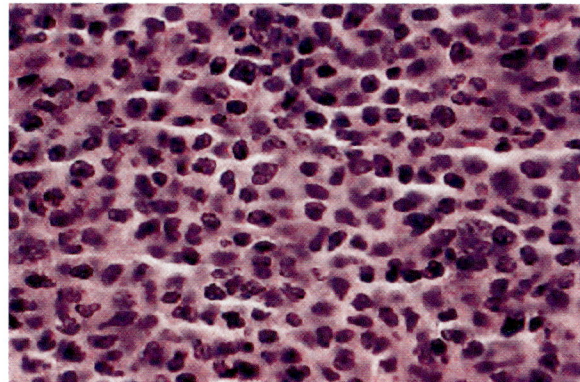

Figure 13-10

FOLLICULAR LYMPHOMA

Left: The internal aspects of the neoplastic follicles are composed of atypical lymphoid cells of various sizes and shapes. No tingible body macrophages are present.

Right: This neoplastic follicle contains a more monotonous population of lymphoid cells with cleaved nuclear contours.

In accord with the heterogeneous nature of the neoplastic cells in the follicles, CFL may be subclassified into predominantly small cleaved cell, mixed large and small cell, or predominantly large cell types, which correspond to three biological grades. Mann and Berard (94) codified this segregation by assigning grade I to those tumors with 5 percent or fewer large cells; grade II to lesions with 6 to 15 percent large cells; and grade III to follicular neoplasms containing more than 15 percent large cells.

Immunophenotyping of follicular lymphomas is the best way of separating them from benign reactive lymphoid infiltrates in the skin that may contain germinal centers. Neoplastic follicular cells are reactive for CD20, CD45RA, and CD79, and variably positive for CD10; conversely, they usually lack T-cell–related markers such as CD5 and CD43 (41,55,57). CD23 and cyclin D1 are also absent in CFL (57). Controversy has surrounded the question of whether the bcl-2 and bcl-6 proteins are present in primary CFLs, and similar comments apply to the t(14;18) chromosomal translocation (54,83,88). Those markers characterize follicular lymphomas that arise in lymph nodes (88). Some investigators have concluded that primary CFLs lack these markers (54, 83,88); however, Lawnicki et al. (88) provided a dissenting opinion in a recent study, and showed that bcl-2 and t(14;18) are observed preferentially in a subset of low-grade lesions. We have had a similar experience with such tumors (fig.

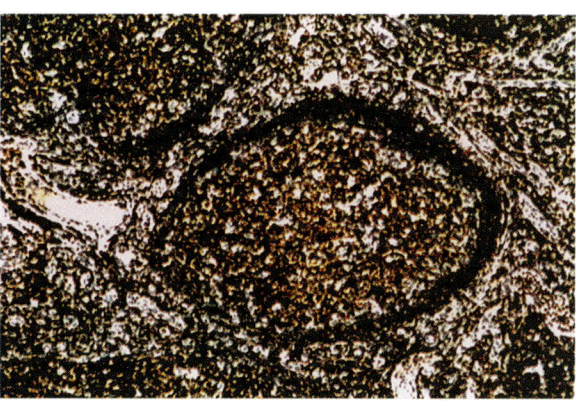

Figure 13-11

FOLLICULAR LYMPHOMA

Immunoreactivity for bcl-2 protein is apparent within the neoplastic follicles of this cutaneous follicular lymphoma.

13-11). As Lawnicki and colleagues have outlined, this apparent discrepancy probably relates to differing morphologic criteria for the definition of CFL, as related to the WHO, REAL, Kiel, and International Working Formulation classification systems for lymphoma (102). Such dissimilarities are beyond the scope of this discussion, and interested readers should consult other sources that deal exclusively with hematopathology for a more complete elaboration of them.

Differential Diagnosis. There are really only two differential diagnostic considerations in cases of CFL. The first is atypical follicular lymphoid hyperplasia (AFLH) of the skin. That condition may be idiopathic, or it may relate to infection with organisms such as *Borrelia* (64, 89). AFLH is typified by follicular aggregates of lymphoid cells that closely resemble the image of CFL. There is more cellular heterogeneity in the former disorder, however, often with a polarity to the follicles and considerable variation in their size and shape. Germinal centers are seen at least focally in AFLH, complete with tingible body macrophages, mitotic activity, and apoptotic cells. Special stains are helpful in making the diagnostic distinction. Silver impregnation methods may demonstrate the presence of spirochetes in infection-related AFLH, and immunostains show a consistent lack of reactivity for bcl-2 protein, CD10, bcl-6 protein, and MT2 in the follicular lymphoid aggregates in that condition (41,55). There are more admixed mature T cells in AFLH than in CFL, and these label for CD3, CD5, CD7, and CD43. Finally, it has been our experience that stains for Ki-67/Mib-1 show well-demarcated groups of immunoblastic elements in the follicular centers of AFLH, whereas that is not usually the case in examples of CFL (125). Demonstrable infection is not always a reliable indicator of a benign nature with regard to follicular lymphoid lesions of the skin. Rare examples of CFL have been linked to infection with hepatitis C virus and other agents (124).

The second diagnostic alternative to CFL is extranodal marginal zone lymphoma (related to mucosa-associated lymphoma) of the skin. Those two malignancies are similar morphologically, and, as outlined by de Leval and colleagues (57), immunohistologic studies are often necessary in order to distinguish them. The expression of bcl-6 protein, CD10, and bcl-2 protein favors a diagnosis of CFL, particularly when seen in lymphoid populations that also lack CD21, a marker for selected B lymphocytes and dendritic cells. Extranodal marginal zone lymphoma consistently lacks CD10 and bcl-6.

Diffuse Large B-Cell Lymphoma

Clinical Features. *Diffuse large B-cell lymphoma* (LBCL) is composed of large neoplastic cells of B-cell lineage. LBCL can arise de novo or through the transformation of another type of lymphoma, such as follicular lymphoma or marginal zone lymphoma (67). As a group, these tumors account for 30 to 40 percent of adult non-Hodgkin's lymphomas (67). Up to 40 percent present in extranodal sites, the gastrointestinal tract being the most common. The skin can serve as either a primary or a secondary site for these tumors.

Several clinical and histopathologic variants have been described. Two of the most important, from a dermatopathologic point of view, are *LBCL of the leg* and *T-cell–rich B-cell lymphoma*. Despite a broad age range, these variants are primarily tumors of older adults, with a slight male predominance (36). LBCL of the leg is more common in women (123). Epstein-Barr virus (EBV) may play a role in some cases of LBCL, particularly among immunosuppressed individuals (47,118), and one case has been linked to *Borrelia burgdorferi* infection (75).

Primary cutaneous lesions arise most commonly in the head and neck regions or on the legs (69); lesions on the trunk have also been reported (49). Primary lesions are most often described as single or multiple erythematous nodules or plaques. One leg lesion was described as a nonhealing ulcer (66), and a case of T-cell–rich B-cell lymphoma was accompanied by erythroderma and lymphadenopathy (118). The described rapidity of growth of cutaneous lesions has been variable.

Treatment includes local radiation therapy or chemotherapy (123), interferon alpha-2a (129, 130), or the monoclonal antibody to CD20, rituximab (32,66). Antibiotics were used successfully in the case linked to *Borrelia burgdorferi* infection. Sentinel node biopsy has been employed for staging and treatment planning (116). LBCL is considered to be an aggressive tumor, although potentially curable with chemotherapy (67). Patients with primary cutaneous tumors appear to have a generally excellent prognosis; this is particularly the case for those with solitary or localized skin lesions (62,90,111).

Over the years, it has been recognized that patients with LBCL arising on the leg tend to have a worse prognosis than those with lesions presenting in other cutaneous sites, with a 5-year survival rate of 58 percent (123). As a result, members of the EORTC created a separate category for primary cutaneous large B-cell lymphoma of the leg (LBCL of the leg) (127). The status of

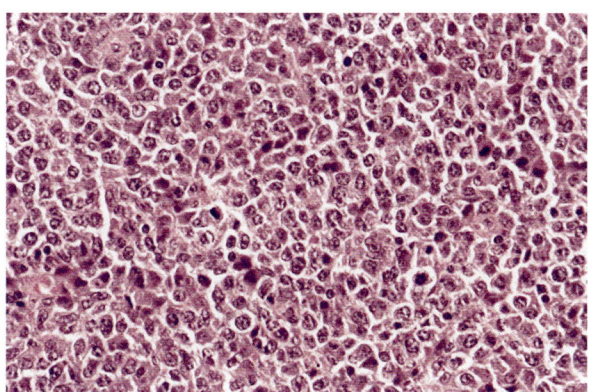

Figure 13-12

DIFFUSE LARGE B-CELL LYMPHOMA

There is diffuse growth of medium-sized to large atypical lymphoid cells.

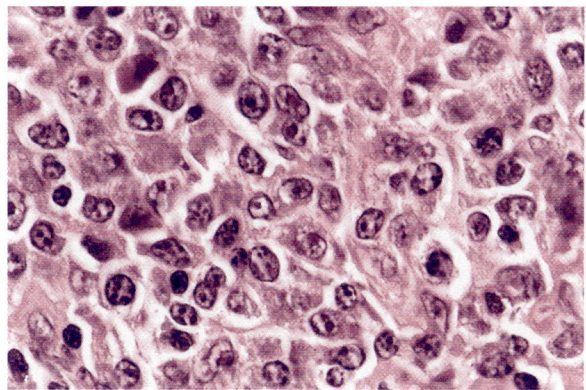

Figure 13-13

DIFFUSE LARGE B-CELL LYMPHOMA

Relatively sparse cytoplasm and oval to round nuclei with one or more nucleoli.

LBCL of the leg as a distinct entity is controversial, however, since the number of cases is small and the duration of follow-up has been limited. In addition, patients with LBCL consisting of multiple lesions or involving multiple sites other than the leg can have an equally guarded prognosis (102,110). One characteristic feature of the tumor cells of LBCL of the leg is bcl-2 expression, seen also in secondary cutaneous LBCL but uncommonly in primary cutaneous LBCL arising in other sites (49,69). Bcl-2 expression, or rearrangement of the associated oncogene, is an adverse prognostic variable in terms of disease-free survival (67,102). Therefore, although cases of LBCL of the leg should be given special consideration, it is doubtful that these tumors merit an entirely separate classification.

Pathologic Findings. There is typically diffuse growth of medium-sized to large atypical lymphoid cells (fig. 13-12). Most often, these cells have the characteristics of centroblasts, with scant, amphophilic to basophilic cytoplasm and oval to round, vesicular nuclei, sometimes with several nucleoli (fig. 13-13). At times, the nuclei are multilobated. Other variants include immunoblastic, featuring cells with generous amounts of basophilic cytoplasm and centrally placed nucleoli; anaplastic, with particularly large cells with bizarre nuclei that may show cohesive growth arrangements (67); and spindled, with small amounts of cytoplasm and dispersed nuclear chromatin (49). Centroblasts comprise at least a small proportion of these other tumor variants. In the T-cell–rich B-cell lymphoma, there are large numbers of reactive T cells with only a small component (less than 10 percent) of large, neoplastic B cells, which are partly obscured by the dense T-cell component (90). Other less common variants of LBCL include a signet ring type, a plasmablastic type that presents in the oral cavity in association with HIV infection, and tumors with myxoid or sclerotic stroma (49,67).

Consonant with the B-cell origin of LBCL, these tumors are usually positive for CD19, CD20, CD22, and CD79a (60), and the cells possess surface or cytoplasmic immunoglobulin (67). Up to half of the tumors express CD10 and bcl-2, although, as mentioned previously, bcl-2 expression is often not observed among primary cutaneous tumors arising in locations other than the legs (69). CD5 is positive in 10 percent of tumors; cyclin D1 is negative (67). Bcl-6 is often positive, as is the proliferation marker Ki-67 (97). There is sometimes staining for p53 and the plasma cell marker CD138 (67). There is also occasional CD30 positivity, and the cells of the anaplastic type are regularly CD30 positive (106). Cells of the immunoblastic type may express the anaplastic large cell lymphoma kinase (ALK) protein (67). The T-cell component of T-cell–rich B-cell lymphoma is positive for CD3 and CD45RO (111). An adverse prognosis is associated with tumors with a high proliferative rate (97), bcl-2 expression (102), and p53 overexpression (128).

Light chain restriction has been specifically mentioned in connection with the ALK-positive variants and T-cell–rich B-cell lymphoma (67,111). B-cell clonality can be demonstrated in LBCL by immunoglobulin heavy or light chain gene rearrangements (62,90,111). In cases of T-cell–rich B-cell lymphoma, clonal rearrangements of the T-cell receptor gamma (γ) gene are typically not identified (90,111). There was one case report of an angiocentric T-cell–rich B-cell lymphoma in which there were rearrangements of both the immunoglobulin heavy chain and T-cell receptor genes (70). A t(14;18) translocation of the *BCL2* gene is seen in some cases, but in one study this was detected only in some secondary cutaneous lesions but in none of five primary cutaneous lesions (69). A t(8;14) translocation was also detected in one case of LBCL; this anomaly can be seen in Burkitt's lymphoma as well as other non-Hodgkin's lymphomas (47). Abnormalities of 3q27 involving *BCL6* have also been reported (67).

Differential Diagnosis. The morphologic atypia observed in the neoplastic cells of LBCL usually permits distinction from reactive infiltrates or lymphocytoma cutis, and this can be further supported by the demonstration of light chain restriction or clonality of the immunoglobulin heavy or light chain genes. The anaplastic variant of LBCL, with cohesive cellular aggregates, resembles poorly differentiated squamous cell carcinoma, but can be readily distinguished since the tumor cells are cytokeratin negative while expressing B-cell antigens such as CD20. When LBCL cells express CD30, problems may arise in the distinction from anaplastic CD30-positive large cell lymphoma, but the latter is of cytotoxic T-cell derivation, and therefore is distinguishable from this B-cell–derived tumor. Similarly, the T-cell–rich B-cell variant of LBCL can be distinguished from peripheral T-cell lymphoma, since T cells in the former lack significant morphologic atypia, while the large atypical cells are of B-cell lineage and show light chain restriction (111). When multinucleated cells or small B cells are present, LBCL can resemble Hodgkin's disease. Classic Reed-Sternberg cells are not seen in LBCL, however, while Hodgkin's disease rarely presents in skin in the absence of established nodal disease. In addition, except for the anaplastic variant, the cells of LBCL are often CD30 negative (111). Some examples of LBCL may have large numbers of plasma cells that demonstrate monoclonality, and therefore can resemble extramedullary plasmacytoma or immunocytoma, although in other respects the clinical presentation of these entities is distinctive. The large, centroblast-like cells of LBCL are distinct from the cells usually encountered in plasmacytoma, including plasmablasts, and in contrast to most cases of LBCL, plasmacytomas tend to lack the pan-B-cell antigens CD19 and CD20 (73). Unlike the blastoid variants of mantle cell lymphoma, an uncommon tumor in skin, the occasional examples of LBCL that express CD5 are cyclin D1 negative (67).

As noted above, LBCL can sometimes arise through transformation in another type of lymphoma. Transitions from lymphomatoid granulomatosis to LBCL are described, and this occurrence has been incorporated into the classification scheme of lymphomatoid granulomatosis (92).

Intravascular Large B-Cell Lymphoma

Clinical Features. *Intravascular large B-cell lymphoma* was once termed *malignant angioendotheliomatosis* because of a presumed intravascular proliferation of neoplastic endothelial cells. This was in contrast to another condition, termed *reactive angioendotheliomatosis,* a rare, self-limited disorder in which intravascular endothelial cell proliferation and thrombosis accompany infectious diseases (e.g., subacute bacterial endocarditis) or hypersensitivity states. During the 1980s, morphologic, ultrastructural, and immunohistochemical studies showed that the malignant process is actually a form of *intravascular lymphomatosis* that is clearly separable, clinically and histopathologically, from reactive angioendotheliomatosis (44,61,126,133). Intravascular lymphomatosis is now classified as intravascular large B-cell lymphoma (ILBCL) in the WHO classification system.

ILBCL is a disease of adults, affecting both men and women in the sixth decade and beyond. It is a multifocal disease with a particular propensity to target the skin and central nervous system (53). Other organs can also be involved, including lung, kidney, and bone marrow (85). Symptoms and clinical presentations vary considerably, since many of the findings result from small

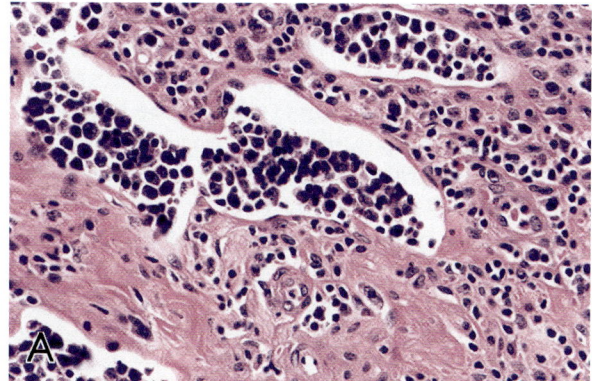
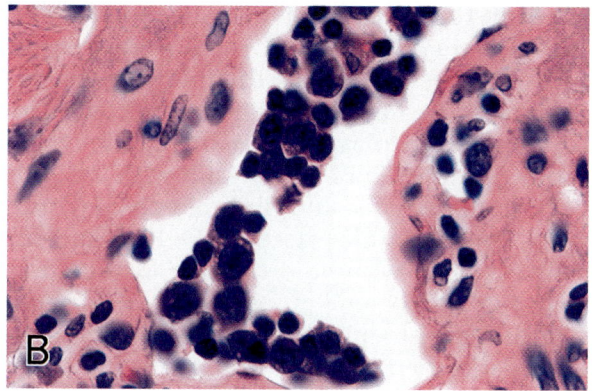
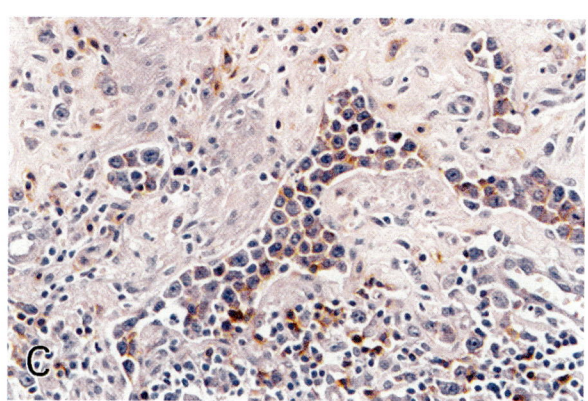

Figure 13-14

INTRAVASCULAR LARGE B-CELL LYMPHOMA

A: Atypical lymphoid cells are present in small vessels.
B: The cells have large vesicular nuclei, and some display prominent nucleoli.
C: The neoplastic cells in this lesion are CD45RA positive.

vessel occlusion. Dementia, hypertension, nephrotic syndrome, and disseminated intravascular coagulation are among the presenting findings (68). Skin lesions are typically erythematous or purpuric macules, papules, and nodules (53,86,113). Chemotherapy is used to manage these patients, but generally the response is poor and death typically ensues rapidly (59,86). An occasional case confined to the skin may have a prolonged clinical course (53).

Pathologic Findings. Atypical lymphoid cells are present in small cutaneous blood vessels, sometimes associated with fibrin thrombi. These cells have large vesicular nuclei and prominent nucleoli, and mitotic figures can be found (fig. 13-14) (68). Tumor cells are leukocyte common antigen (CD45) positive (fig. 13-14C). In most cases, they express B-cell lineage antigens, such as CD20, CD22, and CD79a. Occasionally, they also express CD5, an antigen usually associated with T cells but also occurring in several subsets of B-cell lymphoma. The cells of ILBCL are CD23 and cyclin D1 negative, in contrast to other CD5-positive B-cell lesions, namely, chronic lymphocytic leukemia/small cell lymphoma and mantle cell lymphoma (85). Rarely, ILBCL is composed of T cells that express CD3 and CD45RO (37). Staining for factor VIII is sometimes observed, but this is considered to be most likely due to nonspecific absorption of the molecule rather than its expression by lymphoma cells (68). Light chain restriction has been demonstrated among tumor cells (86). Immunoglobulin heavy chain gene rearrangements are regularly demonstrated in B-cell tumors that are studied by this method (53,85, 114). T-cell receptor gene rearrangements have rarely been reported (87,105). EBV infection has been detected in both the B-cell and T-cell varieties of ILBCL, using in situ hybridization and PCR methods (37,81).

The lymphoma cells of ILBCL have been reported to express lymphocyte function–associated antigens 1 alpha (CD11a) and 1 beta (CD18), and the integrin, VLA-4 (CD49d), while endothelial cells express the CD11a ligand, ICAM-1 (CD54), and the CD49d ligand, CD106 (81,113). The cells lack CD29 (beta-1 integrin) and CD54

(ICAM-1), two molecules involved in transvascular migration and lymphocyte trafficking (107). These studies suggest that defects in transvascular migration or interaction of adhesion molecules on lymphocytes with their ligands on endothelial cells may explain the peculiar intravascular localization of these tumors.

Differential Diagnosis. The chief differential diagnostic issue is the exclusion of other intravascular tumors, including metastatic malignancies. The key to the diagnosis of ILBCL is the identification of tumor cells as lymphocytes by immunohistochemical methods. This is also a critical factor in the exclusion of reactive angioendotheliomatosis. The latter is composed of bland-appearing intravascular cells. Despite the occasional presence of factor VIII-related antigen in ILBCL, the cells of this intravascular lymphoma regularly express leukocyte common antigen (CD45) and B-cell (or, rarely, T-cell) antigens, and are negative for *Ulex europaeus* lectin or blood group isoantigens. The reverse is the case in reactive angioendotheliomatosis (126).

Lymphomatoid Granulomatosis

Clinical Features. *Lymphomatoid granulomatosis* is an extranodal, angiocentric lymphoproliferative disorder that is currently classified as a B-cell proliferation of uncertain malignant potential. Evolution to diffuse large B-cell lymphoma may occur. The principal target organ is the lung, but the skin represents the most common extrapulmonary site (42). Other affected organs include the central nervous system, kidney, and liver. Lymphoid granulomatosis is believed to be due to proliferations of B cells that have been transformed by EBV (96). Immunodeficiency often plays a role in lymphomatoid granulomatosis, and may manifest either in the form of overt disease, such as HIV infection (74), or as a detectable laboratory abnormality (115).

Lymphomatoid granulomatosis most commonly presents in adults, with a male predominance (82). Presenting symptoms are usually referable to pulmonary involvement, and include cough, dyspnea, and chest pain (78). Skin lesions, however, may be the initial (98,131), or apparently the only (119), manifestation of the disease. Lesions include papules, nodules, plaques, ulcers, or maculopapular eruptions (42, 79,131). Unusual cutaneous manifestations include annular (45) or necrobiosis lipoidica-like (34) lesions, crusted lesions, facial edema, and folliculitis-like eruptions (48). In one study, patients with early cutaneous changes were also prone to central nervous system and joint involvement (79). Although spontaneous regression of lesions has been reported (42) and remissions with chemotherapy are possible (45), an aggressive clinical course is the more usual scenario, often with death resulting from pulmonary complications (82).

Pathologic Findings. Changes are concentrated in the deep dermis and subcutis (42,84), where there is a distinctly angiocentric infiltrative process. Typically, the infiltrate is polymorphous, including small lymphocytes, macrophages, and plasma cells or plasmacytoid forms. Infiltration of vessel walls with vascular occlusion, necrosis, and fibrinoid change indicate "lymphocytic vasculitis." In some instances, larger lymphoid cells are identified as well (fig. 13-15).

Immunohistochemical staining shows a predominance of T cells, mostly of helper (CD4) phenotype (42,48,96,119), a fact which early on led investigators to suspect a primary T-cell abnormality; however, the larger, atypical cells are B cells, expressing CD20 and sometimes CD79a and CD30 (78,96,119). EBV RNA has been identified in lesions by in situ hybridization, and colabeling has shown that its expression is restricted to B cells (42,96). It has been more difficult to demonstrate EBV in skin lesions than in the lung (35,42,119). PCR studies have shown clonal rearrangements of the immunoglobulin heavy chain gene (42,96) but no rearrangements of the T-cell receptor gene (96). It is now apparent that lymphomatoid granulomatosis is in fact a T-cell–rich B-cell lymphoproliferative disorder. Ultrastructural study has demonstrated lymphocyte-mediated small vessel necrosis, occlusion, and endothelial regeneration (101).

The proportion of atypical lymphoid cells varies from case to case, and this has formed the basis of a grading system. Few, if any, atypical cells can be identified in grade I lesions. Progression from grade I to grade III is accompanied by an increasing proportion of large, atypical, EBV-positive B cells; fewer reactive cells; and a correspondingly worse prognosis (78).

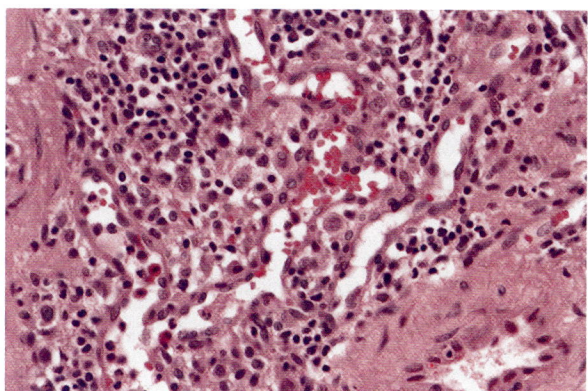
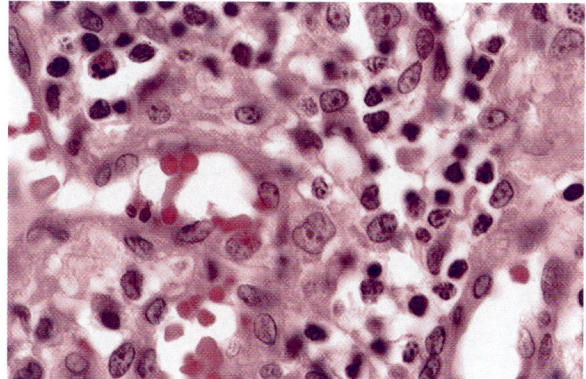

Figure 13-15

LYMPHOMATOID GRANULOMATOSIS

Left: There is a polymorphic infiltrate involving vessels in the deep dermis.
Right: In addition to small lymphocytes with irregular nuclear contours, there are larger lymphoid cells. With immunohistochemical staining, the latter cells are shown to be B cells.

Differential Diagnosis. Several considerations arise in the differential diagnosis of lymphomatoid granulomatosis. Examples with polymorphic infiltrates can be confused with benign forms of lymphocytic vasculitis. This is a term for a heterogeneous group of reactive conditions characterized by infiltration of vessel walls by lymphocytes and, less commonly, fibrinoid necrosis of vessels. Among the best-known examples of lymphocytic vasculitis are pityriasis lichenoides, forms of pigmented purpura, gyrate erythemas, and viral exanthems. These conditions can generally be excluded by clinical data or by findings on routine microscopic study. In particular, they tend to show more superficial dermal infiltrates than would be the case for lymphomatoid granulomatosis; for example, pityriasis lichenoides shows a superficial to mid-dermal, wedge-shaped infiltrate, interface changes of the epidermis, and varying degrees of exocytosis and epidermal necrosis. The infiltrates of pigmented purpuric eruptions tend to involve papillary dermal vessels and are accompanied by capillary proliferation, extravasated erythrocytes, and hemosiderin deposition. In the inflammatory conditions characterized by lymphocytic vasculitis, infiltrates tend to be mild to moderate, and cytologic atypia is minimal; furthermore, B-cell clonality would not be demonstrable (T-cell receptor gene rearrangements have been identified in cases of pityriasis lichenoides).

The angiocentricity of lymphomatoid granulomatosis is similar to that of extranodal NK/T-cell lymphoma, nasal type (see below), and in fact these disorders were formerly linked. Both are associated with EBV. Extranodal NK/T-cell lymphoma, nasal type, has a predilection for sinonasal and nasopharyngeal tissues, and is a lesion comprised of NK/T cells that are positive for CD2, CD56, and CD3, as well as for cytotoxic granule proteins (77).

In high-grade lesions of lymphomatoid granulomatosis, the atypical lymphoid cells can resemble cells of Hodgkin's disease. Cutaneous involvement in Hodgkin's disease is rare, and angiocentricity is not as striking. Classic Reed-Sternberg cells are not identified in lymphomatoid granulomatosis. In addition, the atypical B cells of the latter are CD15 negative (78).

Other B-Cell Lymphomas Involving the Skin

Chronic lymphocytic leukemia/small lymphocytic lymphoma is considered in the section on leukemias.

Precursor B-Cell Lymphoblastic Lymphoma. This is an uncommon lymphoma, representing 10 percent of cases of lymphoblastic lymphoma. It is defined as a lymphoma rather than a leukemia when presenting as a mass lesion with less than 25 percent lymphoblasts in the bone marrow. The skin is a common site of involvement, along with bone, soft tissue, and lymph nodes (46). It is primarily a disease of children

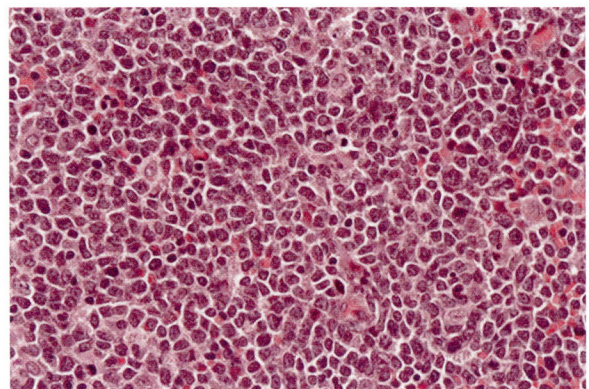 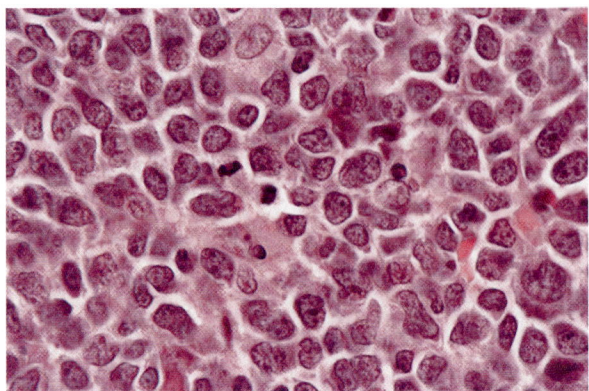

Figure 13-16

PRECURSOR B LYMPHOBLASTIC LYMPHOMA
Left: Diffuse growth of small to medium-sized lymphoid cells.
Right: Mitotic activity, dispersed chromatin, and multiple small nucleoli are seen.

and young adults (80,91). Cutaneous lesions consist of multiple nodules (46). The tumor can follow an aggressive clinical course, although there is a relatively high remission rate, with good response to chemotherapy (91).

Microscopically, there is diffuse dermal growth of small to medium-sized lymphoid cells, with dispersed chromatin, multiple inconspicuous nucleoli, and numerous mitotic figures (fig. 13-16) (91). The common immunohistochemical profile is positivity for CD19, CD20 (variable), CD79a, CD10, and HLA-DR. Virtually all cases are terminal deoxynucleotidyl transferase (TdT) positive (80,93). Several cytogenetic abnormalities have been detected, and these may have a significant bearing on prognosis (46).

The differential diagnosis includes several other lymphomas that are uncommon in skin, specifically Burkitt's lymphoma and blastoid mantle cell lymphoma, but lymphoblastic lymphoma is the only lymphoma that shows nuclear TdT positivity (46).

Mantle Cell Lymphoma. This lymphoma is believed to be derived from pre-germinal center B cells, and a role for chronic antigenic stimulation has been proposed (63). Mantle cell lymphoma represents 3 to 10 percent of non-Hodgkin's lymphomas, and usually presents in middle-aged adults with lymph node, spleen, and/or bone marrow disease. The most common extranodal sites are the gastrointestinal tract and Waldeyer's ring (63,117). Cutaneous involvement is rare (95,100,112). Overall, the median survival period is 3 to 5 years (117).

Histopathologic changes include infiltrates of small to medium-sized lymphocytes with irregular nuclear contours that have the appearance of centrocytes. Nucleoli are inconspicuous. Scattered epithelioid macrophages can create a "starry sky" appearance (fig. 13-17). A common immunohistochemical profile is positivity for CD5, CD20, FMC-7 (which recognizes a subpopulation of B cells), CD43, bcl-2, and cyclin D1 (fig. 13-18) (95,100,117). Marti et al. (95) found expression of cutaneous lymphocyte-associated antigen (CLA) in examples of mantle cell lymphoma with cutaneous involvement, an unusual and possibly important result since CLA is normally associated with T cells and cutaneous T-cell lymphomas. Despite the possibility of a starry sky appearance resembling Burkitt's lymphoma, there are significant cytologic and immunohistochemical differences between the two tumors: Burkitt cells are generally larger, with rounded nuclei and deeply basophilic cytoplasm with lipid vacuoles, and are CD5 and bcl-2 negative (117).

Burkitt's Lymphoma. This is a highly aggressive tumor of germinal center origin that is often associated with bulky disease due to its rapid doubling time. It is a common malignancy of childhood, especially in its endemic and sporadic forms. It can also be associated with immunodeficiency, especially with HIV infection,

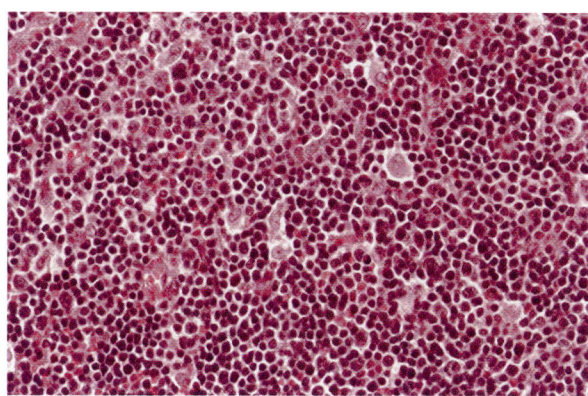 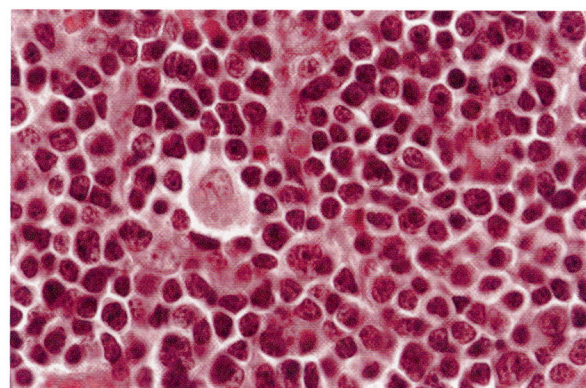

Figure 13-17

MANTLE CELL LYMPHOMA

Left: There is a diffuse infiltrate of small to medium-sized lymphocytes. Scattered epithelioid histiocytes (macrophages) create a "starry sky" appearance.

Right: Note the irregular nuclear contours and inconspicuous nucleoli. A macrophage is identified left of center.

and has a significant association with EBV (58). It often presents in extranodal sites. Specific cutaneous involvement is rare (38,108), although the skin can be secondarily involved, for example, with disease of the jaw or breast. Despite its aggressive clinical course, cure is possible with intensive chemotherapy (58).

Microscopically, there are diffuse infiltrates of medium-sized cells with basophilic cytoplasm containing lipid vacuoles, round nuclei, and clumped chromatin. Mitotic figures are numerous. Scattered macrophages within the lesion can give it a "starry sky" appearance (fig. 13-19). The immunohistochemical profile is positivity for CD19, CD20, CD22, CD10, and bcl-6, and negativity for CD5, CD23, TdT, and bcl-2. As might be expected of such a rapidly replicating tumor, most cells are Ki-67 positive (58). There are clonal rearrangements of the immunoglobulin heavy and light chain genes, and translocations involving the *MYC* gene are expected (104).

T-CELL AND NK-CELL NEOPLASMS

Precursor T-Cell Lymphoblastic Lymphoma

Clinical Features. *Precursor T lymphoblastic lymphoma* is composed of T-lineage lymphoblasts. It is essentially the same disorder as *precursor T lymphoblastic leukemia*, except that the lymphoma presents as a mass lesion with less than 25 percent lymphoblasts in the bone marrow (169).

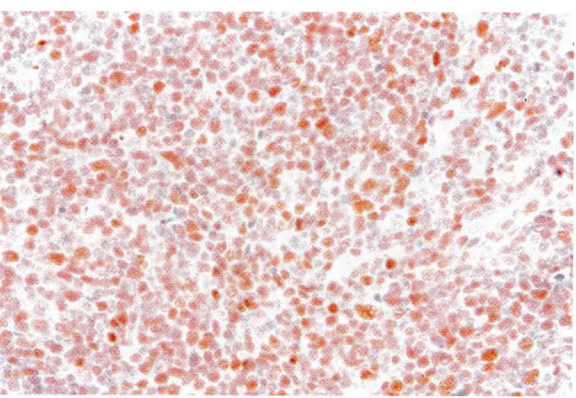

Figure 13-18

MANTLE CELL LYMPHOMA

Immunohistochemical staining shows cyclin D1 expression.

Precursor T lymphoblastic lymphoma primarily occurs in adolescent males. It presents most often as a rapidly growing mediastinal mass with pleural effusion. Extranodal sites include the liver, spleen, Waldeyer's ring, central nervous system, and skin. A peculiarity of this lymphoma is that, although it represents the vast majority of all lymphoblastic lymphomas, it apparently involves the skin less often than does precursor B lymphoblastic lymphoma (189,366). Cutaneous involvement most often consists of one or more tumor nodules, with a particular predilection for the head and neck (189,313,366). Responses

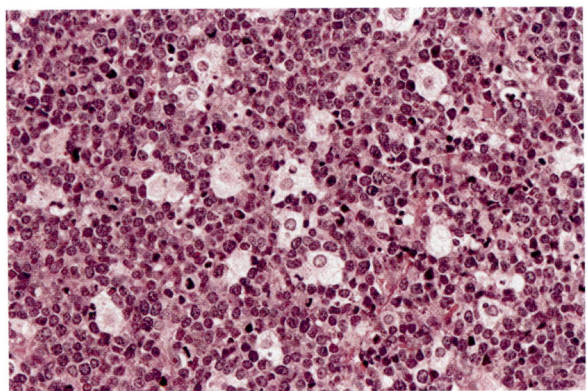
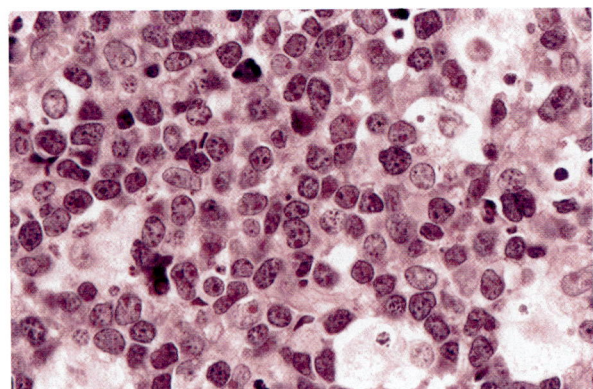

Figure 13-19

BURKITT'S LYMPHOMA

Left: There is a diffuse infiltrate of medium-sized cells. Scattered macrophages create a starry sky appearance.
Right: The cells have vacuolated cytoplasm, rounded nuclei, and clumped chromatin.

to therapy are comparable to those of precursor B lymphoblastic lymphoma.

Pathologic Findings. Findings include a dense, diffuse infiltrate of medium-sized lymphoid cells with a high nuclear to cytoplasmic ratio. These cells feature rounded to convoluted nuclei with dispersed to condensed chromatin and inconspicuous nucleoli (fig. 13-20) (169,189). Mitotic figures are readily identified. Scattered macrophages can produce a starry sky appearance. Several authors have emphasized that there are few, if any, morphologic differences between precursor T lymphoblastic lymphoma and its B-cell counterpart (189,366).

Immunohistochemistry confirms the T-cell nature of the process, as tumor cells commonly express CD2, CD3, CD4, CD5, CD7, and CD8. Blastic cells may co-express CD4 and CD8 (169). As is characteristic of B lymphoblastic lymphoma, cells are TdT positive. Other antigens that are sometimes expressed are CD10, CD79a, and the myeloid markers CD13 and CD33 (169, 189). With the possible exception of CD79a, B-cell markers are negative (189). Clonal rearrangement of T-cell receptor genes can be detected. Translocations that involve T-cell receptor loci and an assortment of partner genes, including several transcription factors, are seen (169,328).

Differential Diagnosis. The starry sky appearance of some examples can mimic Burkitt's lymphoma or variants of mantle cell lymphoma, both uncommon in skin. Nuclear TdT positivity, however, confirms the diagnosis of lymphoblastic lymphoma. Differential B- and T-cell staining can be used to determine the precise lineage of the neoplastic cells.

Adult T-Cell Leukemia/Lymphoma

Clinical Features. *Adult T-cell leukemia/lymphoma* (ATLL) is characterized by the infiltration of a variety of organs by highly pleomorphic lymphoid cells, induced by the retrovirus, human T lymphotrophic virus (HTLV)-1. ATLL is endemic in certain regions of the world, particularly in Japan but also in the Caribbean and Central Africa, regions with a high prevalence of HTLV-1. Cases have also been reported in the United States (256). It is encountered most often in middle-aged or older adults, with a slight male predominance. ATLL typically shows widespread involvement of lymph nodes and peripheral blood as well as a variety of organs, including spleen, lung, liver, and gastrointestinal tract. Cutaneous involvement is common, and the skin is the most common extralymphatic site for this lymphoma (275).

ATLL has been divided into four clinical types: *acute, lymphomatous, chronic,* and *smoldering* (383). These types reflect a spectrum of clinical and laboratory abnormalities. The acute type, the leukemic phase of the disorder, is associated with lymphadenopathy, hepatosplenomegaly, constitutional symptoms, leukocytosis, immunodeficiency (with a proneness to opportunistic infections), hypercalcemia, and elevated lactate dehydrogenase levels. At the other end of

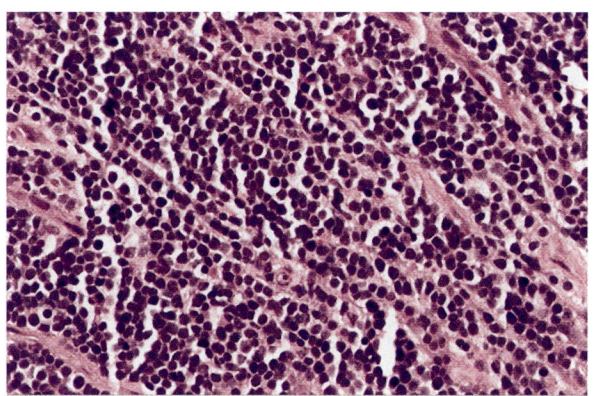 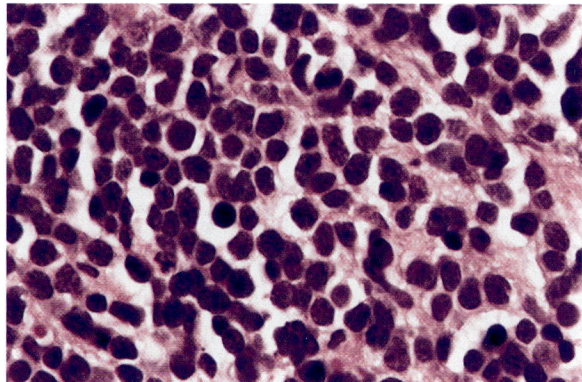

Figure 13-20

PRECURSOR T-CELL LYMPHOBLASTIC LYMPHOMA

Left: There is a dense, diffuse infiltrate of medium-sized lymphoid cells.

Right: The cells are characterized by a high nuclear:cytoplasmic ratio. The nuclei are rounded to convoluted, have dispersed to condensed chromatin, and have inconspicuous nucleoli. There are few morphologic differences from the B-cell counterpart of this disorder.

the spectrum, the smoldering variety features normal white blood cell counts, fewer than 5 percent circulating neoplastic cells, frequent cutaneous or pulmonary lesions, and no hypercalcemia (275,383). The diagnosis may be aided by identifying serum antibody to HTLV-associated antigen (180,276,393).

The overall prognosis of patients with ATLL is poor, but there can be significant variations in survival that correlate to some extent with the clinical types. Survival periods for patients with the acute and lymphomatous types are from 6 to 10 months, while for those with chronic and smoldering types, they range from 14 to 24 months (379,383). Unfortunately, chronic or smoldering ATLL can progress to the acute form of the disease.

Cutaneous lesions include erythematous to purpuric papules, nodules (including subcutaneous nodules), and plaques (180,222,300,379, 393). Other reported changes are erythroderma (263), ulcerated or necrotic nodules (180,241), pompholyx-like vesicular eruptions (180), and nodular eruptions mimicking the d'emblee variant of mycosis fungoides (263). Pruritus may be a major complaint (180). The precise clinical type of ATLL does not always correlate with the cutaneous manifestations, although "rash" has been described in the acute type and exfoliative dermatitis in the chronic type (275). Skin involvement is sometimes noted before the onset of a leukemic phase (276), and several reports have documented clonal integration of the HTLV-1 provirus and T-cell receptor gene rearrangements in skin and not in peripheral lymphocytes (207,222,300). Such findings suggest that the disease can originate in the skin (276). There is also some evidence that patients with the smoldering type of ATLL with skin involvement may have a worse prognosis than those with the same type without skin involvement (379).

Pathologic Findings. The usual microscopic feature of ATLL is a dermal infiltrate of atypical lymphoid cells with irregular nuclei. Epidermal infiltration with the formation of Pautrier's microabscesses can occur (275). The infiltrates may be angiocentric and angiodestructive (241,299, 301). The infiltrating lymphoid cells vary from medium to large, with irregularly shaped or polylobated nuclei containing coarse chromatin and prominent nucleoli, to small lymphoid cells with varying degrees of nuclear pleomorphism (fig. 13-21). This appears to correlate to some extent with the clinical type: the larger cells are seen in the acute and lymphomatous varieties, while smaller cells with lesser degrees of atypia are encountered in the chronic and smoldering types (275). In a case reported by Maeda et al. (300), there were cerebriform cells in the upper dermis and large lymphoid cells in the lower dermis. The neoplastic cells tend to have deeply basophilic cytoplasm. Lymphoblastoid

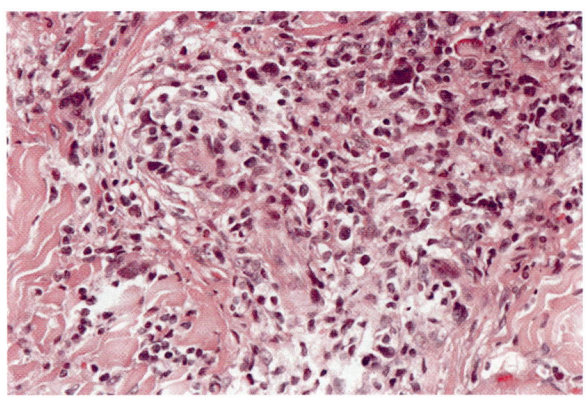 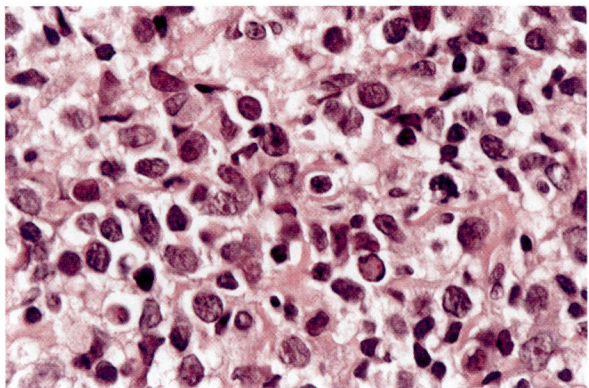

Figure 13-21

ADULT T-CELL LEUKEMIA/LYMPHOMA

Left: There are medium to large lymphoid cells in the dermis.
Right: These cells possess nuclei with markedly irregular shapes, coarse chromatin, and prominent nucleoli.

cells possessing nuclei with dispersed chromatin are sometimes observed (275,300). Epithelioid granulomas similar to those seen in Lennert's lymphoma have been reported in one case that was associated with prolonged survival (380).

The usual immunophenotype of the infiltrating cells of ATLL is positivity for CD2, CD3, CD4, CD5, and CD25, and negativity for CD7, CD8, and granzyme B (275,319). There appears to be a discrepancy in immunophenotype among cells in different organs; for example, neoplastic cells in skin are CD45RA negative, CD45RO and CD29 (integrin β1) positive, while those in the peripheral blood are CD45RA positive, CD45RO and CD29 negative (319). Large lymphoblastoid cells are CD30 positive, ALK-1 negative (275, 300). Although usually the cells of ATLL are CD4 positive, CD8 negative, co-expression of these two antigens also occurs, and there are also examples of CD4 negative, CD8 positive infiltrates (275, 300). There may also be expression of CD38, T9, and leu-8 (299). There has also been a report of sialyl Lewis X antigen expression in ATLL associated with skin involvement (220).

Genetic analysis shows both monoclonal integration of HTLV proviral DNA and T-cell receptor gene rearrangements in the infiltrating cells of ATLL (146,207,222,271,299,393, 440). In some cases, these findings are detected in skin but not in peripheral lymphocytes (207, 222). In situ hybridization may be a more effective technique than PCR in identifying HTLV-1 proviral DNA in paraffin-embedded tissues (146). Viral particles within or budding from neoplastic lymphoid cells have been identified by electron microscopy (241,440).

Differential Diagnosis. The major differential diagnostic consideration is cutaneous T-cell lymphoma (CTCL). Both can present with cutaneous plaques, nodules, or erythroderma (263). ATLL, however, is more likely to present with extensive systemic disease, including lymph node and bone marrow involvement, and hepatosplenomegaly (319). Although the microscopic configuration of these two conditions can be quite similar in skin, a higher proportion of neoplastic to non-neoplastic cells is seen in the perivascular zones in ATLL, and the cells of that condition are more apt to possess deeply basophilic cytoplasm (demonstrable with the Giemsa stain). Giant cells with irregularly contoured nuclei are characteristic of ATLL but not CTCL (240). Skin lesions of ATLL have higher levels of interleukin-2 receptor alpha genomic RNA than is the case in CTCL lesions (327). A definitive diagnosis of ATLL can be made by identifying HTLV-1 proviral DNA in tissues (146,217).

Angiocentric lesions of ATLL can resemble two other angiocentric lymphomas, lymphomatoid granulomatosis or extranodal NK/T-cell lymphoma, nasal type. In lymphomatoid granulomatosis, the perivascular T cells are morphologically bland and the atypical lymphocytes mark as B cells. B-cell rather than T-cell clonality is demonstrable, and there is an association with EBV rather than HTLV-1 (although demonstration of EBV in skin lesions of lymphomatoid granulomatosis can be difficult). Unlike ATLL, extranodal NK/T-cell lymphoma, nasal type, tends to involve sinonasal tissues, is composed of NK cells that are CD56 positive and possess cytotoxic granule proteins (including granzyme B), and is associated with EBV (257).

Extranodal NK/T-Cell Lymphoma, Nasal Type

Clinical Features. The lymphoma phenotype that now carries the designation of *NK/T-cell lymphoma, nasal type,* was formerly called *lethal midline granuloma* or *lethal midline disease* (254). As the latter terms suggest, this disorder is associated with substantial tissue destruction in the midfacial region, including the nose, paranasal sinuses, and oral cavity. Purely extracranial lesions are also encountered in some patients, such that the diagnosis of *primary cutaneous NK/T-cell sinonasal-type lymphoma* (NKTSTL) is now accepted in the realm of dermatopathology (143, 150,187,257,259). Involvement of the skin may also occur secondarily (272,356). As detailed subsequently, this disease is recognizable only through the application of strict morphologic and immunophenotypic requirements. Otherwise, its presentation in the integument is usually indistinguishable from that of malignant lymphomas in general (143,257,272). Indeed, Hwang and colleagues (249) have described a clinical image of NKTSTL that simulated that of mycosis fungoides.

NKTSTL is most common in Asians, but geographic concentrations of this disease also exist in Central and South America and in native American communities (259); thus, it appears that a non-African-American, non-Caucasian heritage somehow predisposes to this disorder (150,259). De Campos-Lima et al. (199) have suggested that the prevalence of HLA-A11 in such populations may be contributory, since it is associated with interference of the immune response to EBV, an agent that is indisputably and strongly linked to NKTSTL (221,238,259). Canioni et al. (175) described a case wherein co-infection with HIV and EBV was associated with this tumor.

A common abnormality relating to the regulation of apoptosis has been detected in the cells of NKTSTL: deletion of *FAS* gene sequences that code for cell death domains (382). That event confers an "immune privilege" to the neoplastic lymphoid cells in this disorder. Although no consistent cytogenetic aberrations have been connected to NKTSTL, several appear to occur more often than chance would predict: DNA losses at chromosomes 6q, 11q, 13q, and 17p, and DNA gains at 1p, 6p, 11q, 12q, 17q, 19p, 20q, and Xp (387). Importantly, and in contrast to most other non-Hodgkin's lymphomas, NKTSTL cases typically demonstrate no evidence of T-cell receptor or immunoglobulin heavy chain gene rearrangements, and instead exhibit a germ-line genotype (143,367).

Patients with this form of non-Hodgkin's lymphoma have an unfavorable prognosis; NKTSTL is only partially responsive to radiotherapy and generally fails to remit after chemotherapy (187,356), possibly because of the expression of multidrug-resistance gene products (259). The skin and subcutis are common sites of relapse for systemic NKTSTL, and a hemophagocytic syndrome may accompany the tumor (187, 259). The aerodigestive tract, gonad, soft tissue, and spleen may also be involved concomitantly with the skin or at another time, but lymph nodes are usually spared (367).

Pathologic Findings. The basic microscopic image of NKTSTL in the skin is that of a variably atypical dermal lymphoid infiltrate that is usually accompanied by geographic or "en masse" necrosis. The latter feature was initially felt to reflect the presence of angiocentricity and angioinvasion by the neoplastic cells, with attendant occlusion of vascular lumens and microinfarction of the skin. However, vascular permeation is not always observed in cutaneous NKTSTL (fig. 13-22), and it is now felt that the chemokines IP-10 and Mig, which are related to EBV, may instead be responsible for the necrotizing nature of this lesion (259).

As cited above, the cytologic attributes of this lymphoma morphotype are heterogeneous. At the bland pole of the spectrum, the neoplastic lymphoid cells may be small (fig. 13-23) and admixed with numerous inflammatory elements; this image was called *polymorphic reticulosis* in the past literature, especially that dealing with midline tumors in the head and neck (411). The other extreme of the morphologic picture of NKTSTL features sheets of large, pleomorphic, obviously anaplastic lymphocytes with many apoptotic figures and mitoses (fig. 13-24). There is obviously a continuum between the poles,

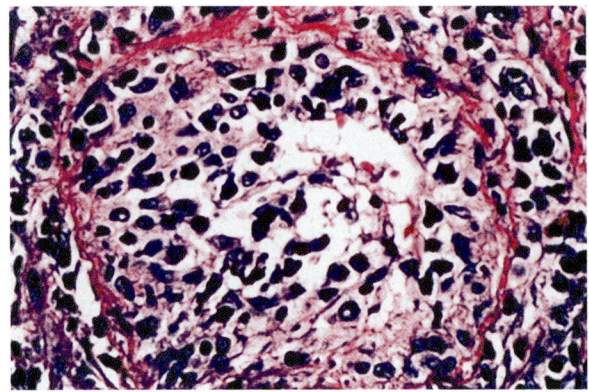

Figure 13-22

EXTRANODAL NK/T-CELL LYMPHOMA, NASAL TYPE

Angioinvasion is apparent in this example.

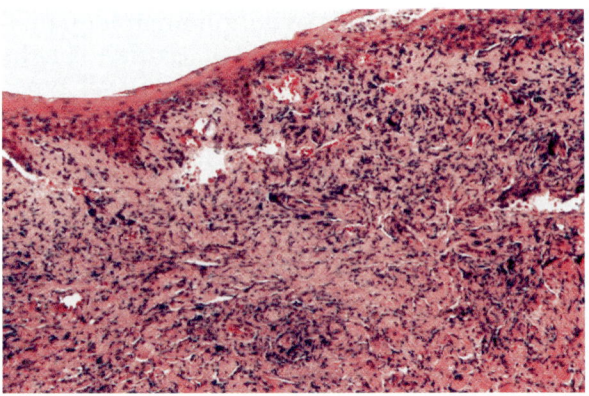

Figure 13-23

EXTRANODAL NK/T-CELL LYMPHOMA, NASAL TYPE

Relatively bland lymphoid cells dissect randomly through the dermal collagen.

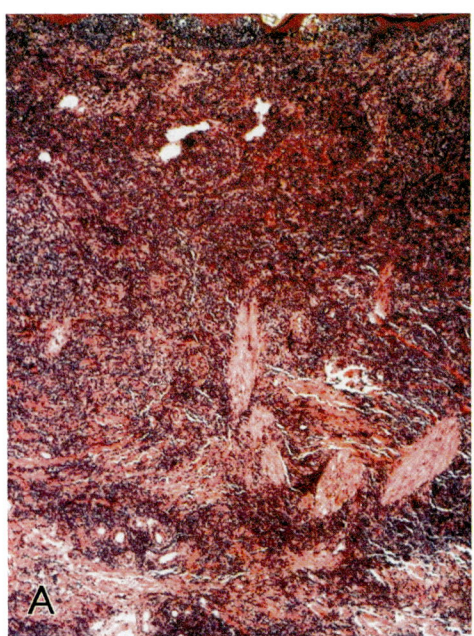

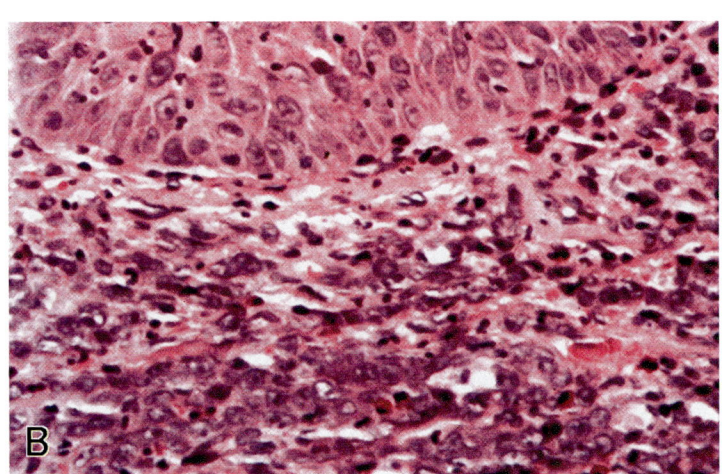

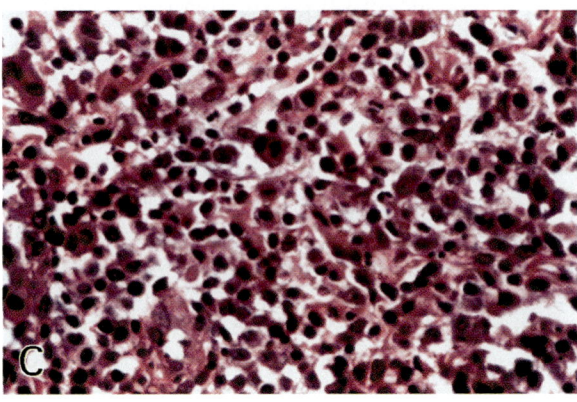

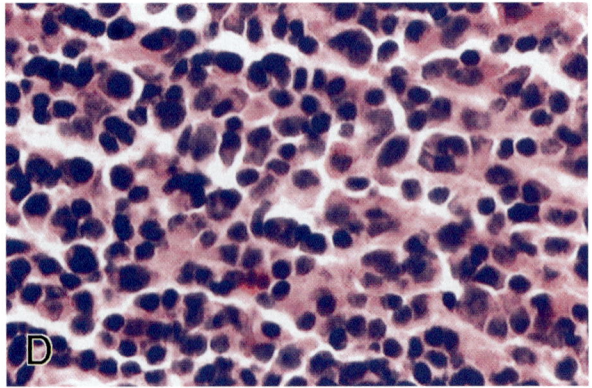

Figure 13-24

EXTRANODAL NK/T-CELL LYMPHOMA, NASAL TYPE

Obviously atypical lymphoid cells are in the dermis.

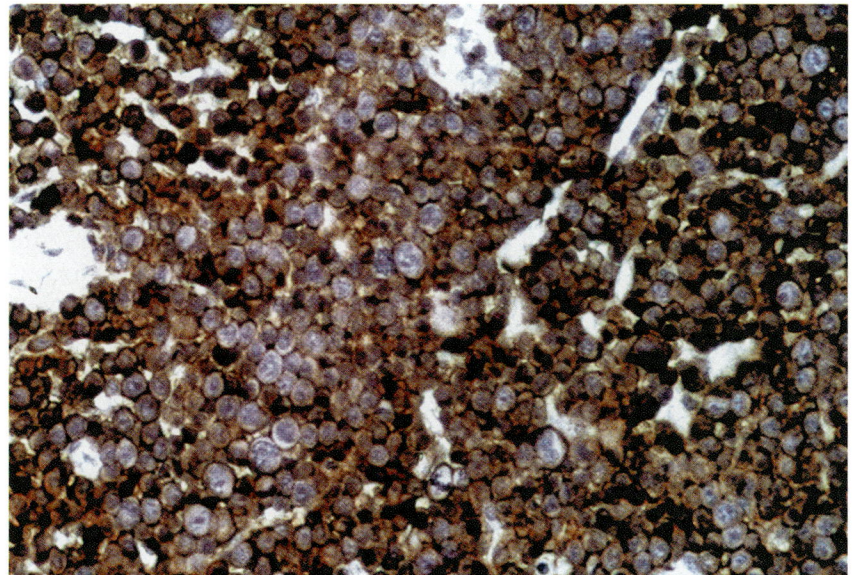

Figure 13-25

EXTRANODAL NK/T-CELL LYMPHOMA, NASAL TYPE

Diffuse immunoreactivity for CD56 is shown.

and the middle ground is occupied by lesions with variable numbers of the large, poorly differentiated lymphoid elements in an inflammatory background.

The immunophenotype of NKTSTL is characterized by reactivity for CD2, CD3, CD3-epsilon, CD56 (fig. 13-25), perforin, TIA-1, and granzyme-B, but CD16 and CD57 are usually absent (259, 367). Stains for EBV-latent membrane protein are only variably reactive, but in situ hybridization or PCR studies for EBV nucleic acid in the tumor cells are virtually always positive (221,238). Blakolmer et al. (162) have found that occasional examples of NKTSTL may aberrantly label for CD20 and CD79a, both of which are regarded as B-cell markers. We also have encountered cases that were CD45 negative. These observations reinforce the need for extended immunohistologic panels in the evaluation of such lesions.

Differential Diagnosis. The principal differential diagnostic possibilities in cases of NKTSTL in the skin are lymphomatoid granulomatosis (angiocentric immunoproliferative lesion) and aggressive NK-cell leukemia/lymphoma (blastoid NK-cell lymphoma) (259,367). Lymphomatoid granulomatosis has many morphologic and mechanistic similarities to NKTSTL, including an association with EBV, but it is a peculiar angiocentric form of a T-cell–rich B-cell lymphoproliferation. The kidneys and central nervous system are commonly involved by this lesion, but not by NKTSTL (259).

Blastoid NK-cell lymphoma has an immunophenotype that differs slightly from that of NKTSTL: variable positivity for CD2, reactivity for CD56, and a lack of labeling for CD3, CD16, CD57, and EBV-related markers (227). Clinically, blastoid NK-cell lymphoma also is singular in its systemic nature, with regular involvement of multiple lymph nodes and the bone marrow. Jaffe et al. (259) have suggested that the latter tumor type is most closely related to lymphoblastic lymphoma, but with commitment to an NK-cell lineage.

Another potential diagnostic trap is represented by a case reported by Taddesse-Heath and coworkers (392). They encountered a patient who had nasal infection with herpes simplex II virus, and a highly atypical, NKTSTL-like lymphoproliferative response to the virus that featured immunoreactivity for CD3, CD4, CD5, and CD56. Additional studies for EBV infection were negative. It remains to be seen whether these findings could be recapitulated in cases of cutaneous viral infection.

Subcutaneous Panniculitis-Like T-Cell Lymphoma

Clinical Features. As the name implies, *subcutaneous panniculitis-like T-cell lymphoma* (SPTCL) primarily involves the subcutis. It is composed most often of cells with the cytotoxic phenotype. SPTCL affects patients of a broad age range, although many patients are young adults (261), and children have been reported (139,184). Among the minority of patients whose T cells are of the gamma/delta (γδ) subtype, immunosuppression may be an important factor in the pathogenesis of the disease (148).

Patients present with erythematous subcutaneous nodules, especially on the trunk and extremities, but also in the head and neck region (151,252,326). Plaques (416) and woody infiltration of the skin (149) have also been described. The lesions are reported to be either asymptomatic or tender (326), and nodules may undergo ulceration and necrosis. Involvement is generally restricted to the subcutis until late in the course of the disease. Some cases, however, are associated with a hemophagocytic syndrome, with associated pancytopenia, fever, weight loss, and hepatosplenomegaly (184,261,304,326, 441). SPTCL is an aggressive neoplasm, and the hemophagocytic syndrome can have an especially fulminant course. Some individuals respond to combination chemotherapy (151,261, 362), and survival periods of greater than 5 years have been reported (304,362).

There has been some discussion in the literature regarding the relationship of SPTCL to a condition called *cytophagic histiocytic panniculitis* (CHP). First described as such in 1980 by Winkelmann and Bowie (431), CHP presents as ulcerating subcutaneous nodules associated with consumptive coagulopathy, peripheral cytopenia, and hepatosplenomegaly. Microscopically, there is a lobular panniculitis with a mixed inflammatory infiltrate and clusters of large "histiocytes" engaged in cytophagocytosis; atypical cells are classically not observed. CHP tends to be an aggressive disorder that is sometimes responsive to antineoplastic therapy. Although some cases have a favorable outcome and might conceivably represent a non-neoplastic, infection-associated hemophagocytic syndrome, most examples prove to be manifestations of a lymphoid malignancy, particularly cutaneous T-cell lymphoma (415). It is now widely recognized that CHP and SPTCL are closely related (239,304, 424,441) and probably represent ends of a spectrum of disease, with frequent biologic progression from a picture of CHP to frank SPTCL (239). A likely explanation for lesions with the microscopic features of CHP is the existence of a lymphoid clone, difficult to detect by routine morphology, that activates macrophages and stimulates phagocytic activity through the secretion of mediators such as interferon gamma and macrophage inflammatory protein-1-alpha (424).

Pathologic Findings. Microscopically, SPTCL shows a lobular subcutaneous infiltrate consisting of pleomorphic lymphoid elements, ranging from small cells with rounded nuclei and inconspicuous nucleoli to large cells with pale cytoplasm and hyperchromatic nuclei (fig. 13-26) (261,362). Rimming of lipocytes by neoplastic lymphocytes is a characteristic feature (151,261, 285), and angioinvasion has been noted in a number of cases (261,362,416). Karyorrhexis is common (362,439), and necrosis may be extensive (fig. 13-26A) (362,416). Histiocytes (macrophages) are present and may phagocytize cellular material (252,416,441) and form granulomas (362). These are sometimes described as "bean-bag" cells (fig. 13-27). Several reports have described lipomembranous (membranocystic) lesions in the subcutis (326,417), consisting of thickened, undulating membranes that form cysts and papillary configurations. These structures are believed to derive from degenerated cell membranes of lipocytes or macrophages, and are comprised of ceroid, an oxidation product of unsaturated fatty acids. Lipomembranous change is generally considered nonspecific, although it is prone to develop in forms of panniculitis associated with degrees of vascular compromise. It is typical of SPTCL that the epidermis and dermis are spared, although involvement of these components has been reported in cases of SPTCL of T γδ origin (285).

The immunohistochemical findings in SPTCL vary, depending upon whether the neoplasm derives from cells of the T alpha/beta (αβ) receptor subtype (about 75 percent of cases) or the T γδ receptor subtype (about 25 percent of cases). The typical immunohistochemical profile of the lymphocytes in T αβ SPTCL is CD4 negative, CD8 positive, and CD56 negative, while that in T γδ SPTCL is CD4 negative, CD8 negative, and CD56 positive (261,285,304,362). Both types are positive for CD3, CD45RO, and CD43, as well as for the cytotoxic granule-associated proteins granzyme B, perforin, and TIA-1 (T-cell intracellular antigen) (261,285,315,416).

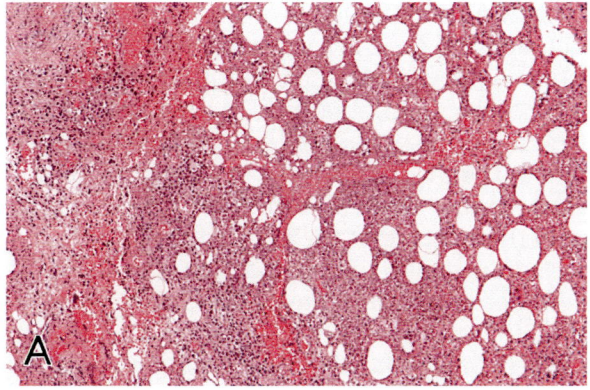
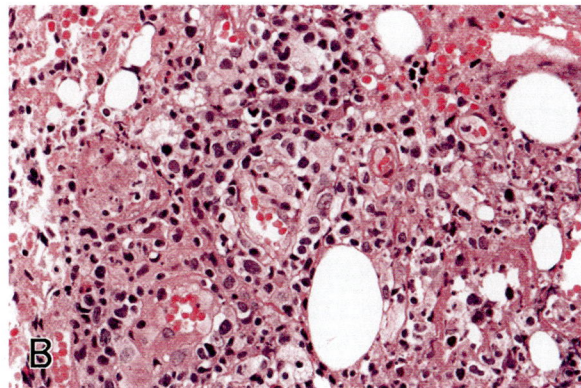
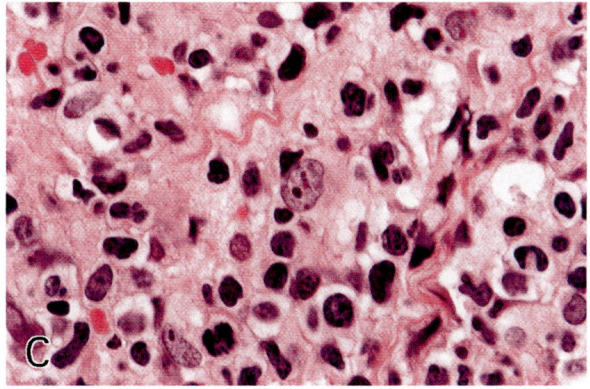

Figure 13-26

SUBCUTANEOUS PANNICULITIS-LIKE T-CELL LYMPHOMA

A: The lobular subcutaneous infiltrate is associated with considerable necrosis.

B: Atypical lymphoid elements permeate the subcutis. Lymphocytes tend to form rims around lipocytes.

C: There is a predominance of small cells with irregular nuclear contours.

The majority of cases are negative for EBV sequences by a variety of methods (285,362), but EBV genetic material has been found in some cases (239,416). Iwatsuki et al. (253) suggested that EBV infection is detected in cases of SPTCL associated with hemophagocytic syndrome, but is not identified in the uncommon, nonfatal CHP cases. T-cell receptor gene rearrangements are commonly identified (285,304,362). Ultrastructural studies have shown membrane-bound granules resembling those of cytotoxic T lymphocytes (197) and phagocytosis of apoptotic bodies by macrophages (bean-bag cells) (252).

Differential Diagnosis. The chief considerations in the differential diagnosis of SPTCL are benign forms of panniculitis and other T-cell lymphomas that sometimes present with subcutaneous infiltrates. In addition to showing a more polymorphous infiltrate and a lack of significant cytologic atypia, ordinary forms of panniculitis show mixtures of CD4- and CD8-positive T cells as well as CD20-positive B cells (285). Differential diagnostic problems may arise when examples of CHP have insufficient microscopic evidence to permit a diagnosis of lymphoma,

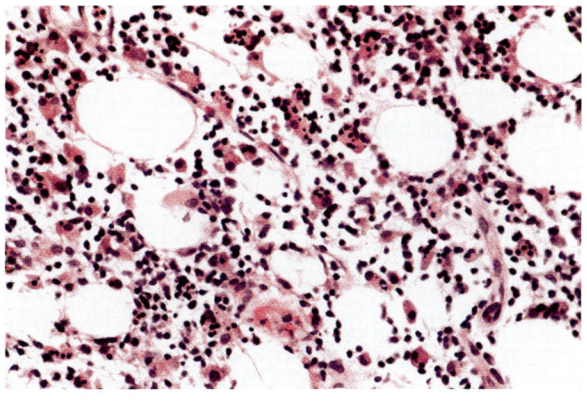

Figure 13-27

SUBCUTANEOUS PANNICULITIS-LIKE T-CELL LYMPHOMA (CYTOPHAGIC HISTIOCYTIC PANNICULITIS)

The cytophagic activity by macrophages is evident. These are sometimes termed "bean-bag" cells.

but nevertheless these should have demonstrable cytophagocytic activity. Gene rearrangement studies can be attempted, but a negative result does not rule out a subclinical lymphoma that is simply not detectable by current methods

(424). In such cases, close clinical follow-up is indicated to permit the earliest possible detection of a transition to SPTCL. Other forms of peripheral T-cell lymphoma can involve the subcutis, but these are prone to involve the epidermis and dermis, are likely to form solid sheets of tumor in preference to the rimming of individual lipocytes seen in SPTCL, and may express CD4 among neoplastic cells (285).

The majority of examples of SPTCL are not difficult to distinguish from extranodal NK/T-cell lymphoma, nasal type, since the latter tumor has a predilection for sinonasal regions and is CD56 positive, CD8 negative, and EBV positive. However, SPTCL of the T γδ subtype tends to have this same profile, and other overlapping features include CD-epsilon positivity (with staining of the cytoplasm rather than the cell membrane) and expression of cytotoxic granule proteins (186,439). Extranodal NK/T-cell lymphoma, nasal type, is perhaps more likely to involve the dermis as well as the subcutis, and is particularly angiocentric (186). In addition, this lymphoma usually shows a germline configuration of T-cell receptor genes (261). As a practical matter, differentiation between the two lymphomas may make little difference. Both are potentially aggressive tumors, although thus far extranodal NK/T-cell lymphomas involving the subcutis appear to be uniformly so, and are unresponsive to chemotherapy (186).

Mycosis Fungoides

Clinical Features. Initially described by Alibert in 1806, *mycosis fungoides* seems to be an inappropriate term for a cutaneous lymphoma in this modern era. Nevertheless, the term is ingrained in the literature, and it clearly has assumed a more specific meaning than cutaneous T-cell lymphoma, which can be applied to a number T-cell lymphomas with differing clinical, histopathologic, and immunohistochemical characteristics.

Mycosis fungoides is the most common primary cutaneous T-cell lymphoma. It is derived from a mature, post-thymic peripheral T cell (232,346). The incidence and mortality rates of mycosis fungoides are increasing (418), although overall it is still considered a rare disease, representing less than 0.5 percent of all non-Hodgkin lymphomas (278). It can affect patients of widely ranging ages, although it most commonly arises in adult life. Men are affected more often than women (346). There is frequently a preceding history of an erythematous, scaling dermatitis, which may be present for years before the development of overt features of lymphoma. In some cases, contact dermatitis may be suspected as the underlying cause of the dermatitis.

Other, specific precursor dermatoses have been termed *parapsoriases*. Several types of lesions have received this designation, and two of these, *large plaque parapsoriasis (parapsoriasis en plaque)* and the rare *retiform (reticulated, or net-like) parapsoriasis (parapsoriasis variegata)* are considered to be frequent precursors of mycosis fungoides (286,287). Up to 30 percent of patients with large plaque parapsoriasis, and almost all patients with retiform parapsoriasis, are reported to develop mycosis fungoides (286, 287). In addition to erythema and scale, these forms of parapsoriasis may show degrees of atrophy, mottling of pigmentation, and telangiectasia (poikiloderma atrophicans vasculare). As is further discussed below, there are close clinical, histopathologic, and genetic similarities between parapsoriasis en plaque and early mycosis fungoides. It has therefore been suggested that parapsoriasis en plaque be regarded as an early stage of mycosis fungoides (385). This apparently has become the case in actual clinical practice, at least for the atrophic form of parapsoriasis en plaque, the diagnosis of which is now widely regarded as tantamount to a diagnosis of early mycosis fungoides (265).

There is greater controversy regarding the condition known as *small plaque parapsoriasis (chronic superficial dermatitis, digitate dermatosis)*. This persistent dermatosis is not characterized by progression to lymphoma. A dominant T-cell clone has been detected in some cases, also a feature of two other disorders frequently characterized by a benign clinical course: pityriasis lichenoides and lymphomatoid papulosis (234). This, as well as other clinical and histopathologic evidence, has led some authors to consider small plaque parapsoriasis either an abortive cutaneous T-cell lymphoma (171) or a true variant of mycosis fungoides (279).

The clinical history of mycosis fungoides is usually that of an erythematous, scaly eruption of long duration, with transition to limited patches or plaques often localized to the trunk. The disease may persist in this form for years, but eventually progresses to generalized infiltrative plaques or tumors, sometimes with ulceration. Erythroderma can develop, in some cases with the full clinical picture of Sézary's syndrome (see below), but in others, without the typical Sézary cells in the peripheral blood. Rarely, the disease begins with cutaneous tumors, the so called *d'emblee variant*, although it may be that some of these cases represent other types of T-cell lymphoma that involve the skin (e.g., subcutaneous panniculitis-like T-cell lymphoma) (346). There is a unilesional variant of mycosis fungoides, which by the very nature of its clinical presentation can create considerable diagnostic consternation. Although these lesions are often responsive to local therapy, recurrence and distant cutaneous spread can occur (244,330). Unusual cutaneous manifestations of mycosis fungoides include hypopigmented lesions, which are prone to occur in childhood and adolescence (212,421); bullous lesions (270); and lesions mimicking perioral dermatitis (432). Bullous pemphigoid has developed in mycosis fungoides lesions following ultraviolet therapy (334).

Another issue is the relationship between mycosis fungoides and *follicular mucinosis*. The latter, in the clinical form designated *alopecia mucinosa*, has historically been regarded as a benign dermatosis, characterized clinically by the development of boggy, hairless cutaneous plaques and microscopically by the accumulation of mucin within follicular epithelium. Progression to mycosis fungoides, however, has been reported in some cases of follicular mucinosis (164,224). Cerroni et al. (178) evaluated cases of follicular mucinosis with and without associated mycosis fungoides, and found that lymphoma-associated follicular mucinosis was more likely to occur in a slightly older age group (although with some overlap) and to present in body sites other than the head and neck. Lesions that were solitary at the time of presentation were uncommon in the lymphoma group. As had previously been reported (224), these authors found no obvious histopathologic differences between cases of follicular mucinosis with and without lymphoma, but they were able to find T-cell receptor γ gene rearrangements in half the patients from each group. This suggested to the authors that follicular mucinosis may represent a localized form of T-cell lymphoma in skin. There is also a *follicular variant* of mycosis fungoides that may not show the microscopic changes of follicular mucinosis. Clinically, follicular mycosis fungoides has presented as infiltrative plaques with dilated, comedo-like openings (283) or as lesions resembling dissecting cellulitis of the scalp (225).

A *syringotropic mycosis fungoides* has also been described (442). As in the case of follicular mucinosis, syringotropic mycosis fungoides bears a close relationship to a dermatosis known as *syringolymphoid hyperplasia*. The latter presents as brownish papules or patches, sometimes associated with alopecia or anhidrosis (395,401). Syringolymphoid hyperplasia can be idiopathic, coexist with established mycosis fungoides, or show T-cell receptor gene rearrangements (236,395,401).

Most often, extracutaneous dissemination of mycosis fungoides appears to be a late event, occurring with advanced cutaneous disease (278). Lymph nodes, liver, spleen, lung, and peripheral blood are involved; bone marrow involvement is rare (346). A sensitive PCR assay has detected malignant cells in morphologically uninvolved extracutaneous tissues (blood, lymph node, and/or bone marrow) from patients who had been classified clinical stage I (disease confined to the skin) (409). This suggests that covert extracutaneous involvement may be present even in early disease.

The prognosis of patients with mycosis fungoides depends upon the extent of disease, reflected in part by the clinical stage. Patients with cutaneous plaques only, and no systemic involvement, have an overall survival period of greater than 12 years (368), and those with limited plaque disease have survival periods that approach those of age-matched controls. Those with more advanced disease, including tumors, ulcers, and extracutaneous dissemination, have a less favorable prognosis. Patients with advanced cutaneous disease, with involvement of lymph nodes and peripheral blood but without node effacement or visceral involvement, have a median survival period of 5 years, and those with node effacement or visceral involvement have a median survival period of 2.5 years (368). Transformation to large cell lymphoma is generally associated with a markedly diminished survival period (179). Other clinical and laboratory features that are associated with an adverse prognosis include elevated lactate dehydrogenase levels, older age, African-American ethnicity, previous malignancy, or Sézary's syndrome at the time of diagnosis (346, 418). Certain microscopic and immunophenotypic characteristics may also influence prognosis; these are discussed below.

The etiology of mycosis fungoides has been of great interest. It has long been believed that chronic antigenic stimulation can trigger the disease, possibly through a breakdown in immune surveillance (394,398). This idea receives circumstantial support from the frequent clinical history of a preceding dermatitis or of potential exposure to toxins or allergens in industry (287). On the other hand, it is recognized that mycosis fungoides can itself mimic virtually every known inflammatory reaction pattern (381). This, plus the detection of T-cell gene rearrangements in early or precursor lesions, suggests that malignant cells are present from the very beginning, but are capable of eliciting a host inflammatory response that simultaneously obscures and helps to control the neoplastic process (232). This "chicken-egg" problem remains to be resolved.

The association of HTLV-1 with adult T-cell leukemia/lymphoma has stimulated interest in its possible role in mycosis fungoides. In one study, HTLV pol and/or tax proviral sequences were found in peripheral blood mononuclear cells in 92 percent of tested patients, and five patients lacking antibodies to HTLV-I/II structural proteins were seropositive for tax (333); however, no proviral integration of HTLV-I was detected in lesional skin of patients in a European study (163). It is apparent that further studies are needed to investigate the potential role of HTLV or other viruses in mycosis fungoides.

Pathologic Findings. Early lesions that in the past were designated parapsoriasis en plaque show foci of parakeratosis, mild acanthosis, and a superficial dermal infiltrate that can be mild and perivascular or somewhat more dense and band-like. Frequently, the band-like infiltrate is separated from the junctional zone by an ill-defined grenz zone of thickened papillary dermal collagen (fig. 13-28A). In later stages, parapsoriasis lesions show epidermal atrophy, with effacement of the rete ridges, vacuolar degeneration of the basilar layer with superficial dermal pigment deposition, telangiectasia, and a band-like lymphocytic infiltrate; these are changes that have been described as *poikiloderma atrophicans vasculare* (fig. 13-28B) (140,308). Some of the lymphocytes in these atrophic lesions possess convoluted nuclei, and as previously mentioned, this has contributed to the widely held view that atrophic large plaque parapsoriasis is in fact early patch stage mycosis fungoides (265,363).

A key finding in early mycosis fungoides is lymphocytic permeation of the epidermis in the face of minimal discernable spongiosis (fig. 13-28C) (236,381). If spongiosis is present, it may be due, in part, to an osmotic gradient created by the presence of intraepidermal, intercellular mucin (322). Lymphocytes may appear to line up along the basilar layer (323) or to migrate individually or in small groups into more superficial portions of the epidermis. Individual cells may reside within lacunae; these have been termed haloed cells (fig. 13-29A) (363, 388). Collections of lymphocytes within the epidermis are termed Pautrier's microabscesses, and when present are considered characteristic for mycosis fungoides (fig. 13-29B). The superficial dermal infiltrate often appears to permeate thickened, wiry, papillary dermal collagen (fig. 13-29C) (232,323,363).

In early stages, atypia among lymphocytes is often minimal, but this does not necessarily prevent a diagnosis of mycosis fungoides provided other configurational changes are present (363). In later stage patch lesions, there are increasing numbers of small to medium-sized lymphocytes with irregular or cerebriform nuclear contours. Early lesions often have admixtures of other cell types, including reactive lymphocytes, plasma cells, and eosinophils (323,346). Granulomatous inflammation is sometimes encountered, but this does not define a unique subset of cases (147) (however, see the discussion of granulomatous slack skin below).

In the more infiltrative, plaque stage lesions, the epidermal changes are accompanied by increasingly dense dermal infiltrates that tend to be band-like in the superficial dermis and patchy in the deep dermis (fig. 13-30A). These infiltrates contain increasing percentages of

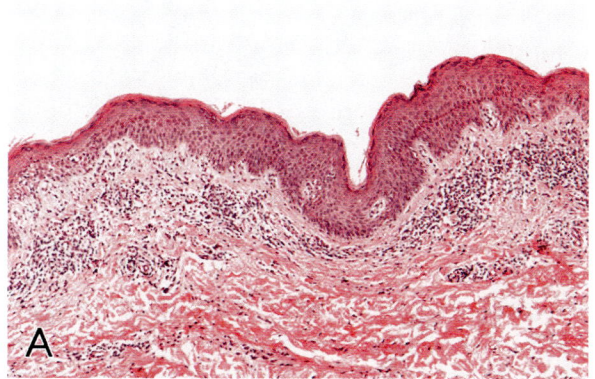

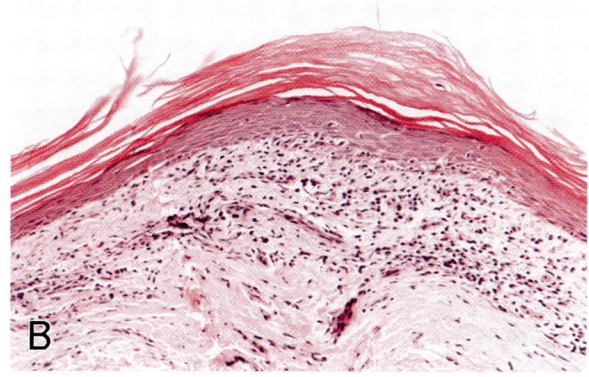

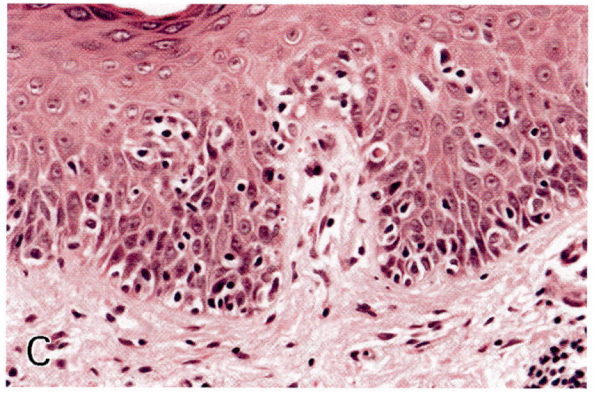

Figure 13-28

EARLY MYCOSIS FUNGOIDES (PARAPSORIASIS EN PLAQUE)

A: The band-like infiltrate in the superficial dermis is separated from the junctional zone by a grenz zone of thickened papillary dermal collagen.

B: This lesion has the configuration of poikiloderma atrophicans vasculare. Some atypical lymphocytes are present in the dermal infiltrate.

C: In this lesion that shows early evolution to mycosis fungoides, scattered solitary lymphocytes permeate the epidermis in the absence of spongiosis.

Figure 13-29

MYCOSIS FUNGOIDES, PATCH STAGE

A: Individual lymphocytes line up along the basilar layer and migrate singly into the epidermis. These cells appear to reside within small lacunae, and have been termed haloed cells.

B: Collections of atypical lymphocytes within the epidermis are termed Pautrier's microabscesses.

C: In the superficial dermis, lymphocytes appear to permeate thickened, wiry, papillary dermal collagen.

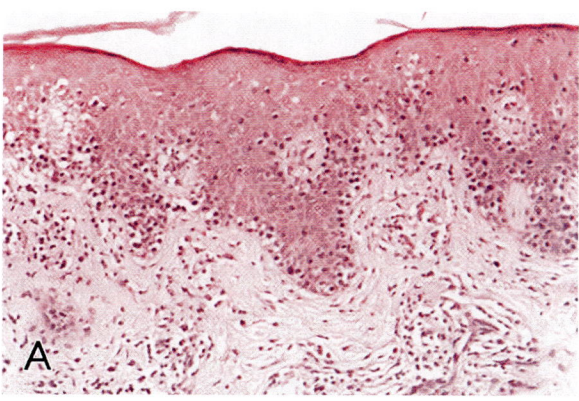

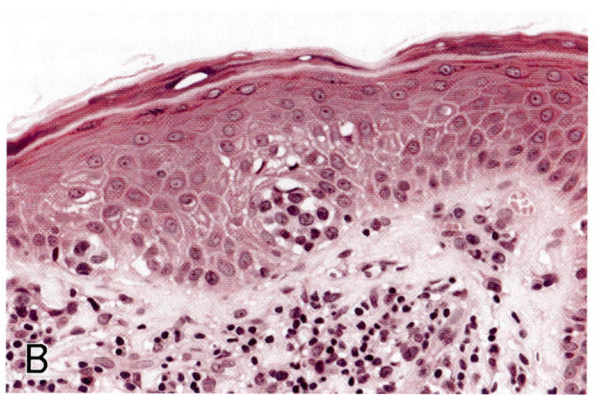

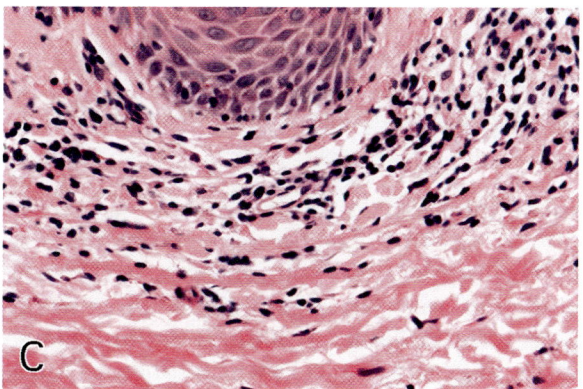

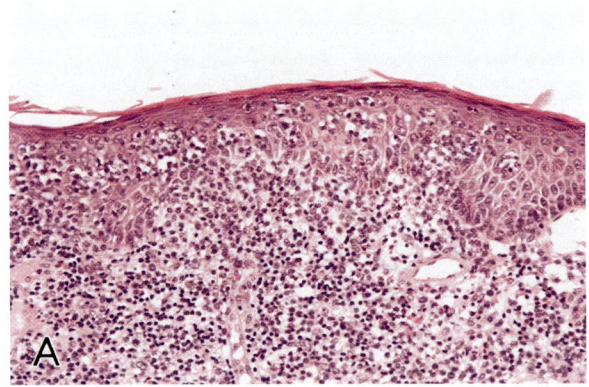
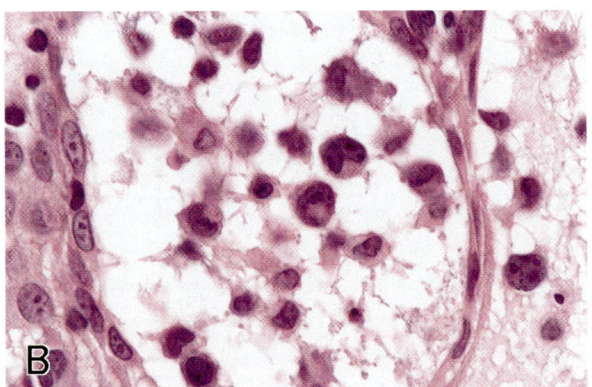
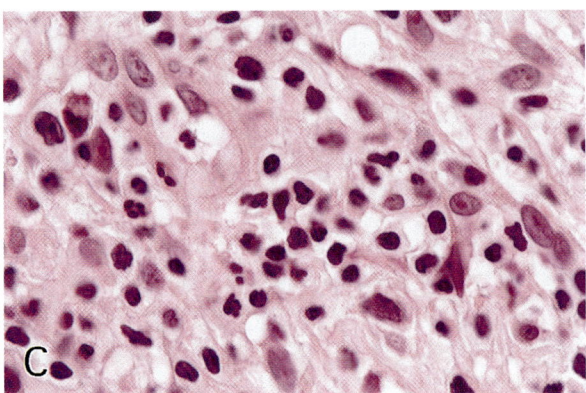

Figure 13-30

MYCOSIS FUNGOIDES, PLAQUE STAGE

Epidermotropism is pronounced, and there is a more prominent dermal infiltrate (A). Lymphocytes within the epidermis (B) are often larger than are those in the dermis (C).

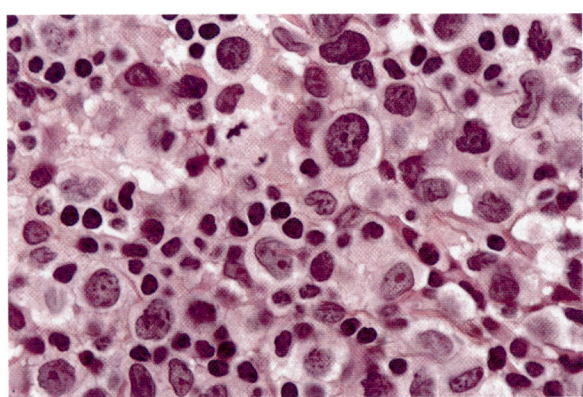

Figure 13-31

MYCOSIS FUNGOIDES, TUMOR STAGE

This lesion has undergone transformation. Note the predominance of large, pleomorphic lymphoid cells.

small, intermediate, and sometimes large lymphocytes with hyperchromatic, convoluted or cerebriform nuclei. Lymphocytes within the epidermis are often larger than are those in the dermis (fig. 13-30B,C) (388). In tumor stage lesions, large, atypical cells with numerous mitoses predominate and epidermal involvement diminishes (248). Transformation to large cell malignant lymphoma can occur and typically reflects a more aggressive clinical course. The cell morphology of transformed tumors includes medium to large-sized pleomorphic, immunoblastic, large cell anaplastic, and other unclassified types (fig. 13-31) (179).

Lymph nodes often show changes of dermatopathic lymphadenopathy, including paracortical expansion by macrophages and interdigitating cells, lipid accumulation in these cells, and melanin or hemosiderin deposition (371). A few scattered cells with cerebriform nuclei can be identified. In more advanced disease, clusters of lymphocytes with cerebriform nuclei are present that can partly or completely efface the normal architecture of the node (fig. 13-32) (193,346).

In follicular mucinosis, there is mucin accumulation within the follicular epithelium, frequently resulting in separation among keratinocytes, with microcyst formation. There is a surrounding inflammatory infiltrate composed of lymphocytes, macrophages, and eosinophils.

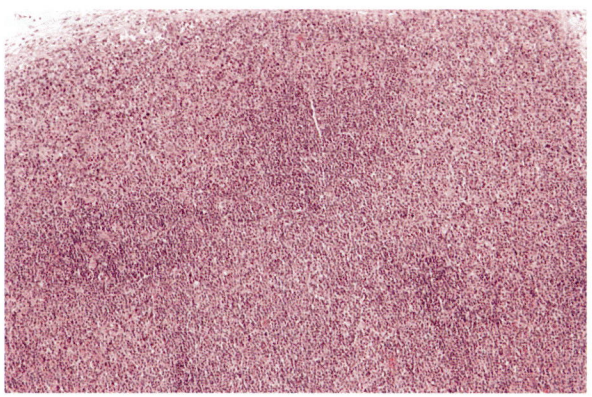
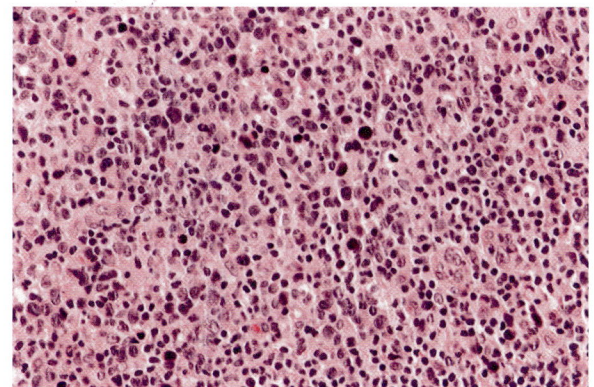

Figure 13-32

MYCOSIS FUNGOIDES INVOLVING LYMPH NODE

Left: The normal nodal architecture is effaced.
Right: There are numerous atypical lymphocytes with cerebriform nuclei.

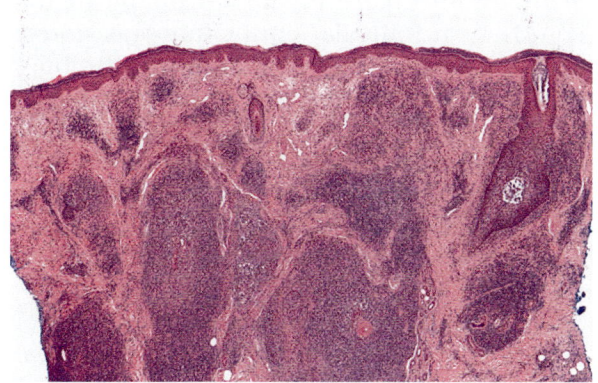
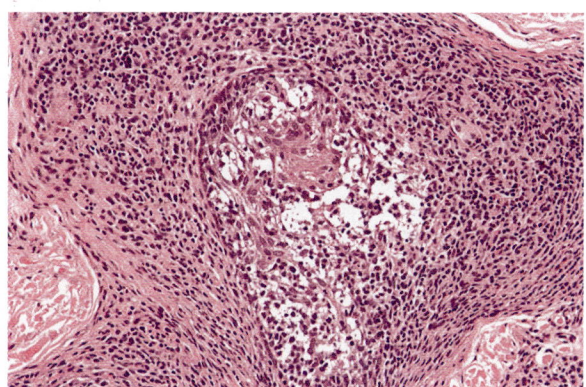

Figure 13-33

MYCOSIS FUNGOIDES, FOLLICULAR VARIANT

Left: There is pronounced follicular infiltration, in the absence of epidermal involvement.
Right: Folliculotropism can be associated with varying degrees of follicular mucinosis.

Follicular involvement in mycosis fungoides may combine the changes of follicular mucinosis with atypical lymphocytic infiltrates (fig. 13-33) (164). There is also a follicular variant of mycosis fungoides that lacks mucinous changes in the follicles but shows folliculotropism of atypical cells (including Pautrier's microabscess formation) in the absence of epidermotropism (283). Syringolymphoid hyperplasia shows hyperplastic eccrine glandular and ductal epithelium, periglandular lymphocytic infiltrates, and syringotropism (401,442).

The neoplastic cells in mycosis fungoides are T cells, usually of the T-helper (CD4 positive) phenotype. The most common immunohistochemical profile is therefore positivity for CD2, CD3, CD4, CD5, and TCRβ and negativity for CD8 (346,414). CD7 deficiency or "dropout" is a frequent finding in mycosis fungoides (346,435) and has been increasingly used as a diagnostic tool, particularly with the availability of an antibody that can now be used in paraffin-embedded tissues. CD7 deficiency can also be identified in early mycosis fungoides (parapsoriasis en plaque), but since it has been seen in benign cutaneous infiltrates, this feature in isolation is of limited value (292,344). However, CD7 counts as a percentage of total lymphocytes are significantly lower for patch stage mycosis fungoides than for benign inflammatory diseases (318). Furthermore, when used together with other morphologic, immunohistochemical, or genetic features, CD7 deficiency can be quite helpful. For example, the combination of CD7 deletion and T-cell receptor γ gene rearrangements is highly specific for mycosis fungoides (331). In addition, discordance of dermal and epidermal expression of pan-T-cell antigens, including CD5, CD7, and TCRβ (expression in the dermis, but not in the epidermis) is seen in mycosis fungoides and not in inflammatory skin diseases (312).

A recent study has shown absent or weak surface CD26 expression in peripheral blood T cells from patients with mycosis fungoides and Sézary's syndrome, allowing better separation from normal peripheral blood T cells than could be achieved by analyzing CD7 expression (188). It will be interesting to assess the utility of CD26 staining in formalin-fixed, paraffin-embedded tissues.

CD8 positivity can occur in two settings: as a rare variant of mycosis fungoides, or as a population of reactive T-cytotoxic cells. CD8-positive tumors may be rapidly progressive and show a poor response to therapy (138,342), although there are also indolent variants of CD8-positive mycosis fungoides (209,423). Among CD8-positive cases, there may be differences in biologic behavior related to the phenotypic profile of the neoplastic cells. Thus, in one study, patients who experienced rapid progression of the disease bore the phenotype CD8 positive, CD4 negative, CD2 negative, CD3 positive, and CD7 positive, whereas those who had chronic disease (more typical of CD4-positive mycosis fungoides) had the phenotype CD8 positive, CD4 negative, CD2 positive, CD3 positive, and CD7 negative (138).

There is some dispute regarding the role of tumor-infiltrating CD8-positive lymphocytes in the prognosis of patients with mycosis fungoides. Earlier studies concluded that the presence of CD8-positive cells did not correlate with response to topical treatment or subsequent clinical course of pretumoral mycosis fungoides (414). On the other hand, more recent studies have found that in each stage of the disease, patients with a larger proportion of CD8-positive cells had improved survival rates, implying that these cells may indeed exert antitumor effects (246).

Additional antigens expressed by the neoplastic cells in mycosis fungoides include HECA-452, an antigen associated with lymphocyte homing to the skin (427); CD44v6, a glycoprotein involved in cell-cell and cell-matrix interactions, and associated with aggressive behavior of cutaneous T-cell lymphomas (206); and cytotoxic granule-associated proteins, which are expressed to a greater degree in the tumor stage of the disease (410). Examples of mycosis fungoides in which the neoplastic cells express γ/δ receptors have been reported (154). In a study of follicular mycosis fungoides, upregulation of intercellular adhesion molecule (ICAM)-1 on follicular epithelium was noted, providing a possible explanation for the preferential follicular homing of adjacent, lymphocyte function-associated antigen (LFA)-1–positive lymphoma cells (225).

Electron microscopy has been used to enhance diagnostic accuracy. This has been accomplished by developing formulae to express degrees of nuclear contour irregularity. McNutt and Crain (310) accomplished this by calculating a nuclear contour index (NCI), representing the nuclear profile circumference divided by the square root of the nuclear area. Using this measurement, these authors found that a diagnosis of mycosis fungoides could be made with a mean NCI of 6.1 or greater and at least 6 percent of lymphocytes with an NCI of 9.0 or greater. There was a low false-positive rate, and a 50 percent false-negative rate for early mycosis fungoides.

T-cell receptor gene rearrangements are found in mycosis fungoides (331,346). Other reported genetic abnormalities include *p16 (INK4a)* gene alterations, more common in tumor stage than in plaque stage lesions (321), and loss of heterozygosity on 10q and microsatellite instability, again in advanced stages of the disease (370).

Differential Diagnosis. The most important differential diagnostic problem in mycosis fungoides is its distinction in early stages from benign reactive inflammatory processes. These inflammatory conditions can show rather dense dermal infiltrates and exocytosis of lymphocytes, including collections of cells within the epidermis that can mimic Pautrier's microabscess, although they are usually present within the context of spongiosis, an ingredient that is often absent in mycosis fungoides (135). Activated T cells with small but irregularly shaped nuclei can be seen in chronic inflammatory processes, such as contact dermatitis, while at the same time the degree of cytologic atypia in early mycosis fungoides is often minimal (363).

Despite these problems, it is generally recognized that the traditional light microscopic diagnosis is the "gold standard" for the early diagnosis of mycosis fungoides (323). Therefore, numerous studies have been undertaken to establish morphologic criteria for diagnosis. Reviews of large numbers of cases of mycosis fungoides have emphasized the diagnostic importance of lymphocytes, singly and in small clusters, within the epidermis (in the absence of spongiotic vesiculation). Other important findings include lacunae around intraepidermal lymphocytes (haloed cells), lymphocytes singly distributed along a broad front of basilar epidermis, a dermal infiltrate that includes plasma cells and eosinophils as well as lymphocytes, and papillary dermal fibrosis, with singly dispersed lymphocytes permeating wiry collagen (323,363). The significance of these features has been supported in a statistical analysis of the histopathologic features of mycosis fungoides (388), along with the presence of hyperconvoluted intraepidermal lymphocytes that are larger than dermal lymphocytes (388). Pautrier's microabscesses, when found, are diagnostically useful, but they are present only in a minority of cases (346,388).

Despite the widespread knowledge of these microscopic features, there has continued to be a lack of diagnostic agreement among pathologists (329). In an attempt to standardize pathology reports of mycosis fungoides, Guitart et al. (232) have recently developed a microscopic grading system. Major criteria are based upon the density of the dermal infiltrate, prominence of epidermotropism, and degree of cytologic atypia, and minor criteria are related to papillary dermal fibroplasia, atypia of intraepidermal lymphocytes, and lack of inflammatory features. In this system, a score of 7 or more is considered diagnostic for mycosis fungoides.

Computer-assisted morphometric analysis has been employed to enhance the evaluation of nuclear irregularities in cutaneous infiltrates. Such an analysis can improve the ability to discriminate early mycosis fungoides from a traditionally difficult inflammatory dermatosis, contact dermatitis (351). Immunohistochemistry can also be of value. An infiltrate comprised of 70 percent or greater T cells (as assessed by pan-T-cell markers), with a CD4 to CD8 ratio 6 or higher, permits a high level of discrimination between cutaneous T-cell lymphoma and other disorders (414). Although there are problems regarding the specificity of CD7 deficiency, as noted above, this finding can gain significance when combined with other immunohistochemical features or gene rearrangement studies (331).

There are several other disorders that can be confused with mycosis fungoides. One of these, actinic reticuloid, is a chronic photodermatitis associated with erythema, induration, and demonstrable sensitivity to a variety of wavelengths of light. Microscopically, actinic reticuloid can closely resemble mycosis fungoides, including exocytosis and formation of Pautrier-like microabscesses. There is a predominance of CD8-positive cells in the epidermis in actinic reticuloid, a finding that differs from most cases of mycosis fungoides. The demonstration of photosensitivity or T-cell receptor gene rearrangements supports the diagnosis of actinic reticuloid or mycosis fungoides, respectively. Two patients, however, have recently been reported with photosensitivity and lack of T-cell receptor gene rearrangements who progressed to microscopic and genotypic mycosis fungoides (200). A study is needed that provides a detailed comparison of the lymphocyte antigen profile of these two conditions.

A mycosis fungoides-like dermatosis also occurs in association with phenytoin or carbamazepine therapy. This can present as a Sézary-like erythroderma or as plaque type lesions (196,353). Microscopically, the findings are quite similar to those of mycosis fungoides, and numerous lymphocytes with cerebriform nuclei are observed. The immunohistochemical profile shows a marked CD4 predominance (353). Keys to the diagnosis include an absence of T-cell receptor gene rearrangements (167) and often rapid resolution of the dermatosis upon discontinuation of the offending drug (167,196,353,433).

Pagetoid Reticulosis

Clinical Features. *Pagetoid reticulosis* is a limited form of cutaneous T-cell lymphoma that generally follows an indolent clinical course and displays marked epidermotropism of atypical lymphocytes. The name *localized epidermotropic reticulosis* has also been applied to this condition (302), although this designation is not widely used. Two forms of the disease are known. The best accepted is *Woringer-Kolopp disease*, characterized by solitary or localized lesions. A disseminated form, *Ketron-Goodman disease*, may be difficult if not impossible to distinguish from mycosis fungoides, and therefore it is not widely accepted as a form of pagetoid reticulosis.

Localized pagetoid reticulosis, or Woringer-Kolopp disease, presents as an erythematous, scaly to verrucous plaque that characteristically arises on the distal extremities (235,302,438). A possible example involving the palms and soles has been reported (309), and a lesion on the tongue has been described (235). It occurs most often in middle-aged adults but can arise in young persons; males are affected more often than females (235,302). Untreated, these lesions may persist for years, but generally they respond well to therapy, particularly surgical excision or radiation therapy (302). Lesions can recur after treatment or following spontaneous resolution (235). The development of disseminated lesions after apparently successful removal of a localized lesion has also been reported (438). A disseminated, or Ketron-Goodman variant, has been reported from time to time (160,194,295). It may be that these cases actually represent mycosis fungoides with extensive epidermotropism, but this remains a controversial issue (354). The argument that disseminated examples are not mycosis fungoides because the lesions may lack CD4 expression is not convincing, since CD4-negative cases of mycosis fungoides have been reported, some of which are characterized by rapid progression (138).

Pathologic Findings. The epidermis is variably hyperkeratotic and acanthotic. There is extensive infiltration of the epidermis by atypical lymphocytes arranged in a pagetoid configuration. These may be particularly numerous in lower portions of the epidermis (302). The lymphocytes feature hyperchromatic, convoluted nuclei and often reside within lacunae (haloed cells) (fig. 13-34A,B). Nuclear convolutions are particularly striking in ultrathin sections, and nucleoli are prominent (437). The dermal infiltrate may be rather sparse, and is composed of bland-appearing, reactive lymphocytes and macrophages (fig. 13-34C); eosinophils are not commonly observed (235,309,437).

Pagetoid reticulosis is characterized immunohistochemically by phenotypic heterogeneity. Although some cases show a predominance of CD4-positive cells, many other examples are CD8 positive, thereby expressing the phenotype of cytotoxic T lymphocytes (172,195,204, 235,298,309). CD4-, CD8-negative cases have also been reported (235). There may be reduced expression of CD7 and leu-8, with preservation of other pan-T-cell markers such as CD2, CD3, and CD5 (172). CD30 expression has been detected (235,389), as has the proliferation marker Ki-67 (235). The neoplastic T cells express the adhesion molecules cutaneous lymphocyte antigen and alpha-E-beta 7 (208,309). These molecules interact with E-selectin and E-cadherin on epithelial cells, and their expression may explain, in part, the pagetoid growth pattern and unique biologic behavior of these tumors (208). On ultrastructural examination, the infiltrating lymphocytes display cerebriform nuclei, resembling those of mycosis fungoides (204,302,389). T-cell receptor gene rearrangements have been found in pagetoid reticulosis (235,309), but not invariably (172).

Differential Diagnosis. The major consideration in the differential diagnosis of pagetoid reticulosis is its distinction from mycosis fungoides, and in particular, from unilesional mycosis fungoides. Although this distinction may not be possible in all cases, pagetoid reticulosis is typified by a particular clinical and histopathologic profile that usually permits its recognition; this information has been summarized by Haghighi et al. (235). Verrucoid plaques localized to distal extremities are more likely to represent pagetoid reticulosis. Microscopic changes favoring pagetoid reticulosis over mycosis fungoides include: neoplastic cells confined to the epidermis, a dermal infiltrate restricted to reactive cells with a sparsity or absence

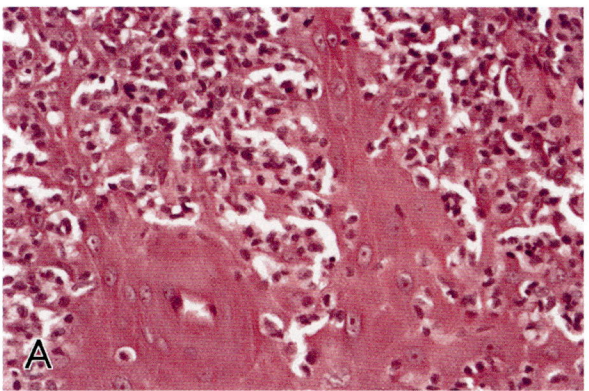
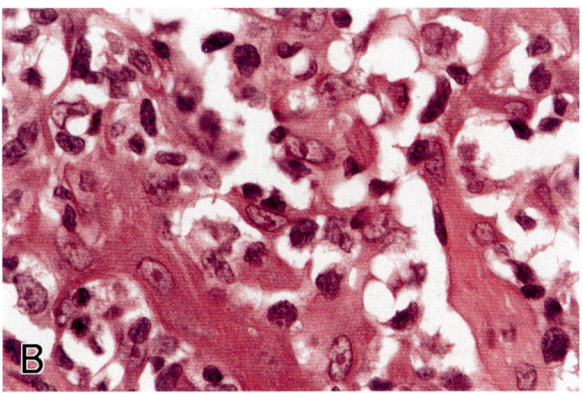
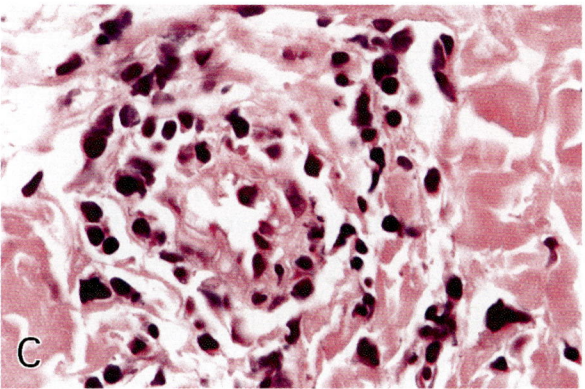

Figure 13-34

PAGETOID RETICULOSIS

A: The epidermis is permeated by atypical lymphocytes. A few haloed cells are noted.

B: The lymphoid cells possess hyperchromatic, convoluted nuclei.

C: The dermal infiltrate is sparse, and is comprised mainly of bland-appearing, reactive lymphocytes.

of eosinophils, and neoplastic T cells that are more likely to be CD8 positive or CD4, CD8 negative, to express CD30, and to demonstrate a high proliferation rate via Ki-67 positivity.

Granulomatous Slack Skin

Clinical Features. *Granulomatous slack skin* is an usual form of cutaneous T-cell lymphoma in which exaggerated folds of erythematous skin develop in flexural sites, associated with a granulomatous as well as an atypical lymphocytic infiltrate. Less than 40 cases have been reported. This condition appears predominantly to develop in middle-aged adults, but children have also been affected (174,324). Lesions begin as erythematous patches and plaques that evolve into areas of lax, pendulous skin (152,288,324). These are located especially in the axillae, groin, and abdomen. The condition tends to be relatively indolent, but progression to systemic lymphoma has occurred (290,407), and an association with Hodgkin's disease has been reported on several occasions (201,288,324). The lesions of granulomatous slack skin can be controlled with a variety of therapies, including surgery, radiation therapy, systemic corticosteroids, and interferon-alpha (288,324).

Pathologic Findings. There is a diffuse dermal and subcutaneous infiltrate of lymphocytes with convoluted nuclei (290,403); epidermotropism is present (288). The unique feature of granulomatous slack skin is the presence of a widespread granulomatous infiltrate with numerous multinucleated giant cells (404); the giant cells may contain numerous nuclei (fig. 13-35) (290). Special stains demonstrate elastolysis, with extensive loss of elastic fibers (290, 324,403) explaining the laxity of skin noted clinically. The infiltrating lymphocytes are T cells that display the helper T-cell phenotype (174,243,289,403,434); the granulomatous component of the infiltrate is CD68 and variably MAC387 positive (174,243,403).

On ultrastructural study, the giant cells possess villous processes and lysosomes, features associated with macrophages (403). In one study, the lysosomes had unusual configurations, including small vacuoles that fused with

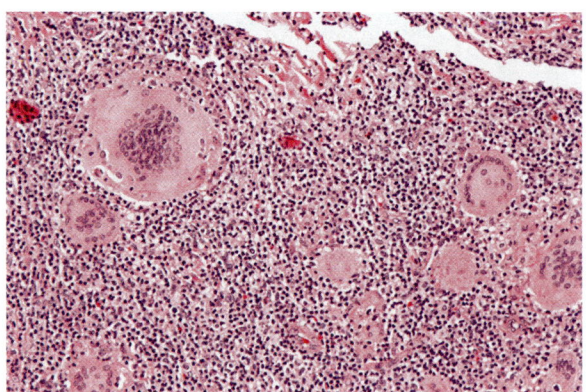 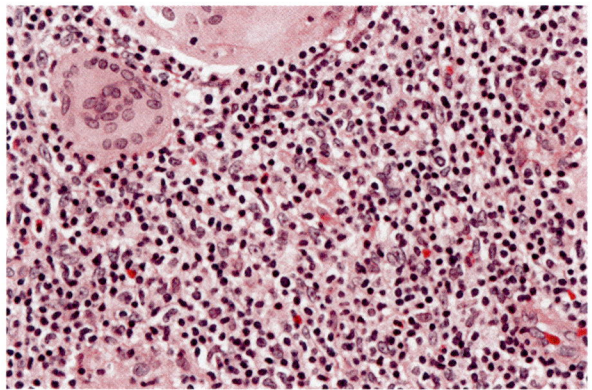

Figure 13-35

GRANULOMATOUS SLACK SKIN

Left: There are giant cells containing multiple nuclei, associated with a diffuse dermal lymphoid infiltrate.
Right: The lymphoid infiltrate is composed of cells with irregular nuclear contours.

mitochondria and cup-shaped forms that produced a resemblance to Birbeck granules (404). Clonal rearrangements of the T-cell receptor gene have been repeatedly demonstrated (174,230,289,407). Trisomy of chromosome 8 was found in one case (230).

Differential Diagnosis. The clinical features of granulomatous slack skin are distinctive. The demonstration of an atypical lymphoid infiltrate with epidermotropism allows differentiation from inflammatory granulomatous disorders. On microscopic grounds, a distinction from granulomatous mycosis fungoides unassociated with the typical clinical features of granulomatous slack skin could be difficult. Permeation of the entire dermis and subcutis by lymphocytes, even distribution of granulomas and giant cells, and complete dermal elastolysis are features that favor the diagnosis of granulomatous slack skin (290). It remains to be seen whether this distinction makes any consistent difference in terms of the ultimate prognosis of the associated lymphoma.

Sézary's Syndrome

Clinical Features. *Sézary's syndrome* is a form of T-cell lymphoma consisting of erythroderma, lymphadenopathy, and circulating atypical T cells in the peripheral blood. It is often considered the leukemic variant of mycosis fungoides (412). It is primarily a disease of adults (427), but childhood cases have been reported (250, 311). The erythroderma is accompanied by severe pruritus. Palmoplantar keratoderma and nail dystrophy are also observed in some cases (173). Among the unusual cutaneous manifestations that sometimes occur is an eruption of seborrheic keratoses (251). This has been considered to be a variant of the sign of Leser-Trelat, an eruption of seborrheic keratoses associated with internal malignant neoplasms. Some experts do not accept this designation, however, since seborrheic keratoses can develop in erythrodermas that are not associated with malignant processes. The cutaneous changes are associated with lymphadenopathy and at least 1,000 atypical cells (Sézary cells) per mm^3 of blood (346). It has been proposed that the diagnosis of Sézary's syndrome should also be supported by demonstration of a clonal T-cell population in the peripheral blood (360). Erythrodermic mycosis fungoides also occurs; these cases lack the circulating atypical T cells (277).

Sézary's syndrome follows an aggressive clinical course, with an overall 5-year survival rate ranging from 10 to 33 percent (158,427). Clinical and laboratory findings that unfavorably affect prognosis include a previous history of mycosis fungoides, age over 65 years, advanced lymph node stage, high number of circulating leukocytes, Sézary cells in the peripheral blood, and elevated serum lactate dehydrogenase levels (158,277). Treatment includes the use of topical and systemic chemotherapy (237), monoclonal antibodies, retinoids, cyclosporin, interferon, and extracorporeal photopheresis (426).

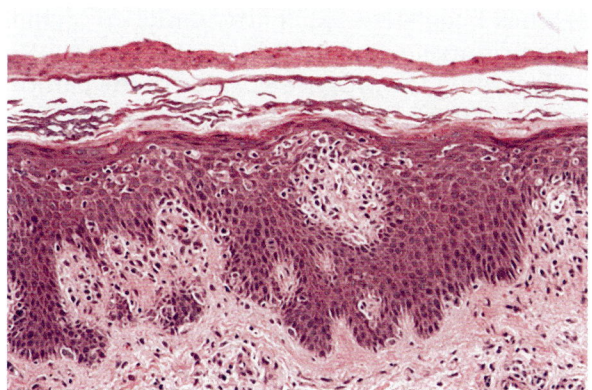 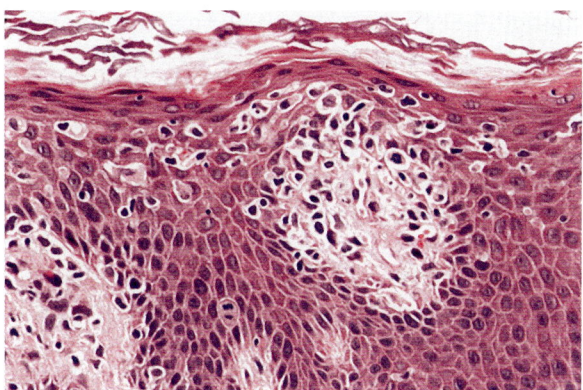

Figure 13-36

SÉZARY'S SYNDROME

Left: Confluent parakeratosis and acanthosis are seen.
Right: Epidermotropism is extensive.

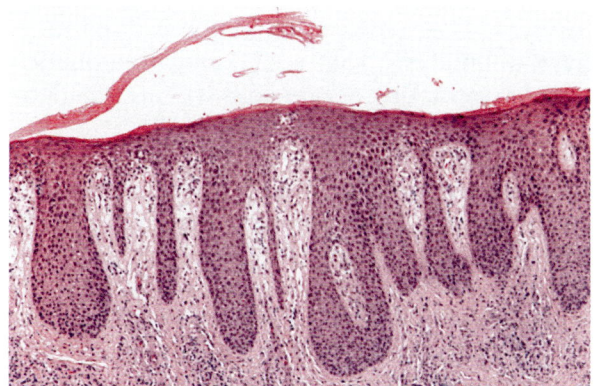 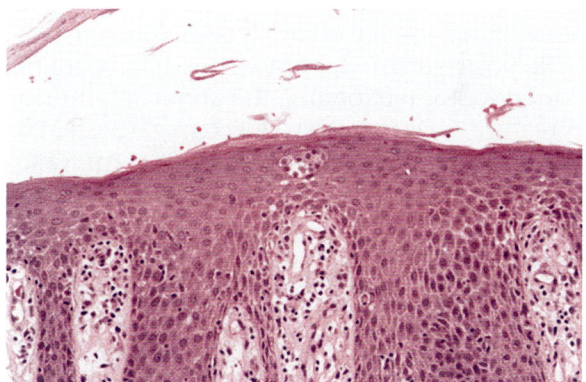

Figure 13-37

SÉZARY'S SYNDROME

Left: Low-power findings are those of a spongiotic psoriasiform dermatitis.
Right: On high-power magnification, rare Pautrier's microabscesses are seen.

Pathologic Findings. In the classic form of the disease, there is a band-like subepidermal lymphocytic infiltrate containing varying proportions of atypical cells that possess cerebriform nuclei (170). Epidermotropism can be present (fig. 13-36), and Pautrier's microabscesses are sometimes observed (426). When present, the latter structures are of great help in distinguishing Sézary's syndrome from benign forms of erythroderma (378). In some studies, only a minority of cases showed epidermal involvement of the type seen in traditional mycosis fungoides (170). When compared to patch and plaque stages of mycosis fungoides, erythrodermic cases tend to show comparatively less epidermotropism and fewer lymphocytes lining up along the basilar layer of the epidermis (284). At the same time, when compared to patch and plaque stage mycosis fungoides, skin biopsies in Sézary's syndrome show greater degrees of parakeratosis and acanthosis, more cells with convoluted nuclei in the dermis, and greater degrees of papillary dermal fibrosis and telangiectasia (284). Unfortunately, features of nonspecific chronic dermatitis predominate in 17 to 33 percent of cases (170,402) and accompany more diagnostic changes in others (378), creating significant diagnostic difficulties (fig. 13-37). In one case, granulomas resembling those of sarcoidosis were found in both skin and lymph nodes (231). In contrast to mycosis fungoides, Sézary's syndrome shows early nodal involvement. Lymph nodes show infiltration by varying numbers of lymphocytes with cerebriform nuclei; the changes have been classified in three grades, depending upon the degree of effacement of lymph node tissue (173).

As is the case for mycosis fungoides, Sézary's syndrome usually consists of a proliferation of lymphocytes that mark as helper T cells, and are therefore CD4 positive (158,210,245,278, 412). There is usually a predominance over CD8-positive, cytotoxic T cells, with CD4 to CD8 ratios ranging from 2 to 1 to greater than 10 to 1 (338,412); however, a case with a predominance of cytotoxic T cells (presumably CD8 positive) in the epidermis has been reported (338). Frequently, the atypical lymphocytes are CD4 positive, CD7 negative (210, 278,360), but this is not invariably the case. Clonal populations of cells can also be CD4, CD7-positive (210). Using flow cytometry on blood lymphocytes, Vonderheid et al. (412) showed that CD7 expression did not clearly segregate into two distinct CD7-positive or CD7-negative subgroups, and in some cases CD4-, CD7-positive tumor populations became CD4 positive, CD7 negative over time. The neoplastic cells may be positive for CD2, CD3, CD5, and CD45RO (210). Use of monoclonal antibodies to T-cell receptor variable regions on the beta chain (Vβ) has shown significant expansion of malignant cell populations, beyond what would be expected by morphology or traditional phenotypic markers alone (242).

Ultrastructural studies demonstrate tumor cells with high nuclear contour indices, allowing distinction from reactive lymphocytes or those of other lymphocytic leukemias (335). A close association between atypical lymphocytes and dendritic cells has been observed by electron microscopy, suggesting a possible pathogenetic relationship between these cells (358). T-cell receptor gene rearrangements are regularly demonstrated (210,278), best by PCR methods (360). Cytogenetic studies show aneuploidy (426), and a variety of clonal abnormalities has been detected, particularly involving chromosomes 1 and 8 (397).

Regarding the prognostic value of the pathologic findings, there is little or no correlation between prognosis and histopathologic pattern or degree of lymph node involvement (170, 173). PAS-positive cytoplasmic inclusions and large circulating Sézary cells have been found to be independent adverse prognostic factors (158). Large cell transformation (i.e., cells that are four or more times larger than a normal lymphocyte), forming microscopic nodules or involving more than 25 percent of an infiltrate, is associated with diminished survival. Elevated levels of β2-microglobulin and lactate dehydrogenase are predictive of transformation (205). The importance of CD7 expression is a matter of controversy. In one study, CD7 expression on blood lymphocytes did not correlate with survival (412), while another showed, by multivariate analysis, that a CD7-negative phenotype of circulating Sézary cells was an independent adverse prognostic factor (158).

Differential Diagnosis. The diagnosis of Sézary's syndrome is not a major problem when erythroderma, lymphadenopathy, and characteristic circulating atypical lymphocytes in the peripheral blood are accompanied by skin biopsies that show atypical, band-like cutaneous infiltrates, epidermotropism, and Pautrier's microabscesses. Unfortunately, the cutaneous changes may be nonspecific, resembling those of a variety of forms of chronic dermatitis (170,284,402). Occasionally, benign forms of erythroderma can have microscopic features suggesting Sézary's syndrome (378); this is particularly the case in some pseudolymphomas due to phenytoin therapy (196). Circulating cells with morphologic characteristics of Sézary cells can be observed in patients with contact or atopic dermatitis, or exfoliative psoriasis (211). In these difficult circumstances, close clinical follow-up, repeat biopsies, and evaluations of blood and lymph nodes are important (378,402). The demonstration of a clonal T-cell population through T-cell receptor gene analysis is a key criterion for diagnosis (360,402). In cases of pseudolymphoma due to phenytoin therapy, discontinuation of the drug is associated with dramatic and sustained remission of signs and symptoms (196).

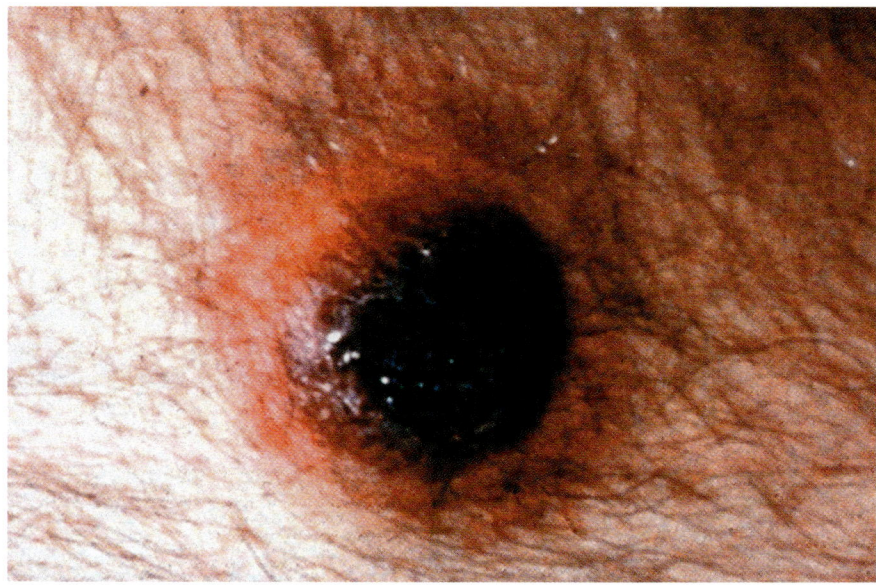

Figure 13-38

ANAPLASTIC LARGE CELL LYMPHOMA

An ulcerated red-violet nodule is in the skin of the leg.

Primary and Secondary Cutaneous Anaplastic Large Cell Lymphoma

Clinical Features. Malignant lymphomas composed of large cells have the potential to simulate other poorly differentiated tumors in the skin, such as high-grade carcinomas and malignant melanomas. The neoplasm that is now known as *anaplastic large cell non-Hodgkin's lymphoma* (ALCL) is one of the most able morphologic masqueraders in this category of tumors (137,153,190,267,281,314,340,396). It is also important because it has become a controversial entity regarding a definitive diagnostic distinction, or lack thereof, among Hodgkin's disease, non-Hodgkin's lymphoma, and malignant histiocytosis (141,202,219,291,359).

Clinically, the primary disease in the skin is often indolent, with lesions that may regress spontaneously. The tumor disseminates systemically only late in the clinical course, if at all. The appearance of ALCL is typical of malignant hematopoietic diseases of the skin in general, with violaceous or reddish plaques and nodules that may ulcerate (fig. 13-38).

The "purity" of ALCL as a pathologic entity has been questioned (336), since some of these lesions are T-cell tumors, and others are apparent null cell neoplasms. Moreover, there is a great deal of pathologic and immunologic similarity (but clinical discordance) between lymph node–based (systemic) ALCL that involves the skin, and several other immunophenotypically related primary cutaneous tumors. The latter include regressing atypical histiocytosis, malignant histiocytosis, lymphomatoid papulosis, and transformed (dedifferentiated) mycosis fungoides (with the latter being considered a form of secondary ALCL), all of which are CD30 positive (137,153,190,267,273,281,314,340,361,396).

Systemic cutaneous ALCL does behave in a predictable fashion, however, in the 40 percent to 60 percent of patients with systemic disease who have involvement of the skin. It tends to be an adverse-prognosis tumor that is often of high stage at presentation and responds relatively poorly to chemotherapy regardless of T-cell or null-cell lineage (213). In addition, it demonstrates a nonrandom karyotypic abnormality, with a t(2;5)(p23;q35) chromosomal translocation, and corresponding expression of the ALK-1 gene product in roughly 60 percent of cases (177,282,305). On the other hand, primary cutaneous ALCL (showing no systemic involvement) usually lacks the t(2;5) and is ALK-1 negative (213).

Pathologic Findings. Tumors in the ALCL group demonstrate a great deal of cellular heteromorphism, including large bizarre pleomorphic elements, multinucleated forms with "wreath" configurations of peripheralized nuclei, monomorphic large or small epithelioid cells (figs. 13-39–13-41), and even sarcomatoid

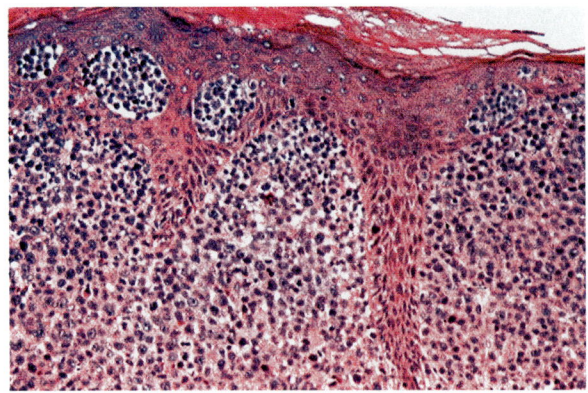

Figure 13-39
ANAPLASTIC LARGE CELL LYMPHOMA
Scanning power photomicrograph demonstrates effacement of the dermis by large, pleomorphic, obviously atypical tumor cells, whose lymphoid lineage is not immediately apparent morphologically.

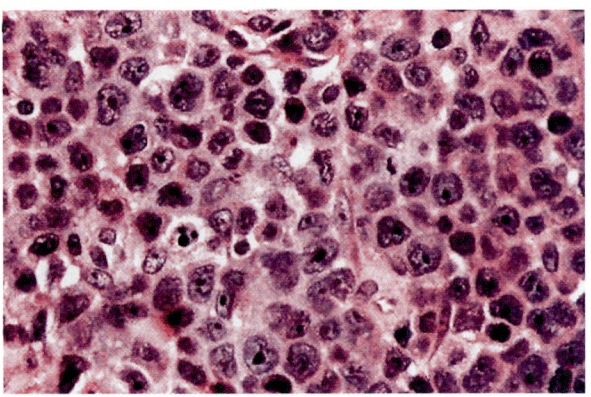

Figure 13-40
ANAPLASTIC LARGE CELL LYMPHOMA
The large epithelioid elements could easily be mistaken for those of a carcinoma or melanoma.

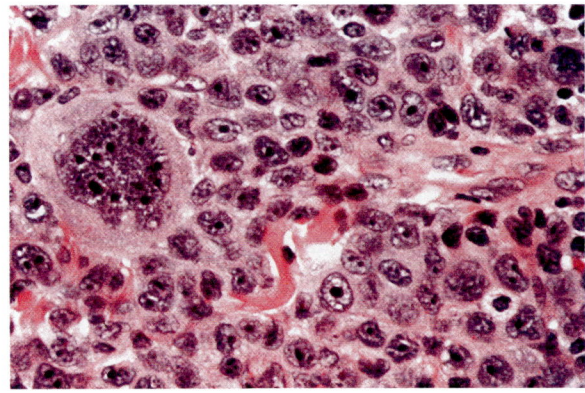

Figure 13-41
ANAPLASTIC LARGE CELL LYMPHOMA
Striking cytologic pleomorphism is evident, with gigantiform cells demonstrating multiple "wreath-like" nuclei.

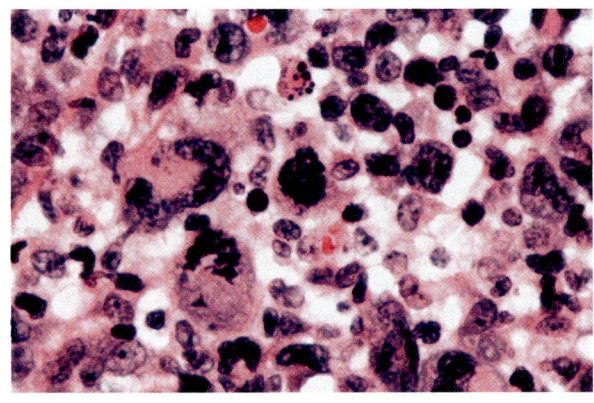

Figure 13-42
ANAPLASTIC LARGE CELL LYMPHOMA
Pathologically shaped mitotic figures are seen.

cells that assume a bluntly fusiform appearance and may be associated with myxoid stroma. Interposed reactive (non-neoplastic) inflammatory cells, including plasma cells, eosinophils, and neutrophils, also may be prominent. Recognized variants include *lymphohistiocytic, small cell, giant cell,* and *signet ring cell ALCL* (137,153,181, 183,190,267,281,314,336,340,341,396). Mitoses are numerous and are often atypically shaped (fig. 13-42); unlike other forms of lymphoma, ALCL also may exhibit large zones of geographic necrosis. Some of these lesions correspond to tumors that were formerly called *anemone cell lymphomas* or *microvillous lymphomas* (280). The latter were defined at an ultrastructural level as hematopoietic proliferations that demonstrate very elaborate, "bushy," cell surface projections that resemble the spines of a sea anemone. It has now been shown by several authors that ALCL may lack leukocyte common antigen (CD45) while paradoxically expressing epithelial membrane antigen (fig. 13-43), and well-documented examples have even shown aberrant keratin immunoreactivity (208,214,218,233). Given

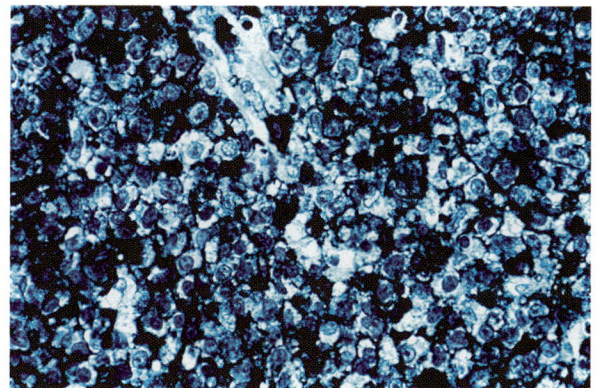

Figure 13-43

ANAPLASTIC LARGE CELL LYMPHOMA

There is "aberrant" immunoreactivity for epithelial membrane antigen.

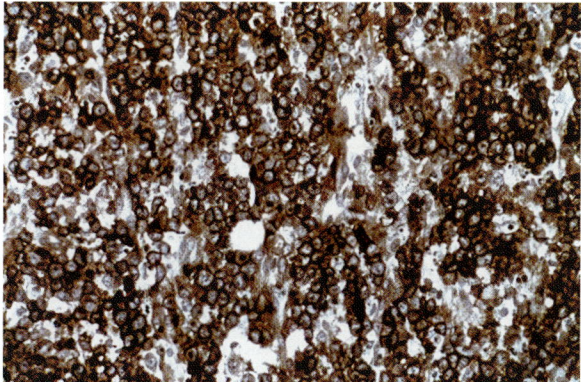

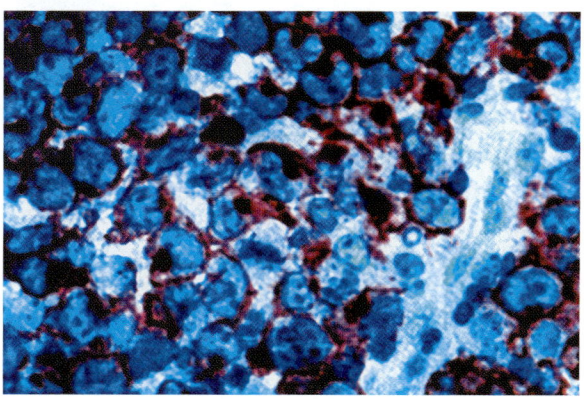

Figure 13-44

ANAPLASTIC LARGE CELL LYMPHOMA

Top: Immunoreactivity for CD30 is observed in virtually all tumor cells

Bottom: Cellular labeling involves both the plasmalemmae and the Golgi zones of the neoplastic lymphoid cells.

the fact that these determinants form the basic framework of the approach to separating carcinomas and lymphomas, occasional examples of ALCL are misdiagnosed as epithelial tumors. There is no facile remedy to this problem, except for the routine application of antibody panels, and the routine inclusion of reagents that recognize CD30 antigens (i.e., Ki-1, BerH2) (fig. 13-44) as well as keratin and CD45. Fortunately, the aberrant expression of epithelial determinants is rare in primary cutaneous ALCL.

Differential Diagnosis. Approximately 75 percent of cases of ALCL in the skin express CD45, and over 90 percent lack keratin. Almost all cases show CD30 immunoreactivity, and some authors require the presence of that marker for a diagnosis. Metastatic embryonal (germ cell) carcinoma is the only truly epithelial neoplasm known to be capable of showing a similar phenotype, so other appropriate markers (such as antiplacental alkaline phosphatase [anti-PLAP], a germ cell determinant) are used to avoid confusion of these two tumor types.

Parenthetically, it should be remembered that the CD30 antigen is nothing more than an "activation" marker that happens to be shared by ALCL, lymphomatoid papulosis, other non-Hodgkin's lymphoma morphotypes, and nonlymphocyte-predominant Hodgkin's lymphoma (390). The question of why some subsets of those neoplasms express that determinant is unanswered at the present time. Some benign reactive lymphoproliferative conditions, such as those seen in EBV infections and other florid immunoblastic viral reactions, may likewise express CD30 and, therefore, this determinant should never be utilized by itself as an indicator of malignancy.

The latter point is crucial when considering whether ALCL and selected forms of Hodgkin's disease, particularly the syncytial nodular sclerosing variant (which is extraordinarily rare in the skin), are related or not. CD15, CD30, CD45, CD117, EBV-related markers, and fascin are not reliable as discriminants between these neoplasms (141,176,215), and they are also potentially seen in lymphomatoid papulosis (266). Therefore, tissue should routinely be submitted for cytogenetic analysis and ALK-1 immunostaining if ALCL is a potential diagnostic consideration. Despite its relative insensitivity,

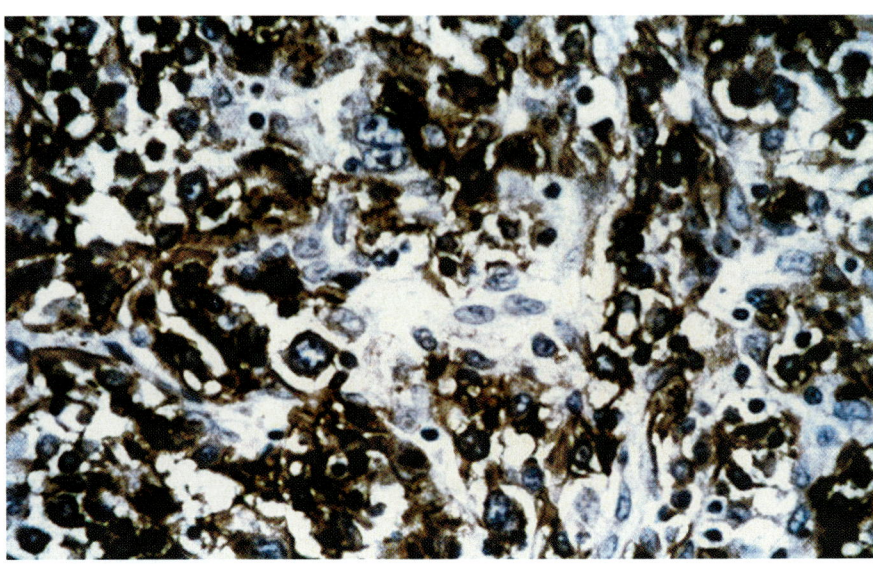

Figure 13-45

ANAPLASTIC LARGE CELL LYMPHOMA

Diffuse immunolabeling for the ALK-1 gene product.

ALK-1 expression does appear to be restricted to ALCL (fig. 13-45), and its presence in systemic ALCL is said to be associated with a better prognosis as compared with cases that are ALK-1 negative (213). Clusterin, a cell aggregating protein encoded by a gene on chromosome 8p21, is similarly present in ALCL but not in Hodgkin's disease (266).

Regarding the synonymity, or lack thereof, between malignant histiocytosis and ALCL, it is certainly true that the latter entity was confused in the past with histiocytic cutaneous tumors (216,425). It is now generally accepted that malignant proliferations of macrophage-related cells are rare, if they exist at all, and virtually all lesions formerly diagnosed as malignant histiocytosis actually represent examples of ALCL. In particular, some CD30-positive neoplasms appear to be especially capable of inducing reactive erythrophagocytosis by non-neoplastic histiocytes that are admixed with (and possibly recruited by) the tumor cells (see section on panniculitis-like T-cell lymphoma of the skin).

Peripheral T-Cell Lymphoma, Not Further Specified (Including Lennert's Lymphoma)

According to the WHO and REAL classification schemes, T-cell neoplasms are categorized according to their particular anatomic preferences and genotypic-molecular characteristics. Those that affect the skin have been presented in that manner in this chapter. Nonetheless, a group of lesions remains that defies the predefined labels of current nosologic systems, and these tumors are simply designated as *peripheral T-cell lymphomas, not further specified* (PTCL) (226).

Clinical Features. Because this category is somewhat heterogeneous biologically, it is logical to expect that the manifestations of these tumors also vary clinically. Most PTCLs present in a nondescript fashion as nodular, red-violet plaques or nodules in the skin, which are often multiple, and develop over the course of weeks or months. Virtually any skin site may be affected, and patients of all ages are encountered (223,226,229,320). Rare examples are associated with peripheral blood eosinophilia, with or without pruritus, polyclonal hypergammaglobulinemia, or hypercalcemia (223,320). Rencic et al. (349) described a dermatomyositis-like eruption in association with PTCL; granuloma annulare-like and prurigo nodularis-like presentations have been documented as well (161,375).

Treatment must be aggressive and based on systemic chemotherapy (229,320). A sizable proportion of patients with PTCL enter remission with that approach, but relapse is seen in at least 50 percent of cases (223). Most patients with PTCL that initially involves only the skin develop systemic disease if they are not treated promptly.

Pathologic Findings. In contrast to cutaneous T-cell lymphoma, PTCL shows no involvement of the epidermis. Instead, infiltrates composed of variable mixtures of medium-sized or large atypical lymphoid cells are present in the deep dermis and subcutis, with displacement

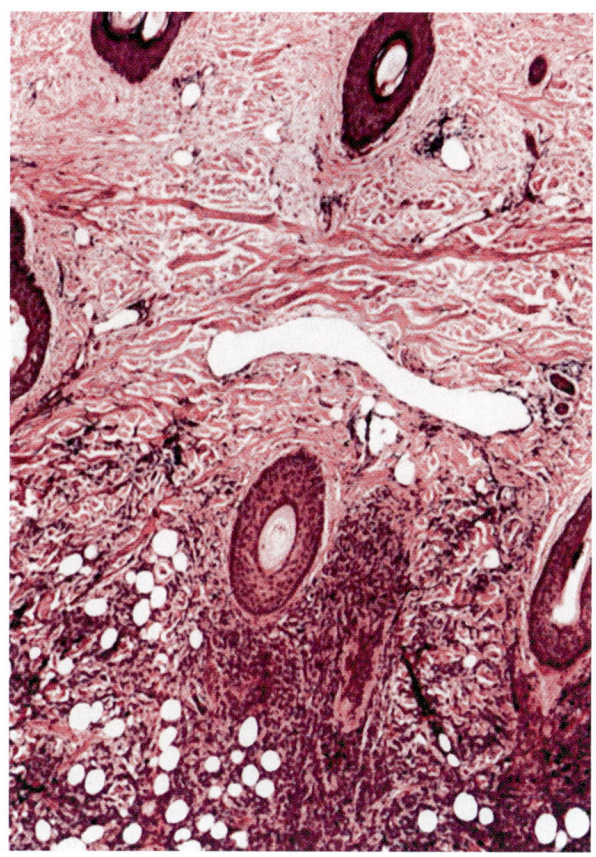

Figure 13-46

PERIPHERAL T-CELL LYMPHOMA

This tumor presents in the deep dermis as a diffuse and randomly disposed cellular infiltrate.

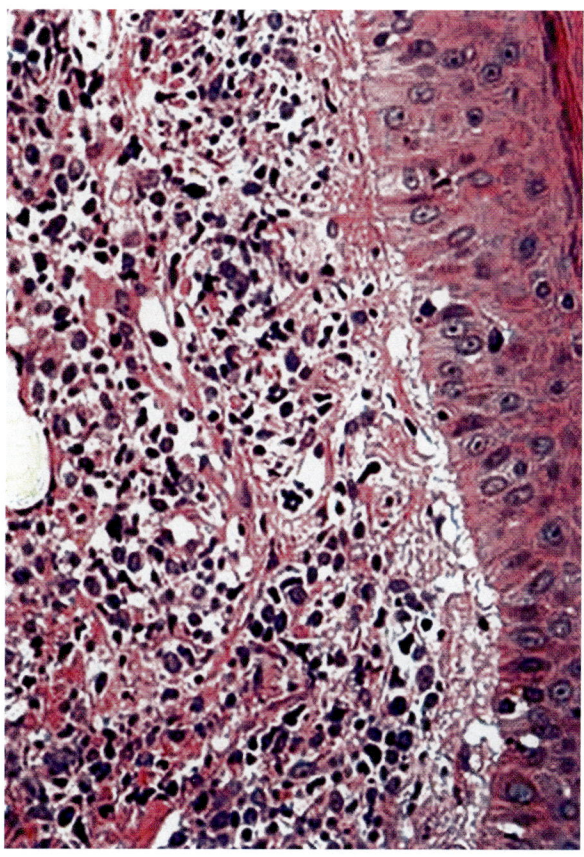

Figure 13-47

PERIPHERAL T-CELL LYMPHOMA

Cutaneous involvement is completely dermal and subcutaneous in its localization, or nearly so.

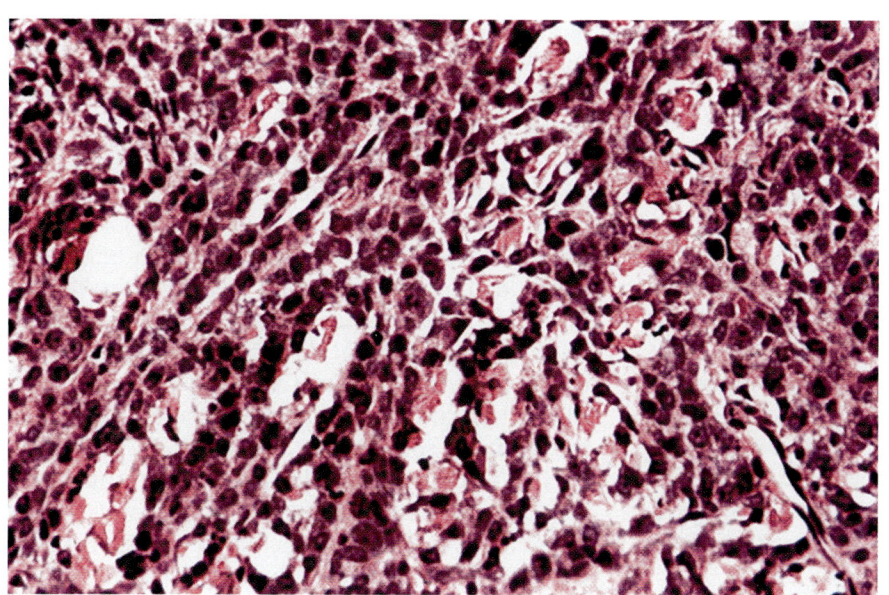

Figure 13-48

PERIPHERAL T-CELL LYMPHOMA

Irregular permeation of the dermal collagen is apparent.

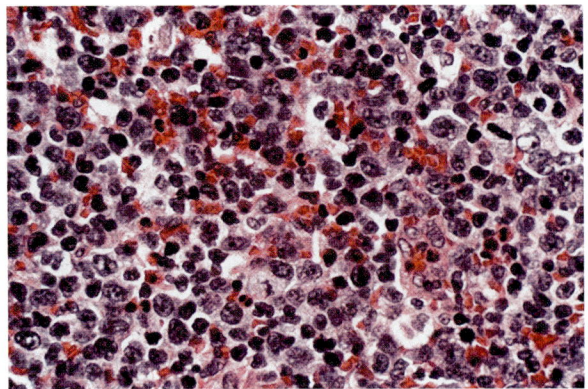

Figure 13-49

PERIPHERAL T-CELL LYMPHOMA

Cellular heterogeneity includes large and small lymphoid cells with variable nuclear appearances.

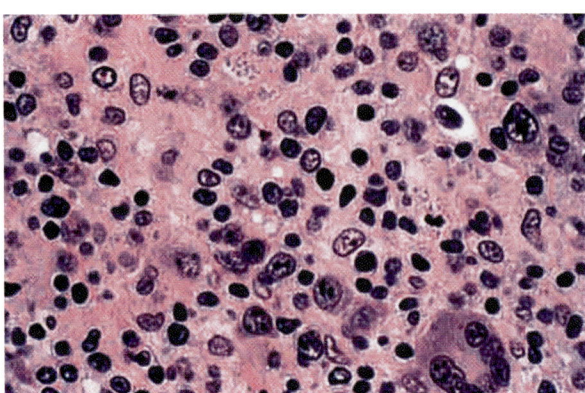

Figure 13-51

PERIPHERAL T-CELL LYMPHOMA

The notable epithelioid-histiocytic infiltrate (so-called Lennert's lymphoma) is complete with Langhans-type multinucleated giant cells. This lesion may be confused with granulomatous infectious diseases.

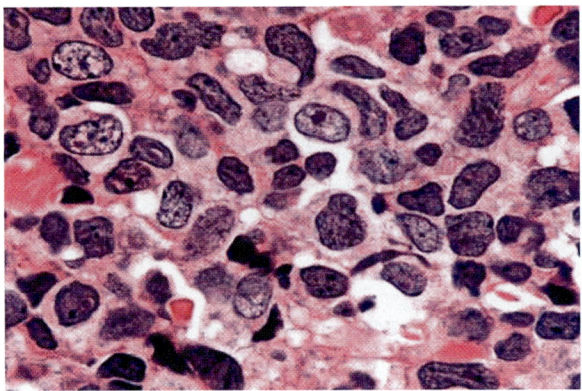

Figure 13-50

PERIPHERAL T-CELL LYMPHOMA

The tumor cells are inconsistently nucleolated and vary considerably in size; some show irregular nuclear membranes.

or effacement of appendages (figs. 13-46–13-49). Nuclear contours may be either round or irregular, nucleoli are variably seen, and mitotic activity varies greatly (fig. 13-50). Some of the tumor cells resemble Reed-Sternberg cells in selected cases, and a background population of eosinophils, plasma cells, and histiocytes further heightens a morphologic resemblance to Hodgkin's lymphoma. Stromal fibrosis is not usually notable, but may be marked in rare examples. Angiocentricity, angioinvasion, and a panniculitis-like image should not be present if the diagnostic label of PTCL, not further specified, is used.

Uncommon examples of this tumor type include randomly dispersed aggregates of epithelioid histiocytes that form vague granulomatoid clusters (fig. 13-51). This feature is not unique to T-cell proliferations, as discussed by Scarabello et al. (369); the name *Lennert's lymphoma* has been used in the past for PTCL which demonstrates this particular finding (161,226,375).

Vaillant and colleagues (406) described an unusual form of cutaneous PTCL in which the neoplastic lymphoid cells contained cytoplasmic vacuoles, yielding a signet ring cell–like appearance. Ultrastructurally, these spaces were occupied by microvesicles. This observation extends the biologic spectrum of signet ring cell lymphoma, which is more typically associated with B-cell differentiation.

Immunophenotypically, the neoplastic cells in PTCL may or may not express pan-T-cell determinants such as CD2, CD3, CD5, CD7, and CD43. Indeed, the selective deletion of one of those antigens can be used as presumptive evidence of a neoplastic infiltrate if that point is in doubt (223,226). Although most cases of PTCL have a CD4-positive/CD8-negative profile, other combinations of those two markers are seen in selected instances (229,320). Epithelioid histiocytes in lesions with granulomatous features are reactive for CD68.

Molecular studies typically reveal rearrangement of T-cell receptor genes in PTCL; no single rearrangement is characteristic (443). Similarly, there is no consistent karyotypic abnormality in this group of cutaneous lymphomas; however, Schlegelberger et al. (372) found that deletions of chromosome 6q, trisomy of 7q, and monosomy of 13 were most often observed in biologically aggressive lesions in this tumor cluster.

Differential Diagnosis. The differential diagnostic possibilities in cases of PTCL are several, even when other, more restricted variants of T-cell lymphoma have been excluded. Selected B-cell lymphomas may imitate the morphologic image of PTCL virtually perfectly, a fact that initially led Jaffe to coin the term "pseudo-T-cell lymphoma" to describe them (255). Some of those tumors are particularly difficult to recognize because they are dominated by reactive T-cell infiltrates, and can rightly be designated as T-cell–rich B-cell lymphomas of the skin (365). As stated earlier, immunophenotyping and genotypic studies for possible T-cell receptor gene or immunoglobulin heavy-chain gene rearrangements are required to confirm the lineage of PTCLs and also to recognize their morphologic simulants.

Another important diagnostic consideration is cutaneous granulocytic sarcoma (extramedullary acute leukemia). This lesion can present in the skin even when the bone marrow and peripheral blood are completely normal, and its histologic features may be remarkably similar to those of T-cell proliferations (355). In our experience with cutaneous granulocytic sarcoma, histochemical staining for chloroacetate esterase (with the von Leder method) is an unacceptably insensitive technique for its recognition; Goldstein et al. (228) have shown that stains for myeloperoxidase, CD15, and lysozyme are helpful in labeling this tumor, after the application of routine lymphoid markers has indicated that the tumor is a diagnostic potentiality. In paraffin sections, isolated reactivity for CD43 in the atypical hematopoietic cells is a particularly useful clue to this ultimate interpretation (377).

Cases of Lennert's lymphoma rarely are so dominated by epithelioid granulomas that an infectious condition is suspected (369). In such examples, histochemical stains for microorganisms will, of course, produce negative results. Close attention to the cytologic attributes of dermal lymphoid cells should then stimulate a necessary level of suspicion that the process is neoplastic.

As stated above, PTCL also may imitate Hodgkin's lymphoma. Again, immunophenotyping and genotypic analysis are capable of distinguishing these conditions; tumor cells in PTCL express at least one pan-T-cell marker as well as CD45, whereas all of those determinants are lacking in typical Reed-Sternberg cells and their variants in Hodgkin's lymphoma. Similarly, the latter neoplasm shows no rearrangements of T-cell receptor genes.

Angioimmunoblastic T-Cell Lymphoma

Clinical Features. Angioimmunoblastic T-cell lymphoma (AITCL) is now widely regarded as a form of peripheral T-cell lymphoma, although initially it was thought to be a reactive process, triggered in some cases by drugs, which could evolve into lymphoma (159). This is reflected in the original names for the condition, *angioimmunoblastic lymphadenopathy* and *angioimmunoblastic lymphadenopathy with dysproteinemia*. There continues to be a viewpoint that AITCL is a prelymphomatous process, associated with oligoclonal T-cell receptor gene rearrangement patterns (373).

AITCL is generally a disease of middle-aged to elderly adults (260), with a slight male predominance (384). A case has been reported in a 13-year-old girl (374). There is acute onset of fever, pruritus, edema, and lymphadenopathy, sometimes associated with hepatosplenomegaly, pleural effusion, arthritis, and ascites (348,384). Immunodeficiency can be demonstrated (260). Laboratory findings include polyclonal hyperglobulinemia, Coombs-positive hemolytic anemia, antinuclear and antismooth muscle antibodies, and cryoglobulins (384). Skin involvement is seen in about 40 percent of cases, and presents prior to or simultaneously with lymphadenopathy (307,376). Unfortunately, in many reports this is described simply as a rash. The most frequently described pattern of eruption is maculopapular, and can be generalized (307) or concentrated over the trunk (303) or extremities (374). Other cutaneous changes include erythroderma (157,376), papulonodules or plaques (157,303), purpuric or urticarial lesions (303), or petechiae (376). The median

Figure 13-52
ANGIOIMMUNOBLASTIC T-CELL LYMPHOMA

A: Superficial dermal edema is pronounced and there is a dense, deep dermal infiltrate.

B: There can be a variety of cell types in these lesions. Vascular proliferation accompanies the process.

C: High-power view shows a number of atypical lymphocytes, including cells with the characteristics of immunoblasts.

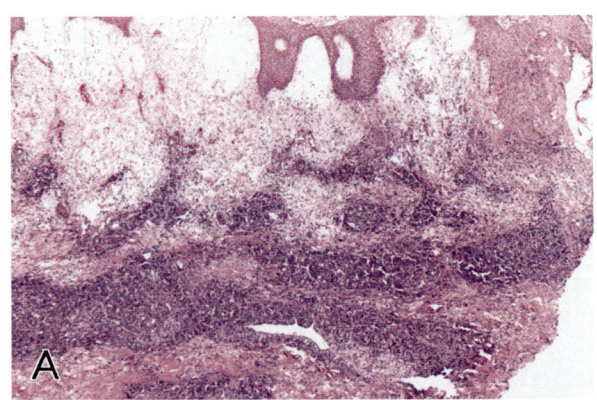
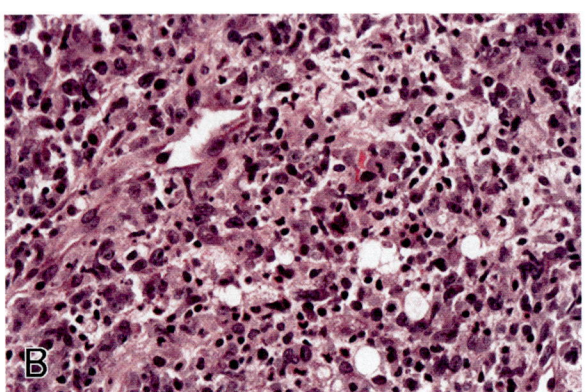
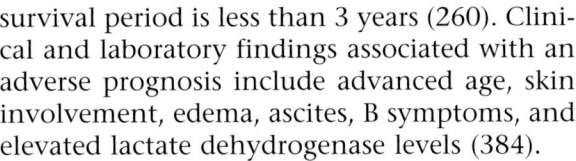
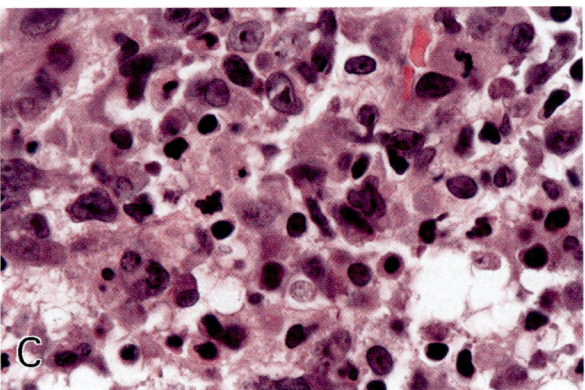

survival period is less than 3 years (260). Clinical and laboratory findings associated with an adverse prognosis include advanced age, skin involvement, edema, ascites, B symptoms, and elevated lactate dehydrogenase levels (384).

Pathologic Findings. The most characteristic histopathologic changes of AITCL are identified in lymph nodes, which show diffuse infiltrates of small to medium lymphocytes (260). Many of these cells have the characteristics of immunoblasts, showing generous amounts of pale to clear cytoplasm and round to oval, vesicular nuclei with one or more eosinophilic nucleoli. Reed-Sternberg–like cells are sometimes identified (343). To varying degrees, these lymphocytes efface the normal lobular architecture of the node (373), although hyperplastic germinal centers with ill-defined borders have been described in some cases (348). This process is associated with arborizing postcapillary venules (260,317,373) and interstitial deposits of eosinophilic material.

Findings on skin biopsy include a superficial and deep, dermal and subcutaneous, perivascular and (according to some descriptions) periadnexal infiltrate (168,373,374,376). This is comprised primarily of lymphocytes, with varying admixtures of plasma cells, histiocytes (macrophages), or eosinophils (374,376). Although these infiltrates may appear to be nonspecific, particularly in maculopapular lesions (159,303), cutaneous changes are said to be similar to, if less well developed than, those in involved lymph nodes (157,376). Accordingly, atypical lymphocytes can also be observed, including cells with the characteristics of centroblasts and immunoblasts (fig. 13-52) (168,317, 373,374). Vascular proliferation and erythrocyte extravasation accompany the process (307, 374,376). A more apparent lymphomatous picture can be observed in plaque-type lesions (303).

The neoplastic lymphocytes are mainly T cells, with a predominance of CD4- over CD8-positive cells (260,317); CD3, CD43, and CD45RO are also positive (343). CD20-positive B lymphocytes accumulate, possibly activated by the CD4-positive cell population (157). The plasma cells are polyclonal (260). In lymph nodes, CD21-positive dendritic cells surround the arborizing vessels, and there is also a network of desmin-positive reticulum cells that are characterized by long cytoplasmic processes (264). The Reed-Sternberg–like cells are CD30- and CD15-positive, and sometimes express CD20 (343).

An association with EBV has been repeatedly demonstrated, using PCR for EBV DNA, in situ hybridization for EBV-encoded small nuclear RNA, and immunohistochemistry for EBV-encoded latent membrane protein (142). The number of infected cells varies from study to study, and such cells are more frequently detected in lymph nodes than in skin lesions (303). Viral sequences are found most often in B cells, but they can also be detected in T cells (142,419) and have been found in the Reed-Sternberg–like cells (343). The presence of EBV may be a reflection of the diminished immunocompetence of these individuals (419).

As expected, T-cell receptor gene rearrangements are common (317,325,343), and identical rearrangements are seen in skin and lymph nodes of affected individuals (303); however, rearrangements of the immunoglobulin heavy chain gene are also sometimes detected (293, 325,343). The presence of EBV may explain the expansion of B-cell clones and the occasional occurrence of secondary B-cell lymphomas in cases of AITCL (134,419).

Differential Diagnosis. Since the cutaneous changes in AITCL often appear to be nonspecific, resembling a variety of inflammatory dermatoses, the diagnosis of this lymphoma requires a high index of suspicion and a full knowledge of the clinical features. Since more diagnostic changes are usually seen in affected lymph nodes, lymph node biopsy is essential. Fortunately for the purposes of diagnosis, T-cell receptor gene rearrangements can be found even when clinical and histopathologic changes are nonspecific (303). Among the changes in lymph nodes, perivascular proliferations of CD21-positive follicular dendritic cells and networks of desmin-positive reticulum cells are highly characteristic of AITCL (264). The presence of Reed-Sternberg–like cells can lead to an erroneous diagnosis of Hodgkin's disease, and therefore the constellation of other morphologic features and T-cell clonality should be evaluated in order to permit the correct diagnosis. It may well be that the proliferations of EBV-infected cells seen in some cases of AITCL could serve as a model for the reported development of Hodgkin's disease in some T-cell lymphomas (343).

Lymphomatoid Papulosis

Clinical Features. During the 1960s, it was increasingly recognized that there were examples of a self-healing cutaneous eruption clinically resembling a well-established benign cutaneous disease, *pityriasis lichenoides et varioliformis acuta (Mucha-Habermann disease)*, but, in contrast to that disorder, showing remarkable cytologic atypia on biopsy. Macaulay (296,297) set this condition apart and named it in 1968. Since then, it has been recognized as a distinctive T-cell lymphoproliferative disorder, though of uncertain malignant potential (258). Ironically, the idea of a relationship between lymphomatoid papulosis and pityriasis lichenoides has been renewed, prompted in part by the discovery that both show similar T-cell receptor gene rearrangements (337).

Lymphomatoid papulosis primarily affects adults of a mean age of 43 years (399), although children have also developed the disorder (352,408). There is a slight male predominance. The condition consists of recurrent crops of papulonodules, particularly on the trunk and extremities. These may ulcerate or form pustules (364), and they heal with characteristic varioliform scars.

Lymphomatoid papulosis most often persists for years, unaccompanied by other malignant lymphoid processes. A percentage of individuals (the range most often quoted is 10 to 20 percent), however, develop malignant lymphoma (268). The most common associated malignancies are mycosis fungoides, Hodgkin's disease, and CD30-positive anaplastic large cell lymphoma (191, 427), although other lymphomas, and even a case of acute myeloblastic leukemia, have also been reported (294,364). Rarely, lymphomatoid papulosis lesions present concurrently with, or are preceded by, other cutaneous lymphomas (144, 269,352). Uncomplicated lymphomatoid papulosis follows a benign clinical course, and can be controlled or improved, although not cured, by several therapies, including methotrexate and PUVA (psoralen and ultraviolet A light) (345). Since at present there is no certain way to determine which cases will progress to lymphoma, close clinical follow-up is warranted.

Figure 13-53
LYMPHOMATOID PAPULOSIS, TYPE A LESION

A: The dermal infiltrate is wedge shaped. The epidermis shows spongiosis and exocytosis, and there is an overlying scale-crust.

B: There is a mixture of inflammatory and neoplastic cells.

C: Neoplastic cells have pale cytoplasm; large vesicular nuclei with clumped, marginated chromatin; and prominent nucleoli.

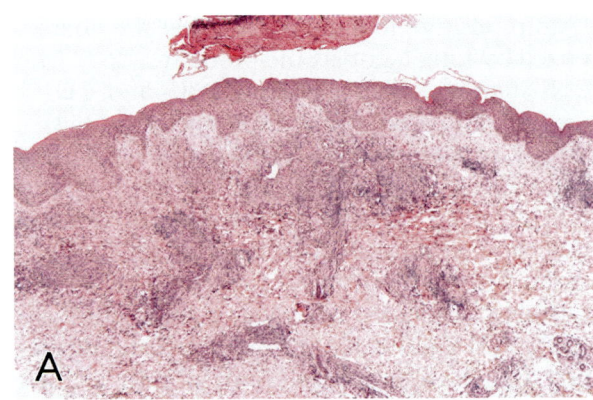
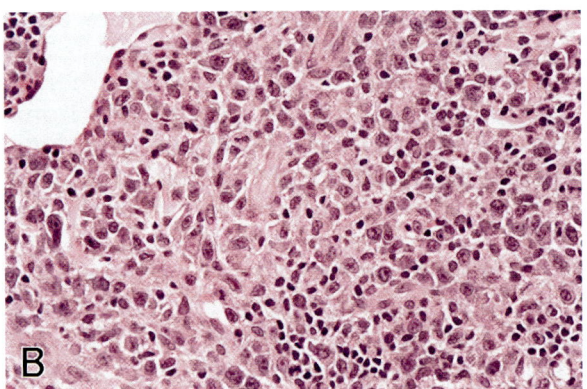
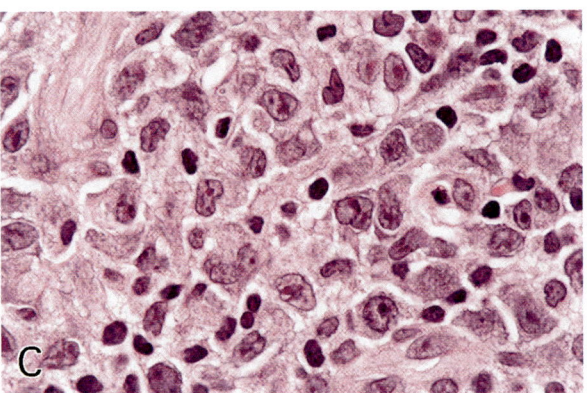

Pathologic Findings. The classic histopathologic picture of lymphomatoid papulosis is that of a wedge-shaped dermal infiltrate. This is composed of varying proportions of atypical cells, with the base of the wedge near the dermal-epidermal interface and the point of the wedge in the deep dermis (fig. 13-53A) (192,400). The epidermis shows varying degrees of spongiosis, exocytosis, and necrosis, and ulceration may be present. These epidermal changes are dependent to a large extent upon lesion sampling; early- or late-stage lesions may show minimal epidermal involvement. Infiltrates concentrated around follicles or ruptured follicular cysts have also been reported (339,350).

Three types of lesions have been delineated by Willemze and colleagues (428–430), depending upon the morphologic and immunohistochemical features of the constituent atypical cells. *Type A lymphomatoid papulosis* shows a proportion of cells with generous amounts of pale basophilic cytoplasm, large vesicular nuclei with clumped chromatin along the nuclear membranes, and large nucleoli; cells resembling Reed-Sternberg cells are also identified. These cells closely resemble those of anaplastic large cell lymphoma or Hodgkin's disease (fig. 13-53). In this type of lymphomatoid papulosis, there is a significant admixture of inflammatory cell types, including small lymphocytes, neutrophils, eosinophils, and macrophages (345). In *type B lymphomatoid papulosis*, the neoplastic cells vary in size (although large cells are commonly identified) and feature hyperchromatic, convoluted or cerebriform nuclei. The infiltrates may be dense and band-like, and contain fewer inflammatory cells (345,413). The atypical cells resemble those of mycosis fungoides (fig. 13-54). Transitional forms with features of both types A and B are observed (428). A third type, *type C*, has been described. This form of lymphomatoid papulosis has characteristic clinical features, but microscopically, there are solid sheets of atypical cells resembling those of anaplastic large cell lymphoma (427). Lesions heal with dermal scarring. The accompanying inflammatory infiltrates suggest a role for cell-mediated immunity in the regression of lymphomatoid papulosis lesions (136).

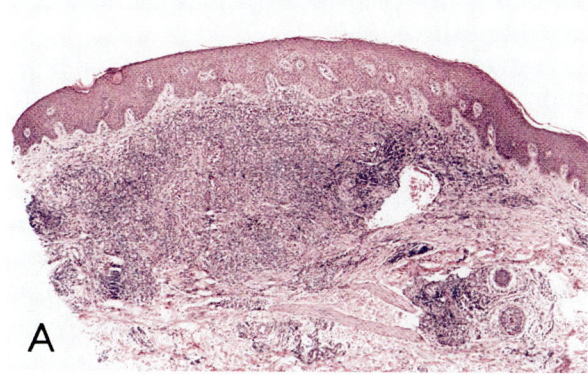
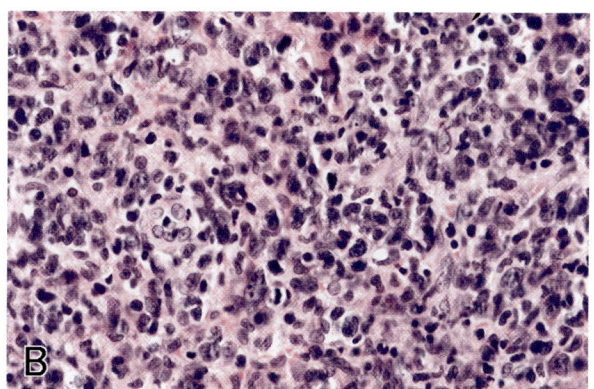
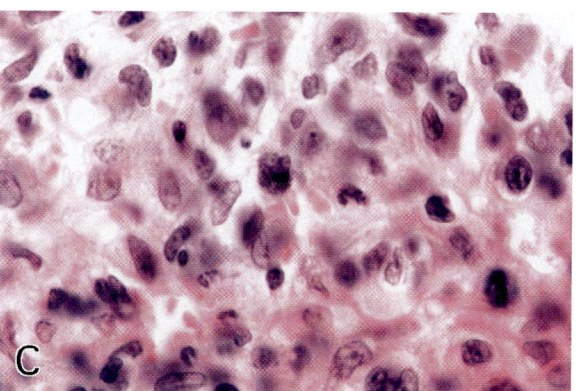

Figure 13-54

LYMPHOMATOID PAPULOSIS, TYPE B LESION

A: Low-power view shows a dense, somewhat band-like dermal infiltrate. Epidermal involvement is minimal in this case.
B: Atypical lymphoid cells with mitotic activity can be identified.
C: The neoplastic cells have hyperchromatic, convoluted nuclei.

By immunohistochemistry, the atypical cells of lymphomatoid papulosis are often CD4 positive, CD8 negative, and may show a loss of pan-T-cell antigens (198,347). However, there can be variability in T-cell antigen expression: CD4-, CD8-negative cases have been reported (156), and in one study, less than 10 percent of infiltrating lymphocytes were CD4 positive (262). There has also been a case with a nature killer (NK) cell phenotype (156). The cells resembling those of anaplastic large cell lymphoma, predominant in type A and type C lesions, are CD30 positive (400, 422,427). These cells have been shown to be of T-cell lineage (191). The infiltrating cells express activation or proliferation markers, such as CD25 or Ki-67 (347). At least one of the cytotoxic granule proteins (from among TIA-1, granzyme B, and perforin) is expressed by a high percentage of the neoplastic cells (165). Ultrastructural study has shown a close association between atypical lymphoid cells and Langerhans cells (247), and immunoelectron microscopy has shown evidence of a possible transition between T lymphocytes and large Reed-Sternberg–like cells (198).

Rearrangements of the T-cell receptor genes are found in about half of the cases of lymphomatoid papulosis, most often in type B or mixed cases (422). Multiclonal examples have also been described in some patients, with different rearrangements of β, γ, and/or δ T-cell receptor genes (420,422). In other patients, a single dominant clone has been identified in separate lesions with different histopathologic features; in some individuals who eventually developed frank lymphoma, the same clone was detected in both the lymphomatoid papulosis lesions and the resulting lymphoma (191). The t(2;5) translocation, with resulting expression of a fusion protein containing the catalytic domain of ALK, is found in many anaplastic CD30-positive large cell lymphomas of extracutaneous origin. Neither the translocation nor the expression of ALK have been detected in cases of lymphomatoid papulosis (436).

In situ hybridization has not demonstrated evidence of EBV infection (262), and PCR methods have not supported an association with herpesviruses 6, 7, or 8 (274). In one study, HTLV-1 antibodies were detected in some patients (399), however, another investigation failed to demonstrate HTLV-1 proviral sequences in patients with lymphomatoid papulosis (332).

Differential Diagnosis. An accurate diagnosis of lymphomatoid papulosis is dependent upon a combination of clinical features: recurrent, self-healing lesions, often in an otherwise healthy individual, with the typical microscopic findings. Accordingly, knowledge of the clinical presentation is essential. Although biopsy findings alone (including a wedge-shaped dermal infiltrate composed of atypical lymphocytes) may be highly suggestive, typical microscopic changes of lymphomatoid papulosis can occasionally be observed in cases that present clinically as solitary skin tumors, a picture more characteristic of anaplastic large cell lymphoma (155).

The clinical presentation of pityriasis lichenoides et varioliformis acuta (PLEVA) is similar to that of lymphomatoid papulosis, and the conditions share similar microscopic configurations (a wedge-shaped infiltrate and varying degrees of epidermal involvement and necrosis). Lymphocyte markers can be exploited in the differential diagnosis; for example, there are differences between the two disorders in degrees of CD8, CD79, and cutaneous lymphocyte-associated antigen (CLA) expression, and CD30 expression is seen only in lymphomatoid papulosis (262). In our experience, such detailed analysis is rarely necessary, since, in contrast to PLEVA, the degree of cytologic atypia in lymphomatoid papulosis is profound.

The Reed-Sternberg–like cells in type A lymphomatoid papulosis can raise the possibility of cutaneous Hodgkin's disease (see below). The history of recurrent, self-healing lesions is not typical of Hodgkin's disease with cutaneous involvement. As previously noted, however, Hodgkin's disease can evolve from lymphomatoid papulosis, and a histogenetic relationship between these disorders and anaplastic CD30-positive lymphoma has been proposed (198, 268) There may also be a rare primary cutaneous variant of Hodgkin's disease that presents as spontaneously regressing lesions. This condition differs from lymphomatoid papulosis in that the Reed-Sternberg cells are CD30 and CD15 positive, CD45R negative, while the morphologically similar cells of lymphomatoid papulosis are CD30 positive, CD15 negative, CD45R positive (386).

Primary cutaneous anaplastic large cell lymphoma usually lacks the wedge-shaped infiltrate and admixtures of inflammatory cell types of type A lymphomatoid papulosis, while displaying a higher percentage of CD30-positive cells. The rare type C variant of lymphomatoid papulosis does show confluent sheets of CD30-positive cells, and could be difficult to distinguish from anaplastic large cell lymphoma in the absence of clinical data.

Other T-Cell and NK-Cell Lymphomas Involving the Skin

Blastic NK-cell lymphoma is a condition that has only recently come into focus as a distinct entity. It most commonly arises in middle-aged to elderly individuals. Cutaneous nodules often constitute the presenting finding (182,405). Skin lesions are sometimes described as rash or exanthem (145,316), and in one case lesions were said to resemble angiosarcoma (405). Disseminated disease is often present, with lymphadenopathy, anemia, and liver, spleen, and bone marrow involvement (166,306,316). This is a particularly aggressive lymphoma, with deaths usually occurring several months to 3 years following diagnosis (306,337).

Microscopically, there are infiltrates of medium-sized cells with fine chromatin and lymphoblastic characteristics (fig. 13-55) (182,316). Although there is some variability in the reported immunophenotype, neoplastic cells are regularly CD56 positive, usually CD4 and CD43 positive, and negative for surface CD3; they are also negative for markers of myeloid lineage (145,182,185,337). T-cell receptor genes are germline (185,337,405). In contrast to NK/T-cell lymphoma, nasal type, these cases are negative for EBV (185,306,316,391,405).

CUTANEOUS INVOLVEMENT IN HODGKIN'S DISEASE

Cutaneous manifestations are found in about 25 percent of patients with Hodgkin's disease. Nonspecific changes are most common, and may precede the diagnosis by months or years. There is a lengthy list of such changes, but the most common and significant include pruritus, addisonian hyperpigmentation, acquired ichthyosis,

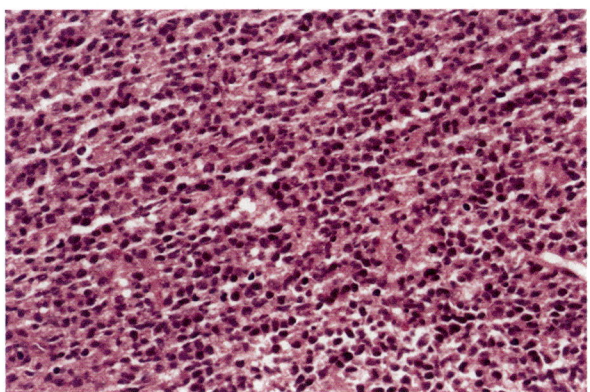 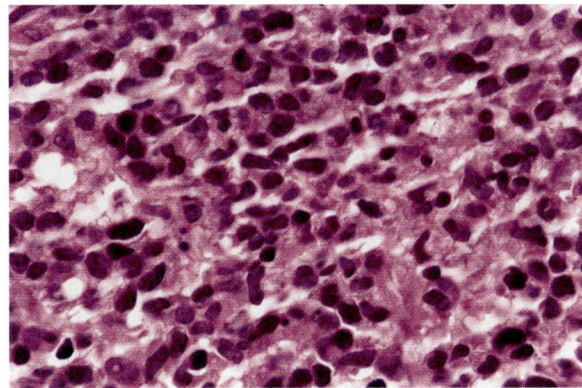

Figure 13-55

BLASTIC NK-CELL LYMPHOMA

Left: Within the dermis are sheets of atypical lymphoid cells.
Right: There are medium-sized cells with moderate amounts of cytoplasm and irregularly shaped nuclei. Nucleoli are not readily identifiable in this preparation. (Courtesy of E. C. Parlette, LT, MC, USNR, San Diego, CA.)

infectious complications such as herpes zoster, erythroderma, and various hypersensitivity phenomena (457). Specific skin lesions are uncommon, with reported incidences ranging from 0.5 to 7.5 percent (444,461,464). They most often present as papules, plaques, nodules, or larger tumors that may ulcerate (445). Rarely, exfoliative dermatitis accompanying Hodgkin's disease shows specific histopathologic features. Bullous lesions have also been described (450). Granulomatous slack skin is associated with Hodgkin's disease in some cases (455).

The usual mechanism of skin involvement is via retrograde lymphatic spread distal to involved lymph nodes (451,461,464). Other, less common mechanisms include direct extension from an underlying nodal focus and hematogenous dissemination. In some instances, there are specific skin lesions at the time of first presentation of the disease, with lymph node involvement detected at the same time or shortly thereafter (451,463,464). Hodgkin's disease has been preceded by lymphomatoid papulosis (446,466), and has been accompanied or followed by mycosis fungoides (446,448). Usually, the presence of specific cutaneous lesions indicates stage IV disease and carries an adverse prognosis (461,464).

Clinical Features. The following discussion concerns the classic form of Hodgkin's disease. Hodgkin's disease is a lymphoma that consists of a particular type of atypical cell, the Hodgkin cell, and its variants (the Reed-Sternberg cell and lacunar cell), together with a mixed inflammatory cell infiltrate and, sometimes, stromal changes. This disorder has a bimodal age of incidence, with one peak occurring in early adult life and another in later life. Typically, Hodgkin's disease presents with lymphadenopathy, particularly cervical, mediastinal, axillary, para-aortic, or inguinal-femoral (457,462). Intermittent fever, night sweats, weight loss, and anemia can accompany the lymphadenopathy. Treatment involves radiation and chemotherapy. Over the years, there has been progressive improvement in the prognosis, and now cures are possible in many cases. The stage of the disease and associated symptoms are better predictors of outcome than the histopathologic type (457,462). The neoplastic cells of Hodgkin's disease are believed to most often arise from a germinal center B cell (454), but a T-cell derivation is also possible (446,458). EBV is detected in a number of cases and may play a pathogenetic role, particularly in patients who are immunosuppressed (462).

There are also rare instances of *primary cutaneous Hodgkin's disease* (464). Lesions have most often been isolated cutaneous or subcutaneous nodules (449,452,459), but there have also been papules or nodules that have undergone spontaneous involution (460). The diagnosis of primary cutaneous Hodgkin's disease requires the presence of typical histopathologic and immunohistochemical features and a negative workup

Figure 13-56
CUTANEOUS INVOLVEMENT IN HODGKIN'S DISEASE

A: There is a dense dermal infiltrate with overlying acanthosis. In this case, cutaneous involvement was detected just prior to the discovery of regional nodal disease.

B: A polymorphous infiltrate is present. A centrally located Hodgkin cell shows light-staining cytoplasm, a large rounded nucleus, and a single prominent nucleolus.

C: In another field, a characteristic Reed-Sternberg cell is observed.

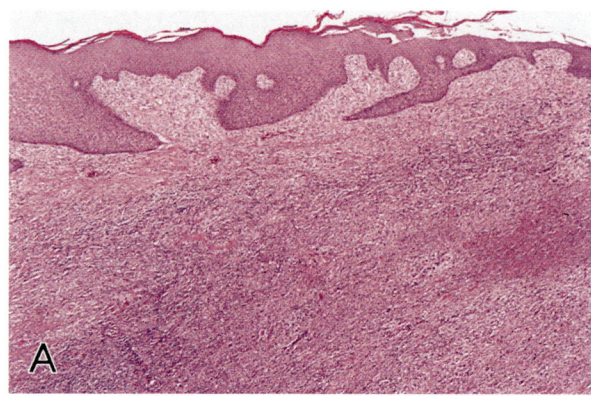

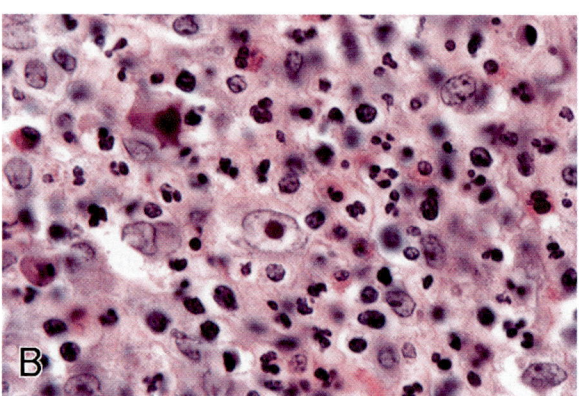

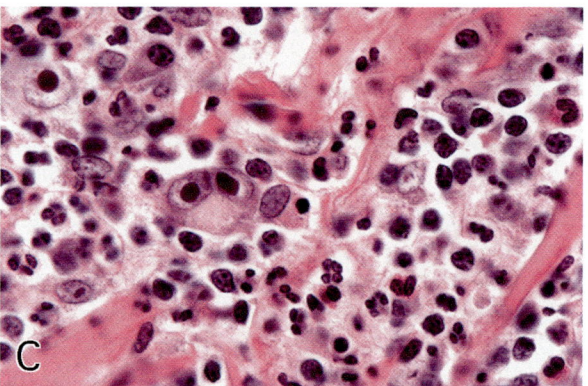

for systemic disease (449,460). In contrast to the usual situation of cutaneous lesions developing secondarily in established disease, primary cutaneous Hodgkin's disease has a more favorable prognosis, and some cases persist in the skin for years without systemic findings (460). Nevertheless, typical nodal involvement may eventually occur, at intervals ranging from several months to 6 years following the diagnosis of the cutaneous disease (449,459,460).

Pathologic Findings. As in lymph nodes and other tissues, a diagnosis of cutaneous involvement by Hodgkin's disease (fig. 13-56A) depends upon finding atypical cells with the characteristics of Hodgkin or Reed-Sternberg cells. This often occurs in the setting of a polymorphous infiltrate that includes lymphocytes, macrophages, neutrophils, and eosinophils (445,460,463). The Hodgkin cell displays generous amounts of lightly basophilic cytoplasm and a large rounded nucleus with a single prominent acidophilic nucleolus (fig. 13-56B). The Reed-Sternberg cell possesses a bilobed nucleus, each lobe containing a prominent acidophilic nucleolus (fig. 13-56C) (462). A lacunar cell, such as seen the nodular sclerosis subtype of Hodgkin's disease, has also been described in cutaneous lesions (445). This is a Hodgkin or Reed-Sternberg cell with retraction of the cytoplasmic membrane, creating the appearance of a cell residing in a space or lacuna (462). To a certain extent, the patterns of cutaneous infiltration can mimic those of the established nodal subtypes of the disease, and accordingly, nodular sclerosis, mixed cellularity, and lymphocyte depleted configurations have been observed in skin (445, 451,464). The cutaneous pattern frequently reflects that in the involved lymph nodes (445). In one study, the cutaneous pattern was always in the same or a prognostically worse histopathologic category than that displayed in the proximal nodal focus of disease (464).

The neoplastic cells in Hodgkin's disease are CD30 positive, CD15 positive, and CD45 negative (445,449,456,460). A substantial minority of the cells express CD20 to varying degrees of intensity (462). They also frequently express B-cell–specific activator protein (447); however,

T-cell antigens have been expressed on Reed-Sternberg cells in some cases (453). EBV encoded latent membrane protein (LMP-1) is found in some cases (462). Overexpression of cytokines and their receptors by the neoplastic cells may account for the admixture of inflammatory cells so often observed in Hodgkin's disease (462). Immunoglobulin gene rearrangements are found in most cases, but there are rare cases in which T-cell receptor gene rearrangements have been detected (458). Most often, gene rearrangements are detected in isolated Hodgkin or Reed-Sternberg cells rather than in whole tissue specimens (462).

Differential Diagnosis. Cutaneous lesions with heavy mixed infiltrates can be confused with a variety of inflammatory dermatoses, unless the characteristic cells of Hodgkin's disease are identified. This is less likely to be a problem in established nodal or systemic disease.

The neoplastic cells of Hodgkin's disease closely resemble the atypical cells of type A lymphomatoid papulosis. Lymphomatoid papulosis can precede the onset of Hodgkin's disease, while rare cases of primary cutaneous Hodgkin's disease present with self-healing papulonodular lesions that clinically mimic lymphomatoid papulosis. Although the atypical cells of lymphomatoid papulosis are also CD30 positive, they are usually CD15 negative, CD45 positive, in contrast to Hodgkin and Reed-Sternberg cells.

Anaplastic CD30-positive large cell lymphoma may resemble Hodgkin's disease microscopically. However, the polymorphous inflammatory infiltrate of Hodgkin's disease is distinctive (460). In contrast to anaplastic large cell lymphoma, the neoplastic cells of Hodgkin's disease are positive for B-cell–specific activator protein and are negative for epithelial membrane antigen (EMA) and the ALK protein (447, 462). The latter two staining results are helpful in making a distinction from systemic anaplastic large cell lymphoma but not from the primary cutaneous form of the disease, since the latter tumor cells are usually also EMA and ALK negative. The neoplastic cells of primary cutaneous anaplastic large cell lymphoma are usually CD4 positive (465). When present, positivity for EBV latent membrane protein also favors Hodgkin's disease (462). A distinction from anaplastic large B-cell lymphoma may not always be possible, but this is not likely to be a major issue in cases of cutaneous Hodgkin's disease, particularly when all the clinical and histopathologic features are taken into account.

LEUKEMIA CUTIS

Clinical Features. Skin involvement in patients with leukemia can be categorized as specific leukemic infiltrates and nonspecific manifestations. The discussion that follows concentrates on specific lesions of leukemia cutis. Aside from the morbidity they produce, nonspecific lesions are a possible source of clinical confusion with true leukemic infiltrates, a manifestation of complications related to the leukemia (e.g., purpura due to thrombocytopenia, cutaneous infection due to immunosuppression), or a reactive process with a close association with leukemia. Some of the latter include generalized pruritus, Sweet's syndrome, pyoderma gangrenosum (476), and drug eruptions (496). More recently, there have been reports of insect bite-like reactions in patients with leukemias and lymphomas (470).

Specific cutaneous lesions have been associated with most of the leukemias, including acute myeloid leukemia (M1-3 in the French-American-British [FAB] classification), acute myelomonocytic leukemia (M4), acute monocytic leukemia (M5), acute erythroleukemia (M6), acute lymphoblastic leukemia, chronic myelogenous leukemia, chronic myelomonocytic leukemia, chronic lymphocytic leukemia, adult T-cell leukemia, T-cell prolymphocytic leukemia, and hairy cell leukemia (488). The lymphomatous counterparts of the following have already been discussed: acute lymphoblastic leukemia (precursor B lymphoblastic lymphoma), adult T-cell leukemia/lymphoma, and precursor T lymphoblastic leukemia/lymphoma. Aggressive NK-cell leukemia will be considered briefly, but it may represent the leukemic form of extranodal NK/T-cell lymphoma, nasal type (477).

The frequency of specific lesions of leukemia cutis varies, depending upon the type of leukemia. Cutaneous involvement is common in monocytic leukemia, occurring in 10 to 50 percent of cases (473). It is also frequent in chronic lymphocytic leukemia, particularly in T-cell subtypes, such as T-cell chronic lymphocytic leukemia (488) and T-cell large granular lymphocytic leukemia (468,483). Specific skin lesions are less common in other varieties, such as acute lymphoblastic leukemia, myeloid leukemia, and hairy cell leukemia (467,486,488).

The lesions of leukemia cutis are most often papules and nodules. Plaques, ulcers, and purpuric lesions also occur (473,492,493). Unusual manifestations include erythroderma (479,488) and bullous lesions (493). Gingival hypertrophy is associated with monocytic and myelomonocytic leukemias. The chloroma (granulocytic sarcoma), a green to greenish gray tumor, is a characteristic if uncommon lesion associated with acute myeloid leukemia. Its greenish color is due to the presence of high concentrations of myeloperoxidase in infiltrating myeloblasts (473). Lesions appearing at arterial and venous puncture sites have been reported in acute promyelocytic leukemia (M3) (489).

There is a strong association between cutaneous lesions of leukemia and the involvement of other extramedullary sites (469,490). As might be expected, the appearance of cutaneous lesions of leukemia is associated with a poor prognosis (490,493). *Aleukemic leukemia cutis* refers to the occurrence of leukemic skin lesions prior to the detection of peripheral blood or bone marrow involvement. Although uncommon, there are numerous reports of this phenomenon, most of which involve cases of acute monocytic or myelomonocytic leukemia (471,475,482,484, 487). It has also been reported in acute lymphoblastic leukemia (495).

Pathologic Findings. Most varieties of leukemia cutis feature a dense dermal infiltrate of atypical cells that permeates collagen bundles (474). A grenz zone frequently separates the infiltrate from the overlying epidermis in the non-T-cell leukemias (fig. 13-57A) (488,497). The atypical cells are often present in a perivascular and/or periadnexal distribution (486,488). Infiltration and destruction of adnexal structures, vessels, nerves, and muscle are seen, particularly in myeloid, monocytic, and myelomonocytic leukemias (fig. 13-57B) (474,488), and examples of leukemic vasculitis have been described (485). A Kaposi's sarcoma–like pattern has been reported in myeloid leukemia, in which myeloblasts appear to line slit-like, blood-filled spaces (fig. 13-57C) (497). T-cell variants of chronic lymphocytic leukemia show epidermotropism (488). The cells of chronic lymphocytic leukemia can also appear, apparently incidentally, in other types of cutaneous lesions (472), where they are recognized by the formation of varying sized clusters of monotonous, small to medium-sized cells (fig. 13-58).

Recognition of the cytologic characteristics of the cells is important in refining the diagnosis. The myeloblasts of acute myeloid leukemia are large cells with round to oval nuclei, fine to coarse (when minimally differentiated) chromatin, and scant basophilic cytoplasm (fig. 13-57D). Chronic myeloid leukemia features a much more varied cell population, including atypical myelocytes, metamyelocytes, eosinophil precursors, and mature neutrophils. In monocytic leukemia, monocytoid forms have indented nuclei, with fine to lacy chromatin and one or more distinct nucleoli. In acute lymphoblastic leukemia, the cells are medium to large with fine to reticulated chromatin and scant to moderate amounts of cytoplasm (fig. 13-59). Lymphocytes are smaller and relatively mature in appearance in chronic lymphocytic leukemia (fig. 13-60). In the case of hairy cell leukemia, the characteristic cytoplasmic projections are not seen in routinely processed skin specimens, and imprints are required in order to see this feature (488). Fresh specimens are needed to demonstrate staining with tartrate-resistant acid phosphatase (481).

Histochemistry and immunohistochemistry can be of great help in reaching a specific diagnosis of the type of leukemia cutis. Among the most useful stains for formalin-fixed, paraffin-embedded tissues are chloroacetate esterase (Leder stain [CAE]) and the immunostains, myeloperoxidase, lysozyme, and CD20, CD30, CD43, CD45, CD45RO, and CD68 (488). Ratnam et al. (488) have provided a detailed schema for using some of these antibodies in the workup of atypical dermal infiltrates. Cells of myeloid leukemia express lysozyme and CAE. Myeloperoxidase is found in myeloid and myelomonocytic leukemia. Monocytic and myelomonocytic leukemias are positive for CD43 and CD68 (475,478,491). In acute lymphoblastic leukemia, the usual profile is positivity for CD19, CD20 (variable), CD79a, CD10, and HLA-DR. In formalin-fixed skin specimens, the most noteworthy practical finding is that neoplastic cells are

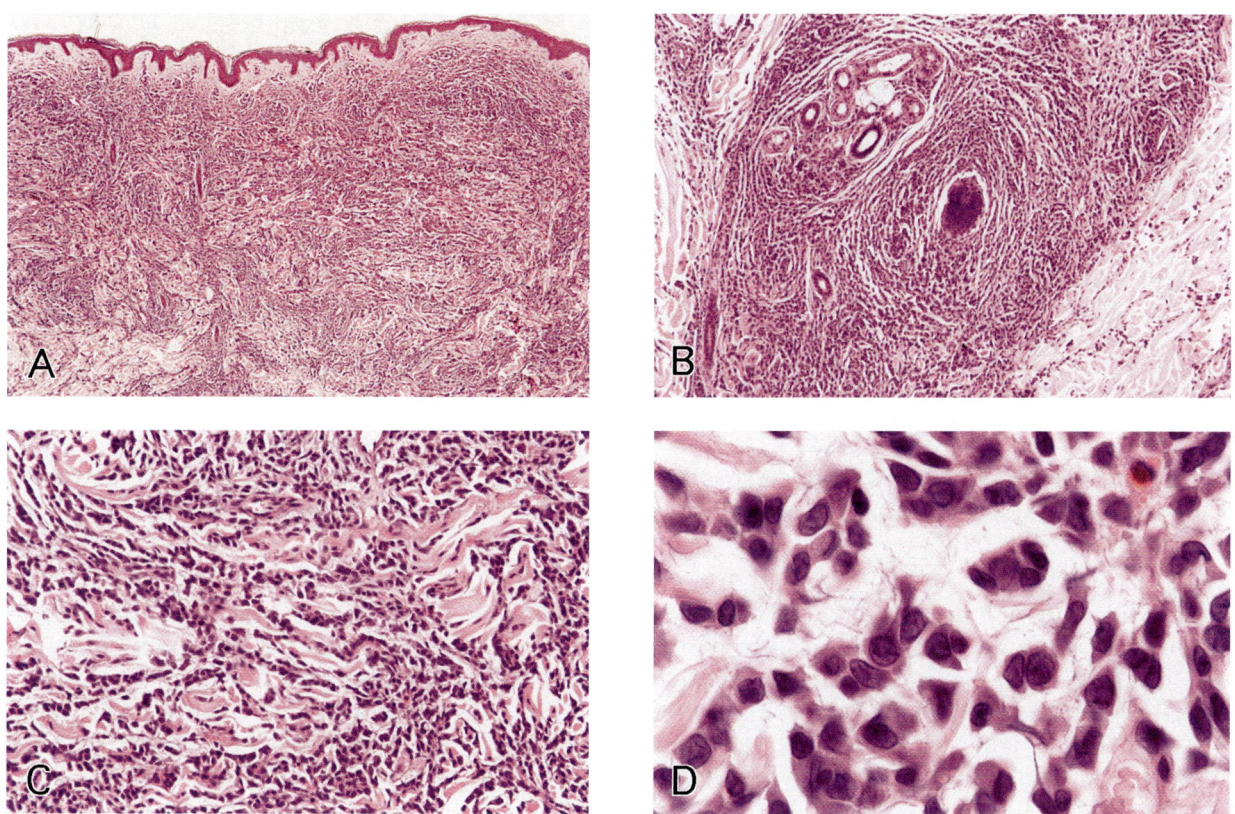

Figure 13-57

LEUKEMIA CUTIS: ACUTE MYELOID LEUKEMIA

A: A dense dermal infiltrate of atypical myeloid cell is separated from the overlying epidermis by a grenz zone.
B: Infiltration of adnexal structures (eccrine sweat coil and portion of hair matrix) is apparent.
C: Myeloblasts appear to line slit-like spaces, which do not appear blood-filled in this example.
D: The neoplastic cells have scant cytoplasm, round to oval nuclei, and coarse chromatin.

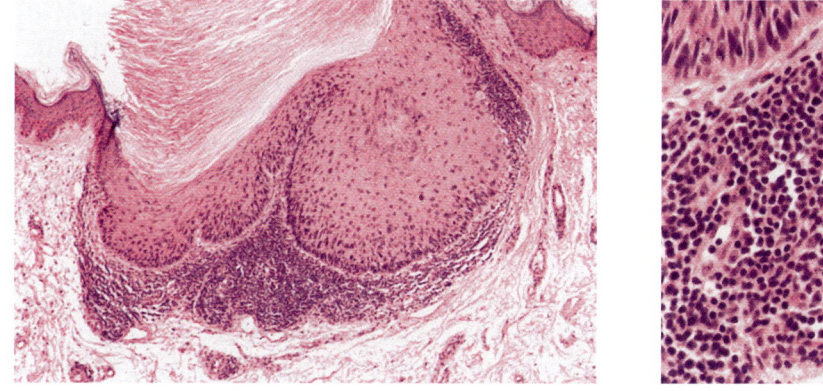 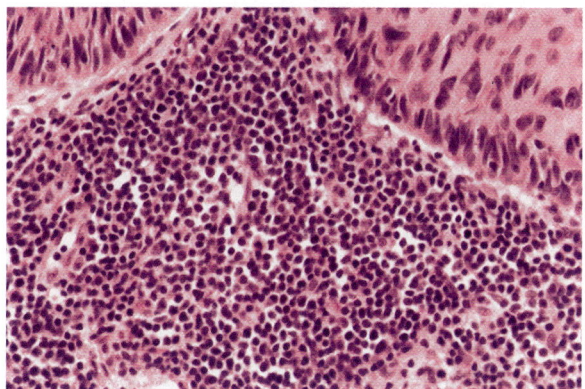

Figure 13-58

CELLS OF CHRONIC LYMPHOCYTIC LEUKEMIA ASSOCIATED WITH HYPERTROPHIC ACTINIC KERATOSIS

Left: The neoplastic cells underlie hypertrophic actinic keratosis.
Right: They are recognizable by their small size, monotony, and sharp separation from the overlying epidermis.

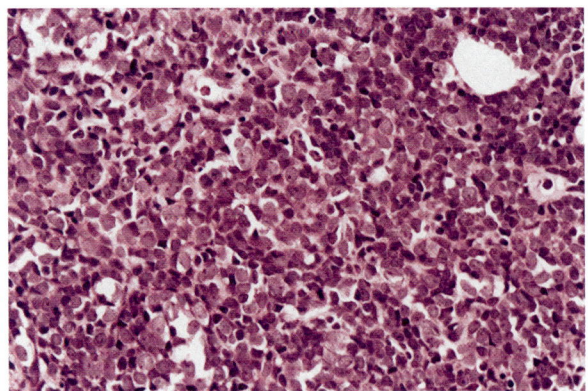

Figure 13-59

LEUKEMIA CUTIS: ACUTE LYMPHOBLASTIC LEUKEMIA
There are medium sized cells with fine chromatin and scant cytoplasm.

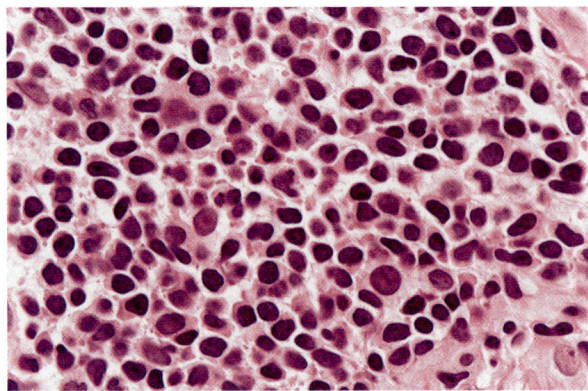

Figure 13-60

LEUKEMIA CUTIS: CHRONIC LYMPHOCYTIC LEUKEMIA
The neoplastic lymphocytes have a small and relatively mature appearance.

weakly positive or negative for CD20 and, among the other common lymphocyte markers, may only express CD45 (488). CD20 is also negative or weakly expressed in B-cell chronic lymphocytic leukemia (488). Recently, Dorfman et al. (480) demonstrated that CD99, representing the E21/MIC2 gene product, is regularly positive in skin lesions of acute lymphoblastic leukemia and in a high percentage of those of acute myeloid leukemia. In a case of aggressive NK-cell leukemia involving the skin, the neoplastic cells were positive for CD2, CD8, CD56, TIA-1, granzyme B, EBV (by in situ hybridization), and were negative for CD3, CD4, CD16, and CD57 (494). In T-cell large granular lymphocytic leukemia, the infiltrating cells are CD3 positive, CD4 negative, CD8 positive, and EBV infection may be demonstrable (468).

Differential Diagnosis. The presence of atypical cutaneous infiltrates with the morphologic changes outlined above suggests the possibility of leukemia cutis. A more detailed clinical and laboratory investigation should then follow, with a specific diagnosis depending upon findings in bone marrow and peripheral blood. In the case of aleukemia cutis, close clinical follow-up is indicated to detect the early development of systemic manifestations of the disease. A distinction from cutaneous lymphoma could be a major challenge, but a number of these disorders (adult T-cell leukemia/lymphoma, acute lymphoblastic leukemia/precursor B lymphoblastic lymphoma) actually have both leukemic and nonleukemic phases. The diagnosis may be challenging when there are only a few atypical cells obscured by a dense, reactive infiltrate, as has been described in some lesions resembling Sweet's syndrome or pyoderma gangrenosum (497).

EXTRAMEDULLARY HEMATOPOIESIS

Clinical Features. *Cutaneous hematopoiesis* normally occurs in the 8-cm embryo, and ceases by 34 to 38 weeks' gestation (499). Otherwise, cutaneous hematopoiesis is distinctly unusual, arising in two major settings: in neonates, associated with abnormalities that have begun in utero, and in adults, usually associated with myelofibrosis and often following splenectomy (503).

Neonatal hematopoiesis is associated with congenital viral infections, specifically rubella, cytomegalovirus, and Coxsackie virus B-2; twin transfusion syndrome; Rh hemolytic disease of the newborn; and hereditary spherocytosis (498,499,502,510). It has also been reported in diffuse hemangiomatosis in a newborn (500). The cutaneous eruption (unassociated with hemangiomas) can consist of petechiae; purpuric macules, papules, and plaques; and ecchymotic lesions; the more purpuric of these are often referred to as "blueberry muffin" lesions (499,504). There is a predilection for involvement of the head, neck, and trunk (499). The ultimate prognosis depends upon the underlying condition and its resulting complications. Skin lesions tend to fade within 3 to 6 weeks of birth (499).

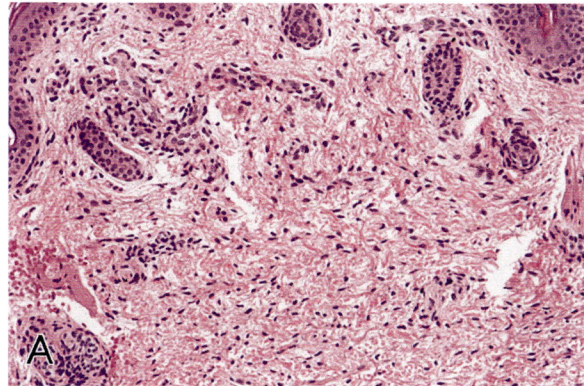
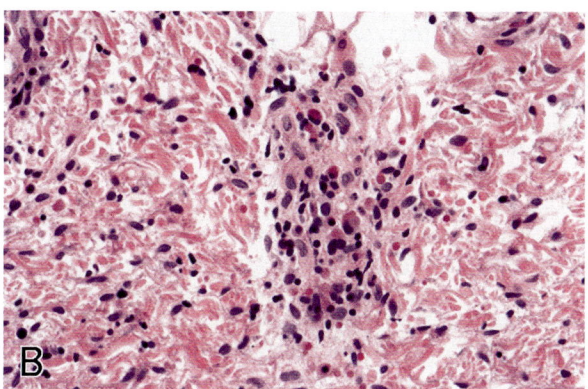

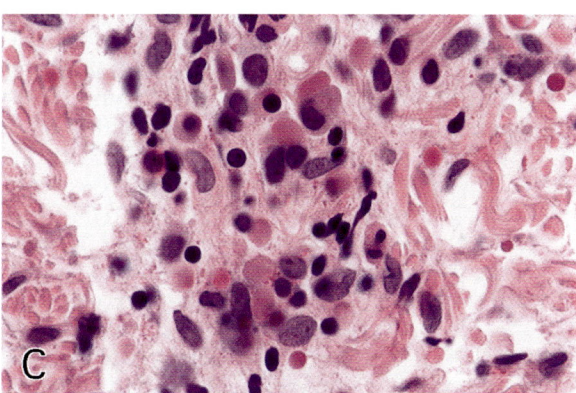

Figure 13-61

EXTRAMEDULLARY HEMATOPOIESIS

A: There is a loosely organized interstitial dermal infiltrate.

B: Myeloid cells, including cells of eosinophil lineage, and erythroid precursors are seen.

C: Nucleated erythrocytes are apparent.

Most adults with cutaneous extramedullary hematopoiesis have myelofibrosis (503,505–508, 511), but sporadic cases have been associated with agnogenic myeloid metaplasia, polycythemia vera, and chronic myelogenous leukemia (501). Lesions consist of erythematous to purpuric papulonodules (505,507,508), and a patient with bilateral leg ulcers has been described (506). Head and neck, trunk, and extremities are involved. The prognosis depends upon the course of the underlying disease. Skin lesions show a variable response to hydroxyurea (503,509). In one case, electron beam therapy helped to control the eruption (503), and in another, danazol and alpha-interferon given for the underlying myelofibrosis did not have an impact on the cutaneous lesions (505).

Pathologic Findings. There is an infiltrate of varying intensity in the dermis and subcutis, both in a perivascular and interstitial distribution. The infiltrate includes varying combinations of myeloid and erythroid elements as well as megakaryocytes. Myeloid cells in different stages of maturation are present; in some reports, there has been an increase in cells of eosinophil lineage (505,507). Nucleated erythrocytes may be observed (fig. 13-61) (499). Large, atypical cells with pale eosinophilic cytoplasm and multiple or multilobated nuclei constitute megakaryocytes (505,509). The neonatal cases frequently contain only erythrocyte precursors, and myeloid cells are only occasionally present. For this reason, the term *cutaneous erythropoiesis* is sometimes applied to examples in newborns (499). All three elements are present in some adult cases (508, 511), but a number of reports have indicated a lack of erythrocyte precursors (505). Fairly numerous fibroblasts accompany the process. By using the Wilder or other methods, reticulin can be shown to surround megakaryocytes (505).

Myeloid cells stain red with CAE and also stain with MAC387. Megakaryocytes and scattered fibroblast-like cells are factor XIIIa positive, and megakaryocytes also express factor VIII–related antigen (505). The characteristics of the cells of erythroid and myeloid lineage can be identified ultrastructurally (504).

Differential Diagnosis. In neonates, the microscopic features of cutaneous extramedullary hematopoiesis provide a clue to an underlying systemic condition, particularly a congenital infection or hematologic abnormality. In adults, extramedullary hematopoiesis can be difficult to differentiate from chronic myelogenous leukemia. This is a particular problem in the setting of myelofibrosis, which has a number of features in common with chronic myelogenous leukemia. Myelofibrosis, however, is not associated with the Philadelphia chromosome (505). Erythroid precursors, when present, help in the recognition of extramedullary hematopoiesis. A predominance of megakaryocytes has also been reported in several cases of extramedullary hematopoiesis, and this also aids in the distinction between the two disorders (505,509).

REFERENCES

Lymphocytoma Cutis

1. Albrecht S, Hofstadter S, Artsob H, Chaban O, From L. Lymphadenosis benigna cutis resulting from Borrelia infection (Borrelia lymphocytoma). J Am Acad Dermatol 1991;24:621–5.
2. Bachelez H, Hadida F, Parizot C, et al. Oligoclonal expansion of HIV-specific cytotoxic CD8 T lymphocytes in the skin of HIV-1-infected patients with cutaneous pseudolymphoma. J Clin Invest 1998;101:2506–16.
3. Bafverstedt B. Lymphadenosis benigna cutis. Acta Derm Venereol 1968;48:1–6.
4. Baldassano MF, Bailey EM, Ferry JA, Harris NL, Duncan LM. Cutaneous lymphoid hyperplasia and cutaneous marginal zone lymphoma: comparison of morphologic and immunophenotypic features. Am J Surg Pathol 1999;23:88–96.
5. Braddock SW, Harrington D, Vose J. Generalized nodular cutaneous pseudolymphoma associated with phenytoin therapy. Use of T-cell receptor gene rearrangement in diagnosis and clinical review of cutaneous reactions to phenytoin. J Am Acad Dermatol 1992;27(Pt 2):337–40.
6. Burg G, Braun-Falco O, Hoffman-Fezer O, et al. Differentiation between pseudolymphomas and malignant B cell lymphomas of the skin. In: Christopher E, Goos M, eds. Lymphoproliferative diseases of the skin. Berlin: Springer-Verlag; 1982:101.
7. Caro WA, Helwig HB. Cutaneous lymphoid hyperplasia. Cancer 1969;24:487–502.
8. Crowson AN, Magro CM. Antidepressant therapy. A possible cause of atypical cutaneous lymphoid hyperplasia. Arch Dermatol 1995;131:925–9.
9. D'Incan M, Souteyrand P, Bignon YJ, Fonck Y, Roger H. Hydantoin-induced cutaneous pseudolymphoma with clinical, pathologic, and immunologic aspects of Sezary syndrome. Arch Dermatol 1992;128:1371–4.
10. Duncan SC, Evans HL, Winkelmann RK. Large cell lymphocytoma. Arch Dermatol 1980;116:1142–6.
11. Fan K, Kelly R, Kendrick V. Nonclonal lymphocytic proliferation in cutaneous lymphoid hyperplasia: a flow-cytometric and morphological analysis. Dermatology 1992;185:113–9.
12. Hovmark A, Asbrink E, Olsson I. The spirochetal etiology of lymphadenosis benigna cutis solitaria. Acta Derm Venereol 1986;66:479–84.
13. Jaffe ES, Harris NL, Stein H, Vardiman JW. Summary of the WHO classification of tumours of haematopoietic and lymphoid tissues. In: Jaffe ES, Harris NL, Stein H, Vardiman JW, eds. Pathology and genetics of tumours of haematopoietic and lymphoid tissues. Lyon: IARC Press; 2001:10–3.
14. Jubert C, Cosnes A, Wechsler J, Andre P, Revuz J, Bagot M. Anetoderma may reveal cutaneous plasmacytoma and benign cutaneous lymphoid hyperplasia. Arch Dermatol 1995;131:365–6.
15. Kuo TT, Lo SK, Chan HL. Immunohistochemical analysis of dermal mononuclear cell infiltrates in cutaneous lupus erythematosus, polymorphous light eruption, lymphocytic infiltration of Jessner, and cutaneous lymphoid hyperplasia: a comparative differential study. J Cutan Pathol 1994;21:430–6.
16. Lanzafame S, Micali G. [Cutaneous lymphoid hyperplasia (pseudolymphoma) secondary to vaccination.] Pathologica 1993;85:555–61. (Italian.)
17. LeBoit PE, McNutt NS, Reed JA, Jacobson M, Weiss LM. Primary cutaneous immunocytoma. A B-cell lymphoma that can easily be mistaken for cutaneous lymphoid hyperplasia. Am J Surg Pathol 1994;18:969–78.
18. Magro CM, Crowson AN. Drugs with antihistaminic properties as a cause of atypical cutaneous lymphoid hyperplasia. J Am Acad Dermatol 1995;32:419–28.
19. Medeiros LJ, Picker LJ, Abel EA, et al. Cutaneous lymphoid hyperplasia. Immunologic characteristics and assessment of criteria recently proposed as diagnostic of malignant lymphoma. J Am Acad Dermatol 1989;21(Pt 1):929–42.

20. Miracco C, Spina D, Santopietro R, et al. Apoptotic index: discriminant feature for the differentiation of cutaneous diffuse malignant follicular center cell lymphomas from lymphoid hyperplasia. J Invest Dermatol 1993;100:699–704.
21. Norton AJ. Classification of cutaneous lymphoma: a critical appraisal of recent proposals. Am J Dermatopathol 1999;21:279–87.
22. Patterson JW. Lymphomas. Dermatol Clin 1992;10:235–51.
23. Rijlaarsdam JU, Meijer CJ, Willemze R. Differentiation between lymphadenosis benigna cutis and primary cutaneous follicular center cell lymphomas. A comparative clinicopathologic study of 57 patients. Cancer 1990;65:2301–6.
24. Roo E, Villegas C, Lopez-Bran E, Jimenez E, Valle P, Sanchez-Yus E. Postzoster cutaneous pseudolymphoma. Arch Dermatol 1994;130:661–3.
25. Sander CA, Flaig MJ, Kaudewitz P, Jaffe ES. The revised European-American Classification of Lymphoid Neoplasms (REAL): a preferred approach for the classification of cutaneous lymphomas. Am J Dermatopathol 1999;21:274–8.
26. Schmid U, Eckert F, Griesser H, et al. Cutaneous follicular lymphoid hyperplasia with monotypic plasma cells. A clinicopathologic study of 18 patients. Am J Surg Pathol 1995;19:12–20.
27. Shelley WB, Wood MG, Wilson JF, Goodman R. Premalignant lymphoid hyperplasia preceding and coexisting with malignant lymphoma in the skin. Arch Dermatol 1981;117:500–3.
28. Slater DN. Recent developments in cutaneous lymphoproliferative disorders. J Pathol 1987;153:5–19.
29. Spina D, Miracco C, Santopietro R, et al. Distinction between diffuse cutaneous malignant follicular center cell lymphoma and lymphoid hyperplasia by computerized nuclear image analysis. Am J Dermatopathol 1993;15:415–22.
30. Toyota N, Matsuo S, Iizuka H. Immunohistochemical differential diagnosis between lymphocytoma cutis and malignant lymphoma in paraffin-embedded sections. J Dermatol 1991;18:586–91.
31. Willemze R, Meijer CJ. EORTC classification for primary cutaneous lymphomas: the best guide to good clinical management. European Organization for Research and Treatment of Cancer. Am J Dermatopathol 1999;21:265–73.

B-Cell Neoplasms

32. Aboulafia DM. Primary cutaneous large B-cell lymphoma of the legs: a distinct clinical pathologic entity treated with CD20 monoclonal antibody (rituximab). Am J Clin Oncol 2001;24:237–40.
33. Aguilera NS, Tomaszewski MM, Moad JC, Bauer FA, Taubenberger JK, Abbondanzo SL. Cutaneous follicle center lymphoma: a clinicopathologic study of 19 cases. Mod Pathol 2001;14:828–35.
34. Akagi M, Taniguchi S, Ozaki M, et al. Necrobiosis-lipoidica-like skin manifestation in lymphomatoid granulomatosis (Liebow). Dermatologica 1987;174:84–92.
35. Angel CA, Slater DN, Royds JA, Nelson SN, Bleehen SS. Epstein-Barr virus in cutaneous lymphomatoid granulomatosis. Histopathology 1994;25:545–8.
36. Armitage JO, Weisenburger DD. New approach to classifying non-Hodgkin's lymphomas: clinical features of the major histologic subtypes. Non-Hodgkin's Lymphoma Classification Project. J Clin Oncol 1998;16:2780–95.
37. Au WY, Shek WH, Nicholls J, Tse KM, Todd D, Kwong YL. T-cell intravascular lymphomatosis (angiotropic large cell lymphoma): association with Epstein-Barr viral infection. Histopathology 1997;31:563–7.
38. Bachmeyer C, Bazarbachi A, Rio B, et al. Specific cutaneous involvement indicating relapse of Burkitt's lymphoma. Am J Hematol 1997;54:176.
39. Bailey EM, Ferry JA, Harris NL, Mihm MC Jr, Jacobson JO, Duncan LM. Marginal zone lymphoma (low-grade B-cell lymphoma of mucosa-associated lymphoid tissue type) of skin and subcutaneous tissue: a study of 15 patients. Am J Surg Pathol 1996;20:1011–23.
40. Baldassano MF, Bailey EM, Ferry JA, Harris NL, Duncan LM. Cutaneous lymphoid hyperplasia and cutaneous marginal zone lymphoma: comparison of morphologic and immunophenotypic features. Am J Surg Pathol 1999;23:88–96.
41. Barcus ME, Karageorge LS, Veloso YL, Kornstein MJ. CD10 expression in follicular lymphoma versus reactive follicular hyperplasia: evaluation in paraffin-embedded tissue. Appl Immunohistochem Mol Morphol 2000;8:263–6.
42. Beaty MW, Toro J, Sorbara L, et al. Cutaneous lymphomatoid granulomatosis: correlation of clinical and biologic features. Am J Surg Pathol 2001;25:1111–20.
43. Bergman R, Kurtin PJ, Gibson LE, Hull PR, Kimlinger TK, Schroeter AL. Clinicopathologic, immunophenotypic, and molecular characterization of primary cutaneous follicular B-cell lymphoma. Arch Dermatol 2001;137:432–9.
44. Bhawan J, Wolff SM, Ucci AA, Bhan AK. Malignant lymphoma and malignant angioendotheliomatosis: one disease. Cancer 1985;55:570–6.
45. Brodell RT, Miller CW, Eisen AZ. Cutaneous lesions of lymphomatoid granulomatosis. Arch Dermatol 1986;122:303–6.

46. Brunning RD, Borowitz M, Matutes E, et al. Precursor B lymphoblastic leukaemia/lymphoblastic lymphoma (precursor B-cell acute lymphoblastic leukaemia. In: Jaffe ES, Harris NL, Stein H, Vardiman JW, eds. Pathology and genetics of tumours of haematopoietic and lymphoid tissues. Lyon: IARC Press; 2001:111–14.
47. Busschots AM, Geerts ML, Mecucci C, Stul M, Cassiman JJ, van den Berghe H. A translocation (8;14) in a cutaneous large B-cell lymphoma. Am J Clin Pathol 1993;99:615–21.
48. Carlson KC, Gibson LE. Cutaneous signs of lymphomatoid granulomatosis. Arch Dermatol 1991;127:1693–8.
49. Cerroni L, El-Shabrawi-Caelen L, Fink-Puches R, LeBoit PE, Kerl H. Cutaneous spindle-cell B-cell lymphoma: a morphologic variant of cutaneous large B-cell lymphoma. Am J Dermatopathol 2000;22:299–304.
50. Cerroni L, Kerl H. Primary cutaneous follicle center cell lymphoma. Leuk Lymphoma 2001;42:891–900.
51. Cerroni L, Signoretti S, Hofler G, et al. Primary cutaneous marginal zone B-cell lymphoma: a recently described entity of low-grade malignant cutaneous B-cell lymphoma. Am J Surg Pathol 1997;21:1307–15.
52. Cerroni L, Zochling N, Putz B, Kerl H. Infection by Borrelia burgdorferi and cutaneous B-cell lymphoma. J Cutan Pathol 1997;24:457–61.
53. Chang A, Zic JA, Boyd AS. Intravascular large cell lymphoma: a patient with asymptomatic purpuric patches and a chronic clinical course. J Am Acad Dermatol 1998;39(Pt 2):318–21.
54. Child FJ, Russell-Jones R, Woolford AJ, et al. Absence of the t(14;18) chromosomal translocation in primary cutaneous B-cell lymphoma. Br J Dermatol 2001;144:735–44.
55. Chimenti S, Cerroni L, Zenahlik P, Peris K, Kerl H. The role of MT2 and anti-bcl-2 protein antibodies in the differentiation of benign from malignant cutaneous infiltrates of B-lymphocytes with germinal center formation. J Cutan Pathol 1996;23:319–22.
56. de la Fouchardiere A, Balme B, Chouvet B, et al. Primary cutaneous marginal zone B-cell lymphoma: a report of 9 cases. J Am Acad Dermatol 1999;41(Pt 1):181–8.
57. de Leval L, Harris NL, Longtine J, Ferry JA, Duncan LM. Cutaneous b-cell lymphomas of follicular and marginal zone types: use of Bcl-6, CD10, Bcl-2, and CD21 in differential diagnosis and classification. Am J Surg Pathol 2001;25:732–41.
58. Diebold J, Jaffe ES, Raphael M, Warnke RA. Burkitt lymphoma. In: Jaffe ES, Harris NL, Stein H, Vardiman JW, eds. Pathology and genetics of tumours of haematopoietic and lymphoid tissues Lyon: IARC Press; 2001:181–4.
59. DiGiuseppe JA, Nelson WG, Seifter EJ, Boitnott JK, Mann RB. Intravascular lymphomatosis: a clinicopathologic study of 10 cases and assessment of response to chemotherapy. J Clin Oncol 1994;12:2573–9.
60. Doggett RS, Wood GS, Horning S, et al. The immunologic characterization of 95 nodal and extranodal diffuse large cell lymphomas in 89 patients. Am J Pathol 1984;115:245–52.
61. Dominguez FE, Rosen LB, Kramer HC. Malignant angioendotheliomatosis proliferans. Report of an autopsied case studied with immunoperoxidase. Am J Dermatopathol 1986;8:419–25.
62. Dommann SN, Dommann-Scherrer CC, Zimmerman D, Dours-Zimmermann MT, Hassam S, Burg G. Primary cutaneous T-cell-rich B-cell lymphoma. A case report with a 13-year follow-up. Am J Dermatopathol 1995;17:618–24.
63. Du MQ, Diss TC, Xu CF, Wotherspoon AC, Isaacson PG, Pan LX. Ongoing immunoglobulin gene mutations in mantle cell lymphomas. Br J Haematol 1997;96:124–31.
64. Duray PH. The surgical pathology of human Lyme disease. An enlarging picture. Am J Surg Pathol 1987;11(Suppl 1):47–60.
65. Franco R, Fernandez-Vazquez A, Mollejo M, et al. Cutaneous presentation of follicular lymphomas. Mod Pathol 2001;14:913–9.
66. Garbea A, Dippel E, Hildenbrand R, Bleyl U, Schadendorf D, Goerdt S. Cutaneous large B-cell lymphoma of the leg masquerading as a chronic venous ulcer. Br J Dermatol 2002;146:144–7.
67. Gatter KC, Warnke RA. Diffuse large B-cell lymphoma. In: Jaffe ES, Harris NL, Stein H, Vardiman JW, eds. Pathology and genetics of tumours of haematopoietic and lymphoid tissues. Lyon: IARC Press; 2001:171–4.
68. Gatter KC, Warnke RA. Intravascular large B-cell lymphoma. In: Jaffe ES, Harris NL, Stein H, Vardiman JW, eds. Pathology and genetics of tumours of haematopoietic and lymphoid tissues. Lyon: IARC Press; 2001:177–8.
69. Geelen FA, Vermeer MH, Meijer CJ, et al. bcl-2 protein expression in primary cutaneous large B-cell lymphoma is site-related. J Clin Oncol 1998;16:2080–5.
70. Gogstetter D, Brown M, Seab J, Scott G. Angiocentric primary cutaneous T-cell-rich B-cell lymphoma: a case report and review of the literature. J Cutan Pathol 2000;27:516–25.

71. Goodlad JR, Davidson MM, Hollowood K, Batstone P, Ho-Yen DO. Borrelia burgdorferi-associated cutaneous marginal zone lymphoma: a clinicopathological study of two cases illustrating the temporal progression of B. burgdorferi-associated B-cell proliferation in the skin. Histopathology 2000;37:501–8.
72. Goodlad JR, Krajewski AS, Batstone PJ, et al. Primary cutaneous follicular lymphoma: a clinicopathologic and molecular study of 16 cases in support of a distinct entity. Am J Surg Pathol 2002;26:733–41.
73. Grogan TM, Van Camp B, Kyle RA, Muller-Hermelink HK, Harris NL. Plasma cell neoplasms [myeloma]. In: Jaffe ES, Harris NL, Stein H, Vardiman JW, eds. Tumours of haematopoietic and lymphoid tissues. Lyon: IARC Press; 2001:142–56.
74. Haque AK, Myers JL, Hudnall SD, et al. Pulmonary lymphomatoid granulomatosis in acquired immunodeficiency syndrome: lesions with Epstein-Barr virus infection. Mod Pathol 1998;11:347–56.
75. Hofbauer GF, Kessler B, Kempf W, Nestle FO, Burg G, Dummer R. Multilesional primary cutaneous diffuse large B-cell lymphoma responsive to antibiotic treatment. Dermatology 2001;203:168–70.
76. Isaacson PG, Muller-Hermelink HK, Piris MA, et al. Extranodal marginal zone B-cell lymphoma of mucosa-associated lymphoid tissue (MALT lymphoma). In: Jaffe ES, Harris NL, Stein H, Vardiman JW, eds. Pathology and genetics of tumours of haematopoietic and lymphoid tissues. Lyon: IARC Press; 2001:157–60.
77. Jaffe ES, Chan JK, Su IJ, et al. Report of the Workshop on Nasal and Related Extranodal Angiocentric T/Natural Killer Cell Lymphomas. Definitions, differential diagnosis, and epidemiology. Am J Surg Pathol 1996;20:103–11.
78. Jaffe ES, Wilson WH. Lymphomatoid granulomatosis. In: Jaffe ES, Harris NL, Stein H, Vardiman JW, eds. Pathology and genetics of tumours of haematopoietic and lymphoid tissue. Lyon: IARC Press; 2001:185–7.
79. James WD, Odom RB, Katzenstein AL. Cutaneous manifestations of lymphomatoid granulomatosis. Report of 44 cases and a review of the literature. Arch Dermatol 1981;117:196–202.
80. Kahwash SB, Qualman SJ. Cutaneous lymphoblastic lymphoma in children: report of six cases with precursor B-cell lineage. Pediatr Dev Pathol 2002;5:45–53.
81. Kanda M, Suzumiya J, Ohshima K, Tamura K, Kikuchi M. Intravascular large cell lymphoma: clinicopathological, immuno-histochemical and molecular genetic studies. Leuk Lymphoma 1999;34:569–80.
82. Katzenstein AL, Carrington CB, Liebow AA. Lymphomatoid granulomatosis: a clinicopathologic study of 152 cases. Cancer 1979;43:360–73.
83. Kerl H, Cerroni L. Controversies in cutaneous lymphomas. Semin Cutan Med Surg 2000;19:157–60.
84. Kessler S, Lund HZ, Leonard DD. Cutaneous lesions of lymphomatoid granulomatosis. Comparison with lymphomatoid papulosis. Am J Dermatopathol 1981;3:115–27.
85. Khalidi HS, Brynes RK, Browne P, Koo CH, Battifora H, Medeiros LJ. Intravascular large B-cell lymphoma: the CD5 antigen is expressed by a subset of cases. Mod Pathol 1998;11:983–8.
86. Kiyohara T, Kumakiri M, Kobayashi H, Shimizu T, Ohkawara A, Ohnuki M. A case of intravascular large B-cell lymphoma mimicking erythema nodosum: the importance of multiple skin biopsies. J Cutan Pathol 2000;27:413–8.
87. Lakhani SR, Hulman G, Hall JM, Slack DN, Sloane JP. Intravascular malignant lymphomatosis (angiotropic large-cell lymphoma). A case report with evidence for T-cell lineage with polymerase chain reaction analysis. Histopathology 1994;25:283–6.
88. Lawnicki LC, Weisenburger DD, Aoun P, Chan WC, Wickert RS, Greiner TC. The t(14;18) and bcl-2 expression are present in a subset of primary cutaneous follicular lymphoma: association with lower grade. Am J Clin Pathol 2002;118:765–72.
89. LeBoit PE, McNutt NS, Reed JA, Jacobson M, Weiss LM. Primary cutaneous immunocytoma. A B-cell lymphoma that can easily be mistaken for cutaneous lymphoid hyperplasia. Am J Surg Pathol 1994;18:969–78.
90. Li S, Griffin CA, Mann RB, Borowitz MJ. Primary cutaneous T-cell-rich B-cell lymphoma: clinically distinct from its nodal counterpart? Mod Pathol 2001;14:10–3.
91. Lin P, Jones D, Dorfman DM, Medeiros LJ. Precursor B-cell lymphoblastic lymphoma: a predominantly extranodal tumor with low propensity for leukemic involvement. Am J Surg Pathol 2000;24:1480–90.
92. Lipford EH Jr, Margolick JB, Longo DL, Fauci AS, Jaffe ES. Angiocentric immunoproliferative lesions: a clinicopathologic spectrum of post-thymic T-cell proliferations. Blood 1988;72:1674–81.
93. Maitra A, McKenna RW, Weinberg AG, Schneider NR, Kroft SH. Precursor B-cell lymphoblastic lymphoma. A study of nine cases lacking blood and bone marrow involvement and review of the literature. Am J Clin Pathol 2001;115:868–75.

94. Mann RB, Berard CW. Criteria for the cytologic subclassification of follicular lymphomas: a proposed alternative method. Hematol Oncol 1983;1:187–92.
95. Marti RM, Campo E, Bosch F, Palou J, Estrach T. Cutaneous lymphocyte-associated antigen (CLA) expression in a lymphoblastoid mantle cell lymphoma presenting with skin lesions. Comparison with other clinicopathologic presentations of mantle cell lymphoma. J Cutan Pathol 2001;28:256–64.
96. McNiff JM, Cooper D, Howe G, et al. Lymphomatoid granulomatosis of the skin and lung. An angiocentric T-cell-rich B-cell lymphoproliferative disorder. Arch Dermatol 1996;132:1464–70.
97. Miller TP, Grogan TM, Dahlberg S, et al. Prognostic significance of the Ki-67-associated proliferative antigen in aggressive non-Hodgkin's lymphomas: a prospective Southwest Oncology Group trial. Blood 1994;83:1460–6.
98. Minars N, Kay S, Escobar MR. Lymphomatoid granulomatosis of the skin. A new clinocopathologic entity. Arch Dermatol 1975;111:493–6.
99. Mirza I, Macpherson N, Paproski S, et al. Primary cutaneous follicular lymphoma: an assessment of clinical, histopathologic, immunophenotypic, and molecular features. J Clin Oncol 2002;20:647–55.
100. Moody BR, Bartlett NL, George DW, et al. Cyclin D1 as an aid in the diagnosis of mantle cell lymphoma in skin biopsies: a case report. Am J Dermatopathol 2001;23:470–6.
101. Murphy GF, Harrist TJ, Sato S, Mihm MC Jr. Microvascular injury in lymphomatoid granulomatosis involving the skin. An ultrastructural study. Arch Dermatol 1981;117:804–8.
102. Norton AJ. Classification of cutaneous lymphoma: a critical appraisal of recent proposals. Am J Dermatopathol 1999;21:279–87.
103. Ott G, Katzenberger T, Greiner A, et al. The t(11;18)(q21;q21) chromosome translocation is a frequent and specific aberration in low-grade but not high-grade malignant non-Hodgkin's lymphomas of the mucosa-associated lymphoid tissue (MALT-) type. Cancer Res 1997;57:3944–8.
104. Pelicci PG, Knowles DM 2nd, Magrath I, Dalla-Favera R. Chromosomal breakpoints and structural alterations of the c-myc locus differ in endemic and sporadic forms of Burkitt lymphoma. Proc Natl Acad Sci U S A 1986;83:2984–8.
105. Perniciaro C, Winkelmann RK, Daoud MS, Su WP. Malignant angioendotheliomatosis is an angiotropic intravascular lymphoma. Immunohistochemical, ultrastructural, and molecular genetics studies. Am J Dermatopathol 1995;17:242–8.
106. Piris M, Brown DC, Gatter KC, Mason DY. CD30 expression in non-Hodgkin's lymphoma. Histopathology 1990;17:211–8.
107. Ponzoni M, Arrigoni G, Gould VE, et al. Lack of CD 29 (beta1 integrin) and CD 54 (ICAM-1) adhesion molecules in intravascular lymphomatosis. Hum Pathol 2000;31:220–6.
108. Rogge T. [Burkitt's lymphoma with skin infiltrates.] Hautarzt 1975;26:379–82. (German.)
109. Roggero E, Zucca E, Mainetti C, et al. Eradication of Borrelia burgdorferi infection in primary marginal zone B-cell lymphoma of the skin. Hum Pathol 2000;31:263–8.
110. Sander CA, Flaig MJ, Kaudewitz P, Jaffe ES. The revised European-American Classification of Lymphoid Neoplasms (REAL): a preferred approach for the classification of cutaneous lymphomas. Am J Dermatopathol 1999;21:274–8.
111. Sander CA, Kaudewitz P, Kutzner H, et al. T-cell-rich B-cell lymphoma presenting in skin. A clinicopathologic analysis of six cases. J Cutan Pathol 1996;23:101–8.
112. Sarikaya I, Patel M, Holder L. Cutaneous mantle cell lymphoma detected with Ga-67 Citrate. Clin Nucl Med 2000;25:849–51.
113. Setoyama M, Mizoguchi S, Orikawa T, Tashiro M. A case of intravascular malignant lymphomatosis (angiotropic large-cell lymphoma) presenting memory T cell phenotype and its expression of adhesion molecules. J Dermatol 1992;19:263–9.
114. Sleater JP, Segal GH, Scott MD, Masih AS. Intravascular (angiotropic) large cell lymphoma: determination of monoclonality by polymerase chain reaction on paraffin-embedded tissues. Mod Pathol 1994;7:593–8.
115. Sordillo PP, Epremian B, Koziner B, Lacher M, Lieberman P. Lymphomatoid granulomatosis: an analysis of clinical and immunologic characteristics. Cancer 1982;49:2070–6.
116. Starz H, Balda BR, Bachter D, Buchels H, Vogt H. Secondary lymph node involvement from primary cutaneous large B-cell lymphoma of the leg: sentinel lymph nodectomy as a new strategy for staging circumscribed cutaneous lymphomas. Cancer 1999;85:199–207.
117. Swerdlow SH, Berger F, Isaacson PI, et al. Mantle cell lymphoma. In: Jaffe ES, Harris NL, Stein H, Vardiman JW, eds. Pathology and genetics of tumours of haematopoietic and lymphoid tissues. Lyon: IARC Press; 2001:168–70.
118. Take H, Kubota K, Fukuda T, Shinonome S, Ishikawa O, Shirakura T. An indolent type of Epstein-Barr virus-associated T-cell-rich B-cell lymphoma of the skin: report of a case. Am J Hematol 1996;52:221–3.

119. Tas S, Simonart T, Dargent J, et al. [Primary and isolated cutaneous lymphomatoid granulomatosis following heart-lung transplantation.] Ann Dermatol Venereol 2000;127:488–91. (French.)
120. Thieblemont C, Berger F, Dumontet C, et al. Mucosa-associated lymphoid tissue lymphoma is a disseminated disease in one third of 158 patients analyzed. Blood 2000;95:802–6.
121. Tomaszewski MM, Abbondanzo SL, Lupton GP. Extranodal marginal zone B-cell lymphoma of the skin: a morphologic and immunophenotypic study of 11 cases. Am J Dermatopathol 2000;22:205–11.
122. Valdez R, Finn WG, Ross CW, Singleton TP, Tworek JA, Schnitzer B. Waldenstrom macroglobulinemia caused by extranodal marginal zone B-cell lymphoma: a report of six cases. Am J Clin Pathol 2001;116:683–90.
123. Vermeer MH, Geelen FA, van Haselen CW, et al. Primary cutaneous large B-cell lymphomas of the legs. A distinct type of cutaneous B-cell lymphoma with an intermediate prognosis. Dutch Cutaneous Lymphoma Working Group. Arch Dermatol 1996;132:1304–8.
124. Viguier M, Rivet J, Agbalika F, et al. B-cell lymphomas involving the skin associated with hepatitis C virus infection. Int J Dermatol 2002;41:577–82.
125. Wick MR, Ritter JH, Humphrey PA, Swanson PE. Immunopathology of nonneoplastic skin disease: a brief review. Am J Clin Pathol 1996;105:417–29.
126. Wick MR, Rocamora A. Reactive and malignant "angioendotheliomatosis": a discriminant clinicopathological study. J Cutan Pathol 1988;15:260–71.
127. Willemze R, Meijer CJ. EORTC classification for primary cutaneous lymphomas: the best guide to good clinical management. European Organization for Research and Treatment of Cancer. Am J Dermatopathol 1999;21:265–73.
128. Wilson WH, Teruya-Feldstein J, Fest T, et al. Relationship of p53, bcl-2, and tumor proliferation to clinical drug resistance in non-Hodgkin's lymphomas. Blood 1997;89:601–9.
129. Wollina U. Complete response of a primary cutaneous T-cell-rich B cell lymphoma treated with interferon alpha2a. J Cancer Res Clin Oncol 1998;124:127–9.
130. Wollina U, Mentzel T, Graefe T. Large B-cell lymphoma of the leg—complete remission with perilesional interferon alpha. Dermatology 2001;203:165–7.
131. Wood ML, Harrington CI, Slater DN, Rooney N, Clark A. Cutaneous lymphomatoid granulomatosis: a rare cause of recurrent skin ulceration. Br J Dermatol 1984;110:619–25.
132. Wotherspoon AC, Finn TM, Isaacson PG. Trisomy 3 in low-grade B-cell lymphomas of mucosa-associated lymphoid tissue. Blood 1995;85:2000–4.
133. Wrotnowski U, Mills SE, Cooper PH. Malignant angioendotheliomatosis. An angiotropic lymphoma? Am J Clin Pathol 1985;83:244–8.

T-Cell and NK-Cell Neoplasms

134. Abruzzo LV, Schmidt K, Weiss LM, et al. B-cell lymphoma after angioimmunoblastic lymphadenopathy: a case with oligoclonal gene rearrangements associated with Epstein-Barr virus. Blood 1993;82:241–6.
135. Ackerman AB, Breza TS, Capland L. Spongiotic simulants of mycosis fungoides. Arch Dermatol 1974;109:218–20.
136. Agnarsson BA, Kadin ME. Host response in lymphomatoid papulosis. Hum Pathol 1989;20:747–52.
137. Agnarsson BA, Kadin ME. Ki-1 positive large cell lymphoma. A morphologic and immunologic study of 19 cases. Am J Surg Pathol 1988;12:264–74.
138. Agnarsson BA, Vonderheid EC, Kadin ME. Cutaneous T cell lymphoma with suppressor/cytotoxic (CD8) phenotype: identification of rapidly progressive and chronic subtypes. J Am Acad Dermatol 1990;22:569–77.
139. Ali SK, Othman NM, Tagoe AB, Tulba AA. Subcutaneous panniculitic T cell lymphoma mimicking histiocytic cytophagic panniculitis in a child. Saudi Med J 2000;21:1074–7.
140. Altman J. Parapsoriasis: a histopathologic review and classification. Semin Dermatol 1984;3:14–21.
141. Anagnostopoulos I, Herbst H, Niedobitek G, Stein H. Demonstration of monoclonal EBV genomes in Hodgkin's disease and Ki-1-positive anaplastic large cell lymphoma by combined Southern blot and in situ hybridization. Blood 1989;74:810–6.
142. Anagnostopoulos I, Hummel M, Finn T, et al. Heterogeneous Epstein-Barr virus infection patterns in peripheral T-cell lymphoma of angioimmunoblastic lymphadenopathy type. Blood 1992;80:1804–12.
143. Ansai S, Maeda K, Yamakawa M, et al. CD56-positive (nasal-type T/NK cell) lymphoma arising on the skin. Report of two cases and review of the literature. J Cutan Pathol 1997;24:468–76.
144. Aoki M, Niimi Y, Takezaki S, Azuma A, Seike M, Kawana S. CD30+ lymphoproliferative disorder: primary cutaneous anaplastic large cell lymphoma followed by lymphomatoid papulosis. Br J Dermatol 2001;145:123–6.

145. Aoyama Y, Yamane T, Hino M, et al. Blastic NK-cell lymphoma/leukemia with T-cell receptor gamma rearrangement. Ann Hematol 2001;80:752–4.
146. Arai E, Chow KC, Li CY, Tokunaga M, Katayama I. Differentiation between cutaneous form of adult T cell leukemia/lymphoma and cutaneous T cell lymphoma by in situ hybridization using a human T cell leukemia virus-1 DNA probe. Am J Pathol 1994;144:15–20.
147. Argenyi ZB, Goeken JA, Piette WW, Madison KC. Granulomatous mycosis fungoides. Clinicopathologic study of two cases. Am J Dermatopathol 1992;14:200–10.
148. Arnulf B, Copie-Bergman C, Delfau-Larue MH, et al. Nonhepatosplenic gammadelta T-cell lymphoma: a subset of cytotoxic lymphomas with mucosal or skin localization. Blood 1998;91:1723–31.
149. Ashworth J, Coady AT, Guy R, Breathnach SM. Brawny cutaneous induration and granulomatous panniculitis in large cell non-Hodgkin's (T suppressor/cytotoxic cell) lymphoma. Br J Dermatol 1989;120:563–9.
150. Au WY, Liang R. Peripheral T-cell lymphoma. Curr Oncol Rep 2002;4:434–42.
151. Au WY, Ng WM, Choy C, Kwong YL. Aggressive subcutaneous panniculitis-like T-cell lymphoma: complete remission with fludarabine, mitoxantrone and dexamethasone. Br J Dermatol 2000;143:408–10.
152. Balus L, Bassetti F, Gentili G. Granulomatous slack skin. Arch Dermatol 1985;121:250–2.
153. Banerjee SS, Heald J, Harris M. Twelve cases of Ki-1 positive anaplastic large cell lymphoma of skin. J Clin Pathol 1991;44:119–25.
154. Barzilai A, Goldberg I, Shibi R, Kopolovic J, Trau H. Mycosis fungoides expressing gamma/delta T-cell receptors. J Am Acad Dermatol 1996;34 (Pt 1):301–2.
155. Bekkenk MW, Geelen FA, van Voorst Vader PC, et al. Primary and secondary cutaneous CD30(+) lymphoproliferative disorders: a report from the Dutch Cutaneous Lymphoma Group on the long-term follow-up data of 219 patients and guidelines for diagnosis and treatment [lymphomatoid papulosis]. Blood 2000;95:3653–61.
156. Bekkenk MW, Kluin PM, Jansen PM, Meijer CJ, Willemze R. Lymphomatoid papulosis with a natural killer-cell phenotype. Br J Dermatol 2001;145:318–22.
157. Bernengo MG, Levi L, Zina G. Skin lesions in angioimmunoblastic lymphadenopathy: histological and immunological studies. Br J Dermatol 1981;104:131–9.
158. Bernengo MG, Quaglino P, Novelli M, et al. Prognostic factors in Sezary syndrome: a multivariate analysis of clinical, haematological and immunological features. Ann Oncol 1998;9:857–63.
159. Bernstein JE, Soltani K, Lorincz AL. Cutaneous manifestations of angioimmunoblastic lymphadenopathy. J Am Acad Dermatol 1979;1:227–32.
160. Berti E, Cerri A, Cavicchini S, et al. Primary cutaneous gamma/delta T-cell lymphoma presenting as disseminated pagetoid reticulosis. J Invest Dermatol 1991;96:718–23.
161. Bhushan M, Craven NM, Armstrong GR, Chalmers RJ. Lymphoepithelioid cell lymphoma (Lennert's lymphoma) presenting as atypical granuloma annulare. Br J Dermatol 2000;142:776–80.
162. Blakolmer K, Vesely M, Kummer JA, Jurecka W, Mannhalter C, Chott A. Immunoreactivity of B-cell markers (CD79a, L26) in rare cases of extranodal cytotoxic peripheral T- (NK/T-) cell lymphomas. Mod Pathol 2000;13:766–72.
163. Boni R, Davis-Daneshfar A, Burg G, Fuchs D, Wood GS. No detection of HTLV-I proviral DNA in lesional skin biopsies from Swiss and German patients with cutaneous T-cell lymphoma. Br J Dermatol 1996;134:282–4.
164. Bonta MD, Tannous ZS, Demierre MF, Gonzalez E, Harris NL, Duncan LM. Rapidly progressing mycosis fungoides presenting as follicular mucinosis. J Am Acad Dermatol 2000;43:635–40.
165. Boulland ML, Wechsler J, Bagot M, Pulford K, Kanavaros P, Gaulard P. Primary CD30-positive cutaneous T-cell lymphomas and lymphomatoid papulosis frequently express cytotoxic proteins. Histopathology 2000;36:136–44.
166. Bower CP, Standen GR, Pawade J, Knechtli CJ, Kennedy CT. Cutaneous presentation of steroid responsive blastoid natural killer cell lymphoma. Br J Dermatol 2000;142:1017–20.
167. Braddock SW, Harrington D, Vose J. Generalized nodular cutaneous pseudolymphoma associated with phenytoin therapy. Use of T-cell receptor gene rearrangement in diagnosis and clinical review of cutaneous reactions to phenytoin. J Am Acad Dermatol 1992;27(Pt 2):337–40.
168. Brown HA, Macon WR, Kurtin PJ, Gibson LE. Cutaneous involvement by angioimmunoblastic T-cell lymphoma with remarkable heterogeneous Epstein-Barr virus expression. J Cutan Pathol 2001;28:432–8.
169. Brunning RD, Borowitz M, Matutes E, et al. Precursor T lymphoblastic leukaemia/lymphoblastic lymphoma (precursor T-cell acute lymphoblastic leukemia). In: Jaffe ES, Harris NL, Stein H, Vardiman JW, eds. Pathology and genetics of tumours of haematopoietic and lymphoid tissues. Lyon: IARC Press; 2001:115–7.

170. Buechner SA, Winkelmann RK. Sezary syndrome. A clinicopathologic study of 39 cases. Arch Dermatol 1983;119:979–86.
171. Burg G, Dummer R. Small plaque (digitate) parapsoriasis is an 'abortive cutaneous T-cell lymphoma' and is not mycosis fungoides. Arch Dermatol 1995;131:336–8.
172. Burns MK, Chan LS, Cooper KD. Woringer-Kolopp disease (localized pagetoid reticulosis) or unilesional mycosis fungoides? An analysis of eight cases with benign disease. Arch Dermatol 1995;131:325–9.
173. Buzzanga J, Banks PM, Winkelmann RK. Lymph node histopathology in Sezary syndrome. J Am Acad Dermatol 1984;11(Pt 1):880–8.
174. Camacho FM, Burg G, Moreno JC, Campora RG, Villar JL. Granulomatous slack skin in childhood. Pediatr Dermatol 1997;14:204–8.
175. Canioni D, Arnulf B, Asso-Bonnet M, Raphael M, Brousse N. Nasal natural killer lymphoma associated with Epstein-Barr virus in a patient infected with human immunodeficiency virus. Arch Pathol Lab Med 2001;125:660–2.
176. Carbone A, Gloghini A, Volpe R, Boiocchi M, Tirelli U. High frequency of Epstein-Barr virus latent membrane protein-1 expression in acquired immunodeficiency syndrome-related Ki-1 (CD30)-positive anaplastic large-cell lymphomas. Italian Cooperative Group on AIDS and Tumors. Am J Clin Pathol 1994;101:768–72.
177. Cataldo KA, Jalal SM, Law ME, et al. Detection of t(2;5) in anaplastic large cell lymphoma: comparison of immunohistochemical studies, FISH, and RT-PCR in paraffin-embedded tissue. Am J Surg Pathol 1999;23:1386–92.
178. Cerroni L, Fink-Puches R, Back B, Kerl H. Follicular mucinosis: a critical reappraisal of clinicopathologic features and association with mycosis fungoides and Sezary syndrome. Arch Dermatol 2002;138:182–9.
179. Cerroni L, Rieger E, Hodl S, Kerl H. Clinicopathologic and immunologic features associated with transformation of mycosis fungoides to large-cell lymphoma. Am J Surg Pathol 1992;16:543–52.
180. Chan HL, Su IJ, Kuo TT, et al. Cutaneous manifestations of adult T cell leukemia/lymphoma. Report of three different forms. J Am Acad Dermatol 1985;13(Pt 1):213–9.
181. Chan JK, Buchanan R, Fletcher CD. Sarcomatoid variant of anaplastic large-cell Ki-1 lymphoma. Am J Surg Pathol 1990;14:983–8.
182. Chan JK, Jaffe ES, Ralfkiaer E. Blastic NK-cell lymphoma. In: Jaffe ES, Harris NL, Stein H, Vardiman JW, eds. Pathology and genetics of tumours of hematopoietic and lymphoid tissues. Lyon: IARC Press; 2001:214–5.
183. Chan JK, Ng CS, Hui PK, et al. Anaplastic large cell Ki-1 lymphoma. Delineation of two morphological types. Histopathology 1989;15:11–34.
184. Chan YF, Lee KC, Llewellyn H. Subcutaneous T-cell lymphoma presenting as panniculitis in children: report of two cases. Pediatr Pathol 1994;14:595–608.
185. Chang SE, Choi HJ, Huh J, et al. A case of primary cutaneous CD56+, TdT+, CD4+, blastic NK-cell lymphoma in a 19-year-old woman. Am J Dermatopathol 2002;24:72–5.
186. Chang SE, Huh J, Choi JH, Sung KJ, Moon KC, Koh JK. Clinicopathological features of CD56+ nasal-type T/natural killer cell lymphomas with lobular panniculitis. Br J Dermatol 2000;142:924–30.
187. Chang SE, Yoon GS, Huh J, et al. Comparison of primary and secondary cutaneous CD56+ NK/T cell lymphomas. Appl Immunohistochem Mol Morphol 2002;10:163–70.
188. Child FJ, Russell-Jones R, Woolford AJ, et al. Absence of the t(14;18) chromosomal translocation in primary cutaneous B-cell lymphoma. Br J Dermatol 2001;144:735–44.
189. Chimenti S, Fink-Puches R, Peris K, et al. Cutaneous involvement in lymphoblastic lymphoma. J Cutan Pathol 1999;26:379–85.
190. Chott A, Kaserer K, Augustin I, et al. Ki-1-positive large cell lymphoma. A clinicopathologic study of 41 cases. Am J Surg Pathol 1990;14:439–48.
191. Chott A, Vonderheid EC, Olbricht S, Miao NN, Balk SP, Kadin ME. The dominant T cell clone is present in multiple regressing skin lesions and associated T cell lymphomas of patients with lymphomatoid papulosis. J Invest Dermatol 1996;106:696–700.
192. Cockerell CJ, Stetler LD. Accuracy in diagnosis of lymphomatoid papulosis. Am J Dermatopathol 1991;13:20–5.
193. Colby TV, Burke JS, Hoppe RT. Lymph node biopsy in mycosis fungoides. Cancer 1981;47:351–9.
194. Cotten H, Janin A, Gross S, Bombart M, Thomas P, Gosselin B. [Strictly epidermotropic "Ketron Goodman"-type lymphoma. Immunohistochemical and ultrastructural analysis of a case.] Ann Pathol 1991;11:117–21. (French.)
195. Crowson AN, Magro CM. Woringer-Kolopp disease. A lymphomatoid hypersensitivity reaction. Am J Dermatopathol 1994;16:542–8.
196. D'Incan M, Souteyrand P, Bignon YJ, Fonck Y, Roger H. Hydantoin-induced cutaneous pseudolymphoma with clinical, pathologic, and immunologic aspects of Sezary syndrome. Arch Dermatol 1992;128:1371–4.

197. Dargent JL, Roufosse C, Delville JP, et al. Subcutaneous panniculitis-like T-cell lymphoma: further evidence for a distinct neoplasm originating from large granular lymphocytes of T/NK phenotype. J Cutan Pathol 1998;25:394–400.
198. Davis TH, Morton CC, Miller-Cassman R, Balk SP, Kadin ME. Hodgkin's disease, lymphomatoid papulosis, and cutaneous T-cell lymphoma derived from a common T-cell clone. N Engl J Med 1992;326:1115–22.
199. de Campos-Lima PO, Levitsky V, Brooks J, et al. T cell responses and virus evolution: loss of HLA A11-restricted CTL epitopes in Epstein-Barr virus isolates from highly A11-positive populations by selective mutation of anchor residues. J Exp Med 1994;179:1297–305.
200. De Silva BD, McLaren K, Kavanagh GM. Photosensitive mycosis fungoides or actinic reticuloid? Br J Dermatol 2000;142:1221–7.
201. DeGregorio R, Fenske NA, Glass LF. Granulomatous slack skin: a possible precursor of Hodgkin's disease. J Am Acad Dermatol 1995;33:1044–7.
202. del Mistro A, Leszl A, Bertorelle R, et al. A CD30-positive T cell line established from an aggressive anaplastic large cell lymphoma, originally diagnosed as Hodgkin's disease. Leukemia 1994;8:1214–9.
203. Delsol G, Al Saati T, Gatter KC, et al. Coexpression of epithelial membrane antigen (EMA), Ki-1, and interleukin-2 receptor by anaplastic large cell lymphomas. Diagnostic value in so-called malignant histiocytosis. Am J Pathol 1988;130:59–70.
204. Deneau DG, Wood GS, Beckstead J, Hoppe RT, Price N. Woringer-Kolopp disease (pagetoid reticulosis). Four cases with histopathologic, ultrastructural, and immunohistologic observations. Arch Dermatol 1984;120:1045–51.
205. Diamandidou E, Colome-Grimmer M, Fayad L, Duvic M, Kurzrock R. Transformation of mycosis fungoides/Sezary syndrome: clinical characteristics and prognosis. Blood 1998;92:1150–9.
206. Dommann SN, Ziegler T, Dommann-Schener CC, Meyer J, Panizzon R, Burg G. CD44v6 is a marker for systemic spread in cutaneous T-cell lymphomas. A comparative study between nodal and cutaneous lymphomas. J Cutan Pathol 1995;22:407–12.
207. Dosaka N, Tanaka T, Miyachi Y, Imamura S, Kakizuka A. Examination of HTLV-I integration in the skin lesions of various types of adult T-cell leukemia (ATL): independence of cutaneous-type ATL confirmed by Southern blot analysis. J Invest Dermatol 1991;96:196–200.
208. Drillenburg P, Bronkhorst CM, van der Wal AC, Noorduyn LA, Hoekzema R, Pals ST. Expression of adhesion molecules in pagetoid reticulosis (Woringer-Kolopp disease). Br J Dermatol 1997;136:613–6.
209. Dummer R, Kamarashev J, Kempf W, Haffner AC, Hess-Schmid M, Burg G. Junctional CD8+ cutaneous lymphomas with nonaggressive clinical behavior: a CD8+ variant of mycosis fungoides? Arch Dermatol 2002;138:199–203.
210. Dummer R, Nestle FO, Niederer E, et al. Genotypic, phenotypic and functional analysis of CD4+CD7+ and CD4+CD7- T lymphocyte subsets in Sezary syndrome. Arch Dermatol Res 1999;291:307–11.
211. Duncan SC, Winkelmann RK. Circulating Sezary cells in hospitalized dermatology patients. Br J Dermatol 1978;99:171–8.
212. El-Shabrawi-Caelen L, Cerroni L, Medeiros LJ, McCalmont TH. Hypopigmented mycosis fungoides: frequent expression of a CD8+ T-cell phenotype. Am J Surg Pathol 2002;26:450–7.
213. Falini B. Anaplastic large cell lymphoma: pathological, molecular and clinical features. Br J Haematol 2001;114:741–60.
214. Falini B, Pileri S, Stein H, et al. Variable expression of leucocyte-common (CD45) antigen in CD30 (Ki1)-positive anaplastic large-cell lymphoma: implications for the differential diagnosis between lymphoid and nonlymphoid malignancies. Hum Pathol 1990;21:624–9.
215. Fan G, Kotylo P, Neiman RS, Braziel RM. Comparison of fascin expression in anaplastic large cell lymphoma and Hodgkin disease. Am J Clin Pathol 2003;119:199–204.
216. Flynn KJ, Dehner LP, Gajl-Peczalska KJ, Dahl MV, Ramsay N, Wang N. Regressing atypical histiocytosis: a cutaneous proliferation of atypical neoplastic histiocytes with unexpectedly indolent biologic behavior. Cancer 1982;49:959–70.
217. Fouchard N, Mahe A, Huerre M, et al. Cutaneous T cell lymphomas: mycosis fungoides, Sezary syndrome and HTLV-I-associated adult T cell leukemia (ATL) in Mali, West Africa: a clinical, pathological and immunovirological study of 14 cases and a review of the African ATL cases. Leukemia 1998;12:578–85.
218. Frierson HF Jr, Bellafiore FJ, Gaffey MJ, McCary WS, Innes DJ Jr, Williams ME. Cytokeratin in anaplastic large cell lymphoma. Mod Pathol 1994;7:317–21.
219. Frizzera G. The distinction of Hodgkin's disease from anaplastic large cell lymphoma. Semin Diagn Pathol 1992;9:291–6.
220. Furukawa Y, Tara M, Ohmori K, Kannagi R. Variant type of sialyl Lewis X antigen expressed on adult T cell leukemia cells is associated with skin involvement. Cancer Res 1994;54:6533–8.

221. Gaal K, Weiss LM, Chen WG, Chen YY, Arber DA. Epstein-Barr virus nuclear antigen (EBNA)-1 carboxy-terminal and EBNA-4 sequence polymorphisms in nasal natural killer/T-cell lymphoma in the United States. Lab Invest 2002;82:957–62.
222. Gessain A, Moulonguet I, Flageul B, et al. Cutaneous type of adult T cell leukemia/lymphoma in a French West Indian woman. Clonal rearrangement of T-cell receptor beta and gamma genes and monoclonal integration of HTLV-I proviral DNA in the skin infiltrate. J Am Acad Dermatol 1990;23(Pt 2):994–1000.
223. Giam YC, Ong BH. Clinicopathological and immunohistological correlation of malignant lymphomas of the skin. Ann Acad Med Singapore 1994;23:412–7.
224. Gibson LE, Muller SA, Leiferman KM, Peters MS. Follicular mucinosis: clinical and histopathologic study. J Am Acad Dermatol 1989;20:441–6.
225. Gilliam AC, Lessin SR, Wilson DM, Salhany KE. Folliculotropic mycosis fungoides with large-cell transformation presenting as dissecting cellulitis of the scalp. J Cutan Pathol 1997;24:169–75.
226. Gilliam AC, Wood GS. Primary cutaneous lymphomas other than mycosis fungoides. Semin Oncol 1999;26:290–306.
227. Ginarte M, Abalde MT, Peteiro C, Fraga M, Alonso N, Toribio J. Blastoid NK cell leukemia/lymphoma with cutaneous involvement. Dermatology 2000;201:268–71.
228. Goldstein NS, Ritter JH, Argenyi ZB, Wick, MR. Granulocytic sarcoma: potential diagnostic clues from immunostaining patterns seen with "anti-lymphoid" antibodies. Int J Surg Pathol 1995;2:199–206.
229. Gordon BG, Weisenburger DD, Warkentin PI, et al. Peripheral T-cell lymphoma in childhood and adolescence. A clinicopathologic study of 22 patients. Cancer 1993;71:257–63.
230. Grammatico P, Balus L, Scarpa S, et al. Granulomatous slack skin: cytogenetic and molecular analyses. Cancer Genet Cytogenet 1994;72:96–100.
231. Gregg PJ, Kantor GR, Telang GH, Lessin SR, Nowell PC, Vonderheid EC. Sarcoidal tissue reaction in Sezary syndrome. J Am Acad Dermatol 2000;43(Pt 2):372–6.
232. Guitart J, Kennedy J, Ronan S, Chmiel JS, Hsiegh YC, Variakojis D. Histologic criteria for the diagnosis of mycosis fungoides: proposal for a grading system to standardize pathology reporting. J Cutan Pathol 2001;28:174–83.
233. Gustmann C, Altmannsberger M, Osborn M, Griesser H, Feller AC. Cytokeratin expression and vimentin content in large cell anaplastic lymphomas and other non-Hodgkin's lymphomas. Am J Pathol 1991;138:1413–22.
234. Haeffner AC, Smoller BR, Zepter K, Wood GS. Differentiation and clonality of lesional lymphocytes in small plaque parapsoriasis. Arch Dermatol 1995;131:321–4.
235. Haghighi B, Smoller BR, LeBoit PE, Warnke RA, Sander CA, Kohler S. Pagetoid reticulosis (Woringer-Kolopp disease): an immunophenotypic, molecular, and clinicopathologic study. Mod Pathol 2000;13:502–10.
236. Haller A, Elzubi E, Petzelbauer P. Localized syringolymphoid hyperplasia with alopecia and anhidrosis. J Am Acad Dermatol 2001;45:127–30.
237. Hamminga L, Hartgrink-Groeneveld CA, van Vloten WA. Sezary's syndrome: a clinical evaluation of eight patients. Br J Dermatol 1979;100:291–6.
238. Harabuchi Y, Imai S, Wakashima J, et al. Nasal T-cell lymphoma causally associated with Epstein-Barr virus: clinicopathologic, phenotypic, and genotypic studies. Cancer 1996;77:2137–49.
239. Harada H, Iwatsuki K, Kaneko F. Detection of Epstein-Barr virus genes in malignant lymphoma with clinical and histologic features of cytophagic histiocytic panniculitis. J Am Acad Dermatol 1994;31(Pt 2):379–83.
240. Hasui K, Sato E, Tokudome T, Tokunaga M, Setoyama M, Tashiro M. A comparative microphotometric analysis of adult T-cell leukemia/lymphoma (ATLL) in the skin and mycosis fungoides (MF). Acta Pathol Jpn 1987;37:1405–14.
241. Haynes BF, Miller SE, Palker TJ, et al. Identification of human T cell leukemia virus in a Japanese patient with adult T cell leukemia and cutaneous lymphomatous vasculitis. Proc Natl Acad Sci U S A 1983;80:2054–8.
242. Heald P, Yan SL, Edelson R. Profound deficiency in normal circulating T cells in erythrodermic cutaneous T-cell lymphoma. Arch Dermatol 1994;130:198–203.
243. Helm KF, Cerio R, Winkelmann RK. Granulomatous slack skin: a clinicopathological and immunohistochemical study of three cases. Br J Dermatol 1992;126:142–7.
244. Hodak E, Phenig E, Amichai B, et al. Unilesional mycosis fungoides: a study of seven cases. Dermatology 2000;201:300–6.
245. Hofman FM, Meyer PR, Yanagihara E, et al. Demonstration of a subpopulation of Ia+ T-helper cells in mycosis fungoides and the Sezary syndrome. Am J Dermatopathol 1983;5:135–43.
246. Hoppe RT, Medeiros LJ, Warnke RA, Wood GS. CD8-positive tumor-infiltrating lymphocytes influence the long-term survival of patients with mycosis fungoides. J Am Acad Dermatol 1995;32:448–53.

247. Horiguchi Y, Horiguchi M, Toda K, Mitani T, Imamura S. The ultrastructural observation of a case of lymphomatoid papulosis. Acta Derm Venereol 1984;64:308–15.
248. Horiuchi Y, Tone T, Umezawa A, Takezaki S. Large cell mycosis fungoides at the tumor stage. Unusual T8, T4, T6 phenotypic expression. Am J Dermatopathol 1988;10:54–8.
249. Hwang DK, Kwon HM, Park JW, Yu HJ, Park YW. TCR gene-rearranged, extranodal NK/T-cell lymphoma, nasal type, presenting as gyrate patches. J Dermatol 2002;29:648–52.
250. Ikai K, Uchiyama T, Maeda M, Takigawa M. Sezary-like syndrome in a 10-year-old girl with serologic evidence of human T-cell lymphotropic virus type I infection. Arch Dermatol 1987;123:1351–5.
251. Ikari Y, Ohkura M, Morita M, Seki K, Kubota Y, Mizoguchi M. Leser-Trelat sign associated with Sezary syndrome. J Dermatol 1995;22:62–7.
252. Ikeda E, Endo M, Uchigasaki S, et al. Phagocytized apoptotic cells in subcutaneous panniculitis-like T-cell lymphoma. J Eur Acad Dermatol Venereol 2000;15:159–62.
253. Iwatsuki K, Harada H, Ohtsuka M, Han G, Kaneko F. Latent Epstein-Barr virus infection is frequently detected in subcutaneous lymphoma associated with hemophagocytosis but not in nonfatal cytophagic histiocytic panniculitis. Arch Dermatol 1997;133:787–8.
254. Jaffe ES. Lymphoid lesions of the head and neck: a model of lymphocyte homing and lymphomagenesis. Mod Pathol 2002;15:255–63.
255. Jaffe ES. Post-thymic T-cell lymphomas surgical pathology of the lymph nodes and related organs, 2nd ed. Philadelphia: WB Saunders; 1995:344–89.
256. Jaffe ES, Blattner WA, Blayney DW, et al. The pathologic spectrum of adult T-cell leukemia/lymphoma in the United States. Human T-cell leukemia/lymphoma virus-associated lymphoid malignancies. Am J Surg Pathol 1984;8:263–75.
257. Jaffe ES, Chan JK, Su IJ, et al. Report of the Workshop on Nasal and Related Extranodal Angiocentric T/Natural Killer Cell Lymphomas. Definitions, differential diagnosis, and epidemiology. Am J Surg Pathol 1996;20:103–11.
258. Jaffe ES, Harris NL, Stein H, Vardiman JW. Summary of the WHO classification of tumours of haematopoietic and lymphoid tissues. In: Jaffe ES, Harris NL, Stein H, Vardiman JW, eds. Pathology and genetics of tumours of haematopoietic and lymphoid tissues. Lyon: IARC Press; 2001:10–3.
259. Jaffe ES, Krenacs L, Kumar S, Kingma DW, Raffeld M. Extranodal peripheral T-cell and NK-cell neoplasms. Am J Clin Pathol 1999;111 (Suppl 1):S46–55.
260. Jaffe ES, Ralfkiaer E. Angioimmunoblastic T-cell lymphoma. In: Jaffe ES, Harris NL, Stein H, Vardiman JW, eds. Pathology and genetics of tumours of haematopoietic and lymphoid tissues. Lyon: IARC Press; 2001:225–6.
261. Jaffe ES, Ralfkiaer E. Subcutaneous panniculitis-like T-cell lymphoma. In: Jaffe ES, Harris NL, Stein H, Vardiman JW, eds. Pathology and genetics of tumours of haematopoietic and lymphoid tissues. Lyon: IARC Press; 2001:212–3.
262. Jang KA, Choi JC, Choi JH. Expression of cutaneous lymphocyte-associated antigen and TIA-1 by lymphocytes in pityriasis lichenoides et varioliformis acuta and lymphomatoid papulosis: immunohistochemical study. J Cutan Pathol 2001;28:453–9.
263. Johno M, Ono T. [Clinicopathological differential diagnosis of mycosis fungoides/Sezary syndrome from the cutaneous type of adult T-cell leukemia/lymphoma.] Nippon Rinsho 2000;58:660–4. (Japanese.)
264. Jones D, Jorgensen JL, Shahsafaei A, Dorfman DM. Characteristic proliferations of reticular and dendritic cells in angioimmunoblastic lymphoma. Am J Surg Pathol 1998;22:956–64.
265. Jones RE Jr. Questions to the Editorial Board and other authorities. Am J Dermatopathol 1986;8:534–45.
266. Kadin M, Nasu K, Sako D, Said J, Vonderheid E. Lymphomatoid papulosis. A cutaneous proliferation of activated helper T cells expressing Hodgkin's disease-associated antigens. Am J Pathol 1985;119:315–25.
267. Kadin ME. Ki-1-positive anaplastic large-cell lymphoma: a clinicopathologic entity? J Clin Oncol 1991;9:533–6.
268. Kadin ME. Lymphomatoid papulosis, Ki-1+ lymphoma, and primary cutaneous Hodgkin's disease. Semin Dermatol 1991;10:164–71.
269. Kardashian JL, Zackheim HS, Egbert BM. Lymphomatoid papulosis associated with plaque-stage and granulomatous mycosis fungoides. Arch Dermatol 1985;121:1175–80.
270. Kartsonis J, Brettschneider F, Weissmann A, Rosen L. Mycosis fungoides bullosa. Am J Dermatopathol 1990;12:76–80.
271. Kato N, Sugawara H, Aoyagi S, Mayuzumi M. Lymphoma-type adult T-cell leukaemia-lymphoma with a bulky cutaneous tumour showing multiple human T-lymphotropic virus-1 DNA integration. Br J Dermatol 2001;144:1244–8.
272. Kato N, Yasukawa K, Onozuka T, Kikuta H. Nasal and nasal-type T/NK-cell lymphoma with cutaneous involvement. J Am Acad Dermatol 1999;40(Pt 2):850–6.

273. Kaudewitz P, Stein H, Dallenbach F, et al. Primary and secondary cutaneous Ki-1+ (CD30+) anaplastic large cell lymphomas. Morphologic, immunohistologic, and clinical-characteristics. Am J Pathol 1989;135:359–67.
274. Kempf W, Kadin ME, Kutzner H, et al. Lymphomatoid papulosis and human herpesviruses—a PCR-based evaluation for the presence of human herpesvirus 6, 7 and 8 related herpesviruses. J Cutan Pathol 2001;28:29–33.
275. Kikuchi M, Jaffe ES, Ralfkiaer E. Adult T-cell leukaemia/lymphoma. In: Jaffe ES, Harris NL, Stein H, Vardiman JW, eds. Pathology and genetics of tumours of haematopoietic and lymphoid tissues. Lyon: IARC Press; 2001:200–3.
276. Kikuchi M, Mitsui T, Kozuru M, Uike N, Kurata T, Katsuta Y. Case report of adult T-cell leukemia with preceding long-standing cutaneous involvement. Jpn J Clin Oncol 1983;13(Suppl 2):201–7.
277. Kim YH, Bishop K, Varghese A, Hoppe RT. Prognostic factors in erythrodermic mycosis fungoides and the Sezary syndrome. Arch Dermatol 1995;131:1003–8.
278. Kim YH, Hoppe RT. Mycosis fungoides and the Sezary syndrome. Semin Oncol 1999;26:276–89.
279. King-Ismael D, Ackerman AB. Guttate parapsoriasis/digitate dermatosis (small plaque parapsoriasis) is mycosis fungoides. Am J Dermatopathol 1992;14:518–30; discussion 531–5.
280. Kinney MC, Glick AD, Stein H, Collins RD. Comparison of anaplastic large cell Ki-1 lymphomas and microvillous lymphomas in their immunologic and ultrastructural features. Am J Surg Pathol 1990;14:1047–60.
281. Kinney MC, Greer JP, Glick AD, Salhany KE, Collins RD. Anaplastic large-cell Ki-1 malignant lymphomas. Recognition, biological and clinical implications. Pathol Annu 1991;26(Pt 1):1–24.
282. Kinney MC, Kadin ME. The pathologic and clinical spectrum of anaplastic large cell lymphoma and correlation with ALK gene dysregulation. Am J Clin Pathol 1999;111 (Suppl 1):S56–67.
283. Klemke CD, Dippel E, Assaf C, et al. Follicular mycosis fungoides. Br J Dermatol 1999;141: 137–40.
284. Kohler S, Kim YH, Smoller BR. Histologic criteria for the diagnosis of erythrodermic mycosis fungoides and Sezary syndrome: a critical reappraisal. J Cutan Pathol 1997;24:292–7.
285. Kumar S, Krenacs L, Medeiros J, et al. Subcutaneous panniculitic T-cell lymphoma is a tumor of cytotoxic T lymphocytes. Hum Pathol 1998;29:397–403.
286. Lambert WC, Everett MA. The nosology of parapsoriasis. J Am Acad Dermatol 1981;5:373–95.
287. Lazar AP, Caro WA, Roenigk HH Jr, Pinski KS. Parapsoriasis and mycosis fungoides: the Northwestern University experience, 1970 to 1985. J Am Acad Dermatol 1989;21(Pt 1):919–23.
288. LeBoit PE. Granulomatous slack skin. Dermatol Clin 1994;12:375–89.
289. LeBoit PE, Beckstead JH, Bond B, Epstein WL, Frieden IJ, Parslow TG. Granulomatous slack skin: clonal rearrangement of the T-cell receptor beta gene is evidence for the lymphoproliferative nature of a cutaneous elastolytic disorder. J Invest Dermatol 1987;89:183–6.
290. LeBoit PE, Zackheim HS, White CR Jr. Granulomatous variants of cutaneous T-cell lymphoma. The histopathology of granulomatous mycosis fungoides and granulomatous slack skin. Am J Surg Pathol 1988;12:83–95.
291. Leoncini L, Del Vecchio MT, Kraft R, et al. Hodgkin's disease and CD30-positive anaplastic large cell lymphomas—a continuous spectrum of malignant disorders. A quantitative morphometric and immunohistologic study. Am J Pathol 1990;137:1047–57.
292. Lindae ML, Abel EA, Hoppe RT, Wood GS. Poikilodermatous mycosis fungoides and atrophic large-plaque parapsoriasis exhibit similar abnormalities of T-cell antigen expression. Arch Dermatol 1988;124:366–72.
293. Lipford EH, Smith HR, Pittaluga S, Jaffe ES, Steinberg AD, Cossman J. Clonality of angioimmunoblastic lymphadenopathy and implications for its evolution to malignant lymphoma. J Clin Invest 1987;79:637–42.
294. Lish KM, Ramsay DL, Raphael BG, Jacobson M, Gottesman SR. Lymphomatoid papulosis followed by acute myeloblastic leukemia. J Am Acad Dermatol 1993;29:112–5.
295. Luther H, Bacharach-Buhles M, Schultz-Ehrenburg U, Altmeyer P. [Pagetoid reticulosis of the Ketron-Goodman type.] Hautarzt 1989;40:530–5. (German.)
296. Macaulay WL. Lymphomatoid papulosis update. A historical perspective. Arch Dermatol 1989;125:1387–9.
297. Macaulay WL. Lymphomatoid papulosis. A continuing self-healing eruption, clinically benign—histologically malignant. Arch Dermatol 1968;97:23–30.
298. Mackie RM, Turbitt ML. A case of pagetoid reticulosis bearing the T cytotoxic suppressor surface marker on the lymphoid infiltrate: further evidence that pagetoid reticulosis is not a variant of mycosis fungoides. Br J Dermatol 1984;110:89–94.

299. Maeda K, Takahashi M. Characterization of skin infiltrating cells in adult T-cell leukaemia/lymphoma (ATLL): clinical, histological and immunohistochemical studies on eight cases. Br J Dermatol 1989;121:603–12.
300. Maeda K, Yamana K, Takahashi H, Jimbow K. Dual surface makers and HTLV-I proviral DNA in a cutaneous tumour nodule in a case of adult T cell leukaemia/lymphoma. Br J Dermatol 1987;117:561–8.
301. Manabe T, Hirokawa M, Sugihara K, Sugihara T, Kohda M. Angiocentric and angiodestructive infiltration of adult T-cell leukemia/lymphoma (ATLL) in the skin. Report of two cases. Am J Dermatopathol 1988;10:487–96.
302. Mandojana RM, Helwig EB. Localized epidermotropic reticulosis (Woringer-Kolopp disease). J Am Acad Dermatol 1983;8:813–29.
303. Martel P, Laroche L, Courville P, et al. Cutaneous involvement in patients with angioimmunoblastic lymphadenopathy with dysproteinemia: a clinical, immunohistological, and molecular analysis. Arch Dermatol 2000;136:881–6.
304. Marzano AV, Berti E, Paulli M, Caputo R. Cytophagic histiocytic panniculitis and subcutaneous panniculitis-like T-cell lymphoma: report of 7 cases. Arch Dermatol 2000;136:889–96.
305. Mason DY, Bastard C, Rimokh R, et al. CD30-positive large cell lymphomas ('Ki-1 lymphoma') are associated with a chromosomal translocation involving 5q35. Br J Haematol 1990;74:161–8.
306. Matano S, Nakamura S, Nakamura S, et al. Monomorphic agranular natural killer cell lymphoma/ leukemia with no Epstein-Barr virus association. Acta Haematol 1999;101:206–8.
307. Matloff RB, Neiman RS. Angioimmunoblastic lymphadenopathy. A generalized lymphoproliferative disorder with cutaneous manifestations. Arch Dermatol 1978;114:92–4.
308. McMillan EM, Wasik R, Martin D, Donaldson M, Everett MA. Immuno-electron microscopy of "T" cells in large plaque parapsoriasis. J Cutan Pathol 1981;8:385–92.
309. McNiff JM, Schechner JS, Crotty PL, Glusac EJ. Mycosis fungoides palmaris et plantaris or acral pagetoid reticulosis? Am J Dermatopathol 1998;20:271–5.
310. McNutt NS, Crain WR. Quantitative electron microscopic comparison of lymphocyte nuclear contours in mycosis fungoides and in benign infiltrates in skin. Cancer 1981;47:698–709.
311. Meister L, Duarte AM, Davis J, Perez JL, Schachner LA. Sezary syndrome in an 11-year-old girl. J Am Acad Dermatol 1993;28:93–5.
312. Michie SA, Abel EA, Hoppe RT, Warnke RA, Wood GS. Discordant expression of antigens between intraepidermal and intradermal T cells in mycosis fungoides. Am J Pathol 1990;137:1447–51.
313. Millot F, Robert A, Bertrand Y, et al. Cutaneous involvement in children with acute lymphoblastic leukemia or lymphoblastic lymphoma. The Children's Leukemia Cooperative Group of the European Organization of Research and Treatment of Cancer (EORTC). Pediatrics 1997;100:60–4.
314. Miyake K, Yoshino T, Sarker AB, Teramoto N, Akagi T. CD30 antigen in non-Hodgkin's lymphoma. Pathol Int 1994;44:428–34.
315. Mizutani Y, Iwamasa K, Arai J, Sakai I, Yasukawa M, Fujita S. [Subcutaneous panniculitic T-cell lymphoma with chromosomal abnormalities and large granular lymphocytes morphology.] Rinsho Ketsueki 2000;41:519–23. (Japanese.)
316. Mukai HY, Kojima H, Suzukawa K, et al. High-dose chemotherapy with peripheral blood stem cell rescue in blastoid natural killer cell lymphoma. Leuk Lymphoma 1999;32:583–8.
317. Murakami T, Ohtsuki M, Nakagawa H. Angioimmunoblastic lymphadenopathy-type peripheral T-cell lymphoma with cutaneous infiltration: report of a case and its gene expression profile. Br J Dermatol 2001;144:878–84.
318. Murphy M, Fullen D, Carlson JA. Low CD7 expression in benign and malignant cutaneous lymphocytic infiltrates: experience with an antibody reactive with paraffin-embedded tissue. Am J Dermatopathol 2002;24:6–16.
319. Nagatani T, Miyazawa M, Matsuzaki T, et al. Comparative study of cutaneous T-cell lymphoma and adult T-cell leukemia/lymphoma. Semin Dermatol 1994;13:216–22.
320. Nakamura S, Suchi T, Koshikawa T, et al. Clinicopathologic study of 212 cases of peripheral T-cell lymphoma among the Japanese. Cancer 1993;72:1762–72.
321. Navas IC, Ortiz-Romero PL, Villuendas R, et al. p16(INK4a) gene alterations are frequent in lesions of mycosis fungoides. Am J Pathol 2000;156:1565–72.
322. Nickoloff BJ. Epidermal mucinosis in mycosis fungoides. J Am Acad Dermatol 1986;15:83–6.
323. Nickoloff BJ. Light-microscopic assessment of 100 patients with patch/plaque-stage mycosis fungoides. Am J Dermatopathol 1988;10:469–77.
324. Noto G, Pravata G, Miceli S, Arico M. Granulomatous slack skin: report of a case associated with Hodgkin's disease and a review of the literature. Br J Dermatol 1994;131:275–9.

325. O'Connor NT, Crick JA, Wainscoat JS, et al. Evidence for monoclonal T lymphocyte proliferation in angioimmunoblastic lymphadenopathy. J Clin Pathol 1986;39:1229–32.
326. Ohtake N, Shimada S, Mizoguchi S, Setoyama M, Kanzaki T. Membranocystic lesions in a patient with cytophagic histiocytic panniculitis associated with subcutaneous T-cell lymphoma. Am J Dermatopathol 1998;20:276–80.
327. Oishi M, Johno M, Ono T, Honda M. Differences in IL-2 receptor levels between mycosis fungoides and cutaneous type adult T-cell leukemia/lymphoma in the early stages of the disease. J Invest Dermatol 1994;102:710–5.
328. Okuda T, Fisher R, Downing JR. Molecular diagnostics in pediatric acute lymphoblastic leukemia. Mol Diagn 1996;1:139–51.
329. Olerud JE, Kulin PA, Chew DE, et al. Cutaneous T-cell lymphoma. Evaluation of pretreatment skin biopsy specimens by a panel of pathologists. Arch Dermatol 1992;128:501–7.
330. Oliver GF, Winkelmann RK. Unilesional mycosis fungoides: a distinct entity. J Am Acad Dermatol 1989;20:63–70.
331. Ormsby A, Bergfeld WF, Tubbs RR, Hsi ED. Evaluation of a new paraffin-reactive CD7 T-cell deletion marker and a polymerase chain reaction-based T-cell receptor gene rearrangement assay: implications for diagnosis of mycosis fungoides in community clinical practice. J Am Acad Dermatol 2001;45:405–13.
332. Ortiz Romero PL, Vallejo A, Lopez Estebaranz JL, Garcia Saiz A, Fernandez V, Iglesias Diez L. Absence of HTLV-1 proviral sequences in patients with lymphomatoid papulosis. J Invest Dermatol 1997;109:817–8.
333. Pancake BA, Zucker-Franklin D, Coutavas EE. The cutaneous T cell lymphoma, mycosis fungoides, is a human T cell lymphotropic virus-associated disease. A study of 50 patients. J Clin Invest 1995;95:547–54.
334. Patterson JW, Ali M, Murray JC, Hazra TA. Bullous pemphigoid. Occurrence in a patient with mycosis fungoides receiving PUVA and topical nitrogen mustard therapy. Int J Dermatol 1985;24:173–6.
335. Payne CM, Glasser L. Ultrastructural morphometry in the diagnosis of Sezary syndrome. Arch Pathol Lab Med 1990;114:661–71.
336. Penny RJ, Blaustein JC, Longtine JA, Pinkus GS. Ki-1-positive large cell lymphomas, a heterogenous group of neoplasms. Morphologic, immunophenotypic, genotypic, and clinical features of 24 cases. Cancer 1991;68:362–73.
337. Petrella T, Dalac S, Maynadie M, et al. CD4+ CD56+ cutaneous neoplasms: a distinct hematological entity? Groupe Francais d'Etude des Lymphomes Cutanes (GFELC). Am J Surg Pathol 1999;23:137–46.
338. Piepkorn M, Marty J, Kjeldsberg CR. T cell subset heterogeneity in a series of patients with mycosis fungoides and Sezary syndrome. J Am Acad Dermatol 1984;11:427–32.
339. Pierard GE, Ackerman AB, Lapiere CM. Follicular lymphomatoid papulosis. Am J Dermatopathol 1980;2:173–80.
340. Pileri S, Bocchia M, Baroni CD, et al. Anaplastic large cell lymphoma (CD30+/Ki-1+): results of a prospective clinico-pathological study of 69 cases. Br J Haematol 1994;86:513–23.
341. Pileri S, Falini B, Delsol G, et al. Lymphohistiocytic T-cell lymphoma (anaplastic large cell lymphoma CD30+/Ki-1+ with a high content of reactive histiocytes). Histopathology 1990;16:383–91.
342. Quarterman MJ, Lesher JL Jr, Davis LS, Pantazis CG, Mullins S. Rapidly progressive CD8-positive cutaneous T-cell lymphoma with tongue involvement. Am J Dermatopathol 1995;17:287–91.
343. Quintanilla-Martinez L, Fend F, Moguel LR, et al. Peripheral T-cell lymphoma with Reed-Sternberg-like cells of B-cell phenotype and genotype associated with Epstein-Barr virus infection. Am J Surg Pathol 1999;23:1233–40.
344. Ralfkiaer E. Immunohistological markers for the diagnosis of cutaneous lymphomas. Semin Diagn Pathol 1991;8:62–72.
345. Ralfkiaer E, Delsol G, Willemze R, Jaffe ES. Primary cutaneous CD30-positive T-cell lymphoproliferative disorders. In: Jaffe ES, Harris NL, Stein H, Vardiman JW, eds. Pathology and genetics of tumours of haematopoietic and lymphoid tissues. Lyon: IARC Press; 2001:221–4.
346. Ralfkiaer E, Jaffe ES. Mycosis fungoides and Sezary syndrome. In: Jaffe ES, Harris NL, Stein H, Vardiman JW, eds. Pathology and genetics of tumours of haematopoietic and lymphoid tissues. Lyon: IARC Press; 2001:216–20.
347. Ralfkiaer E, Stein H, Wantzin GL, Thomsen K, Ralfkiaer N, Mason DY. Lymphomatoid papulosis. Characterization of skin infiltrates by monoclonal antibodies. Am J Clin Pathol 1985;84:587–93.
348. Ree HJ, Kadin ME, Kikuchi M, et al. Angioimmunoblastic lymphoma (AILD-type T-cell lymphoma) with hyperplastic germinal centers. Am J Surg Pathol 1998;22:643–55.
349. Rencic A, Laman S, Nousari HC. Peripheral T cell lymphoma presenting as dermatomyositis-like eruption. J Cutan Med Surg 2002;6:218–20.
350. Requena L, Sanchez M, Coca S, Sanchez Yus E. Follicular lymphomatoid papulosis. Am J Dermatopathol 1990;12:67–75.

351. Rieger E, Smolle J, Hoedl S, Juettner FM, Kerl H. Morphometrical analysis of mycosis fungoides on paraffin-embedded sections. J Cutan Pathol 1989;16:7–13.
352. Rifkin S, Valderrama E, Lipton JM, Karayalcin G. Lymphomatoid papulosis and Ki-1+ anaplastic large cell lymphoma occurring concurrently in a pediatric patient. J Pediatr Hematol Oncol 2001;23:321–3.
353. Rijlaarsdam U, Scheffer E, Meijer CJ, Kruyswijk MR, Willemze R. Mycosis fungoides-like lesions associated with phenytoin and carbamazepine therapy. J Am Acad Dermatol 1991;24(Pt 1):216–20.
354. Ringel E, Medenica M, Lorincz A. Localized mycosis fungoides not manifesting as Woringer-Kolopp disease. Arch Dermatol 1983;119:756–60.
355. Ritter JH, Goldstein NS, Argenyi Z, Wick MR. Granulocytic sarcoma: an immunohistologic comparison with peripheral T-cell lymphoma in paraffin sections. J Cutan Pathol 1994;21:207–16.
356. Rodriguez J, Romaguera JE, Manning J, et al. Nasal-type T/NK lymphomas: a clinicopathologic study of 13 cases. Leuk Lymphoma 2000;39:139–44.
357. Rogers M. Pityriasis lichenoides and lymphomatoid papulosis. Semin Dermatol 1992;11:73–9.
358. Romagnoli P, Moretti S, Fattorossi A, Giannotti B. Dendritic cells in the dermal infiltrate of Sezary syndrome. Histopathology 1986;10:25–36.
359. Rosso R, Paulli M, Magrini U, et al. Anaplastic large cell lymphoma, CD30/Ki-1 positive, expressing the CD15/Leu-M1 antigen. Immunohistochemical and morphological relationships to Hodgkin's disease. Virchows Arch A Pathol Anat Histopathol 1990;416:229–35.
360. Russell-Jones R, Whittaker S. T-cell receptor gene analysis in the diagnosis of Sezary syndrome. J Am Acad Dermatol 1999;41(Pt 1):254–9.
361. Salhany KE, Cousar JB, Greer JP, Casey TT, Fields JP, Collins RD. Transformation of cutaneous T cell lymphoma to large cell lymphoma. A clinicopathologic and immunologic study. Am J Pathol 1988;132:265–77.
362. Salhany KE, Macon WR, Choi JK, et al. Subcutaneous panniculitis-like T-cell lymphoma: clinicopathologic, immunophenotypic, and genotypic analysis of alpha/beta and gamma/delta subtypes. Am J Surg Pathol 1998;22:881–93.
363. Sanchez JL, Ackerman AB. The patch stage of mycosis fungoides. Criteria for histologic diagnosis. Am J Dermatopathol 1979;1:5–26.
364. Sanchez NP, Pittelkow MR, Muller SA, Banks PM, Winkelmann RK. The clinicopathologic spectrum of lymphomatoid papulosis: study of 31 cases. J Am Acad Dermatol 1983;8:81–94.
365. Sander CA, Kaudewitz P, Kutzner H, et al. T-cell-rich B-cell lymphoma presenting in skin. A clinicopathologic analysis of six cases. J Cutan Pathol 1996;23:101–8.
366. Sander CA, Medeiros LJ, Abruzzo LV, Horak ID, Jaffe ES. Lymphoblastic lymphoma presenting in cutaneous sites. A clinicopathologic analysis of six cases. J Am Acad Dermatol 1991;25(Pt 1):1023–31.
367. Santucci M, Pimpinelli N, Massi D, et al. Cytotoxic/natural killer cell cutaneous lymphomas. Report of EORTC Cutaneous Lymphoma Task Force Workshop. Cancer 2003;97:610–27.
368. Sausville EA, Eddy JL, Makuch RW, et al. Histopathologic staging at initial diagnosis of mycosis fungoides and the Sezary syndrome. Definition of three distinctive prognostic groups. Ann Intern Med 1988;109:372–82.
369. Scarabello A, Leinweber B, Ardigo M, et al. Cutaneous lymphomas with prominent granulomatous reaction: a potential pitfall in the histopathologic diagnosis of cutaneous T- and B-cell lymphomas. Am J Surg Pathol 2002;26:1259–68.
370. Scarisbrick JJ, Woolford AJ, Russell-Jones R, Whittaker SJ. Loss of heterozygosity on 10q and microsatellite instability in advanced stages of primary cutaneous T-cell lymphoma and possible association with homozygous deletion of PTEN. Blood 2000;95:2937–42.
371. Scheffer E, Meijer CJ, Van Vloten WA. Dermatopathic lymphadenopathy and lymph node involvement in mycosis fungoides. Cancer 1980;45:137–48.
372. Schlegelberger B, Himmler A, Godde E, Grote W, Feller AC, Lennert K. Cytogenetic findings in peripheral T-cell lymphomas as a basis for distinguishing low-grade and high-grade lymphomas. Blood 1994;83:505–11.
373. Schmuth M, Ramaker J, Trautmann C, et al. Cutaneous involvement in prelymphomatous angioimmunoblastic lymphadenopathy. J Am Acad Dermatol 1997;36(Pt 2):290–5.
374. Schotte U, Megahed M, Jansen T, et al. [Angioimmunoblastic lymphadenopathy with cutaneous manifestations in a 13-year-old girl.] Hautarzt 1992;43:728–34. (German.)
375. Seeburger J, Anderson-Wilms N, Jacobs R. Lennert's lymphoma presenting as prurigo nodularis. Cutis 1993;51:355–8.
376. Seehafer JR, Goldberg NC, Dicken CH, Su WP. Cutaneous manifestations of angioimmunoblastic lymphadenopathy. Arch Dermatol 1980;116:41–5.
377. Segal GH, Stoler MH, Tubbs RR. The "CD43 only" phenotype. An aberrant, nonspecific immunophenotype requiring comprehensive analysis for lineage resolution. Am J Clin Pathol 1992;97:861–5.

378. Sentis HJ, Willemze R, Scheffer E. Histopathologic studies in Sezary syndrome and erythrodermic mycosis fungoides: a comparison with benign forms of erythroderma. J Am Acad Dermatol 1986;15:1217–26.
379. Setoyama M, Katahira Y, Kanzaki T. Clinicopathologic analysis of 124 cases of adult T-cell leukemia/lymphoma with cutaneous manifestations: the smouldering type with skin manifestations has a poorer prognosis than previously thought. J Dermatol 1999;26:785–90.
380. Setoyama M, Katahira Y, Kanzaki T, Kerdel FA, Byrnes JJ. Adult T-cell leukemia/lymphoma associated with noninfectious epithelioid granuloma in the skin: a clinicopathologic study. Am J Dermatopathol 1997;19:591–5.
381. Shapiro PE, Pinto FJ. The histologic spectrum of mycosis fungoides/Sezary syndrome (cutaneous T-cell lymphoma). A review of 222 biopsies, including newly described patterns and the earliest pathologic changes. Am J Surg Pathol 1994;18:645–67.
382. Shen L, Liang AC, Lu L, et al. Frequent deletion of Fas gene sequences encoding death and transmembrane domains in nasal natural killer/T-cell lymphoma. Am J Pathol 2002;161:2123–31.
383. Shimoyama M. Diagnostic criteria and classification of clinical subtypes of adult T- cell leukaemia-lymphoma. A report from the Lymphoma Study Group (1984-87). Br J Haematol 1991;79:428–37.
384. Siegert W, Nerl C, Agthe A, et al. Angioimmunoblastic lymphadenopathy (AILD)-type T-cell lymphoma: prognostic impact of clinical observations and laboratory findings at presentation. The Kiel Lymphoma Study Group. Ann Oncol 1995;6:659–64.
385. Simon M, Flaig MJ, Kind P, Sander CA, Kaudewitz P. Large plaque parapsoriasis: clinical and genotypic correlations. J Cutan Pathol 2000;27:57–60.
386. Sioutos N, Kerl H, Murphy SB, Kadin ME. Primary cutaneous Hodgkin's disease. Unique clinical, morphologic, and immunophenotypic findings. Am J Dermatopathol 1994;16:2–8.
387. Siu LL, Chan JK, Kwong YL. Natural killer cell malignancies: clinicopathologic and molecular features. Histol Histopathol 2002;17:539–54.
388. Smoller BR, Bishop K, Glusac E, Kim YH, Hendrickson M. Reassessment of histologic parameters in the diagnosis of mycosis fungoides. Am J Surg Pathol 1995;19:1423–30.
389. Smoller BR, Stewart M, Warnke R. A case of Woringer-Kolopp disease with Ki-1 (CD30)+ cytotoxic/suppressor cells. Arch Dermatol 1992;128:526–9.
390. Stein H, Mason DY, Gerdes J, et al. The expression of the Hodgkin's disease associated antigen Ki-1 in reactive and neoplastic lymphoid tissue: evidence that Reed-Sternberg cells and histiocytic malignancies are derived from activated lymphoid cells. Blood 1985;66:848–58.
391. Suzuki R, Nakamura S. Malignancies of natural killer (NK) cell precursor: myeloid/NK cell precursor acute leukemia and blastic NK cell lymphoma/leukemia. Leuk Res 1999;23:615–24.
392. Taddesse-Heath L, Feldman JI, Fahle GA, et al. Florid CD4+, CD56+ T-cell infiltrate associated with herpes simplex infection simulating nasal NK-/T-cell lymphoma. Mod Pathol 2003;16:166–72.
393. Takahashi K, Tanaka T, Fujita M, Horiguchi Y, Miyachi Y, Imamura S. Cutaneous-type adult T-cell leukemia/lymphoma. A unique clinical feature with monoclonal T-cell proliferation detected by Southern blot analysis. Arch Dermatol 1988;124:399–404.
394. Tan RS, Butterworth CM, McLaughlin H, Malka S, Samman PD. Mycosis fungoides—a disease of antigen persistence. Br J Dermatol 1974;91:607–16.
395. Tannous Z, Baldassano MF, Li VW, Kvedar J, Duncan LM. Syringolymphoid hyperplasia and follicular mucinosis in a patient with cutaneous T-cell lymphoma. J Am Acad Dermatol 1999;41(Pt 2):303–8.
396. Tashiro K, Kikuchi M, Takeshita M, Yoshida T, Ohshima K. Clinicopathological study of Ki-1-positive lymphomas. Pathol Res Pract 1989;185:461–7.
397. Thangavelu M, Finn WG, Yelavarthi KK, et al. Recurring structural chromosome abnormalities in peripheral blood lymphocytes of patients with mycosis fungoides/Sezary syndrome. Blood 1997;89:3371–7.
398. Thiers BH. Controversies in mycosis fungoides. J Am Acad Dermatol 1982;7:1–16.
399. Thomsen K, Wantzin GL. Lymphomatoid papulosis. A follow-up study of 30 patients. J Am Acad Dermatol 1987;17:632–6.
400. Tomaszewski MM, Lupton GP, Krishnan J, May DL. A comparison of clinical, morphological and immunohistochemical features of lymphomatoid papulosis and primary cutaneous CD30(Ki-1)-positive anaplastic large cell lymphoma. J Cutan Pathol 1995;22:310–8.
401. Tomaszewski MM, Lupton GP, Krishnan J, Welch M, James WD. Syringolymphoid hyperplasia with alopecia. A case report. J Cutan Pathol 1994;21:520–6.

402. Trotter MJ, Whittaker SJ, Orchard GE, Smith NP. Cutaneous histopathology of Sezary syndrome: a study of 41 cases with a proven circulating T-cell clone. J Cutan Pathol 1997;24:286–91.
403. Tsang WY, Chan JK, Loo KT, Wong KF, Lee AW. Granulomatous slack skin. Histopathology 1994;25:49–55.
404. Tsuruta D, Kono T, Kutsuna H, Yashiro N, Ishii M. Granulomatous slack skin: an ultrastructural study. J Cutan Pathol 2001;28:44–8.
405. Uchiyama N, Ito K, Kawai K, Sakamoto F, Takaki M, Ito M. CD2-, CD4+, CD56+ agranular natural killer cell lymphoma of the skin. Am J Dermatopathol 1998;20:513–7.
406. Vaillant L, Monegier du Sorbier C, Arbeille B, de Muret A, Lorette G. Cutaneous T cell lymphoma of signet ring cell type: a specific clinico-pathologic entity. Acta Derm Venereol 1993;73:255–8.
407. van Haselen CW, Toonstra J, van der Putte SJ, van Dongen JJ, van Hees CL, van Vloten WA. Granulomatous slack skin. Report of three patients with an updated review of the literature. Dermatology 1998;196:382–91.
408. Van Neer FJ, Toonstra J, Van Voorst Vader PC, Willemze R, Van Vloten WA. Lymphomatoid papulosis in children: a study of 10 children registered by the Dutch Cutaneous Lymphoma Working Group. Br J Dermatol 2001;144:351–4.
409. Veelken H, Wood GS, Sklar J. Molecular staging of cutaneous T-cell lymphoma: evidence for systemic involvement in early disease. J Invest Dermatol 1995;104:889–94.
410. Vermeer MH, Geelen FA, Kummer JA, Meijer CJ, Willemze R. Expression of cytotoxic proteins by neoplastic T cells in mycosis fungoides increases with progression from plaque stage to tumor stage disease. Am J Pathol 1999;154:1203–10.
411. Vidal RW, Devaney K, Ferlito A, Rinaldo A, Carbone A. Sinonasal malignant lymphomas: a distinct clinicopathological category. Ann Otol Rhinol Laryngol 1999;108:411–9.
412. Vonderheid EC, Bigler RD, Kotecha A, et al. Variable CD7 expression on T cells in the leukemic phase of cutaneous T cell lymphoma (Sezary syndrome). J Invest Dermatol 2001;117:654–62.
413. Vonderheid EC, Sajjadian A, Kadin ME. Methotrexate is effective therapy for lymphomatoid papulosis and other primary cutaneous CD30-positive lymphoproliferative disorders. J Am Acad Dermatol 1996;34:470–81.
414. Vonderheid EC, Tan E, Sobel EL, Schwab E, Micaily B, Jegasothy BV. Clinical implications of immunologic phenotyping in cutaneous T cell lymphoma. J Am Acad Dermatol 1987;17:40–52.
415. Wang CY, Su WP, Kurtin PJ. Subcutaneous panniculitic T-cell lymphoma. Int J Dermatol 1996;35:1–8.
416. Wang L, Yang Y, Liu W, et al. [Subcutaneous panniculitis-like T-cell lymphoma: expression of cytotoxic-granule-associated protein TIA-1 and its relation with Epstein-Barr virus infection.] Zhonghua Bing Li Xue Za Zhi 2000;29:103–6. (Chinese.)
417. Weenig RH, Ng CS, Perniciaro C. Subcutaneous panniculitis-like T-cell lymphoma: an elusive case presenting as lipomembranous panniculitis and a review of 72 cases in the literature. Am J Dermatopathol 2001;23:206–15.
418. Weinstock MA, Horm JW. Population-based estimate of survival and determinants of prognosis in patients with mycosis fungoides. Cancer 1988;62:1658–61.
419. Weiss LM, Jaffe ES, Liu XF, Chen YY, Shibata D, Medeiros LJ. Detection and localization of Epstein-Barr viral genomes in angioimmunoblastic lymphadenopathy and angioimmunoblastic lymphadenopathy-like lymphoma. Blood 1992;79:1789–95.
420. Weiss LM, Wood GS, Trela M, Warnke RA, Sklar J. Clonal T-cell populations in lymphomatoid papulosis. Evidence of a lymphoproliferative origin for a clinically benign disease. N Engl J Med 1986;315:475–9.
421. Whitmore SE, Simmons-O'Brien E, Rotter FS. Hypopigmented mycosis fungoides. Arch Dermatol 1994;130:476–80.
422. Whittaker S, Smith N, Jones RR, Luzzatto L. Analysis of beta, gamma, and delta T-cell receptor genes in lymphomatoid papulosis: cellular basis of two distinct histologic subsets. J Invest Dermatol 1991;96:786–91.
423. Whittam LR, Calonje E, Orchard G, Fraser-Andrews EA, Woolford A, Russell-Jones R. CD8-positive juvenile onset mycosis fungoides: an immunohistochemical and genotypic analysis of six cases. Br J Dermatol 2000;143:1199–204.
424. Wick MR, Patterson JW. Cytophagic histiocytic panniculitis—a critical reappraisal. Arch Dermatol 2000;136:922–4.
425. Wick MR, Sanchez NP, Crotty CP, Winkelmann RK. Cutaneous malignant histiocytosis: a clinical and histopathologic study of eight cases, with immunohistochemical analysis. J Am Acad Dermatol 1983;8:50–62.
426. Wieselthier JS, Koh HK. Sezary syndrome: diagnosis, prognosis, and critical review of treatment options. J Am Acad Dermatol 1990;22:381–401.

427. Willemze R, Kerl H, Sterry W, et al. EORTC classification for primary cutaneous lymphomas: a proposal from the Cutaneous Lymphoma Study Group of the European Organization for Research and Treatment of Cancer. Blood 1997;90:354–71.
428. Willemze R, Meyer CJ, Van Vloten WA, Scheffer E. The clinical and histological spectrum of lymphomatoid papulosis. Br J Dermatol 1982;107:131–44.
429. Willemze R, Scheffer E. Clinical and histologic differentiation between lymphomatoid papulosis and pityriasis lichenoides. J Am Acad Dermatol 1985;13:418–28.
430. Willemze R, Scheffer E, Ruiter DJ, van Vloten WA, Meijer CJ. Immunological, cytochemical and ultrastructural studies in lymphomatoid papulosis. Br J Dermatol 1983;108:381–94.
431. Winkelmann RK, Bowie EJ. Hemorrhagic diathesis associated with benign histiocytic, cytophagic panniculitis and systemic histiocytosis. Arch Intern Med 1980;140:1460–3.
432. Wolf P, Cerroni L, Kerl H. Mycosis fungoides mimicking perioral dermatitis. Clin Exp Dermatol 1992;17:132–4.
433. Wolf R, Kahane E, Sandbank M. Mycosis fungoides-like lesions associated with phenytoin therapy. Arch Dermatol 1985;121:1181–2.
434. Wollina U, Graefe T, Fuller J. Granulomatous slack skin or granulomatous mycosis fungoides—a case report. Complete response to percutaneous radiation and interferon alpha. J Cancer Res Clin Oncol 2002;128:50–4.
435. Wood GS, Abel EA, Hoppe RT, Warnke RA. Leu-8 and Leu-9 antigen phenotypes: immunologic criteria for the distinction of mycosis fungoides from cutaneous inflammation. J Am Acad Dermatol 1986;14:1006–13.
436. Wood GS, Hardman DL, Boni R, et al. Lack of the t(2;5) or other mutations resulting in expression of anaplastic lymphoma kinase catalytic domain in CD30+ primary cutaneous lymphoproliferative disorders and Hodgkin's disease. Blood 1996;88:1765–70.
437. Wood WS, Killby VA, Stewart WD. Pagetoid reticulosis (Woringer-Kolopp disease). J Cutan Pathol 1979;6:113–23.
438. Yagi H, Hagiwara T, Shirahama S, Tokura Y, Takigawa M. Disseminated pagetoid reticulosis: need for long-term follow-up. J Am Acad Dermatol 1994;30(Pt 2):345–9.
439. Yamashita Y, Tsuzuki T, Nakayama A, Fujino M, Mori N. A case of natural killer/T cell lymphoma of the subcutis resembling subcutaneous panniculitis-like T cell lymphoma. Pathol Int 1999;49:241–6.
440. Yoshinaga H. [A case of adult T-cell leukemia (ATL)—various skin eruptions and virus-like particles in the fresh tumor cells.] Nippon Hifuka Gakkai Zasshi 1989;99:25–35. (Japanese.)
441. Yung A, Snow J, Jarrett P. Subcutaneous panniculitic T-cell lymphoma and cytophagic histiocytic panniculitis. Australas J Dermatol 2001;42:183–7.
442. Zelger B, Sepp N, Weyrer K, Grunewald K, Zelger B. Syringotropic cutaneous T-cell lymphoma: a variant of mycosis fungoides? Br J Dermatol 1994;130:765–9.
443. Zelickson BD, Peters MS, Muller SA, et al. T-cell receptor gene rearrangement analysis: cutaneous T cell lymphoma, peripheral T cell lymphoma, and premalignant and benign cutaneous lymphoproliferative disorders. J Am Acad Dermatol 1991;25(Pt 1):787–96.

Hodgkin's Disease

444. Benninghoff DL, Medina A, Alexander LL, Camiel MR. The mode of spread of Hodgkin's disease to the skin. Cancer 1970;26:1135–40.
445. Cerroni L, Beham-Schmid C, Kerl H. Cutaneous Hodgkin's disease: an immunohistochemical analysis. J Cutan Pathol 1995;22:229–35.
446. Davis TH, Morton CC, Miller-Cassman R, Balk SP, Kadin ME. Hodgkin's disease, lymphomatoid papulosis, and cutaneous T-cell lymphoma derived from a common T-cell clone. N Engl J Med 1992;326:1115–22.
447. Foss HD, Reusch R, Demel G, et al. Frequent expression of the B-cell-specific activator protein in Reed-Sternberg cells of classical Hodgkin's disease provides further evidence for its B-cell origin. Blood 1999;94:3108–13.
448. Geldenhuys L, Radhi J, Hull PR. Mycosis fungoides and cutaneous Hodgkin's disease in the same patient: a case report. J Cutan Pathol 1999;26:311–4.
449. Guitart J, Fretzin D. Skin as the primary site of Hodgkin's disease: a case report of primary cutaneous Hodgkin's disease and review of its relationship with non-Hodgkin's lymphoma. Am J Dermatopathol 1998;20:218–22.
450. Hanno R, Bean SF. Hodgkin's disease with specific bullous lesions. Am J Dermatopathol 1980;2:363–6.
451. Heyd J, Weissberg N, Gottschalk S. Hodgkin's disease of the skin. A case report. Cancer 1989;63:924–9.
452. Kadin ME. Lymphomatoid papulosis, Ki-1+ lymphoma, and primary cutaneous Hodgkin's disease. Semin Dermatol 1991;10:164–71.

453. Kadin ME, Muramoto L, Said J. Expression of T-cell antigens on Reed-Sternberg cells in a subset of patients with nodular sclerosing and mixed cellularity Hodgkin's disease. Am J Pathol 1988;130:345–53.
454. Marafioti T, Hummel M, Foss HD, et al. Hodgkin and reed-sternberg cells represent an expansion of a single clone originating from a germinal center B-cell with functional immunoglobulin gene rearrangements but defective immunoglobulin transcription. Blood 2000;95:1443–50.
455. Noto G, Pravata G, Miceli S, Arico M. Granulomatous slack skin: report of a case associated with Hodgkin's disease and a review of the literature. Br J Dermatol 1994;131:275–9.
456. Pagliaro JA, White SI. Specific skin lesions occurring in a patient with Hodgkin's lymphoma. Australas J Dermatol 1999;40:41–3.
457. Patterson JW, Blaylock WK. Hodgkin's disease. In: Demis DJ, Dobson RL, McGuire J, eds. Clinical dermatology, vol. 4. Hagerstown: Harper and Row; 1985:Unit 20-8, pp. 1–9.
458. Seitz V, Hummel M, Marafioti T, Anagnostopoulos I, Assaf C, Stein H. Detection of clonal T-cell receptor gamma-chain gene rearrangements in Reed-Sternberg cells of classic Hodgkin disease. Blood 2000;95:3020–4.
459. Silverman CL, Strayer DS, Wasserman TH. Cutaneous Hodgkin's disease. Arch Dermatol 1982;118:918–21.
460. Sioutos N, Kerl H, Murphy SB, Kadin ME. Primary cutaneous Hodgkin's disease. Unique clinical, morphologic, and immunophenotypic findings. Am J Dermatopathol 1994;16:2–8.
461. Smith JL Jr, Butler JJ. Skin involvement in Hodgkin's disease. Cancer 1980;45:354–61.
462. Stein H, Delsol G, Pileri S, et al. Classical Hodgkin lymphoma. In: Jaffe ES, Harris NL, Stein H, Vardiman JW, eds. Pathology and genetics of tumours of haematopoietic and lymphoid tissues. Lyon: IARC Press; 2001:244–53.
463. Torne R, Umbert P. Hodgkin's disease presenting with superficial lymph nodes and tumors of the scalp. Dermatologica 1986;172:225–8.
464. White RM, Patterson JW. Cutaneous involvement in Hodgkin's disease. Cancer 1985;55:1136–45.
465. Willemze R, Kerl H, Sterry W, et al. EORTC classification for primary cutaneous lymphomas: a proposal from the Cutaneous Lymphoma Study Group of the European Organization for Research and Treatment of Cancer. Blood 1997;90:354–71.
466. Zackheim HS, LeBoit PE, Gordon BI, Glassberg AB. Lymphomatoid papulosis followed by Hodgkin's lymphoma. Differential response to therapy. Arch Dermatol 1993;129:86–91.

Leukemia Cutis

467. Arai E, Ikeda S, Itoh S, Katayama I. Specific skin lesions as the presenting symptom of hairy cell leukemia. Am J Clin Pathol 1988;90:459–64.
468. Asada H, Okada N, Tei H, et al. Epstein-Barr virus-associated large granular lymphocyte leukemia with cutaneous infiltration. J Am Acad Dermatol 1994;31(Pt 1):251–5.
469. Baer MR, Barcos M, Farrell H, Raza A, Preisler HD. Acute myelogenous leukemia with leukemia cutis. Eighteen cases seen between 1969 and 1986. Cancer 1989;63:2192–200.
470. Barzilai A, Shpiro D, Goldberg I, et al. Insect bite-like reaction in patients with hematologic malignant neoplasms. Arch Dermatol 1999;135:1503–7.
471. Blaustein JC, Narang S, Palutke M, Karanes C. Extramedullary (skin) presentation of acute monocytic leukemia resembling cutaneous lymphoma: morphological and immunological features. J Cutan Pathol 1987;14:232–7.
472. Bonvalet D, Foldes C, Civatte J. Cutaneous manifestations in chronic lymphocytic leukemia. J Dermatol Surg Oncol 1984;10:278–82.
473. Braverman IM. Skin signs of systemic disease, 2nd ed. Philadelphia: WB Saunders; 1981.
474. Buechner SA, Li CY, Su WP. Leukemia cutis. A histopathologic study of 42 cases. Am J Dermatopathol 1985;7:109–19.
475. Canioni D, Fraitag S, Thomas C, Valensi F, Griscelli C, Brousse N. Skin lesions revealing neonatal acute leukemias with monocytic differentiation. A report of 3 cases. J Cutan Pathol 1996;23:254–8.
476. Caughman W, Stern R, Haynes H. Neutrophilic dermatosis of myeloproliferative disorders. Atypical forms of pyoderma gangrenosum and Sweet's syndrome associated with myeloproliferative disorders. J Am Acad Dermatol 1983;9:751–8.
477. Chan JK. Natural killer cell neoplasms. Anat Pathol 1998;3:77–145.
478. Daoud MS, Snow JL, Gibson LE, Daoud S. Aleukemic monocytic leukemia cutis. Mayo Clin Proc 1996;71:166–8.
479. De Coninck A, De Hou MF, Peters O, Van Camp B, Roseeuw DI. Aleukemic leukemia cutis. An unusual presentation of acute myelomonocytic leukemia. Dermatologica 1986;172:272–5.
480. Dorfman DM, Kraus M, Perez-Atayde AR, Barnhill RL, Pinkus GS, Granter SR. CD99 (p30/32MIC2) immunoreactivity in the diagnosis of leukemia cutis. Mod Pathol 1997;10:283–8.
481. Finan MC, Su WP, Li CY. Cutaneous findings in hairy cell leukemia. J Am Acad Dermatol 1984;11(Pt 1):788–97.

482. Gil-Mateo MP, Miquel FJ, Piris MA, Sanchez M, Martin-Aragones G. Aleukemic "leukemia cutis" of monocytic lineage. J Am Acad Dermatol 1997;36(Pt 2):837–40.
483. Helm KF, Peters MS, Tefferi A, Leiferman KM. Pyoderma gangrenosum-like ulcer in a patient with large granular lymphocytic leukemia. J Am Acad Dermatol 1992;27(Pt 2):868–71.
484. Horlick HP, Silvers DN, Knobler EH, Cole JT. Acute myelomonocytic leukemia presenting as a benign-appearing cutaneous eruption. Arch Dermatol 1990;126:653–6.
485. Jones D, Dorfman DM, Barnhill RL, Granter SR. Leukemic vasculitis: a feature of leukemia cutis in some patients. Am J Clin Pathol 1997; 107:637–42.
486. Lawrence DM, Sun NC, Mena R, Moss R. Cutaneous lesions in hairy-cell leukemia. Case report and review of the literature. Arch Dermatol 1983;119:322–5.
487. Ohno S, Yokoo T, Ohta M, et al. Aleukemic leukemia cutis. J Am Acad Dermatol 1990;22(Pt 2):374–7.
488. Ratnam KV, Khor CJ, Su WP. Leukemia cutis. Dermatol Clin 1994;12:419–31.
489. Sanz MA, Larrea L, Sanz G, et al. Cutaneous promyelocytic sarcoma at sites of vascular access and marrow aspiration. A characteristic localization of chloromas in acute promyelocytic leukemia? Haematologica 2000;85:758–62.
490. Shaikh BS, Frantz E, Lookingbill DP. Histologically proven leukemia cutis carries a poor prognosis in acute nonlymphocytic leukemia. Cutis 1987;39:57–60.
491. Sires UI, Mallory SB, Hess JL, Keating JP, Bloomberg G, Dehner LP. Cutaneous presentation of juvenile chronic myelogenous leukemia: a diagnostic and therapeutic dilemma. Pediatr Dermatol 1995;12:364–8.
492. Stawiski MA. Skin manifestations of leukemias and lymphomas. Cutis 1978;21:814–8.
493. Su WP, Buechner SA, Li CY. Clinicopathologic correlations in leukemia cutis. J Am Acad Dermatol 1984;11:121–8.
494. Takai K, Sanada M. [Aggressive NK cell leukemia/lymphoma: an autopsy case]. Rinsho Ketsueki 2001;42:621–6. (Japanese.)
495. Taniguchi S, Hamada T, Kutsuna H, Ishii M. Lymphocytic aleukemic leukemia cutis. J Am Acad Dermatol 1996;35(Pt 2):849–50.
496. Verhagen C, Stalpers LJ, de Pauw BE, Haanen C. Drug-induced skin reactions in patients with acute non-lymphocytic leukaemia. Eur J Haematol 1987;38:225–30.
497. Wong TY, Suster S, Bouffard D, et al. Histologic spectrum of cutaneous involvement in patients with myelogenous leukemia including the neutrophilic dermatoses. Int J Dermatol 1995;34:323–9.

Extramedullary Hematopoiesis

498. Argyle JC, Zone JJ. Dermal erythropoiesis in a neonate. Arch Dermatol 1981;117:492–4.
499. Bowden JB, Hebert AA, Rapini RP. Dermal hematopoiesis in neonates: report of five cases. J Am Acad Dermatol 1989;20:1104–10.
500. Evole-Buselli M, Hernandez-Marti MJ, Gasco-Lacalle B, Esquembre Menor C, Mascunan-Diaz I, Sorni-Valls G. Neonatal dermal hematopoiesis associated with diffuse neonatal hemangiomatosis. Pediatr Dermatol 1997;14:383–6.
501. Green LK, Klima M, Burns TR. Extramedullary hematopoiesis occurring in a hemangioma of the skin. Arch Dermatol 1988;124:1720–1.
502. Hebert AA, Esterly NB, Gardner TH. Dermal erythropoiesis in Rh hemolytic disease of the newborn. J Pediatr 1985;107:799–801.
503. Hocking WG, Lazar GS, Lipsett JA, Busuttil RW. Cutaneous extramedullary hematopoiesis following splenectomy for idiopathic myelofibrosis. Am J Med 1984;76:956–8.
504. Hodl S, Aubock L, Reiterer F, Soyer HP, Muller WD. [Blueberry muffin baby: the pathogenesis of cutaneous extramedullary hematopoiesis.] Hautarzt 2001;52:1035–42. (German.)
505. Hoss DM, McNutt NS. Cutaneous myelofibrosis. J Cutan Pathol 1992;19:221–5.
506. Kuo T. Cutaneous extramedullary hematopoiesis presenting as leg ulcers. J Am Acad Dermatol 1981;4:592–6.
507. Kwon KS, Lee JB, Jang HS, Chung TA, Oh CK. A case of cutaneous extramedullary hematopoiesis in myelofibrosis with a preponderance of eosinophilic precursor cells. J Dermatol 1999;26:379–84.
508. Mizoguchi M, Kawa Y, Minami T, Nakayama H, Mizoguchi H. Cutaneous extramedullary hematopoiesis in myelofibrosis. J Am Acad Dermatol 1990;22(Pt 2):351–5.
509. Schofield JK, Shun JL, Cerio R, Grice K. Cutaneous extramedullary hematopoiesis with a preponderance of atypical megakaryocytes in myelofibrosis. J Am Acad Dermatol 1990;22(Pt 2):334–7.
510. Schwartz JL, Maniscalco WM, Lane AT, Currao WJ. Twin transfusion syndrome causing cutaneous erythropoiesis. Pediatrics 1984;74:527–9.
511. Tagami H, Tashima M, Uehara N. Myelofibrosis with skin lesions. Br J Dermatol 1980;102:109–12.

SUPPLEMENTAL REFERENCES

Lymphoid Infiltrates and Lymphomas

Willemze R, Jaffe ES, Burg G, et al. WHO-EORTC classification for cutaneous lymphomas. Blood 2005; 105:3768–85.

Lymphocytoma Cutis

Colli C, Leinweber B, Mullegger R, Chott A, Kerl H, Cerroni L. Borrelia burgdorferi-associated lymphocytoma cutis: clinicopathologic, immunophenotypic, and molecular study of 106 cases. J Cutan Pathol 2004;31:232–40.

Gutermuth J, Audring H, Roseeuw D. Disseminated cutaneous B-cell lymphoma mimicking pseudolymphoma over a period of six years. Am J Dermatopathol 2004;26:225–9.

Muche JM, Toppe E, Sterry W, Haas N. Palpable arciform migratory erythema in an HIV patient, a CD8+ pseudolymphoma. J Cutan Pathol 2004;31:379–82.

Cutaneous Marginal Zone Lymphoma

Arai E, Shimizu M, Hirose T. A review of 55 cases of cutaneous lymphoid hyperplasia: reassessment of the histopathologic findings leading to reclassification of 4 lesions as cutaneous marginal zone lymphoma and 19 as pseudolymphomatous folliculitis. Hum Pathol 2005;36:505–11.

Demirkesen C, Tuzuner N, Su O, Esckazan AE, Soysal T, Onsun N. Primary cutaneous immunocytoma/marginal zone B-cell lymphoma: a case with unusual course. Am J Dermatopathol 2004;26:119–22.

Espinet B, Gallardo F, Pujol RM, Estrach T, Servitje O, Sole F. Absence of MALT1 translocations in primary cutaneous marginal zone B-cell lymphoma. Haematologica 2004;89:ELT14.

May SA, Netto G, Domiati-Saad R, Kasper C. Cutaneous lymphoid hyperplasia and marginal zone B-cell lymphoma following vaccination. J Am Acad Dermatol 2005;53:512–6.

Schreuder MI, Hoefnagel JJ, Jansen PM, van Krieken JH, Willemze R, Hebeda KM. FISH analysis of MALT lymphoma-specific translocations and aneuploidy in primary cutaneous marginal zone lymphoma. J Pathol 2005;205:302–10.

Follicular Lymphoma

Goodlad JR, MacPherson S, Jackson R, Batstone P, White J; Scotland and Newcastle Lymphoma Group. Extranodal follicular lymphoma: a clinicopathological and genetic analysis of 15 cases arising at non-cutaneous extranodal sites. Histopathology 2004;44:268–76.

Kazakov DV, Palmedo G, Mukensnabl P, Hes O, Kempf W, Michal M. Follicular lymphoma of the skin and superficial soft tissues associated with a prominent follicular dendritic cell proliferation: an unusual pattern which may represent a diagnostic pitfall. Pathol Res Pract 2004;200:557–65.

Diffuse Large B-Cell Lymphoma

Bubala H, Maldyk J, Wlodarska I, Sonta-Jakimczyk D, Szczepanski T. ALK-positive diffuse large B-cell lymphoma. Pediatr Blood Cancer 2005 April 25. [Epub ahead of print.]

Dargent JL, Lespagnard L, Feoli F, Debusscher L, Greuse M, Bron D. De novo CD5-positive diffuse large B-cell lymphoma of the skin arising in chronic limb lymphedema. Leuk Lymphoma 2005;46:775–80.

Fu K, Iqbal J, Chan WC. Recent advances in the molecular diagnosis of diffuse large B-cell lymphoma. Expert Rev Mol Diagn 2005;5:397–408.

Hedvat CV, Teruya-Feldstein J, Puig P, et al. Expression of p63 in difuse large B-cell lymphoma. Appl Immunohistochem Mol Morphol 2005;13:237–42.

Rossi D, Gaidano G. Molecular heterogeneity of diffuse large B-cell lymphoma: implications for disease management and prognosis. Hematology 2002;7:239–52.

Zu Y, Steinberg SM, Campo E, et al. Validation of tissue microarray immunohistochemistry staining and interpretation in diffuse large B-cell lymphoma. Leuk Lymphoma 2005;46:693–701.

Intravascular Large B-Cell Lymphoma

Cerroni L, Zalaudek I, Kerl H. Intravascular large B-cell lymphoma colonizing cutaneous hemangiomas. Dermatology 2004;209:132–4.

Nixon BK, Kussick SJ, Carlon MJ, Rubin BP. Intravascular large B-cell lymphoma involving hemangiomas: an unusual presentation of a rare neoplasm. Mod Pathol 2005;18:1121–6.

Seki K, Miyakoshi S, Lee GH, et al. Prostatic acid phosphatase is a possible tumor marker for intravascular large B-cell lymphoma. Am J Surg Pathol 2004;28:1384–8.

Lymphomatoid Granulomatosis

Agarwal V, Agarwal A, Pal L, Misra R. Arthritis in lymphomatoid granulomatosis: report of a case and review of literature. Indian J Med Sci 2004;58:67–71.

Other B-Cell Lymphomas Involving the Skin

Bertoni F, Zucca E, Cavalli F. Mantle cell lymphoma. Curr Opin Hematol 2004;11:411–8.

Bociek RG. Adult Burkitt's lymphoma. Clin Lymphoma 2005;6:11–20.

Dodiuk-Gad RP, Dann EJ, Bergman R. Insect bite-like reaction associated with mantle cell lymphoma: a report of two cases and review of the literature. Int J Dermatol 2004;43:754–8.

Pott C, Schrader C, Bruggemann M, et al. Blastoid variant of mantle cell lymphoma: late progression from classical mantle cell lymphoma and quantitation of minimal residual disease. Eur J Haematol 2005;74:353–8.

Ruchlemer R, Parry-Jones N, Brito-Babapulle V, et al. B-prolymphocytic leukaemia with t(11;14) revisited: a splenomegalic form of mantle cell lymphoma evolving with leukaemia. Br J Haematol 2004;125:330–6.

Shigekiyo T, Ohmori H, Chohraku M, et al. Unusual skin reactions after mosquito bites and Epstein-Barr virus reactivation in a patient with mantle cell lymphoma. Intern Med 2004;43:986–9.

van den Bosch CA. Is endemic Burkitt's lymphoma an alliance between three infections and a tumour promoter? Lancet Oncol 2004;5:738–46.

Precursor T-Lymphoblastic Lymphoma

Feldman AL, Berthold F, Arceci RJ, et al. Clonal relationship between precursor T-lymphoblastic leukaemia/lymphoma and Langerhans-cell histiocytosis. Lancet Oncol 2005;6:435–7.

Adult T-Cell Leukemia/Lymphoma

Mahieux R, Gessain A. HTLV-1 and associated adult T-cell leukemia/lymphoma. Rev Clin Exp Hematol 2003;7:336–61.

Nicot C. Current views in HTLV-I-associated adult T-cell leukemia/lymphoma. Am J Hematol 2005;78:232–9.

Shimauchi T, Hirokawa Y, Tokura Y. Purpuric adult T-cell leukaemia/lymphoma: expansion of unusual CD4/CD8 double-negative malignant T cells expressing CCR4 but bearing the cytotoxic molecule granzyme B. Br J Dermatol 2005;152:350–2.

Sugita K, Shimauchi T, Tokura Y. Chronic actinic dermatitis associated with adult T-cell leukemia. J Am Acad Dermatol 2005;52(2 Suppl 1):38–40.

Yamaguchi T, Ohshima K, Karube K, et al. Clinicopathological features of cutaneous lesions of adult T-cell leukaemia/lymphoma. Br J Dermatol 2005;152:76–81.

Yamaguchi T, Ohshima K, Tsuchiya T, et al. The comparison of expression of cutaneous lymphocyte-associated antigen (CLA), and Th1- and Th2-associated antigens in mycosis fungoides and cutaneous lesions of adult T-cell leukemia/lymphoma. Eur J Dermatol 2003;13:553–9.

Extranodal NK/T-Cell Lymphoma, Nasal Type

Kase S, Adachi H, Osaki M, et al. Epstein-Barr virus-infected malignant T/NK-cell lymphoma in a patient with hypersensitivity to mosquito bites. Int J Surg Pathol 2004;12:265–72.

Ko YH, Cho EY, Kim JE, et al. NK and NK-like T-cell lymphoma in extranasal sites: a comparative clinicopathological study according to site and EBV status. Histopathology 2004;44:480–9.

Subcutaneous Panniculitis-Like T-Cell Lymphoma

Bregman SG, Yeaney GA, Greig BW, Vnencak-Jones CL, Hamilton KS. Subcutaneous panniculitic T-cell lymphoma in a cardiac allograft recipient. J Cutan Pathol 2005;32:366–70.

Cassis TB, Fearneyhough PK, Callen JP. Subcutaneous panniculitis-like T-cell lymphoma with vacuolar interface dermatitis resembling lupus erythematosus panniculitis. J Am Acad Dermatol 2004;50:465–9.

Ghobrial IM, Weenig RH, Pittlekow MR, et al. Clinical outcome of patients with subcutaneous panniculitis-like T-cell lymphoma. Leuk Lymphoma 2005;46:703–8.

Go RS, Wester SM. Immunophenotypic and molecular features, clinical outcomes, treatments, and prognostic factors associated with subcutaneous panniculitis-like T-cell lymphoma: a systematic analysis of 156 patients reported in the literature. Cancer 2004;101:1404–13.

Manosca F, Ariga R, Bengana C, Reddy VB, Loew J, Gattuso P. Fine-needle aspiration of subcutaneous panniculitis-like T-cell lymphoma. Diagn Cytopathol 2004;31:338–9.

Mycosis Fungoides

Foss F. Mycosis fungoides and the Sezary syndrome. Curr Opin Oncol 2004;16:421–8.

Franck N, Carlotti A, Gorin I, Buffet M, Mateus C, Dupin N. Mycosis fungoides-type cutaneous T-cell lymphoma and neutrophilic dermatosis. Arch Dermatol 2005;141:353–6.

Girardi M, Heald PW, Wilson LD. The pathogenesis of mycosis fungoides. N Engl J Med 2004;350:1978–88.

Hodak E, Akerman L, David M, et al. Cytokine gene polymorphisms in patch-stage mycosis fungoides. Acta Derm Venereol 2005;85:109–12.

Kazakov DV, Burg G, Kempf W. Clinicopathological spectrum of mycosis fungoides. J Eur Acad Dermatol Venereol 2004;18:397–415.

Kossard S, Weller P. Pseudotumorous folliculotropic mycosis fungoides. Am J Dermatopathol 2005;27:224–7.

Magro CM, Crowson AN, Kovatich AJ, Burns F. Drug-induced reversible lymphoid dyscrasia: a clonal lymphomatoid dermatitis of memory and activated T cells. Hum Pathol 2003;34:119–29.

Massone C, Kodama K, Kerl H, Cerroni L. Histopathologic features of early (patch) lesions of mycosis fungoides: a morphologic study on 745 biopsy specimens from 427 patients. Am J Surg Pathol 2005;29:550–60.

Cutaneous CD8-Positive T-Cell Lymphoma

Heliot-Hosten I, Versapuech J, Vergier B, Taieb A, Delaunay M. [Cutaneous CD8+ squamous T-cell bullous lymphoma.] Ann Dermatol Venereol 2005;132:359–61. (French.)

Wenzel J, Gutgemann I, Distelmaier M, et al. The role of cytotoxic skin-homing CD8+ lymphocytes in cutaneous cytotoxic T-cell lymphoma and pityriasis lichenoides. J Am Acad Dermatol 2005;53:422–7.

Pagetoid Reticulosis

Shiozawa E, Shiokawa A, Shibata M, et al. Autopsy case of CD4/CD8 cutaneous T-cell lymphoma presenting as disseminated pagetoid reticulosis with aggressive granulomatous invasion to the lungs and pancreas. Pathol Int 2005;55:32–9.

Steffen C. Ketron-Goodman disease, Woringer-Kolopp disease, and pagetoid reticulosis. Am J Dermatopathol 2005;27:68–85.

Granulomatous Slack Skin

Gadzia J, Kestenbaum T. Granulomatous slack skin without evidence of a clonal T-cell proliferation. J Am Acad Dermatol 2004;50(Suppl):S4–8.

Sézary's Syndrome

Diwan AH, Prieto VG, Herling M, Duvic M, Jone D. Primary Sezary syndrome commonly shows low-grade cytologic atypia and an absence of epidermotropism. Am J Clin Pathol 2005;123:510–5.

Introcaso CE, Hess SD, Kamoun M, Ubriani R, Gelfand JM, Rook AH. Association of change in clinical status and change in the percentage of the CD4+CD26- lymphocyte population in patients with Sezary syndrome. J Am Acad Dermatol 2005;53:428–34.

Magazin M, Poszepczynska-Guigne E, Bagot M, et al. Sezary syndrome cells unlike normal circulating T lymphocytes fail to migrate following engagement of NT1 receptor. J Invest Dermatol 2004;122:111–8.

Ponti R, Quaglino P, Novelli M, et al. T-cell receptor gamma gene rearrangement by multiplex polymerase chain reaction/heteroduplex analysis in patients with cutaneous T-cell lymphoma (mycosis fungoides/Sezary syndrome) and benign inflammatory disease: correlation with clinical, histological and immunophenotypical findings. Br J Dermatol 2005;153:565–73.

Poszepczynska-Guigne E, Schiavon V, D'Incan M, et al. CD158k/KIR3DL2 is a new phenotypic marker of Sezary cells: relevance for the diagnosis and follow-up of Sezary syndrome. J Invest Dermatol 2004;122:820–3.

Sokolowska-Wojdylo M, Wenzel J, Gaffal E, et al. Circulating clonal CLA(+) and CD4(+) T cells in Sezary syndrome express the skin-homing chemokine receptors CCR4 and CCR10 as well as the lymph node-homing chemokine receptor CCR7. Br J Dermatol 2005;152:258–64.

Vonderheid EC, Bernengo MG. The Sezary syndrome: hematologic criteria. Hematol Oncol Clin North Am 2003;17:1367–89, viii.

Cutaneous Anaplastic Large Cell Lymphoma

Kim HK, Jin SY, Lee NS, Won JH, Park HS, Yang WI. Posttransplant primary cutaneous Ki-1 (CD30)+/CD56+ anaplastic large cell lymphoma. Arch Pathol Lab Med 2004;128:e96–9.

Kumar S, Pittaluga S, Raffeld M, Guerrera M, Seibel NL, Jaffe ES. Primary cutaneous CD30-positive anaplastic large cell lymphoma in childhood: report of 4 cases and review of the literature. Pediatr Dev Pathol 2005;8:52–60.

Lin JH, Lee JY. Primary cutaneous CD30 anaplastic large cell lymphoma with keratoacanthoma-like pseudocarcinomatous hyperplasia and marked eosinophilia and neutrophilia. J Cutan Pathol 2004;31:458–61.

Lucioni M, Ippoliti G, Campana C, et al. EBV positive primary cutaneous CD30+ large T-cell lymphoma in a heart transplanted patient: case report. Am J Transplant 2004;4:1915–20.

Salama S. Primary "cutaneous" T-cell anaplastic large cell lymphoma, CD30+, neutrophil-rich variant with subcutaneous panniculitic lesions, in a post-renal transplant patient: report of unusual case and literature review. Am J Dermatopathol 2005; 27:217–23.

Sasaki K, Sugaya M, Fujita H, et al. A case of primary cutaneous anaplastic large cell lymphoma with variant anaplastic lymphoma kinase translocation. Br J Dermatol 2004;150:1202–7.

Shimauchi T, Onoue A, Yamamoto O, Hino R, Tokura Y. Evidence for polyclonal infection of Epstein-Barr virus in a patient with primary cutaneous anaplastic large cell lymphoma. Clin Exp Dermatol 2004;29:383–6.

Peripheral T-Cell Lymphoma

Kojima H, Hasegawa Y, Suzukawa K, et al. Clinicopathological features and prognostic factors of Japanese patients with "peripheral T-cell lymphoma, unspecified" diagnosed according to the WHO classification. Leuk Res 2004;28:1287–92.

Massone C, Basso M, Rongioletti F. Cutaneous presentation of recurrence of lymphoepithelioid T-cell lymphoma (Lennert's lymphoma). Clin Exp Dermatol 2005;30:155–7.

Okabe S, Miyazawa K, Iguchi T, et al. Peripheral T-cell lymphoma together with myelofibrosis with elevated plasma transforming growth factor-beta1. Leuk Lymphoma 2005;46:599–602.

Vaillo Vinagre A, Gutierrez Martin A, Perez Barrios A, Alberti Masgrau N, Ruiz Liso JM. Lymphoepithelioid cell lymphoma (Lennert's lymphoma). Report of a case with fine needle aspiration cytology. Acta Cytol 2004;48:234–8.

Zettl A, Rudiger T, Konrad MA, et al. Genomic profiling of peripheral T-cell lymphoma, unspecified, and anaplastic large T-cell lymphoma delineates novel recurrent chromosomal alterations. Am J Pathol 2004;164:1837–48.

Angioimmunoblastic T-Cell Lymphoma

Huang CT, Chuang SS. Angioimmunoblastic T-cell lymphoma with cutaneous involvement: a case report with subtle histologic changes and clonal T-cell proliferation. Arch Pathol Lab Med 2004;128:e122–4.

Jones B, Vun Y, Sabah M, Egan CA. Toxic epidermal necrolysis secondary to angioimmunoblastic T-cell lymphoma. Australas J Dermatol 2005;46:187–91.

Willenbrock K, Renne C, Gaulard P, Hansmann ML. In angioimmunoblastic T-cell lymphoma, neoplastic T cells may be a minor cell population. A molecular single-cell and immunohistochemical study. Virchows Arch 2005;446:15–20.

Yamamoto H, Miwa H, Kato Y, Nakamura S, Hara K, Nitta M. Angioimmunoblastic T cell lymphoma with an unusual proliferation of Epstein-Barr virus-associated large B cells arising in a patient with progressive systemic sclerosis. Acta Haematol 2005;114:108–12.

Yuan CM, Vergilio JA, Zhao XF, Smith TK, Harris NL, Bagg A. CD10 and BCL6 expression in the diagnosis of angioimmunoblastic T-cell lymphoma: utility of detecting CD10(+) T cells by flow cytometry. Hum Pathol 2005;36:784–91.

Zhao WL, Mourah S, Mounier N, et al. Vascular endothelial growth factor-A is expressed both on lymphoma cells and endothelial cells in angioimmunoblastic T-cell lymphoma and related to lymphoma progression. Lab Invest 2004;84:1512–9.

Lymphomatoid Papulosis

Gallardo F, Costa C, Bellosillo B, et al. Lymphomatoid papulosis associated with mycosis fungoides: clinicopathological and molecular studies of 12 cases. Acta Derm Venereol 2004;84:463–8.

Nijsten T, Curiel-Lewandrowski C, Kadin ME. Lymphomatoid papulosis in children: a retrospective cohort study of 35 cases. Arch Dermatol 2004;140:306–12.

Perna AG, Jones DM, Duvic M. Lymphomatoid papulosis from childhood with anaplastic large-cell lymphoma of the small bowel. Clin Lymphoma 2004;5:190–3.

Pujol RM, Muret MP, Bergua P, Bordes R, Alomar A. Oral involvement in lymphomatoid papulosis. Report of two cases and review of the literature. Dermatology 2005;210:53–7.

Rassidakis GZ, Georgakis GV, Oyarzo M, Younes A, Medeiros LJ. Lack of c-kit (CD117) expression in CD30+ lymphomas and lymphomatoid papulosis. Mod Pathol 2004;17:946–53.

Rassidakis GZ, Thomaides A, Atwell C, et al. JunB expression is a common feature of CD30+ lymphomas and lymphomatoid papulosis. Mod Pathol 2005 May 6. [Epub ahead of print.]

Schultz JC, Granados S, Vonderheid EC, Hwang ST. T-cell clonality of peripheral blood lymphocytes in patients with lymphomatoid papulosis. J Am Acad Dermatol 2005;53:152–5.

Weinstein A, Mirzabeigi M, Withee M, Vincek V. Lymphomatoid papulosis in an HIV-positive man. AIDS Patient Care STDS 2004;18:563–7.

Wu WM, Tsai HJ. Lymphomatoid papulosis histopathologically simulating angiocentric and cytotoxic T-cell lymphoma: a case report. Am J Dermatopathol 2004;26:133–5.

Other T-Cell and NK-Cell Lymphomas Involving the Skin (Blastic NK-Cell Lymphoma)

Argyrakos T, Rontogianni D, Karmiris T, et al. Blastic natural killer (NK)-cell lymphoma: report of an unusual CD4 negative case and review of the CD4 negative neoplasms with blastic features in the literature. Leuk Lymphoma 2004;45:2127–33.

Kim Y, Kang MS, Kim CW, Sung R, Ko YH. CD4+CD56+ lineage negative hematopoietic neoplasm: so called blastic NK cell lymphoma. J Korean Med Sci 2005;20:319–24.

Liu XY, Atkins RC, Feusner JH, Rowland JM. Blastic NK-cell-like lymphoma with T-cell receptor gene rearrangement. Am J Hematol 2004;75:251–3.

Machet L, De Muret A, Wiezberka E, et al. [Agranular CD4+ CD56+ CD123+ hematodermic neoplasm (blastic NK-cell lymphoma) revealed by cutaneous localization: 2 cases.] Ann Dermatol Venereol 2004;131:969–73. (French.)

Cutaneous Hodgkin's Disease

Jain S, Nigam S, Kumar N, Reddy BS. Cutaneous relapse in Hodgkin's disease: a case report. Acta Cytol 2005;49:191–4.

Jurisic V, Bogunovic M, Colovic N, Colovic M. Indolent course of the cutaneous Hodgkin's disease. J Cutan Pathol 2005;32:176–8.

Leukemia Cutis

Burns CA, Scott GA, Miller CC. Leukemia cutis at the site of trauma in a patient with Burkitt leukemia. Cutis 2005;75:54–6.

Del Pozo J, Martinez W, Pazos JM, Yebra-Pimentel MT, Garcia Silva J, Fonseca E. Concurrent Sweet's syndrome and leukemia cutis in patients with myeloid disorders. Int J Dermatol 2005;44:677–80.

Landers MC, Malempati S, Tilford D, Gatter K, White C, Schroeder TL. Spontaneous regression of aleukemia congenital leukemia cutis. Pediatr Dermatol 2005;22:26–30.

Onozawa M, Hashino S, Kanamori H, et al. Aleukemic leukemia cutis in a patient with Philadelphia chromosome-positive biphenotypic leukemia. Int J Hematol 2004;80:278–80.

Petrella T, Meijer CJ, Dalac S, et al. TCL1 and CLA expression in agranular CD4/CD56 hematodermic neoplasms (blastic NK-cell lymphomas) and leukemia cutis. Am J Clin Pathol 2004;122:307–13.

Extramedullary Hematopoiesis

Brennan LV, Mayer T, Devitt J. Extramedullary hematopoiesis occurring as a nasal polyp in a man with a myeloproliferative disorder. Ear Nose Throat J 2004;83:258–9.

Vega Harring SM, Niyaz M, Okada S, Kudo M. Extramedullary hematopoiesis in a pyogenic granuloma: a case report and review. J Cutan Pathol 2004;31:555–7.

Index*

A

Abdominal/extra-abdominal desmoid tumor, 237
Acantholytic acanthoma, 17, **17**, **18**, 19
Acantholytic dyskeratotic epidermal nevus, 15, 19
Acanthosis nigricans, 16, 17
Acne keloidosis, 232
Acquired elastotic hemangioma, 289, **290**
Acquired immunodeficiency disease/virus and Kaposi's sarcoma, 300, **301**
Acquired tufted angioma, 283, **283**, **284**
Acral arteriovenous tumor, 285, **286**, **287**
Acroangiodermatitis, 309, **311**
Acrochordon, see Fibroepithelial polyp
Acrokeratosis verruciformis of Hopf, 23
Acrosyringeal nevus, see Eccrine syringofibroadenoma
Actinic keratosis, 25, 27, **28-30**
    acantholytic, 29, **29**
    arsenical, 30
    bowenoid, 28, **29**, 34
    hypertrophic, 28, **29**
    lichenoid, 30, **30**
    spreading pigmented, 28
Actinic reticuloid, 463
Adenoid cystic carcinoma, 155, **155-157**
Adenosquamous carcinoma, 44, **45**
Adnexal carcinoma with mixed differentiation, 98, 177, **178**
Adult T-cell leukemia/lymphoma, 448
    clinical features, 448
    differential diagnosis, 450
    genetics, 450
    human T lymphotrophic virus association, 448
    immunohistology, 450
    pathologic findings, 449, **449**, **450**
Alopecia mucinosa, 457
Anaplastic large cell lymphoma (ALCL), 469, **469-472**
    giant cell ALCL, 470
    lymphohistiocytic ALCL, 470
    signet ring cell ALCL, 470
    small cell ALCL, 470
Anaplastic syringoma, see Microcystic adnexal carcinoma
Aneurysmal fibrous histiocytoma, 220, **222**
Angioblastoma of Nakagawa, 283
Angioendotheliomatosis, 291
Angiofibroma, 223, **226**
    angiofibroma of tuberous sclerosis, 223
    digital fibrokeratoma, 223, **225**
    familial myxovascular fibroma, 223
    fibrous papule of the face, 223, **224**
    pearly penile papule, 223, **225**
Angiofollicular lymph node hyperplasia, see Castleman's disease
Angiohistiocytoma, 288, **289**
Angioimmunoblastic lymphadenopathy, see Angioimmunoblastic T-cell lymphoma, 475
Angioimmunoblastic T-cell lymphoma, 475, **476**
    Epstein-Barr virus association, 477
Angiokeratoma, 291, **292**, **293**
Angioleiomyoma, 366, **368**
    epithelioid, 368
Angiolipoleiomyoma, see Angiomyolipoma
Angiolipoma, 351, **351**
    cellular angiolipoma, 351, **352**
Angiolymphoid hyperplasia with eosinophilia, 284, **286**
Angiomatosis, 291
Angiomyofibroblastoma, 249, **251**
Angiomyolipoma, 369, **369**
Angiomyxomas, 249
    aggressive angiomyxoma, 249, **250**
    superficial angiomyxoma, 249, **250**
Angiosarcoma, 304, **305**, **306**, 347
    epithelioid, 308, **308**, **310**
    granular cell, 307, **308**
    lesions that mimic, 313
    minimal deviation type, 307, **308**
    pleomorphic, 307, **309**
    spindle cell, 307, **307**
Apocrine carcinomas, 168
    ductal apocrine adenocarcinoma, 172, **173**, **174**
    ductopapillary apocrine adenocarcinoma, 172
    ductopapillary apocrine carcinoma, 169, **169**, **170**
    Paget's disease, 170, see also Paget's disease
    signet ring cell adenocarcinoma, 174, **175**
Apocrine hidradenoma, 149

*Numbers in boldface indicate table and figure pages.

Apocrine hidrocystoma, 185, **187**
Aprocrine nevus, 184
Arteriovenous hemangioma, 285
Atypical fibroxanthoma, 222, 253, **254**, **255**
    angiomatoid, 254
    clear cell, 254
    myxoid, 254
    spindle cell, 254
    with osteoclast-like giant cells, 254, **255**
Atypical follicular lymphoid hyperplasia, 440

B

B-cell lymphomas, 435, *see individual lymphoma types*
Bacillary angiomatosis, 310, **312**
Bannayan's syndrome, 279
Basal cell carcinoma, 30, 46, **48-55**, 81, 87, 121, 130, 156
    adamantinoid basal cell carcinoma, 53
    adenoid basal cell carcinoma, 50, **50**
    and squamous cell carcinoma, 40
    associated syndromes, 48
    basosebaceous basal cell carcinoma, 51, **51**
    basosquamous basal cell carcinoma, 52, **53**
    carcinosarcomatous basal cell carcinoma, 53
    clear cell basal cell carcinoma, 53, **54**
    clinical features, 46
    differential diagnosis, 55
    fibroepithelioma of Pinkus, 49, **50**
    granular cell basal cell carcinoma, 53
    infiltrative basal cell carcinoma, 52, **52**
    keratotic basal cell carcinoma, 50, **51**
    linear basal cell nevus, 48
    metatypical basal cell carcinoma, 52, **53**
    micronodular basal cell carcinoma, 54
    morpheaform basal cell carcinoma, 51, **52**
    nodulocystic basal cell carcinoma, 48, **48**, **49**
    pathologic findings, 48
    superficial basal cell carcinoma, 48, **48**
    with sebaceous differentiation, 121, 124, **124-126**
Basal cell hamartoma with follicular differentiation, *see* Tumor of the follicular infundibulum
Basaloid follicular hamartoma, 86, **87**, 89, 100
Basosebaceous carcinoma, *see* Basal cell carcinoma with sebaceous differentiation
Becker's nevus, 216
    and smooth muscle hamartoma, 365
Bednar's tumor, 247, **247**

Benign cephalic histiocytosis, 392
Benign proliferating pilar tumor, 5, **5**, 75, **75-77**
Benign trichogenic tumor, *see* Trichoblastoma
Birt-Hogg-Dube syndrome and trichodiscoma, 89
Blastic NK-cell lymphoma, 480, **481**
Blue nevus, 332
Blueberry muffin lesion, 486
Borrelia infection
    and large B-cell lymphoma, 440
    and lymphocytoma cutis, 433
    and marginal zone B-cell lymphoma, 436
Borst-Jadassohn phenomenon, 21, 24, 33, **34**
Bowen's disease, 24, 25, 32, **33-35**
Bowenoid papulosis, 36, **37**
Branchial cleft cyst, 2, 10, **12**
Bronchogenic cyst, 10, **11**
Brooke-Fordyce syndrome, 79
Burkitt's lymphoma, 446, **448**
    Epstein-Barr virus association, 447
    human immunodeficiency virus association, 446
Buschke-Ollendorff syndrome, 216

C

Calcifying aponeurotic fibroma, 379, **380**
Calcifying epithelioma of Malherbe, *see* Pilomatricoma
Capillary hemangioma, 279, **280**
    cellular, 280, **281**
    lobular, 281, **281**, **282**, 285
Carcinoma ex dermal cylindroma, 162, **162**, **163**
Carcinoma ex eccrine spiradenoma, 162, **163**, **164**
Carcinosarcoma, 45, **45**
Castleman's disease, 419, **420**, **421**
Cavernous hemangioma, 279, **280**
Cellular angiolipoma, 351, **352**
Cellular capillary hemangioma, 280, **281**
Cellular schwannoma, 335
Chondroid lipoma, 352
Chondroid syringoma, *see* Cutaneous mixed tumor
Chondroma
    extraskeletal chondroma, 375, **375**, **376**
    extraskeletal with lipoblast-like cells, 375
    periosteal chondroma, 375
Chondrosarcoma, 377
    mesenchymal chondrosarcoma, 377
    myxoid chondrosarcoma, 377, **378**
Chordoma, 377
Ciliated cyst, cutaneous, 8, 10, **11**

Clear cell acanthoma, 25, **25**
Clear cell eccrine carcinoma, 167, **168**
Clear cell papulosis, 26, **26**
Collagenous fibroma, 229
Congenital fibromatosis, *see* Myofibroma
Congenital midline hamartoma, *see* Rhabdomyomatous mesenchymal hamartoma
Congenital self-healing reticulohistiocytosis, *see* Reticulohistiocytosis
Congenital vellus hamartoma, *see* Hair follicle nevus
Connective tissue nevus, 216, **216**, **217**
    Buschke-Ollendorff syndrome, 216
    nevus anelasticus, 216
    nevus elasticus, 216
    papular elastorrhexis, 216
Contact dermatitis, 463
Cowden's disease, 23
Cranial fasciitis, 241, **242**
Cutaneous apudoma, *see* Primary neuroendocrine carcinoma
Cutaneous fibrous histiocytoma, *see* Dermatofibroma
Cutaneous keratocyst, 3
Cutaneous leiomyoma, 222
Cutaneous lymphoid hyperplasia, *see* Lymphocytoma cutis
Cutaneous mastocytosis, *see* Mastocytosis, cutaneous
Cutaneous mixed tumor, 149, **150**, **151**
Cutaneous telangiectasia, 277
    and Osler-Weber-Rendu syndrome, 277
Cysts, *see* Epithelial cysts
Cytophagic histiocytic panniculitis, 454, **455**

D

Dabska's tumor, *see* Papillary endovascular angioendothelioma
Darier's disease, 19, 30
Dendritic fibromyxolipoma, 351
Dermal duct tumor, 141, **142**
Dermal epithelioid nevus, 223, 332, 337, 392
Dermal nerve sheath myxoma, 335, **336**
Dermatofibroma, 218, **218-221**, 239, 244, 246, 368
    aneurysmal fibrous histiocytoma, 220, **222**
    cellular dermatofibroma, 220, **221**
    deep penetrating dermatofibroma, 219, **219**
    epithelioid cell histiocytoma, 220, **221**
    granular cell dermatofibroma, 221
    lipidized dermatofibroma, 219, **220**, 391
Dermatofibrosarcoma protuberans, 222, 244
    clinical features, 244
    differential diagnosis, 246
    fibrosarcomatous with giant rosettes, 245
    giant cell fibroblastoma, 248
    pathologic findings, 244, **245**, **246**
    pigmented (Bednar's tumor), 247, **257**
Dermatomyofibroma, 223, **223**
Dermatosis papulosa nigra, 20, **21**
Dermoid cyst, 7, **7**
Desmoid tumor, abdominal/extra-abdominal, 237
Desmoplastic fibroblastoma, *see* Collagenous fibroma
Desmoplastic trichoepithelioma, 81, **82**, **83**
Digital fibrokeratoma, 223, **225**
Disseminated superficial actinic porokeratosis, 31
Ductal apocrine adenocarcinoma, 172, **173**, **174**
Ductal eccrine adenocarcinoma, 164, **164-167**
    small cell type, 165, **166**
    with fibromyxoid stroma, 164, **166**
    with sarcomatoid change, 165, **167**
Ductopapillary apocrine adenocarcinoma, 172
Ductopapillary apocrine carcinoma, 169, **169**, **170**
Dutcher bodies, 418, 435, 437

E

Ecchondroma, 375
Eccrine acrospiroma, 143, **145-147**
Eccrine angiomatous hamartoma, 184, **185**
Eccrine carcinomas, 152
    adenoid cystic carcinoma, 155, **155-157**
    carcinoma ex dermal cylindroma, 162, **162**, **163**
    carcinoma ex eccrine spiradenoma, 162, **163**, **164**
    clear cell eccrine carcinoma, 167, **167**, **168**
    ductal eccrine adenocarcinoma, 164, *see also* Ductal eccrine adenocarcinoma
    malignant mixed tumor, 168, **169**
    microcystic adnexal carcinoma, 158, **159-161**
    mucinous eccrine carcinoma, 153, **154**, **155**
    mucoepidermoid carcinoma, 161, **162**
    papillary digital eccrine adenocarcinoma, 157, **157-159**
    porocarcinoma, 152, **152-154**
Eccrine cylindroma, 137, **138**, **139**
Eccrine hydrocystoma, 185, **186**
Eccrine nevus, 183, 183
Eccrine porocarcinoma, 152, **152-154**

Eccrine poroma, 139, **142**, **143**
  dermal duct tumor, 141, **142**
  hidroacanthoma simplex, 141, **142**
Eccrine spiradenoma, 138, **139**, **140**
Eccrine syringofibroadenoma, 141, **144**
Elastofibroma dorsi, 233, **234**
Enchondroma, 375
Endometriosis, 9, **9**
Endosalpingiosis, 10
Eosinophilic granuloma, 402
Epidermal cyst, 1, **1**, **2**
Epidermal nevus, 14, **14-16**, 19
  acantholytic dyskeratotic epidermal nevus, 15
  connective tissue nevus, association with, 216
  ichthyosis hystrix, 14
  inflammatory linear verrucous epidermal nevus, 14, **16**
  nevoid hyperkeratosis of nipple, 14, **16**
  nevus comedonicus, 1, 14, **16**
  nevus unius lateris, 14
Epidermolytic acanthoma, 17, **18**
Epidermolytic hyperkeratosis, 17
Epithelial cysts, 1
  branchial cleft cyst, 10, **12**
  bronchogenic cyst, 10, **11**
  ciliated cysts, cutaneous, 8, 10, **11**
  cutaneous keratocyst, 3
  dermoid cyst, 7, **7**
  epidermal cyst, 1, **1**, **2**
  epithelial cyst and Gardner's syndrome, 3, **4**
  eruptive vellus hair cyst, 8, **8**
  human papillomavirus-associated cyst, 2
  median raphe cyst, 12, **13**
  metaplastic synovial cyst, 11, **13**
  milium, 1
  mucinous/ciliated vulvar cyst, 10, **10**
  omphalomesenteric duct polyp, 13, **14**
  pigmented follicular cyst, 3, **3**
  proliferating epidermal cyst, 2, **3**
  proliferating trichilemmal cyst, 5, **5**, *see also* Benign proliferating pilar tumor
  steatocystoma, 6, **6**, 101, **101**
  thymic cyst, 10
  thyroglossal duct cyst, 10, **12**
  trichilemmal cyst, 2, 4, **4**, **5**
Epithelioid cell histiocytoma, 220, **221**
Epithelioid hemangioendothelioma, 294, **295**
Epithelioid hemangioma, 283, **286**

Epithelioid malignant peripheral nerve sheath tumor, 344, **344**
Epithelioid sarcoma, 256, **257**
Epithelioma adenoides cysticum syndrome, and trichoepithelioma, 79, **79**
Epithelioma cuniculatum, 40
Epithelioma, superficial, with sebaceous differentiation, 122, **123**
Epstein-Barr virus
  and angioimmunoblastic T-cell lymphoma, 477
  and Burkitt's lymphoma, 447
  and diffuse large B-cell lymphoma, 440
  and Hodgkin's disease, 481
  and intravascular large B-cell lymphoma, 443
  and lymphomatoid granulomatosis, 444
Epulis gravidarum, 283
Eruptive keratoacanthoma of Grzybowski, 42
Eruptive vellus hair cyst, 8, **8**, 101, **102**
Erythroplasia of Queyrat, 35, **36**
Exostosis, subungual, 376
Extramedullary hematopoiesis, 486, **487**
Extraosseous plasmacytoma, 416, **417**
Extraskeletal chondroma, 375, **375**, **376**
Extraskeletal osteosarcoma, *see* Osteosarcoma, extraskeletal

F

Familial histiocytic dermatoarthritis, 399
Familial myxovascular fibroma, 223
Favre-Racouchot syndrome, 1
Fibroepithelial polyps, 215, **215**
  resemblance to dermatosis papulosa nigra, 20
Fibroepithelioma of Pinkus, 49, **50**
Fibrofolliculoma, 90, **91**
Fibrohistiocytic lipoma, 352, **352**
Fibroma of tendon sheath, 236, **237**
Fibromatosis, 237, **238**
  abdominal/extra-abdominal desmoid tumor, 237
  knuckle pads, 237
  palmar fibromatosis, 237, **238**
  penile fibromatosis, 237
  plantar fibromatosis, 237
Fibromyxoid sarcoma, low-grade, 252, **252**
Fibro-osseous pseudotumor of the digits, 378
Fibrosarcoma, 238, 242, 258, **258**
Fibrous hamartoma of infancy, 217, **217**
Fibrous papule of face, 223, **224**
Flegel's disease, 23

Follicular center cell lymphoma, *see* Follicular lymphoma
Follicular lymphoma, 438, **438**, **439**
Follicular mucinosis, 457
Follicular myxoma, 91, **92**
Folliculosebaceous cystic hamartoma, 78

G

Ganglion cell choristoma, *see* Ganglioneuroma
Ganglioneuroma, 329, **330**
Gardner's syndrome, 1
    and epithelial cysts, 3, **4**
    and pilomatricoma, 83
Generalized eruptive histiocytoma, 394
Giant cell epulis, *see* Peripheral giant cell granuloma
Giant cell fibroblastoma, 248, **248**, **249**
Giant cell tumor of tendon sheath, 234, **235**
    malignant giant cell tumor, 235
Giant hair matrix tumor, *see* Malignant proliferating pilar tumor
Giant lymph node hyperplasia, *see* Castleman's disease
Giant vascular spiradenoma, 138
Glandular lipoma, 349
Glial heterotopia, 347, **347**, **348**
Glomeruloid hemangioma, 291, **291**
Granular cell tumor, 337, **338**, **339**
    malignant granular cell tumor, 345
Granulocytic sarcoma, 475
Granulomatous slack skin, 465, **466**
Grover's disease, 19

H

Hair follicle neoplasms, 71
Hair follicle nevus, 99, **100**
Hand-Schuller-Christian disease, 402
Hemangiomas, 279, 347
    acquired elastotic hemangioma, 289, **290**
    acquired tufted angioma, 283, **283**, **284**
    acral arteriovenous tumor (venous/arteriovenous hemangioma), 285, **286**, **287**
    angioblastoma of Nakagawa, 283
    capillary hemangioma, 279, **280**
    cavernous hemangioma, 279, **280**
    cellular capillary hemangioma, 280, **281**
    epithelioid hemangioma, 283, **286**
    epulis gravidarum, 283
    glomeruloid hemangioma, 291, **291**
    hobnail (targetoid) hemangioma, 287, **287**, **288**
    infantile hemangioendothelioma, 280
    infiltrating hemangioma, 291, **292**
    lobular capillary hemangioma, 281, **281**, **282**, **285**
    microvenular hemangioma, 289, **290**
    sinusoidal hemangioma, 290
    verrucous hemangioma, 291, **291**
Hemangioendotheliomas, 294
    composite hemangioendothelioma, 299
    epithelioid hemangioendothelioma, 294, **295**
    epithelioid sarcoma-like hemangioendothelioma, 299, **300**
    kaposiform hemangioendothelioma, 297, **298**
    retiform hemangioendothelioma, 298, **298**
    spindle cell hemangioendothelioma, 296, **296**, **297**
Hemangiopericytoma, 244
Hematopoiesis, *see* Extramedullary hematopoiesis
Herpesvirus, human
    and hobnail hemangioma, 287
    and Kaposi's sarcoma, 301
    and reactive angioendotheliomatosis, 315
    and retiform hemangioendothelioma, 298
Hibernoma, 353, **353**, **354**
Hidradenoma papilliferum, 148, **148**, **149**
Hidroacanthoma simplex, 141, **142**
    differentiation from nested seborrheic keratosis, 24
Histiocytic lymphoma, 401
Histiocytic medullary reticulosis, *see* Malignant histiocytosis
Histiocytic sarcoma, 401
Histiocytoid hemangioma, *see* Epithelioid hemangioma
Histiocytosis X, *see* Langerhans cell histiocytosis
Hobnail (targetoid) hemangioma, 287, **287**, **288**
Hodgkin's disease, 442, 445, 471, 480
    clinical features, 481
    Epstein-Barr virus association, 481
    general features, 480
    pathologic findings, 482, **482**
    primary cutaneous, 481
Human immunodeficiency virus
    and Burkitt's lymphoma, 446
    and lymphocytoma cutis, 433
Human papilloma virus, 2
    and basal cell carcinoma, 47

and Bowen's disease, 33
and bowenoid papulosis, 36
and erythroplasia of Queyrat, 36
and seborrheic keratosis, 23
and verrucous carcinoma, 41
associated cyst, 2
Human papilloma virus-associated cyst, 2
Human T-cell lymphotrophic virus and adult T-cell leukemia/lymphoma, 448
Hyalinizing spindle cell tumor with giant rosettes, 246, 252
Hypertrophic actinic keratosis, 24

I

Ichthyosis hystrix, 14
Immunocytoma, lymphoplasmacytic type, 418, 435
Indeterminate cell histiocytosis, 404
Infantile digital fibroma, 238, **239**
Infantile digital myofibroblastoma, 238
Infantile hemangioendothelioma, 280
Infantile systemic hyalinosis, 240
Infiltrating hemangioma, 291, **292**
Inflammatory pseudotumor, 230, **232**
Infundibuloma, see Tumor of the follicular infundibulum
Intravascular fasciitis, 241, 242
Intravascular large B-cell lymphoma, 442, **443**
Isthmus-catagen cyst, 4, see also Trichilemmal cyst
Inverted follicular keratosis, 20, 21, 23

J

Jadassohn's nevus, see Nevus sebaceous
Juvenile hyaline fibromatosis, 240, **241**
Juvenile xanthogranuloma, 389, **390-392**, 396, 398, 404
and neurofibromatosis/chronic myelogenous leukemia, 389
and neurofibromatosis type 2, 389

K

Kaposi's sarcoma, 300, 309
African type, 300, **301**
AIDS-related, 300, **301**
associated with immunosuppression, 300
classic type, 300, **300**
clinical features, 300
differential diagnosis, 304, **305**
lesions that mimic, 309
pathologic findings, 301, **302-304**
Kaposiform hemangioendothelioma, 297, **298**
Kasabach-Merritt syndrome, 279
Keloid, 231, **233**
acne keloidalis, 232
Keratoacanthoma, 42, **43**
eruptive keratoacanthoma of Grzybowski, 42
keratoacanthoma centrifugum marginatum, 42
multiple self-healing epithelioma of Ferguson-Smith, 42
Keratoacanthoma centrifugum marginatum, 42
Keratocyst, 3
Ketron-Goodman disease, 464
Kimura's disease, 283, **285**, **286**
Kimura's tumor, see Kimura's disease
Klippel-Trenaunay-Weber syndrome, 277
Knuckle pads, 237

L

Langerhans cell histiocytosis, 391, 396, 398, 402, **403**, 429
eosinophilic granuloma, 402
Hand-Schuller-Christian disease, 402
Letterer-Siwe disease, 402
Langerhans cell sarcoma, 402
Large B-cell lymphoma, diffuse, 440, **441**
Borrelia infection association, 440
Epstein-Barr virus association, 440
of the leg, 440
T-cell-rich B-cell lymphoma, 440
Large B-cell lymphoma, intravascular, 442, **443**
Epstein-Barr virus association, 443
Large cell acanthoma, 24, **25**, 30
Ledderhose's disease, see Plantar fibromatosis
Leiomyoma, 239, 335, 366
angioleiomyoma, 366, **368**
epithelioid angioleiomyoma, 368
leiomyoma of nipple, areola, or genital region, 366
piloleiomyoma, 366, **367**
symplastic leiomyoma, 368
Leiomyosarcoma, 369, 370, **371**
dermal, 370
epithelioid, 370
granular cell, 370
subcutaneous, 370
Lennert's lymphoma, 474
Lentigo maligna, 30

Lethal midline granuloma, *see* NK/T-cell sinonasal-type lymphoma
Letterer-Siwe disease, 402
Leukemia cutis, 483, **485**, **486**
    aleukemic leukemia cutis, 484
Linear basal cell nevus, 48, 100
Lipedema, tumefactive localized, 355, **355**
Lipoblastoma, 353
Lipoid proteinosis, 241
Lipoma, 348, **348**, **349**
    angiolipoma, 351, **351**
        cellular angiolipoma, 351, **352**
    chondroid lipoma, 352
    dendritic fibromyxolipoma, 351
    fibrohistiocytic lipoma, 352, **352**
    glandular lipoma, 349
    metaplastic lipoma, 352
    pleomorphic/atypical lipoma, 350, **350**
    sclerotic lipoma, 228, 351
    spindle cell lipoma, 244, 349, **349**, **350**
Lipomembranous (membranocystic) lesion, 454
Liposarcoma, 353
Lobular capillary hemangioma, 281, **281**, **282**, **285**
Lobular infundibuloisthmicoma, *see* Pilar sheath acanthoma
Localized epidermotropic reticulosis, *see* Pagetoid reticulosis
Localized nodular tenosynovitis, *see* Giant cell tumor of tendon sheath
Lupus erythematosus, 30
Lymphadenosis benigna cutis, *see* Lymphocytoma cutis
Lymphangioma, 278, **278**, **279**
   deep lymphangioma, 278, **278**
   lymphangioma superficialis circumscriptum, 278, **279**
Lymphangioendothelioma, benign, 287, **288**, **304**
Lymphocytoma cutis, 432, 437, 442
   Borrelia infection association, 433
   clinical features, 432
   differential diagnosis, 434
   human immunodeficiency virus association, 433
   pathologic findings, 433, **433**, **434**
Lymphoepithelioma-like carcinoma, 46, **46**, 98, 175, **176**
Lymphoid infiltrates, 431
Lymphoma, 46, 431, 435, *see also individual lymphoma types*
   classifications schemes, 431, **432**
Lymphomatoid granulomatosis, 444, **445**
   Epstein-Barr virus association, 444
Lymphomatoid papulosis, 477, **478**, **479**
   and Hodgkin's disease, 483
   association with pityriasis lichenoides et varioliformis acuta, 477

M

Macroglobulinemia of Waldenström, 417, **418**, **419**
   immunocytoma, lymphoplasmacytic type, 418, 435
   storage papules, 418
Maffucci's syndrome, 277, 279, 296
   and hemangiomas, 279
   and spindle cell hemangioendothelioma, 296, **296**
Malignant angioendotheliomatosis, *see* Large B-cell lymphoma, intravascular
Malignant fibrous histiocytoma, 242, 255, **256**
Malignant giant cell tumor, 235
Malignant granular cell tumor, 345
Malignant histiocytosis, 401, **401**
Malignant mixed tumor, 168, **169**
Malignant peripheral nerve sheath tumor (MPNST), 332, 337, 341, **341-345**
   and von Recklinghausen's disease, 341
   epithelioid MPNST, 344, **344**
   glandular MPNST, 342
   malignant MPNST, 342
   malignant triton tumor, 342
Malignant pilar tumor, *see* Malignant proliferating pilar tumor
Malignant proliferating pilar tumor, 5, 95, **96**, **97**
Malignant rhabdoid tumor, 374, **374**
Malignant trichilemmal cyst, *see* Malignant proliferating pilar tumor
Malignant triton tumor, 342
Mantle cell lymphoma, 446, **447**
Marginal zone B-cell lymphoma, 435, 440
   Borrelia infection association, 436
   clinical features, 436
   differential diagnosis, 437
   pathologic findings, 436, **436**, **437**
Masson's vegetant intravascular hemangioendothelioma, 313
Mastocytoma, 392
Mastocytosis, 425, **427**, **428**
   cutaneous, 426
      fibrous mastocytosis, 426

telangiectasia macularis eruptiva perstans, 426, **426**, **428**
World Health Organization classification, 425, **425**
Median raphe cyst, 12, **13**
Melanoacanthoma, 22, **23**
Melanocytic nevus, 332
Melanoma, 171, 255, 371
   spindle cell melanoma, 343, **344**
Meningoceles, 314, **315**
   rudimentary meningocele, 345, **346**, **347**
Meningotheliomatous hamartoma, 346
Merkel cell carcinoma, 46, 177, **179-182**, 340
Mesenchymal chondrosarcoma, 377
Metaplastic carcinoma, 45
Metaplastic lipoma, 352
Metaplastic synovial cyst, 11, **13**
Metastatic neoplasms to skin, 201
   clinical features, 201, **202-204**
   immunohistochemistry, 209, **210**
   pathologic findings, 203, **204**
   visceral sources, 204
     breast, 207, **208**
     gastrointestinal, 206, **206**, **207**
     kidney, 205
     lung, 204, **205**
     ovarian, 206, **207**, **208**
     salivary gland, 208
Michelin tire baby syndrome
   and nevus lipomatosus, 354
   and smooth muscle hamartoma, 365
Microcystic adnexal carcinoma, 158, **159-161**
Microvenular hemangioma, 289, **290**
Milium, 1
Monsel's solution reaction, 310, **311**
Mucha-Habermann disease, 477
Mucinous/ciliated vulvar cyst, 10, **10**
Mucinous eccrine carcinoma, 153, **154**, **155**
Mucoepidermoid carcinoma, 161, **162**
Mucosa-associated lymphoid tissue (MALT) lymphoma, *see* Marginal zone B-cell lymphoma
Muir-Torre syndrome
   and sebaceoma, 123
   and sebaceous adenoma, 120
Multiple myeloma, 415, **416**
   myeloma with plasmablastic morphology, 415
   nonsecretory myeloma, 415
   plasma cell leukemia, 415
Multiple self-healing epithelioma of Ferguson-Smith, 42
Mycosis fungoides, 456, 464
   clinical features, 456
   etiology, 458
   follicular mucinosis association, 457
   pathologic findings, 458, **459-461**
   precursor lesions, 456
     parapsoriasis en plaque, 456, **459**
     parapsoriasis variegata, 456
   Sézary's syndrome association, 457
   syringotropic mycosis fungoides, 457
Myoepithelioma, 151, **151**
Myofibroma, 238, **240**, 244
Myositis ossificans, 378
Myxoid chondrosarcoma, 377, **378**

N

NAME syndrome, and follicular myxoma, 91
Nasal glioma, *see* Glial heterotopia
Neurilemmoma, 333, **333-335**, 368
   ancient neurilemmoma, 333, **334**
   and von Recklinghausen's disease, 333
   cellular schwannoma, 335
   epithelioid neurilemmoma, 335
   glandular neurilemmoma, 334
   melanotic neurilemmoma, 334, **335**
   plexiform neurilemmoma, 334
   psammomatous-melanotic neurilemmoma, 335
Neurofibroma, 330, **330-333**, 368
   and von Recklinghausen's disease, 330, **331**
   dendritic cell neurofibroma with pseudorosettes, 331
   plexiform neurofibroma, 332, **332**
Neurofollicular hamartoma, 102
Neuroma, 329, **330**
   palisading/encapsulated neuroma, 329
   post-traumatic neuroma, 329
Neurothekeoma, 240, 335, **336**, **337**
   and dermal nerve sheath myxoma, 335, **336**
Nevoid hyperkeratosis of nipple, 14, **16**
Nevus anelasticus, 216
Nevus araneus, 277
Nevus comedonicus, 1, 14, **16**
Nevus elasticus, 216
Nevus, epidermal, *see* Epidermal nevus
Nevus, epidermal, 14, **14-16**, 19
   acantholytic dyskeratotic epidermal nevus, 15
   connective tissue nevus, association with, 216

ichthyosis hystrix, 14
inflammatory linear verrucous epidermal nevus, 14, **16**
nevoid hyperkeratosis of nipple, 14, **16**
nevus comedonicus, 1, 14, **16**
nevus unius lateris, 14
Nevus flammeus, 277, **277**, **278**
Nevus lipomatosus, 353, **354**
and Michelin tire baby syndrome, 354
Nevus sebaceus, 117, **119**, **120**
Nevus unius lateris, 14
NK/T-cell lymphoma, nasal type, 451, **452**, **453**, 456
NK/T-cell sinonasal-type lymphoma, 451
Nodular hidradenoma, see Eccrine acrospiroma
Nodular fasciitis, 241, **242**
cranial fasciitis, 241, **242**
Nodular small cleaved cell lymphoma, see Follicular lymphoma
Non-Hodgkin's lymphoma, 440, 442, 446, 451, 456
Non-Langerhans cell histiocytic proliferations, 389

O

Omphalomesenteric duct polyp, 13, **14**
Organoid nevus, see Nevus sebaceous
Osler-Weber-Rendu syndrome, 277, 279
Ossifying fibromyxoid tumor, 377, **379**
Osteochondroma, subungual, 376
Osteosarcoma, extraskeletal, 379, 380, **380**

P

Paget's disease, 26, 35, 170, **171-173**
extramammary Paget's disease, 170
and sebaceous carcinoma, 128
mammary Paget's disease, 170
Pagetoid reticulosis, 464, **465**
Ketron-Goodman disease, 464
Woringer-Kolopp disease, 464
Pale cell acanthoma, 25, see Clear cell acanthoma
Palmar fibromatosis, 237
Panniculitis-like T-cell lymphoma, subcutaneous, see Subcutaneous panniculitis-like T-cell lymphoma
Papillary digital eccrine adenocarcinoma, 157, **157-159**
Papillary eccrine adenoma, 143, **144**, **145**
Papillary endovascular angioendothelioma, 292, **293**, **294**
Papillary intravascular endothelial hyperplasia, 313, **314**
Papillomatosis, confluent and reticulated, of Gougerot and Carteaud, 16, 17
Papular elastorrhexis, 216
Parachordoma, 376
Parapsoriasis en plaque, see Mycosis fungoides
Parapsoriasis variegata, see Mycosis fungoides
Pautrier's microabscess
and mycosis fungoides, 463
and Sézary's syndrome, 467
Pearly penile papule, 223, **225**
Penile fibromatosis, 237
Perifollicular fibroma, 89, **90**
Perineurioma, 333
subungual, 227
Periosteal chondroma, 375
Peripheral giant cell granuloma, 235, **236**
Peripheral neuroepithelioma/primitive neuroectodermal tumor, 339, **340**, **341**
Peripheral T-cell lymphoma, not further specified, 472, **473**, **474**
Pigmented follicular cyst, 3, **3**
Pigmented villonodular synovitis, 234
Pilar cyst, see Trichilemmal cyst
Pilar leiomyoma, 91, **93**
Pilar leiomyosarcoma, 98
Pilar neurocristic hamartoma, 102, **102**, **103**
Pilar sheath acanthoma, 72, **72**
Pilar tumor, see Benign proliferating pilar tumor
Piloleiomyoma, 366, **367**
Pilomatricoma, 82, **83-85**
Pilomatrix carcinoma, 97, **98**
Pilomatrixoma, see Pilomatricoma
Pityriasis lichenoides et varioliformis acuta, 477, 480
Plantar fibromatosis, 237
Plasma cell leukemia, 415
Pleomorphic fibroma, 227, **228**
Pleomorphic/atypical lipoma, 350, **350**
Plexiform fibrohistiocytic tumor, 226, **226**
POEMS syndrome
and Castleman's disease, 420
and glomeruloid hemangioma, 291
Polyp, omphalomesenteric duct, 13, **14**
Porokeratosis, 31, **32**
and squamous cell carcinoma, 32, **32**
disseminated superficial actinic porokeratosis, 31
porokeratosis of Mibelli, 31
porokeratosis palmaris, plantaris et disseminata, 31

punctate porokeratosis, 31
Poroma, see Eccrine poroma
Port wine stain, see Nevus flammeus
Postirradiation lymphangioma-like papule, 316, **317**
Postoperative spindle cell nodule, 230
Precursor B-cell lymphoblastic lymphoma, 445, **446**
Primitive neuroectodermal tumor/extraskeletal Ewing's sarcoma, 332, 339, **340, 341**
Progressive nodular histiocytosis, 393
Proliferating epidermal cyst, 2, **3**
Proliferating pilar tumor
    benign, see Benign proliferating pilar tumor
    malignant, see Malignant proliferating pilar tumor
Proliferating scar, 310
Proliferating trichilemmal cyst, see Benign proliferating pilar tumor
Proliferating trichilemmal tumor, see Benign proliferating pilar tumor
Proliferative fasciitis, 241, **242**
Proliferative myositis, 241, **242**
Pseudoepitheliomatous hyperplasia, 26, **27**
Pseudolymphoma, see Lymphocytoma cutis
Pseudosarcomatous fibromyxoid tumor, 231
PUVA keratosis, 27
Pyogenic granuloma, 281

R

Reactive angioendotheliomatosis, 314, **315**, 316, 442
Reactive lymphoid infiltrate, see Lymphocytoma cutis
Reticulohistiocytoma, 396, **397, 398**
Reticulohistiocytosis, 396
    congenital self-healing reticulohistiocytosis, 404, **405**
    multicentric reticulohistiocytosis, 396, **399**
    reticulohistiocytoma, 396, **397, 398**
Retiform hemangioendothelioma, 298, **299**
Rhabdomyomatous mesenchymal hamartoma, 372, **372**
Rhabdomyosarcoma, 373
    alveolar, 373, **373**
    embryonal, 373, **373**
    pleomorphic, 373
Rosai-Dorfman disease, 399, **400**

S

Sarcomatoid carcinoma, 45

Schwannoma, see Neurilemmoma
Sclerosing epithelial hamartoma, see Desmoplastic trichoepithelioma
Sclerosing sweat duct carcinoma, 160, see also Microcystic adnexal carcinoma
Sclerotic fibroma, 228, **229**
Sclerotic lipoma, 228, 351
Sebaceoma, 123
Sebaceous adenoma, 119, **121, 122**
    and Muir-Torre syndrome, 120
    poorly differentiated, 123
Sebaceous carcinoma, 126
    basaloid sebaceous carcinoma, 129, **130**
    clinical features, 126, **126, 127**
    differential diagnosis, 130
    grading, 128
    pagetoid sebaceous carcinoma, 128, **129**
    pathologic findings, 127, **127-130**
    sarcomatoid sebaceous carcinoma, 129, **130**
    squamoid sebaceous carcinoma, 129
Sebaceous epithelioma, see Basal cell carcinoma with sebaceous differentiation
Sebaceous hyperplasia, 117, **117, 118**
Sebocrine adenoma, 121
Sebomatricoma, 121, 124
Seborrheic keratosis, 17, 19, **20-23**, 30, **34**
    acanthotic seborrheic keratosis, 20, **20**
    dermatosis papulosa nigra, 20, **21**
    hyperkeratotic seborrheic keratosis, 20, **20**
    inverted follicular keratosis, 21
    irritated seborrheic keratosis, 21, **22**
    melanoacanthoma, 22, **23**
    nested seborrheic keratosis, 21, **23**
    reticulated seborrheic keratosis, 20, **21**
    stucco keratoses, 20
Sézary's syndrome, **466, 467**
    and mycosis fungoides, 462
Signet ring cell adenocarcinoma, 174, **175**
Sinus histiocytosis with massive lymphadenopathy, see Rosai-Dorfman disease
Sinusoidal hemangioma, 290
Skin tag, see Fibroepithelial polyp
Smooth muscle hamartoma, 365, **366**
    and Becker's nevus, 365
    and Michelin tire baby syndrome, 365
Soft fibroma, 215, **216**
Solar keratosis, see Actinic keratosis
Solar lentigo, 30

Solid and cystic hidradenoma, *see* Eccrine acrospiroma
Solitary fibrous tumor, 243, **243**
Spider angioma, 277
Spindle cell angiosarcoma, 304
Spindle cell hemangioendothelioma/hemangioma, 296, **296, 297**
Spindle cell lipoma, 244, 349, **349, 350**
Spindle cell xanthogranuloma, 394
Spitz's nevus, *see* Dermal epithelioid nevus
Squamous cell carcinoma, 7, 24, 27, 37, **38, 39**, 44, 171, 442
   acantholytic squamous cell carcinoma, 38
   adenoid squamous cell carcinoma, 38
   and basal cell carcinoma, 40
   and porokeratosis, 32, **32**
   angiosarcoma-like squamous cell carcinoma, 309, **309**
   desmoplastic squamous cell carcinoma, 39, **39**
   differential diagnosis, 40
   in situ, *see* Bowen's disease
   pathologic findings, 37
   pseudoglandular squamous cell carcinoma, 38, **38**
   pseudovascular adenoid squamous cell carcinoma, 38
   signet ring cell squamous cell carcinoma, 39
   small cell (basaloid) squamous cell carcinoma, 56
   spindle cell squamous cell carcinoma, 39, **39**, 255
Steatocystoma, 6, **6**, 101, **101**
   multiplex, 6, 101, **101**
   simplex, 101
Steinert's syndrome,
   and pilomatricoma, 83
Stewart-Treves syndrome
   and angiosarcoma, 304
Storage papules, 418
Stork bite, *see* Nevus flammeus
Striated muscle hamartoma, *see* Rhabdomyomatous mesenchymal hamartoma
Stucco keratosis, 20
Sturge-Weber syndrome, 277, 279
Subcutaneous panniculitis-like T-cell lymphoma, 453, **455**
   and cytophagic histiocytic panniculitis, 454, **455**
Subungual exostosis, 376
Subungual osteochondroma, 376
Subungual perineurioma, 227
Superficial acral fibromyxoma, 227, **227**

Symplastic leiomyoma, 368
Synovial sarcoma, 244, 258, **258**
Syringoacanthoma, *see* Eccrine poroma
Syringocystadenoma papilliferum, 2, 147, **147, 148**
Syringoid carcinoma, *see* Microcystic adnexal carcinoma
Syringolymphoid hyperplasia, 457
Syringoma, 139, **140, 141**
Syringometaplasia, 184, **185**
Systemic Mastocytosis, 425

T

T-cell lymphomas, 447, *see also individual lymphoma types*
T-cell-rich B-cell lymphoma, 440
Targetoid hemangioma, *see* Hobnail hemangioma
Telangiectasia macularis eruptiva perstans, *see* Mastocytosis, cutaneous
Thymic cyst, 10
Thyroglossal duct cyst, 10, **12**
Trabecular carcinoma, *see* Primary neuroendocrine carcinoma
Trichilemmal carcinoma, 92, **93-96**
Trichilemmal cyst, 2, 4, **4**, 5
Trichilemmoma, 23, 73, **74, 75**
   desmoplastic trichilemmoma, 74, **75**
Trichoadenoma of Nikolowski, 73, **73**
Trichoblastic fibroma, *see* Trichoblastoma
Trichoblastic trichoblastoma, *see* Trichoblastoma
Trichoblastoma, 87, **88**
Trichochlamydocarcinoma, *see* Malignant proliferating pilar tumor
Trichodiscoma, 89, **90**
Trichoepithelioma, 55, 78, 79, **79**
   and epithelioma adenoides cysticum syndrome, 79, **79**
Trichofolliculoma, 77, **78**, 100
   sebaceous trichofolliculoma, 78
Trichogerminoma, 85, **86**
Trichomatricoma, *see* Pilomatricoma
Tubular apocrine adenoma, 149, **150**, *see also* Papillary eccrine adenoma
Tubulopapillary hidradenoma, *see* Papillary eccrine adenoma
Tumor of the follicular infundibulum, 71, **71, 72**, 100
Turner's syndrome and pilomatricoma, 83

U

Urticaria pigmentosa, *see* Mastocytosis, cutaneous

V

Vascular nevus, 277
Venous hemangioma, 285
Verrucous carcinoma, 27, 40, **41**
Verrucous cyst, 2
Verrucous epidermal nevus, 14, **16**
Verrucous hemangioma, 291, **291**
Von Recklinghausen's disease
    and malignant peripheral nerve sheath tumor, 341
    and neurofibroma, 330, **331**
    and neurilemmoma, 333

W

Warty dyskeratoma, 2, 18, **19**
Wattles, 365, 375
Winer's pore, 72
Woringer-Kolopp disease, 464

X

Xanthoma disseminatum, 395, **395**, 404
Xanthosiderohistiocytosis, 395
Xeroderma pigmentosum, 27

Z

Zoon's plasmacellular balanitis, 36